Coronary OCT
A Case-based Approach

"The best way to find yourself is to lose yourself in the service of others."
—Mahatma Gandhi

Coronary OCT
A Case-based Approach

Author

Sridhar Kasturi MD DM FACC FESC FSCAI FICC
Head
Department of Cardiology and Cardiothoracic Surgery
KIMS Sunshine Hospitals, Begumpet
Hyderabad, Telangana, India
Chairman, Interventional Cardiologists Forum

Forewords

Takashi Akasaka
Rajesh M Dave
Shailender Singh
Vijay Kumar Reddy S

JAYPEE

JAYPEE BROTHERS MEDICAL PUBLISHERS
The Health Sciences Publisher
New Delhi | London

Jaypee Brothers Medical Publishers (P) Ltd

Headquarters
Jaypee Brothers Medical Publishers (P) Ltd
EMCA House, 23/23-B
Ansari Road, Daryaganj
New Delhi 110 002, India
Landline: +91-11-23272143, +91-11-23272703
+91-11-23282021, +91-11-23245672
Email: jaypee@jaypeebrothers.com

Corporate Office
Jaypee Brothers Medical Publishers (P) Ltd
4838/24, Ansari Road, Daryaganj
New Delhi 110 002, India
Phone: +91-11-43574357
Fax: +91-11-43574314
Email: jaypee@jaypeebrothers.com

Overseas Office
JP Medical Ltd.
83, Victoria Street, London
SW1H 0HW (UK)
Phone: +44 20 3170 8910
Fax: +44 (0)20 3008 6180
Email: info@jpmedpub.com

Website: www.jaypeebrothers.com
Website: www.jaypeedigital.com

Inquiries for bulk sales may be solicited at: jaypee@jaypeebrothers.com

Coronary OCT: A Case-based Approach

First Edition: **2024**

ISBN: 978-93-5696-390-0

Printed at: Samrat Offset Pvt. Ltd.

Dedicated to

My beloved father Late Sri Kasturi Kashaiah and mother Srimathi Kamala with great respect, thankfulness, gratitude, and love from the bottom of the heart for the unconditional love, support, and affection extended to me. I am truly blessed to have you in my life.

I express my thanks from the bottom of the heart in the pursuit of this project to all my family members; most importantly, I thank Dr Sunitha Kasturi for being my wonderful wife and best friend. You inspired me every day with your discipline, meticulous planning, and straight-forwardness. Your positive constructive criticism always helped me to improve myself. My amazing both sons: Sushrith Kasturi and Shishir Kasturi are the very precious gifts of my life. Your presence made me healthier and happier to work hard and to do more enthusiastically. As sons, you are truly special and thanks for everything.

Contributors

Kunihiro Shimamura MD PhD
Assistant Professor
Department of Cardiovascular Medicine
Wakayama Medical University
Kimiidera, Wakayama, Japan
Email: shimamura_kunihiro_188@yahoo.co.jp

Rajesh M Dave MD FACC FSCAI
Co-Editor-in-Chief
Interventional Cardiology
President
Cardiovascular Experts of Pennsylvania
Advanced Limb Salvage Center
Surgical Center of Cardiovascular Experts
Camp Hill, Pennsylvania, USA
Email: rdintervention@yahoo.com

Takashi Akasaka MD PhD FAPSC FESC FJCS FJCC FJCA FACHD
Coronary Intervention
Emeritus Professor
Department of Cardiovascular Medicine
Wakayama Medical University
Kimiidera, Wakayama, Japan
Email: akasat@wakayama-med.ac.jp
Senior Consultant
Department of Cardiovascular Medicine
Nishinomiya Watanabe Cardiovascular Cerebral Center
Nishinomiya City, Hyogo, Japan
Email: akasakat1955@yahoo.co.jp

Yasutsugu Shiono MD PhD FESC FJCS
Assistant Professor
Department of Cardiovascular Medicine
Wakayama Medical University
Kimiidera, Wakayama, Japan
Email: yshiono2012@gmail.com

Foreword

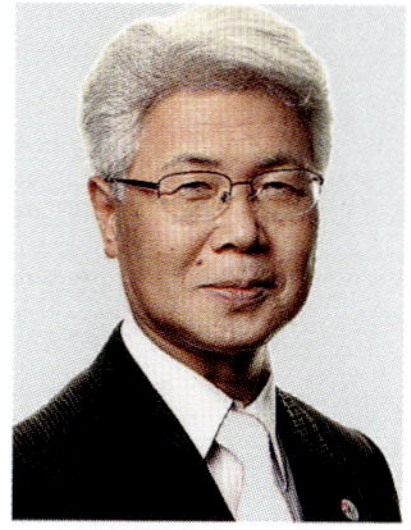

Recent meta-analyses have demonstrated the superiority of intravascular imaging (IVI) guided percutaneous coronary intervention (PCI) to angiography-guided PCI for obtaining better prognosis and avoiding future major adverse cardiovascular events (MACEs). It has been reported that the future MACEs, including myocardial infarction and cardiovascular death could be reduced significantly even in chronic coronary syndrome (CCS) by PCI compared with optimal medical treatment (OMT) in ISCHEMIA trial extend, although there were many provocative discussions after the initial negative results of the usefulness of PCI compared with OMT in the trial. Although there are recommendations of IVI guidance in PCI by several guidelines and expert consensus documents, real-world use of IVI, especially optical coherence tomography (OCT) in our daily clinical practice might be limited all over the world, except for specific institutions or several countries. It should be very important to have some experience how to read images and perform IVI guidance during PCI under the introduction by highly-experienced PCI operators and imaging experts. One impressive experience of IVI-guided PCI or one attractive image during PCI may allow us to understand the importance and usefulness of IVI-guided PCI, especially in complex PCI. Recent OCT system may provide us with high-resolution images (more than 10-micron resolution) as coronary angiography co-registration way with auto-measurement system, three-dimensional reconstruction, and automatic calcium identification by artificial intelligence. Only after several experience, you will realize that "a picture is worth a thousand words" or "seeing is believing", in other words, and confirm that every coronary interventionist needs to know how to use and read intracoronary imaging for PCI optimization and improving the prognosis of the patients.

The present textbook, "Coronary OCT: A Case-based Approach", is demonstrated interesting clinical cases with impressive and attractive images accompanied by an illustrated, up-to-date review of the topic, including the most recent reports, knowledge and practical tips and tricks. All the readers of this book will be provided a great opportunity to "learn to see" and by case-based approach with impressive images enables you to become an expert with ease. Although the textbooks or simple lectures demonstrating the data and the summary of the results of the studies might be sometimes boring to the beginners, case series and discussion with important images and illustrations in this book should be the best method of education and expands the reader's interest.

I am sure that all the authors of this book are highly experienced PCI operators and imaging experts, and the readers will benefit by the study of these cases and images even whether they are well-experienced or early career of OCT-guided PCI. I appreciate the editor, Dr Sridhar Kasturi and the contributing authors of the text for their great effort to complete the book. It is really my great honor and privilege to be able to contribute to them. I sincerely hope this book will contribute to accelerate OCT-guided PCI for optimizing the results and for improving the patients' prognosis as a result.

Takashi Akasaka MD PhD FAPSC FESC FJCS FJCC FJCA FACHD
Coronary Intervention
Emeritus Professor, Department of Cardiovascular Medicine
Wakayama Medical University
Kimiidera, Wakayama, Japan
Email: akasat@wakayama-med.ac.jp
Senior Consultant, Department of Cardiovascular Medicine
Nishinomiya Watanabe Cardiovascular Cerebral Center
Nishinomiya City, Hyogo, Japan
Email: akasakat1955@yahoo.co.jp

Foreword

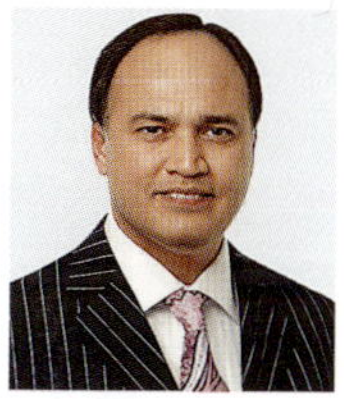

In the journey of percutaneous coronary intervention, we have conquered many challenges such as restenosis, calcification, left main disease to name a few. Despite a great deal of the advances in DES, long term MACE events remain elusive. PCI optimization by use of Imaging and Physiology has provided new hope in improving short and long-term outcomes. Optical Coherence Tomography has proven to be a "high-definition TV" in the world of intracoronary imaging. It is limited in its opportunity only by interpretation experience of the operator. Case series and discussion is the best method of education and expands operator's repertoire.

Sir William Osler once said, "Learn to see, learn to hear, learn to feel, learn to smell and know that by practice alone can you become an expert". This book will provide a great opportunity to "learn to see" and by case review enables you to become an expert. This book is developed from interesting clinical cases accompanied by an illustrated, up to date review of the topic including the most recent literature, knowledge and practical tips and tricks. The contributors to *"Coronary OCT - A Case-based Approach"* are all highly experienced operators and imaging experts. The clarity of their presentation is obvious on every page, and interventionalist whether experienced or early career will benefit by the study of these cases and images.

The year 2024 marks the golden year when our dream of making PCI optimization a routine practice is within reach. Now with exceptional advances in OCT Imaging and Software, OCT will continue to gain wide acceptance in daily interventional practice. This book is a milestone and should be memorialized in OCT development history in India. With the privilege of being a co-editor, I will cherish this book and will continue to rededicate my own efforts to PCI optimization development. I hope that major effort on the part of the editor Dr Sridhar Kasturi and the contributing authors will fill a niche in our field of work. It is my sincere hope that everyone in Interventional Cardiology will read this book and enrich themselves with the techniques of Optical Coherence Tomography.

Rajesh M Dave MD FACC FSCAI
Co-Editor-in-Chief
Interventional Cardiology
President
Cardiovascular Experts of Pennsylvania
Advanced Limb Salvage Center
Surgical Center of Cardiovascular Experts
Camp Hill, Pennsylvania, USA
Email: rdintervention@yahoo.com

Foreword

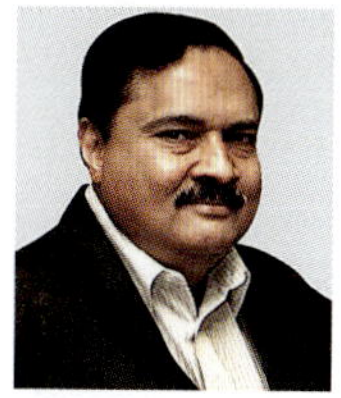

This is indeed a new era in Interventional Cardiology. Dramatic breakthroughs in basic research and exiting result of Interventions both in Coronary and Structural heart disease (with newer devices) have revolutionized cardiovascular care worldwide.

Coronary artery disease is one of the major public health problems, in epidemic proportions in India and worldwide. Complex cardiac Interventional procedures previously available only in developed countries are being done with equal precision and expertise in India and worldwide.

It is in this milieu that Dr Sridhar Kasturi's *Coronary OCT: A Case-based Approach* is so timely and appropriate. It addresses two major issues: Intracoronary imaging and the Clinical benefits of Imaging in achieving excellent results of Interventions. This book addresses both these issues in an outstanding manner and is a private tutorial on outlining a master interventional cardiologists' approach to coronary interventions.

His thesis is (with which I agree) that OCT and IVUS imaging of coronary artery disease forms the foundation upon which management of the patient is built is indeed true. Without such firm basis an optimal intervention of coronary artery disease is not possible. OCT helps not only in the assessment of disease but also on result of intervention both immediate and long-term.

I have the pleasure and honor of working with Dr Sridhar Kasturi over the last decade in Cathlab while treating CAD with interventions. He is an excellent interventional cardiologist and I have cherished my association with him being one of the best in coronary imaging in our country. His enormous wealth of clinical experience in OCT is well reflected in *Coronary OCT: A Case-based Approach* and I believe it is destined to become one of the best (with its illustrative imaging pictures) book for imaging by OCT in CAD.

Shailender Singh MD DM FACC FESC
Senior Interventional Cardiologist
KIMS Sunshine Hospital
Hyderabad, Telangana, India.

Foreword

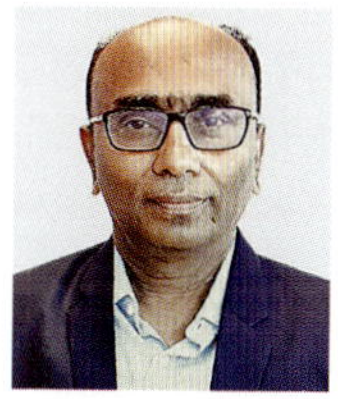

I am honored and have a great pleasure to write the foreword for the state of art book *"Coronary OCT: A Case-based Approach"* by Dr Sridhar Kasturi. This book is the need of the hour due to rapidly advancing Interventional Cardiology both in India and around the world. Over the years, Interventional Cardiology has revolutionized the management of cardiovascular diseases. This book serves as a valuable resource for both aspiring and experienced Interventional Cardiologists. This book dealt with various scenarios with clinical precision and with the latest updates. Dr Sridhar Kasturi spent his valuable time to advancing the practice of precision cardiology with OCT-guided PCI. Each chapter provides a concise yet comprehensive overview of a specific aspect of interventional PCI, supported by clinical evidence.

This is an outstanding book covering all aspects of OCT. The sum of the information provided in this book is a real achievement. Thanks to Dr Sridhar Kasturi for his outstanding contribution. There is no doubt that having this book available will immensely benefit anyone working in the field of interventional cardiology.

The chapters are well outlined, organized, and well written with authentic references. The writing style of every chapter is vivid, concise, practical, and guideline directed. There are excellent graphics and figures that present the relevant information. The printing and binding are of excellent quality.

I congratulate the author Dr Sridhar Kasturi for accomplishing the extraordinary achievement of great book on OCT imaging.

Vijay Kumar Reddy S MD DM FESC
Senior Interventional Cardiologist
KIMS Sunshine Hospital, Begumpet
Hyderabad, Telangana, India

Preface

Current evidence based on recently published studies suggest image guided PCI over Angio guided PCI is associated with improved outcomes, and it is the need of the hour to all interventional cardiologists to know about intravascular imaging to maintain high standard health care practice to provide the best possible outcome to their patients. Image guided PCI is very useful in the pre PCI assessment of plaque, deciding appropriate plaque modification strategy, and sizing of balloons and stents. Post PCI optimization of DES is mainly to identifying and rectifying edge dissection, under-expansion and apposition which are associated with acute and long-term outcomes. OCT due to its high-resolution 3D images helpful in detailed assessment of vessel wall characteristics - type of plaque, plaque burden and identifying vulnerable plaque which is prone for plaque rupture, dissection, and intra & extra mural hematomas. OCT also differentiates intraluminal masses like thrombus (red & white), recanalized thrombus, CN, stent struts, position of guidewires (abluminal position, in relation to stent struts (proximal Vs distal strut crossing) and entrapped broken balloon shafts, guidewires and other intravascular foreign bodies which are very helpful in optimizing PCI results.

I have taken extreme care in drafting this book by picking up proper images within a detailed analysis of OCT and their correlation with Angio images to understand and interpret easily so as to implement proper OCT image-based strategies during day-to-day coronary interventions. I made this book with an intention of providing effective, useful guide to interventional cardiologists who want to learn OCT and also those who are already practicing OCT guided PCI to get additional current concepts with illustrations of high-risk complex PCI with case-based examples with additional tips and tricks. I reviewed literature extensively and thoroughly and tried to incorporate all the relevant current concepts about OCT imaging into appropriate text content within detail analysis of carefully selected very important academic cases of complex PCI which are informative and educative with clear images so as to make it one stops solution to interventional cardiologists who want to learn and understand OCT from simple to complex PCI. I emphasized the usefulness of OCT in PCI subsets with case-based examples - STEMI, bifurcation, multi-vessel, diffuse long lesions, ISR, stent thrombosis and calcified coronary lesions which includes a spectrum of cases in each subset to illustrate the usefulness of OCT for a ready reference and understanding. Two additional chapters with special focus on bifurcation PCI, and current status developments in the field of OCT which are contributed by well-known reputed cardiologist Dr Akasaka (Japan) and one highly educative case reports by Dr Raj Dave (USA) to give some more insights and make it more informative.

I also included recently introduced a new algorithm of OCT workflow during PCI procedures, i.e., MLD MAX to make it simple and effective formula to implement during PCI procedures as a check list for optimization of DES implantation to improve its outcome.

I spent nearly six years to work on this project to design and draft in such way to fulfil the idea what I aimed for i.e., to read and interpret without much difficulty in understanding OCT guided PCI. I feel and believe I reached to the point of focus what I wanted to highlight without compromising the quality and content of the book and you would appreciate the hard work and meticulous designing incorporated into it while reading this book.

I have been using OCT during PCI for 10 years during my 30 years of active interventional cardiology practice. I perform all interventional procedures which include complex coronary PCI, endovascular repair of aortic aneurysms, carotid interventions, renal interventions, upper-limb interventions, aorto-ileac interventions, above and below knee angioplasty non-coronary, valvular interventions, and venous interventions.

I spent many hours in the cathlab while performing high-risk PCI of STEMI with cardiogenic shock during day and night, performed more than 50,000 angiographies and more than 25 interventional procedures including high-risk coronary and non-coronary interventions. Despite having so many years of experience as a high-volume operator and heading the department of cardiology of well-known reputed cardiology center having 14 full time cardiologists and 3 full-time Cardiothoracic surgeons with round the clock emergency cardiology services in a group. Still sometimes I feel it would be very difficult to make decisions based traditional angiography imaging and in such cases intravascular imaging especially OCT due to its high resolution makes things better throws a light in making the right diagnosis, to make the right decision and to implement appropriate strategies.

I presume that this book will meet your expectations, and I am sure you would appreciate our efforts in producing one of the finest OCT books with case-based approach.

Sridhar Kasturi

"Wherever the art of medicine is loved, there is also a love for humanity."

—Hippocrates

Acknowledgments

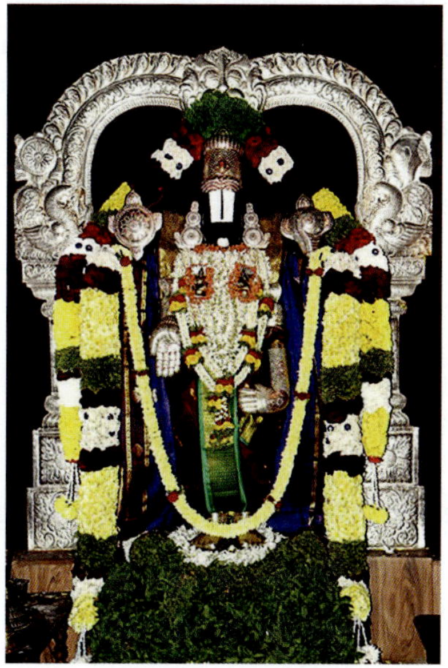

First and foremost, I would like to thank almighty Lord Sri Venkateshwara Swamy, Dharmapuri for giving me the strength, knowledge, ability, and opportunity to carry this latest academic work on Intravascular Imaging Assessment during Angioplasty and Stenting to make it more convenient to read and interpret to implement in day-to-day interventional practice. Without his blessings this work would not have been possible.

Having an idea after writing a book and to make it a real one is a really challenging and rewarding. It involved extensive review of literature, analyzing Angio, OCT images and to arrange them in a sequence for detailed and narrative description of step-by-step approach to make it easy to read, understand and to interpret so as to reach each and every one associated with interventional cardiology is a tough task. This work could not have been possible without the support of my clinical research assistants Mr Manikandhar Pendyala, and Mr Chandrashekar Challa. I express my thanks for their effort to come out with beautiful text, Angio and OCT images, tables, and flowcharts in arranging and re-arranging without compromising quality.

I am extremely thankful to KIMS Sunshine Hospital management, especially Dr Guruva Reddy Annapareddy, Managing Director, Dr Bhavani Annapareddy, all the members of Department of Cardiology of KIMS Sunshine Heart Institute including my colleagues Dr Shailender Singh, Dr S Vijay Kumar Reddy, all other cardiology associates, paramedical and nursing staff of Department of Cardiology.

I am very much pleased to express my big thanks to the entire team of Jaypee Brothers Medical Publications (P) Ltd, New Delhi, India for coming out with one of the finest possible edition and for their timely response and coordinated effort.

"Failure is not fatal, and success is not final: it is the courage to continue that counts."

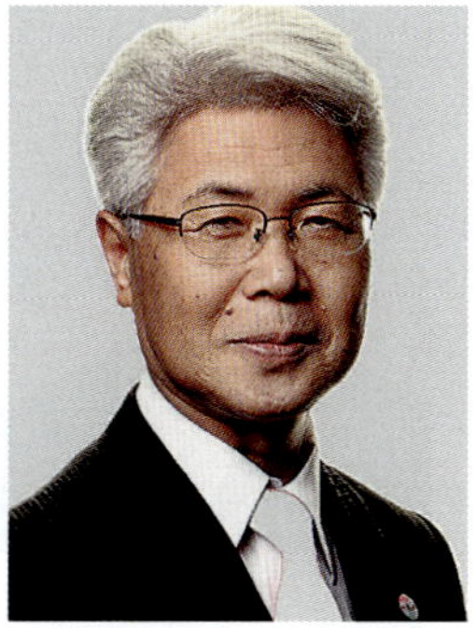

Takashi Akasaka MD PhD FAPSC FESC FJCS FJCC FJCA FACHD
Coronary Intervention
Emeritus Professor
Department of Cardiovascular Medicine
Wakayama Medical University
Kimiidera, Wakayama, Japan
Email: akasat@wakayama-med.ac.jp

Senior Consultant
Department of Cardiovascular Medicine
Nishinomiya Watanabe Cardiovascular Cerebral Center
Nishinomiya City, Hyogo, Japan
Email: akasakat1955@yahoo.co.jp

Words cannot be expressing the gratitude I feel for it. You (Dr Takashi Akasaka, Dr Yasutsugu Shiono and Dr Kunihiro Shimamura) have done so much by contributing two very important chapters which will be very useful in understanding concept of bifurcation PCI and recent developments in OCT imaging. You have been inspiration and wonderful role model all these years for me and so many others.

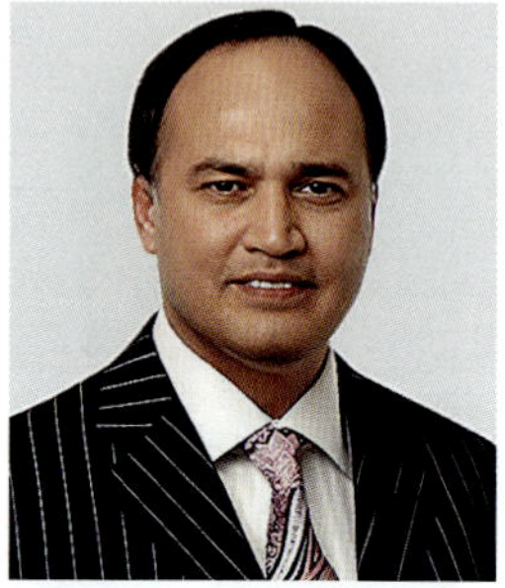

Rajesh M Dave MD FACC FSCAI
Co-Editor-in-Chief
Interventional Cardiology
President
Cardiovascular Experts of Pennsylvania
Advanced Limb Salvage Center
Surgical Center of Cardiovascular Experts
Camp Hill, Pennsylvania, USA
Email: rdintervention@yahoo.com

My heartfelt thanks to Dr Rajesh M Dave for his encouragement and support as and when required in bringing out this book with value added suggestions and his invaluable contribution of two case reports emphasizing role of imaging in understanding stent fracture and ISR with beautiful images.

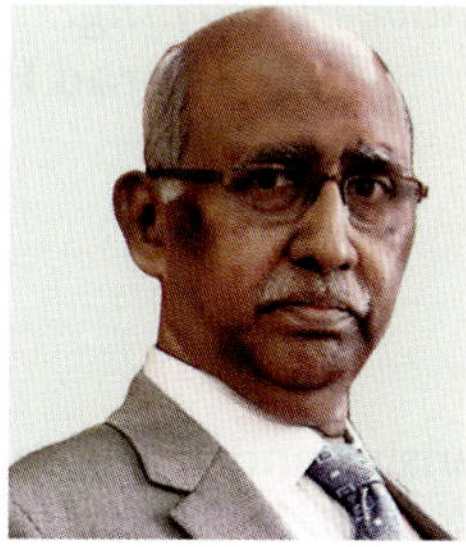

Dr V Dayasagar Rao
MBBS FRCP (Edinburgh) FRCP (Canada) DM (Cardiology)
Senior Consultant Cardiologist
KIMS Hospitals
Secunderabad, Telangana, India

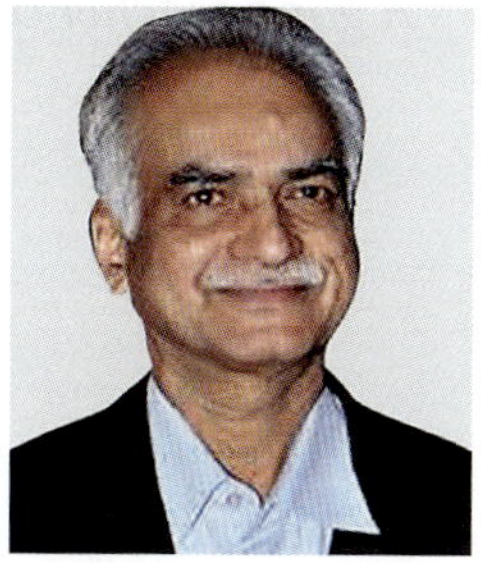

Dr B Somaraju
MBBS MD DM PhD
AIG Hospitals, Gachibowli
Hyderabad, Telangana, India

My big salute and heartfelt thanks
To
My great teachers for motivating and guiding me.

"A good education can change anyone. A good teacher can change everything."

"A good teacher can inspire hope, ignite the imagination, and instill a love of learning."

—Brad Henry

I am extremely thankful to all the Great Teachers of OCT who have inspired me to quest for deep and extensive understanding to develop insights of OCT evaluation of coronaries through their presentations, webinars, review articles, case reports and Lectures.

My Special Thanks to

Dr Akiko Maehara

Dr Gary S Mintz

Dr Giulio Guagliumi

Dr Jonathan Hill

Dr J Wang

Dr Kubo T

Dr Nicolas Amabile

Dr Niels R

Dr Park S-J

Dr Schultz C

Dr Takashi Akasaka

Dr Ziad A Ali

"The chapter you are learning today is going to save someone's life tomorrow – Pay attention."

Contents

Introduction

Traditional angiography being a two-dimensional imaging modality may not be accurate in the assessment of lesion severity, plaque morphology, and plaque burden, especially in patients with diffusely diseased with lack of proper reference segments. Especially, eyeball assessment may result in interventions of functionally insignificant lesions contributing to increased acute and long-term major adverse cardiac events (MACE) rate.[1] In contrast, the intravascular image provides high-resolution three-dimensional images for accurate assessment of plaque morphology, plaque burden, accurate assessment of luminal narrowing, lesion length, and vessel diameter to choose the proper device for plaque modification and selection of proper stent size.

WHAT IS OPTICAL COHERENCE TOMOGRAPHY—BASICS

Optical coherence tomography uses near-infrared light to acquire very good high-resolution intravascular images and it requires clearing of blood from the corresponding blood vessel by either contrast or contrast saline mix flush or saline or dextran as the blood is a poor transmitter of near-infrared rays. Obtaining adequate high resolution requires proper alignment of the guide with a continuous and sustained injection of 4–5 mL/s manually or by injector using 14–16 mL per run at 4–6 atm pressure with continuous purging of OCT catheter. Sometimes, additional usage guide extension catheter or buddy wire technique is useful for placement of OCT catheter in vessels with tortuous anatomy, acute bends, and severe calcification. Careful attention should be paid to avoid forceful advancement or twisting or bending of the catheter, which might cause malfunction of the catheter. Before acquiring an automated pullback, coregistration application is useful for precise planning, especially for the selection of proper landing zones and appropriately sized stent to cover the entire diseased segment by landing in segments with minimal plaque burden or plaque-free zones. It is compatible with the 6Fr guide but ideal to use the 7Fr guide for large vessels or when guide extension is being used for imaging.[2]

BENEFITS OF OPTICAL COHERENCE TOMOGRAPHY TO PATIENTS

Prior to photothermal coherence tomography (PCT) acquisition of OCT images are very useful in assessing plaque morphology, plaque burden, and vulnerability of plaque rupture there it helps in identifying any need for plaque modification, choosing the appropriate plaque modification device, and adequacy of plaque modification before implanting a stent to avoid underexpansion, which is associated with increased stent thrombosis (ST) and in-stent restenosis (ISR).

Poststent implantation: Poststent or device therapy OCT images reveal malapposition, proper expansion of the stent, and significant medial edge dissection. Correction of these factors improve acute and long-term outcomes of drug-eluting stent (DES).

Optical coherence tomography studies suggested that the morphologic features of plaques and serial follow-up with optimal medical therapy may show the evidence of plaque regression or no further progression of plaque. Due to its high resolution, it has an immense role in evaluating ST and ISR lesions, bifurcation lesions, calcific coronary lesions, and diffuse long lesions. Ambiguous lesions on angiography, particularly recanalized thrombus, spontaneous coronary artery dissection (SCAD), dissection/intramural hematoma (IMH), calcific nodule, and intraluminal thrombus.

REFERENCES

1. Nissen SE, Yock P. Intravascular ultrasound: novel pathophysiological insights and current clinical applications. Circulation. 2001;103(4):604-16.
2. Jang I-K. (2013). Who Should Get Optical Coherence Tomography? [online] Available from https://www.acc.org/latest-in-cardiology/articles/2014/07/18/12/55/who-should-get-optical-coherence-tomography [Last accessed February, 2024].

CHAPTER 1

Plaque Morphology

ABSTRACT

Optical coherence tomography (OCT) may allow us to identify tissue characterization of coronary plaques much more easily and more clearly compared with other imaging modalities with very good intra- and interobserver reliabilities and excellent sensitivity and specificity in each plaque. OCT showed a sensitivity of 71–79% and a specificity of 97–98% for fibrous plaques, 95–96% and 97% for fibrocalcific plaques, and 90–94% and 90–92% for lipid-rich plaques. Fibroatheromas are plaques containing lipid pools covered by a fibrous cap. This cap can be thick or thin. It is generally accepted that a thin cap overlying a lipid pool together with the presence of inflammatory cells is the hallmark of a vulnerable plaque. In sudden coronary death cases, hemorrhage into a plaque was most frequent in ruptured plaques but was also observed in lesions with only 40–50% cross-sectional luminal narrowing. Pathologically, "silent plaque rupture (PR) and subsequent healing" or "plaque erosion and thrombosis" contribute to plaque progression. Repeated cycles of rupture and healing might lead to the more stable lesion fibrocalcific plaque. OCT identifies both PR and calcified nodule (CN) with high sensitivity. As the imaging of endothelium is beyond the resolution of current OCT systems, the detection of plaque erosion (PE) is a diagnosis of exclusion.

INTRODUCTION

Assessment of plaque morphology and plaque burden is very much useful for proper planning of coronary interventional procedures. OCT can reveal plaque morphology with a sensitivity of about 75% and a specificity of 98% for fibrous plaques, 96% and 97% for fibrocalcific plaques, and 94% and 92% for lipid-rich plaques, respectively. Fibroatheromas are plaques containing lipid pools covered by a fibrous cap and thickness of the cap varies depending upon the vulnerability of plaque. Thin-cap fibroatheroma (TCFA) with thin cap overlying a lipid pool together with the presence of inflammatory cells is the hallmark of a vulnerable plaque that is responsible for the majority of acute coronary syndrome (ACS) with ST-elevation myocardial infarction (STEMI) cases. Calcific plaque severity and expansion index on imaging helps in choosing various plaque modification strategies and adequacy of modification prior to implanting drug-eluting stent (DES).

Coronary atheroma may manifest like gradual progression of the luminal stenosis or sudden occlusion of the vessel due to thrombus as a result of PR/PE leading to ACS. Presence of plaque is seen as a loss of the three-layered structure (i.e., intima, media, and adventitia) of the vessel wall. OCT can detect earliest phases of atheroma development such as the intimal xanthoma or intimal thickening. Erosions may occur in the early stages of atheroma formation, leading to either asymptomatic healing or ACS presentation. Repeated cycles of rupture and healing might lead to the more stable lesion fibrocalcific plaque.[1] A thin cap atheroma can rupture and directly lead to lesion thrombosis and infarction. Less commonly, dense calcified nodules can penetrate the fibrous cap and cause thrombosis. Fibrocalcific plaques might represent an end stage of the atherosclerosis process and can contain extensive calcifications. Because of a stable fibrous cap and lower lipid content, these lesions rarely cause thrombosis but can cause stable ischemic heart disease because of lumen narrowing **(Figure 1 and Table 1)**.

A stable fibrous cap may prevent rupture of the lesion. If the fibrous cap loses matrix proteins and smooth muscle cells, a thin cap atheroma can result. Intraplaque hemorrhage is also seen frequently in this entity, leading to further enlargement of the lipid core. The risk of plaque rupture is increased as the fibrous cap becomes thin and the lipid core enlarges.[2]

PLAQUE CHARACTERIZATION

Optical coherence tomography (OCT) shows much more clear tissue characterization of coronary plaques compared with intravascular ultrasound (IVUS)/Angio as evident in in vitro and in vivo studies. OCT detects fibrous plaques as signal-rich, homogenous lesions; fibrocalcific plaques as signal-poor, sharp-border lesions; and lipid-rich plaques as signal-poor, diffuse-border lesions.[3] OCT can detect intraluminal thrombus more accurately and compared to IVUS, it can differentiate red thrombus from white thrombi with a high sensitivity and specificity.

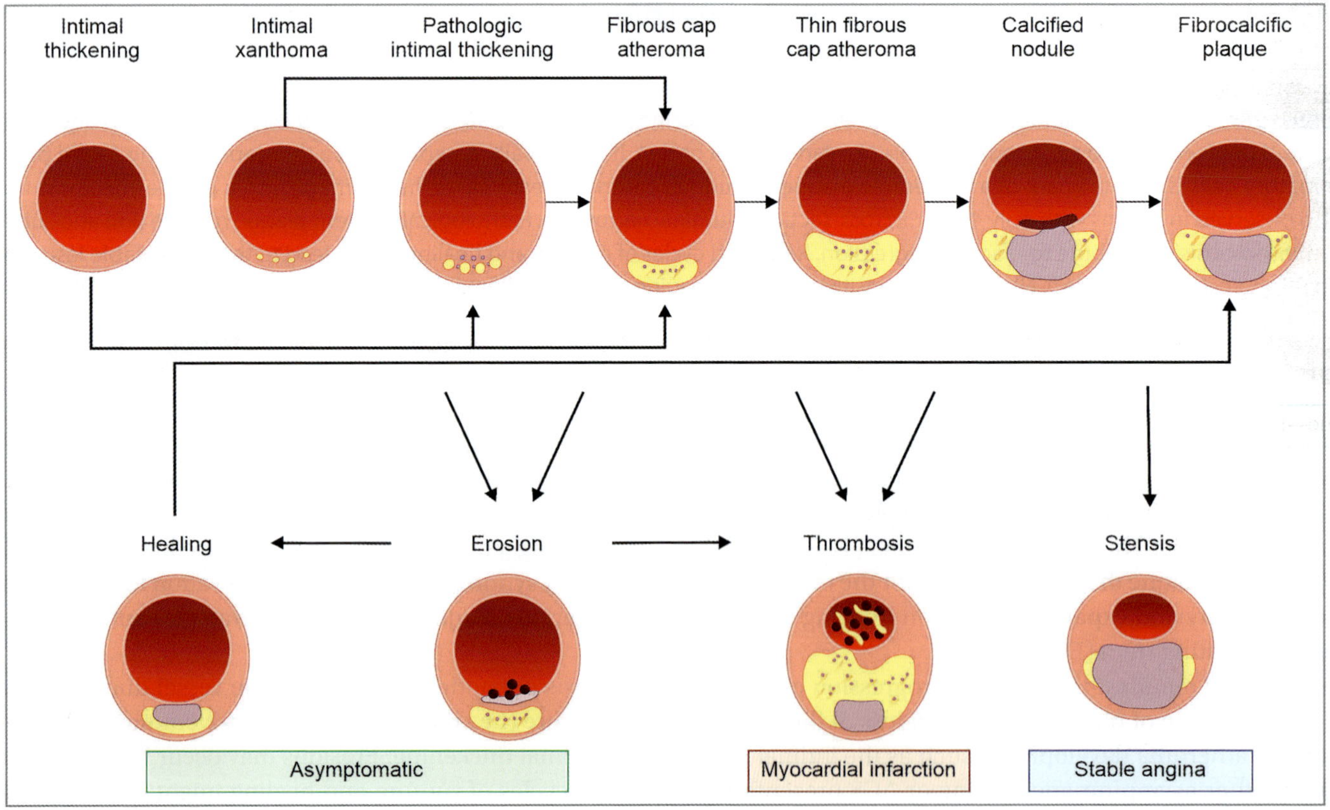

Fig. 1A

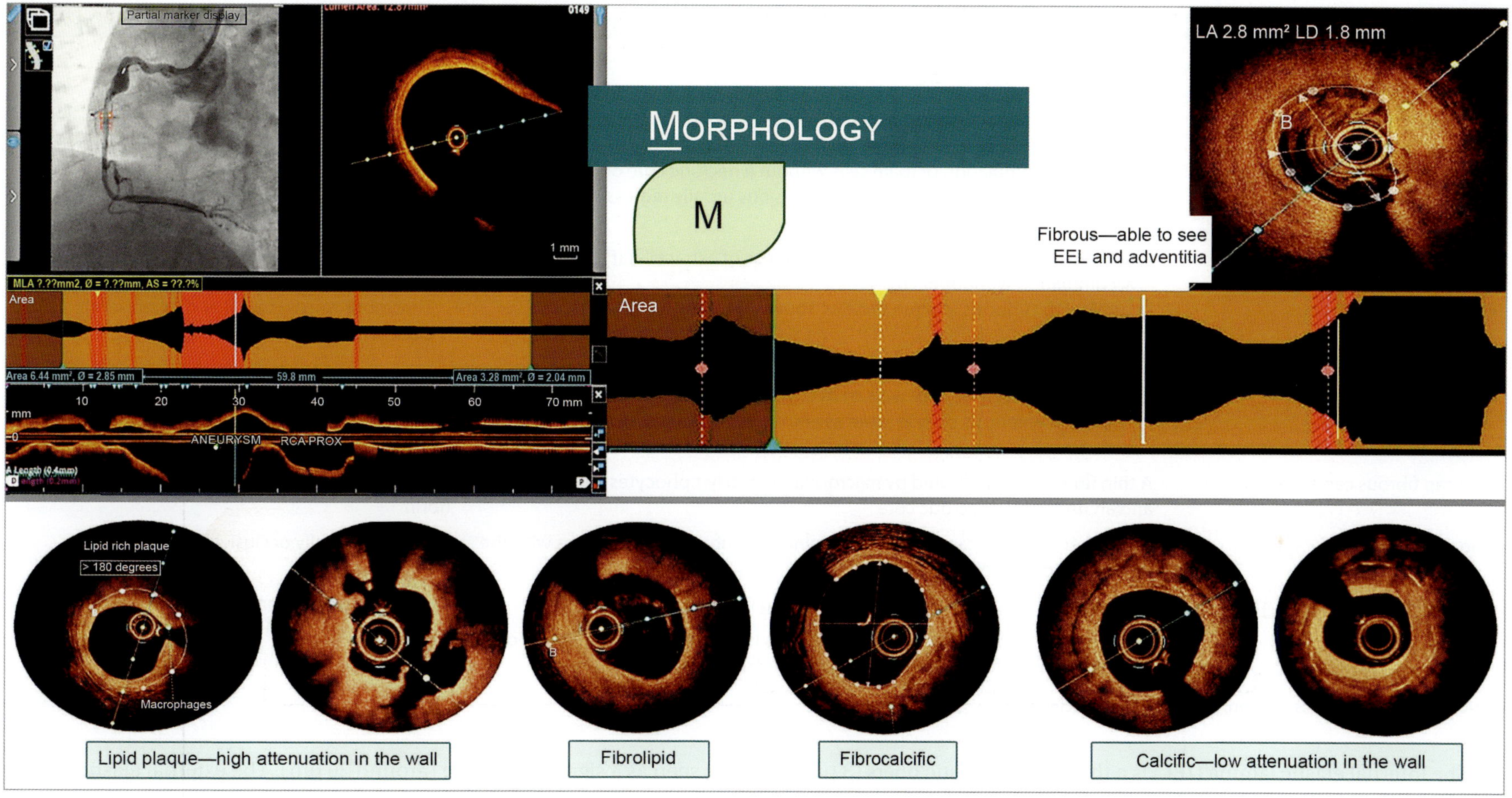

Fig. 1B

Figs. 1A and B: (A) Plaque morphology of various plaques and its clinical presentation Asymptomatic status to ACS; (B) OCT appearance of various plaque morphologies. (EEL: external elastic lamina; LA: luminal area; LD: luminal diameter)

NORMAL CORONARY MORPHOLOGY

Optical coherence tomography shows normal vessel as a tri-layered structure without any plaques **(Figs. 2A and B)** given as follows:

- *Intima:* Signal-rich layer nearest to the lumen
- *Media:* Signal-poor layer in middle of vessel wall (thickness ranges from 125 to 350 μm; mean 200 μm)
- *Adventitia:* Signal-rich outer layer of vessel walls.

TABLE 1: Modified AHA classification based on morphological description.

	Description	***Thrombosis***
Nonatherosclerotic Intimal lesions • Intimal thickening • Intimal xanthoma or fatty streak	 • The normal accumulation of smooth muscle cells in the intima in the absence of lipid or macrophage foam cells • Luminal accumulation of foam cells without a necrotic core or fibrous cap. Based on animal and human data such lesions usually regress	 • Absent • Absent
Progressive atherosclerotic lesions • Pathological intimal thickening • Erosion	 • SMCs in a proteoglycan rich matrix with areas of extracellular lipid accumulation without necrosis • Luminal thrombosis, plaque same as above	 • Absent • Thrombus mostly mural and infrequently occlusive
Fibrous cap atheroma • Erosion	 • Well-formed necrotic core with an overlying fibrous cap • Luminal thrombosis plaque same as above, no communication of thrombus with necrotic core	 • Absent • Thrombus mostly mural and infrequently occlusive
Thin cap fibrous cap atheroma	A thin fibrous cap infiltrated by macrophages and lymphocytes with rare SMCs and an underlying necrotic core	Absent–may contain intra plaque hemorrhage/fibrin
Plaque rupture	Fibroatheroma with cap disruption, luminal thrombus communicates with the underlying necrotic core	Thrombus usually occlusive
Calcified nodule	Eruptive nodular calcification with underlying fibrocalcific plaque	Thrombus usually nonocclusive
Fibrocalcific plaque	Collagen rich plaque with significant stenosis usually contains large areas of calcification with few inflammatory cells, a necrotic core may be present	Absent

(AHA: American Heart Association; SMC: smooth muscle cell)

The internal elastic lamina (IEL) is a thin layer of elastic fibers (3 μm), which is seen as a signal-rich band (around 20 μm). The external elastic lamina (EEL) are a few, often discontinuous layers of short elastic fibers that span a thickness of 3–6 μm, which is seen as a signal-rich band (around 20 μm) between the media and adventitia. The adventitia is a signal-rich, heterogeneously texted outer layer. In the presence of plaque, the media becomes thinner due to accumulation of plaque, resulting in asymmetric expansion of the vessel wall, causing remodeling of the vessel.[4] OCT is poor in assessing large plaques with more plaque burden due to its limited tissue penetration. OCT detects the early stages of atherosclerotic plaque such as intimal thickening, seen as a bright, homogeneous thin rim of tissue and intimal thickness assessment is well correlated with histological examination. Many patients who have an intimal thickening on OCT may show as a normal vessel on angiography.[5]

ATHEROSCLEROTIC INTIMAL LESIONS

Atherosclerotic intimal thickening lesions result from adaptive response to blood flow and intimal xanthomas develop from foam cell accumulations in intima that are nonprogressive **(Fig. 3)**. Intimal thickening is evident on OCT as homogeneous signal-rich intima with a thickness between 300 and 600 μm and a visibility of media in greater than or equal to three quadrants.

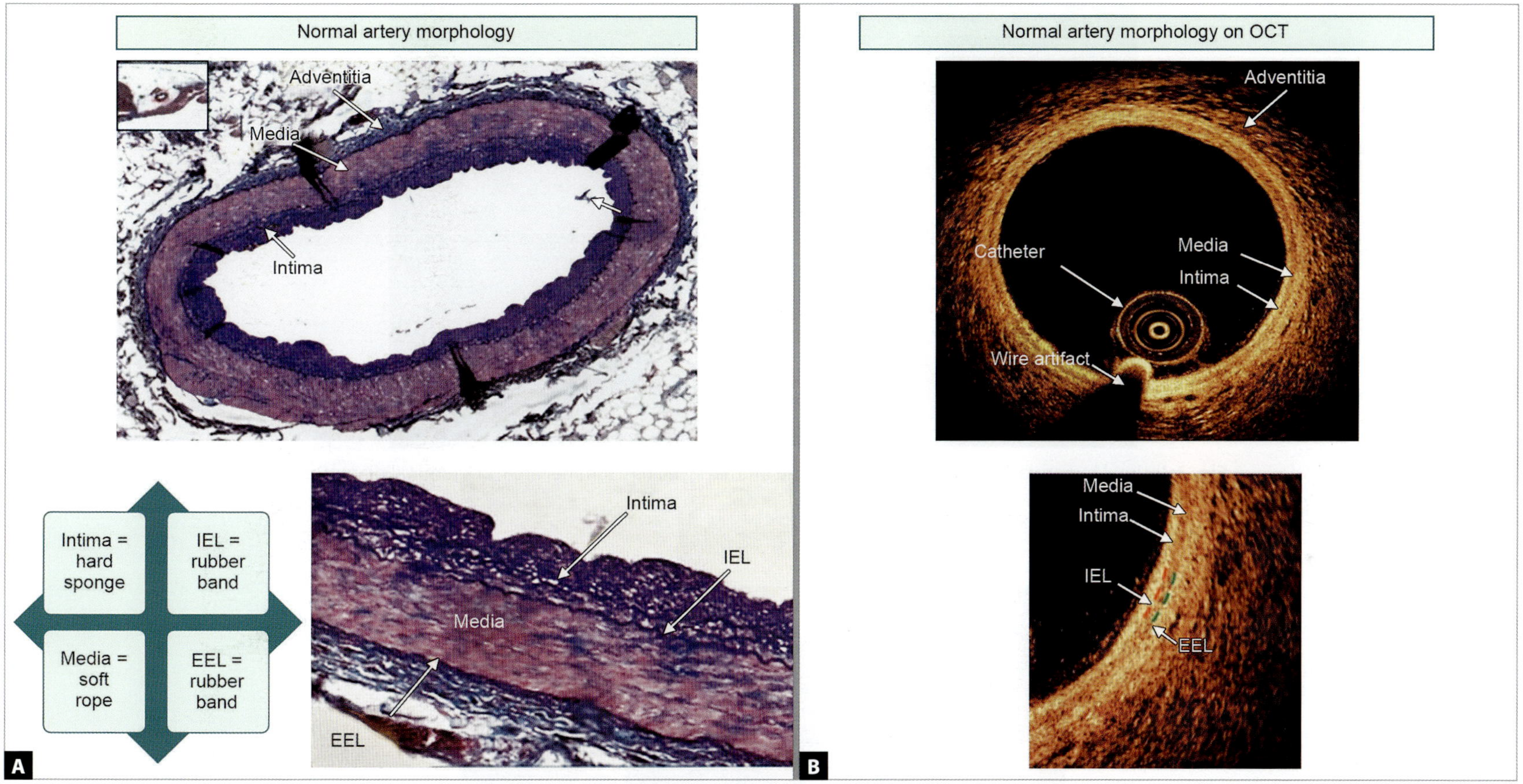

Figs. 2A and B: How the normal vessel looks like and the trilaminar structure. (EEL: external elastic lamina; IEL: internal elastic lamina; OCT: optical coherence tomography)

PROGRESSIVE ATHEROSCLEROTIC LESIONS

Atherosclerotic Plaque

Optical coherence tomography can provide detailed information about plaque morphology, to assess any need for plaque modification strategies, and devices are required or not.[6]

Fibrous Plaque

A fibrous plaque seen as a homogenous, highly backscattering region. Although some lipid or calcified content can be observed in fibrous plaques, these should not occupy more than one quadrant and due to the low attenuation properties of these plaques, it is often possible to see the media more clearly for assessing vessel diameter more accurately **(Fig. 4)**.

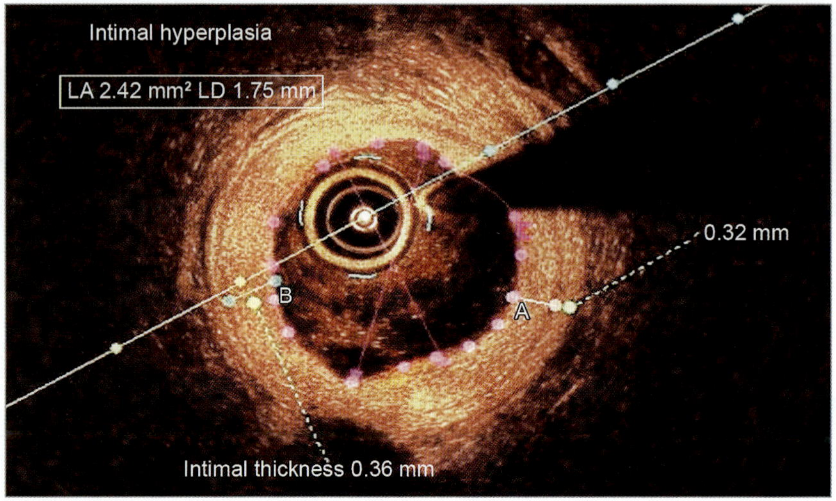

Fig. 3: Intimal hyperplasia and the thickness of the intimal layer. (LA: luminal area; LD: luminal diameter)

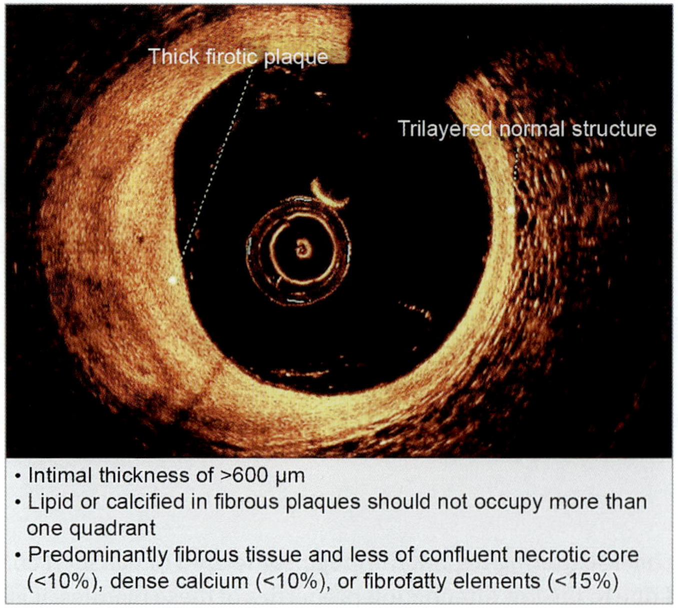

- Intimal thickness of >600 μm
- Lipid or calcified in fibrous plaques should not occupy more than one quadrant
- Predominantly fibrous tissue and less of confluent necrotic core (<10%), dense calcium (<10%), or fibrofatty elements (<15%)

Fig. 4: Fibrous plaque consists of smooth muscle cells in a proteoglycan-collagen matrix, with a variable number of macrophages and lymphocytes.

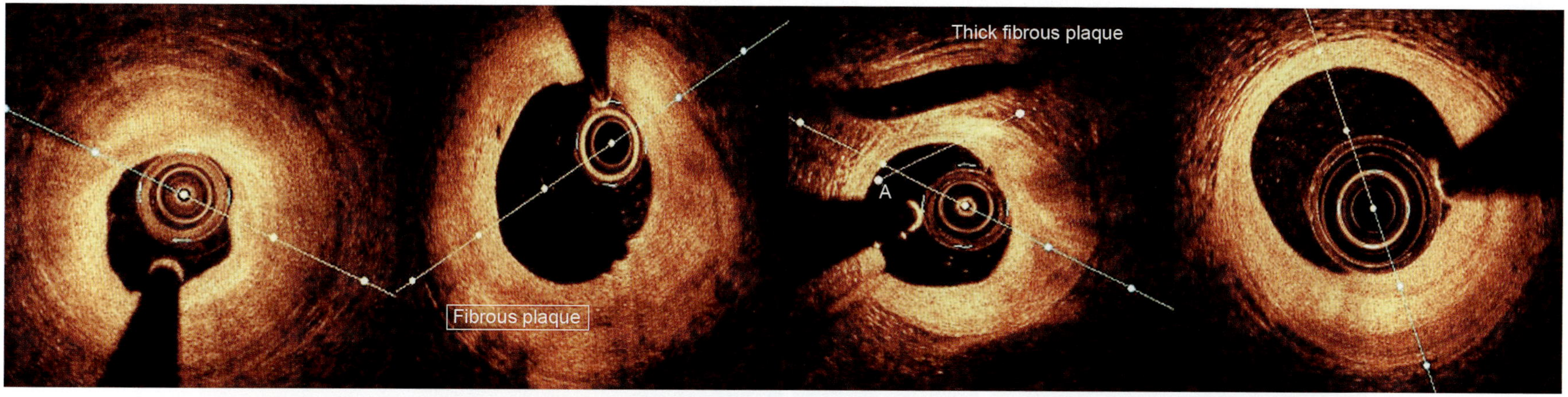

Fig. 5: On OCT imaging, fibrous plaque is defined as a homogenous, signal-rich plaque with low signal attenuation and >600 μm thickness.

Flowchart 1: Fibroatheroma.

Fibroatheroma
(Plaques containing lipid pools covered by a fibrous cap)
(Lipid pool/necrotic core exceeds >1 quadrant)

Thin-cap fibroatheroma
(Lipid pool/necrotic core exceeds >2 quadrant, <65 μm cap thickness)
- More prone to plaque rupture
- More frequent in acute coronary syndrome (ACS)
- More often associated with:
  - Macrophage infiltration
  - Neovascularization
  - Cholesterol crystals

Thick-cap fibroatheroma (>65μm cap thickness)
- Less prone to plaque rupture
- Less frequent in ACS

Fibrous plaques on OCT imaging are seen as signal-rich plaque with low signal attenuation **(Fig. 5)** and >600 μm thickness and it is recognized by IVUS as a plaque that is isoechoic to adventitia and it is shown as a predominantly fibrous tissue and less of confluent necrotic core (<10%), dense calcium (<10%), or fibrofatty elements (<15%).

Fibroatheroma (Flowchart 1)

A fibroatheroma **(Figs. 6A and B)** is a fibrous tissue layer which is often a signal-rich band, overlying a signal-poor region indicating the necrotic core and OCT image shows the necrotic core as signal-poor regions with poorly defined borders, which is similar to that of a lipid pool. The necrotic core is due to conversion of lipid pool from macrophage infiltration and apoptosis.[7]

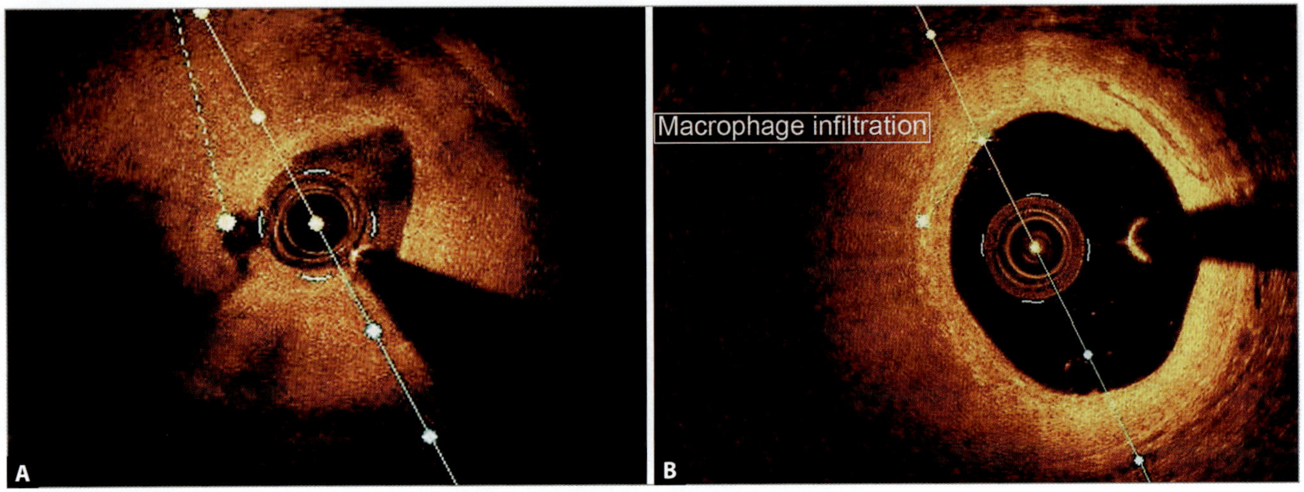

Figs. 6A and B: Fibroatheroma by OCT.

In contrast to early fibroatheromas, late fibroatheromas are associated with significant lumen compromise. OCT imaging also identifies other features of fibroatheromas such as macrophages, microvessels, and spotty calcification.[8]

The number of vulnerable plaques with thin-cap fibroatheroma (TCFA) is more often seen in acute coronary syndrome (ACS) lesions compared to patients with stable ischemic heart disease and more so in culprit vessel versus nonculprit vessels. TCFAs are more frequently seen in the proximal segments of the left coronary artery compared to the distal segment, whereas the distribution of TCFA in right coronary artery is similar throughout the vessel.

Lipid arc was measured every 1 mm; lipid length was measured by calculating the distance between the first and last OCT cross-sections, where lipid was observed **(Figs. 7A and B)** and lipid index was derived as the product of mean lipid arc and lipid length. A plaque with a lipid arc greater than 90° was defined as lipid rich.

Based on postmortem studies and the present pathophysiologic understanding, the following OCT criteria were selected for the definition of vulnerable atherosclerotic plaque:

- MLA at the level of the plaque <3.5 mm^2
- Lipid pool extension inside the plaque >180°
- Fibrous cap thickness <75 µm
- Presence of macrophage inflammatory infiltrate
- Presence of calcific nodules **Table 2 and Fig. 6C (*see* Fig. 16)**
- Presence of neovascularization (vasa vasorum) and/or intraplaque hemorrhage (IPH)
- Presence of cholesterol crystals (within the lipid pool)

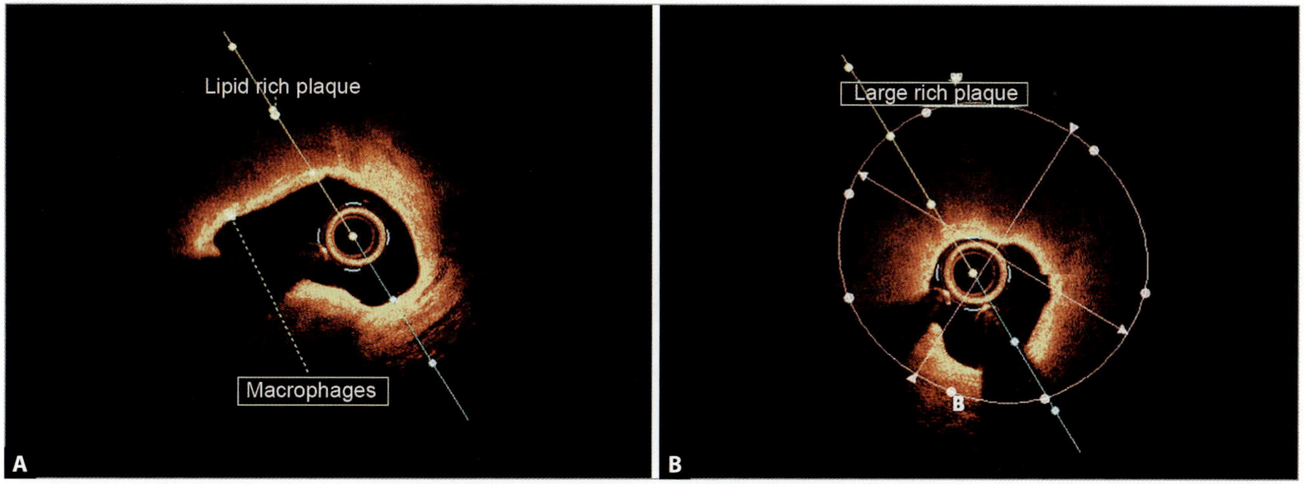

Figs. 7A and B: Lipid rich plaque characteristics by OCT.

TABLE 2: Stable and unstable plaque morphology by optical coherence tomography (OCT).

Fibrous plaque	*Fibrocalcific plaque*	*Fibroatheroma*	*Thin-cap fibroatheroma*	*Macrophages*	*Intimal vasculature*
Signal rich, homogeneous, with low signal attenuation	Signal poor, heterogeneous region, with sharp borders and low signal attenuation	Plaque with necrotic core, defined as a signal-poor region, with diffuse borders and high signal attenuation, and a fibrous cap	Fibroatheroma covered by a thin fibrous cap (65 µm)	Bright reflectance and high signal attenuation	Sharply delineated signal poor voids within the intima

CLIMA Study

The CLIMA study showed the vulnerability OCT criteria of atherosclerotic coronary plaques and predicted the personalized risk score for coronary events **(Fig. 8)**. The CLIMA assessed 1,776 lipid plaques involving untreated proximal left anterior descending (LAD) were evaluated with OCT with 1-year clinical follow-up. Presence of minimum luminal area (MLA) <3.5 mm^2, TCFA <75 µm, lipid arc >180°, presence of macrophages, and cholesterol crystals suggested plaque vulnerability and their positive correlation with hard clinical outcomes such as cardiac death and target vessel myocardial infarction (MI).[9]

Intraplaque Hemorrhage

Intraplaque hemorrhage may be due to the fissuring of the fibrous cap occurring at its thinnest portion, typically at the shoulder region, thereby allowing the entry of blood into the necrotic core and this may also happen as a result of rupture of vasa vasorum, a common feature of advanced lesions with plaque rupture and luminal thrombi. Sometimes, it may contribute to sudden death and acute MI as a consequence of acute luminal compromise **(Fig. 9)**.

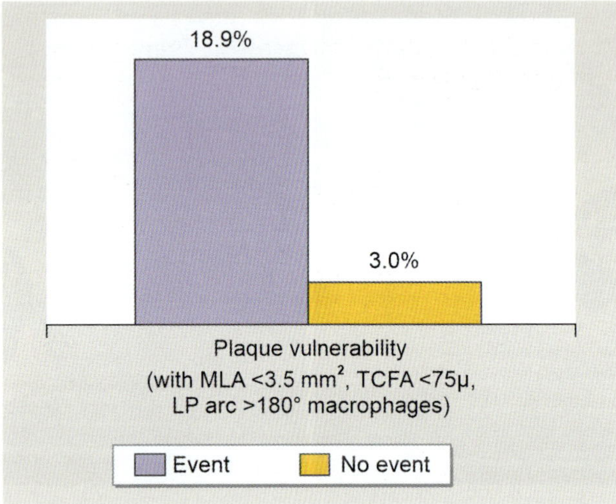

Fig. 8: The CLIMA study: Multicenter international prospective observational registry, to identify and map the vulnerability OCT criteria of atherosclerotic coronary plaques in the individual patient and provide a personalized risk score for coronary events. (LP: lipid; MLA: minimum luminal area; OCT: optical coherence tomography; TCFA: thin-cap fibroatheroma)

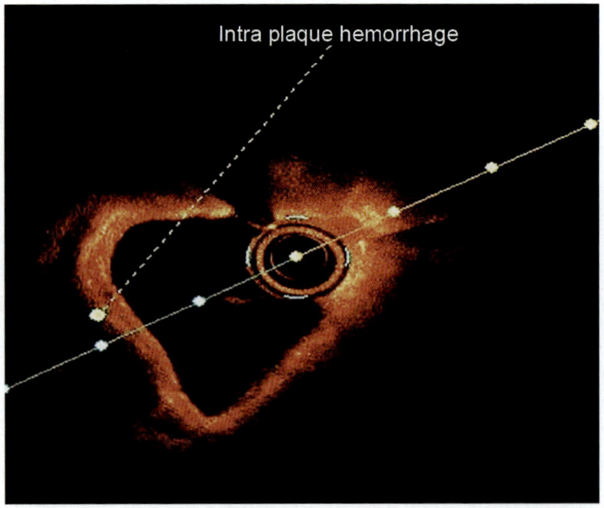

Fig. 9: Intraplaque hemorrhage into a plaque occurs from cracks or fissures originating from the luminal surface.

The prevalence of potential culprit lesion IPH was 11.7% in patients with stable or unstable angina. In OCT and IVUS analyses, more unstable plaque morphologies were observed in lesions with IPH than in those without, and more frequently associated with post-percutaneous coronary intervention (PCI) slow/no-reflow phenomenon and periprocedural MI **(Table 2)**.[10]

HEALED LESIONS

Healed plaque (HP)—when plaque rupture or erosion occurs in a prothrombotic milieu, they are likely to culminate in a symptomatic acute coronary event; otherwise, if thrombosis-resisting factors prevail, thrombus formation is inhibited and plaque healing occurs. Healed erosion as a result of healed previous plaque with erosion and healed lesions with rupture of the fibrous cap (arrowhead) over a necrotic core are due to healing of the plaque overlying the disrupted cap (healed site) **(Fig. 10)**.[10]

Optical coherence tomography is able to detect healed coronary plaques as a multilayered, onion-like appearance, with one or more layers of tissue with different optical signal clearly separated from the underlying plaque. Coronary lesion sites with healed coronary plaques would have a significantly

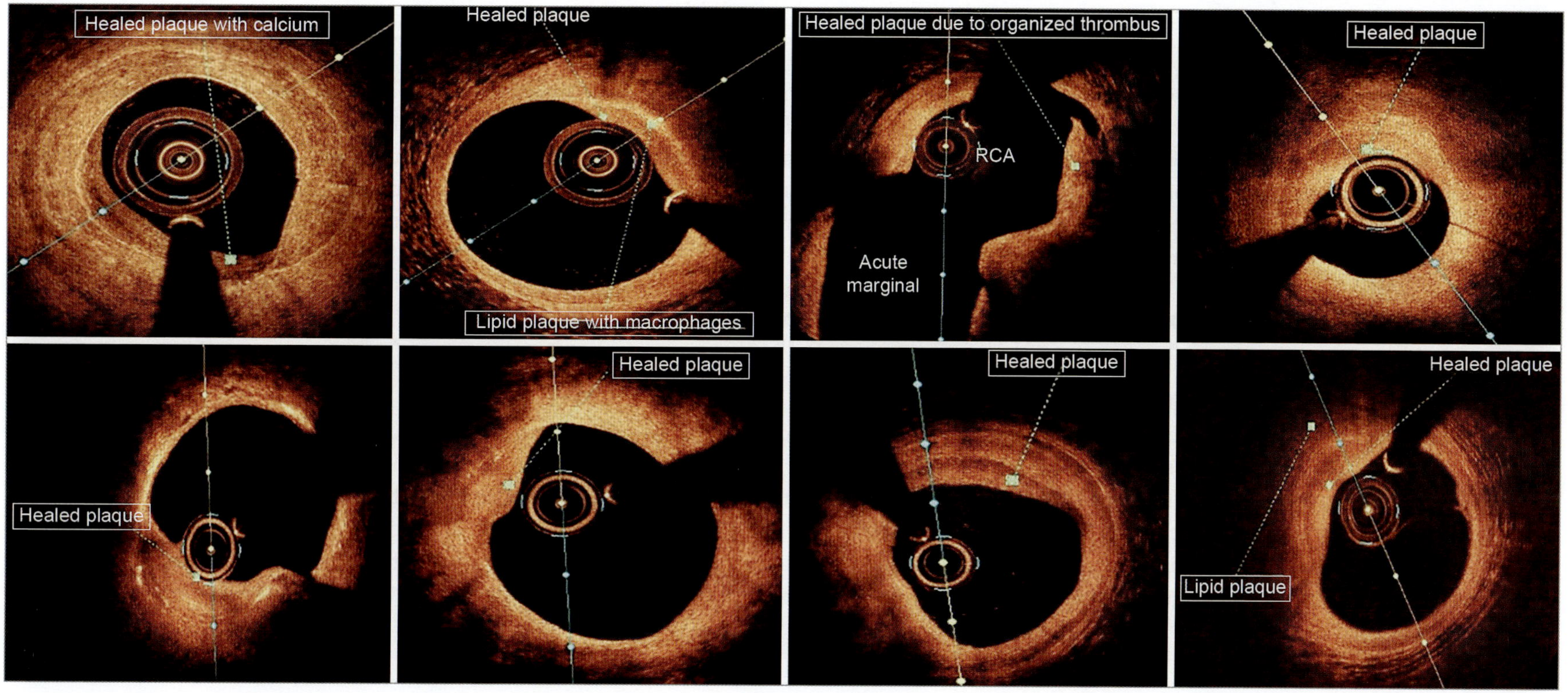

Fig. 10: Healed coronary plaques that typically have a multilayered, onion-like appearance, with one or more layers of tissue with different optical signal clearly separated from the underlying plaque can detect only with OCT imaging. (OCT: optical coherence tomography; RCA: right coronary artery)

smaller mean [standard deviation (SD)] minimal lumen than those without and visible as a different optical resolution with a clear delineation from underlying plaque. HP are more often associated with lipid-rich underlying plaque compared to fibrous plaques.[11]

Healed plaques are seen in 22% of nontreated segments in patients who underwent PCI of culprit vessel and they signal future atherosclerotic plaque progression and with future nonculprit segment-related major adverse cardiovascular events (MACE). Nonculprit segment-related MACE might be due to untreated HP, untreated TCFA, and MLA <3.5 mm^2 in nonculprit plaque (7.42%).

Fibrocalcific Plaque

Fibrocalcific plaque[10] is seen as a signal-poor heterogeneous region with sharp border with low reflectivity and low attenuation. Necrotic lipid pools are less well-delineated than calcifications and exhibit lower signal density and more heterogeneous backscattering than fibrous plaques. Calcified plaque-calcified regions have sharp borders, low signal and low attenuation, permitting deeper penetration **(Fig. 11)**.

Intravascular ultrasound and OCT are superior in detection, localization, and quantification of coronary calcification compared to conventional Angio (75–80% vs. 40%). OCT can evaluate its thickness, arc, and length more accurately than IVUS when the calcium accumulation is located superficially and does not extend into the deeper layers of the vessel wall.[12]

PLAQUE RUPTURE

Ruptured plaques are associated with vulnerable plaques with TCFA and fibrous cap is thinnest at the site of rupture and more often, the luminal thrombus is in communication with the lipid-rich necrotic core.[10] The rupture of an atherosclerotic plaque is visible as the discontinuity of the fibrous cap and the formation of a cavity in the plaque **(Fig. 12)**. An old plaque rupture or with fresh plaque rupture treated with antithrombotic/anticoagulant therapies may not show any evidence of thrombus. Sometimes, multiple plaque ruptures are evident in culprit and nonculprit lesions. However, culprit lesions are associated with the presence of thrombus, smaller luminal area, and greater plaque burden. OCT detects plaque rupture in high percentage of patients (73%) compared to IVUS (40%) and angioscopy (47%).[13]

Plaque Rupture of Thin-cap Fibroatheroma with Lipid-rich Plaque

Plaque Erosion

Plaque erosion is classified as **(Figs. 13 and 14)**:

- *Definite:* No obvious evidence of fibrous cap disruption, in a lesion with more of fibrous nature, with overlying luminal white thrombus.
- *Probable erosion:* No evidence of luminal thrombus but shows an irregular luminal surface or has overlying thrombus with attenuation of the underlying plaque, without evidence of superficial lipid or calcification in the vessel upstream or downstream of the thrombus site.[14]

Plaque erosion is usually associated with lesions with lower percentage of TCFA, smaller lipid burden, and thicker fibrous cap compared to plaque rupture. It tends to occur more often in younger patients, especially premenopausal women, smokers, absence of traditional coronary risk factors, lack of multivessel disease, reduced lesion severity, larger vessel size, and at bifurcation sites. Existing data suggest that PE is associated with better outcomes than plaque rupture.

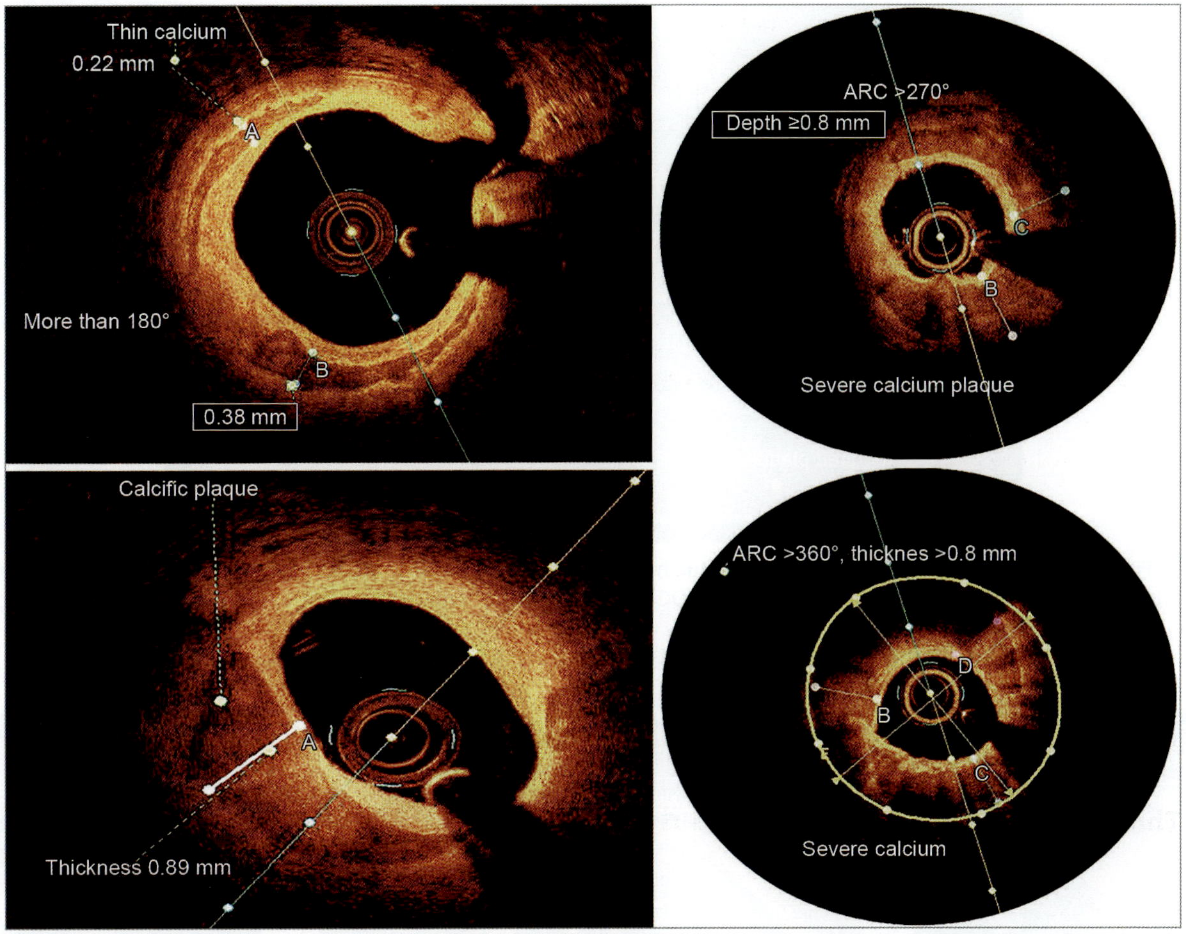

Fig. 11: Calcified plaque-calcified regions having sharp borders, low signal, and low attenuation permitting deeper penetration.

Nodular Calcification

Calcified nodules are more often seen in elderly patients with tortuous arteries. These are formed as a result of fractures of calcium plates due to rotational and excessive motion blood vessels during cardiac motion **(Figures 15A and B)**. Nodular calcium appears similar to calcified nodule (CN) but with intact fibrous cap and no luminal thrombus.

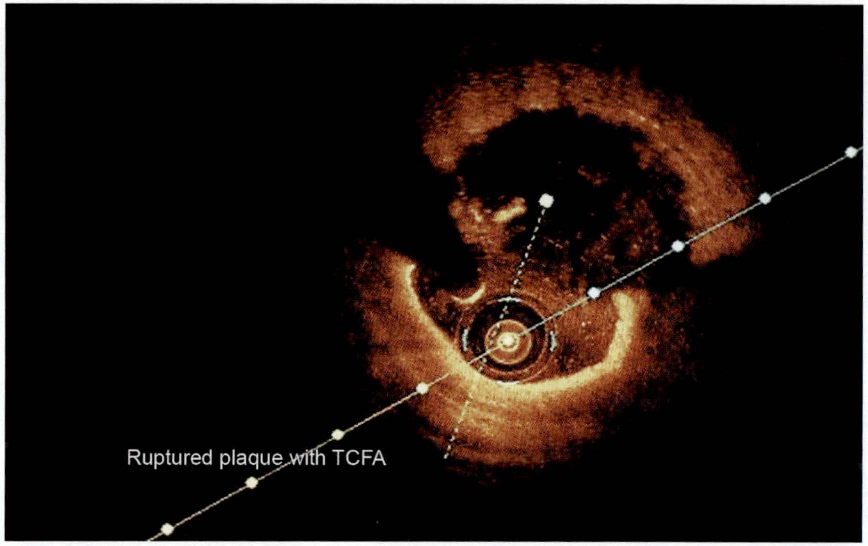

Fig. 12: The rupture of an atherosclerotic plaque has been defined as the discontinuity of the fibrous cap and the formation of a cavity in the plaque can be obtained by OCT. (OCT: optical coherence tomography; TCFA: thin-cap fibroatheroma)

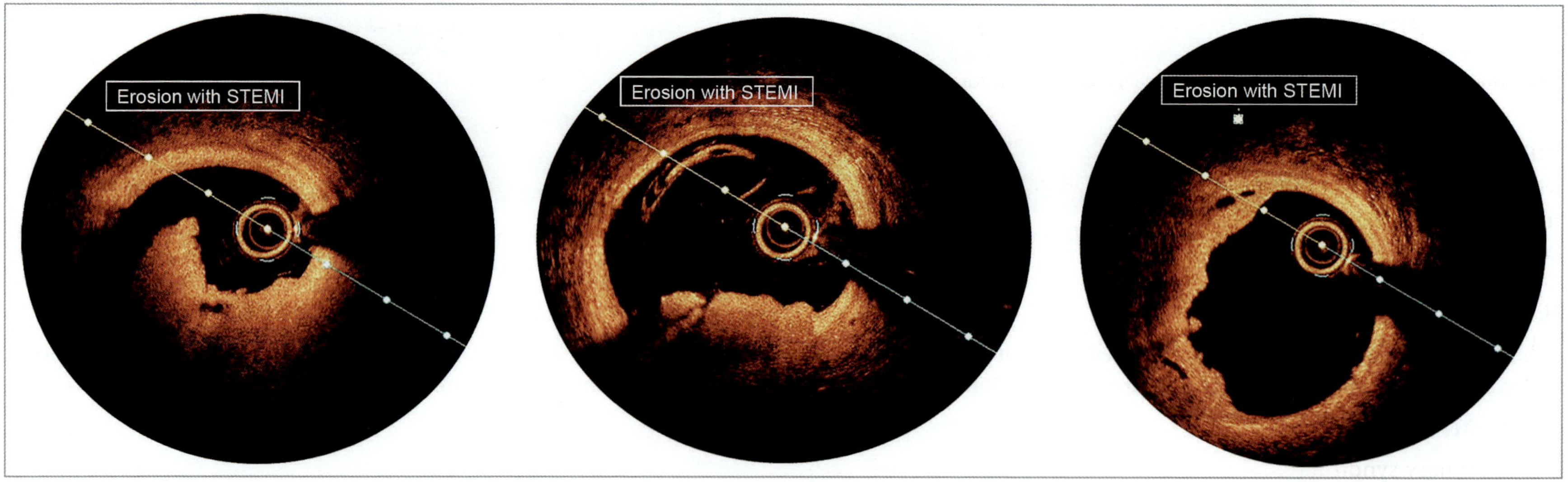

Fig. 13: Plaque erosion is considered "definite" in the absence of fibrous cap disruption, in a lesion frequently composed of fibrous tissue, with overlying luminal white thrombus. (STEMI: ST-elevation myocardial infarction)

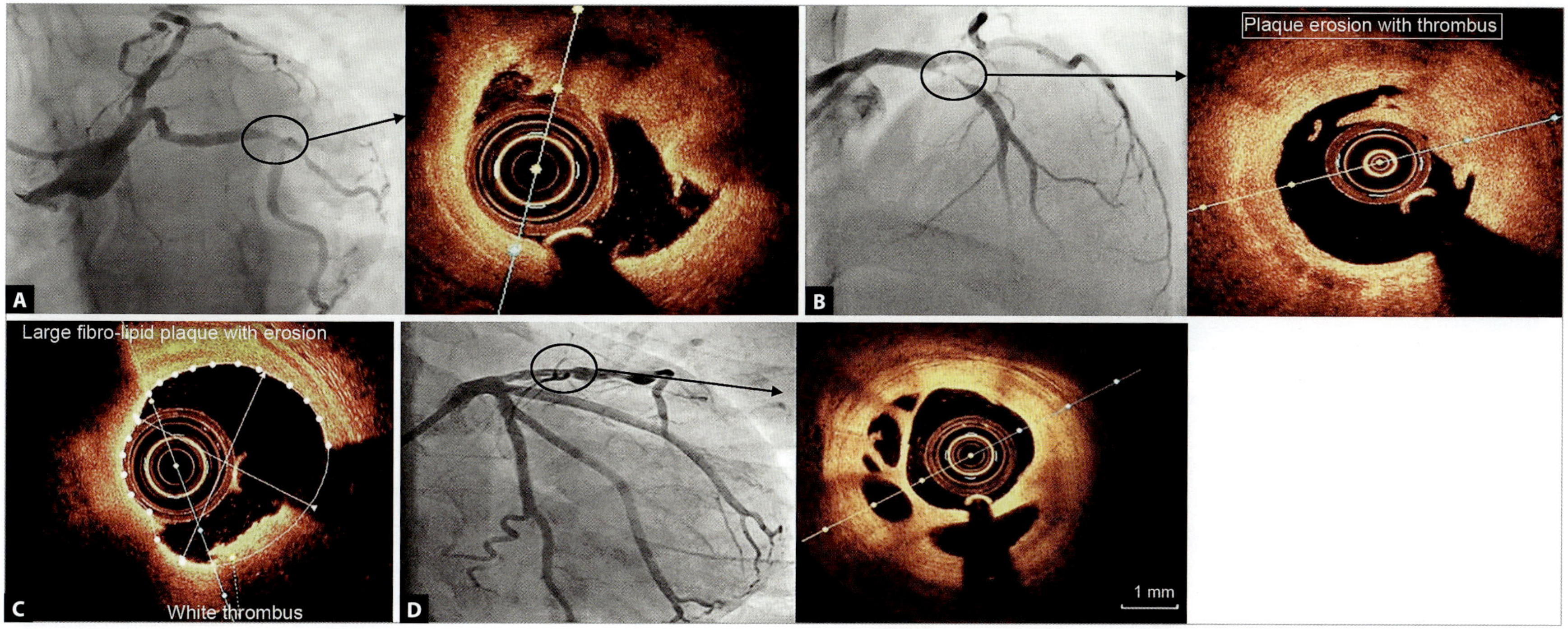

Figs. 14A to D: (A) Optical coherence tomography (OCT) definitive erosion (intact fibrous cap with attached red thrombus); (B) OCT probable erosion [large red thrombus with no adjacent necrotic core/lipid or superficial calcium (not shown in the figure)]; (C) plaque erosion defined by OCT is characterized as intact fibrous cap with thrombosis and underlying plaque structure can be visualized; (D) recanalized thrombus.

Eruptive Calcific Nodule

Eruptive calcific nodule **(Fig. 15A)** seen as a protruding calcification into the lumen and the presence of substantive calcium proximal and/or distal to the lesion with thrombus over the erupted nodule site. It may clinically manifest with ACS and PCI of these lesions are challenging due to significant calcium, leading to underexpansion unless plaques are adequately modified with appropriate calcium modification devices such as scoring balloon/ cutting balloon/ rotational atherectomy (ROTA)/orbital atherectomy (OA)/intravascular lithotripsy (IVL)/excimer laser coronary atherectomy (ELCA). OCT provides higher resolution of thrombus, delineation of superficial and deep calcium in terms of thickness, arc, and length, and plaque disruption. PCI of patients with CN presented with ACS are associated with higher MACE rate. Post-PCI optimization with OCT guidance reduces MACE rate compared to Angio-guided PCI by rectifying malapposition, underexpansion, and medial edge dissections.

LESIONS WITH ACUTE THROMBI

Acute coronary syndrome may be due to thrombus associated with PR/PE/eruptive CN and OCT identifies them with high sensitivity compared to IVUS.[15,16] Out of these three different pathologies, plaque rupture has been reported to be the most frequent (55–60%), plaque erosion to be the second (30–35%), and superficial calcified nodule to be the least (2–7%).

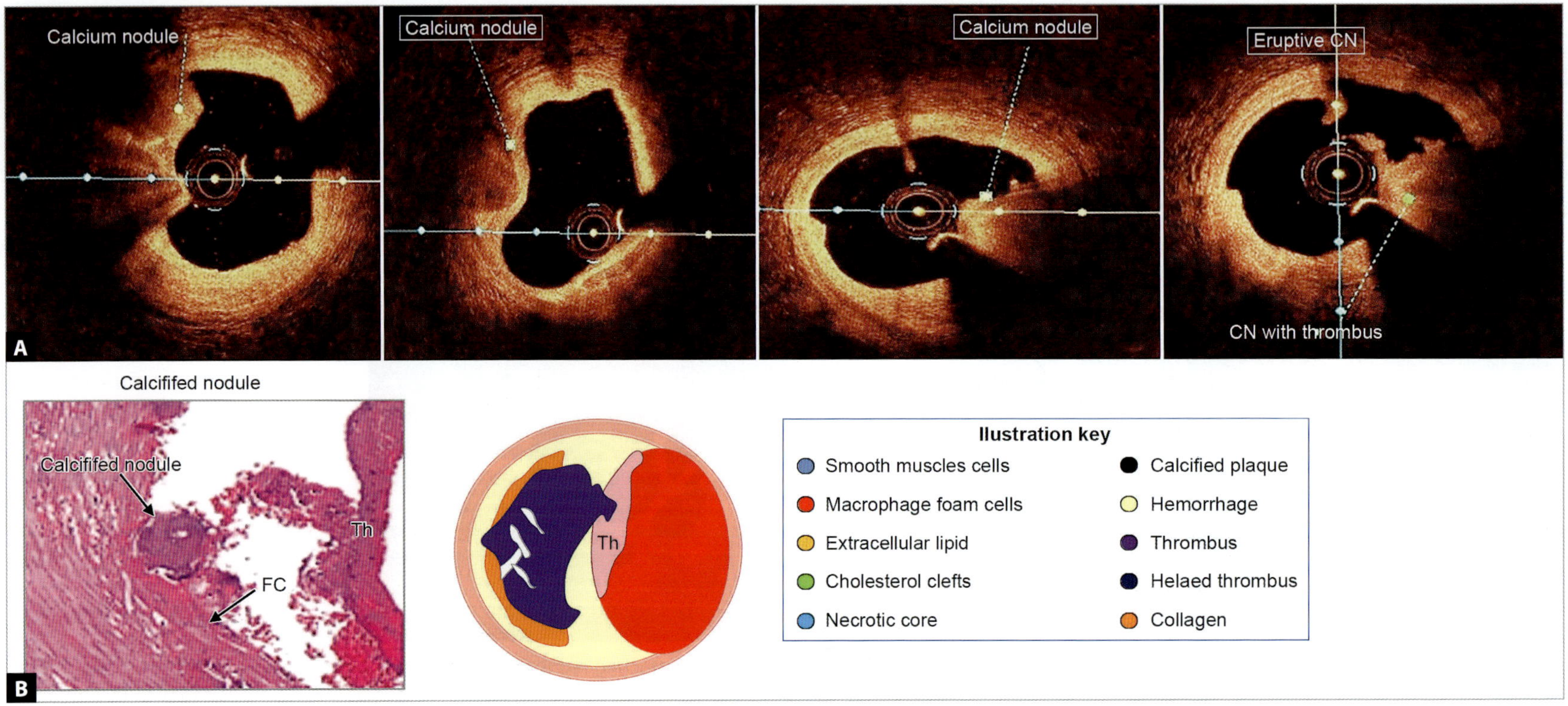

Figs. 15A and B: Calcified nodules (CN) are plaques with luminal thrombi showing calcific nodules protruding into the lumen through a disrupted thin fibrous cap (FC) and nodular calcium appears similar to CN but with intact fibrous cap and no luminal thrombus.

Optical coherence tomography detects thrombus in almost in all cases whereas IVUS in only 33% of patients presenting with acute MI[13] and it differentiates red thrombus from white thrombus. It is very important to discriminate intraluminal thrombus from residual blood due to poor clearance of the vessel.

Red thrombus seen as a high-backscattering protrusion mass with signal-free shadowing inside the vessel lumen and white thrombus is seen as low-backscattering projections. Proper characterization of thrombi may be useful to determine management strategies with appropriate antithrombotic drugs and thrombolytic therapies.

ASSESSMENT OF OCT IN ACS WITH ACUTE THROMBUS (FLOWCHART 2)

- Identify high risk features of vulnerable plaque **Figure 14E (*see* Fig. 18)**.
- Identify source of thrombus—PR/PE/CN/spontaneous coronary artery dissection (SCAD) **(Fig. 15)**.
- Identify calcium thickness, arc, and length—to assess any need for plaque modification **(Figs. 16 and 17)**.

Flowchart 2: Assessment of plaque morphology.

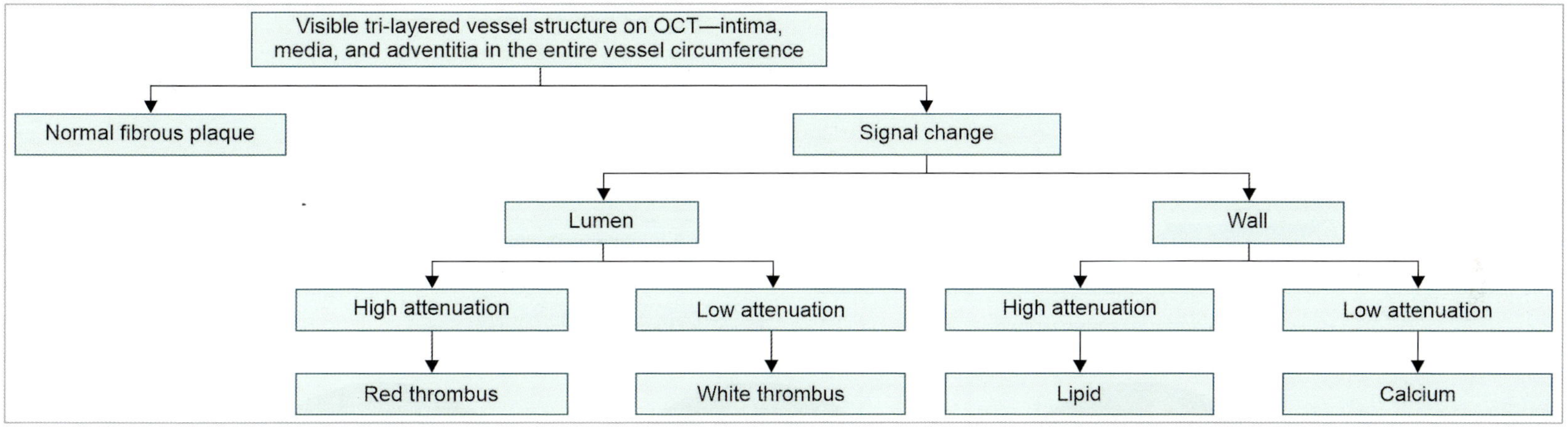

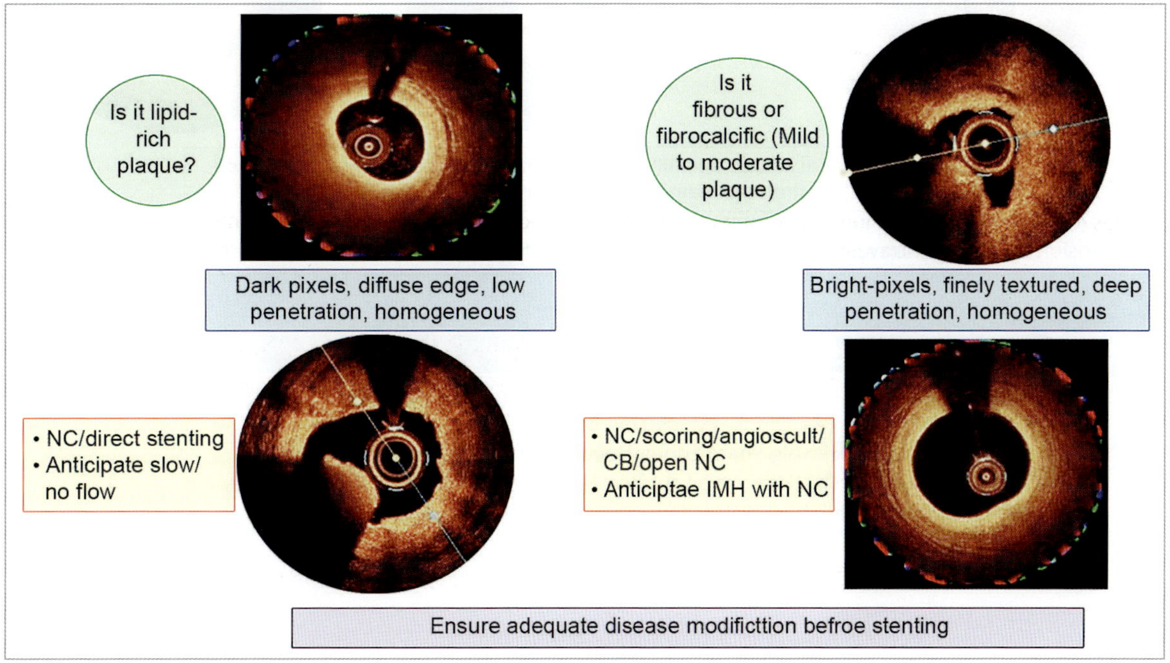

Fig. 16: Plaque morphology. (IMH: intramural hematoma; NC: non-compliant balloon)

- Identify and quantify thrombus load—to assess any need for thrombus aspiration/optimization of medications such as intra-arterial thrombolytic therapy/glycoprotein (GP) IIA and IIIA blockers.
- Identify artifacts and eliminate artifacts as far as possible.
- Good imaging with proper injection and proper alignment of appropriate guide catheter is necessary to get adequate data for proper PCI planning.

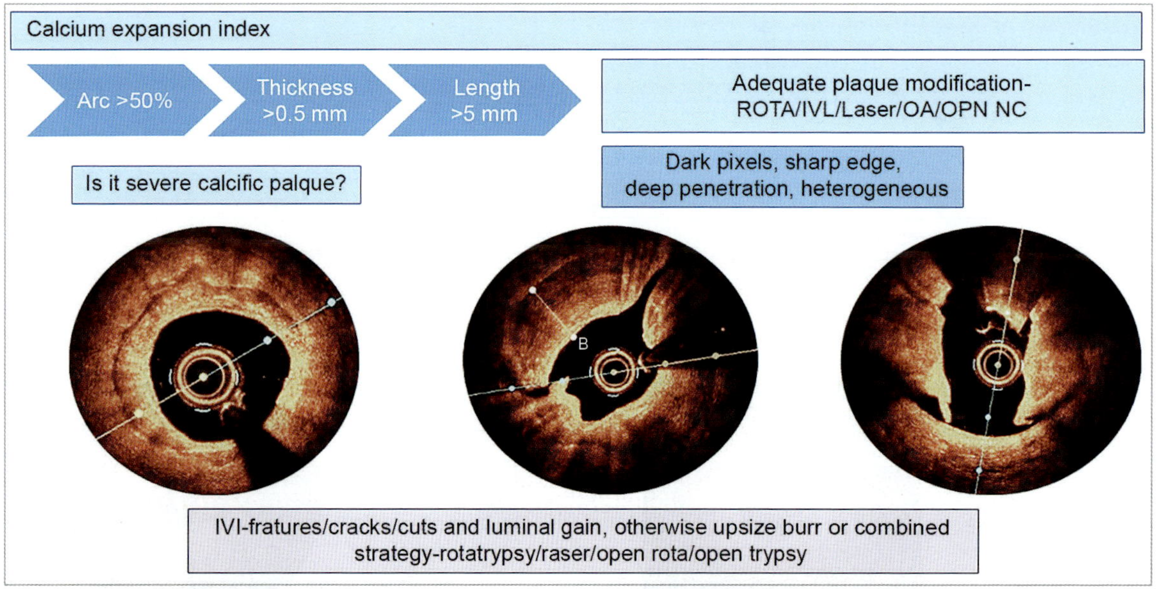

Fig. 17: Calcium expansion index. (IVI: intravascular imaging; IVL: intravascular lithotripsy; OA: orbital atherectomy; ROTA: rotational atherectomy)

Summerized plaque characterization by OCT.

- *Fibrous Plaque:* Bright Pixels, Finely textured, Deep Penetration, and Homogenous
- *Lipd Plaque:* Dark Pixels, Diffuse Edges, Low Penetration, and Homogenous
- *Calcific Plaque:* Dark Pixels, Sharp Edges, Deep Penetration, and Heterogenous
- *Red Thrombus:* High backscatter on surface, High attenuation, and cannot see beyond
- *White Thrombus:* High backscatter, low attenuation, and can be seen beyond

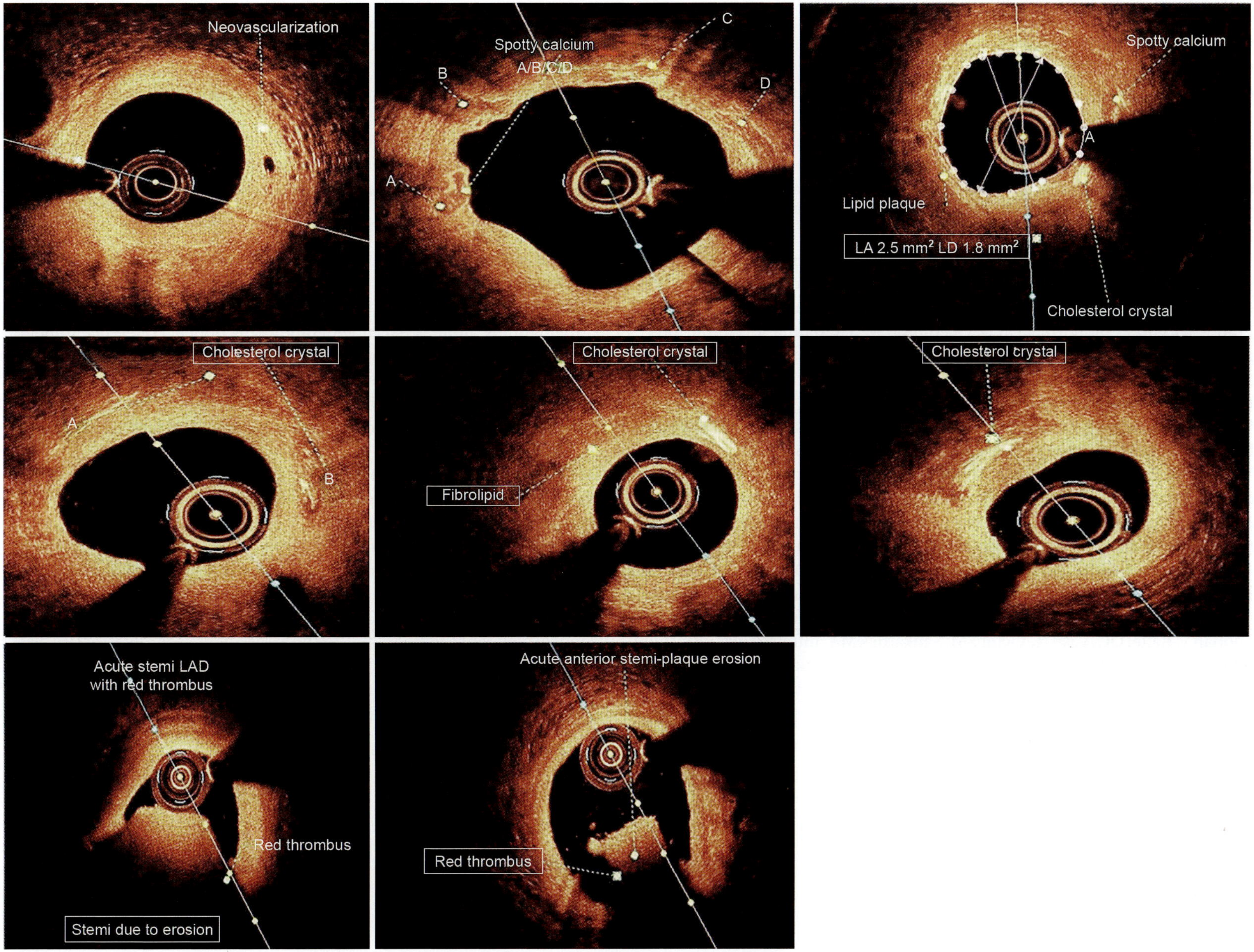

Fig. 18: High risk features of vulnerable plaque assessment by OCT. (LA: luminal area; LAD: left anterior descending; LD: luminal diameter; STEMI: ST-elevation myocardial infarction)

REFERENCES

1. Sandfort V, Lima JA, Bluemke DA. Noninvasive imaging of atherosclerotic plaque progression: status of coronary computed tomography angiography. Circ Cardiovasc Imaging. 2015;8(7):e003316.
2. Carità P, Guaricci AI, Muscogiuri G, Carrabba N, Pontone G. Prognostic value and therapeutic perspectives of coronary CT angiography: A literature review. Biomed Res Int. 2018;2018:6528238.
3. Kubo T, Ino Y, Tanimoto T, Kitabata H, Tanaka A, Akasaka T. Optical coherence tomography imaging in acute coronary syndromes. Cardiol Res Pract. 2011;2011:312978.
4. Prati F, Regar E, Mintz GS, Arbustini E, Di Mario C, Jang IK, et al. Expert review document on methodology, terminology, and clinical applications of optical coherence tomography: physical principles, methodology of image acquisition, and clinical application for assessment of coronary arteries and atherosclerosis. Eur Heart J. 2009;31(4):401-15.
5. Kume T, Uemura S. Current clinical applications of coronary optical coherence tomography. Cardiovasc Interv Ther. 2018;33(1):1-10.
6. Subban V, Raffel OC, Vasu N, Victor SM, Sankardas MA. Intravascular ultrasound and optical coherence tomography for the assessment of coronary artery disease and percutaneous coronary intervention optimization: Specific lesion subsets. Indian Heart J Interv. 2018;1(2):95.
7. Kume T, Kubo T, Akasaka T. Histology Validation of OCT Images. In: Jang I-K (Ed). Cardiovascular OCT Imaging. USA: Springer, Cham; 2015. pp. 39-51.
8. Prati F, Di Vito L, Biondi-Zoccai G, Occhipinti M, La Manna A, Tamburino C, et al. Angiography alone versus angiography plus optical coherence tomography to guide decision-making during percutaneous coronary intervention: the Centro per la Lotta contro l'Infarto-Optimisation of Percutaneous Coronary Intervention (CLI-OPCI) study. EuroIntervention. 2012;8(7):823-9.
9. Romagnoli E, Gatto L, Prati F. The CLIMA study: assessing the risk of myocardial infarction with a new anatomical score. Eur Heart J Suppl. 2019;21(Suppl B):B80-3.
10. Virmani R, Kolodgie FD, Burke AP, Farb A, Schwartz SM. Lessons from sudden coronary death: a comprehensive morphological classification scheme for atherosclerotic lesions. Arterioscler Thromb Vasc Biol. 2000;20(5):1262-75.
11. Vergallo R, Porto I, D'Amario D, Annibali G, Galli M, Benenati S, et al. Coronary atherosclerotic phenotype and plaque healing in patients with recurrent acute coronary syndromes compared with patients with long-term clinical stability: an in vivo optical coherence tomography study. JAMA Cardiol. 2019;4(4):321-9.
12. Räber L, Mintz GS, Koskinas KC, Johnson TW, Holm NR, Onuma Y, et al. Clinical use of intracoronary imaging. Part 1: guidance and optimization of coronary interventions. An expert consensus document of the European Association of Percutaneous Cardiovascular Interventions. Eur Heart J. 2018;39(35):3281-300.
13. Herrero-Garibi J, Cruz-González I, Parejo-Díaz P, Jang IK. Optical coherence tomography: its value in intravascular diagnosis today. Rev Esp Cardiol. 2010;63(8):951-62.
14. Jia H, Abtahian F, Aguirre AD, Lee S, Chia S, Lowe H, et al. In vivo diagnosis of plaque erosion and calcified nodule in patients with acute coronary syndrome by intravascular optical coherence tomography. J Am Coll Cardiol. 2013;62(19):1748-58.
15. Subban V, Raffel OC, Vasu N, Victor SM, Sankardas MA. Intravascular ultrasound and optical coherence tomography for the assessment of coronary artery disease and percutaneous coronary intervention optimization: Specific lesion subsets. Indian Heart J Interv. 2018;1(2):95.
16. Akasaka T, Kubo T, Mizukoshi M, Tanaka A, Kitabata H, Tanimoto T, et al. Pathophysiology of acute coronary syndrome assessed by optical coherence tomography. J Cardiol. 2010;56(1):8-14.

CHAPTER 2

Selection of Optimal Stent Sizing

ABSTRACT

Proper vessel sizing is very important for choosing the balloon, stent length, and diameter to avoid stent underexpansion, which is a strong predictor of early stent thrombosis and restenosis after drug-eluting stent (DES) implantation. Undersized stent is associated with malapposition and underexpansion. Oversized stent is associated with dissection, intramural hematoma, and perforation. Overexpansion of the stent may lead to stent fracture, dissection, and perforation. Select proper landing zones to cover entire diseased segment to maintain better long-term DES outcomes mainly to reduce restenosis and stent thrombosis. Optical coherence tomography (OCT) pre-percutaneous coronary intervention (PCI) allows accurate quantification of stenosis severity and extension characterization of the underlying plaque components and morphometry, helps to locate adequate landing zones for the stent to be implanted, and provides accurate vessel sizing for selection of the stent length and diameter. It also allows up-front anticipation of the need for balloon postdilatation and the type and size of the balloon to be used.

INTRODUCTION

Angiographic assessment of stent sizing is sometimes very difficult in diffuse long lesions, culprit vessel of ST-elevation myocardial infarction (STEMI), distal segment of chronic total occlusion (CTO), myocardial bridge, and segments with remodeling. It would be essential to assess vessel size with optical coherence tomography (OCT) after giving intracoronary nitroglycerin (IC NTG) or nicorandil to rule out any associated vasospasm **(Box 1)**.[1]

As per the OPUS-CLASS study **(Figs. 1A and B)**, Fourier domain OCT (FD-OCT) provided accurate measurements of coronary lumen with excellent intraobserver reproducibility. Compared to FD-OCT, quantitative coronary angiography (QCA) measured smaller lumen diameter and intravascular ultrasound (IVUS) measured larger lumen areas, although the correlations among these three methods were high.[2]

BOX 1: Limitations of coronary angiography.

- Accuracy of angiography for estimating mild lesions (30%) and very severe stenosis (90%) is more, whereas less for intermediate lesions (60%).
- Angio-based decision-making is sometimes difficult when lesions are ambiguous or with complex coronary anatomy such as lesions with thrombus, diffuse disease, calcification, spontaneous dissection, recanalized thrombus, and bifurcation lesions.
- May not be reliable to assess poststenting haziness on angiography, e.g., residual plaque burden in the landing zones, thrombus, medial edge dissection, intramyocardial hemorrhage (IMH), and tissue prolapse.

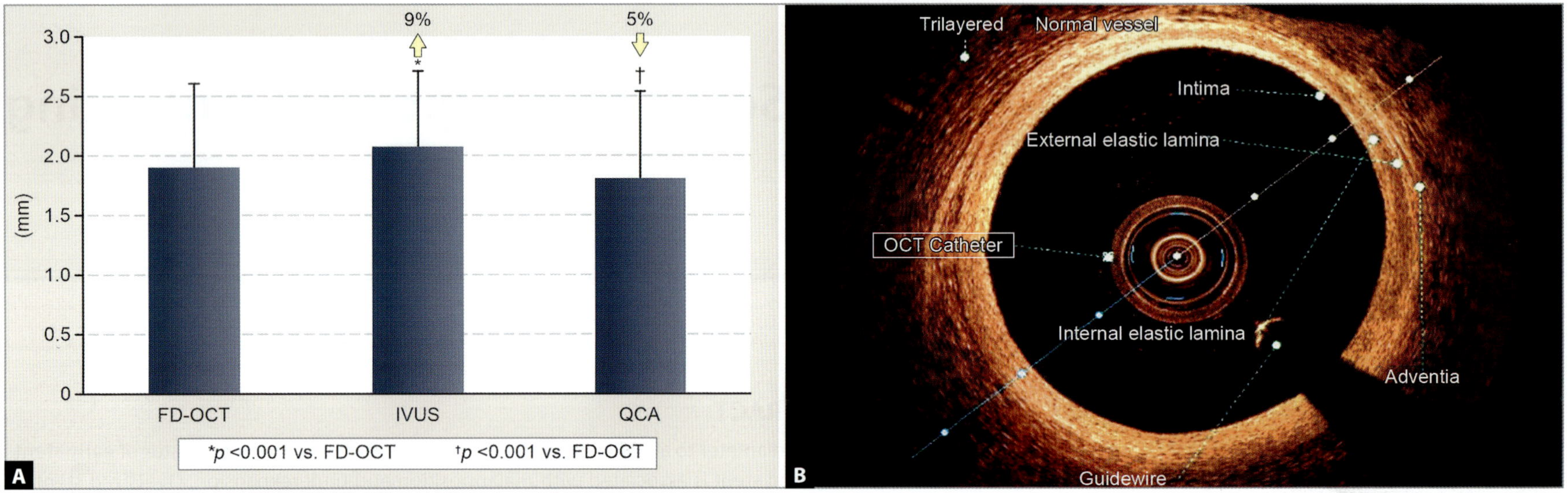

Figs. 1A and B: FD-OCT provided accurate measurements of coronary lumen with excellent intraobserver reproducibility.
(FD-OCT: Fourier domain optical coherence tomography; IVUS: intravascular ultrasound; QCA: quantitative coronary angiography)

SELECTION OF OPTIMAL STENT SIZING AND STENT DIAMETER

Normal artery: The bright-dark bright, three-layered appearance corresponding to intima, media, and adventitia is visualized in the entirety of the vessel circumference. Simplified algorithm for interpretation of OCT images in the native coronary arteries. Common morphologies detected on intracoronary OCT are shown in **Figure 2**.

Stent size is usually based on either distal or proximal or mean of both diameters. While planning percutaneous coronary intervention (PCI) with drug-eluting stent (DES), progressively larger stent diameters would be opted by smallest reference diameter, the mean (average of proximal and distal) reference lumen dimeter, and the largest reference diameter (proximal or distal).[3,4]

INTRAVASCULAR ULTRASOUND VERSUS OPTICAL COHERENCE TOMOGRAPHY FOR SELECTION OF EXTERNAL ELASTIC MEMBRANE VERSUS LUMEN-BASED DIAMETERS ASSESSMENT (TABLE 1)

Operators may face problems in selecting external elastic membrane (EEM) borders with OCT compared to IVUS, particularly when plaque burden is more **(Figs. 3A to D)**. EEM and adventitial layers are easily visible on IVUS compared to OCT, but OCT can detect EEM very clearly when no plaque burden/ plaque burden is less, particularly in the absence of lipid-rich plaque.[5,6]

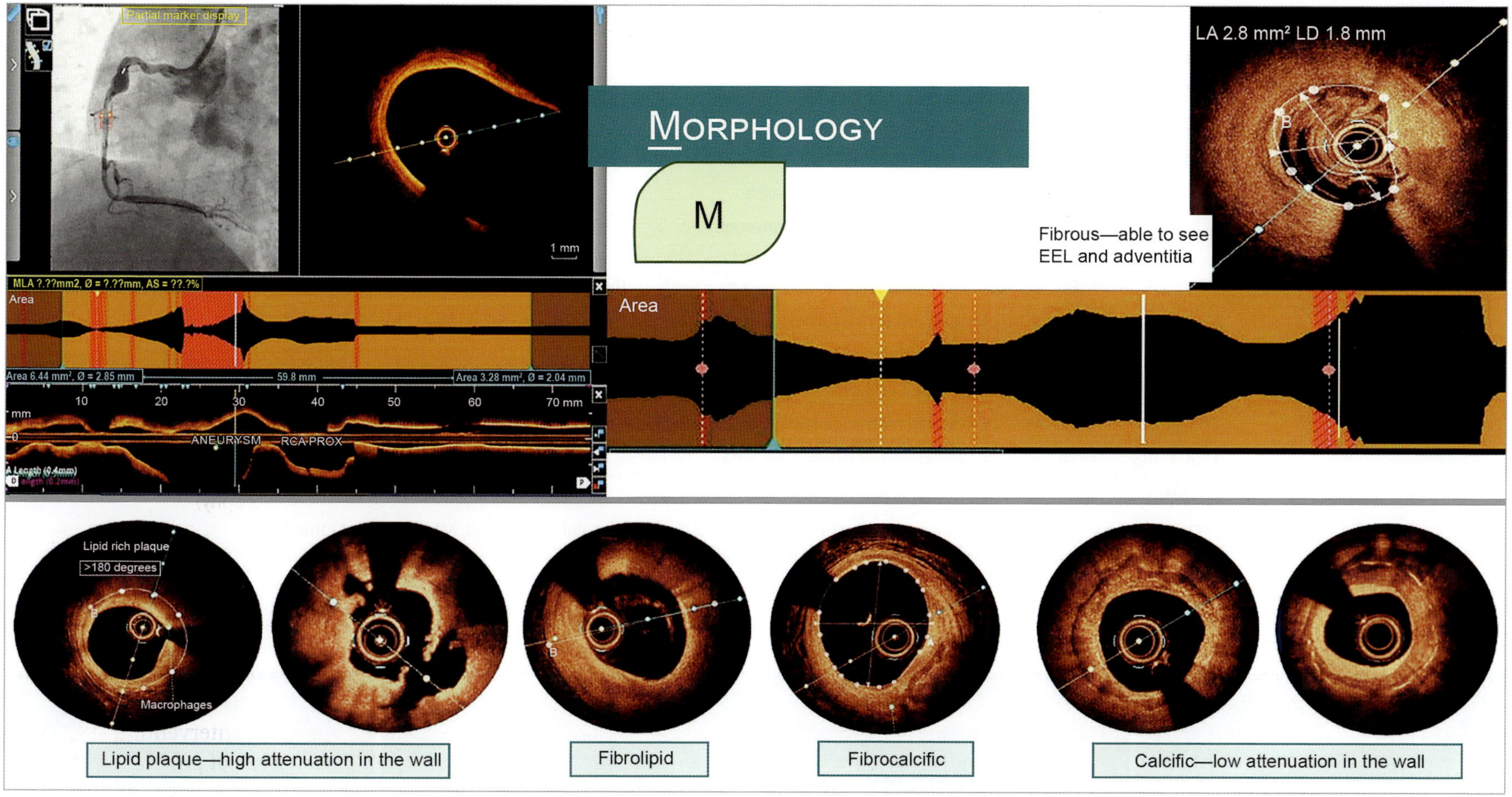

Fig. 2: OCT pre-PCI allows accurate quantification of stenosis severity and extension and characterization of the underlying plaque components and morphometry. (EEL: external elastic lamina; LA: luminal area; LD: luminal diameter; OCT: optical coherence tomography; PCI: percutaneous coronary intervention)

STENT DIAMETER

During PCI, choose proper landing zones with the help of Angio coregistration **(Fig. 4)**, decide distal reference diameter and proximal reference diameter (either EEM or lumen based) by scrolling white marker on the Angio images with corresponding cross-sectional and longitudinal images of OCT, select the stent diameter according to distal reference diameter, and optimize proximal half of the stent with noncompliant (NC) balloon size matching the proximal reference diameter. When applying a lumen-based approach, the use of the mean lumen diameter with up-rounding the stent diameter for 0–0.25 mm was recommended in the OPINION study. Lumen-based stent sizing with OCT results in smaller stent areas compared to that with IVUS, and hence, the recent studies recommend two different approaches. The ILUMIEN III investigators suggested an external elastic lamina- (EEL)-based stent-sizing algorithm.

TABLE 1: IVUS versus OCT for selection of EEM versus lumen-based diameters assessment.

Study	***Target***
IVUS-XPL	MSA >distal reference lumen area
CTO-IVUS	MSA >distal reference lumen area >5 mm^2 at CTO
HOME-DES	MSA >than 5 mm^2 or MSA >80% distal reference lumen area for small vessel
AVID	MSA >90% of distal reference lumen area
TULIP	MLD >80% mean reference lumen diameters MSA >distal reference lumen area
OPTICUS	MSA >90% of mean reference lumen area or >100% of the reference with lowest lumen area
SIPS	MSA >90% of mean reference lumen area or >100% of the reference with lowest lumen area
RESIST	MSA >80% of mean reference lumen area
ILUMEN 3	MSA >90% in proximal and distal reference segments relative to closest reference
OPINION	MSA >90% of average reference lumen area
DOCTORS	MSA >80% of average reference lumen area
OCTACS	MSA >90% of average reference lumen area

(CTO: chronic total occlusion; EEM: external elastic membrane; IVUS: intravascular ultrasound; MLD: minimal lumen diameter; MSA: minimal stent area; OCT: optical coherence tomography)

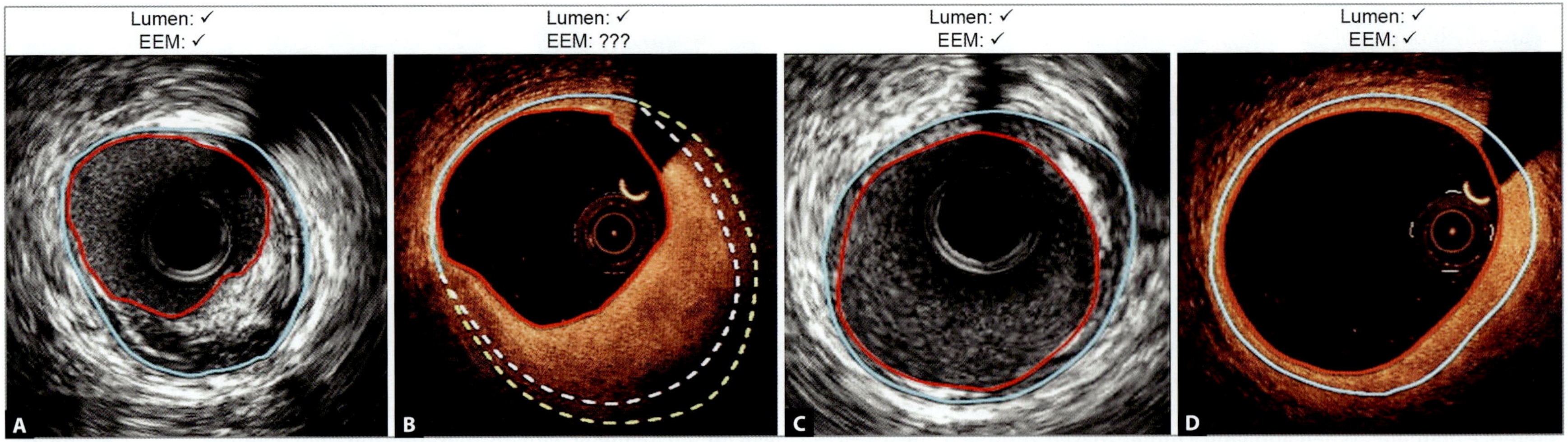

Figs. 3A to D: Difficulty in selecting EEM borders with OCT compared to IVUS, particularly when plaque burden is more.
(EEM: external elastic membrane; IVUS: intravascular ultrasound; OCT: optical coherence tomography)

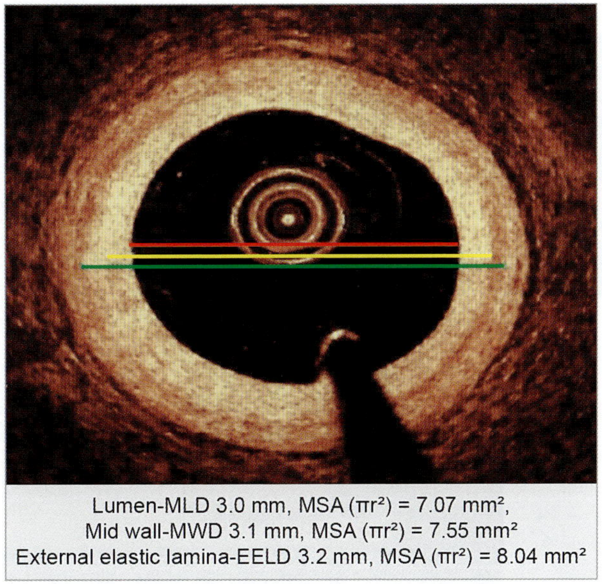

Fig. 4: The OCT compared with IVUS and with angiography to guide coronary stent implantation (ILUMIEN III) study used an EEL-based stent-sizing algorithm. (EEL: external elastic lamina; IVUS: intravascular ultrasound; MLD: minimal lumen diameter; MSA: minimal stent area; OCT: optical coherence tomography)

When the reference segments are healthy and the media is clearly visible all around, maximum and minimum diameters of EEL are measured and the mean EEL diameter of each reference is calculated.

The OPINION trial produced the target vessel failure of 5.2% in OCT-guided PCI versus 4.9% in the IVUS-guided PCI group at 1 year by using luminal-based sizing **(Fig. 5)**.

Increasingly aggressive **(Fig. 6)**—maximum diameter of the smaller reference, average of the maximum diameters of the proximal and distal references, maximum diameter of the largest reference, mid-wall-to-mid-wall diameters (between lumen and media), and media-to-media diameter.

STENT LENGTH (FLOWCHART 1)

Stent length is the distance between proximal and distal reference diameters.

Landing zones are the regions with the largest lumen dimensions proximal and distal to a stenosis, within the same segment, with no major intervening branches **(Figs. 7 and 8)**.

- Avoid landing zone with residual plaque burden (>50%), particularly lipid-rich plaque (TCFA) because of increased SER.
- Plaque with calcium angle of ≥72°.
- Thick fibrotic plaque >50%
- Incomplete stent coverage of lipid pool—an increased risk of postprocedural myocardial infarction (MI).

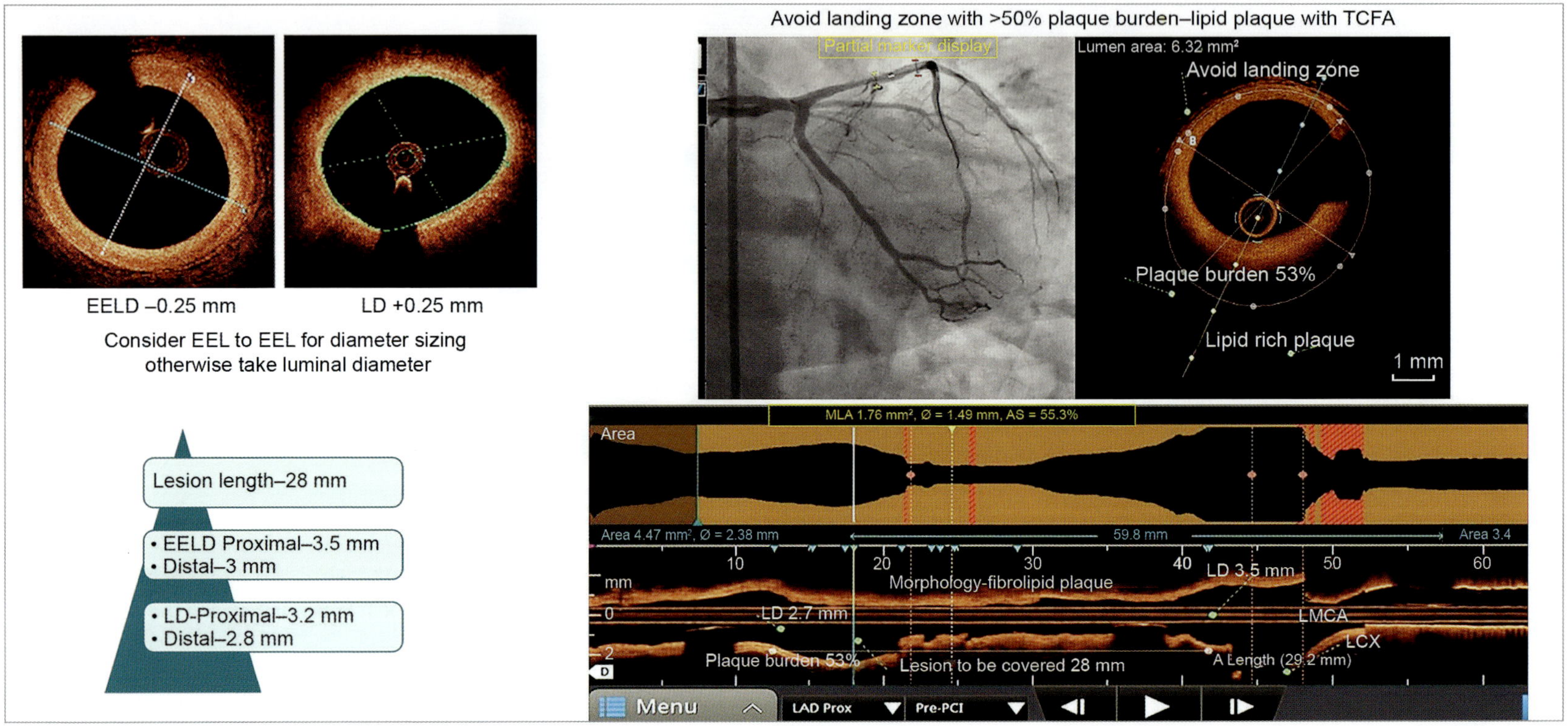

Fig. 5: Case example of sizing of the stent with increased plaque burden in the landing zone based on Angio decision. (EELD: external elastic lamina diameter; IVUS: intravascular ultrasound; LD: lumen diameter; MLA: minimal lumen area; OCT: optical coherence tomography; PROX: proximal; TCFA: thin-cap fibroatheroma)

TABLE 2: Music criteria.

If minimal stent area (MSA) <9.0 mm^2	MSA >90% of the mean reference lumen area or MSA >100% of lumen lowest reference area, proximal stent entrance >90% of proximal reference lumen area
If MSA >9.0 mm^2	MSA >80% of the mean reference area or MSA >90% of lumen lowest reference lumen area
	Symmetric stent expansion defined by stent D_{min}/D_{max} >0.7 complete stent apposition against the vessel wall

Source: Adapted from DeJaegere et al. 1998.

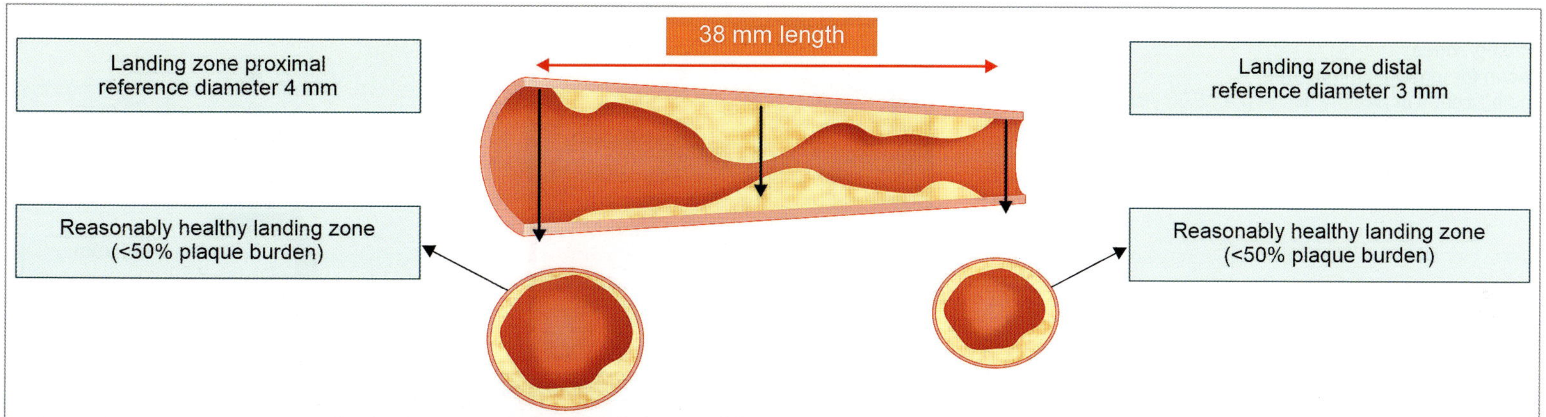

1. Distal lumen reference-based sizing may represent a safe and straightforward approach with subsequent optimization of the mid and proximal stent segments. Specifically, the mean distal lumen diameter with up rounding stent (0–0.25 mm) may be used (e.g., 3.76! 4.0 mm) or the mean EEM (two orthogonal measurements) with down rounding to the nearest 0.25 mm stent size (e.g., 3.76!3.5).
2. Coregistration of angiography and IVUS or OCT is a useful tool to determine stent length and allows for precise stent placement.

Fig. 6: Selecting the stent diameter according to the proximal and distal reference healthy zones. (EEM: external elastic membrane; IVUS: intravascular ultrasound; OCT: optical coherence tomography)

Flowchart 1: OCT stent-sizing algorithm.

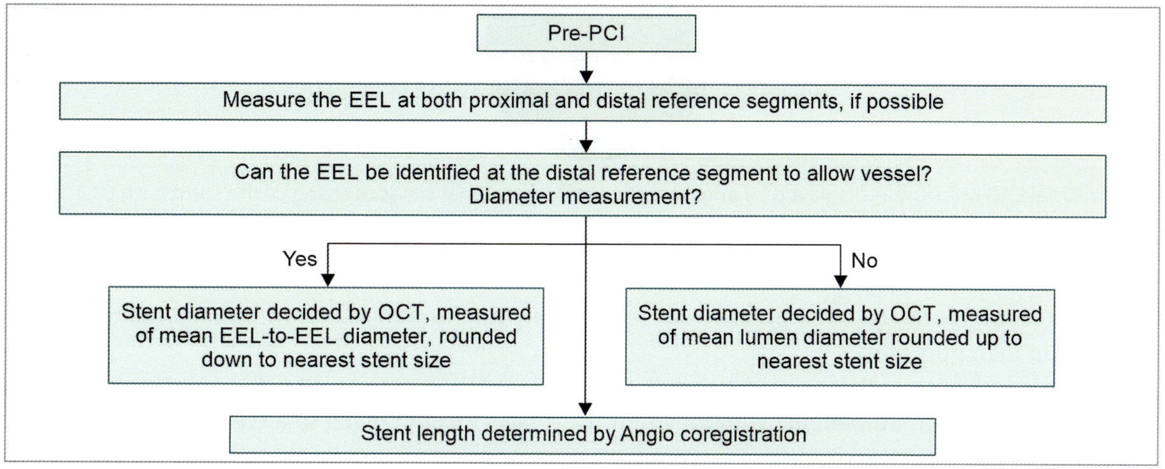

(EEL: external elastic lamina; OCT: optical coherence tomography; PCI: percutaneous coronary intervention)

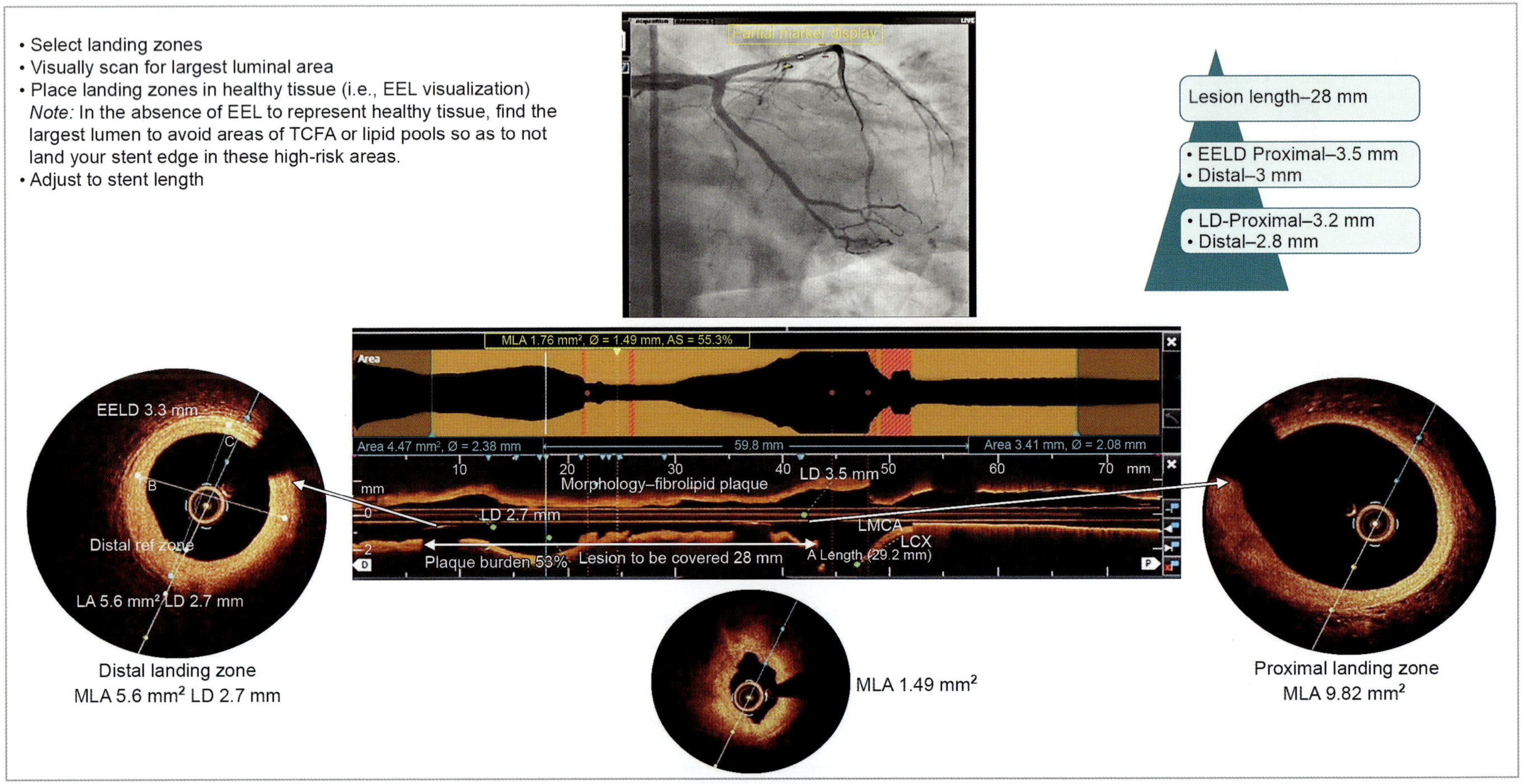

Fig. 7: Illustrative case of a proximal LAD stenosis as displayed by angiography and longitudinal views of sizing of the stent with OCT. (EEL: external elastic lamina; LA: luminal area; LAD: left anterior descending; LD: luminal diameter; MLA: minimal luminal area; REF: reference; TCFA: thin-cap fibroatheroma)

After stenting, postdilatation is recommended in the presence of residual plaque burden >50%, minimal stent area (MSA) was <80% of the distal reference lumen area, and significant malapposition.

Choosing stent with appropriate length is essential to avoid incomplete coverage of the lesion and Angio coregistration is an important tool to facilitate stent length selection and precise implantation. In patients with long lesions, vessels located distal to a CTO or segments involving a myocardial bridge

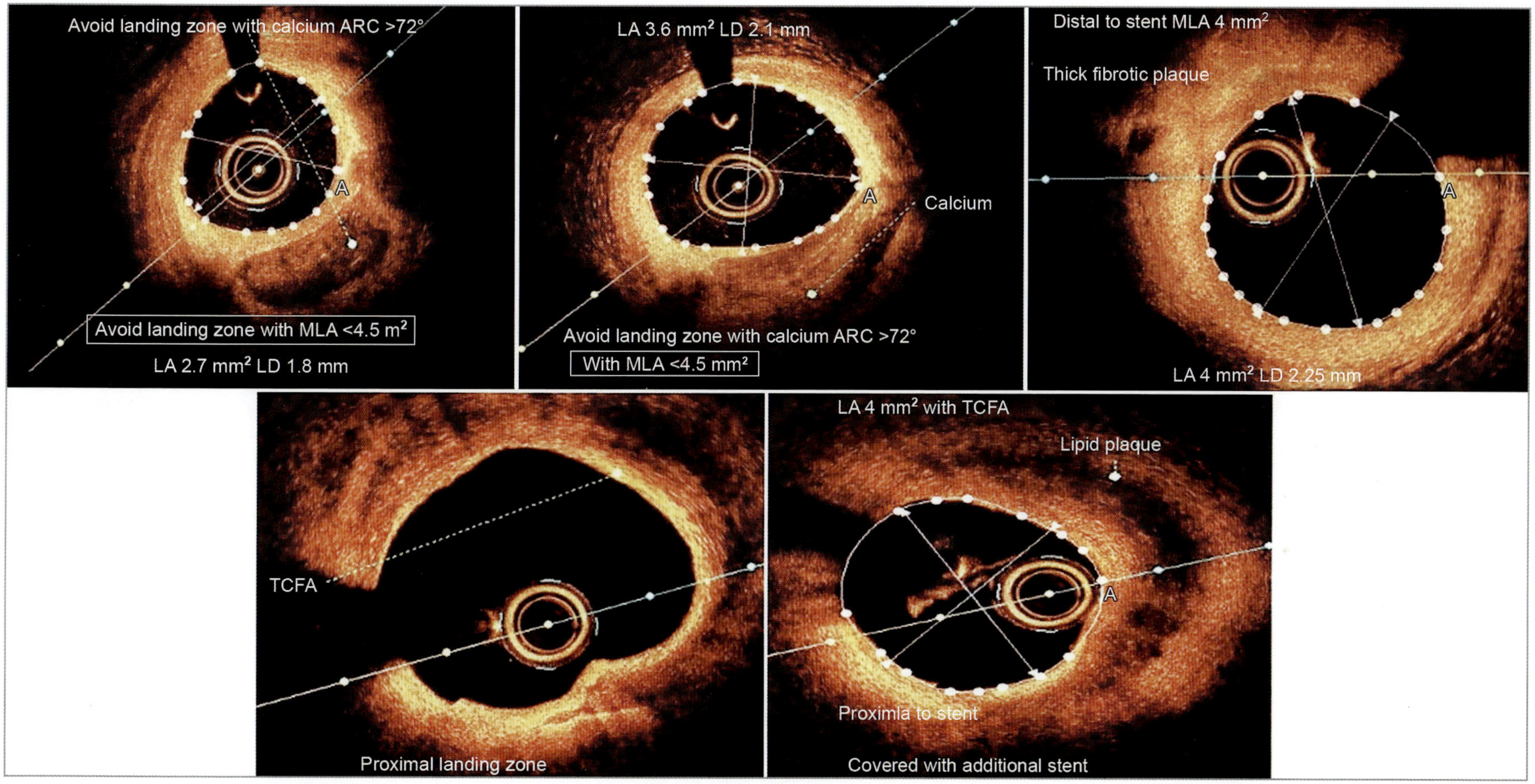

Fig. 8: Avoid landing zones with more plaque burden, especially lipid rich plaques. (LA: luminal area; LD: luminal diameter; MLA: minimal luminal area; TCFA: thin-cap fibroatheroma)

assessment of vessel size may be important to rule out negative vessel remodeling and to ensure that the selected stent size does not lead to the risk of vessel rupture. Intravascular imaging guidance results in larger stent diameter, greater angiographic minimal lumen diameter (MLD) and MSA, and implantation of more and longer stents compared with angiographic guidance.[7]

Angio coregistration is very useful in choosing diameter and length if the stent and optimization of implantation—MLD-MAX algorithm.

REFERENCES

1. Seth A, Gupta S, Singh VP, Kumar V. Expert opinion: optimising stent deployment in contemporary practice: the role of intracoronary imaging and non-compliant balloons. Interv Cardiol Rev. 2017;12(2):81.
2. Räber L, Mintz GS, Koskinas KC, Johnson TW, Holm NR, Onuma Y, et al. Clinical use of intracoronary imaging. Part 1: guidance and optimization of coronary interventions. An expert consensus document of the European Association of Percutaneous Cardiovascular Interventions. Eur Heart J. 2018;39(35):3281-300.
3. Subban V, Raffel OC, Vasu N, Victor SM, Sankardas MA. Intravascular ultrasound and optical coherence tomography for the assessment of coronary artery disease and percutaneous coronary intervention optimization: Specific lesion subsets. Indian Heart J Interv. 2018;1(2):95.
4. Ali ZA, Galougahi KK, Maehara A, Shlofmitz RA, Ben-Yehuda O, Mintz GS, et al. Intracoronary optical coherence tomography 2018: current status and future directions. JACC Cardiovasc Interv. 2017;10(24):2473-87.
5. Ino Y, Kubo T, Matsuo Y, Yamaguchi T, Shiono Y, Shimamura K, et al. Optical coherence tomography predictors for edge restenosis after everolimus-eluting stent implantation. Circ Cardiovasc Interv. 2016;9(10):e004231.
6. https://books.google.co.in/books?id=vKU5DwAAQBAJ&printsec=frontcover&dq=oct+made+easy+hiram&hl=en&sa=X&ved=0ahUKEwiarKLF78bnAhWKXSsKHd7IBoAQ6AEIKDAA#v=onepage&q=oct%20made%20easy%20hiram&f=false
7. Dash D. Stenting of left main coronary artery stenosis: A to Z. Heart Asia. 2013;5(1):18-27.

CASE 1

Device selection and choosing landing zones—provisional stenting of left anterior descending (LAD)/D1 bifurcation.

CLINICAL HISTORY

A 60-year-old male, a known hypertensive and diabetic, presented with coronary artery disease (CAD-unstable angina. Past history of PCI of left circumflex (LCX) in 2019 (2.5 × 38 mm premier element stent). Investigations: Hemoglobin (Hb) 12.5 g/dL, blood urea 23 mg/dL, serum creatinine (S Cr) 1.1 mg/dL, estimated glomerular filtration rate (eGFR) 72 mL/min, random blood sugar (RBS) 137 mg/dL, and troponin I <0.01 ng/mL. Two-dimensional (2D) echo—no regional wall motion abnormalities (RWMA), normal left ventricular (LV) function, and ejection fraction (EF) 62%. CAG: LMCA—normal, LAD—mid 90% stenosis, D1—normal, D2—ostioproximal 50-60% stenosis, LCX—normal with patent stent, and right coronary artery (RCA)—normal **(Figs. 9A to C)**.

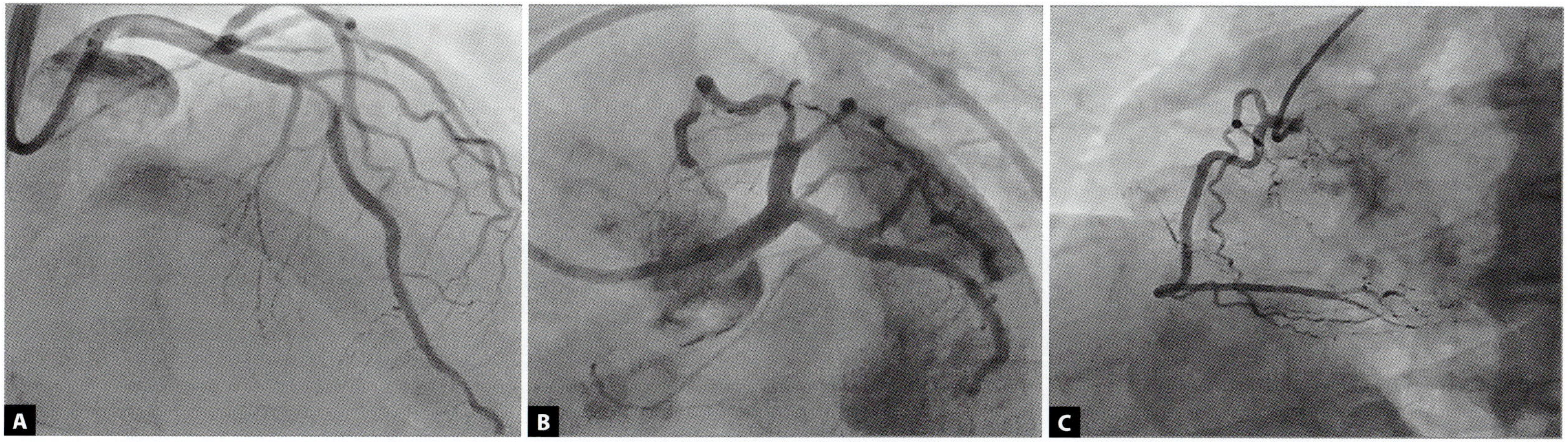

Figs. 9A to C: Coronary angiogram.

PROCEDURE

Route—right radial approach (RRA), using 6 Fr EBU 3.5 guiding catheter, LAD—mid 80-90% lesion which was crossed with 0.014″ Runthrough wire in LAD, and turn track placed in D1. Pre-OCT showed fibrocalcific plaque **(Figs. 10A and B)**. Predilated with 3.0 × 12 mm NC Trek balloon, stenting with

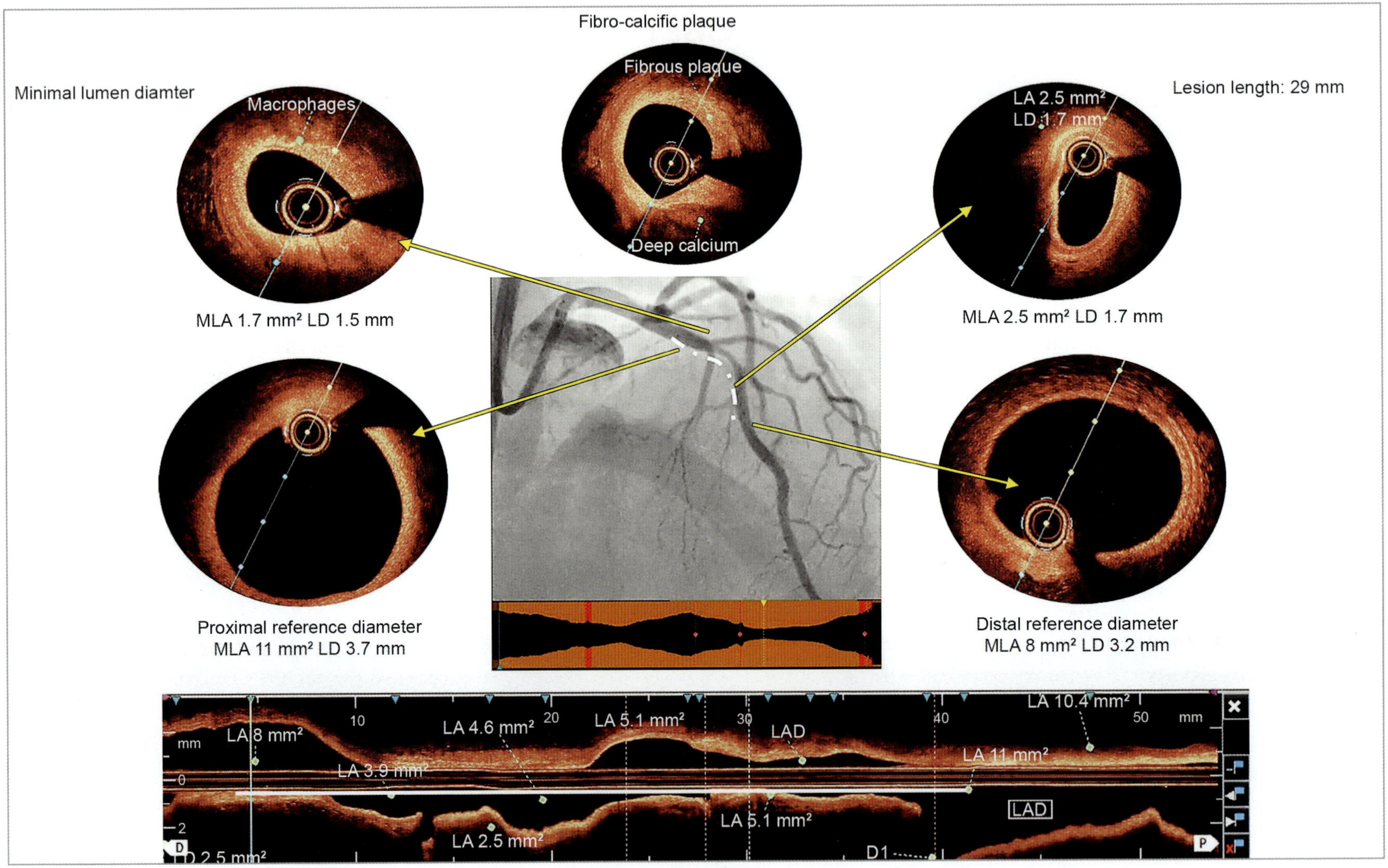

Fig. 10A

- **CB/Scoring balloons- Produces controlled dissections with less inflammation and better MLA gain, less chances of IMH, and No melon seed effect with thick fibrotic lesions**
- **Very useful for dilating Ostial fibrotic and mild to moderate fibrotic plaques**
- **Relatively Expensive compared to NC/Semi compliant balloons.**

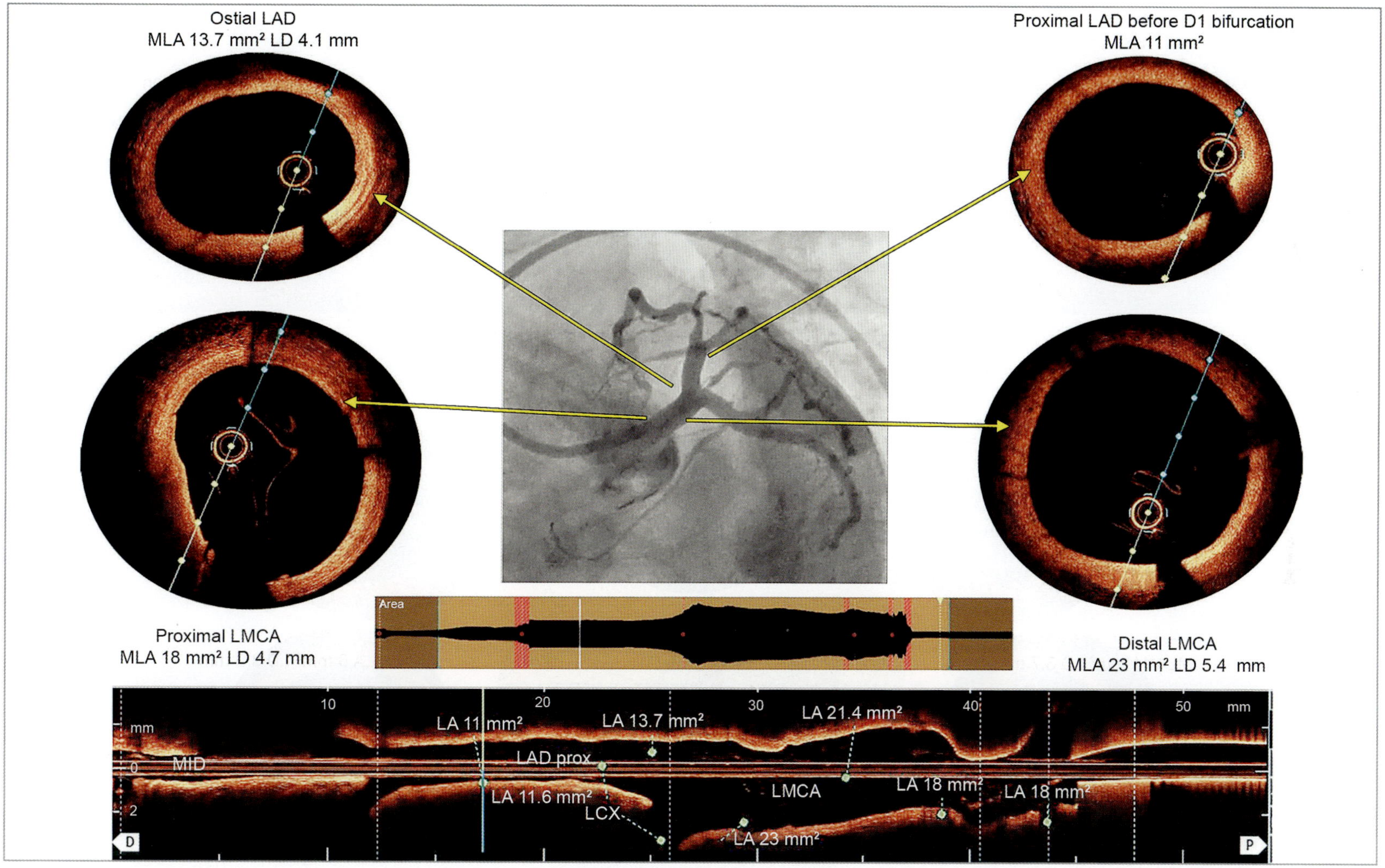

Fig. 10B

Figs. 10A and B: (A) Presenting OCT assessment to select devise size (length and diameter). (B) Assessment of LM and non-LM bifurcation using OCT. (LAD: left anterior descending; LCX: left circumflex; LD: luminal diameter; LM: left main; LMCA: left main coronary artery; MLA: minimal luminal area; OCT: optical coherence tomography)

3.5 × 34 mm Resolute Onyx stent, and postdilatation of LAD was done with 4.0 × 12 mm NC Apollo balloon **(Figs. 11A to D)**. Post-OCT showed well-apposed and expanded stent struts with no edge dissection and no residual thrombus **(Fig. 12)**. Postprocedure Angio view showed well-implanted stents with thrombolysis in myocardial infarction III (TIMI-III) flow without any dissection.

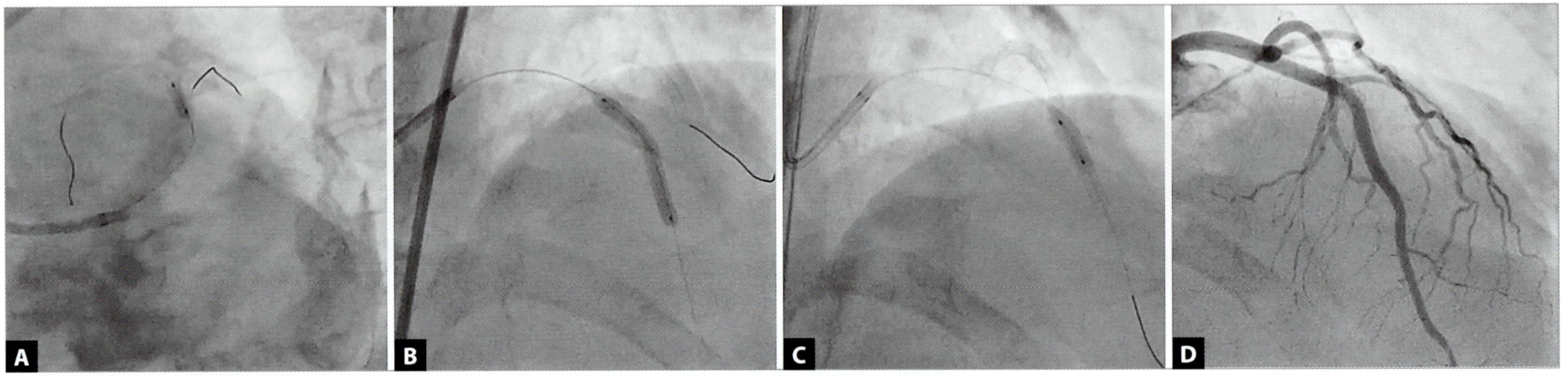

Figs. 11A to D: Predilatation, stenting, postdilatation, and final result.

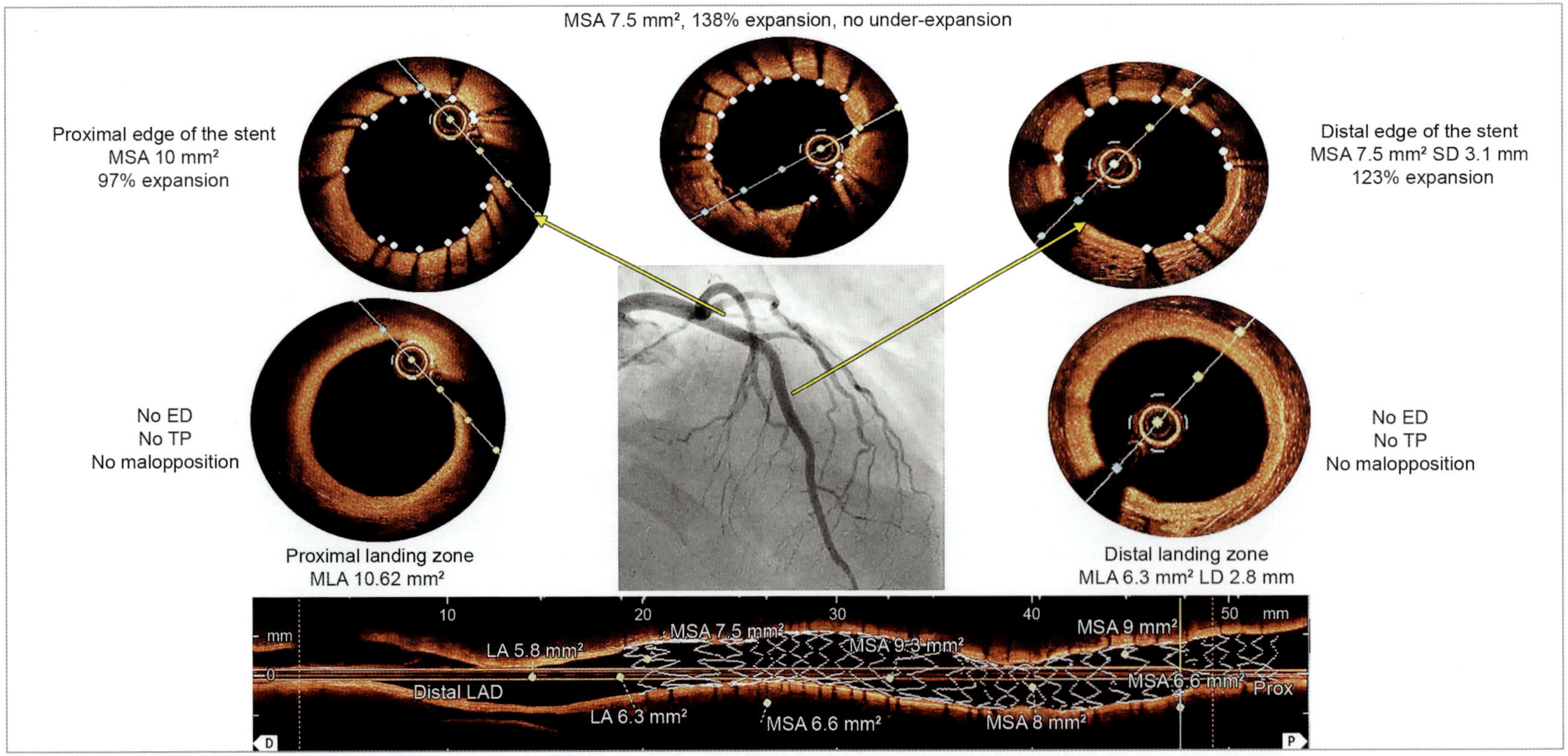

Fig. 12: Poststenting OCT assessment for medial edge dissection, expansion, and apposition of the stent. (LAD: left anterior descending; LD: luminal diameter; MLA: minimal luminal area; MSA: minimal stent area; OCT: optical coherence tomography)

CASE 2

Percutaneous coronary intervention (PCI) with stenting of obtuse marginal (OM)—sizing of the stent (air embolism).

CLINICAL HISTORY

A 40-year-old male, a known hypertensive and diabetic, presented with acute coronary syndrome (ACS) - Unstable Angina (USA). Electrocardiogram (ECG)—ST depression in V4-V6. 2D echo—normal LV function, and EF 60%. Investigations: RBS 143 mg/dL, blood urea 40 mg/dL, S Cr 1.08 mg/dL, and eGFR 85 mL/min. CAG-LMCA—normal, LAD—normal, LCX—normal, OM1—proximal 80% stenosis, RCA—normal **(Figs. 13A and B)**.

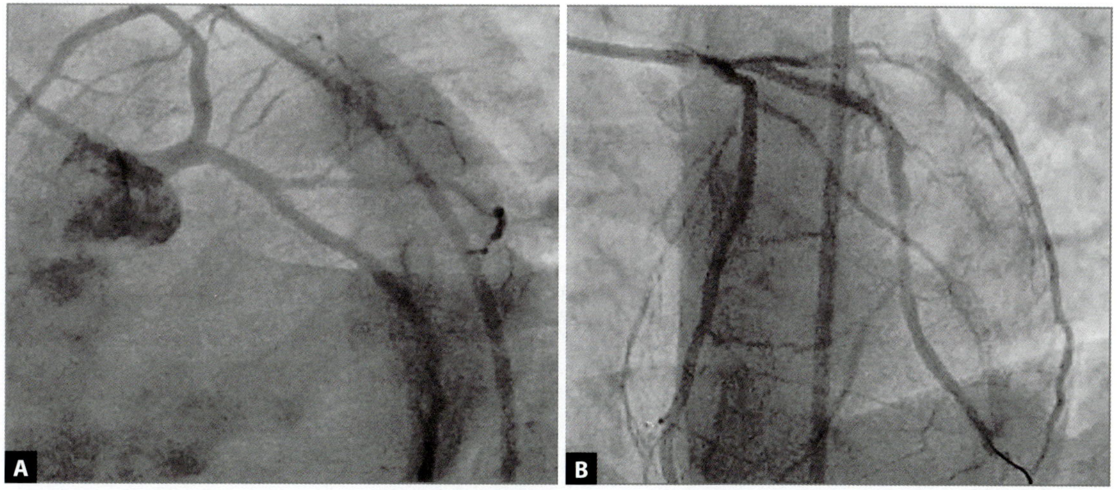

Figs. 13A and B: Coronary angiogram.

PROCEDURE

Route—right femoral artery (RFA), using 6 Fr Judkins Left (JL) 3.5 guiding catheter, obtuse marginal (OM) lesion was crossed with 0.014″ Sion Blue wire. Pre-OCT showed air embolism at the mid lesion with total lesion length 33.1 mm, distal landing zone minimal lumen area (MLA) 3.0 mm^2, MLD 2.2 mm, area of the tight stenosis—MLA 0.98 mm^2, MLD 1.1 mm, proximal landing zone—MLA 4.6 mm^2, MLD 2.4 mm **(Figs. 14A and B)**.

Predilatation done with 2.0 × 10 mm Tazuna balloon. Stenting done with 2.5 × 35 mm Orsiro stent. Proximal portion of stent postdilatation done with 3.5 × 12 mm NC Trek balloon. Distal portion of the stent postdilatation done with 2.5 × 15 mm NC Trek balloon **(Figs. 15A to D)**.

Postprocedure OCT showed distal edge of the stent MLA 4.4 mm^2, MLD 2.4 mm, mid of the lesion MLA 4.7 mm^2, MLD 2.4 mm, proximal edge of the stent MLA 6.0 mm^2, MLD 2.8 mm, well-apposed and expanded stent struts, and no edge dissections **(Fig. 16)**. Postprocedure Angio view showed well-implanted stents with TIMI-III flow without any dissection.

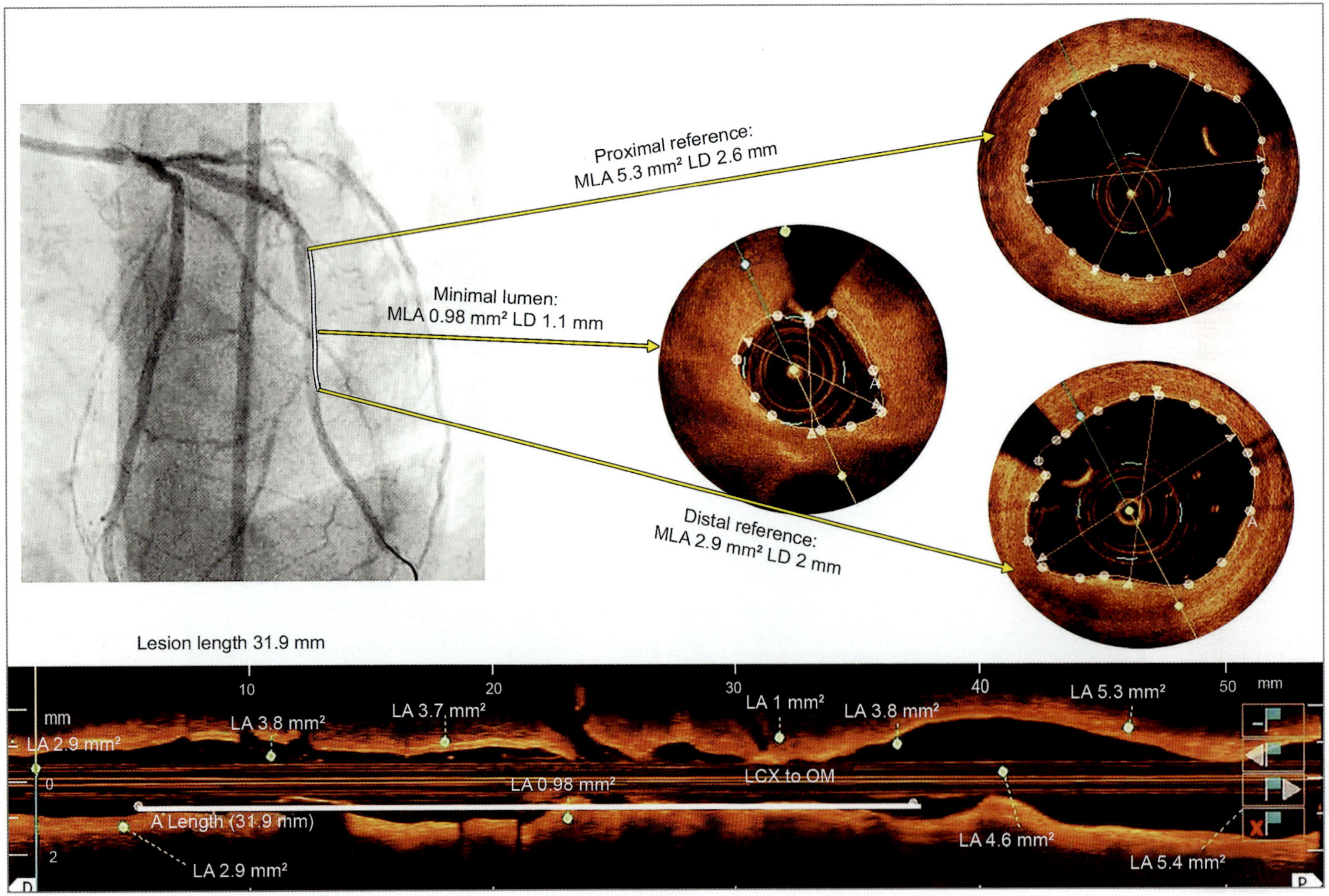

Fig. 14A

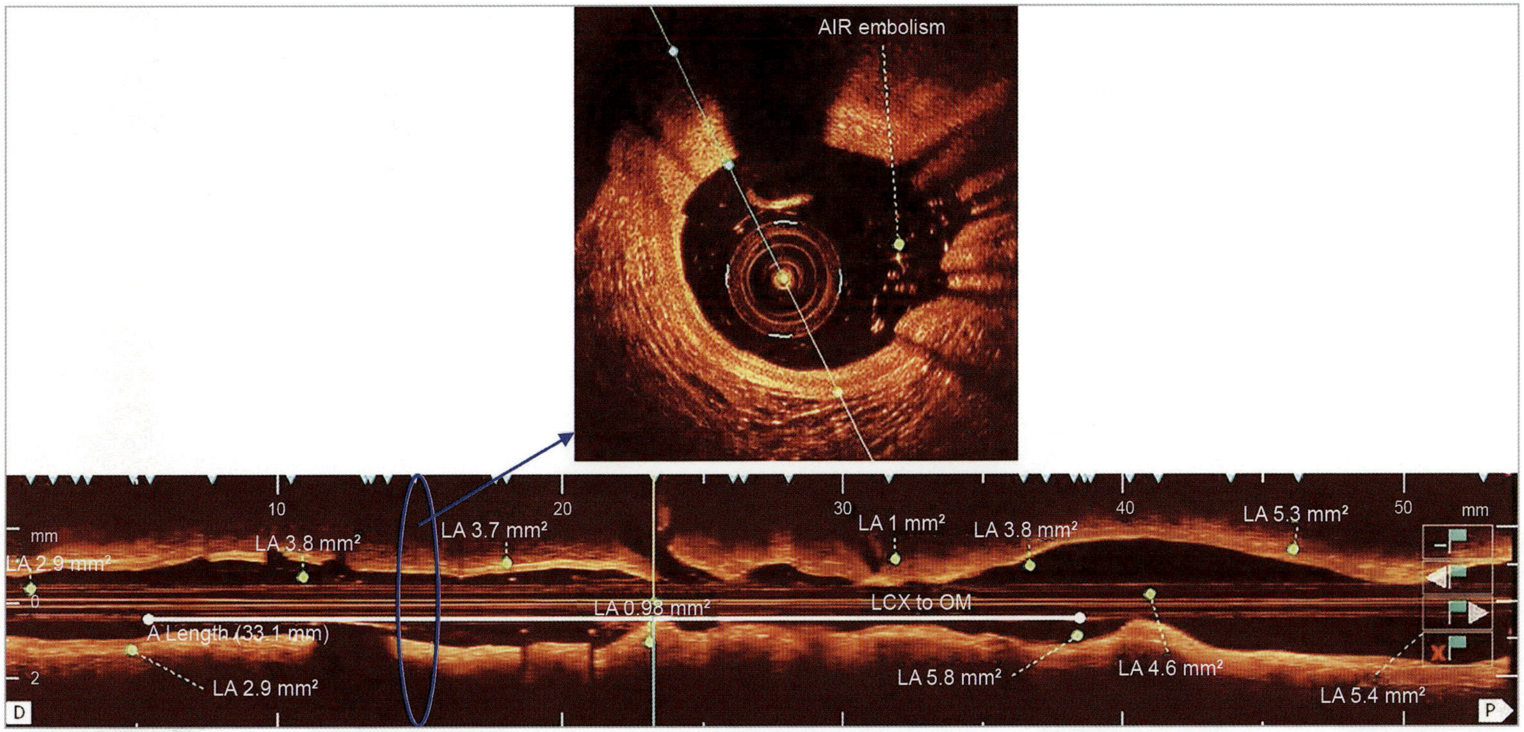

Fig. 14B

Figs. 14A and B: Presenting OCT assessment to select devise size (length and diameter). (B) Detection of air embolism by OCT imaging. (LCX: left circumflex; LD: luminal diameter; MLA: minimal luminal area; OM: obtuse marginal)

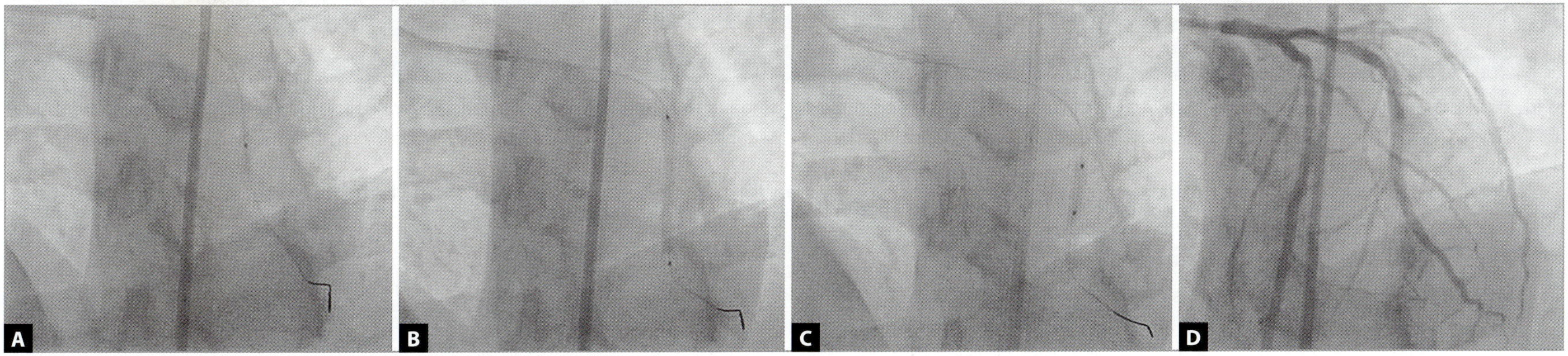

Figs. 15A to D: Predilatation, stenting, postdilatation, and final result.

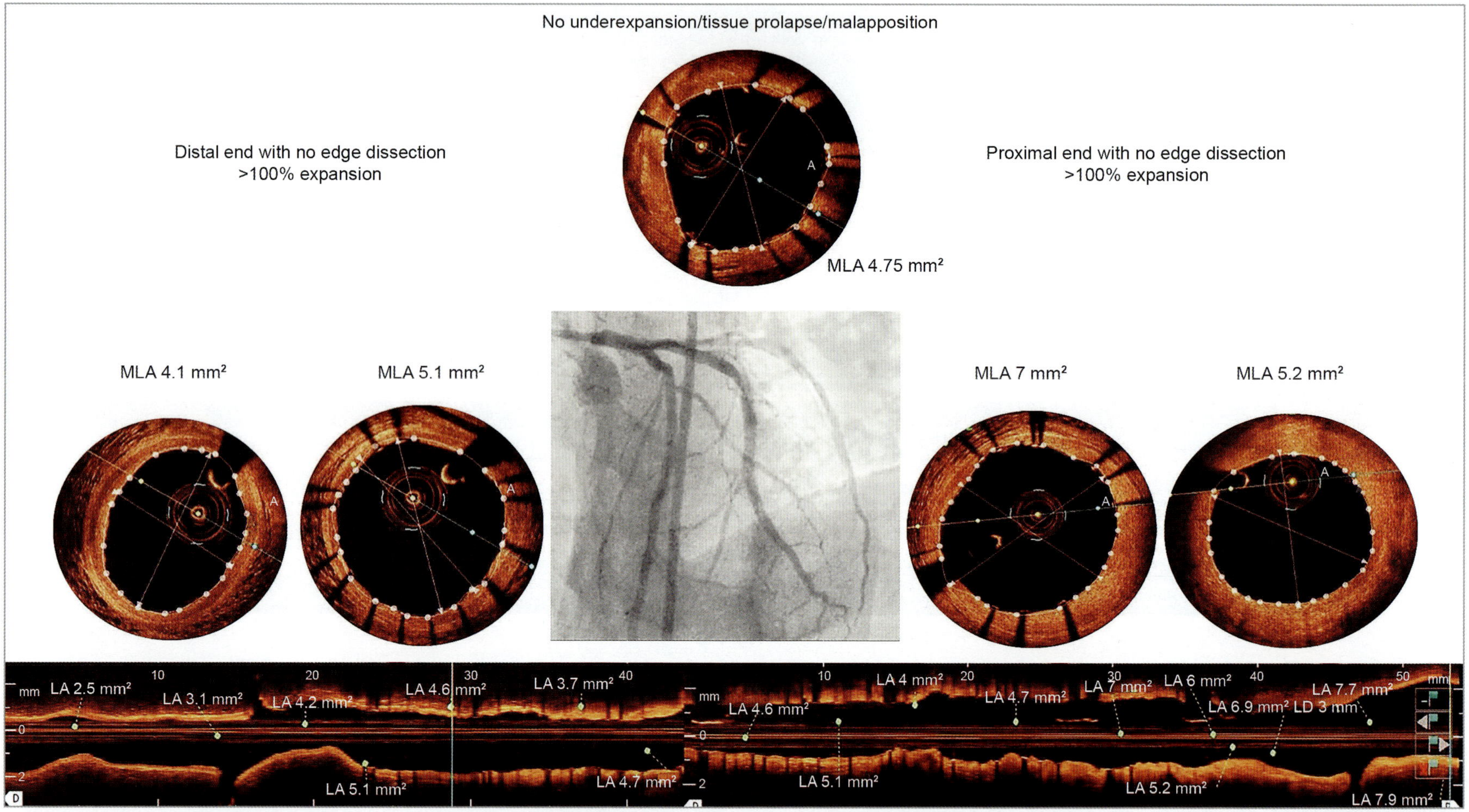

Fig. 16: Poststenting OCT assessment for medial edge dissection, expansion, and apposition of the stent. (LA: luminal area; LD: luminal diameter; MLA: minimal luminal area)

- **Stent Expansion—If the stent is expanding the lumen, holding the lesion close to, or greater than the normal reference segment, the stent expanded.**
- **Acceptable—MSA >80% of Mean reference luminal area.**
- **Optimal—MSA >90% of Mean reference luminal area.**
- **Under expansion—MSA, 70% of Mean reference luminal area.**

CASE 3

PCI of LAD—sizing of stent and selection of landing zones. (LAD: left anterior descending; PCI: percutaneous coronary intervention).

CLINICAL HISTORY

A 62-year-old male, a known hypertensive and diabetic, presented with CAD-unstable angina, chest pain, 2D echo—no RWMA, concentric LV hypertrophy (LVH), normal LV function, EF 64%. Investigations: Troponin I <0.01 ng/mL, S Cr 0.8 mg/dL, cGFR 92 mL/min, blood urea 25 mg/dL, and RBS 163 mg/dL.

Coronary angiography-LMCA—normal, LAD—proximal 60–70% lesion, LCX—normal, RCA—normal. Fractional flow reserve (FFR) study of LAD after intravenous (IV) adenosine infusion for 2 minutes was positive with value of 0.75 indicating significant LAD disease **(Fig. 17)**.

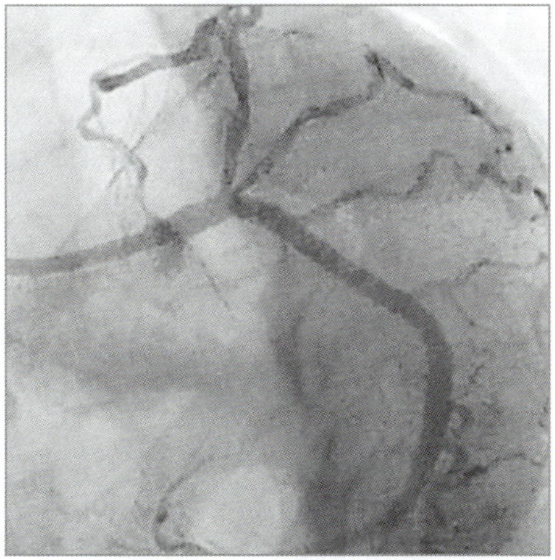

Fig. 17: Coronary angiogram.

PROCEDURE

Route—RFA, 6 Fr EBU 3.5 guiding catheter, LAD lesion was crossed with 0.014″ Runthrough wire, D1 was wired with 0.014″ Sion Blue wire.

Pre-OCT showed long segment fibrocalcific lesion extending from proximal to mid-LAD **(Figs. 18A to C)**.

Predilatation done with 2.5 × 10 mm Tazuna balloon. Stenting done with 3.0 × 38 mm Xience Xpedition Stent. Postdilatation done with 3.0 × 12 mm NC Trek balloon **(Figs. 19A to D)**.

Post-OCT showed edge dissection distal to stent which was covered with **(Fig. 20)** 2.5 × 12 mm Xience Xpedition stent, postdilated with 3.0 × 12 mm NC Trek balloon **(Figs. 21A to D)**.

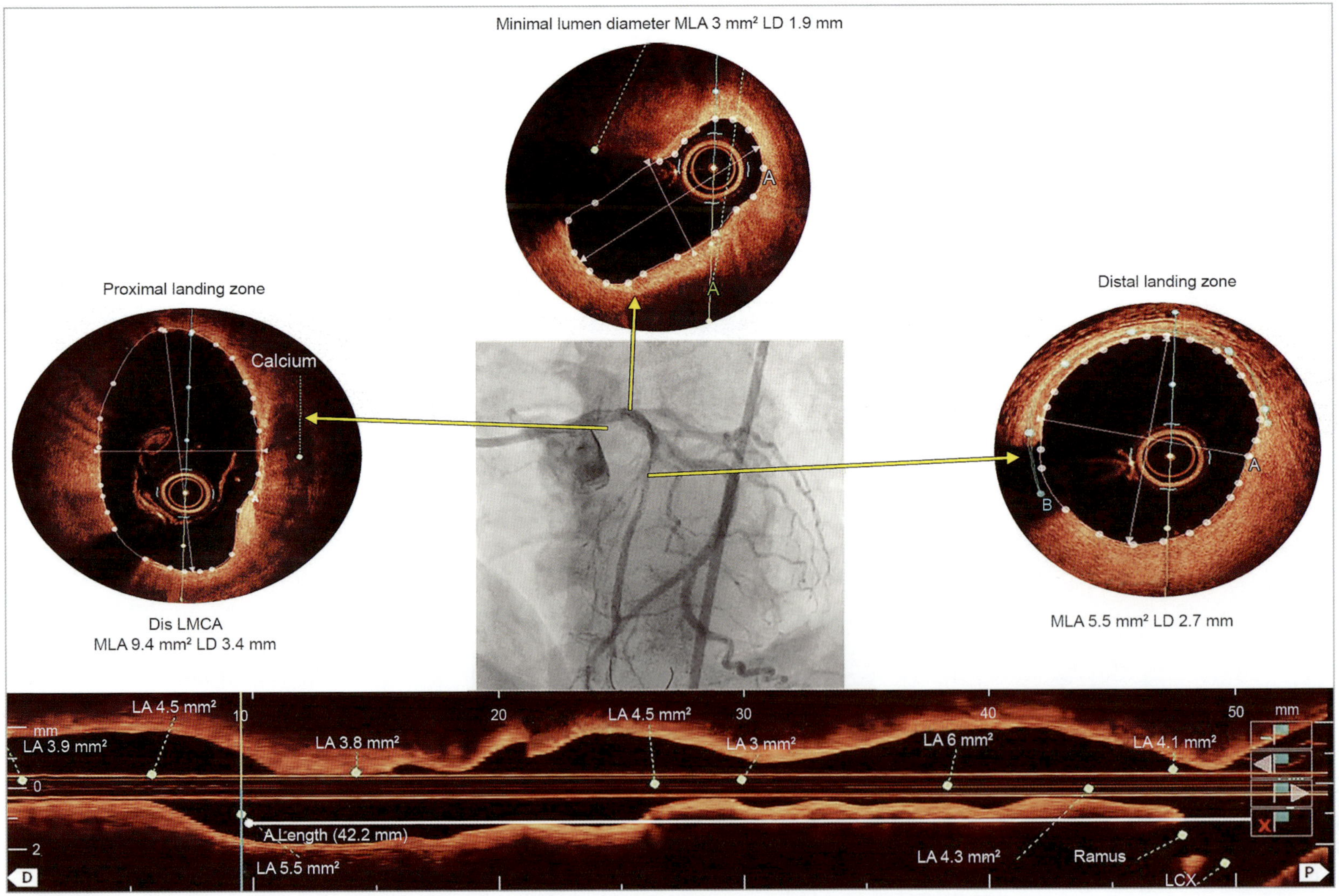

Fig. 18A

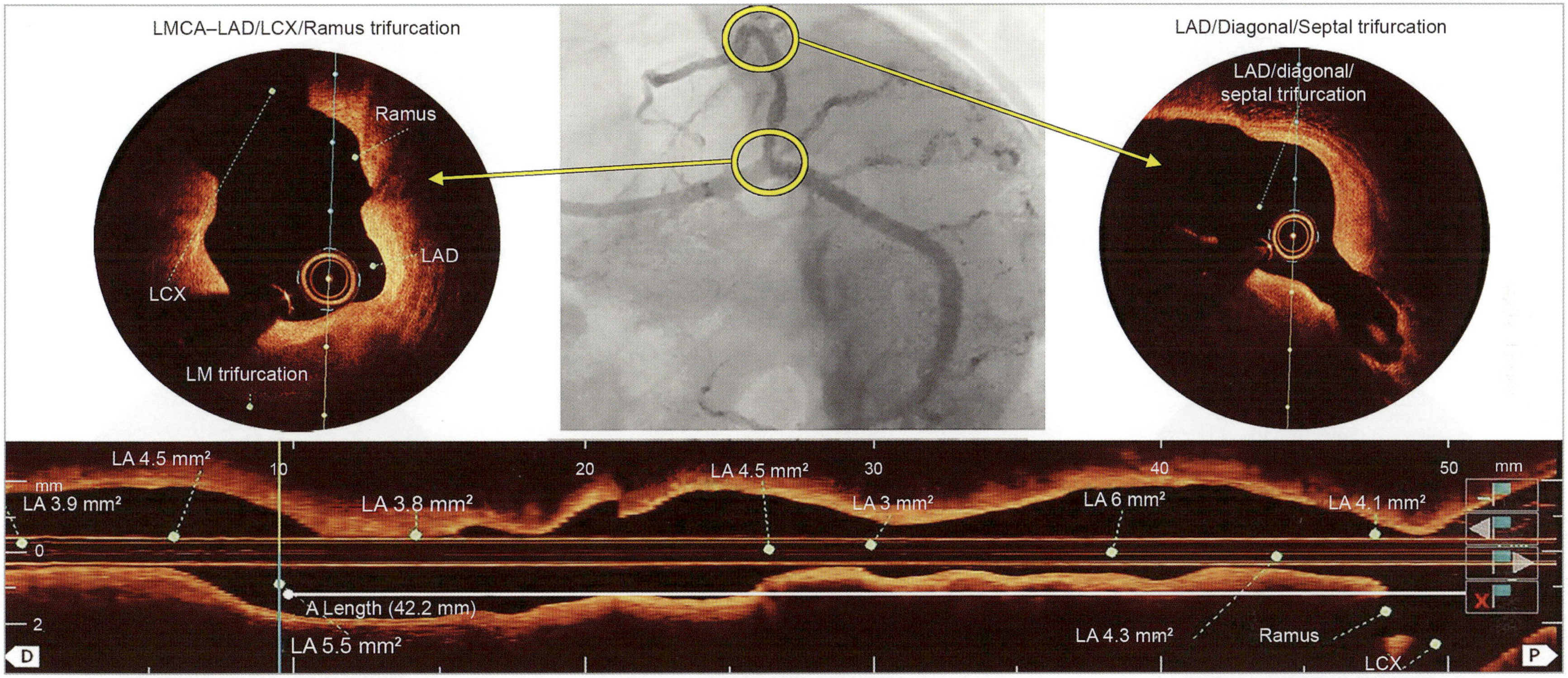

Fig. 18B

Postprocedure Angio view showed well-implanted stents with TIMI-III flow without any dissection **(Fig. 22)**.

IVUS assessment of LMCA significance is based on lumen dimensions, not plaque Burden. OCT lumen dimensions are about 10 to 15% smaller than IVUS.

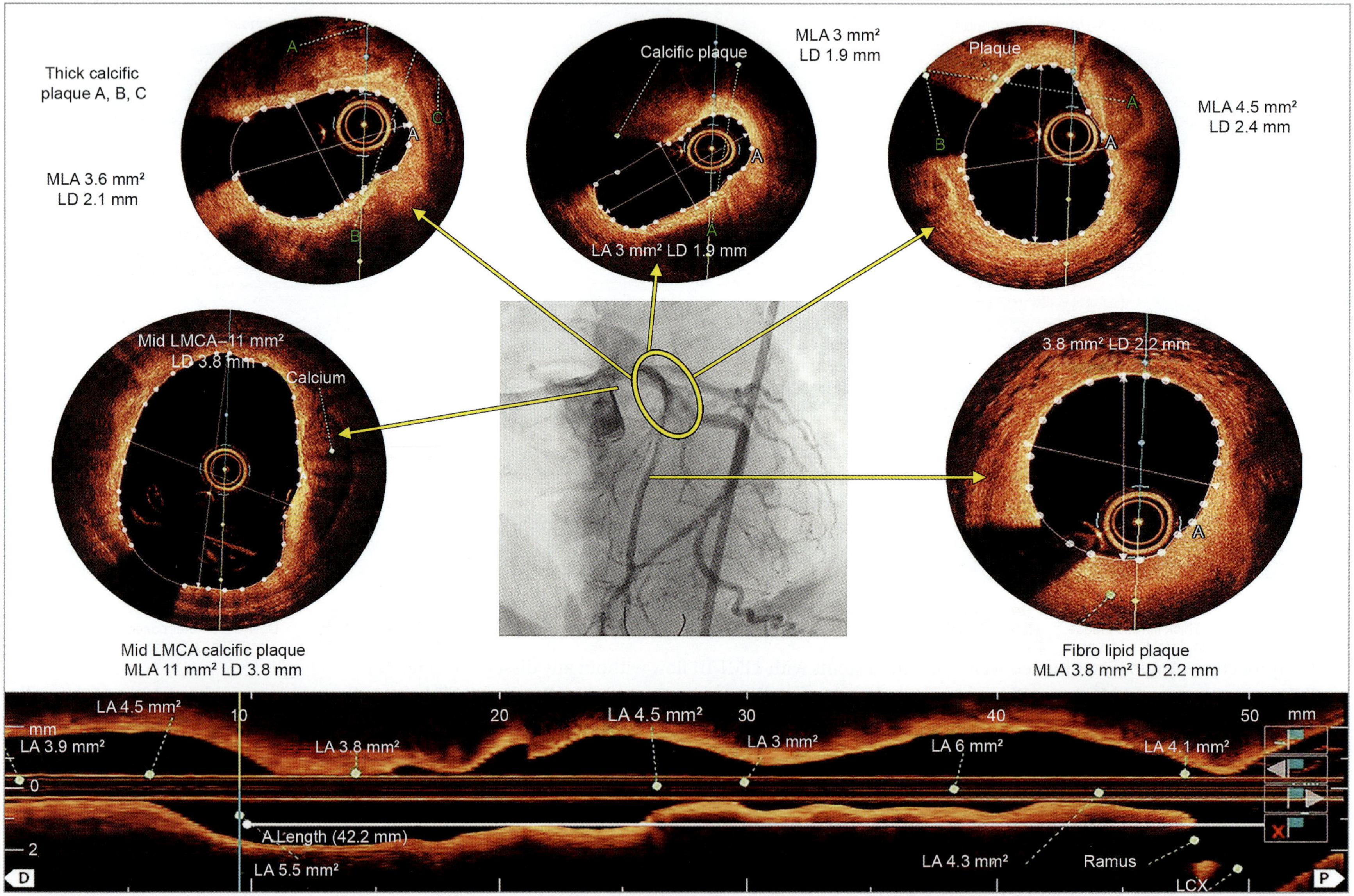

Fig. 18C

Figs. 18A to C: (A) Prestenting OCT assessment to select device size (length and diameter); (B) assessment of LM and non-LM trifurcation using OCT; and (C) morphological assessment of the diseased vessel by OCT imaging. (LA: luminal area; LAD: left anterior descending; LCX: left circumflex; LD: luminal diameter; LM: left main; LMCA: left main coronary artery; MLA: minimal luminal area; OCT: optical coherence tomography)

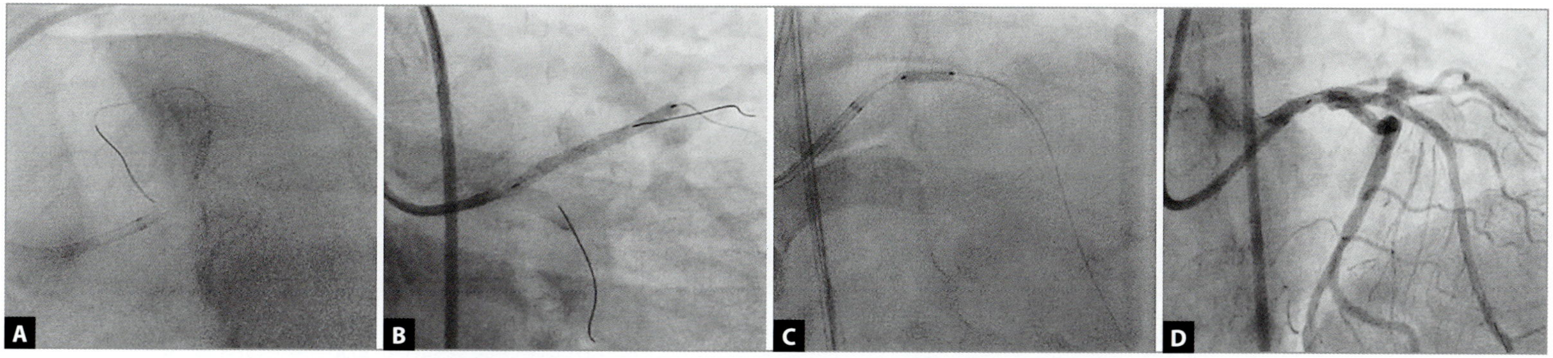

Figs. 19A to D: Predilatation, stenting, postdilatation, and final result.

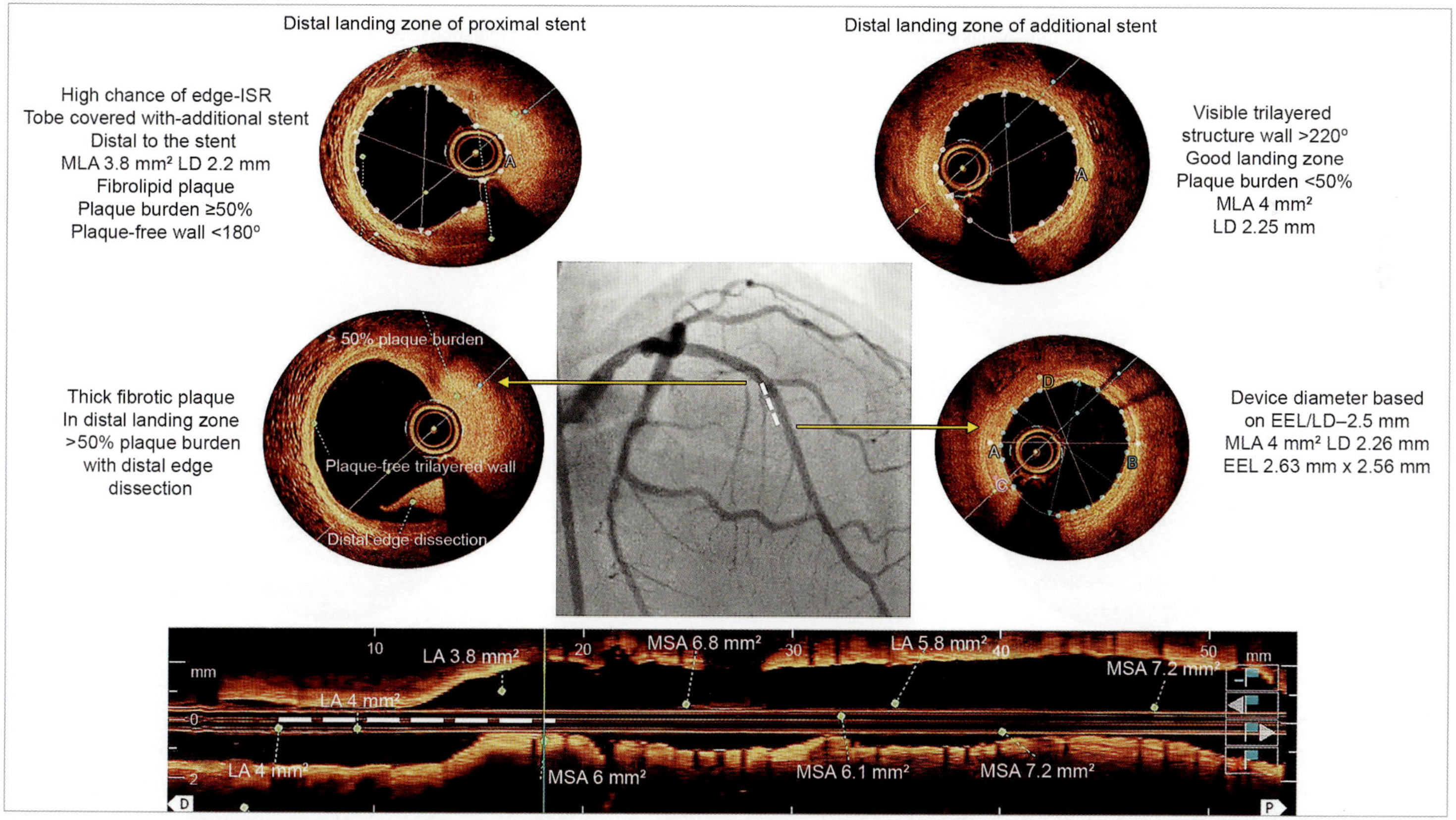

Fig. 20: Poststent OCT is useful in assessing the medial edge dissections at proximal and distal ends for additional stent requirement. (EEL: external elastic lamina; ISR: in-stent restenosis; LA: luminal area; LD: luminal diameter; MLA: minimal luminal area; MSA: minimal stent area; OCT: optical coherence tomography)

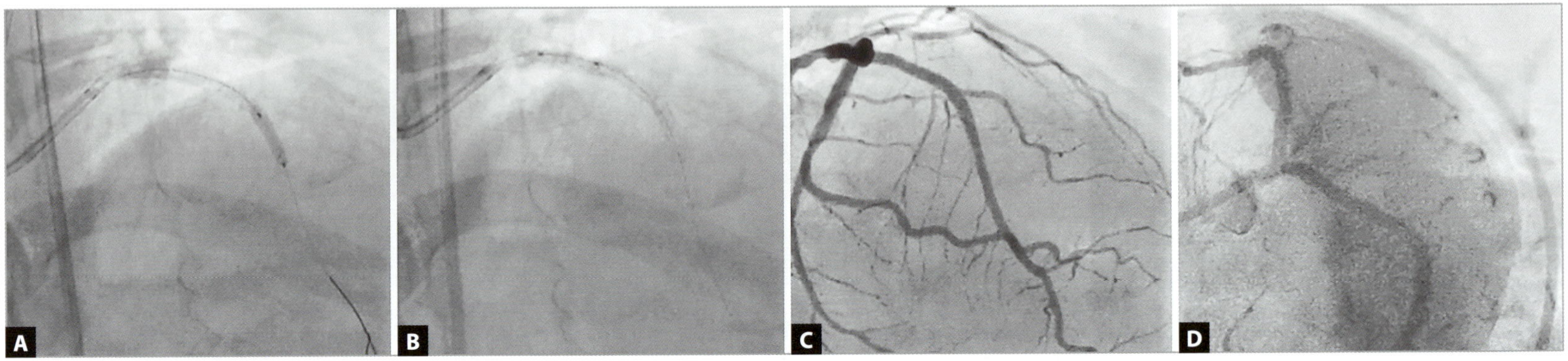

Figs. 21A to D: Distal edge dissection was covered with additional stent.

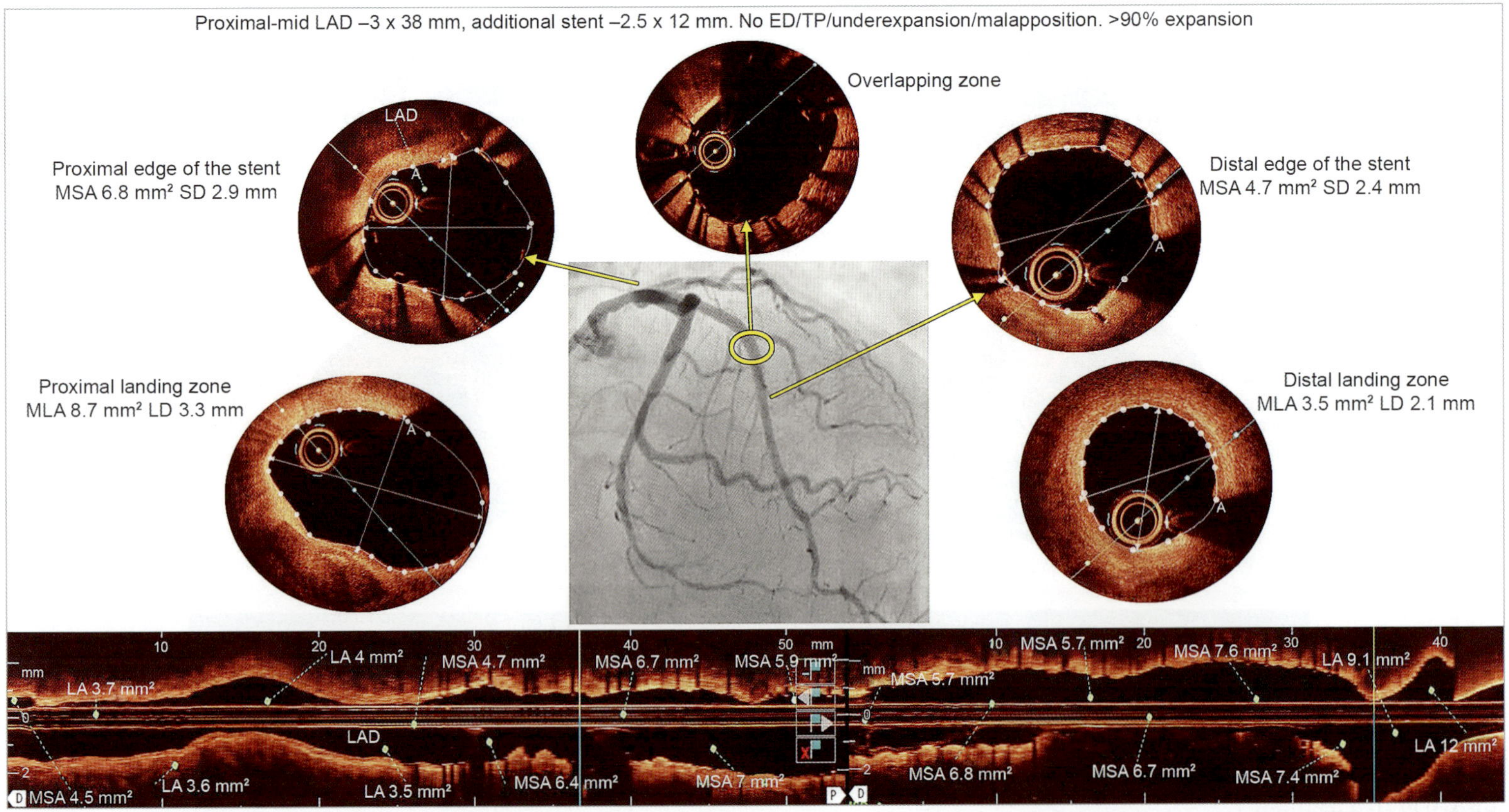

Fig. 22: Poststenting OCT assessment for medial edge dissection, expansion, and apposition of the stent. (LA: luminal area; LAD: left anterior descending; LD: luminal diameter; MLA: minimal luminal area; MSA: minimal stent area; OCT: optical coherence tomography)

CASE 4

Plaque assessment and sizing of stent—PCI of RCA. (PCI: percutaneous coronary intervention; RCA: right coronary artery)

CLINICAL HISTORY

A 68-year-old male, a known hypertensive and diabetic, presented with evolved inferior wall MI (IWMI), postinfarct angina, and chest pain radiating to left arm. 2D echo—inferior wall hypokinesia, mild LV dysfunction, and EF 47%. Investigations: Hb 14.3 g/dL, S Cr 0.99 mg/dL, and RBS 250 mg/dL. CAG-LMCA—normal, LAD—distal mild disease, LCX—normal, and RCA—mid 99% stenosis **(Fig. 23A to C)**.

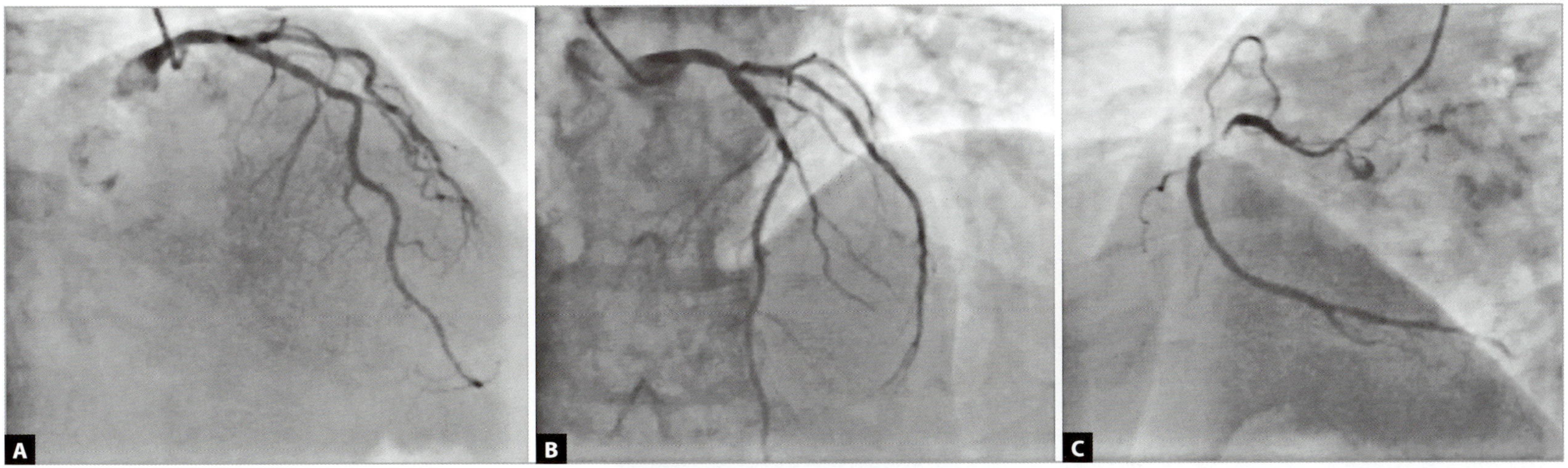

Figs. 23A to C: Coronary angiogram.

PROCEDURE

Route—RRA, 6 Fr JR 3.5 guiding catheter, RCA mid 99% lesion with Runthrough wire, predilated with 1.5 × 10 mm and 2.5 × 15 mm Tazuna using guideliner support. Pre-OCT showed proximal reference vessel MLA 8.6 mm^2, MLD 3.3 mm, mid portion of the lesion minimal lumen vessel MLA 2.8 mm^2,

MLD 1.8 mm, distal reference vessel MLA 9.4 mm^2, and MLD 3.4 mm **(Fig. 24A)** with fibrocalcific lesion **(Fig. 24B)**. OCT showed circumferential calcium (360°), thickness 0.63 mm, length <5 mm with MLA of distal RCA was 4.2 mm^2; hence, stenting was deferred **(Fig. 24C)**.

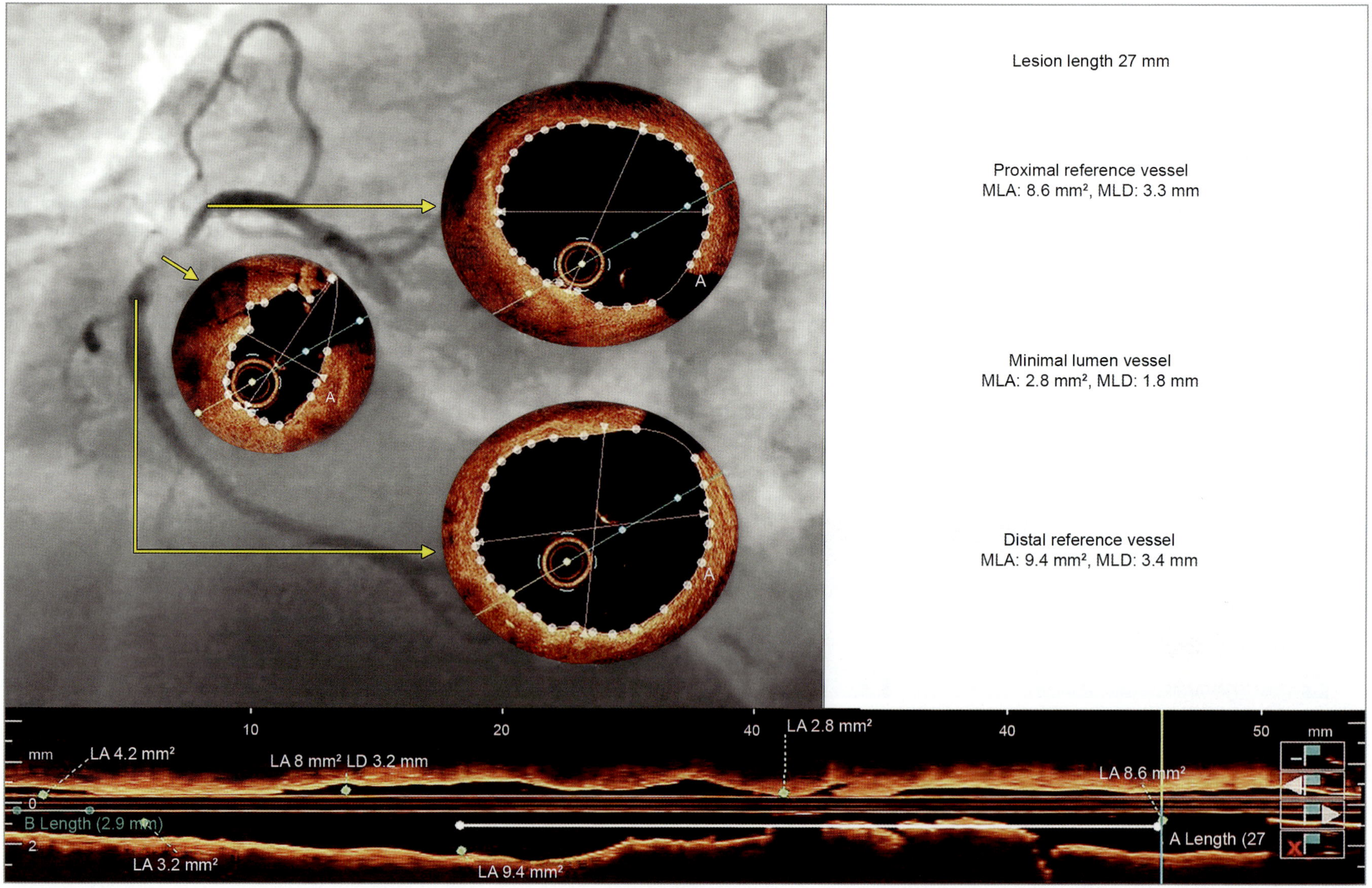

Fig. 24A

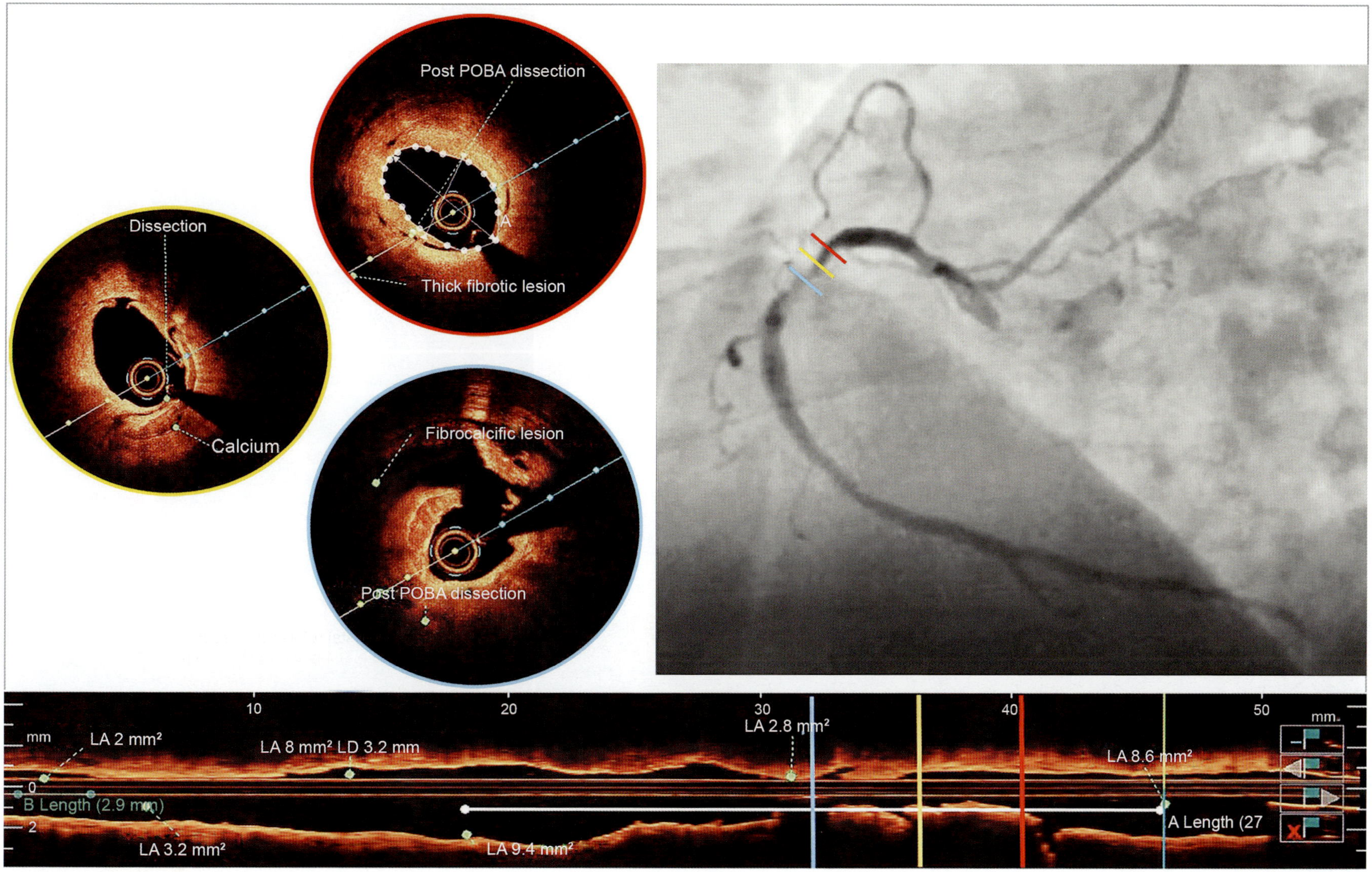
Post POBA dissection
A
Thick fibrotic lesion
Dissection
Calcium
Fibrocalcific lesion
Post POBA dissection
10
20
30
40
50
mm
mm
LA 2 mm²
LA 8 mm² LD 3.2 mm
LA 2.8 mm²
LA 8.6 mm²
0
B Length (2.9 mm)
A Length (27
2
LA 3.2 mm²
LA 9.4 mm²

Fig. 24B

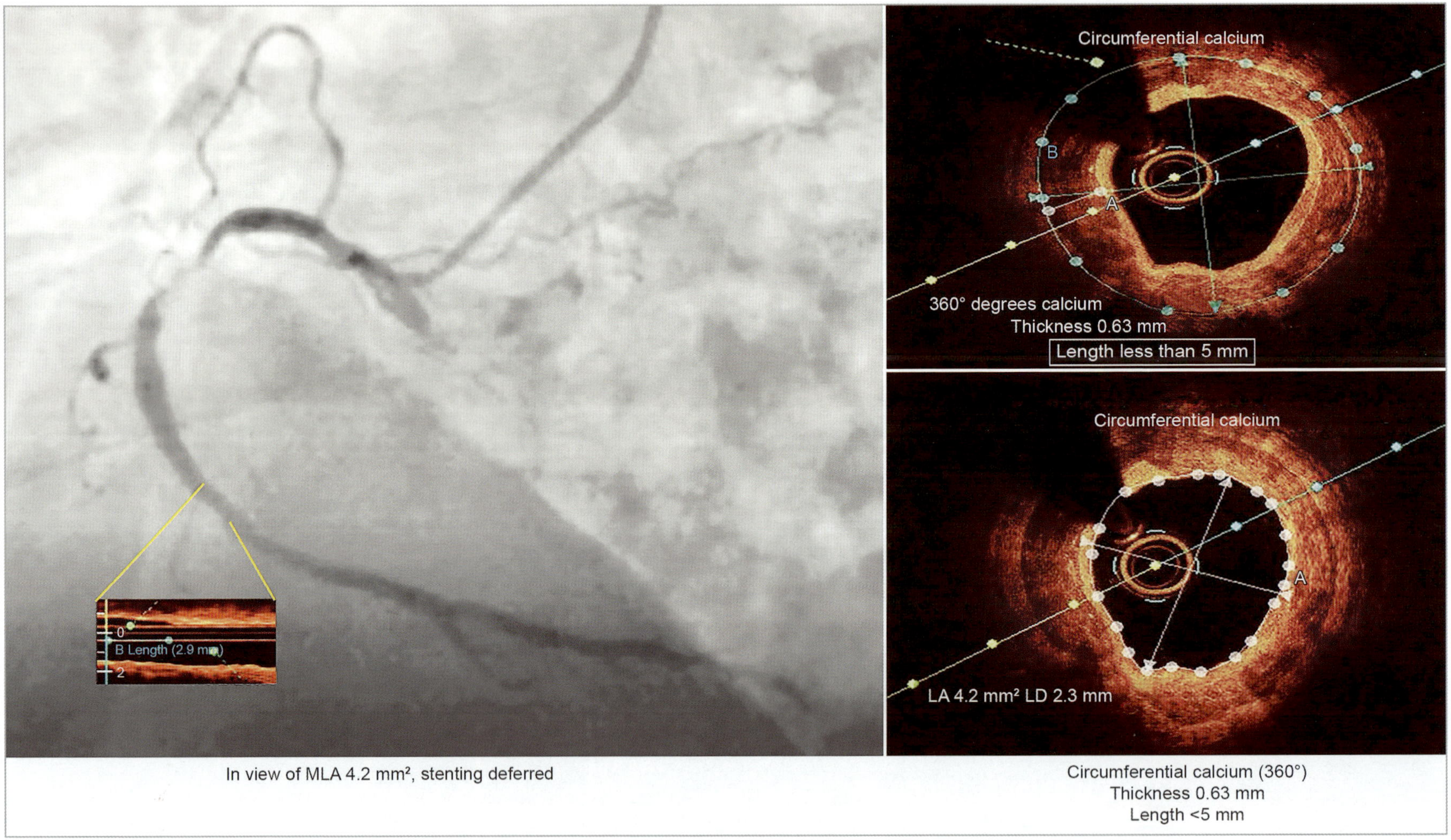

Fig. 24C

Figs. 24A to C: (A) Prestenting OCT assessment to select device size (length and diameter); (B) morphological assessment of the diseased vessel by OCT imaging; and (C) calcific plaque assessment of the diseased vessel by OCT imaging. (LA: luminal area; LD: luminal diameter; MLA: minimal luminal area; MLD: minimal luminal diameter; OCT: optical coherence tomography; POBA: plain old balloon angioplasty)

Predilatation with 1.5 × 10 mm and 2.5 × 15 mm Tazuna with guideliner support, stenting done with 3.5 × 28 mm Xience Xpedition with guideliner support, final result is shown in **Figures 25A to D**.

Postprocedure OCT study showed well-apposed and well-expanded stent struts and no edge dissections **(Fig. 26)**. Postprocedure Angio views showed well-implanted stents with TIMI-III flow without any dissection.

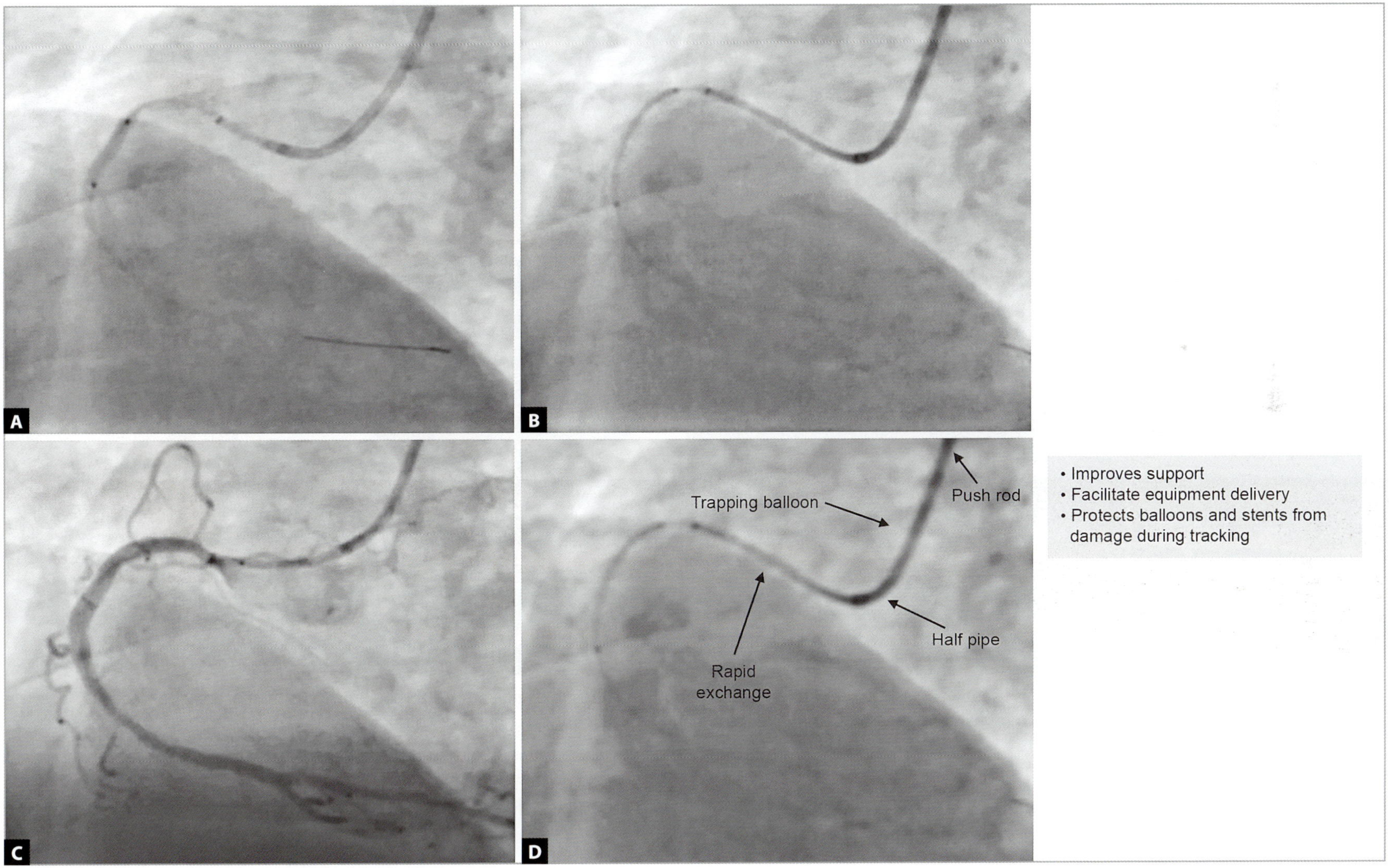

Figs. 25A to D: (A to C) Predilatation, stenting, and final result; (D) Extend the help of guiding catheter.

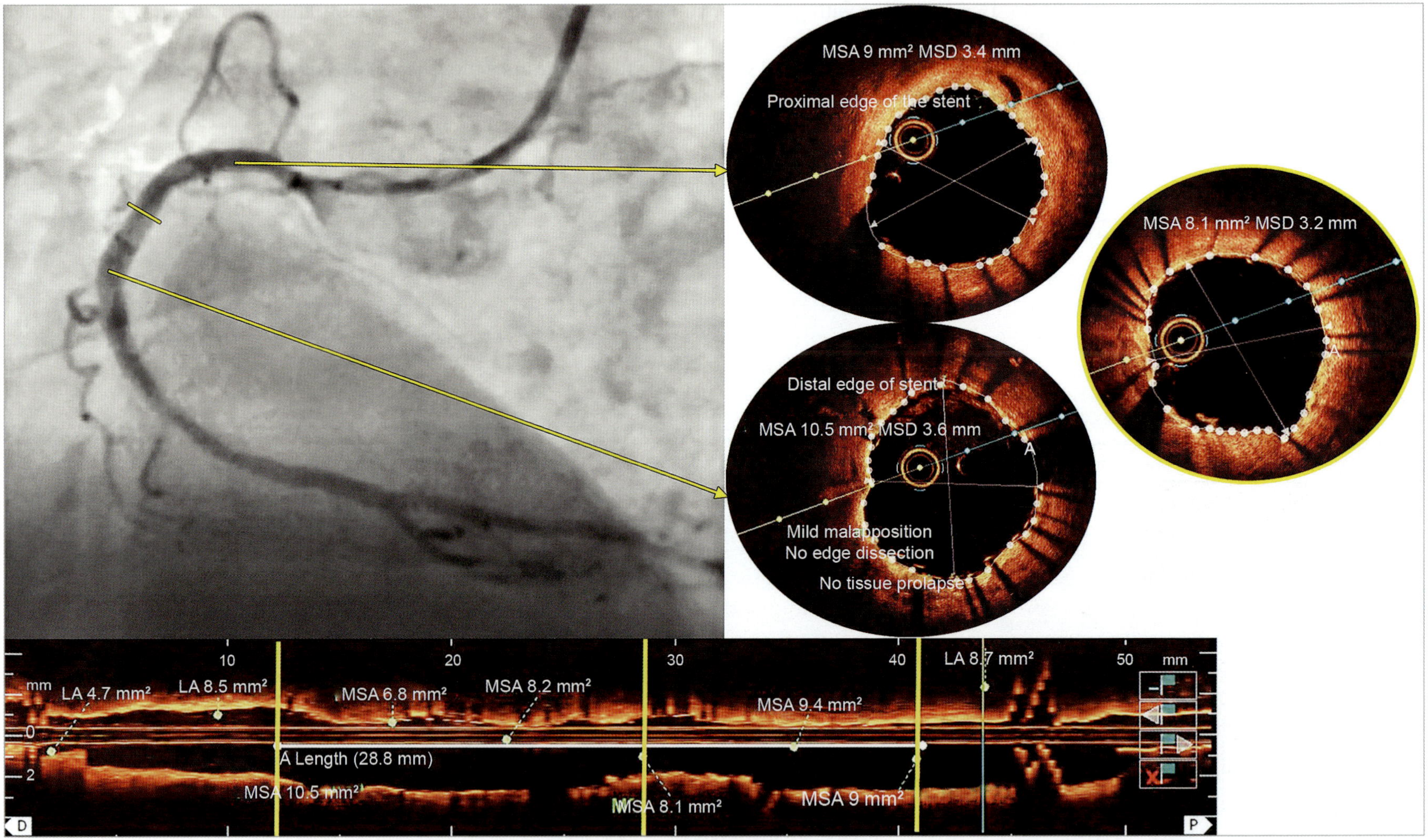

Fig. 26: Poststent OCT is useful in assessing the malapposition at both the ends to decide an upsized balloon. (LA: luminal area; MSA: minimal stent area; MSD: minimal stent diameter; OCT: optical coherence tomography)

If the stent struts are in contact with the artery wall, the stent is apposed. Post dilate the mal-apposed portion of the stent with appropriately sized semi-compliant balloon at low pressure

CASE 5

PCI of LAD—sizing of DES and assessment of landing zones. (DES: drug-eluting stent; LAD: left anterior descending; PCI: percutaneous coronary intervention)

CLINICAL HISTORY

A 55-year-old female, a known hypertensive and diabetic, presented with anterior non-STEMI (NSTEMI) and ECG-anterior ST-depression. 2D echo showed chronic rheumatic heart disease (CRHD), moderate mitral stenosis (MS), mild aortic stenosis (AS), dilated left atrium (LA), no RWMA, normal LV function, and EF 60%. Investigations: RBS 325 mg/dL, blood urea 34 mg/dL, S Cr 0.58 mg/dL, eGFR 104 mL/min. CAG-LMCA—normal, LAD—mid 90% lesion, LCX and RCA—normal **(Figs. 27A to C)**.

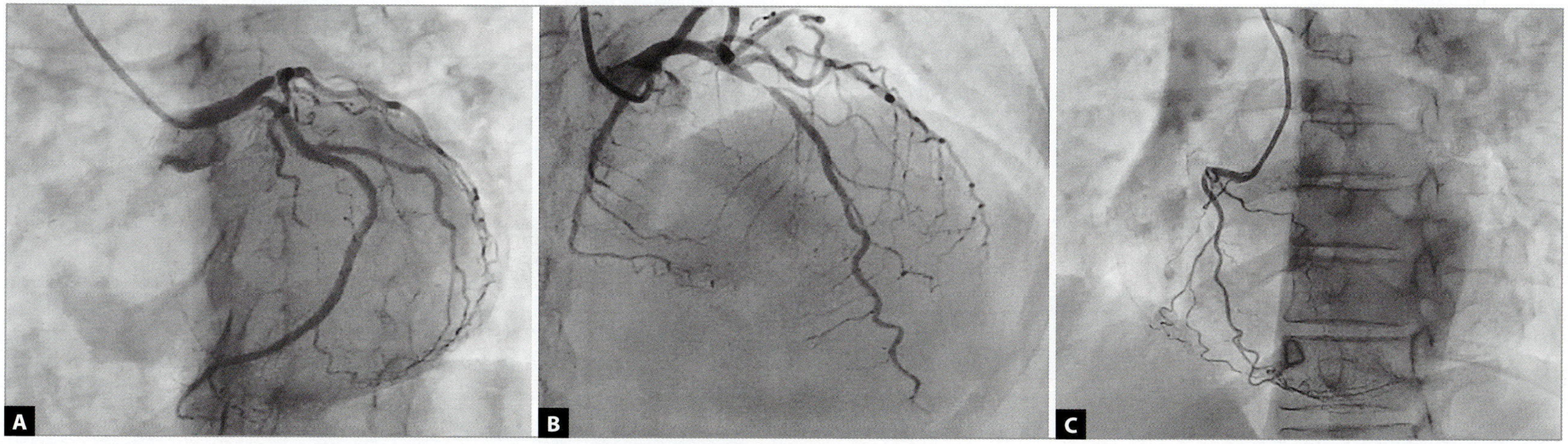

Figs. 27A to C: Coronary angiogram.

PROCEDURE

Route—RFA, 6 Fr EBU 3.5 guiding catheter, LAD lesion was crossed with 0.014″ Sion Blue wire, predilated with 2.0 × 10 mm Tazuna balloon.

Pre-OCT showed proximal LAD thick fibrolipid plaque with tight stenosis before bifurcation with MLA 1.59 mm^2, MLD 1.4 mm, distal landing zone MLA 4.6 mm^2, proximal landing zone—MLA 9.4 mm^2 and MLD 2.7 mm **(Fig. 28A)**.

Pre-OCT showed length of calcific plaque 3.5 mm, arc <90°, thickness of calcific plaque 720 microns. Distal LMCA minimum diameter 3.09 mm, maximum diameter 4.6 mm with MLA 12.9 mm^2 **(Fig. 28B)**.

Predilatation done with 2.0 × 10 mm Tazuna balloon, mid-LAD stenting done with 2.75 × 35 mm Orsiro stent, postdilatation done with 3.0 × 12 mm NC Trek balloon **(Figs. 29A to D)**.

Postprocedure OCT of distal-to-mid LAD showed distal portion of the stent with MLA 4.86 mm^2, maximum dimeter 2.59 mm, and minimum diameter 2.39 mm **(Fig. 30A)**. Postprocedure OCT of mid-LAD-to-LMCA bifurcation showed proximal LAD landing zone MLA 6.65 mm^2, MLD 2.9 mm **(Fig. 30B)**.

Postprocedure Angio showed well-implanted stents with TIMI-III flow without any dissection **(Figs. 29A to D)**.

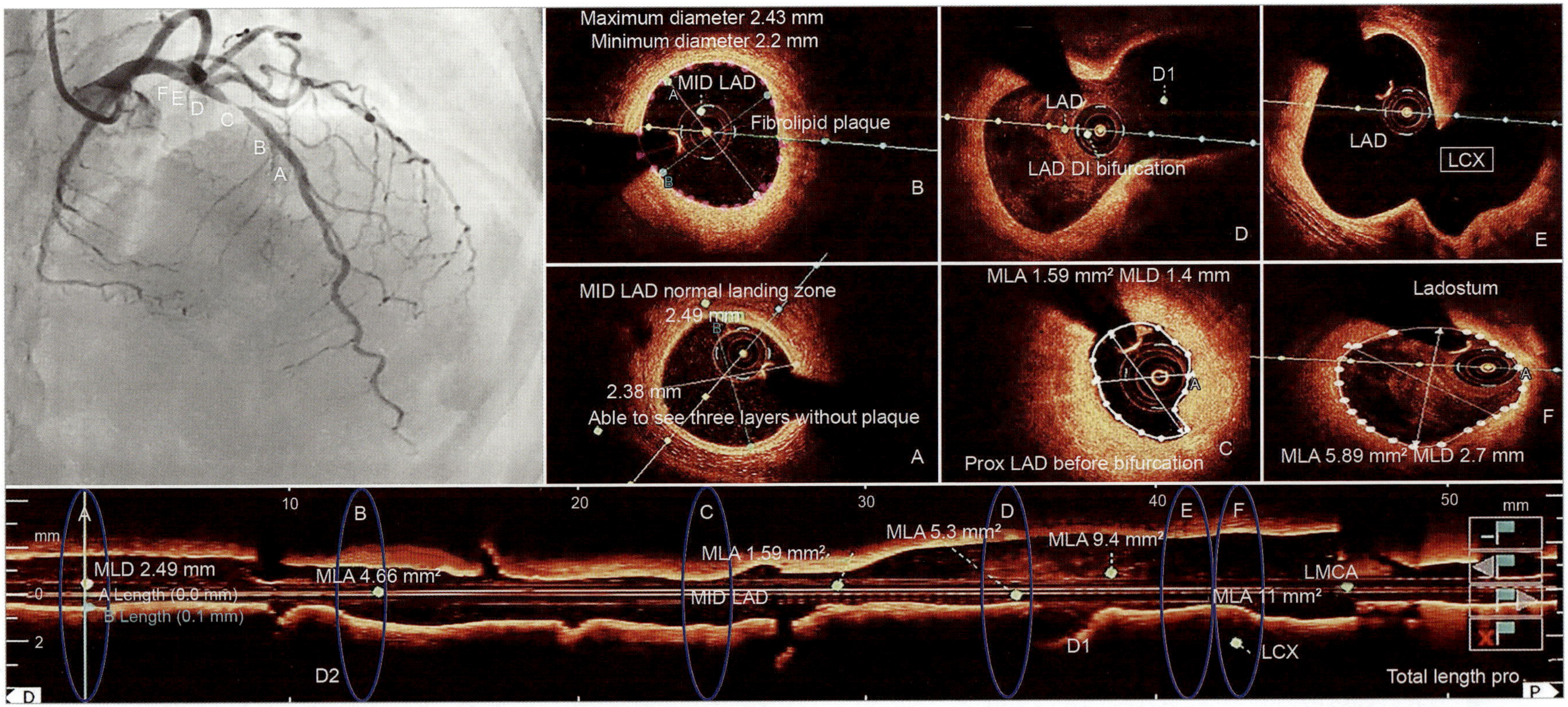

Fig. 28A

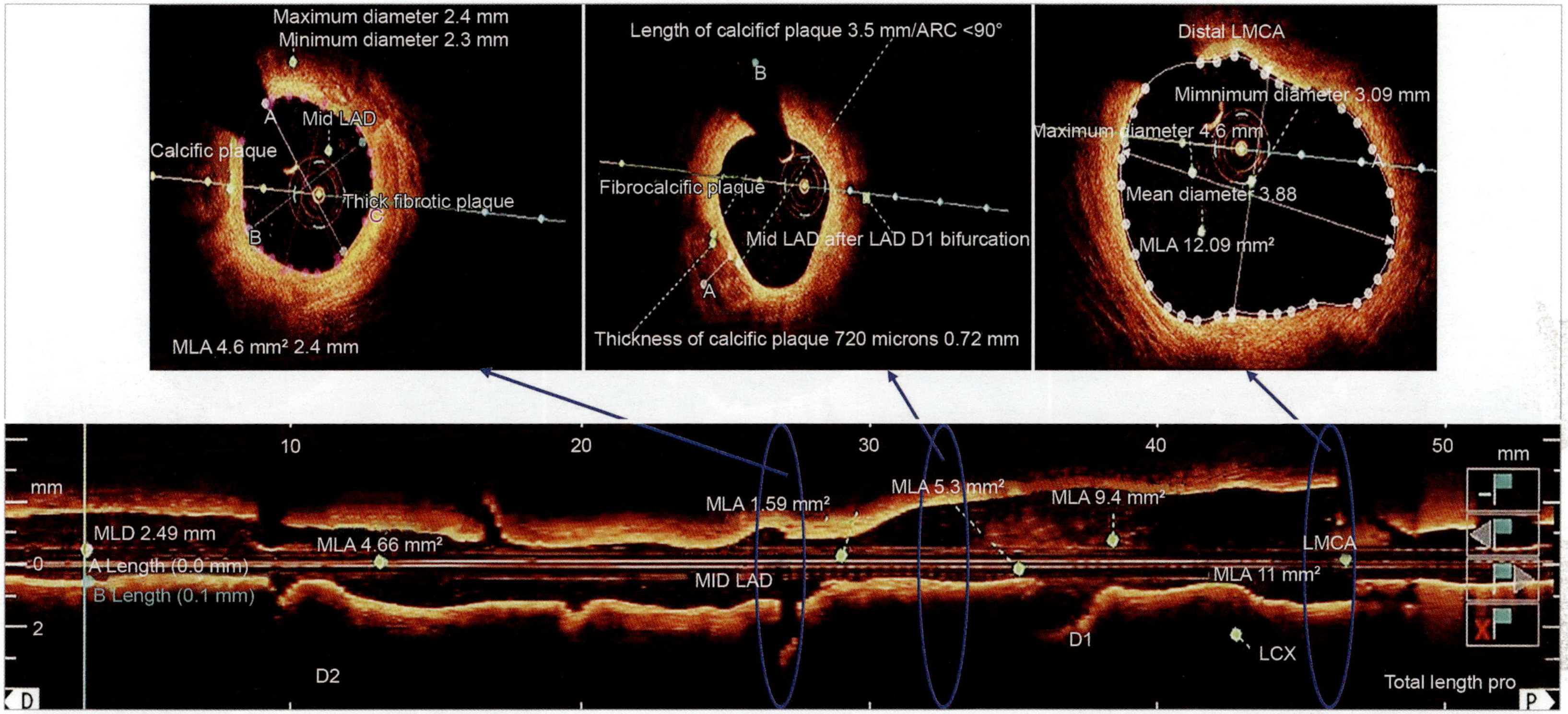

Fig. 28B

Figs. 28A and B: (A) Prestenting OCT assessment to select device size (length and diameter); (B) calcific plaque assessment of the diseased vessel by OCT imaging. (LAD: left anterior descending; LCX: left circumflex; LMCA: left main coronary artery; MLA: minimal luminal area; MLD: minimal luminal diameter; OCT: optical coherence tomography)

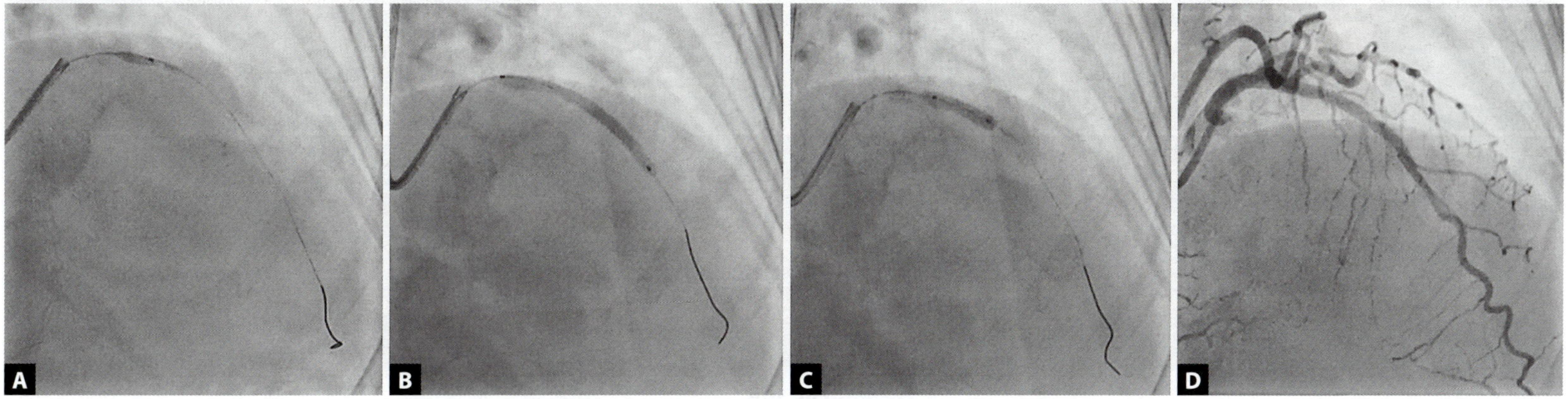

Figs. 29A to D: Predilatation, stenting, postdilatation, and final result.

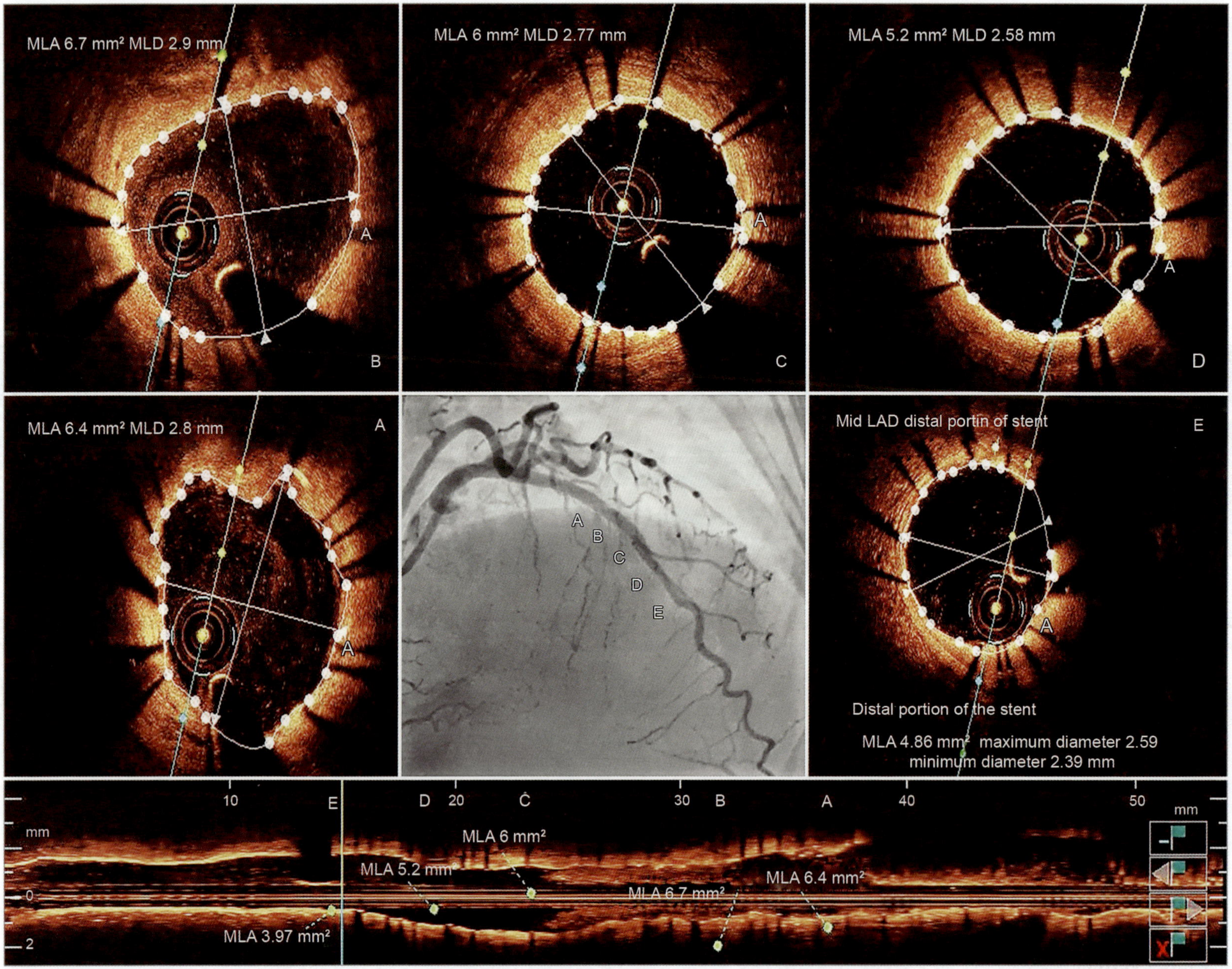
MLA 6.7 mm² MLD 2.9 mm
A
B
MLA 6 mm² MLD 2.77 mm
A
C
MLA 5.2 mm² MLD 2.58 mm
A
D
MLA 6.4 mm² MLD 2.8 mm
A
A
A
B
C
D
E
Mid LAD distal portin of stent
E
A
Distal portion of the stent
MLA 4.86 mm² maximum diameter 2.59
minimum diameter 2.39 mm
10
E
D
20
C
30
B
A
40
50
mm
mm
0
2
MLA 6 mm²
MLA 5.2 mm²
MLA 6.7 mm²
MLA 6.4 mm²
MLA 3.97 mm²

Fig. 30A

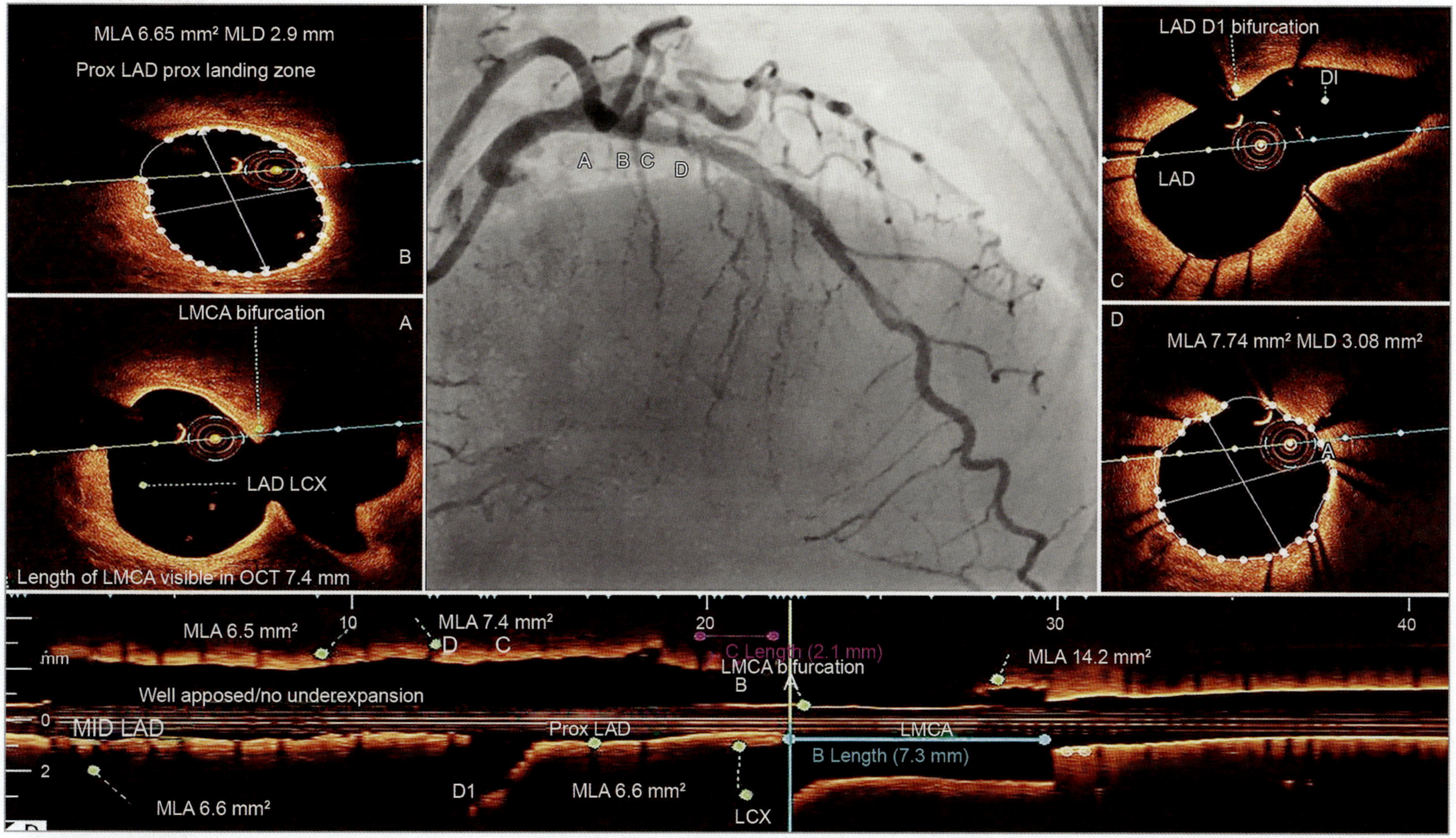

Fig. 30B

Figs. 30A and B: (A) Poststenting OCT assessment for medial edge dissection, expansion, and apposition of distal portion of the stent. (B) Poststenting OCT assessment for medial edge dissection, expansion, and apposition of proximal portion of the stent. (LAD: left anterior descending; LCX: left circumflex; LMCA: left main coronary artery; MLA: minimal luminal area; MLD: minimal luminal diameter; OCT: optical coherence tomography)

Finish the procedure if MAX Criteria is fulfilled , otherwise correct the MAX criteria and repeat the OCT to confirm the fulfilment of MAX criteria before finishing the procedure.

Very late events (beyond a year) were similar between BMS and 2nd generation DES-Approximately 1–2% /year.

By Five years, TLF/TVF with Contemporary DES occurs in nearly 1 in 7 patients.

CASE 6

PCI of LAD in NSTEMI of anterior wall-stent sizing. (LAD: left anterior descending; NSTEMI: non-ST-elevation myocardial infarction; PCI: percutaneous coronary intervention).

CLINICAL HISTORY

A 48-year-old female presented with ACS—anterior NSTEMI, chest pain associated with breathlessness and right hand dragging pain for the past 4 days. ECG—ST-depressions in anterior leads. 2D echo—no RWMA, normal LV systolic function, and EF 60%. Treadmill test (TMT) positive for inducible ischemia. Investigations: RBS 103 mg/dL, blood urea 15 mg/dL, S Cr 0.7 mg/dL, and eGFR 103 mL/min. CAG-LMCA—normal, LAD-proximal LAD 99% lesion, LCX—normal, RCA—normal **(Figs. 31A to C)**.

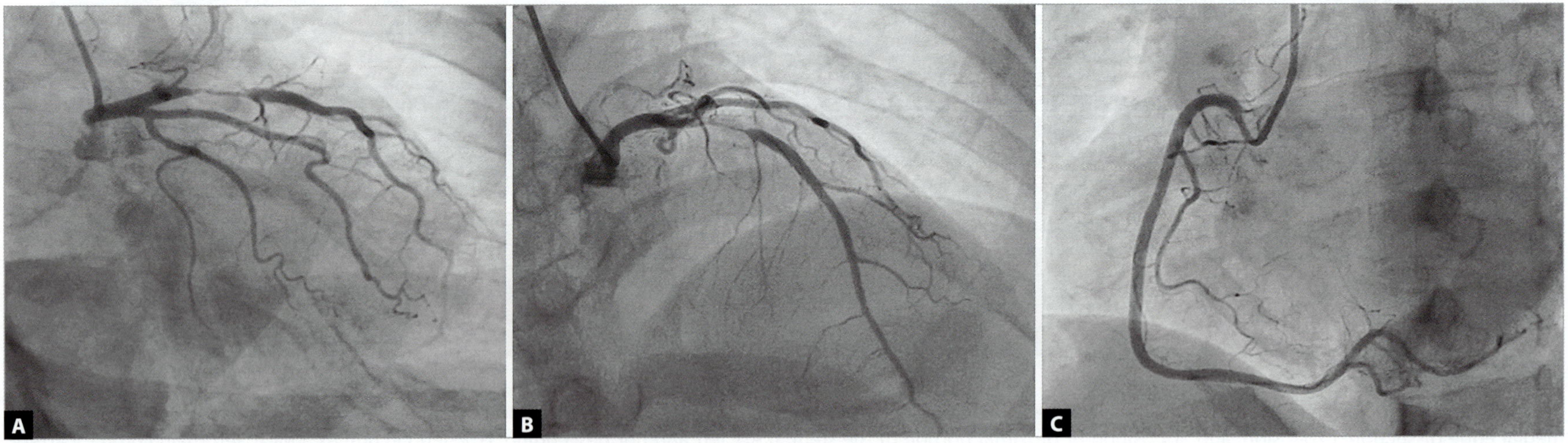

Figs. 31A to C: Coronary angiogram.

PROCEDURE

Procedure performed through right radial artery using 6 Fr EBU 3.5 guiding catheter, LAD lesion was crossed with 0.014″ Sion Blue wire, predilated with 2.0 × 10 mm Tazuna balloon.

Post-plain Old Balloon Angioplasty OCT Study

Post-plain old balloon angioplasty (POBA) OCT—distal landing zone MLA 6.6 mm^2, MLD 2.9 mm, proximal LAD tight stenosis MLA 1.1 mm^2, MLD 1.1 mm, proximal landing zone—MLA 5.4 mm^2, MLD 2.6 mm **(Fig. 32A)** with post-POBA proximal LAD with white thrombus and plaque rupture **(Fig. 32B)**.

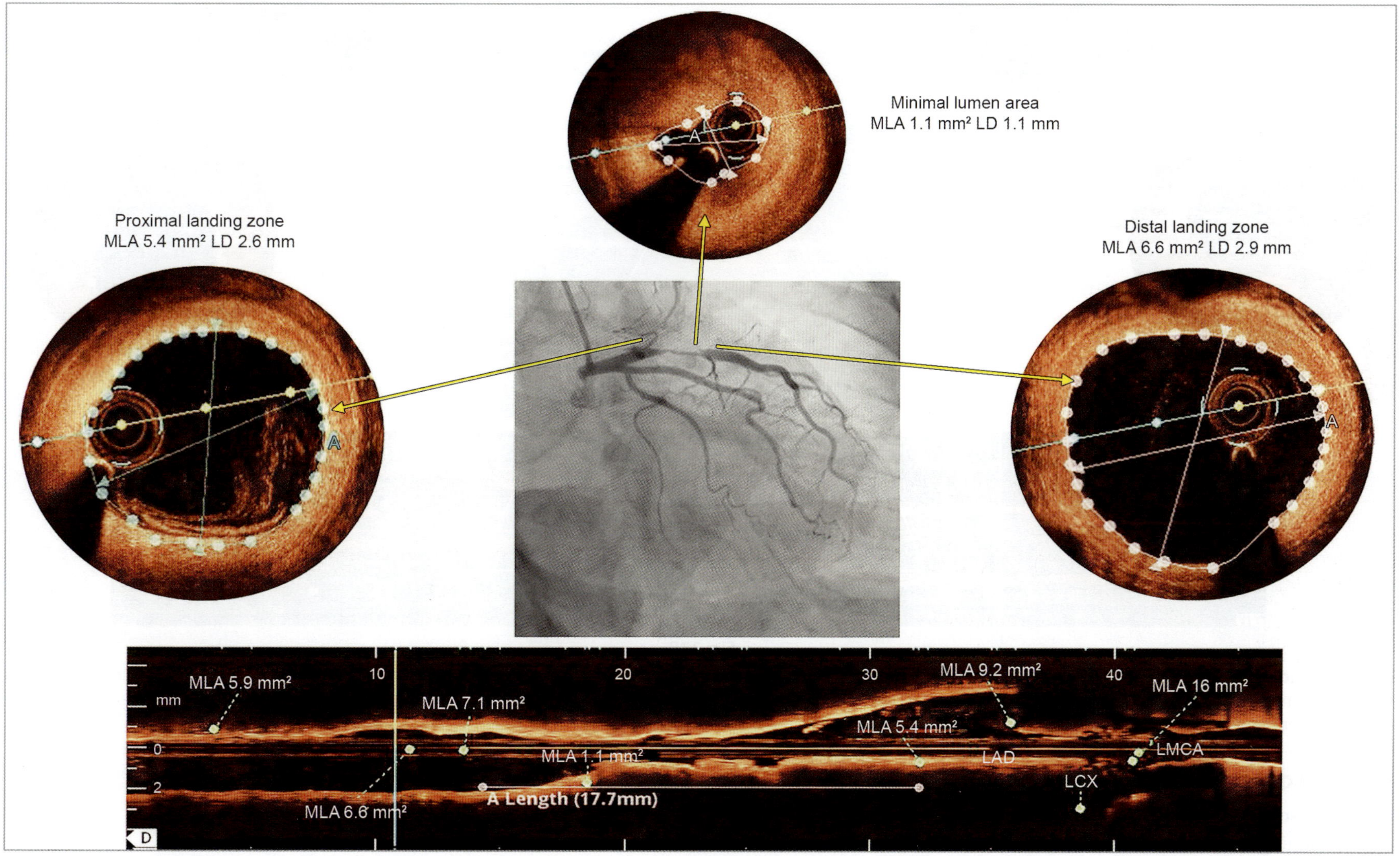

Fig. 32A

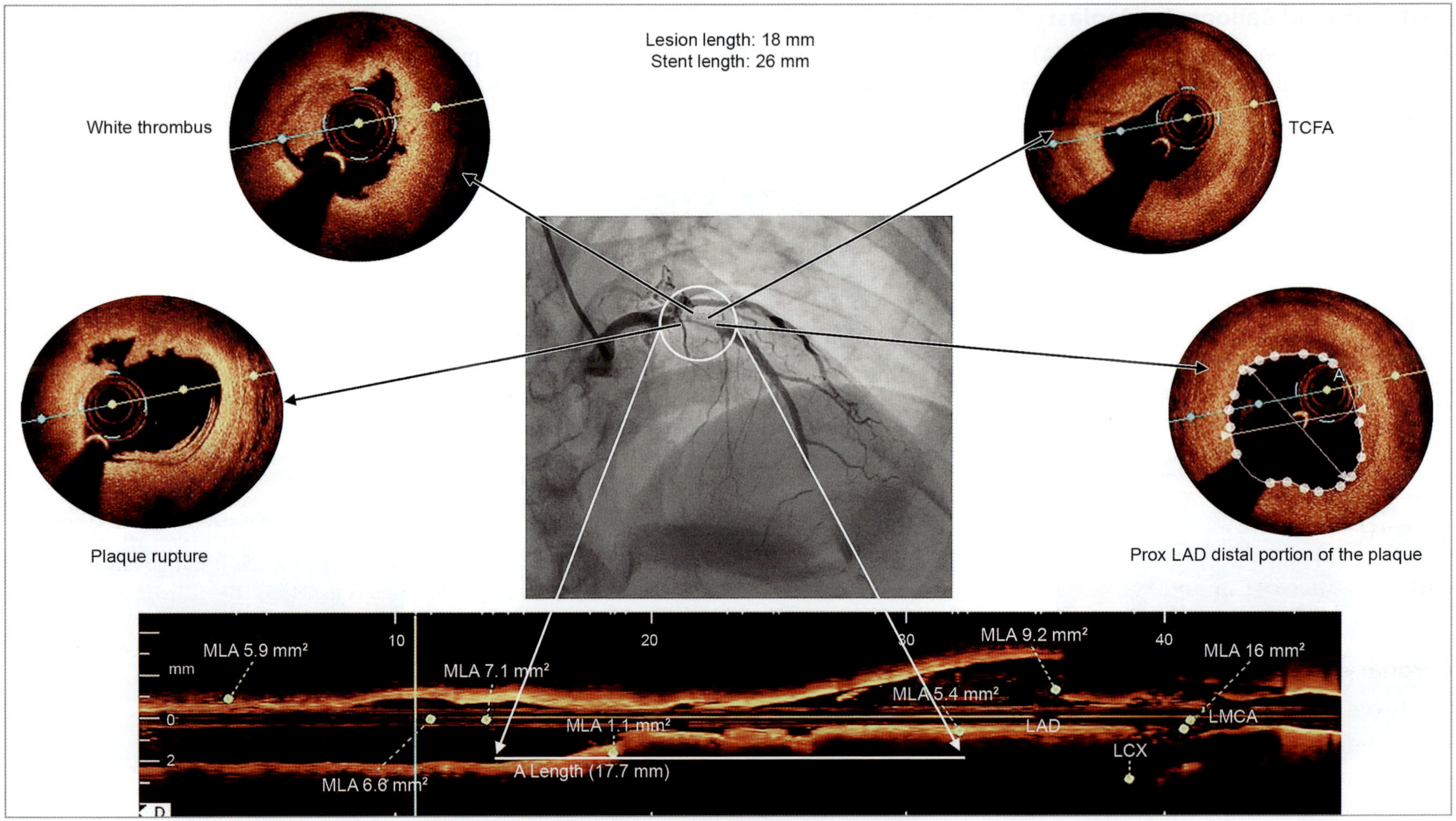

Fig. 32B

Figs. 32A and B: (A) Presenting OCT assessment to select device diameter by choosing healthy landing zones. (B) Presenting OCT assessment to select devise length along with plaque morphology. (LAD: left anterior descending; LCX: left circumflex; LD: luminal diameter; LMCA: left main coronary artery; MLA: minimal luminal area; OCT: optical coherence tomography; TCFA: thin-cap fibroatheroma)

Early IVI observations regarding angiography during PCI that are still true today

- Atherosclerosis is ubiquitous and most of it is angiographically silent.
- The angiogram is often misleading in assessing vessel size and calcification.
- A good angiographic result is not a guarantee of a good anatomic result.

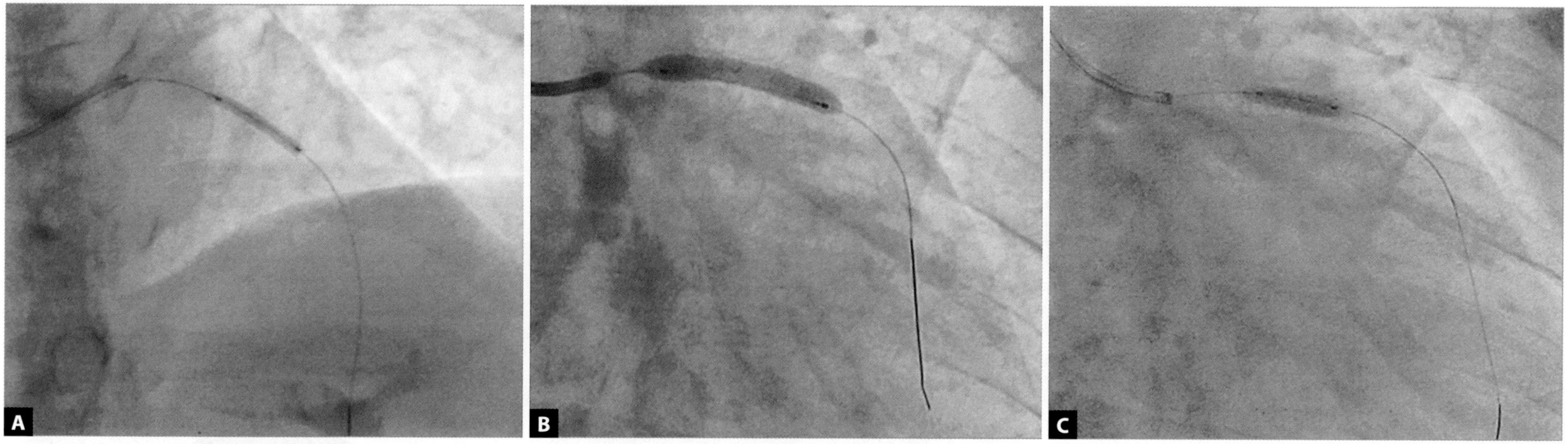

Figs. 33A to C: Predilatation, stenting, and postdilatation.

Predilatation with 2.0 × 10 mm Tazuna balloon, LAD stenting with 3.5 × 26 mm Orsiro stent (DES), and postdilatation done with 3.5 × 12 mm NC Trek balloon **(Figs. 33A to C)**.

Post-OCT—mid LAD distal to the stent MLA 7.5 mm^2, MLD 3.1 mm, distal edge of the stent—MLA 9.4 mm^2, MLD 3.4 mm, mid portion of the proximal LAD stent—MLA 8.7 mm^2, MLD 3.3 mm, and well-apposed and well-expanded stent struts with no edge dissection **(Fig. 34)**.

Postprocedure Angio view showed well-implanted stents with TIMI-III flow without any dissection.

Coronary Balloon Performance

Semi-complaint

- Expand more as pressure increases
- Expand preferentially in areas of least resistance
- Longitudinal growth
- More flexible
- Lower crossing/recrossing profile

Non-complaint

- Expand uniformly even in areas of low resistance
- Exert pressure against focal points of resistance
- More durable
- Less flexible
- Higher crossing/recrossing profile.

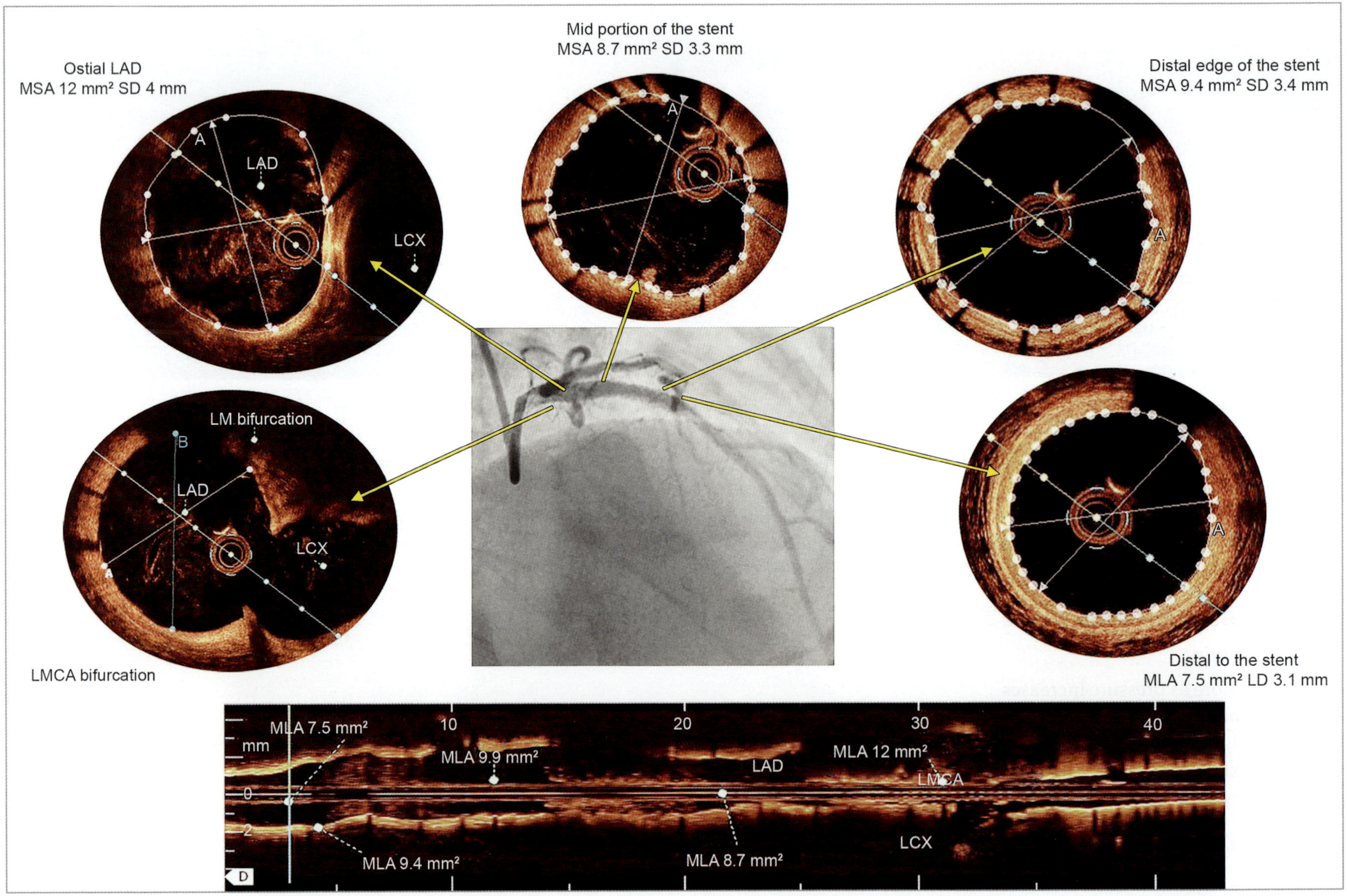

Fig. 34: Poststenting OCT assessment for any medial edge dissections at both the ends, expansion, and apposition of the stent. (LAD: left anterior descending; LCX: left circumflex; LD: luminal diameter; LMCA: left main coronary artery; MLA: minimal luminal area; OCT: optical coherence tomography)

CASE 7

Stent sizing by OCT during PCI of LAD. (LAD: left anterior descending; OCT: optical coherence tomography; PCI: percutaneous coronary intervention).

CLINICAL HISTORY

A 51-year-old male, a known hypertensive and diabetic, presented with CAD—unstable angina, recent onset of exertional chest pain, and shortness of breath (SOB). Investigations: Hb 12.8 g/dL, S Cr 0.8 mg/dL, blood urea 25 mg/dL, 2D echo—no RWMA, normal LV function, and EF 61%. CAG-LMCA—normal, LAD—proximal 80–90% lesion, LCX—proximal 90% lesion **(Figs. 35A and B)**.

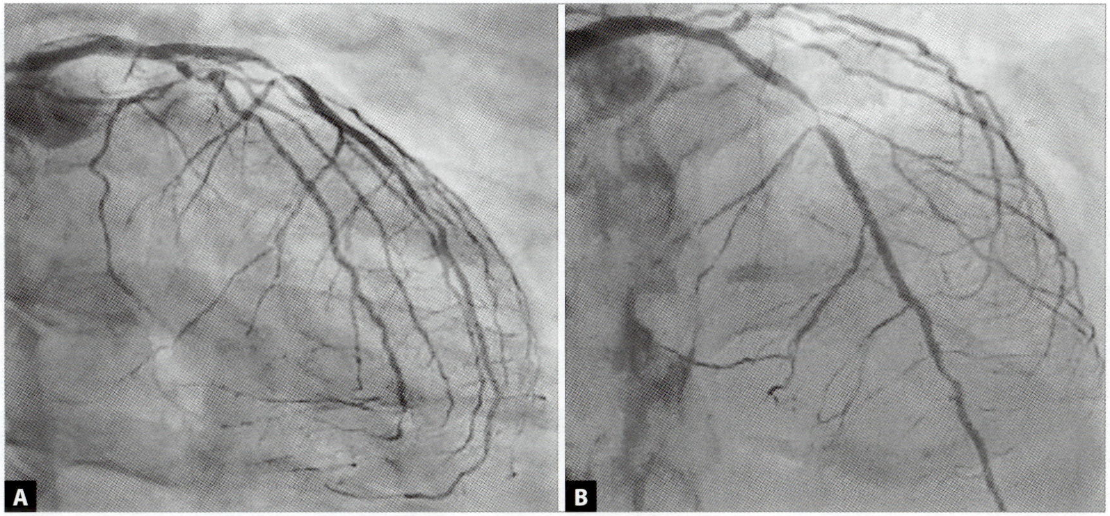

Figs. 35A and B: Coronary angiogram.

PROCEDURE

Percutaneous Coronary Intervention of Left Anterior Descending

Route—RRA, 6 Fr 3.5 EBU guiding catheter. Two 0.014″ Sion Blue wires were placed in LAD and LCX. Predilatation with 2.0 × 10 mm Tazuna balloon. Post-POBA preprocedure OCT showed proximal landing zone—MLA 5.4 mm^2, MLD 2.6 mm, distal landing zone—MLA 5.7 mm^2, MLD 2.7 mm, tight narrowing lesion with MLA 1.2 mm^2, MLD 1.2 mm with long segment diffuse fibrolipid plaque with spotty calcium and microphages of proximal LAD **(Figs. 36A to C)**. Stenting of LAD done with 2.75 × 26 mm Orsiro stent, postdilated with 2.75 × 12 mm NC Trek balloon **(Figs. 37A and B)**. Post-OCT showed proximal portion small edge dissection, which was treated conservatively, proximal landing zone—MLA 5.2 mm^2, MLD 2.6 mm, distal MLA 6.1 mm^2, MLD 2.9 mm, well-apposed and well-expanded stent struts **(Figs. 38A to D)**.

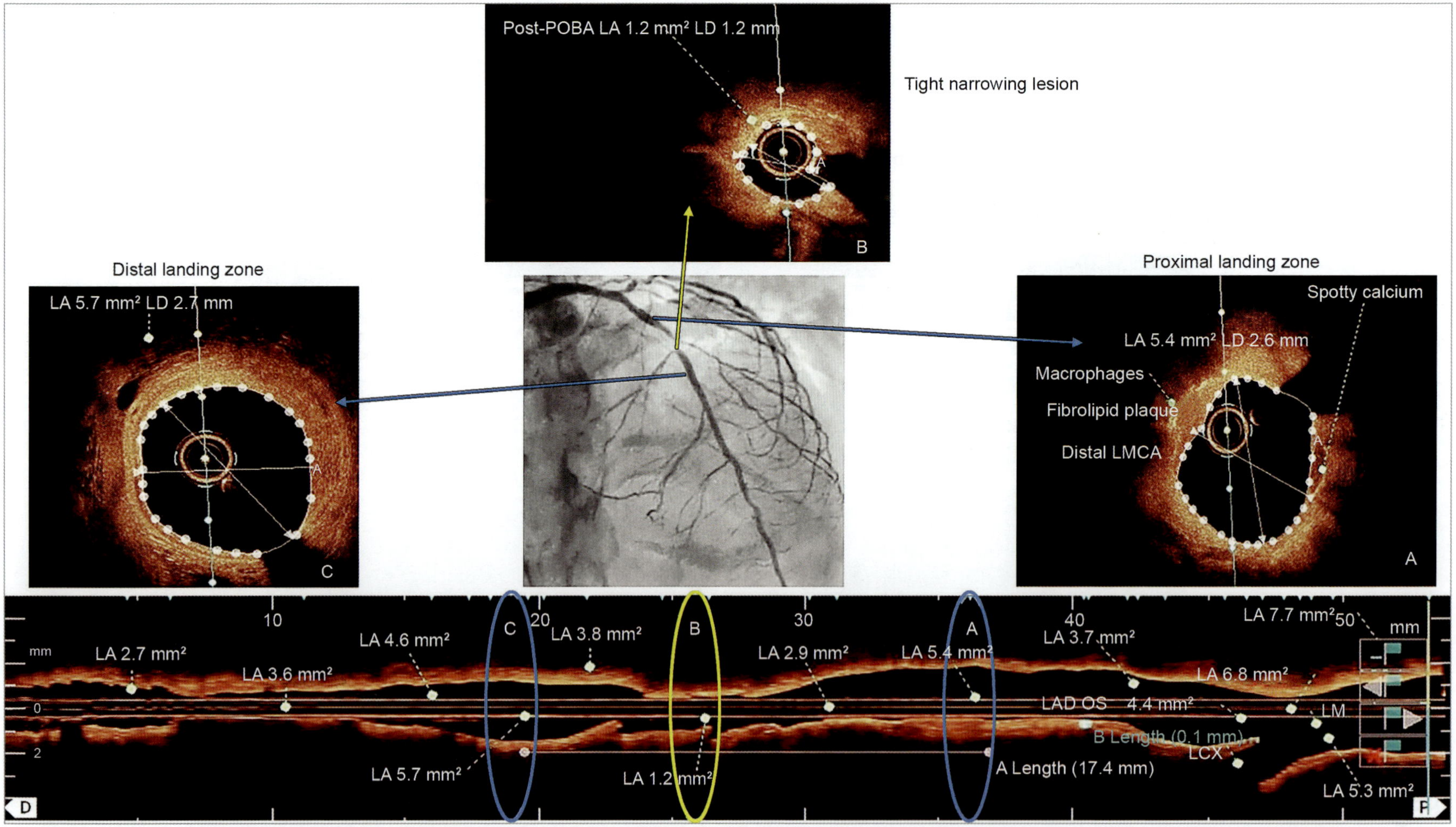

Figs. 36A to C: Prestenting OCT assessment to select device size (length and diameter). (LA: luminal area; LCX: left circumflex; LD: luminal diameter; LM: left main; LMCA: left main coronary artery; OCT: optical coherence tomography; POBA: plain old balloon angioplasty)

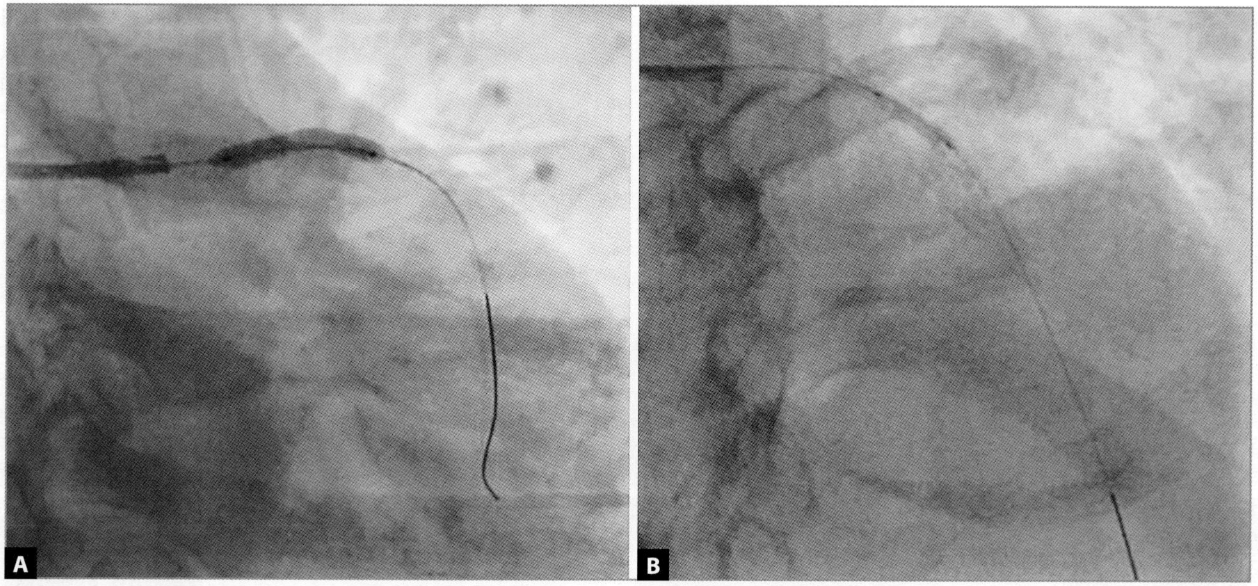

Figs. 37A and B: Stenting, postdilatation, and final result.

Restenosis After Stenting: Causes and Solution

- Causes
  - Recoil and negative remodelling (70%)
  - Neointimal hyperplasia (30%)
- Solution
  - A stent to block recoil and remodelling
  - A therapeutic agent to prevent neointimal hyperplasia.

Very late events (beyond a year) were similar between BMS and 2nd generation DES-approximately 1–2% /year. By five years, TLF/TVF with contemporary DES occurs in nearly 1 in 7 patients.

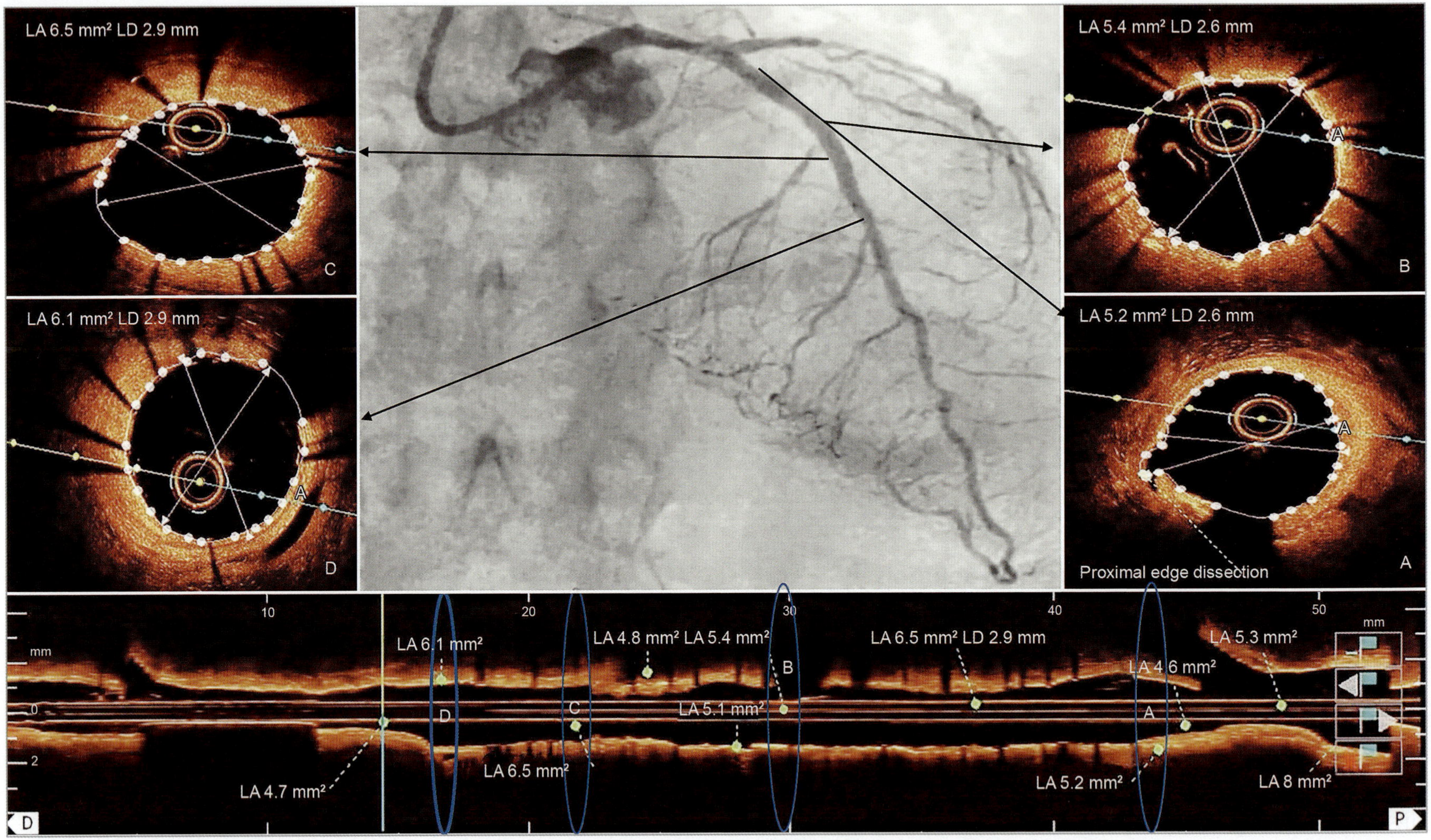

Figs. 38A to D: Poststenting OCT assessment for any medial edge dissections at both the ends, expansion, and apposition of the stent.
(LA: luminal area; LD: luminal diameter; OCT: optical coherence tomography)

CASE 8

PCI with stenting of LAD in anterior STEMI-stent sizing. (LAD: left anterior descending; PCI: percutaneous coronary intervention; STEMI: ST-elevation myocardial infarction).

CLINICAL HISTORY

A 47-year-old male, a known hypertensive and diabetic, presented with acute anterior wall MI (AWMI) and chest pain associated with SOB and sweating. ECG—ST-elevation in anterolateral leads, 2D echo—hypokinetic distal interventricular septum (IVS), apex, anterior wall, moderate LV systolic dysfunction, and EF 41%. CAG-LMCA—normal, LAD—proximal 99% lesion, mid-mild disease, LCX and RCA—normal **(Figs. 39A to C)**.

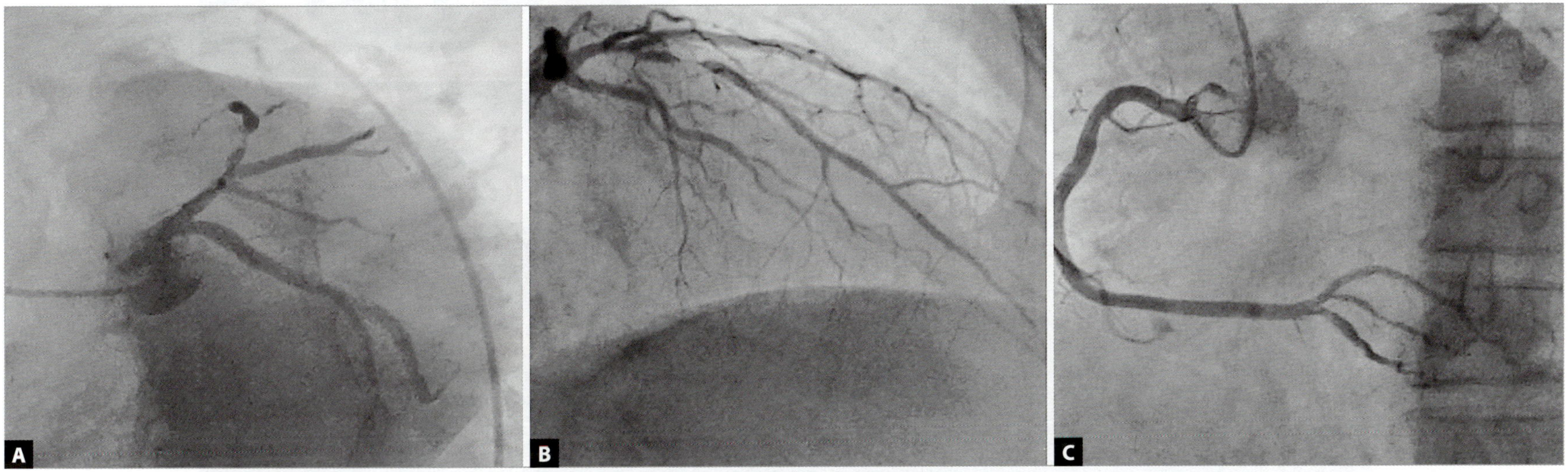

Figs. 39A to C: Coronary angiogram.

PROCEDURE

Route—RFA, using 6 Fr XB 3.5 guiding catheter, 0.014″ Power turn wire placed in LAD, 0.014″ BMW wire was placed in D1. Predilatation of LAD was done with 1.5 × 10 mm Tazuna balloon.

Pre-OCT analysis: Pre-OCT proximal landing zone— external elastic luminal diameter (ELD) 4 mm, luminal diameter (LD) 3.5 mm, distal landing zone—ELD 3.4 mm, LD 3 mm, lesion length 26 mm, device length 3.5 × 26 mm **(Fig. 40A)**, LAD ostium MLA 9.9 mm^2, proximal LAD TCFA with microphages—MLA 2.2 mm^2, MLD 1.7 mm, and tight LAD lesion at D1 origin **(Fig. 40B)**.

Left anterior descending stenting done with 3.5 × 26 mm Orsiro stent, postdilatation done with 3.5 × 12 mm NC Trek balloon, postprocedure Angio views showed well-implanted stents with TIMI-III flow without any dissection **(Figs. 41A to D)**.

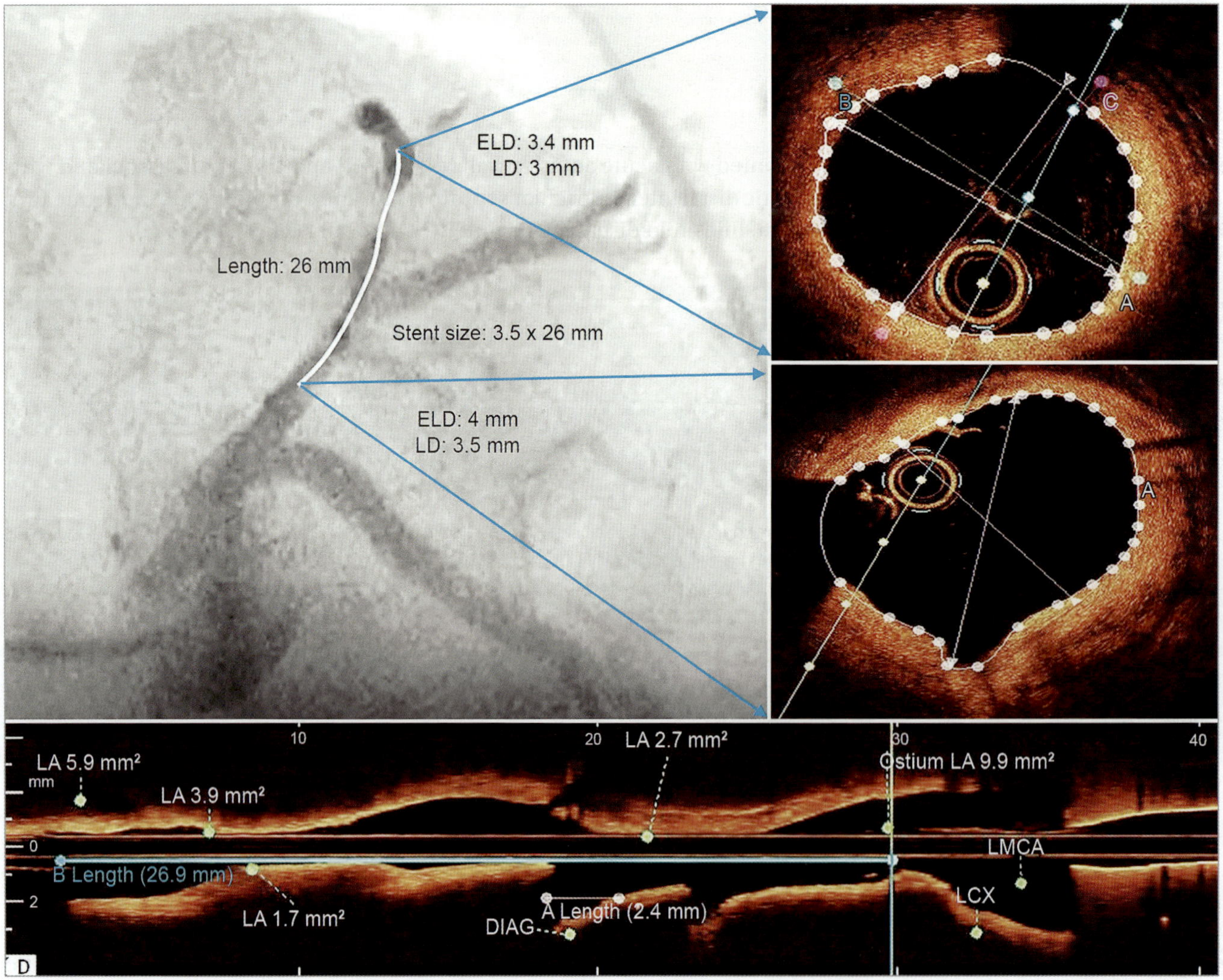

Fig. 40A

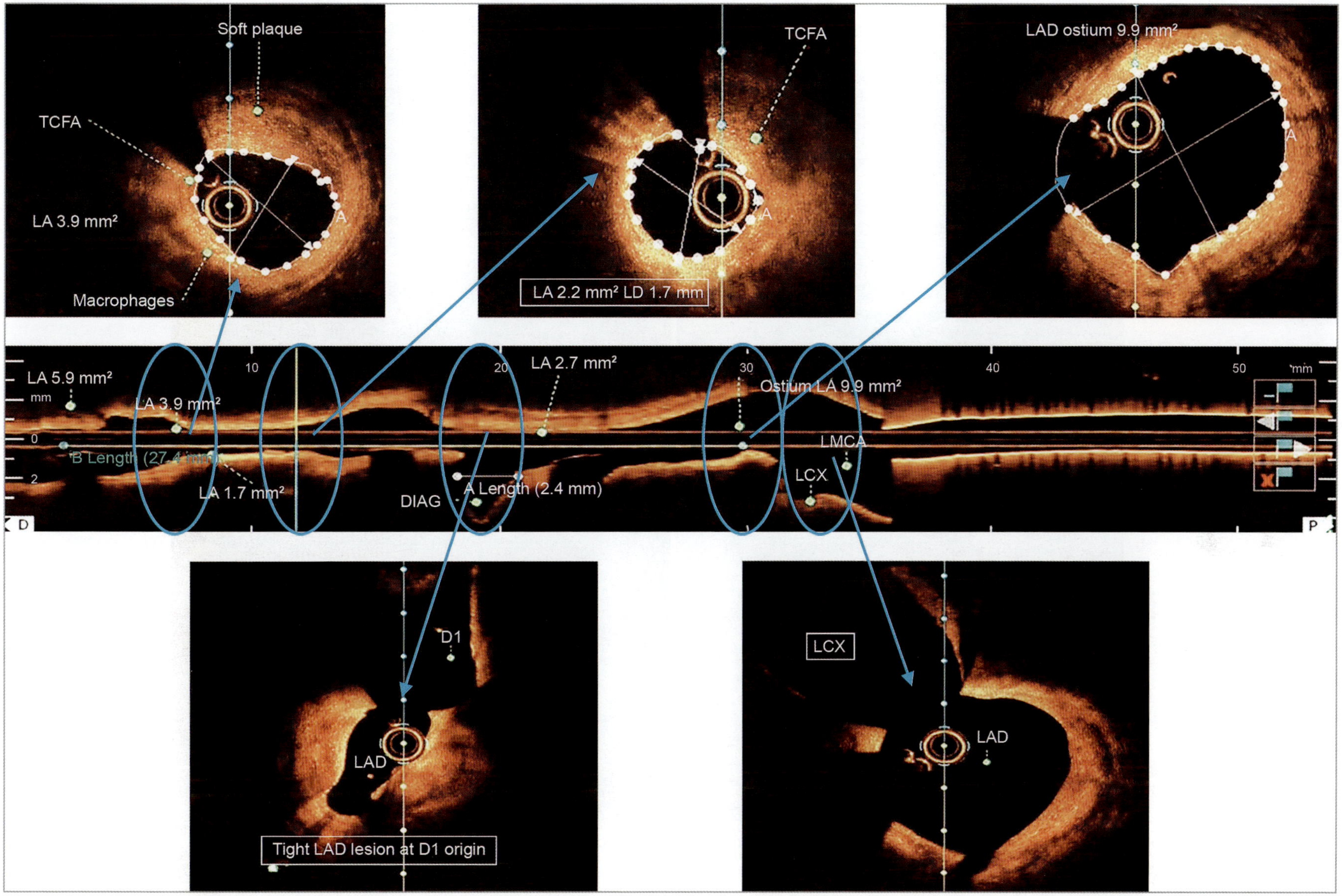

Fig. 40B

Figs. 40A and B: Prestenting OCT assessment to select devise size (length and diameter). (B) Morphological assessment of the diseased vessel by OCT imaging. (ELD: external elastic luminal diameter; LA: luminal area; LAD: left anterior descending; LCX: left circumflex; LD: luminal diameter; LMCA: left main coronary artery; OCT: optical coherence tomography; TCFA: thin-cap fibroatheroma)

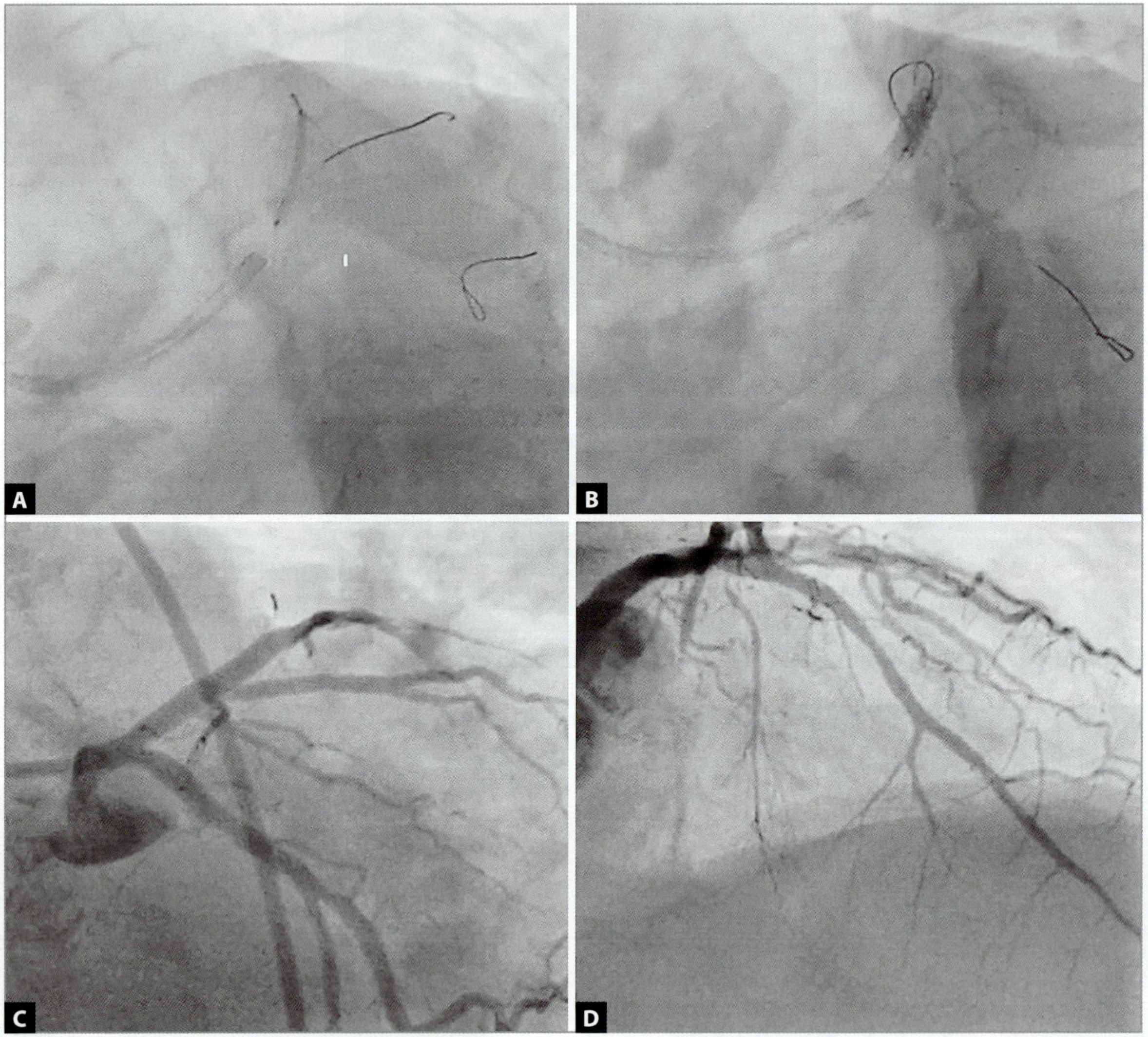

Figs. 41A to D: Stenting, postdilatation, and final result.

Poststenting Optical Coherence Tomography Analysis

Post-OCT showed well-apposed and well-expanded stent with distal mild edge dissection (<60° angle, intimal dissection, <2 mm length, and non-flow limit; hence, additional stenting for esophageal diameter (ED) is deferred) **(Fig. 42)**.

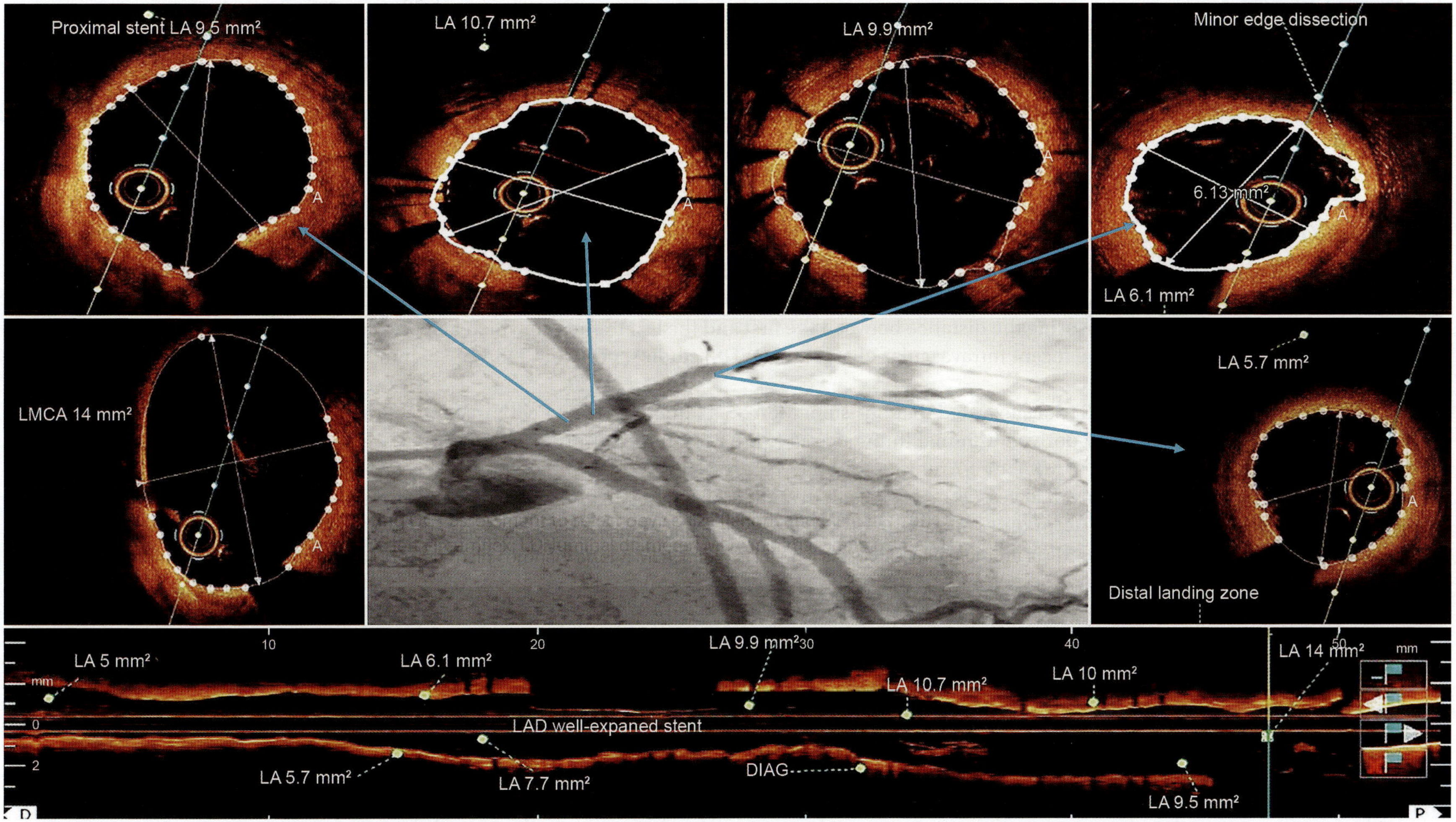

Fig. 42: Poststenting OCT assessment for any medial edge dissections at both the ends, expansion, and apposition of the stent. (LA: luminal area; LAD: left anterior descending; LMCA: left main coronary artery; OCT: optical coherence tomography)

CHAPTER 3

Underexpansion and Malapposition

STENT EXPANSION

Optimal expansion of the stent improves acute and long-term major adverse cardiovascular events (MACE) of drug-eluting stent (DES). Stent expansion is calculated as minimal stent area (MSA) divided by the average reference lumen area multiplied by 100.

The stent length is selected by measuring the distance between the first and the last frames, in which at least 70% of the stent struts are visualized in a single cross-sectional image. As per the recent intravascular ultrasound (IVUS) studies, poststent MSA of 5.5 mm^2 predicted best long-term outcomes in non-left main (LM) lesions **(Fig. 1)**.[1]

As per the evidence, the DOCTORS trial suggested that poststent MSA >5.44 mm^2 correlated with fractional flow reserve (FFR) value >0.90. Similarly, optical coherence tomography (OCT)-derived minimal luminal area (MLA) of 4.5 mm^2 in the CLIOPCI study was associated with improved MACE.[2,3] For LM lesions, recommended values of MSA are >7 mm^2 for distal LM and >8 mm^2 for proximal LM by IVUS to produce favorable outcomes, but these values are not applicable or possible in small vessels or may result in stent undersizing in large vessels where aim for achieving >80–90% of the reference landing zone to provide the best long-term outcomes. As per the ILUMIEN III study, stent length was divided into proximal and distal halves and the optimal expansion was defined as the MSA in each half >90% of the corresponding reference lumen cross-sectional area (CSA) and an achievement of >90% reference lumen CSA might not be possible in majority of the patients and it was achieved in only 40–60% of patients. Contrary to poststent expansion area of >90% of MSA, achievement of 80% average reference lumen is recommended by current consensus group; it can be obtained in the majority of the patients and it is associated with very low MACE rate (1.5% at 1-year follow-up). Expansion area of <70% MSA should be considered as underexpansion which warrants further measures to correct it **(Table 1)**.[4]

MALAPPOSITION

Stent malapposition is manifests as separation of the stent struts from the vessel lumen wall in a region not overlying a side branch and sometimes, it may be associated with underexpansion independently **(Fig. 2)**. There is no consistent evidence of association between acute malapposition (in the absence of underexpansion) and subsequent stent failure and it may resolve spontaneously or persists during follow-up **(Table 2)**.

Incomplete stent apposition (ISA) is expressed at the cross-section level as area and the longitudinal length of ISA can be easily determined.

Malapposition is classified as (1) acute—seen immediately after stenting and (2) late-persistent malapposition—persistent acute stent malapposition seen in nearly 30% of cases during follow-up and it should be distinguished from resolved acute stent malapposition. It is usually related to procedural factors such as mismatch between stent and vessel size, overlapped stents, eccentric vessels (noncircular lumen geometry), coronary aneurysms, and calcified coronary arteries with superficial calcium.[5]

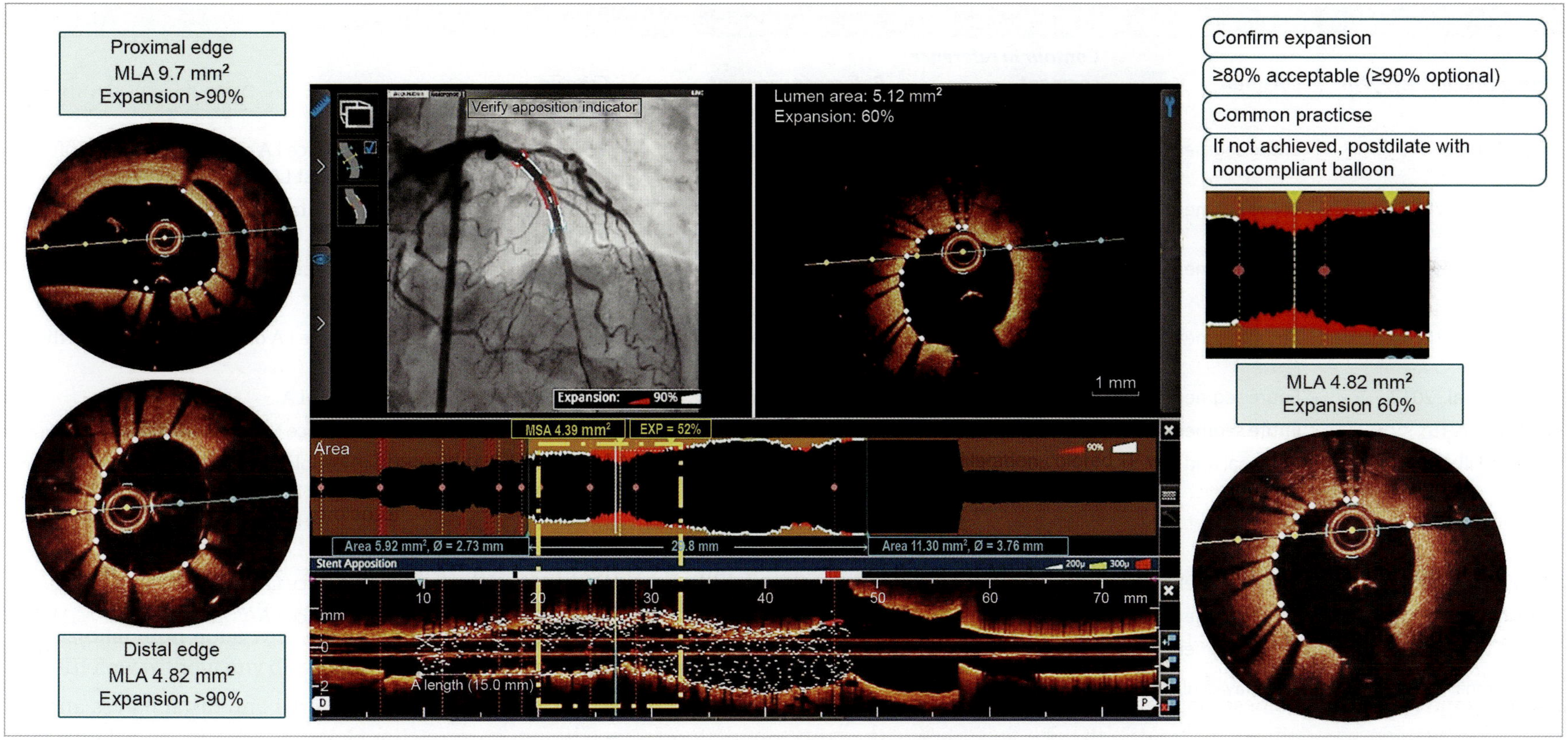

Fig. 1: Determination of expansion. (MLA: minimal luminal area)

Acute malapposition results from one of the three reasons: Undersizing of the stent is very common during percutaneous coronary intervention (PCI) for ST-segment elevation myocardial infarction (STEMI) and chronic total occlusion (CTO), where the vessel may look deceptively small sized as a result of underfilling, coronary spasm, and a layer of thrombus between vessel wall and stent strut. Though intravascular imaging (IVI) helps in identifying true vessel size in the latter situation, it is essential to measure after giving proper doses of coronary vasodilators such as intracoronary (IC) nitroglycerin (NTG)/nicorandil to eliminate spasm-related vessel undersizing. Severely calcified plaque may cause asymmetrical expansion of the stent due to undilatable hard plaque. Sometimes, acute malapposition may fully resolve with reendothelialization of struts, partially resolve, remain stable, or increase in size due to plaque regression of the plaque and positive remodeling. Acute malapposition of optimally expanded stent usually carries good long-term outcomes and it is observed in about 13–65% of cases on OCT evaluation. Size of the malapposition and strut-to-lumen distances are the predictors for the persistence of malapposition and delayed vascular healing.[6-8]

Persistent malapposition: It is usually due to stent underexpansion associated with the presence of severe calcification. Some cases are due to the apposition of the struts over an intimal dissection that does not heal at follow-up.

TABLE 1: Summary of the absolute and relative stent expansion criteria for stent optimization (data from IVUS and OCT studies).

Study/first author, year	*Location*	*Contour in reference segment*	*Reference segment*	*Criteria*
			IVUS studies	
MUSIC, 1998	Entire segment	Lumen	Average reference LA	MSA ≥90% of the average reference LA or ≥100% of the LA of reference segment with the lowest LA
HOME-DES IVUS, 2010	Entire segment	Lumen	Distal reference LA	MSA ≥5.0 mm^2 or >90% of the distal reference lumen MSA for small vessels
IVUS XPL, 2015	Entire segment	Lumen	Distal reference LA	MSA more than the distal reference LA
			OCT studies	
CLI-OPCI, 2012	Entire segment	Lumen	Average reference LA	MSA ≥90% stenosis of the average LA or ≥100% of the LA of the lowest reference LA
Habara et al., 2012	Entire segment	Lumen	Distal reference LA	MSA ≥90% of the distal reference LA
OCTACS, 2015	Entire segment	Lumen	Average reference LA	MSA ≥90% of the average reference LA
ILUMEIN III, OPTIMIZE PCI, 2016	Proximal and distal segment	EEL	Proximal reference EEL–EEL	Proximal MSA >90–95% (acceptable) or ≥95% (optimal) of the proximal reference LA
			Proximal reference EEL–EEL	Distal MSA >90–95% (acceptable) or ≥95% (optimal) of the distal reference LA
DOCTORS, 2016	Entire segment	Lumen	Average reference LA	MSA >80% of the average reference LA
OPINION, 2017	Entire segment	Lumen	Average reference LA	MSA ≥90% of the average reference LA
DETECT-OCT, 2018	Entire segment	Lumen	Distal reference LA	MSA >4.0 mm^2

(EEL: external elastic lamina; IVUS: intravascular ultrasound; LA: luminal area; MSA: minimal stent area; OCT: optical coherence tomography)

Late-acquired malapposition: This is not present at the time of index procedure but developed during follow up as a result of late-positive vascular remodeling without abluminal tissue growth and plaque regression or thrombus dissolution behind the stent struts without vessel remodeling. It may be associated with late ST, especially in the setting of positive remodeling, stent recoiling, areas of large malapposition, and frank aneurysms.[9]

Proposed Causes of Late-acquired Incomplete Stent Apposition

Acute malapposed segments with a strut-to-vessel distance of <100 μm usually heal with reendothelialization at 6-month follow-up. However as per the evidence, the rate of non-reendothelialization of struts increases from 6.1% with malapposition width of 100 and 300 μm to 15.7% with malapposition width of >300 μm.[10]

As the stent strut is a strong reflector of light, OCT shows only the endoluminal side of the stent strut, which results in "blooming" on either side of the strut with the actual strut surface in the middle. Malapposition is said to be present when the distance between the middle of the strut reflection to the lumen surface exceeds the sum of stent strut and polymer thickness. It is commonly expressed as the distance from the strut surface to the surface of the lumen and detects even minor malapposition very clearly. Three-dimensional (3D) OCT with angio-registration systems automatically detects and displays malapposed stent struts both in the cross-sectional and longitudinal views and provides color coding based on the extent of malapposition

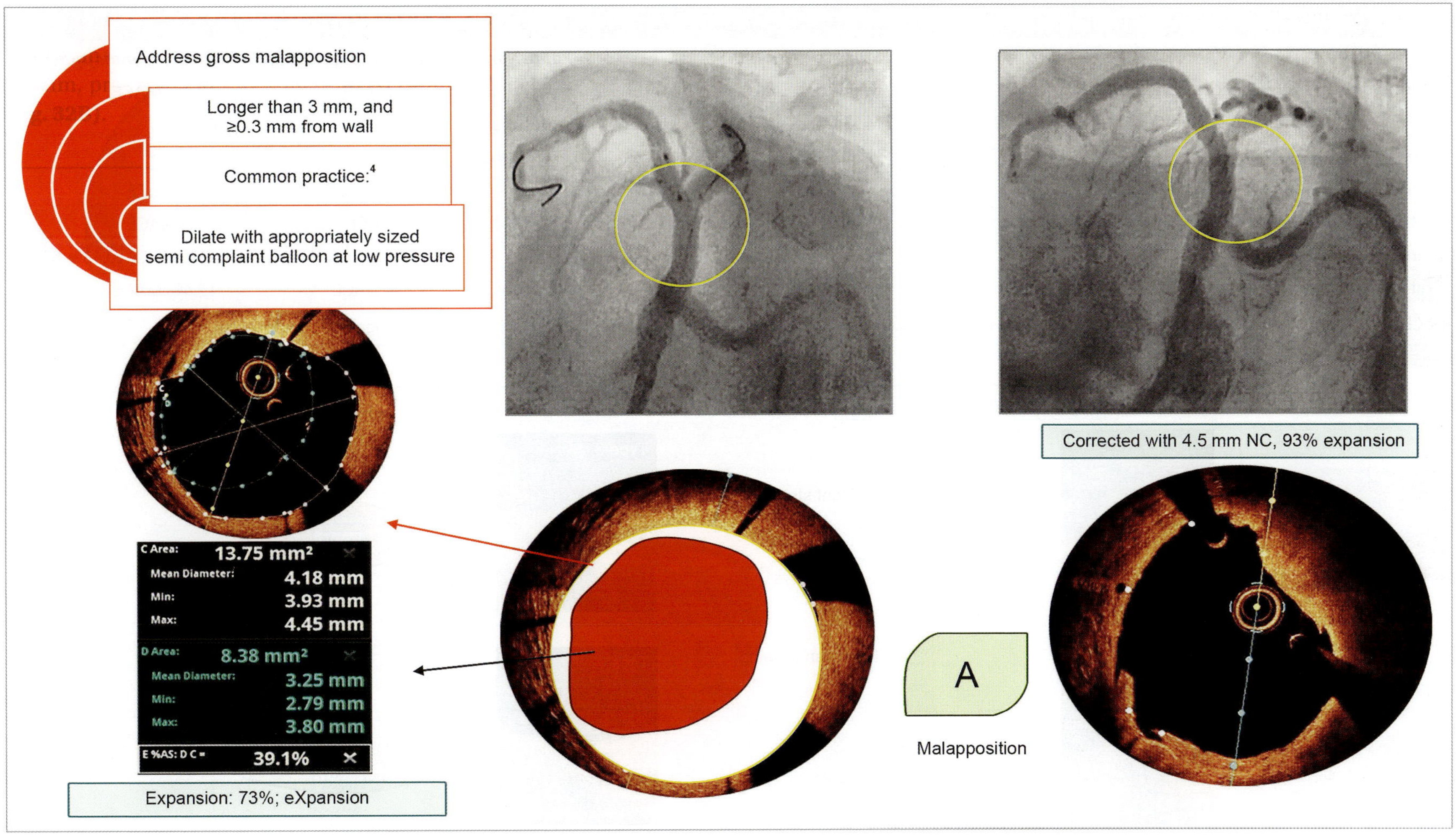

Fig. 2: Poststenting OCT assessment—malapposition and correction. (NC: noncompliant)

circumferentially and longitudinally. The recent consensus statement recommends against treatment of malapposition with ISA distance <400 µm and a length of <1 mm. OCT compared to IVUS is more useful for follow-up evaluation of malapposition in post-PCI patients due to its high resolution.

MALAPPOSITION AT FOLLOW-UP

Management of malapposition at follow-up is only recommended if the cause is correctable and producing a clinical problem (e.g., stent underexpansion in stent thrombosis).

TABLE 2: Events related to acute stent malapposition.

	Study		*Follow-up*	*Acute malapposition*	*No acute malapposition*
Steinberg et al. JACC Cardiovasc Interv. 2010;3:486-94	Combined TAXUS	IVUS	9 months	8.2% MACE	10.7% MACE
Van der Hoven et al. JACC Cardiovasc Interv. 2008;1:192-201	MISSION-AMI	IVUS	9 months	0% ST	0% ST
Guo et al. Circulation. 2010;122:10-77-84	HORIZONS-AMI	IVUS	13 months	0% ST	0% ST
Soeda et al. Circulation. 2015;132:1020-9		OCT	1 year	4.4% DoCE	4.8% DoCE
Prati et al. JACC Cardiovasc Imaging. 2015;8:1297-305	CLI-OPCI-II	OCT	1 year	13% MACE	10% MACE
Wang et al. JAHA, in press	ADAPT-DES	IVUS	2 years	5.2% MACE (0.65% ST)	45% MACE (0.43% ST)
Prati et al. Circ Cardiovasc Interv. 2016:9(12):e003726	CLI-OPCI-ACS	OCT	9 months	12.8% MACE	12.4% MACE

(DoCE: device-oriented composite endpoint; IVUS: intravascular ultrasound; MACE: major adverse cardiovascular events; OCT: optical coherence tomography)

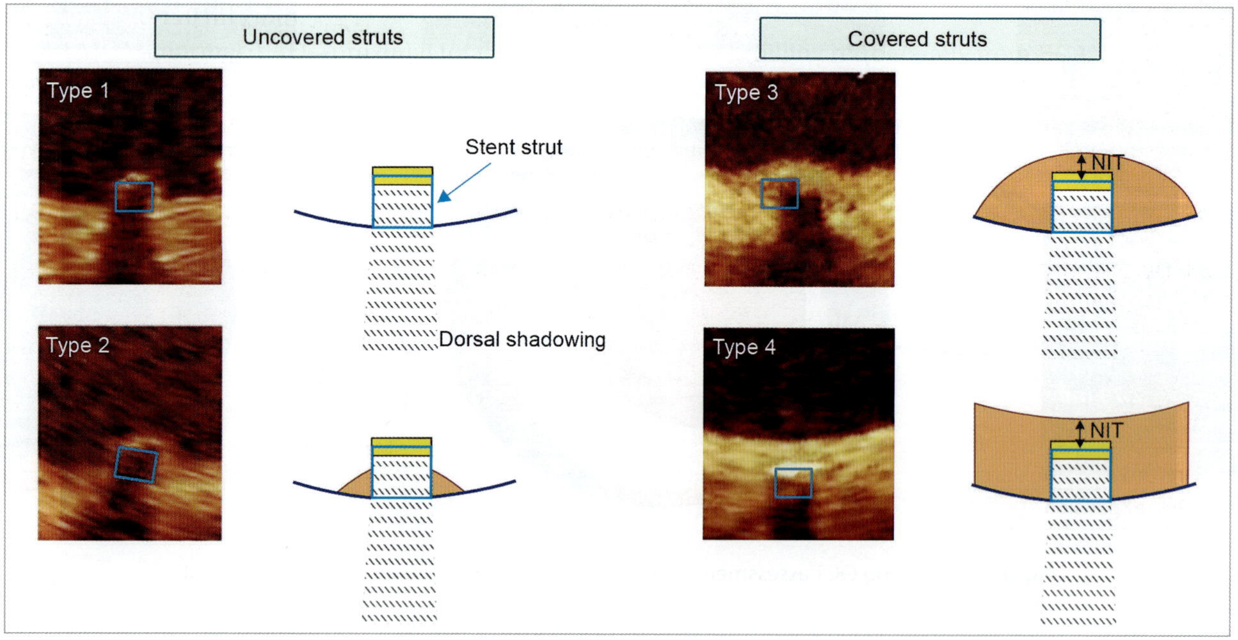

Fig. 3: Uncovered and covered struts by OCT. (NIT: neointimal thickness; OCT: optical coherence tomography)

Classification of tissue coverage of stent struts: The left images show uncovered struts and the right images show covered struts. A strut with surrounding tissue beyond the strut surface is defined as covered. According to the shape of the tissue covering the struts, a covered strut is classified as convex (3) or embedded (4). The neointimal thickness (NIT) was measured from the surface of the neointima covering the strut to the center line of the reflection **(Fig. 3)**.

Stent expansion criteria: While the goal is to achieve acceptable expansion, the goal drives the outcome of the largest MSA possible; consensus document MSA >80% of mean reference area, MSA >5 mm^2 by IVUS and 4.5 mm^2 by OCT.

REFERENCES

1. Russo RJ, Silva PD, Teirstein PS, Attubato MJ, Davidson CJ, DeFranco AC, et al. A randomized controlled trial of angiography versus intravascular ultrasound-directed bare-metal coronary stent placement (the AVID Trial). Circulation: Cardiovasc Interv. 2009;2(2):113-23.
2. Prati F, Romagnoli E, Burzotta F, Limbruno U, Gatto L, La Manna A, et al. Clinical impact of OCT findings during PCI: the CLI-OPCI II study. JACC Cardiovasc Imaging. 2015;8(11):1297-305.
3. Subban V, Raffel OC, Vasu N, Victor SM, Sankardas MA. Intravascular ultrasound and optical coherence tomography for the assessment of coronary artery disease and percutaneous coronary intervention optimization: Specific lesion subsets. Indian Heart J Interv. 2018;1(2):95.
4. Räber L, Mintz GS, Koskinas KC, Johnson TW, Holm NR, Onuma Y, et al. Clinical use of intracoronary imaging. Part 1: guidance and optimization of coronary interventions. An expert consensus document of the European Association of Percutaneous Cardiovascular Interventions. Eur Heart J. 2018;39(35):3281-300.
5. Im E, Kim BK, Ko YG, Shin DH, Kim JS, Choi D, et al. Incidences, predictors, and clinical outcomes of acute and late stent malapposition detected by optical coherence tomography after drug-eluting stent implantation. Circ Cardiovasc Interv. 2014;7(1):88-96.
6. Kubo T, Imanishi T, Kitabata H, Kuroi A, Ueno S, Yamano T, et al. Comparison of vascular response after sirolimus-eluting stent implantation between patients with unstable and stable angina pectoris: a serial optical coherence tomography study. JACC Cardiovasc Imaging. 2008;1(4):475-84.
7. Kume T, Okura H, Miyamoto Y, Yamada R, Saito K, Tamada T, et al. Natural history of stent edge dissection, tissue protrusion and incomplete stent apposition detectable only on optical coherence tomography after stent implantation. Circ J. 2012;76(3):698-703.
8. Kawamori H, Shite J, Shinke T, Otake H, Matsumoto D, Nakagawa M, et al. Natural consequence of post-intervention stent malapposition, thrombus, tissue prolapse, and dissection assessed by optical coherence tomography at mid-term follow-up. Eur Heart J Cardiovasc Imaging. 2013;14(9):865-75.
9. Gonzalo N, Serruys PW, Okamura T, van Beusekom HM, Garcia-Garcia HM, van Soest G, et al. Optical coherence tomography patterns of stent restenosis. Am Heart J. 2009;158(2):284-93.
10. Kang SJ, Mintz GS, Park DW, Lee SW, Kim YH, Lee CW, et al. Late and very late drug-eluting stent malapposition: Serial 2-year quantitative IVUS analysis. Circ Cardiovasc Interv. 2010;3:335-40.

CASE 1

PCI of RCA-OCT assessment of long, tapered vessel (malapposition). (OCT: optical coherence tomography; PCI: percutaneous coronary intervention; RCA: right coronary artery)

CLINICAL HISTORY

A 45-year-old male, a known diabetic, presented with anterolateral STEMI and ongoing chest pain associated with breathlessness. Electrocardiogram (ECG)—anterolateral STEMI. Two-dimensional (2D) echo—mild left ventricular (LV) dysfunction and ejection fraction (EF) 45%.

Coronary angiography-left main coronary artery (CAG-LMCA) and left anterior descending (LAD)—mild disease, left circumflex (LCX)—proximal 100% occlusion, right coronary artery (RCA)—proximal to distal diffuse disease **(Figs. 4A and B)**.

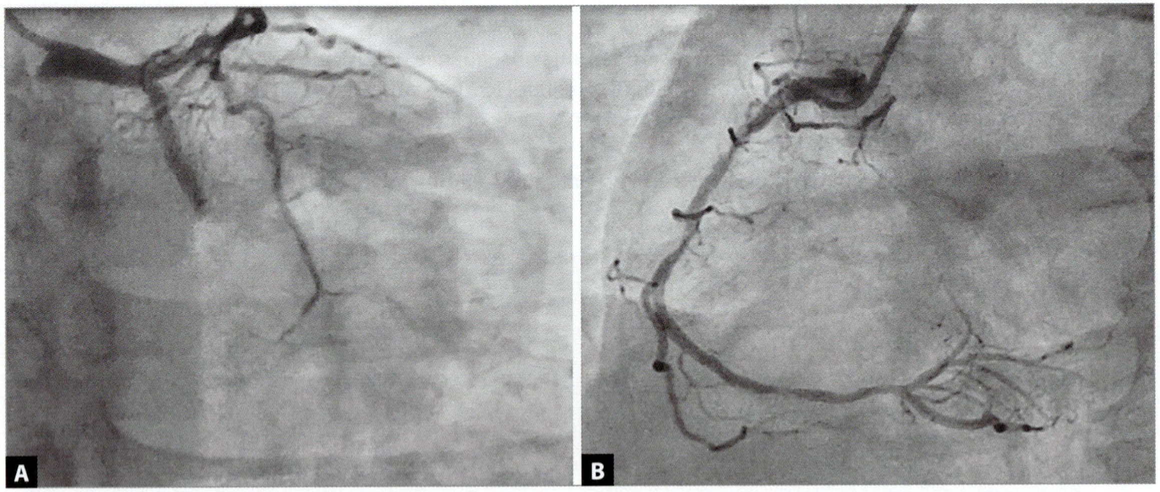

Figs. 4A and B: Coronary angiogram. (A) Left circumflex (LCX) and (B) Right coronary artery (RCA).

PROCEDURE

Percutaneous Coronary Intervention of Left Circumflex

Right radial artery (RRA)—route, using 6 Fr EBU 3.5 guiding catheter. Totally occluded LCX lesion was crossed with 0.014″ Rinato wire. Thrombus aspiration was done with Export AP thrombus aspiration catheter; LCX was stented with 3.0 × 38 mm Xience Xpedition stent (DES) and postdilated with 3.0 × 15 mm

Quantum Maverick balloon. Postprocedure Angio view showed well-implanted stent with thrombolysis in myocardial infarction (TIMI-III) flow without any dissection **(Figs. 5A and B)**.

Percutaneous Coronary Intervention of Right Coronary Artery

Right radial artery—route, using 6 Fr Judkins right (JR) 3.5 guiding catheter, RCA lesion was crossed with 0.014″ Rinato wire, predilated with 2.0 × 15 mm Trek balloon, distal RCA stented with 2.25 × 30 mm Resolute Integrity stent (DES) and proximal RCA stented with 2.75 × 38 mm Xience Xpedition stent **(Figs. 6A and B)**.

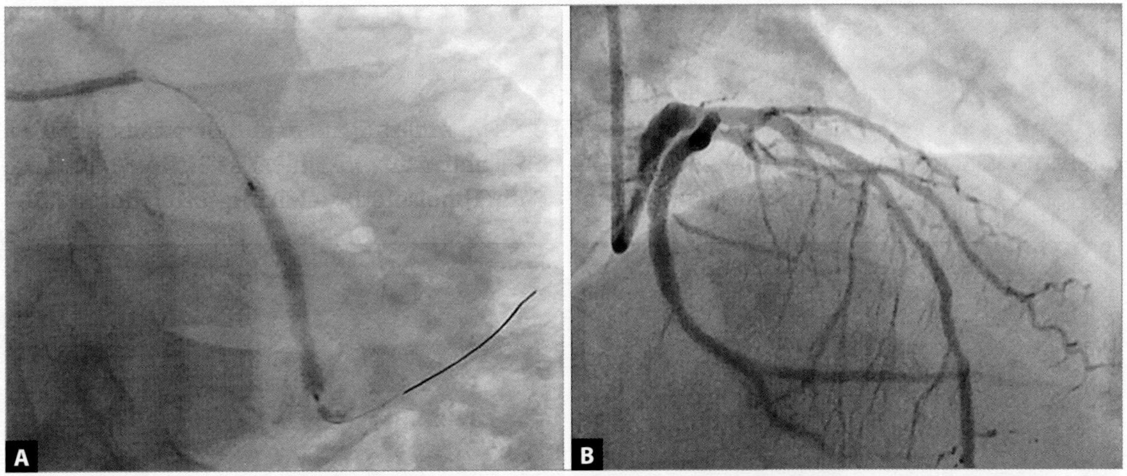

Figs. 5A and B: Stenting of left circumflex (LCX) and final result.

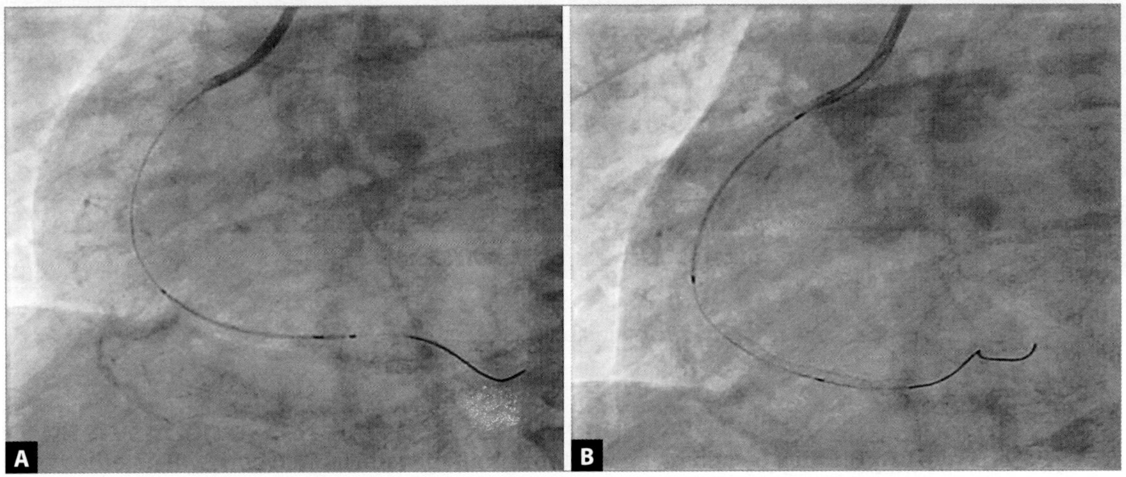

Figs. 6A and B: Stenting of distal and proximal right coronary artery (RCA).

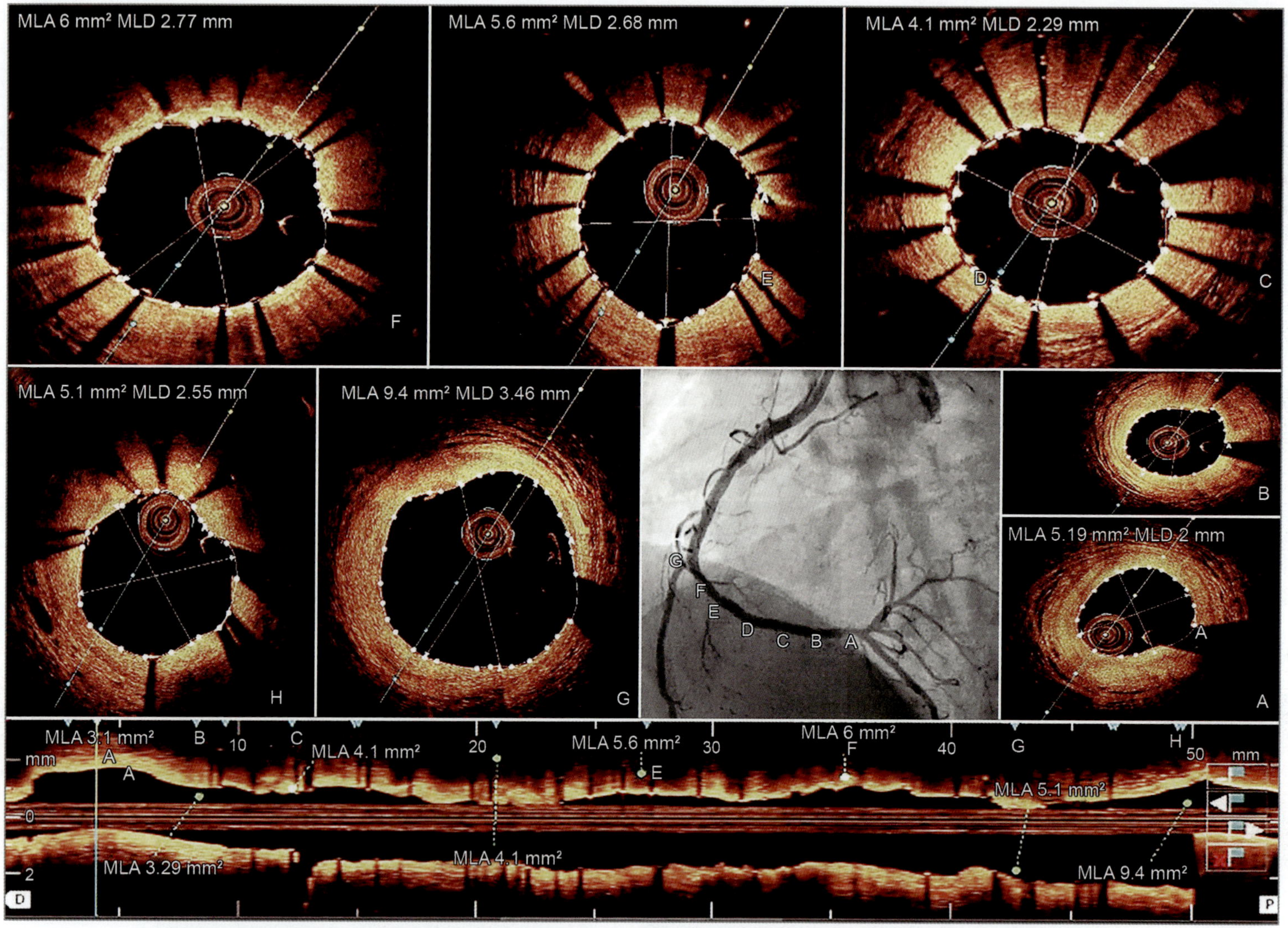

Figs. 7: Assessment of OCT for mid-to-distal RCA vessel. (MLA: minimal luminal area; MLD: minimal luminal diameter; OCT: optical coherence tomography; RCA: right coronary artery)

Poststenting OCT showed distal landing, distal MSA 4.1 mm^2, minimal stent diameter (MSD) 2.3 mm, malapposition in proximal RCA sent **(Fig. 7)**.

Post-OCT study—gross malapposition of the proximal portion of the stent (ring in ring) MSA 4.8 mm^2, MSD 2.47 mm, MLA 7.28 mm^2, minimal luminal diameter (MLD) 3.03 mm, and 33% of malapposition which was **(Fig. 8)** corrected with 3.0 × 15 mm, 3.5 × 18 mm, and 4.0 × 08 mm NC Trek balloons.

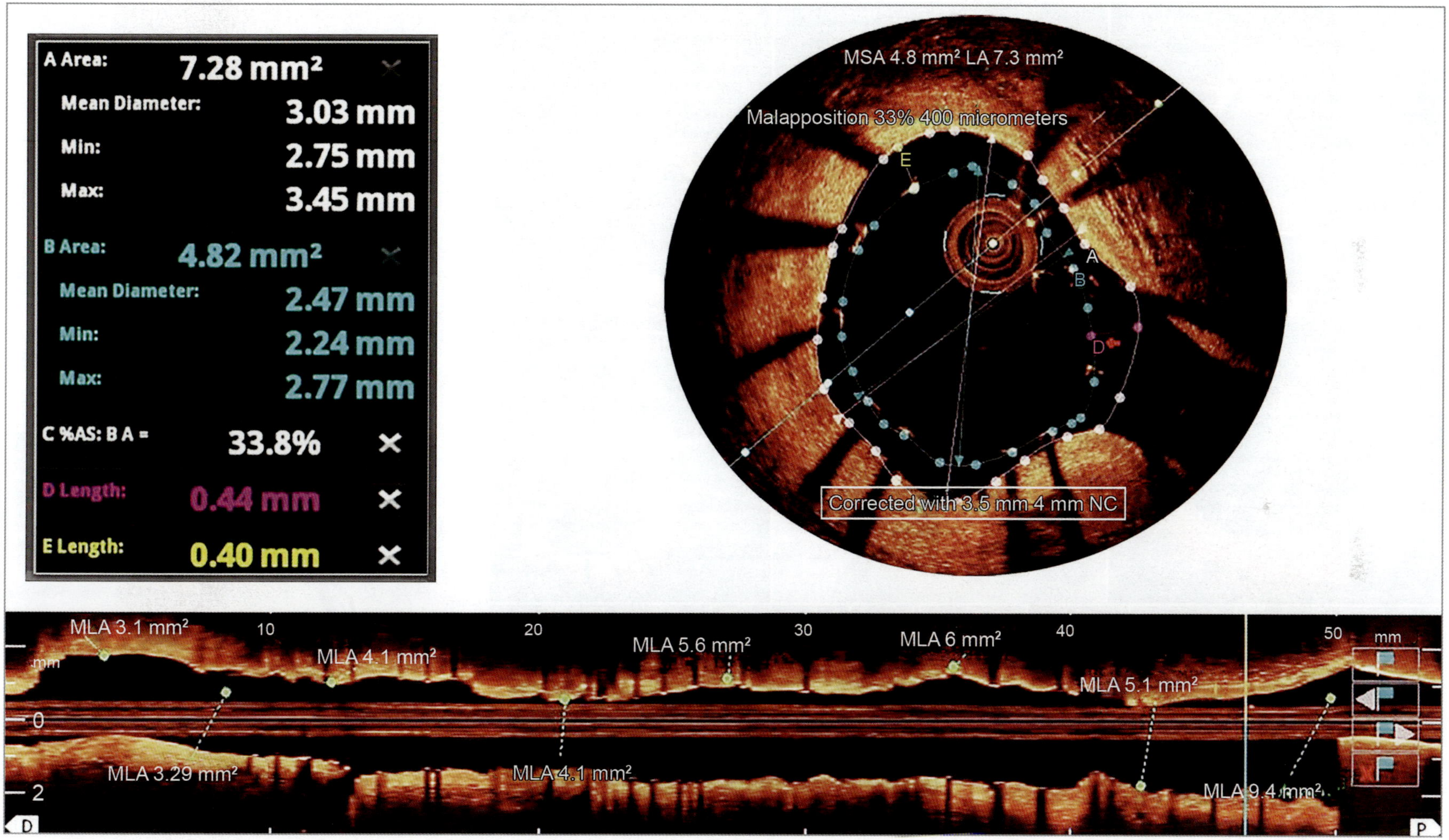

Fig. 8: Detection of malapposition in proximal RCA (ring in ring). (LA: lumen area; MLA: minimal luminal area; MSA: minimal stent area; NC: noncompliant; RCA: right coronary artery)

Repeat OCT showed proximal landing zone, proximal edge of RCA stent fully expanded after 4 NC dilatation with MLA 9.6 mm^2, mean luminal diameter 3.49 mm, minimum diameter 3.26 mm, and maximum diameter 3.80 mm **(Fig. 9)**.

Postprocedure angio view showed well-implanted stents with TIMI-III flow without any dissection **(Fig. 10)**. Patient was discharged on 3rd postprocedure day in a stable status.

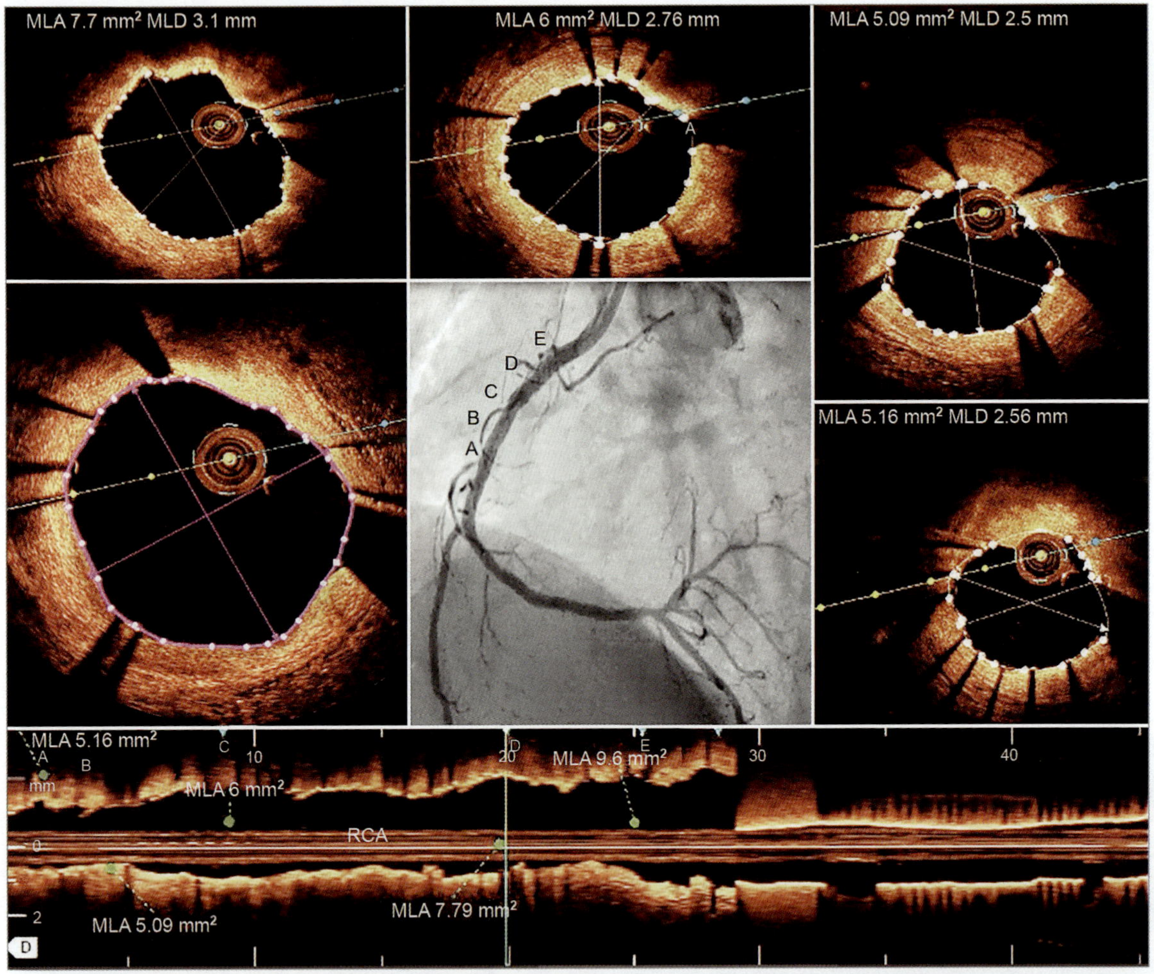

Fig. 9: Assessment of OCT for proximal-to-mid-RCA vessel. (MLA: minimal luminal area; MLD: minimal luminal diameter; OCT: optical coherence tomography; RCA: right coronary artery)

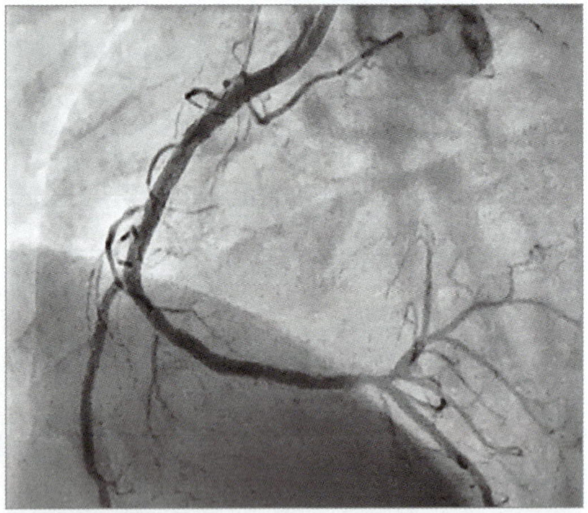

Fig. 10: Final result of right coronary artery (RCA).

Sometimes angio may underestimate and misleads proper lesion preparation with IVI guidance is essential for dealing the complex lesions.

CASE 2

Primary PCI of RCA-STEMI of inferior wall (malapposition). (PCI: percutaneous coronary intervention; RCA: right coronary artery; STEMI: ST-elevation myocardial infarction)

CLINICAL HISTORY

A 38-year-old male, a known hypertensive, presented with acute inferior wall myocardial infarction (MI) (window period—3 hours) with ongoing chest pain. ECG—ST elevation and T inversions in inferior leads. 2D echo—hypokinetic basal inferior wall, regional wall motion abnormalities (RWMA) in RCA territory, fair LV function, and EF 53%.

Investigations: Random blood sugar (RBS) 246 mg/dL, blood urea 20 mg/dL, serum creatinine (S Cr) 1.27 mg/dL, estimated glomerular filtration rate (eGFR) 71 mg/dL, and Troponin I 0.01 ng/dL.

Coronary angiography-LMCA—normal, ostioproximal 50–60% with ectatic proximal LAD lesion, mid-bifurcation 50% lesion. LCX—distal mild disease, and RCA—proximal-to-mid-long segment 99% lesion **(Figs. 11A to C)**.

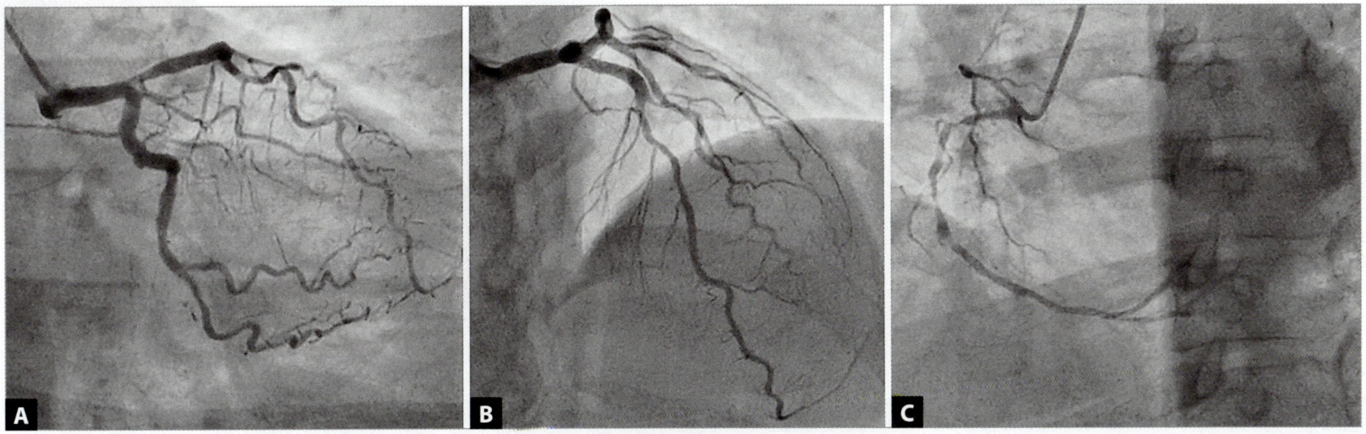

Figs. 11A to C: Coronary angiogram.

PROCEDURE

Left main coronary artery engaged with 6 Fr EBU 3.5 guiding catheter, FFR study of LAD showed 0.97, with injection IC NTG 0.92, intravenous (IV) adenosine infusion (140 μg/kg/min) for 3 minutes—0.84. Hence, LAD-PCI was differed.

Percutaneous Coronary Intervention of Right Coronary Artery

Right radial artery—route, using 6 Fr JR 3.5 guiding catheter, RCA crossed with 0.014" Sion Blue wire.

Pre-OCT showed plaque rupture of RCA due to lipid-rich plaque with thin-cap fibroatheroma (TCFA), tight portion of proximal RCA with MLA 0.9 mm^2, MLD 1.1 mm, RCA near ostium with MLA 6.5 mm^2, MLD 2.9 mm **(Fig. 12)**.

Right coronary artery lesion predilated with 1.25 × 10 mm, 2.5 × 10 mm Tazuna balloons, stented with 3.5 × 48 mm Xience Xpedition stent, and postdilated with 3.5 × 12 mm NC balloon **(Figs. 13A to C)**. OCT showed RCA near-ostium malapposed DES ring-in-ring appearance with MLA 17 mm^2, MLD 4.6 mm, MSA 9.3 mm^2, MSD 3.4 mm well expanded with no edge dissections, and malapposition of proximal portion of the stent which was corrected with 4.5 × 08 mm NC Trek balloon postdilatation **(Figs. 14 and 15)**.

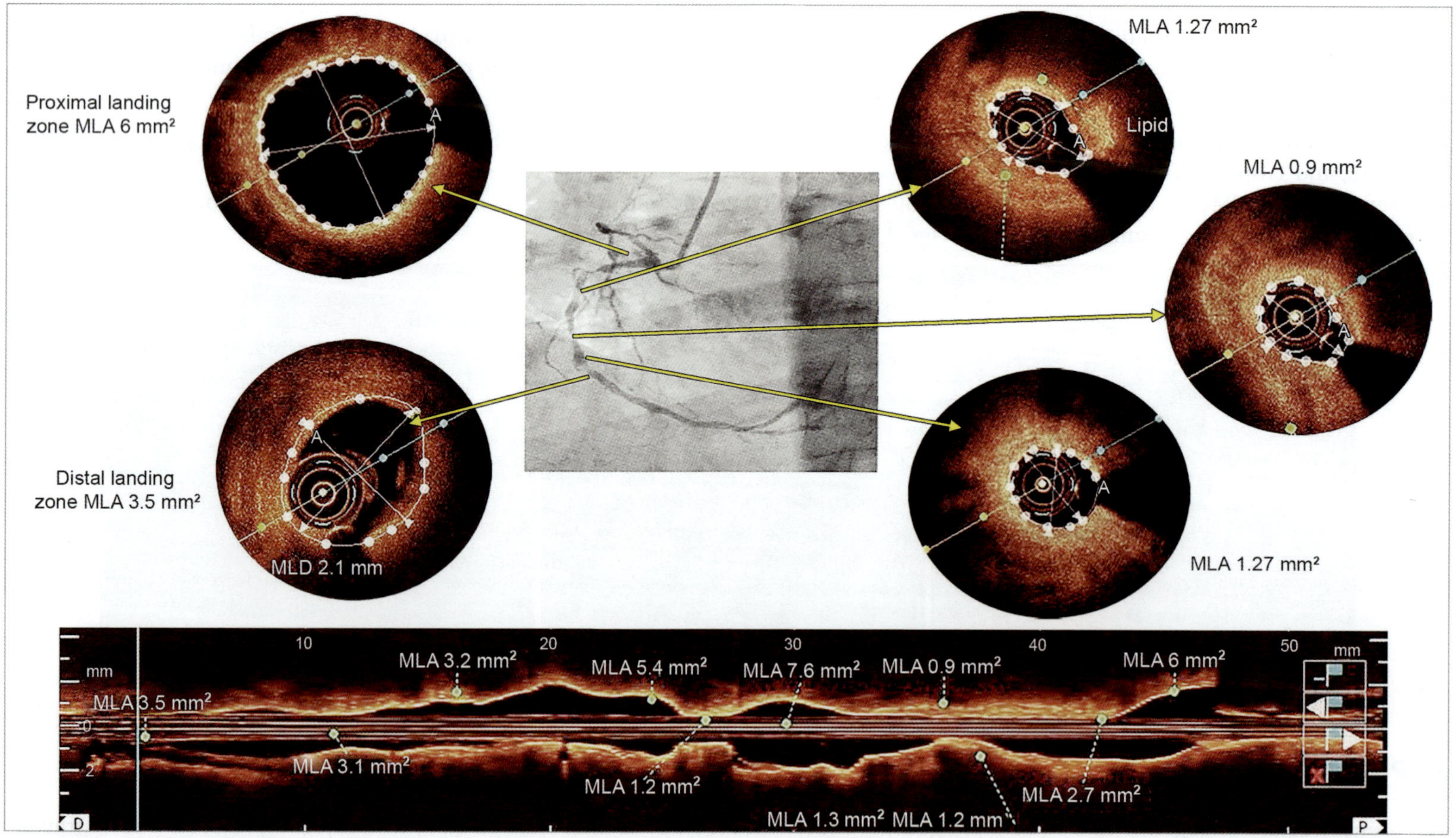

Fig. 12: Prestenting OCT assessment to select the device size. (MLA: minimal luminal area; MLD: minimal luminal diameter; OCT: optical coherence tomography)

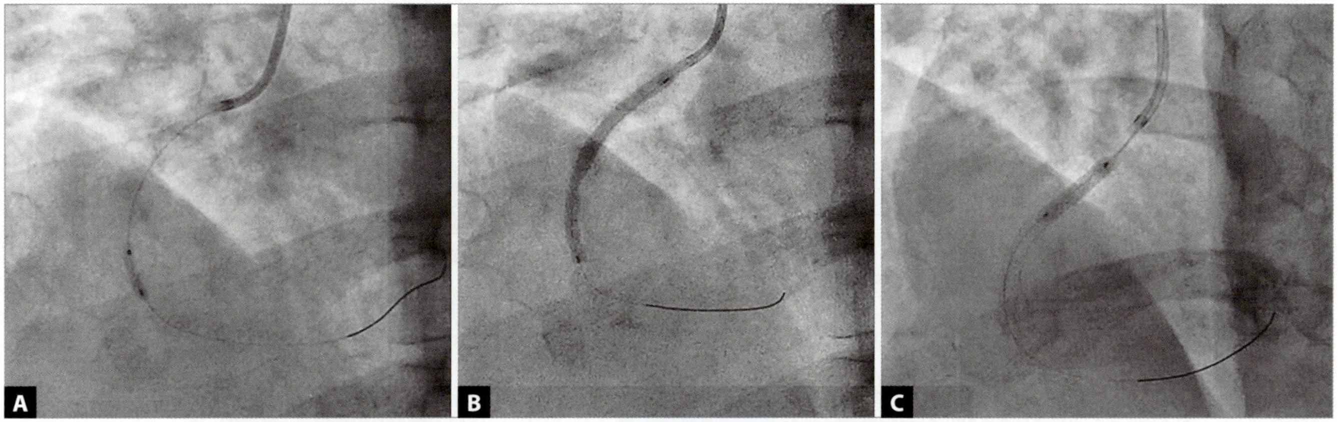

Figs. 13A to C: Predilatation, stenting, and postdilatation.

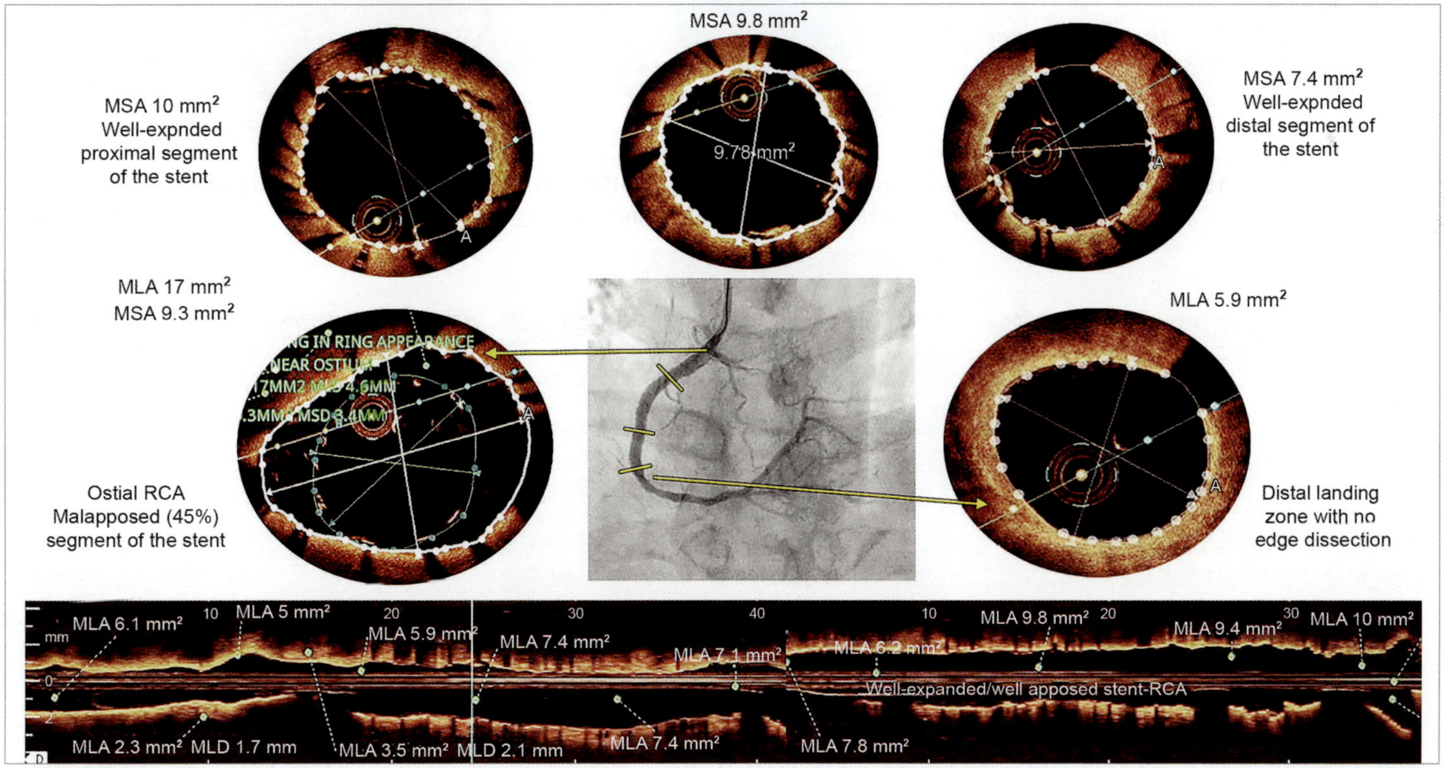

Fig. 14: Poststenting OCT assessment for any medial edge dissections at both ends, expansion, and apposition of stent struts. (MLA: minimal luminal area; MLD: minimal luminal diameter; MSA: minimal stent area; NC: noncompliant; OCT: optical coherence tomography; RCA: right coronary artery)

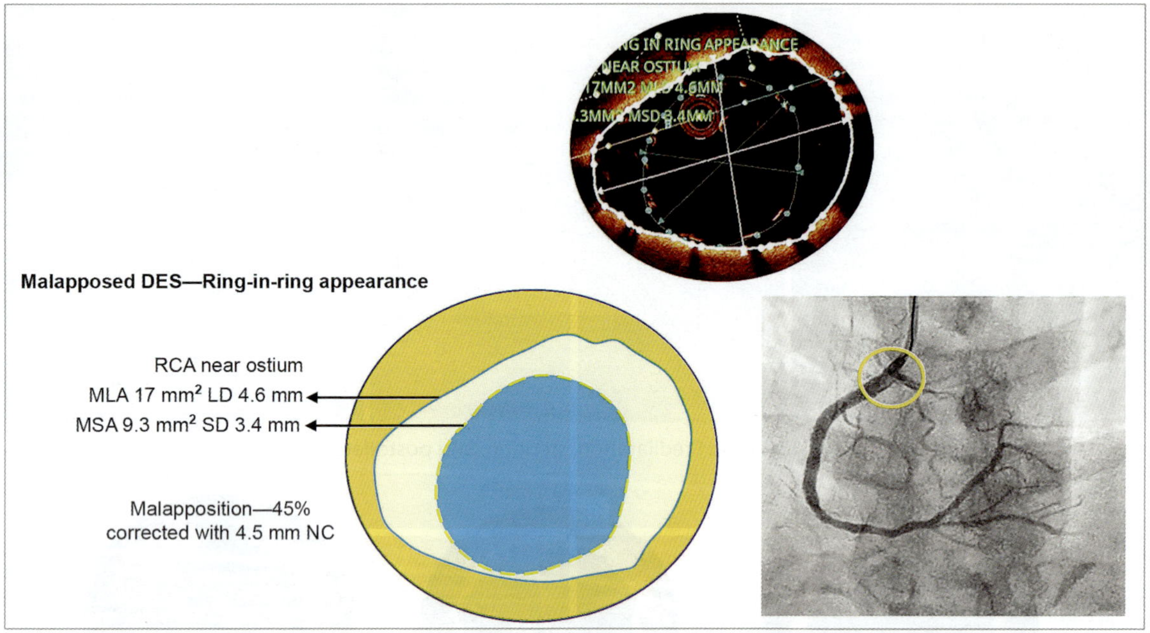

Fig. 15: Detection of malapposition in proximal RCA (ring in ring). (DES: drug-eluting stent; LD: left dominance; MLA: minimal luminal area; MSA: minimal stent area; RCA: right coronary artery)

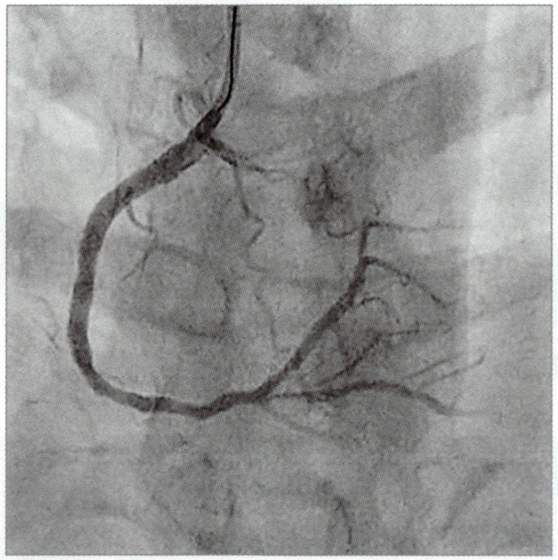

Fig. 16: Final result of right coronary artery (RCA).

Postprocedure angio view showed well-implanted stents with TIMI-III flow without any dissections **(Fig. 16)**. Patient was discharged on 3rd postprocedure day in a stable status.

CASE 3

OCT-guided PCI of LAD malapposition. (LAD: left anterior descending; OCT: optical coherence tomography; PCI: percutaneous coronary intervention)

CLINICAL HISTORY

A 61-year-old male presented with old anterior wall MI (AWMI) and chest pain associated with shortness of breath (SOB). ECG—ST elevation in anterolateral leads, 2D echo—RWMA in LAD territory, severe LV dysfunction, and EF 35%. Myocardial perfusion single-photon emission computed tomography (SPECT) revealed severe LV dysfunction with 50% viable myocardium in LAD territory. CAG-LMCA—normal, LAD—proximal-to-mid 80–90% lesion, LCX—normal, and RCA—normal **(Fig. 17)**. Referred for evaluation and further management of LAD total occlusion.

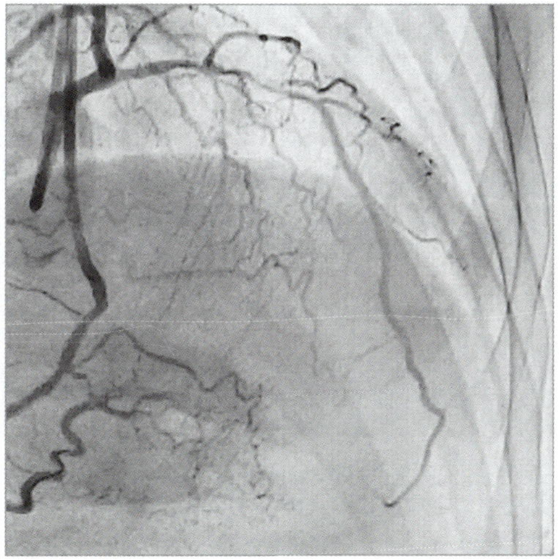

Fig. 17: Coronary angiogram.

PROCEDURE

Procedure performed through route—right femoral artery (RFA), using 6 Fr EBU 3.5 guiding catheter for antegrade approach, LAD lesion was crossed with 0.014″ Sion Blue wire, and RCA was engaged with right Amplatz through right radial route and wired with 0.014″ Runthrough wire for retrograde

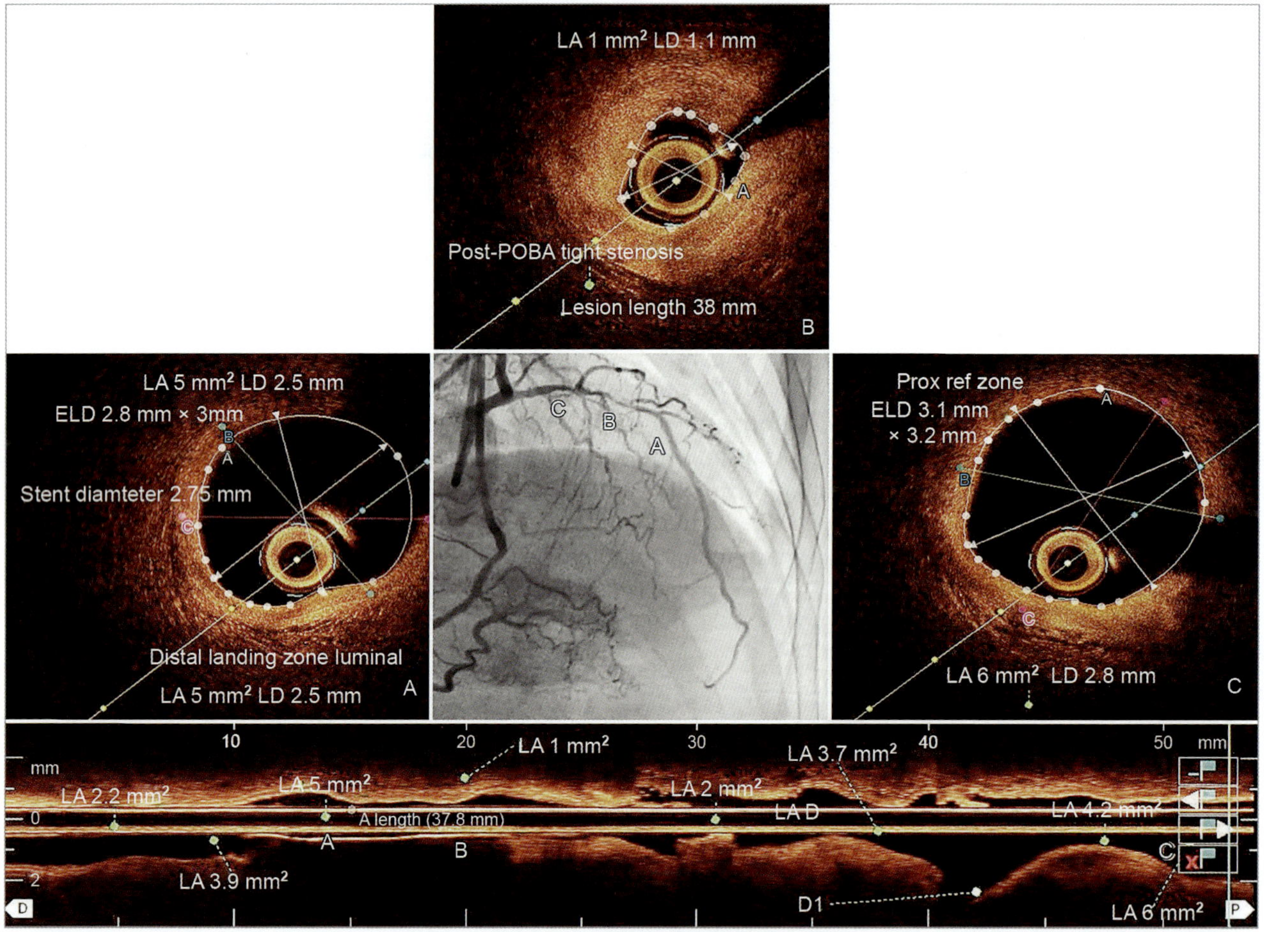

Fig. 18: Prestenting OCT assessment to select the device size. (ELD: external elastic luminal diameter; LA: luminal area; LAD: left anterior descending; LD: luminal diameter; OCT: optical coherence tomography; POBA: plain old balloon angioplasty)

injections. Simultaneous left and right coronary injections showed tight stenosis of proximal LAD with antegrade filling; LAD lesion was crossed with 0.014 Sion Blue wire, and predilated with 2.5 × 15 mm Tazuna balloon.

Pre-OCT of LAD showed distal landing zone MLA 5 mm^2, MLD 2.5 mm, external elastic luminal diameter (ELD) 2.8 × 3 mm, post-plain old balloon angioplasty (POBA) tight, thick fibrotic plaque with MLA 1 mm^2, MLD 1.1 mm, proximal landing zone MLA 6 mm^2, MLD 2.8 mm, ELD 3.1 × 3.2 mm, and total length of the lesion 37.8 mm **(Fig. 18)**.

Mid-LAD stenting done with 2.75 × 24 mm Ultimaster stent, proximal LAD overlapping stenting done with 3.0 × 28 mm Ultimaster stent, and proximal LAD postdilated with 4.0 × 08 mm Accuforce NC and 3.5 × 12 mm NC Trek balloons **(Figs. 19A to C)**.

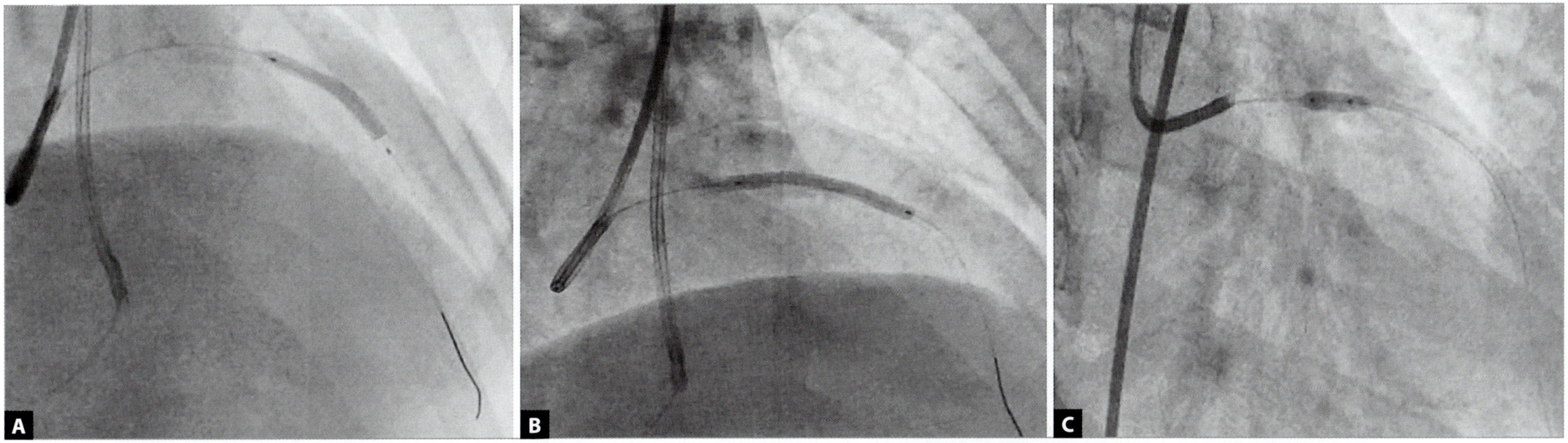

Figs. 19A to C: Predilatation, stenting, and postdilatation.

Post-OCT showed distal landing zone MLA 4.1 mm^2, MLD 2.3 mm, mid portion of the stent MLA 6 mm^2, MLD 2.8 mm, proximal portion of the stent MLA 7.4 mm^2, MLD 3.1 mm **(Figs. 20A and B)**, and malapposition of the stent in LMCA **(Fig. 21)**.

Postdilatation done with 4.0 × 08 mm Accuforce NC and 3.5 × 12 mm NC Trek balloons. Postprocedure angio showed well-implanted stents with TIMI-III flow without any dissection **(Fig. 22)**. Patient was discharged on 3rd postprocedure day in a stable status.

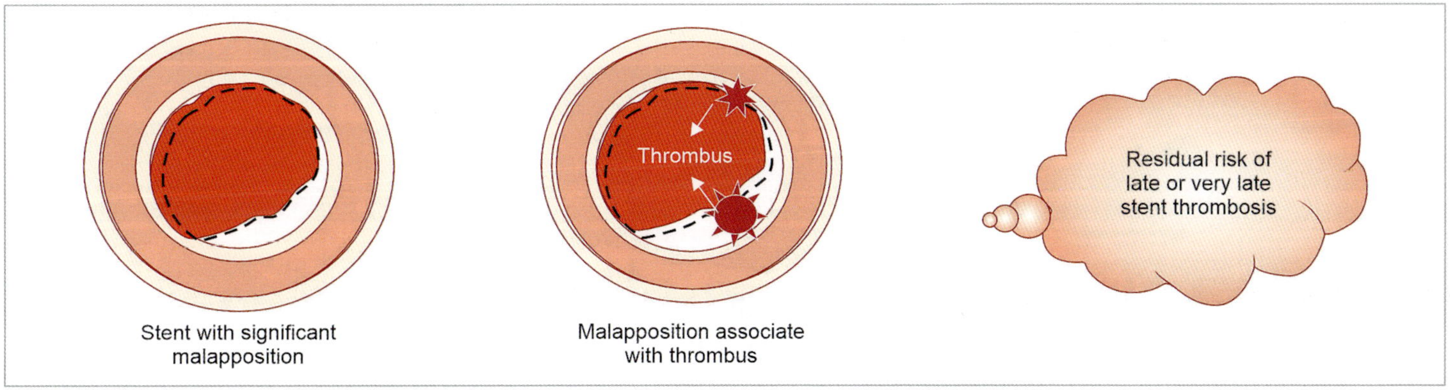

Fig. 20A

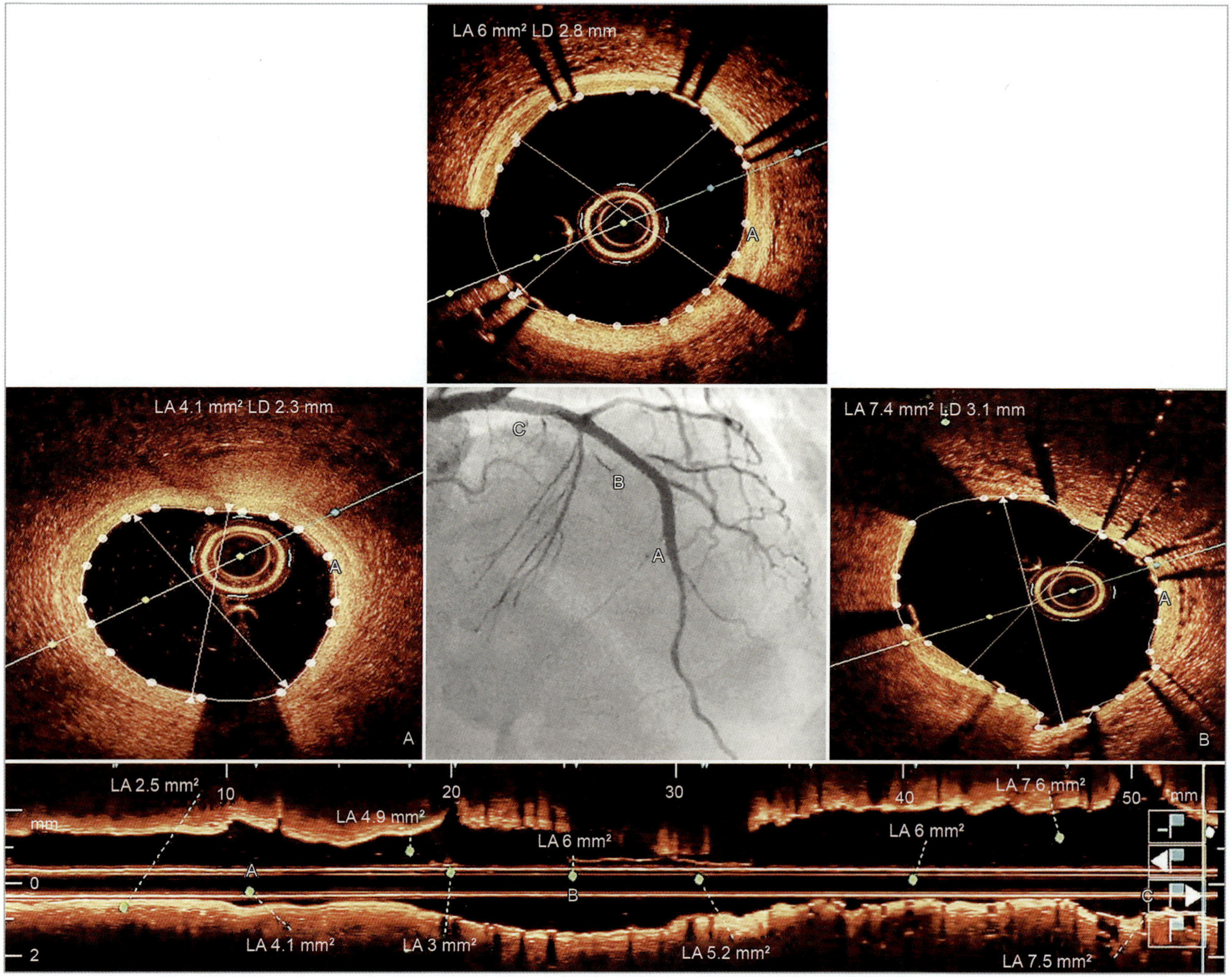

Fig. 20B

Figs. 20A and B: (A) Clinical of implication of significant malapposition; (B) Poststenting OCT assessment for any medial edge dissections at both ends, expansion, and apposition of stent struts. (LA: luminal area; LD: luminal diameter; OCT: optical coherence tomography)

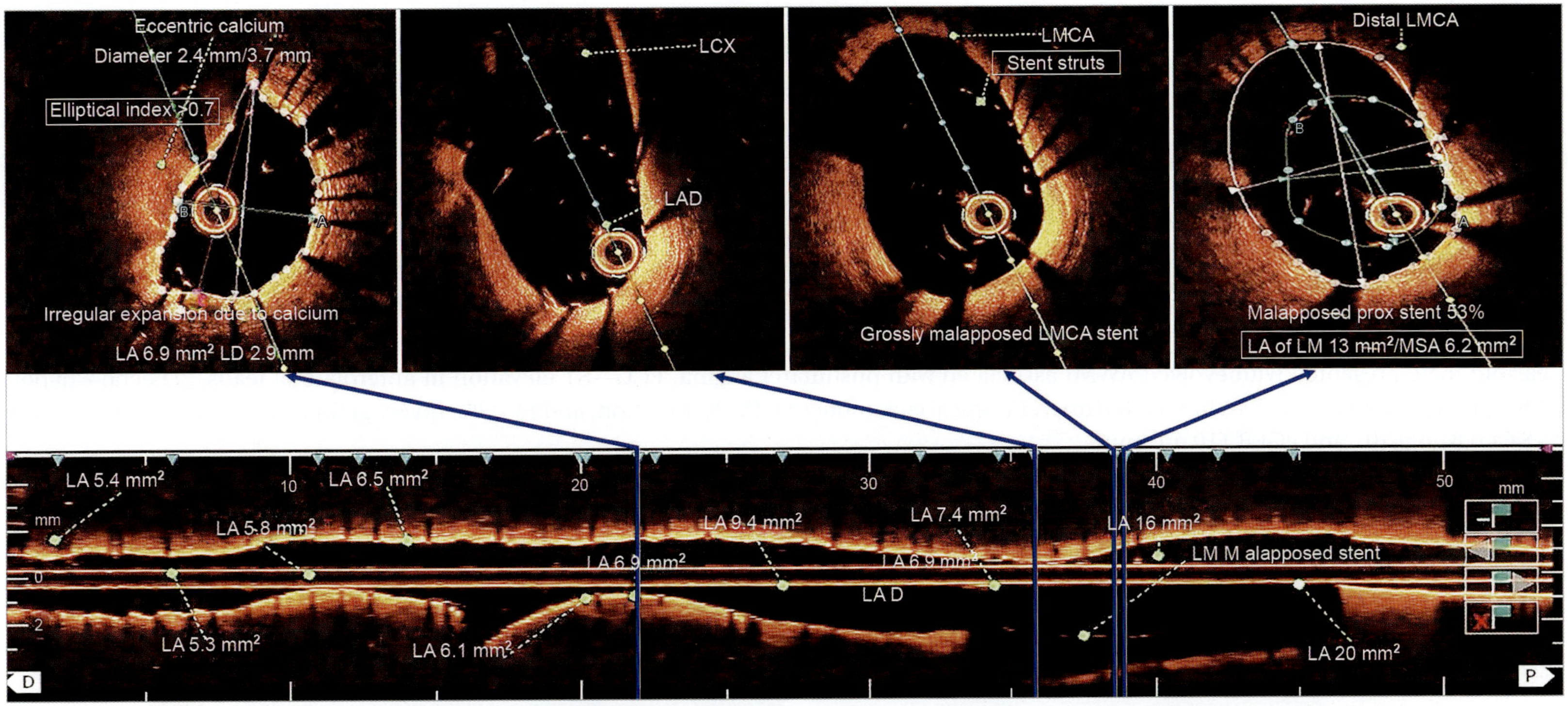

Fig. 21: Detection of malapposition and irregular expansion. (LA: luminal area; LAD: left anterior descending; LCX: left circumflex; LD: luminal diameter; LM: left main; LMCA: left main coronary artery; MSA: minimal stent area)

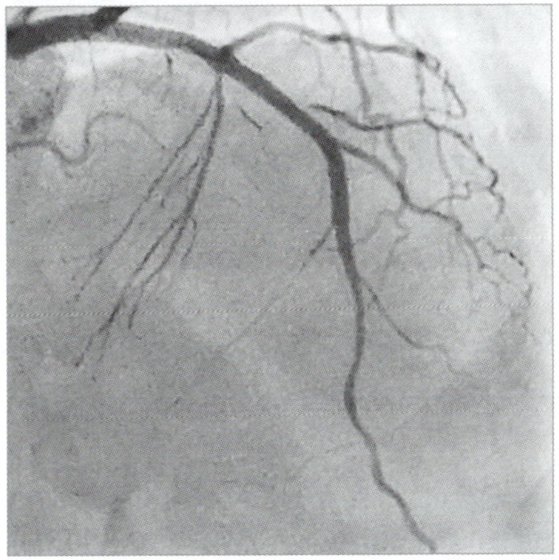

Fig. 22: Final result.

CASE 4

PCI of LAD—malapposition. (LAD: left anterior descending; PCI: percutaneous coronary intervention)

CLINICAL HISTORY

A 37-year-old male presented with evolved AWMI associated with postinfarct angina. ECG—ST elevation in anterolateral leads, 2D echo—hypokinetic distal IVS, apex anterior wall, RWMA in LAD territory, LV apical clot, moderate LV dysfunction, and EF 43%. Investigations: RBS 119 mg/dL, blood urea 43 mg/dL, S Cr 0.87 mg/dL, and eGFR 110 mL/min.

Coronary angiography-LMCA—normal, LAD—proximal total occlusion, distal vessel filling retrogradely from RCA, LCX—proximal mild disease, and RCA—normal **(Figs. 23A and B)**.

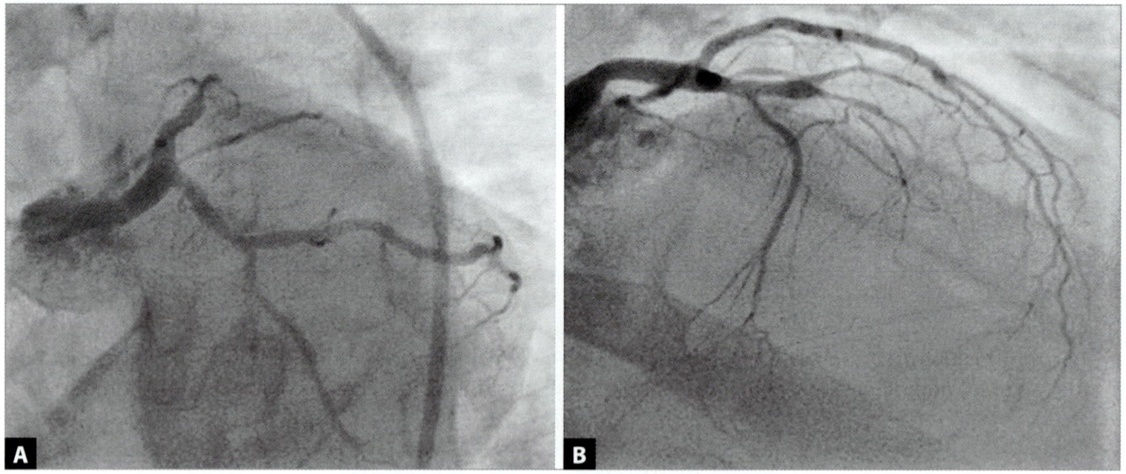

Figs. 23A and B: Coronary angiogram.

PROCEDURE

Procedure performed through route—RFA, 6 Fr XB 3.5 guiding catheter, totally occluded LAD lesion was crossed with 0.014" Sion Blue wire, and D1 was wired with Powerturn wire. Predilated with 1.5 × 10 mm and 2.0 × 10 mm Tazuna balloons, mid-LAD stented with 2.5 × 35 mm Orsiro stent and postdilated with 3.0 × 12 mm NC Trek balloon **(Figs. 24A to C)**.

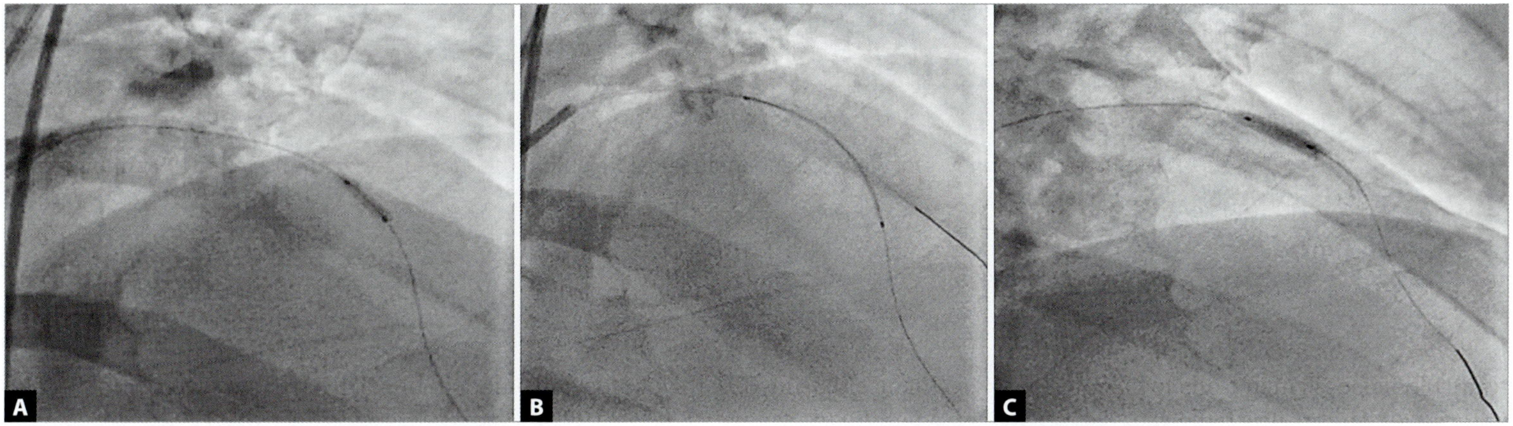

Figs. 24A to C: Predilatation, stenting, and postdilatation.

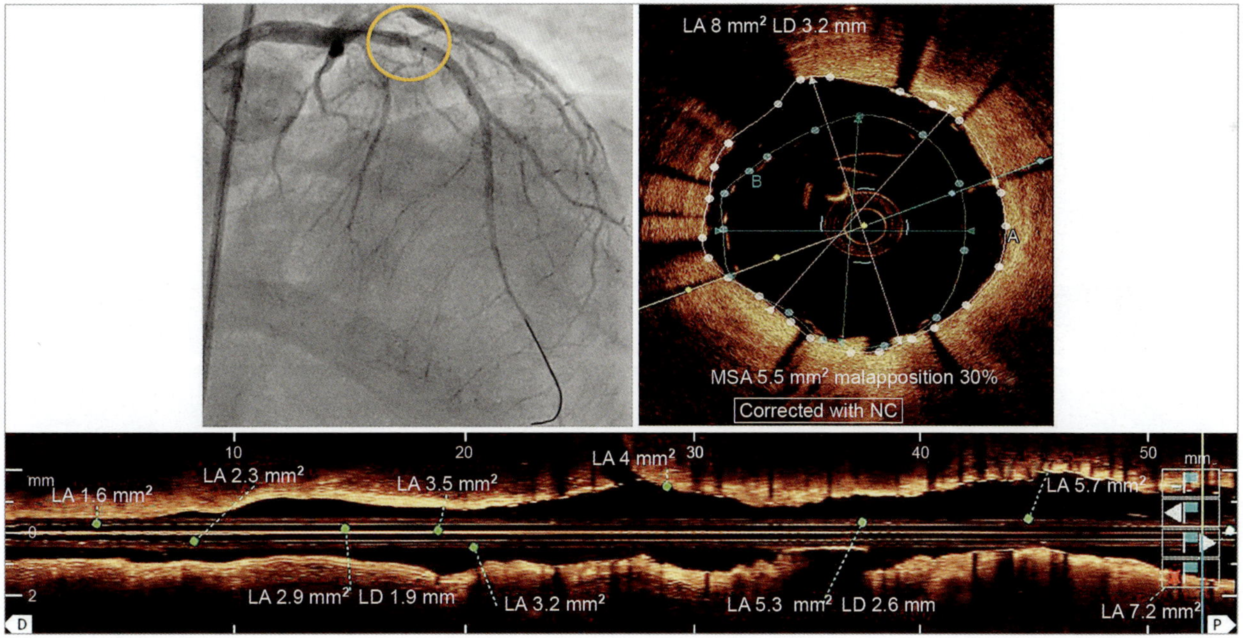

Fig. 25: Detection of stent malapposition at proximal portion. (LA: luminal area; LD: luminal diameter; MSA: minimal stent area; NC: noncompliant)

Post-OCT analysis: Proximal portion of the stent malapposition (MSA 5.5 mm^2) with 30% **(Fig. 25)**, distal landing zone MLA 4.2 mm^2, MLD 2.3 mm, mid portion of the stent MLA 5.2 mm^2, MLD 2.6 mm, proximal landing zone MLA 6.9 mm^2, MLD 3 mm **(Fig. 26)**, and TCFA with calcific lesion at ostium of LAD with MLA 4.7 mm^2 and MLD 2.5 mm **(Fig. 27)**.

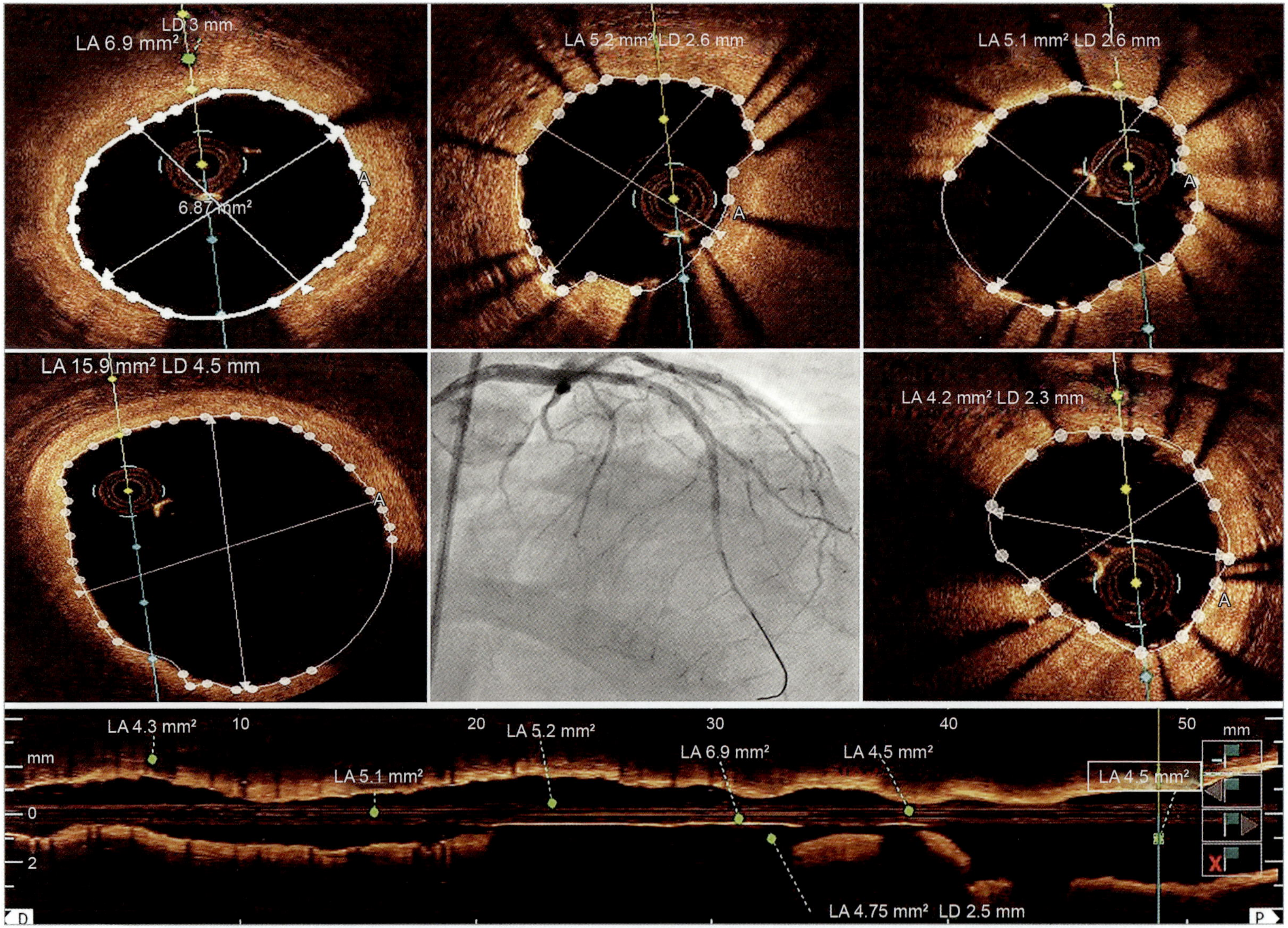

Fig. 26: Poststenting OCT analysis. (LA: luminal area; LD: luminal diameter; LMCA: left main coronary artery; OCT: optical coherence tomography)

Proximal segment postdilatation done with 3.5 × 12 mm NC Apollo balloon. Postprocedure angio view showed well-implanted stents with TIMI-III flow without any dissection **(Figs. 28A and B)**. Patient was discharged on 3rd postprocedure day in a stable status.

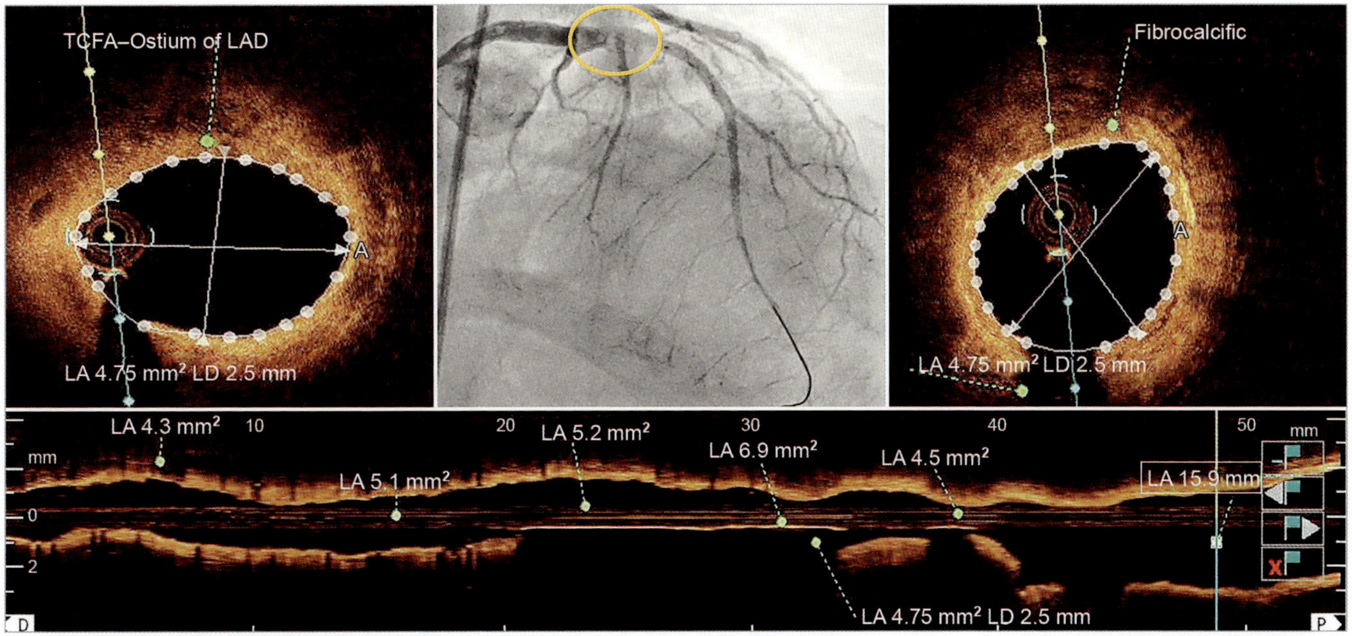

Fig. 27: Plaque burden at ostium LAD. (LA: luminal area; LAD: left anterior descending; LD: luminal diameter; TCFA: thin-cap fibroatheroma)

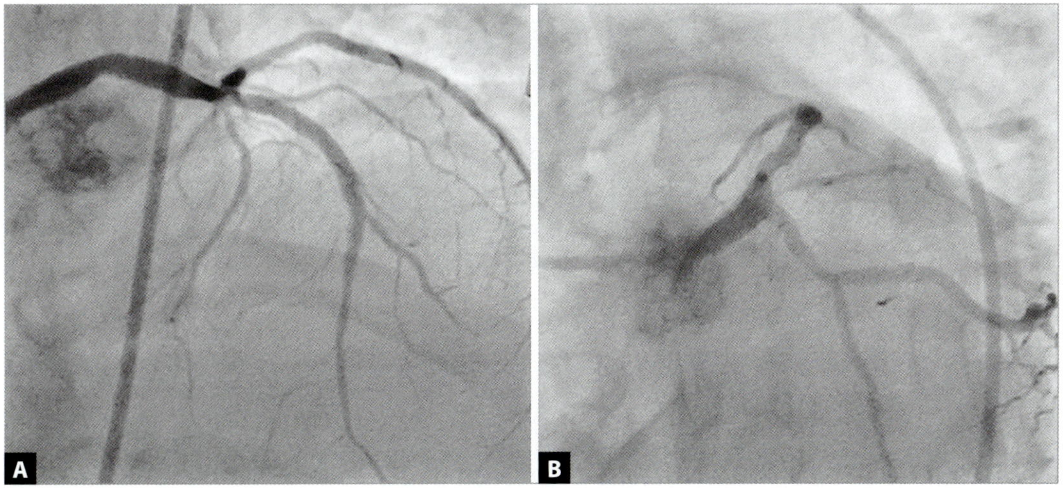

Figs. 28A and B: Final result.

CASE 5

Usefulness of OCT in assessment of LSD and malapposition in distal LMCA and ostial stenting of LAD. (LAD: left anterior descending; LMCA: left main coronary artery; LSD: longitudinal stent deformation; OCT: optical coherence tomography)

CLINICAL HISTORY

A 58-year-old male, a known hypertensive and diabetic, presented with acute coronary syndrome (ACS)-non-STEMI (NSTEMI) of anterior wall and chest heaviness associated with SOB and sweating. History of PCI of D1 in 2016. ECG—ST depressions in anterior leads. 2D echo—good LV function with EF 64%. Investigations: Hemoglobin (Hb) 11.6 g/dL, RBS 125 mg/dL, S Cr 1.37 mg/dL with eGFR 56 mL/min (post S Cr 1.47 mg/dL with eGFR 52 mL/min).

Coronary angiogram revealed double vessel disease with ostioproximal LAD with 90% critical tubular stenosis, in-stent restenosis (ISR) of D1 stent with distal TIMI I flow, and ostioproximal Ramus 80% disease **(Figs. 29A to C)**.

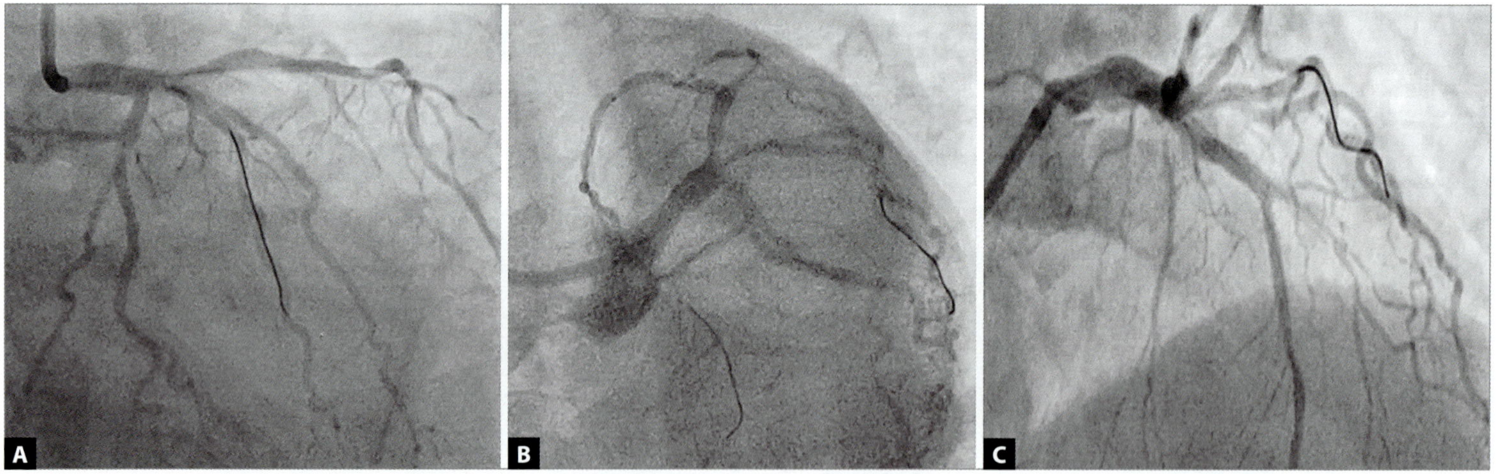

Figs. 29A to C: Coronary angiogram.

PROCEDURE

Procedure was performed through RRA, 7 Fr EBU 3.5 guiding catheter; LAD lesion was crossed with 0.014″ Turntrac wire, and Ramus was crossed with 0.014″ Sion Blue wire and predilated with 2.0 × 10 mm, 2.5 × 15 mm Tazuna balloon.

Pre-OCT showed long-segment fibrous plaque extending from proximal to mid-LAD, ostial LAD with MLA 3.6 mm^2 and MLD 2.1 mm **(Figs. 30A to C)**.

Proximal LAD stented with 2.75 × 28 mm Xience Xpedition stent and mid-LAD was stented with 2.25 × 23 mm Xience Xpedition stent. Postdilated with 3.5 × 15 mm NC Trek balloon and Ramus with 2.0 × 10 mm Tazuna balloon.

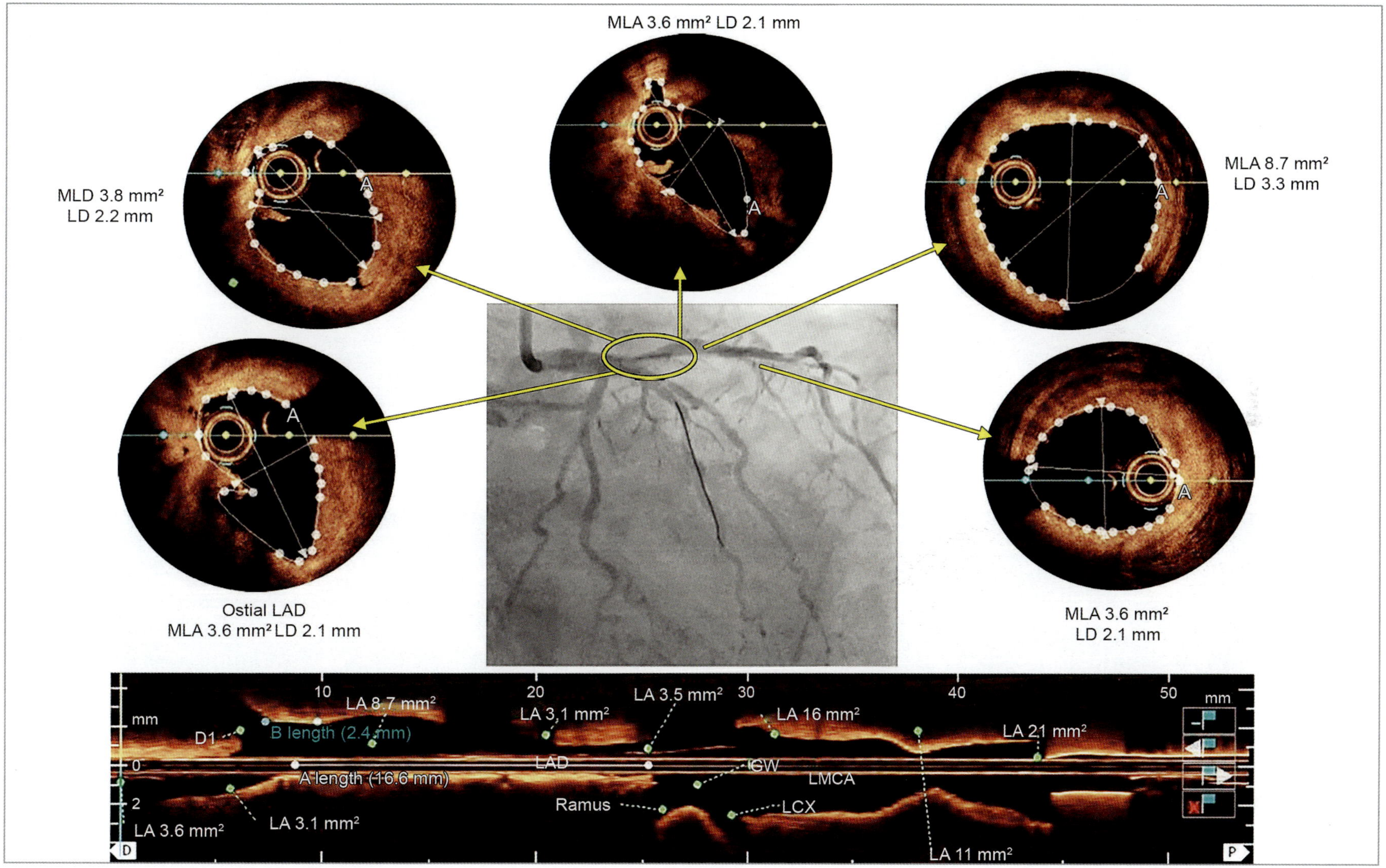

Fig. 30A

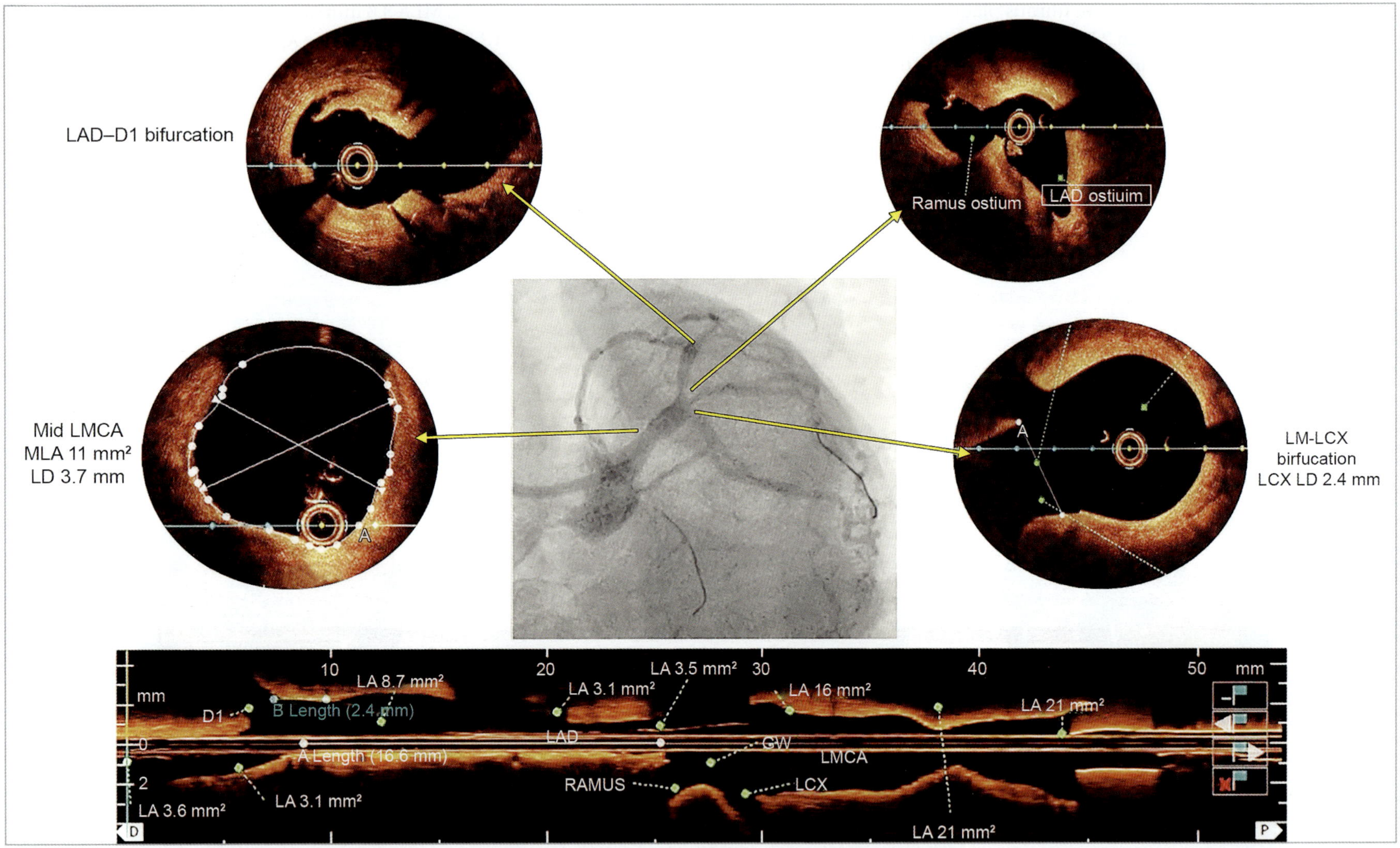

Fig. 30B

Appearance is deceptive—Use IVI when you have doubt or no correlation between angio and clinical findings.

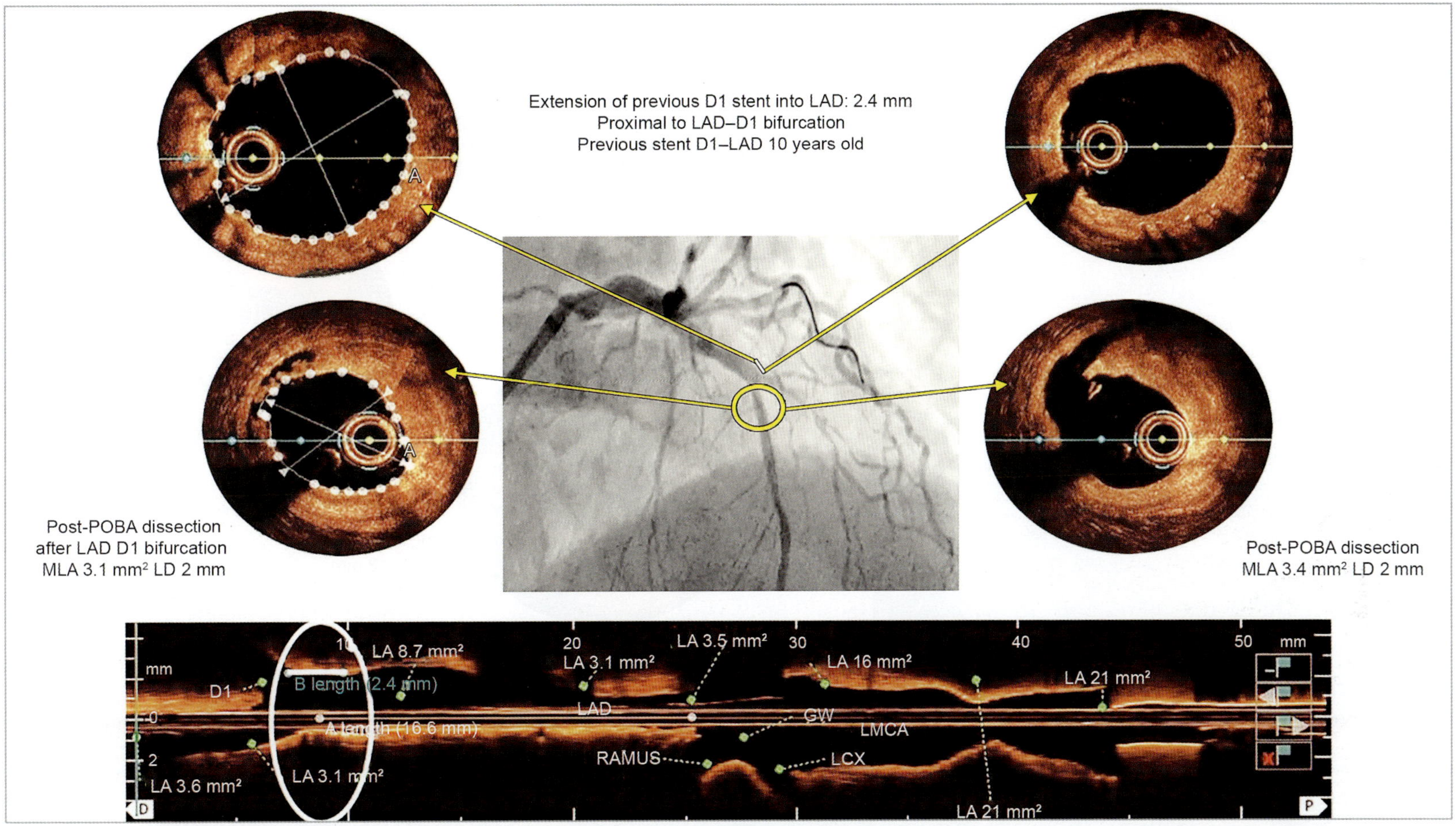

Fig. 30C

Figs. 30A to C: (A) Presenting OCT assessment to select the device size; (B) LM and non-LM bifurcation; and (C) Detection of previous stent in D1 and post-POBA dissection after LAD-D1 bifurcation. (LAD: left anterior descending; LCX: left circumflex; LD: luminal diameter; LM: left main; LMCA: left main coronary artery; MLA: minimal luminal area; OCT: optical coherence tomography; POBA: plain old balloon angioplasty)

Post-OCT showed malapposition of proximal stent of LAD in distal LMCA. During poststenting OCT run, OCT showed passage of OCT catheter through side of the stent strut in the distal LM again entered into true lumen of the stent from the ostium of LAD **(Figs. 31A to D)**. In view of distorted malapposed proximal portion of the stent in distal LMCA, serial dilatations of strut opening (OCT catheter entered through side of the stent strut instead of entering through the center of the stent) were done with 3.0 × 15 mm, 3.5 × 12 mm, and 4.0 × 8 mm NC Trek balloons. Final OCT showed well-expanded stent with longitudinal stent deformation of proximal edge of the stent. Postprocedure angio view showed well-implanted stents with TIMI-III flow without any dissection. Patient was discharged on 3rd postprocedure day in a stable status.

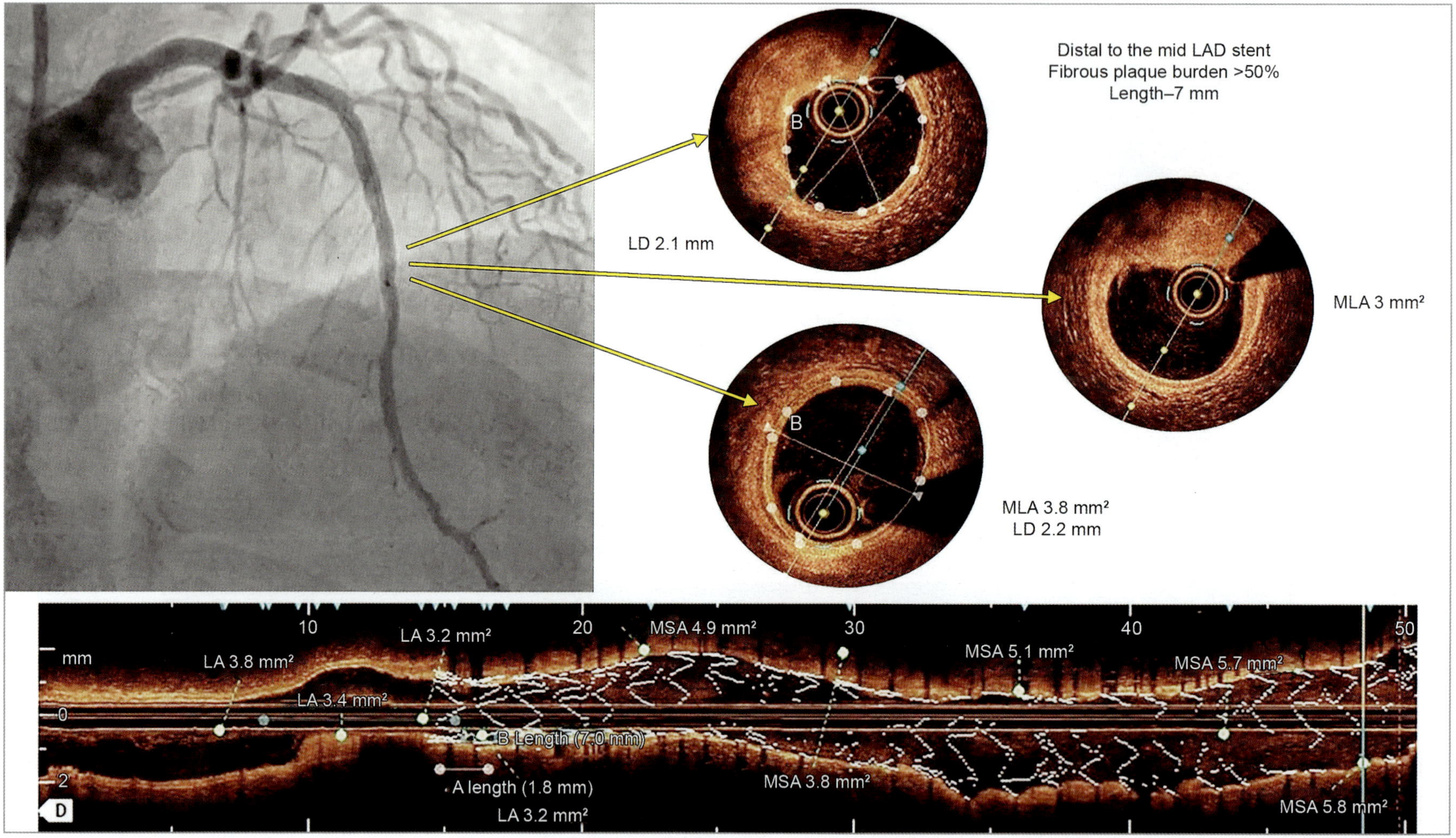

Fig. 31A

Authors/Subjects	*Study/Registry*	*Follow-up (months)*	*Malapposition*	*No Malapposition*
Lm et al./351		24	LPSM vs. LASM: 2.2%, 3.2%, 0% MACE	3.2% MACE
Soeda et al./786	MGH OCT registry	12	1.7% DoCE	2.9% DoCE
Prati et al./832	CLI-OPCI II	12	1.15 % MACE	

Lee SY, Mintz GS, Kim JS, Kim BK, Jang Y, Hong MK. Long-term clinical outcomes of drug-eluting stent malapposition. Korean Circulation Journal. 2020;50(10):880.

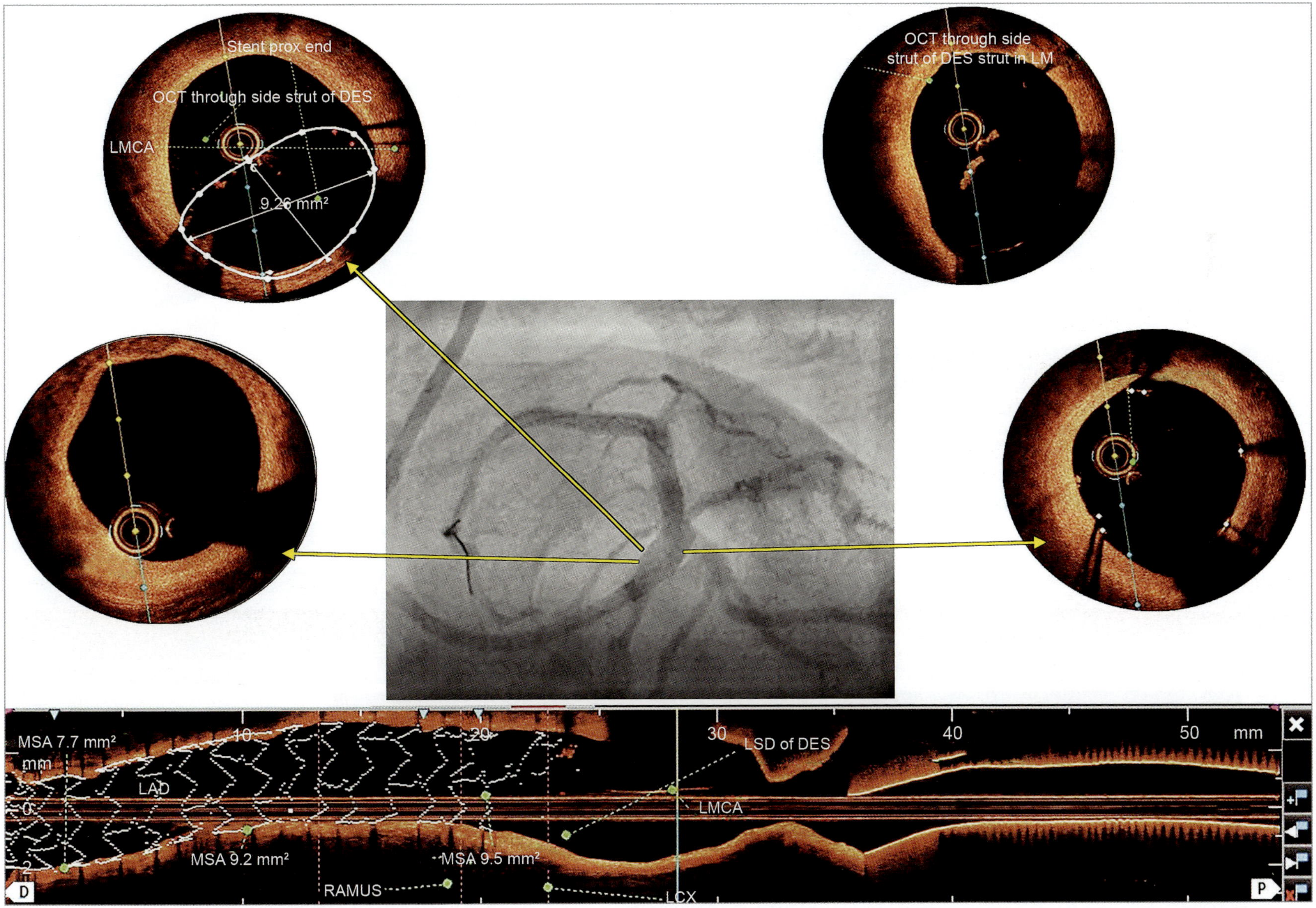

Fig. 31B

Sometimes Angio images may not show under-expansion and malapposition—Use stent boost.

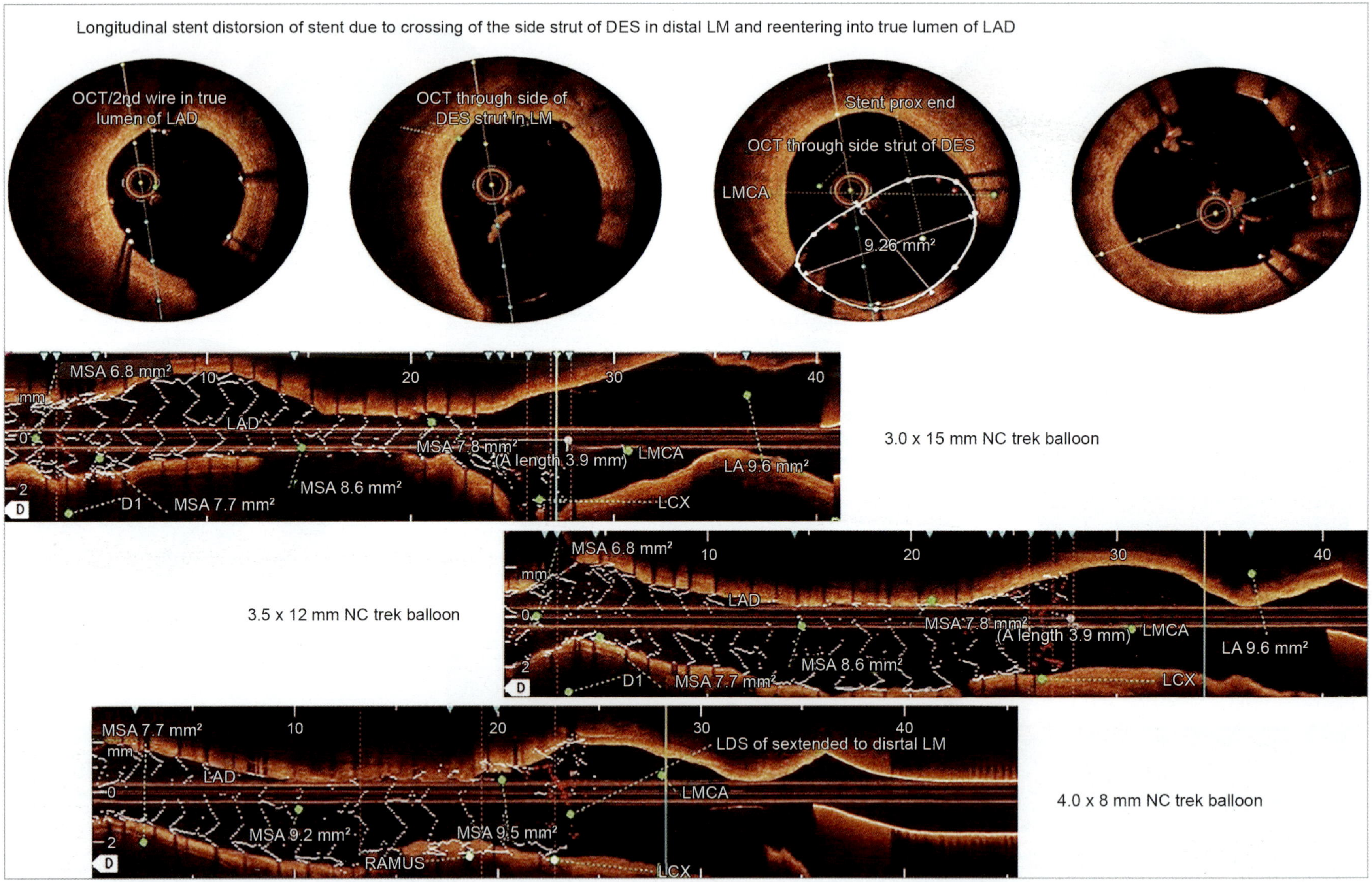

Fig. 31C

Is there any grating feeling or difficulty in placing the balloon while crossing the stent? Suspect under-expansion/LSD.

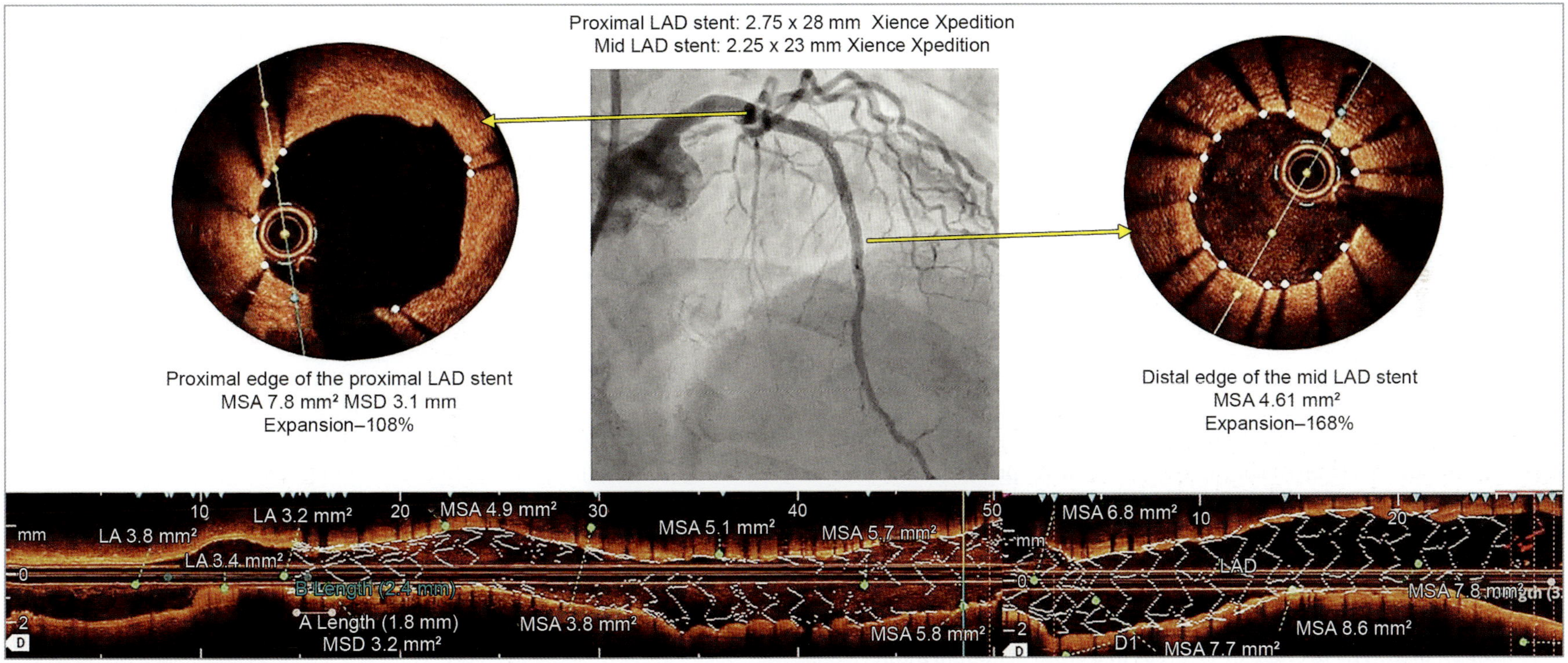

Fig. 31D

Figs. 31A to D: (A) Distal edge plaque burden assessment; (B) LSD of proximal end of the stent; (C) Longitudinal stent deformation of proximal edge of the stent assessment and correction; and (D) Poststenting OCT assessment for any medial edge dissections at both ends, expansion, and apposition of stent struts. (DES: drug-eluting stent; LA: luminal area; LAD: left anterior descending; LCX: left circumflex; LD: luminal diameter; LM: left main; LMCA: left main coronary artery; MLA: minimal luminal area; MSA: minimal stent area; NC: noncompliant; OCT: optical coherence tomography)

About half of the stent deformation was located in the LMCA, resulting in multiple overlapping strut layers within a single stent, often accompanied by stent shortening. In EXCEL, acute LMCA stent deformation was observed in 33 patients (6.6%) and was most commonly located at the LMCA ostium [27/33 (81.8%)]. Any stent can undergo longitudinal stent deformation, either lengthening or shortening; LM stent particularly at ostial site more often prone for longitudinal stent deformation (LSD) due to guide catheter manipulations while engaging, deep intubation of guide catheter hitting the proximal edge of the stent while pulling improperly deflated with large NC balloon, jailed wires, and imaging catheters. LSD at ostial site of LM is associated with increased MACE rate due to its crucial position, which may result in ISR and stent thrombosis of LM compromising blood supply to major myocardial territory. LSD, more often underdiagnosed, can be diagnosed with stent boost or IVI and it needs to be corrected with repeat proximal optimization technique (POT), and if necessary additional stenting.

CHAPTER 4

Tissue Prolapse

INTRODUCTION

Tissue prolapse (TP) is an intraluminal protrusion of tissue toward the lumen between the stent struts. TP is the early predictor of stent thrombosis which is related to adverse short-term prognosis following percutaneous coronary intervention (PCI). Optical coherence tomography (OCT) allows superior visualization of TP compared to intravascular ultrasound (IVUS). The majority of patients who underwent drug-eluting stent (DES) implantation showed TP on OCT, but only half among them showed TP on IVUS. The incidence of TP was lower on IVUS as compared with OCT. This might be due to a higher axial resolution of OCT (up to 10 μm) as compared with IVUS (100–150 μm). TP on OCT 2.5–4 times higher as compared with IVUS.[1]

- *Total TP area:* The sum of TP areas in a cross-sectional image
- *Maximal TP area:* The largest TP area in a cross-sectional frame
- *Mean TP area:* The average of TP areas in a cross-sectional frame
- *TP depth:* The axial diameter between the stent strut and the apex of TP
- *Maximal TP depth:* The longest axial diameter between the stent strut and the apex of TP
- *TP burden:* The percentage of TP area in a stent area
- *Maximal TP burden:* The largest TP burden in a frame
- *TP detection rate:* The percentage of frames with TP within whole frames in a stent.

Corresponding images of OCT and IVUS are shown in **Figures 1A and B**.

Parameters of OCT measurement in a frame are shown in **Figures 2A and B**. Total TP area was defined as the sum of TP area of each frame. Maximal TP area was defined as the largest TP area in a frame (A area among of A–G area). Mean TP area was defined as the average of TP area in a frame (total TP area/number of TP site in a frame). TP depth was defined as the axial diameter between stent strut and apex of TP (a–i distance). Maximal TP depth was defined as the longest axial diameter between stent strut and apex of TP **(Figs. 2A and B)**.

CLASSIFICATION OF TISSUE PROLAPSE

Severity of TP burden is divided into three grades:

1. *Grade I:* TP burden <10%
2. *Grade II:* TP burden >10% and <20%
3. *Grade III:* TP burden >20%

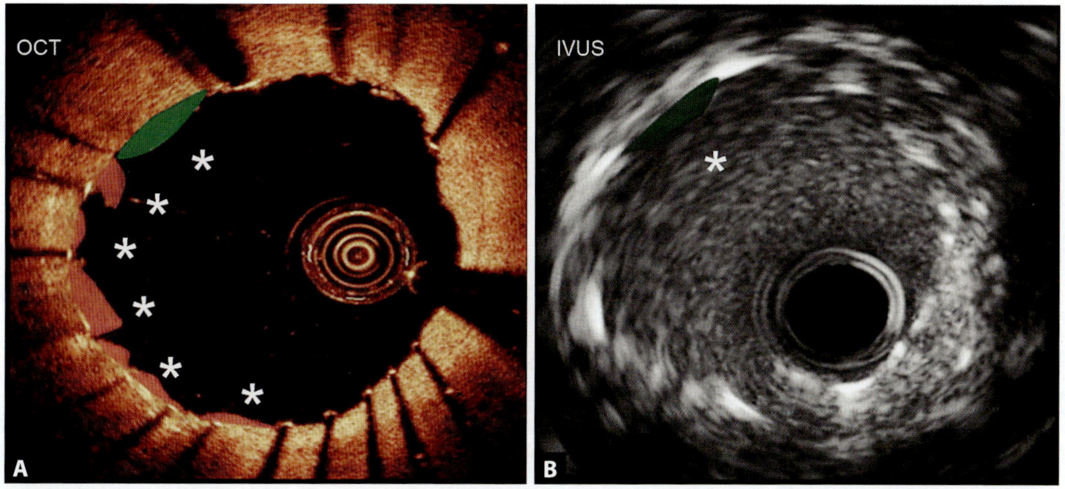

Figs. 1A and B: Many TP (asterisk) were observed by OCT, while only one could be confirmed by IVUS. The green-colored TP was presented both by OCT and IVUS and the pink-colored TP were presented by OCT but not by IVUS. Only a few TP could be seen by IVUS, even though it was observed by OCT. (IVUS: intravascular ultrasound; OCT: optical coherence tomography; TP: tissue prolapse)

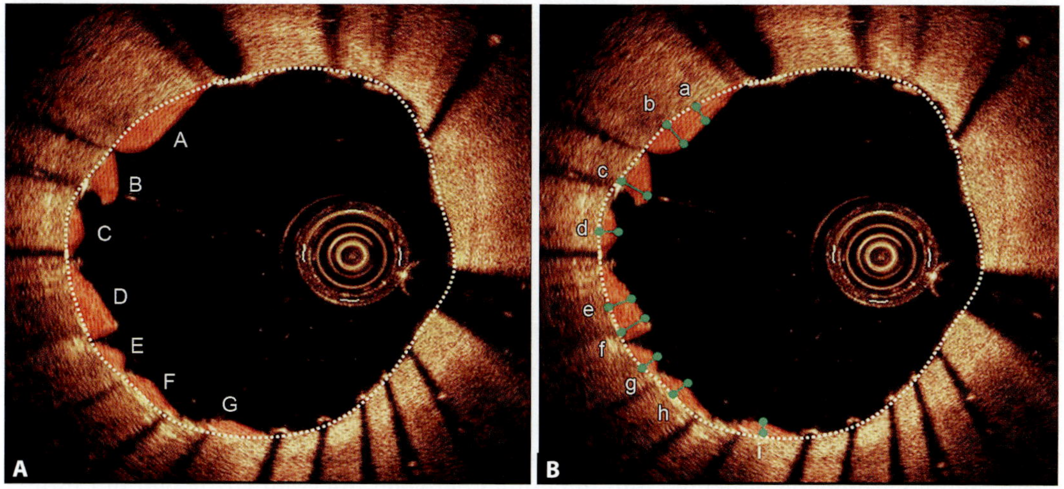

Figs. 2A and B: Parameters of optical coherence tomography (OCT) measurement such as total tissue prolapse and maximal tissue prolapse in a frame.

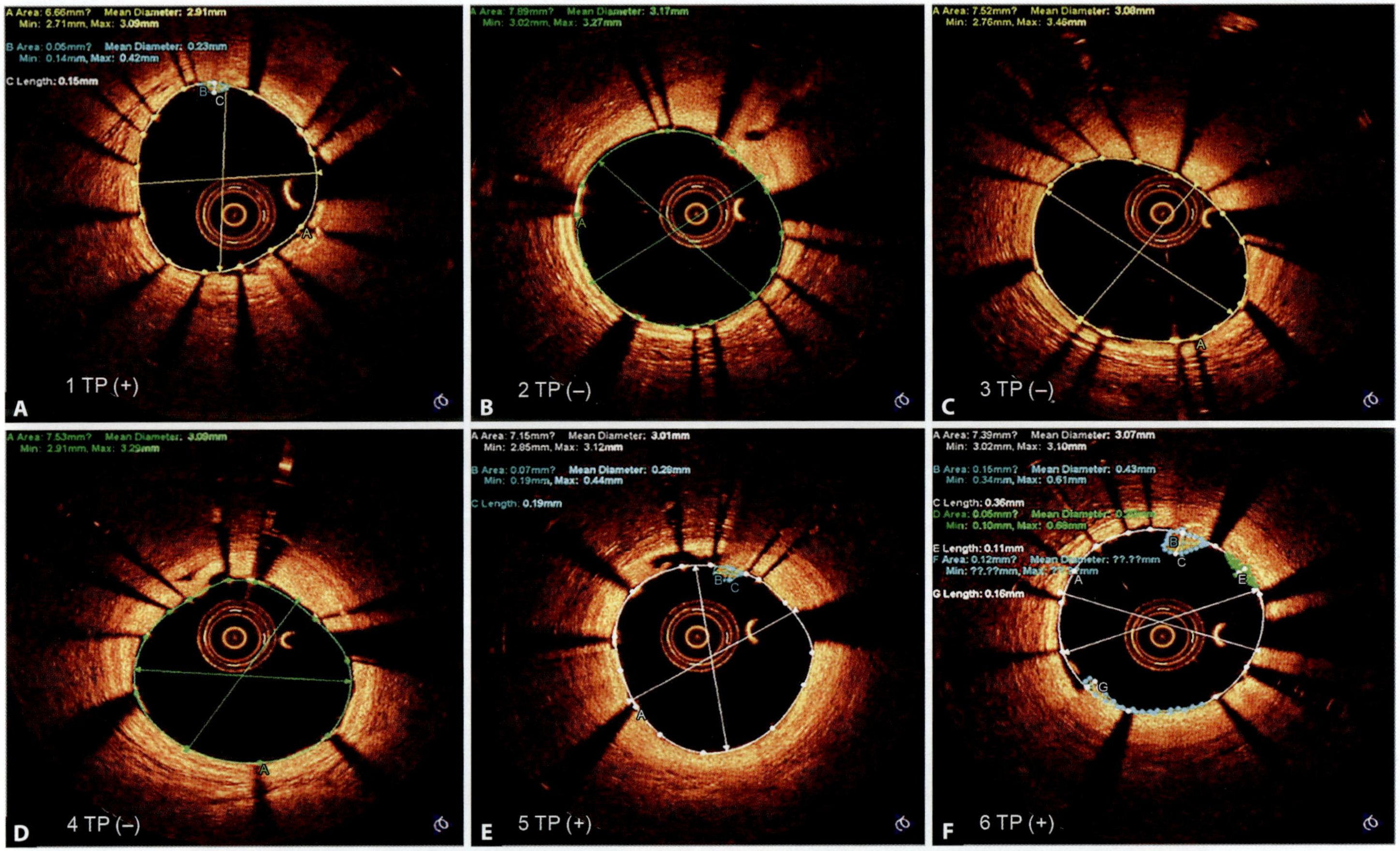

Figs. 3A to F: Tissue prolapse burden measurement in a stent by optical coherence tomography (OCT).

Parameters of OCT measurement in a stent are shown in **Figures 3A to F**. TP burden was defined as the percentage of TP in stent area (total TP area/ stent area 9 100). Maximal TP burden was defined as the largest TP burden in a frame. TP detection rate in a stent was defined as the percentage of frames with TP in a stent.

Soeda et al. categorized in-stent tissue protrusions into three groups claiming to estimate different severities of vessel injury.

- *Smooth protrusion:* They were defined as bowing of plaque into the lumen between the stent struts without intimal disruption and represented minimal vessel injury **(Fig. 4)**.

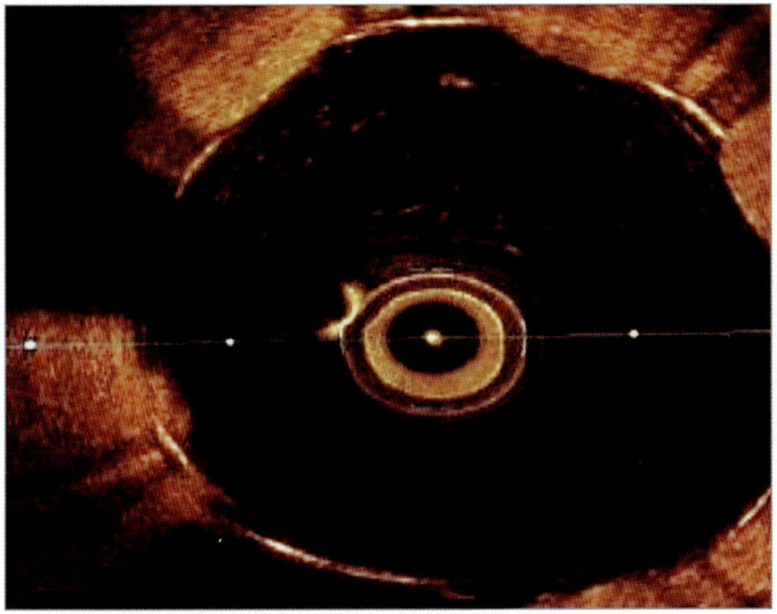

Fig. 4: Smooth protrusion.

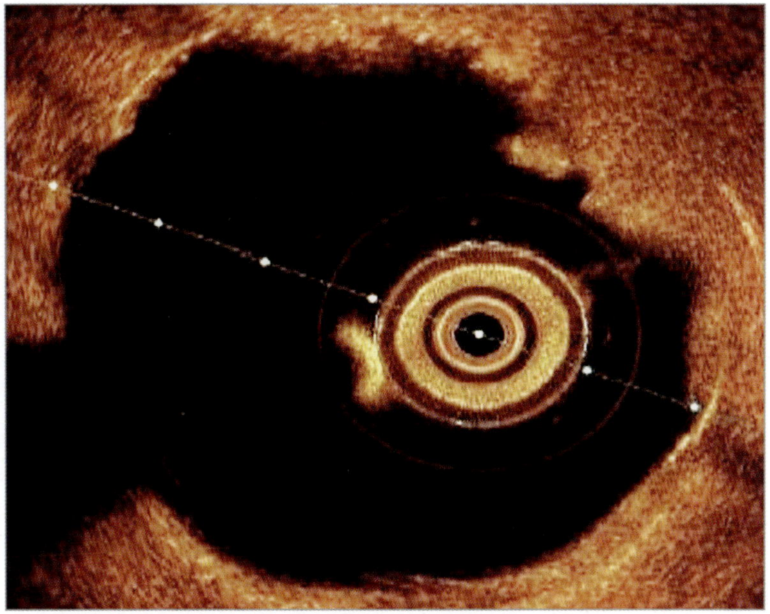

Fig. 5: Irregular protrusions.

- *Disrupted fibrous tissue protrusions:* They (disruption of the underlying fibrous tissue protruding between the struts) represent mild vessel injury
- *Irregular protrusions:* They (protrusion of material with an irregular surface between the struts) indicate moderate-to-severe vessel injury with a high likelihood of medial disruption and lipid core penetration **(Fig. 5)**.
- Bigger the better-Ideal to get MSA of >90% ref area.
- Otherwise aim for achieving MSA of >80% to 90% of Ref area in small vessels or 4.5 mm^2 (OCT)/5.5 mm^2 (IVUS) in large vessels.

Tisue prolapse assessed by planimetry is shown in **Figure 6**.

Incidence of smooth protrusion, disrupted fibrous tissue protrusion, irregular protrusion, and thrombus among stable angina, unstable angina, and acute myocardial infarction (AMI) patients is shown in **Figures 7A to D**.

Patients presenting with AMI had a higher incidence of irregular protrusions (67% vs. 46.7%). Irregular protrusions were identified as independent predictors of device-oriented clinical endpoints (cardiac death, target vessel-related myocardial infarction (MI), target lesion revascularization, and stent thrombosis). Evidence exists that TP in the context of acute coronary syndrome (ACS) is more likely to have consequences than in more stable (non-ACS) clinical setting as suggested by the CLI-OPCI and HORIZONS-AMI substudies.

Presence of positive remodeling, ruptured plaques, thrombus, and longer stent lengths increase the incidence of TP. Minor TP is a common finding with intravascular imaging (IVI) and usually resolves without any consequences. However, major TP may be associated with adverse outcomes. A pathological study linked TP with early-stent thrombosis and an OCT study correlated with extent of TP with periprocedural myonecrosis. In another study, patients with early ST exhibited larger TP volume with significant lumen narrowing (<4 mm^2). In summary, the clinical significance of TP is related to ACS presentation, the amount of prolapse, the extent of lumen compromise, and the severity of vessel wall injury.[2]

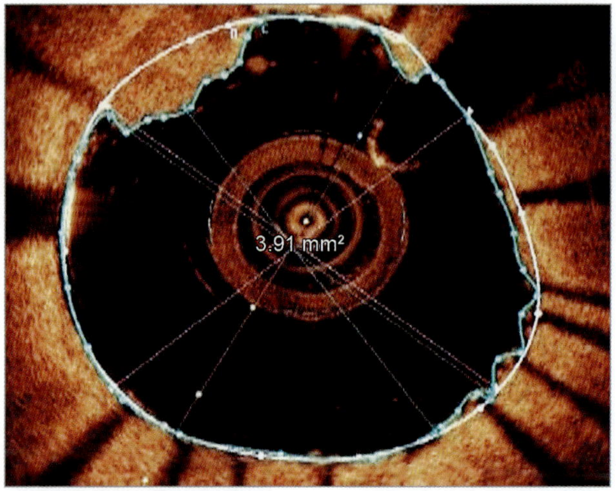

Fig. 6: Tissue planimetry (TP) assessed by planimetry.

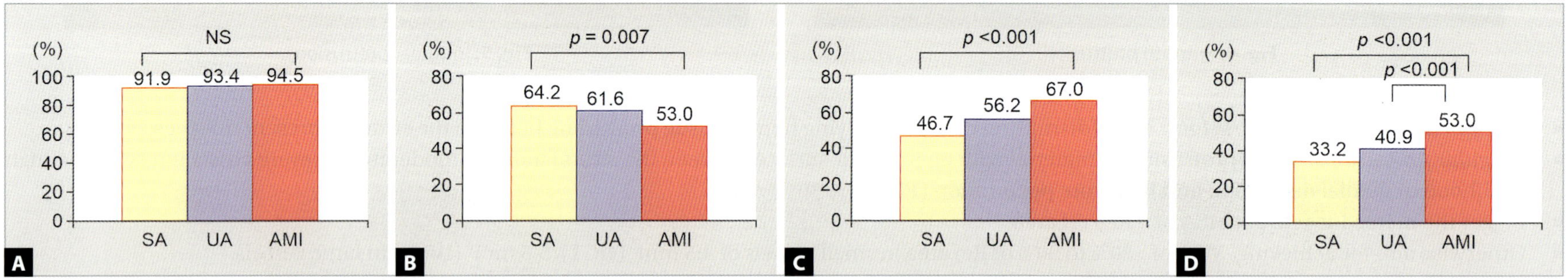

Figs. 7A to D: Incidence of (A) smooth protrusion, (B) disrupted fibrous tissue protrusion, (C) irregular protrusion, and (D) thrombus among stable angina (SA), unstable angina (UA), and acute myocardial infarction (AMI) patients.

REFERENCES

1. Sohn J, Hur SH, Kim IC, Cho YK, Park HS, Yoon HJ, et al. A comparison of tissue prolapse with optical coherence tomography and intravascular ultrasound after drug-eluting stent implantation. Int J Cardiovasc Imaging. 2015;31(1):21-9.
2. Qiu F, Mintz G, Witzenbichler B, Metzger D, Rinaldi M, Duffy P, et al. Clinical Impact Of Tissue Protrusion After Stent Implantation: An ADAPT-DES IVUS Sub study. J Am Coll Cardiol. 2014;63(12 Suppl):A1688.

CASE 1

TP assessment during PCI of LAD. (LAD: left anterior descending; PCI: percutaneous coronary intervention; TP: tissue prolapse)

CLINICAL HISTORY

A 53-year-old male, a known hypertensive and diabetic, presented with ACS-unstable angina and recent onset of chest pain associated with shortness of breath. Electrocardiogram (ECG)—normal sinus rhythm (NSR), no ST-T changes, two-dimensional (2D) echo— regional wall motion abnormality (RWMA) in left anterior descending (LAD) territory, and mild left ventricular (LV) dysfunction with ejection fraction (EF) 46% and routine blood investigations were within normal limits.

Coronary angiography (CAG)-left main coronary artery (LMCA)—normal, LAD—mid 90% thrombotic lesion, left circumflex (LCX)—distal 80-90% lesion, OM1—proximal 70-80%, right coronary artery (RCA)—mild disease **(Figs. 8A to C)**.

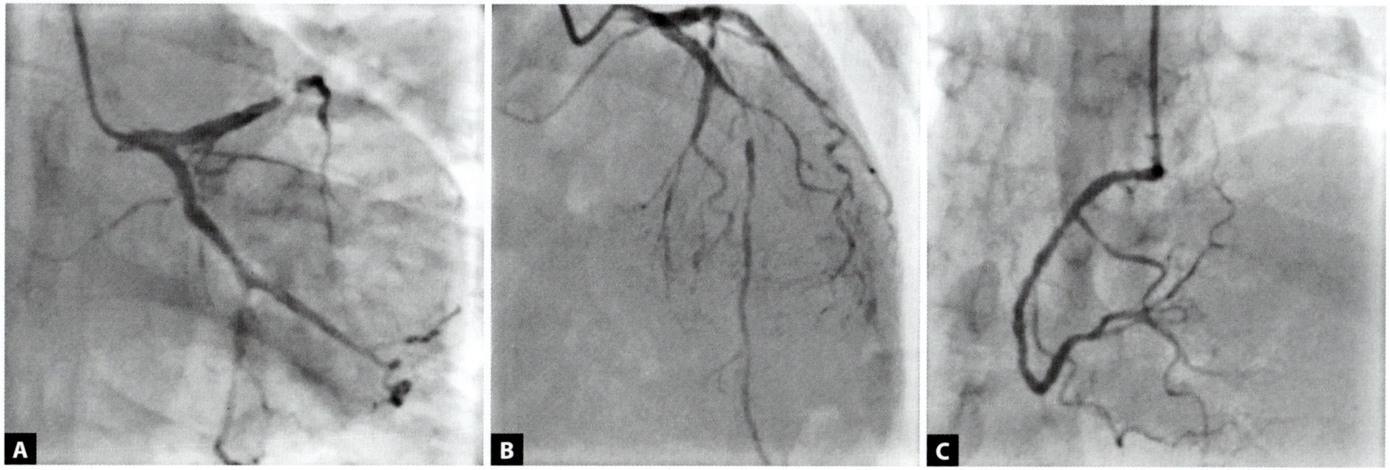

Figs. 8A to C: Coronary angiogram. (A) left circumflex (LCX); (B) left anterior descending (LAD); (C) right coronary artery (RCA).

PROCEDURE

Route—right radial approach (RRA), 6 Fr XB 3.5 guiding catheter, angiogram revealed LAD-mid 90% thrombotic lesion, which was crossed with Sion Blue wire.

Pre-OCT showed long segment fibrolipid plaque extending from proximal to distal LAD, disease segment length 48 mm, proximal landing zone luminal diameter 3.2 mm, and distal landing zone luminal diameter 1.6 mm **(Figs. 9A to C)**.

Distal LAD stenting was done with 2.5 × 33 mm Xience Xpedition stent, mid-LAD stenting was done with 3.0 × 38 mm Xience Xpedition stent, proximal LAD stenting done with 3.5 × 18 mm Xience Xpedition stent **(Figs. 10A to D)** and postdilated with 2.5 and 3.5 mm noncompliant (NC) balloons.

Postprocedure OCT study showed well-apposed stent struts, no residual stenosis, and no thrombosis **(Figs.11A to C)**. Postprocedure angio views showed well-implanted stents with thrombolysis in myocardial infarction (TIMI-III) flow without any dissection.

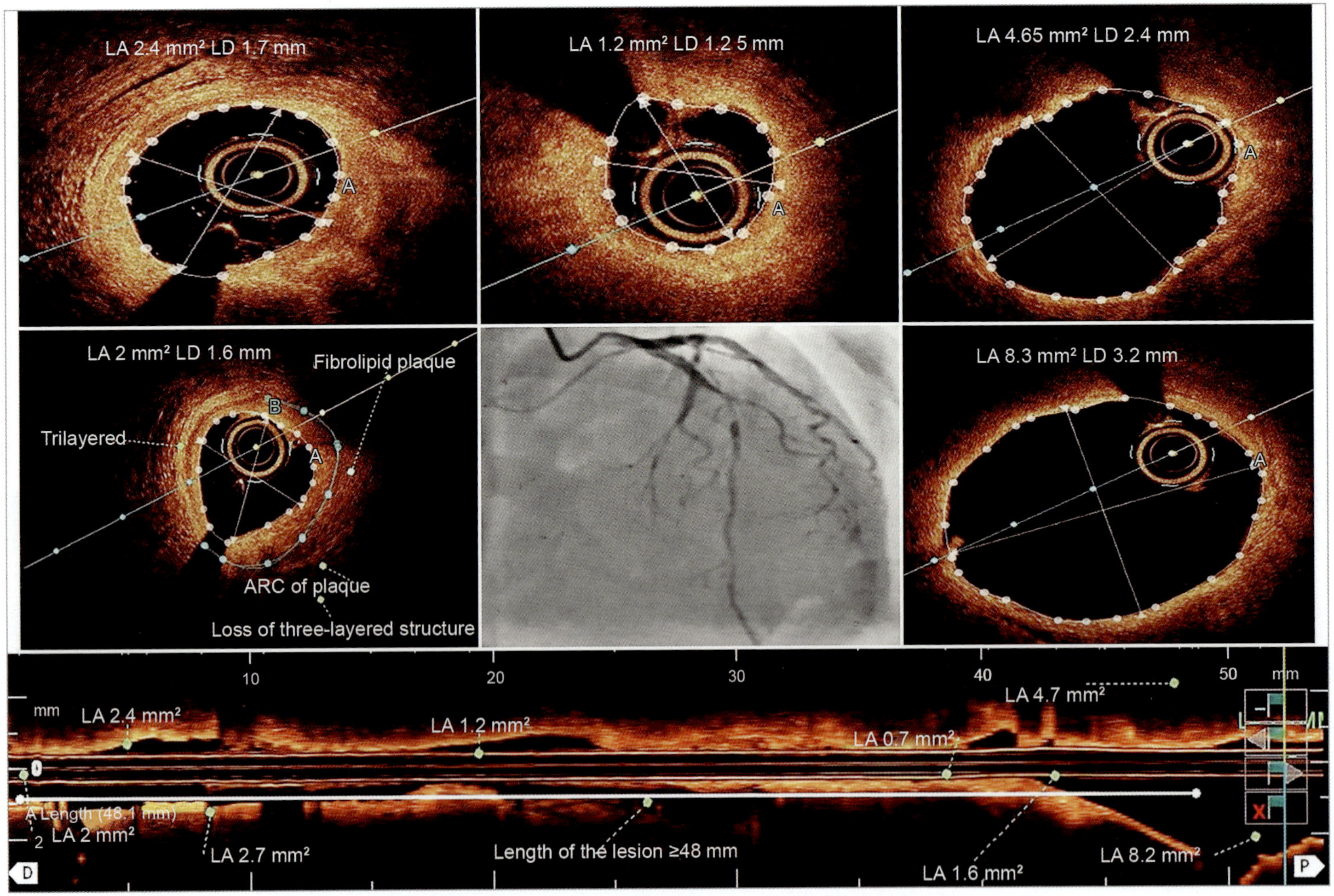

Fig. 9A

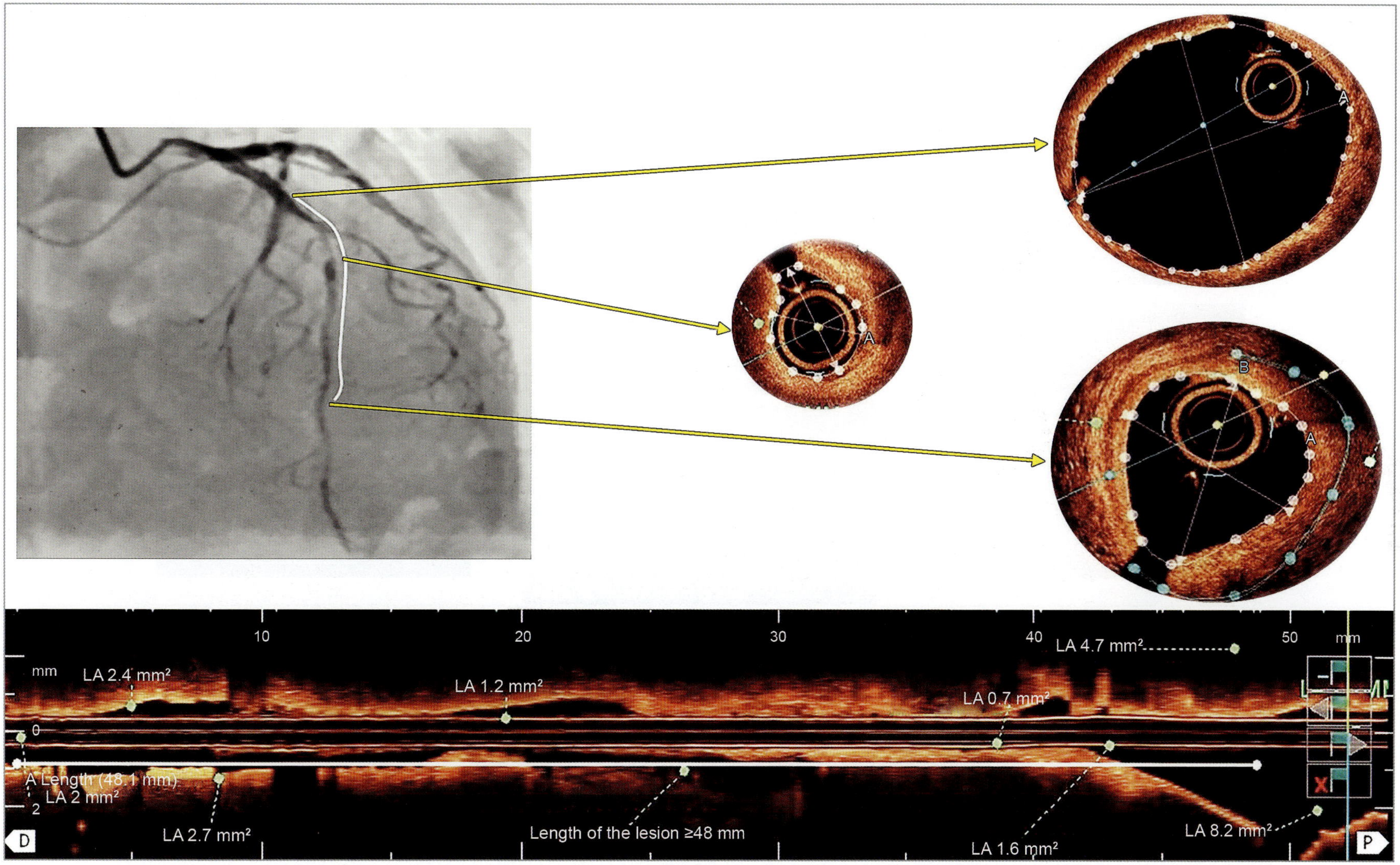

Fig. 9B

Control Guide catheter properly—Inadvertent sucking of the catheter or not co-axial may lead to dissection of the LM.

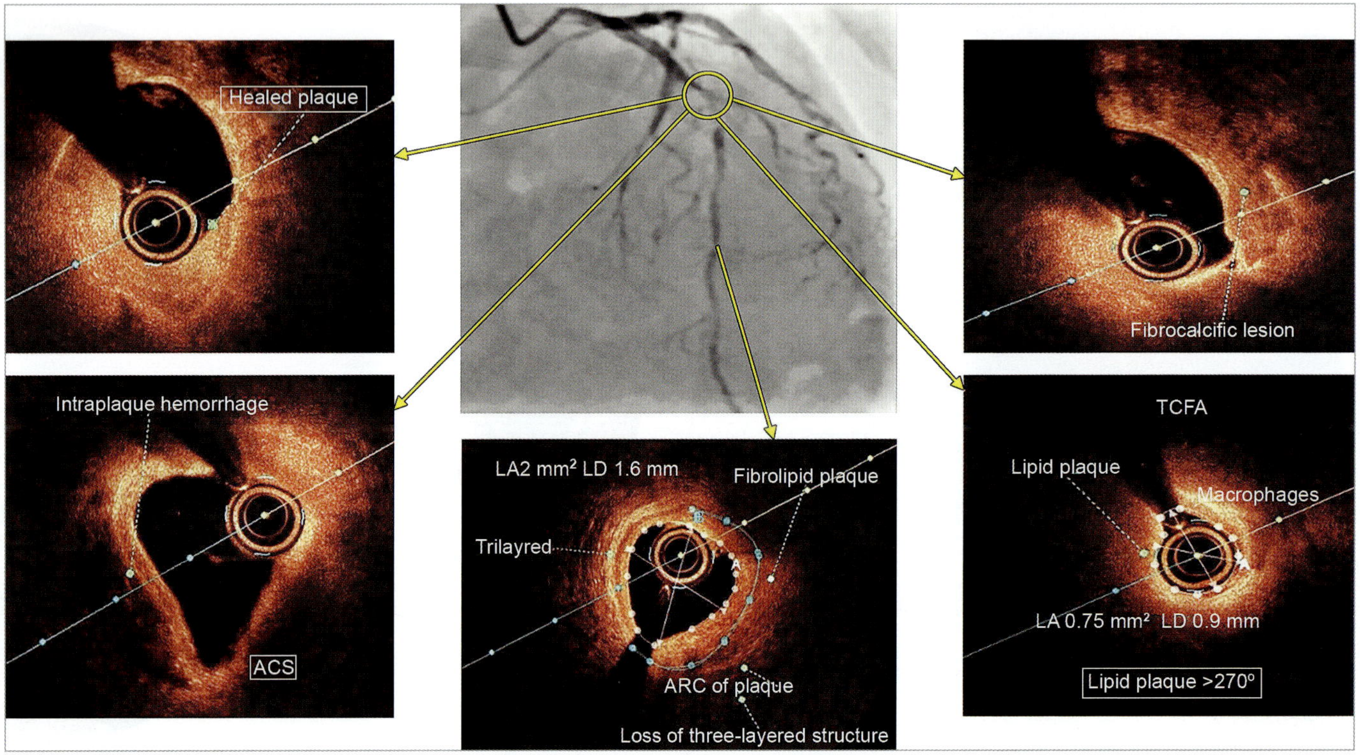

Fig. 9C

Figs. 9A to C: (A) Presenting OCT assessment of diseased vessel; (B) Presenting OCT assessment for device size (length and diameter) selection; and (C) Plaque morphology assessment of the diseased vessel. (LA: luminal area; LD: luminal diameter; OCT: optical coherence tomography; TCFA: thin-cap fibroatheroma)

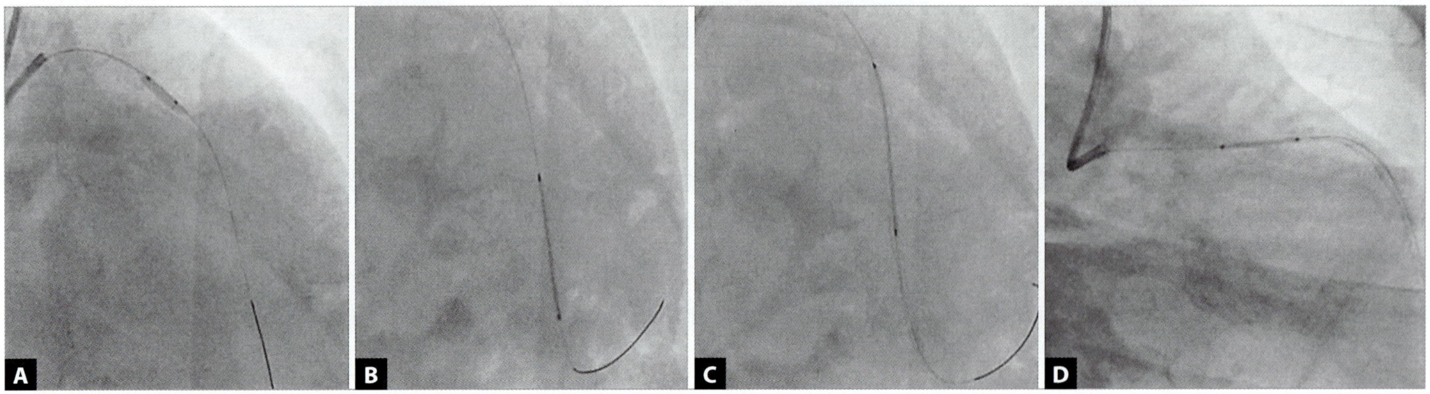

Figs. 10A to D: Distal, mid and proximal LAD stenting.

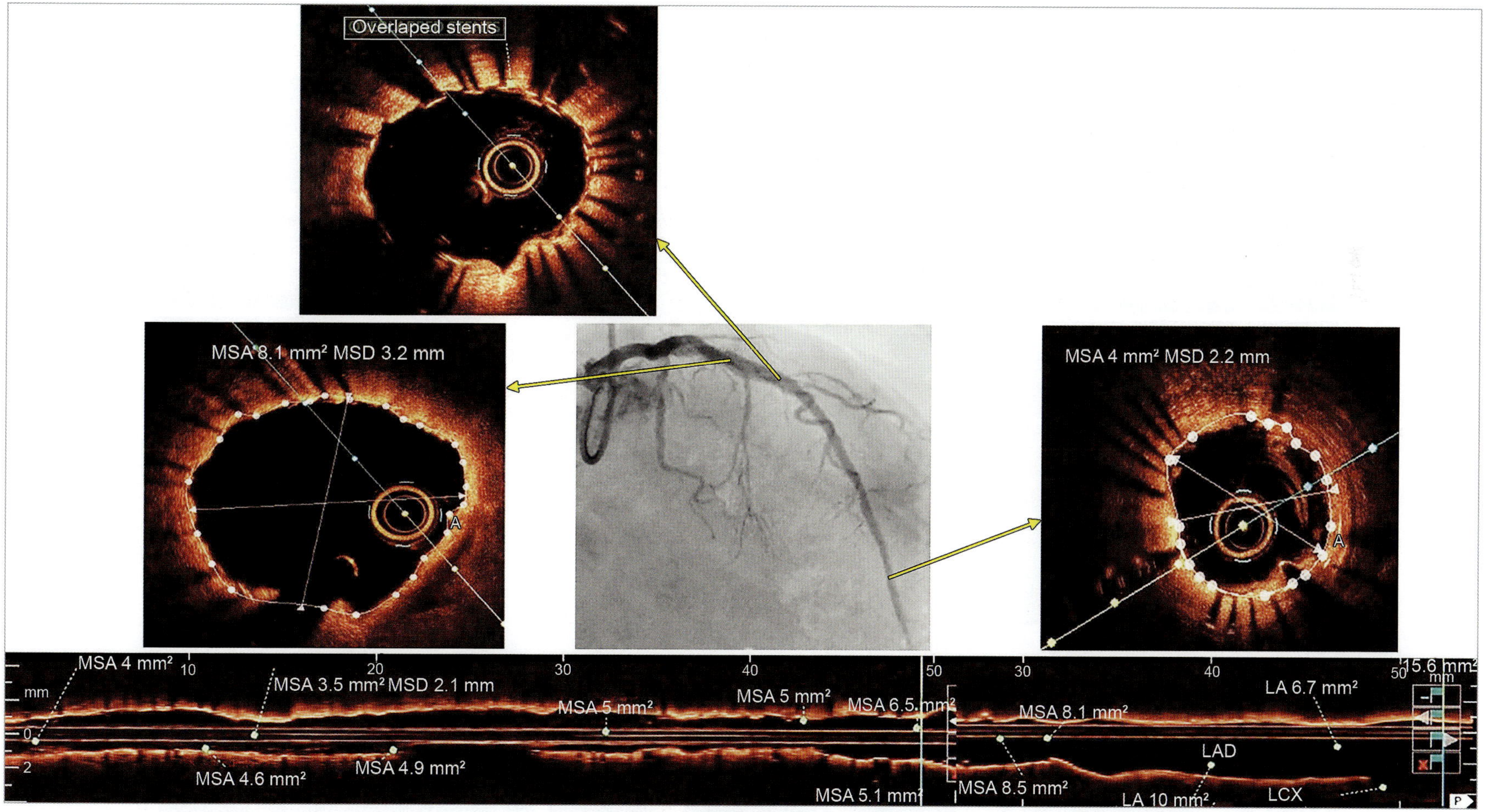
Overlaped stents
MSA 8.1 mm² MSD 3.2 mm
A
MSA 4 mm² MSD 2.2 mm
A
MSA 4 mm²
MSA 3.5 mm² MSD 2.1 mm
MSA 5 mm²
MSA 5 mm²
MSA 6.5 mm²
MSA 4.6 mm²
MSA 4.9 mm²
MSA 5.1 mm²
MSA 8.1 mm²
MSA 8.5 mm²
LA 6.7 mm²
LAD
LA 10 mm²
LCX
15.6 mm²

Fig. 11A

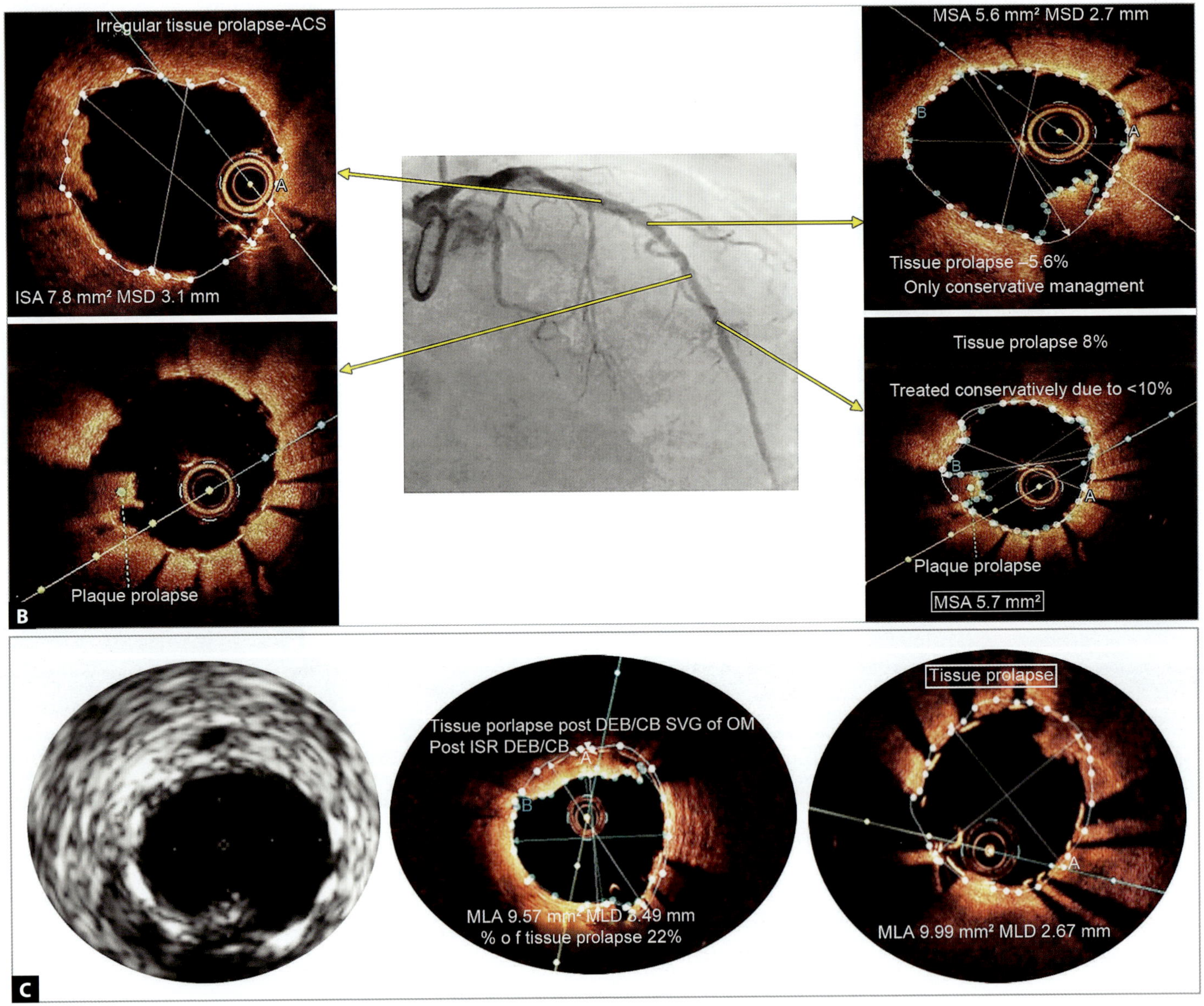

Figs. 11B and C

Figs. 11A and C: (A) Poststenting OCT assessment for any medial edge dissections at both ends, expansion, and apposition of the stent struts. (B) Percentage of tissue prolapse in the stent; (C) An example of Tissue prolapse identification by IVUS and OCT. (LA: luminal area; LAD: left anterior descending; LCX: left circumflex; MSA: minimal stent area; MLD: minimal luminal diameter; MSD: minimal stent diameter; OCT: optical coherence tomography)

CASE 2

PCI of LAD-TP/malapposition. (LAD: left anterior descending; PCI: percutaneous coronary intervention; TP: tissue prolapse)

CLINICAL HISTORY

A 63-year-old male, a known diabetic, presented with ACS-inferoposterior wall MI. On examination (O/E)—pulse rate (PR) 82/min, blood pressure (BP) 120/70 mm Hg, oxygen saturation (SPO_2) 96%, heart—S1+, S2+, S30, S40, investigations—hemoglobin (Hb) 12.4 g%, serum creatinine 0.9 mg/dL, blood urea 17 mg/dL, random blood sugar (RBS) 243 mg/dL, human immunodeficiency virus (HIV), hepatitis B surface antigen (HBsAg), hepatitis C virus (HCV)—negative. ECG—inferior + true posterior MI. 2D echo—RWMA in basal posterior wall, mild LV dysfunction, and EF 48%.

Coronary angiography-LMCA—normal, LAD—mid-total occlusion, diagonal ostioproximal 90% lesion, LCX normal, RCA—mid 99% lesion, posterior descending artery (PDA) proximal stenosis, posterior left ventricular branches (PLVB) normal **(Figs. 12A to C)**.

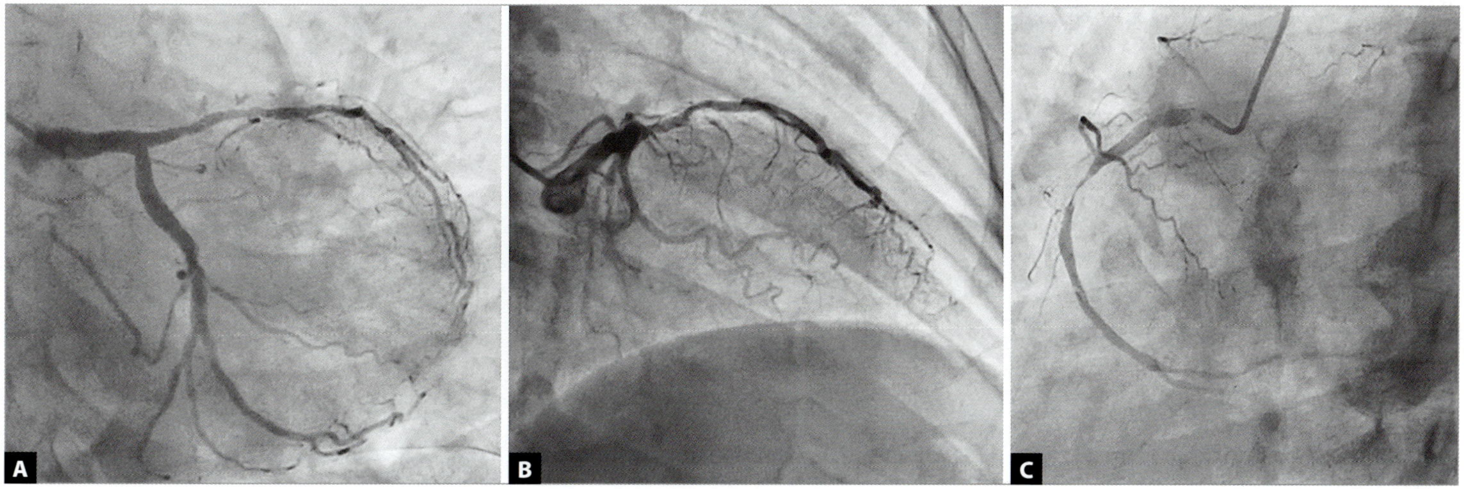

Figs. 12A to C: Coronary angiogram.

PROCEDURE

Percutaneous Coronary Intervention of Right Coronary Artery

Right transradial, 6 Fr Judkins right (JR) 3.5 guiding catheter, RCA mid 99% lesion crossed with 0.014″ Sion Blue wire. Then direct stenting was done with 3.5 × 26 mm Orsiro Stent. The final result was good with TIMI III flow without any complications **(Figs. 13A and B)**.

Percutaneous Coronary Intervention of Left Anterior Descending

Route—right femoral artery (RFA), 7 Fr EBU 3.5 guiding catheter, initially tried to cross the LAD lesions after placing 0.014″ Sion Blue in LAD but could not cross. Finally crossed with Fielder XT wire using microcatheter support.

Pre-Optical Coherence Tomography Analysis

Proximal LAD minimal luminal area (MLA) 6.2 mm^2, minimal luminal diameter (MLD) 2.8 mm, LAD/D1 bifurcation with MLA 4.1 mm^2, MLD 2.25 mm, and distal LAD with MLA 3 mm^2 and MLD 2 mm **(Fig. 14)**.

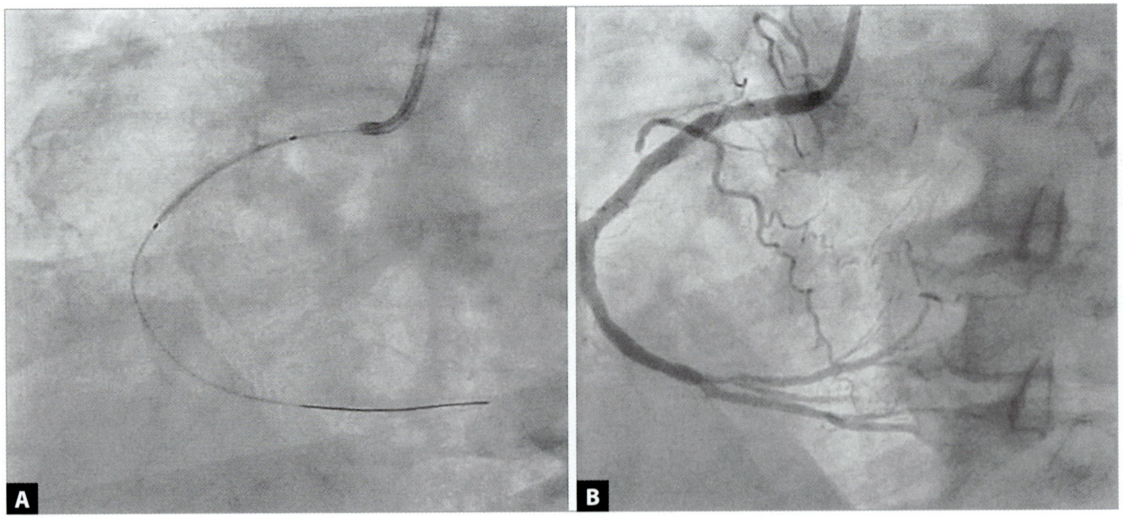

Figs. 13A and B: Coronary angioplasty of right coronary artery (RCA).

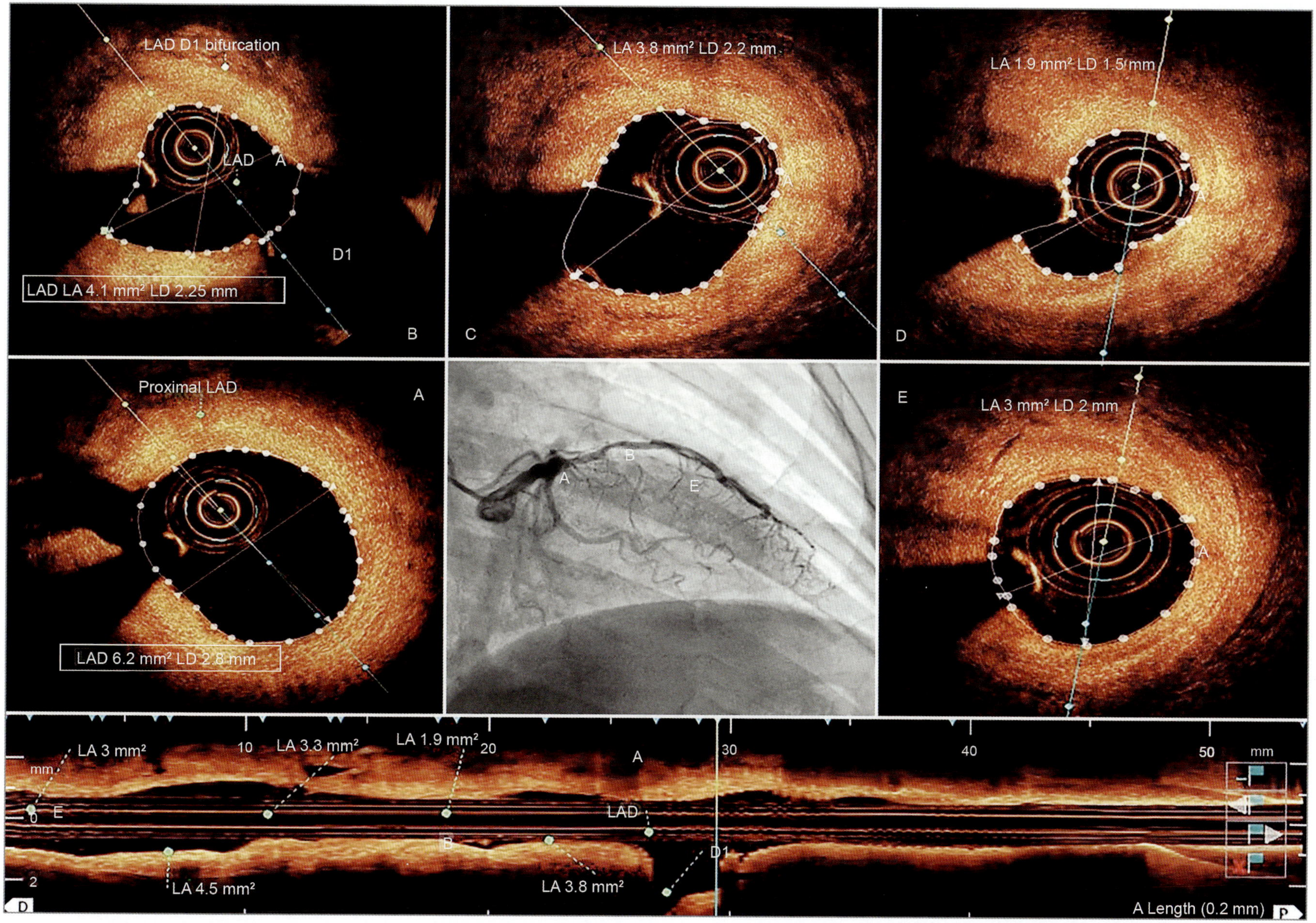

Fig. 14: Presenting OCT assessment of LAD. (LA: luminal area; LAD: left anterior descending; LD: luminal diameter; OCT: optical coherence tomography)

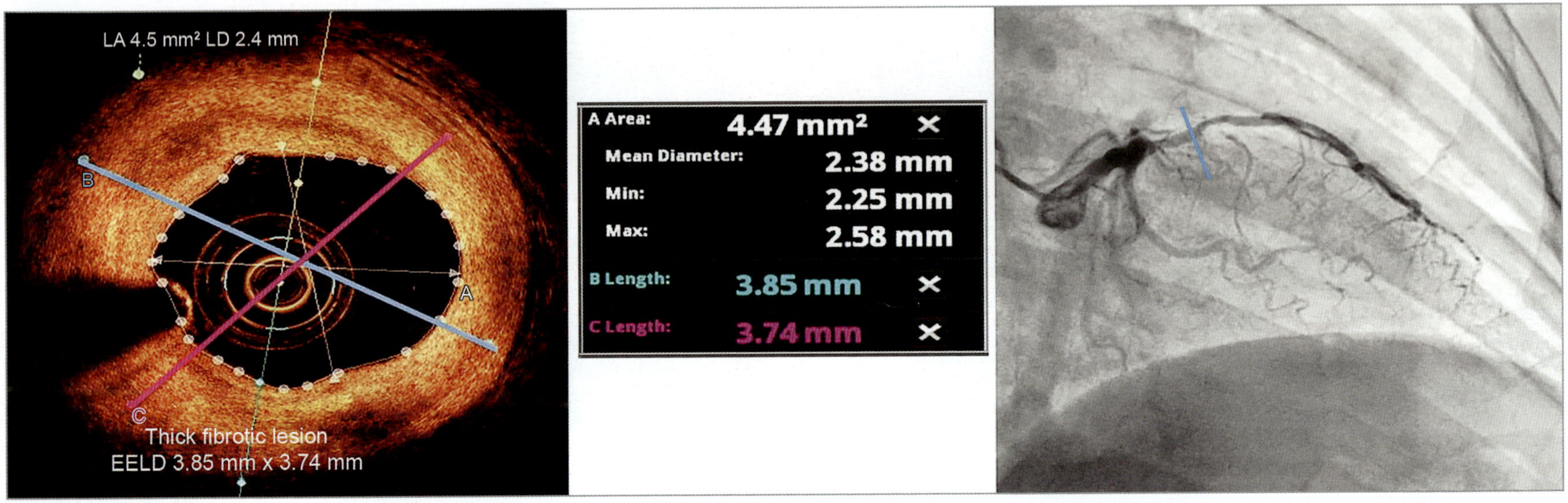

Fig. 15: Fibrotic lesion assessment by OCT. (EELD: external elastic lamina diameter; LA: luminal area; LD: luminal diameter; OCT: optical coherence tomography)

Proximal LAD thick fibrotic lesion with MLA 4.5 mm^2, MLD 2.4 mm, and external elastic lamina diameter (EELD) 3.85 × 3.74 mm **(Fig. 15)**.

Post-plain old balloon angioplasty (POBA) LAD chronic total occlusion (CTO) dissection of tight fibrotic plaque and proximal portion severe narrowing of the disease **(Fig. 16)**.

Predilated with 1.25 × 10 mm and 2.25 × 10 mm Tazuna balloon, proximal LAD stenting was done with 3.0 × 2 mm Yukon Choice Elite stent, mid-LAD overlapping stenting done with 2.75 × 21 mm Yukon Choice Elite stent **(Figs. 17A to C)** postdilated with 3.5 ×12 mm NC Trek balloon.

Post-Optical Coherence Tomography Analysis

Distal landing zone with MLA 4.8 mm^2, MLD 2.47 mm, overlapping stent struts with MLA 8.7mm^2, MLD 3.3 mm, proximal landing zone with MLA 7.1 mm^2, MLD 3 mm, malapposed stent struts 0.34 mm with malapposition 12% **(Fig. 18)**.

Post-OCT showed proximal portion of the stent TP 13% and underexpansion with 8.9 mm diameter **(Fig. 19)** and malapposition **(Fig. 20)**. Postprocedure angio view showed well-implanted stents with TIMI-III flow without any dissection. Patient was discharged on 3rd postprocedure day in a stable status.

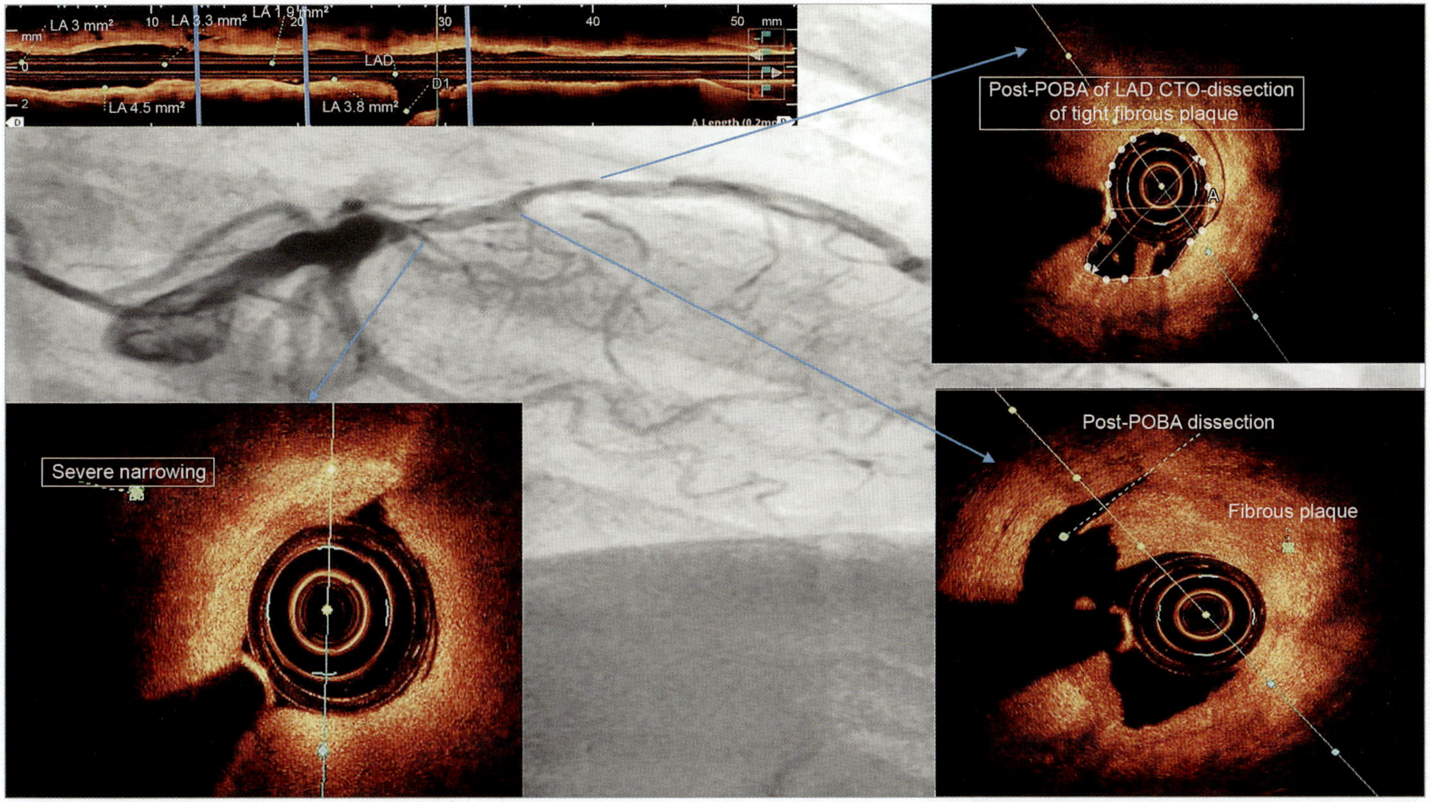

Fig. 16: Post-POBA dissection in the diseased vessel. (CTO: chronic total occlusion; LA: luminal area; LAD: left anterior descending; POBA: plain old balloon angioplasty)

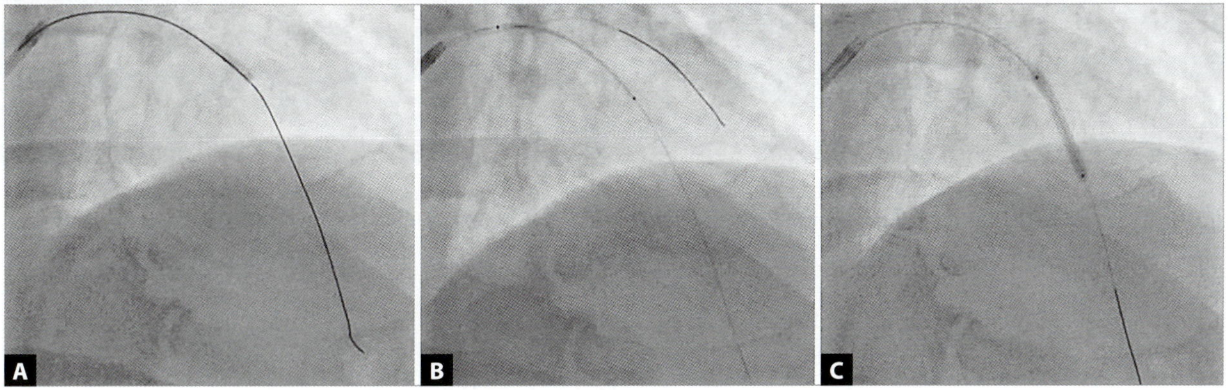

Figs. 17A to C: Coronary angioplasty of left anterior descending (LAD).

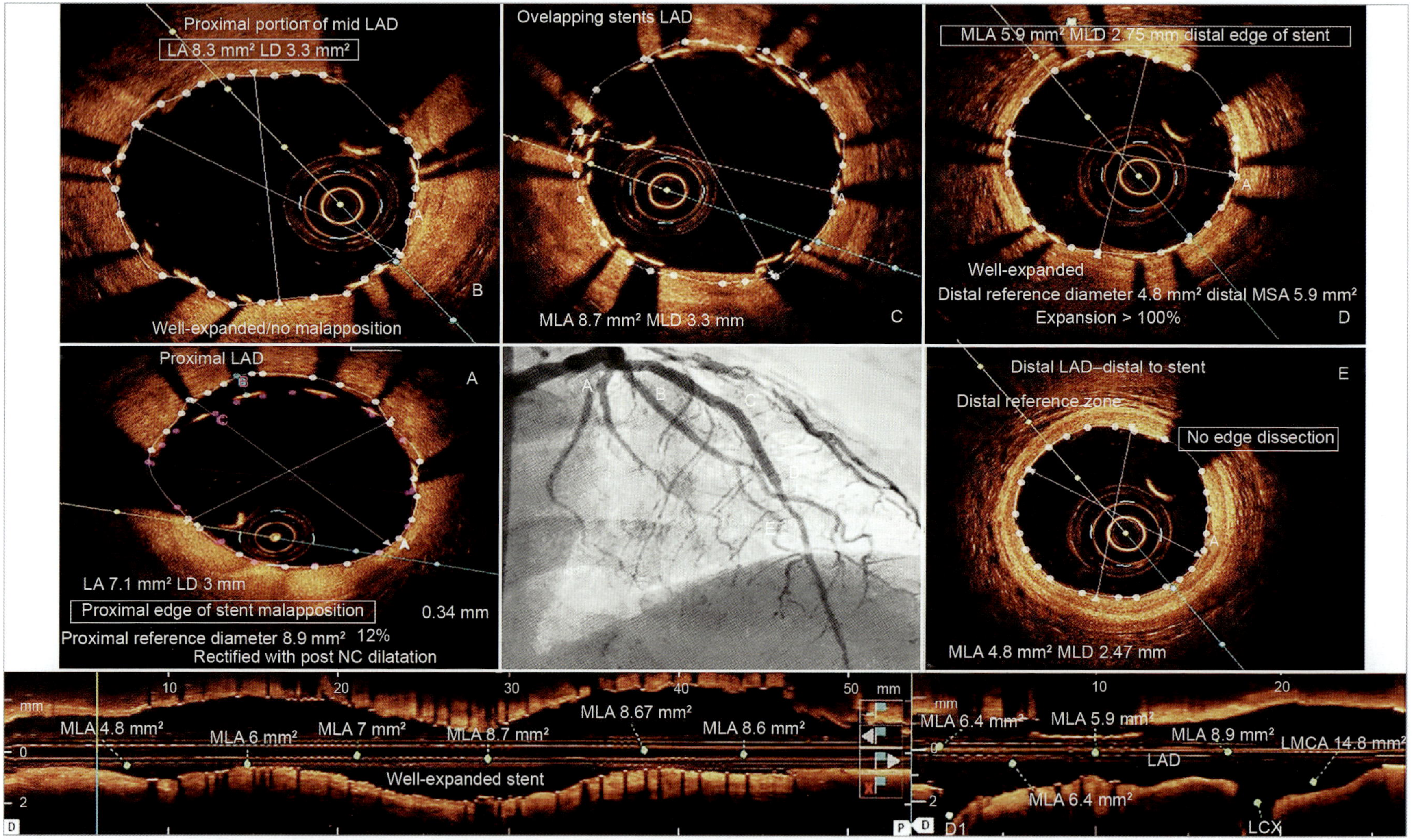

Fig. 18: Poststenting OCT assessment of LAD for medial edge dissections at both ends, expansion, and apposition of the stent struts. (LA: luminal area; LAD: left anterior descending; LCX: left circumflex; LD: luminal diameter; LMCA: left main coronary artery; MLA: minimal luminal area; MLD: minimal luminal diameter; MSA: minimal stent area; NC: noncompliant; OCT: optical coherence tomography)

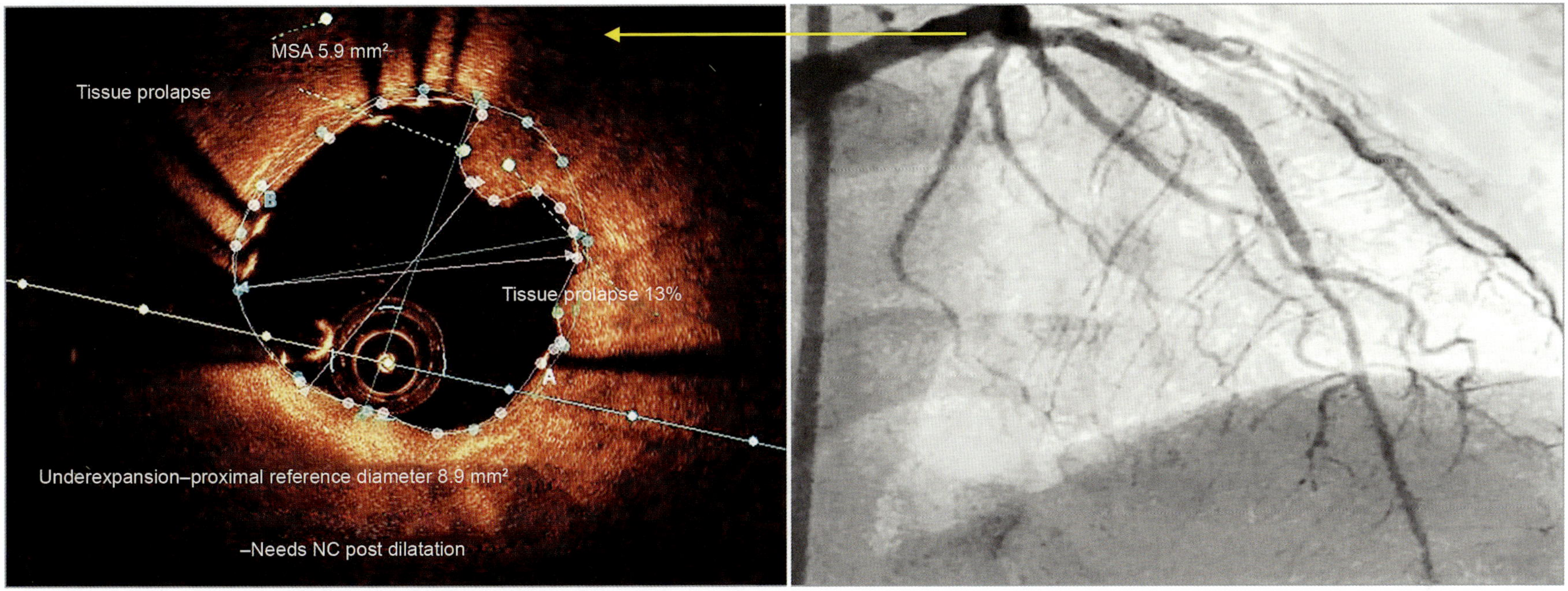

Fig. 19: Detection of underexpansion and tissue prolapse. (MSA: minimal stent area; NC: noncompliant)

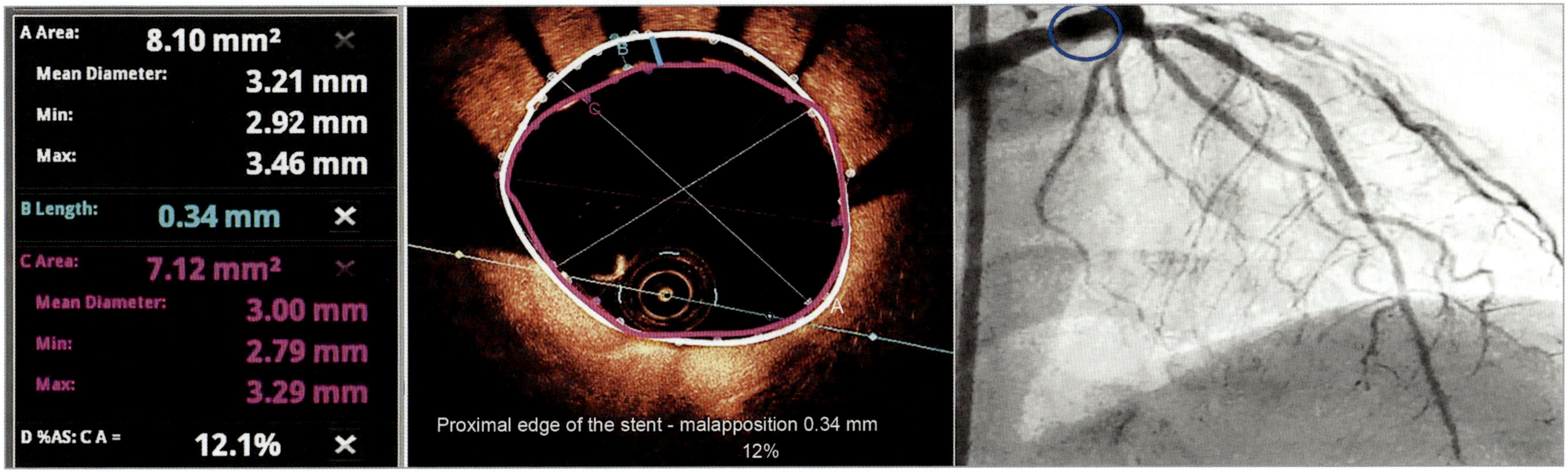

Fig. 20: Malapposition and proximal edge.

CHAPTER 5

Stent Edge Dissection

INTRODUCTION

Stent Edge

Stent Edge is the area 5 mm segment adjacent to the stent margin on either side of the stent.[1]

Stent edge dissection (SED) is usually due to the landing zones with plaque burden >50%, especially with fibrolipid or fibrocalcific lesions **(Fig. 1)**. Edge dissections happen when oversized balloons or stents are used with high-pressure inflation without adequate plaque modification with appropriate modification device. Optical coherence tomography (OCT) detects dissections more precisely in terms of depth, length, and circumferential extent including minor dissections which are frequently missed on conventional angiography. Major flow-limiting dissection is associated with early-stent thrombosis and increased cardiovascular (CV) event rate **(Flowchart 1)**.[2,3]

Major dissection on OCT is characterized by their depth—medial edge dissection (MED), angle >60°, and length >2 mm. Specific morphometric parameters for each flap and cavity were calculated to estimate the magnitude of dissections. The severity of the dissection is also further classified based on the depth of vessel injury as: (1) Intimal—involving intimal alone; (2) medial—involving intima and medial layers; and (3) adventitial—involving intima, media, and extension to the external elastic membrane **(Figs. 2 to 6)**.

Landing zone with increased plaque burden increases the chances of development of MED by six times.

The current consensus document defines significant dissections as follows: Dissection with large residual plaque burden, lateral extent of >60°, longitudinal extent of >2 mm, extension into the media, and located at the distal edge. Dissections with a width >200 µm at the distal stent edge is associated with higher risk of major adverse cardiovascular events (MACE) compared to proximal edge dissections.[4]

Intramural hematoma (IMH) is due to the accumulation of blood with extension in the medial space, displacing the internal elastic membrane inward and the external elastic membrane outward as a consequence of entry of blood through dissection site **(Fig. 7)**.

Flowchart 1: Edge dissection.

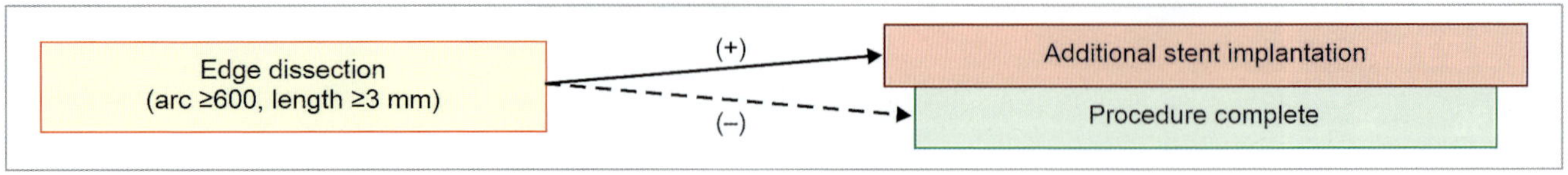

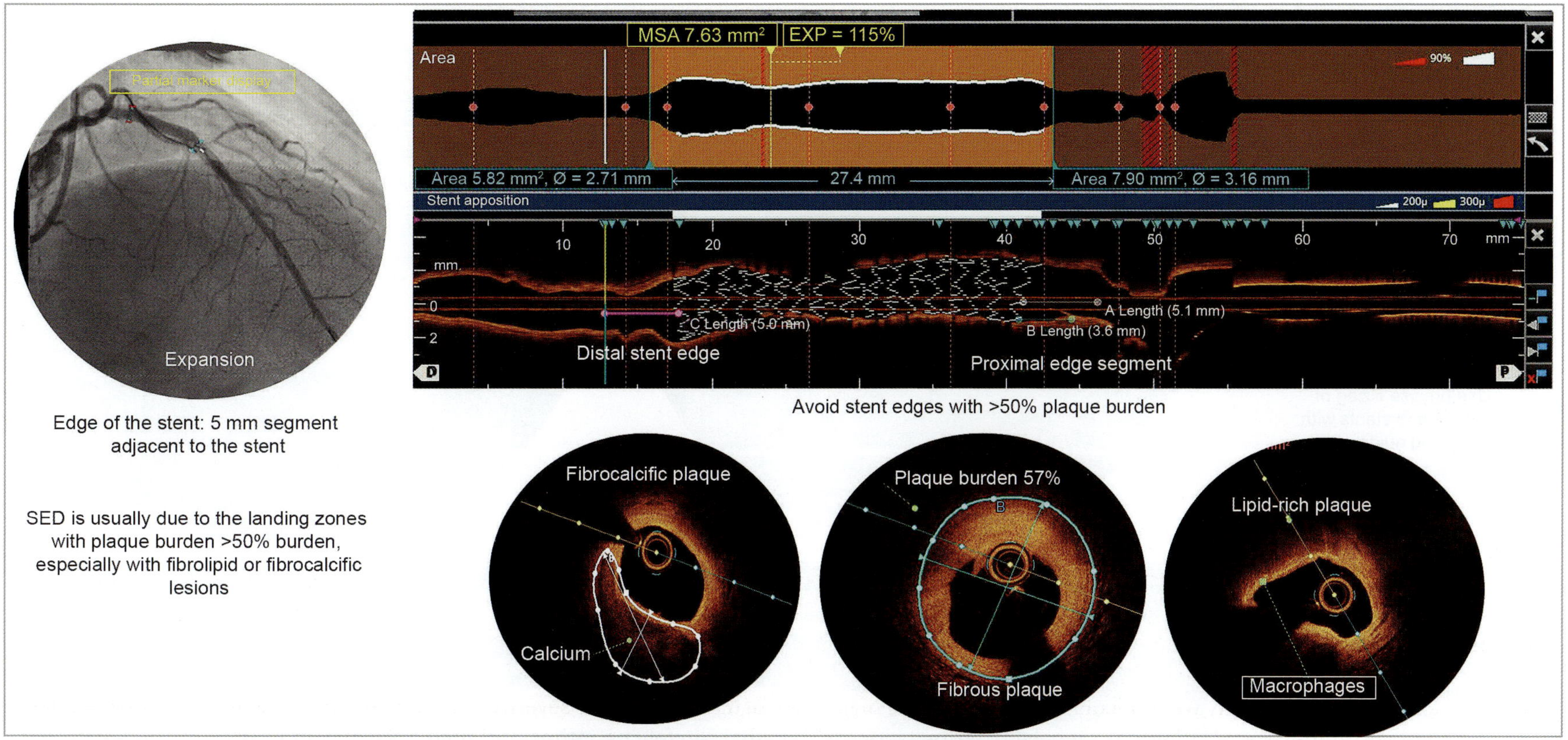

Fig. 1: OCT for the assessment of stent edges and plaque burden. (MSA: minimal stent area; SED: stent edge dissection)

Wherever possible, consider intracoronary imaging during initial PCI for detection of vulnerable plaques particularly in situations with Angio images are uncertain or indeterminate.

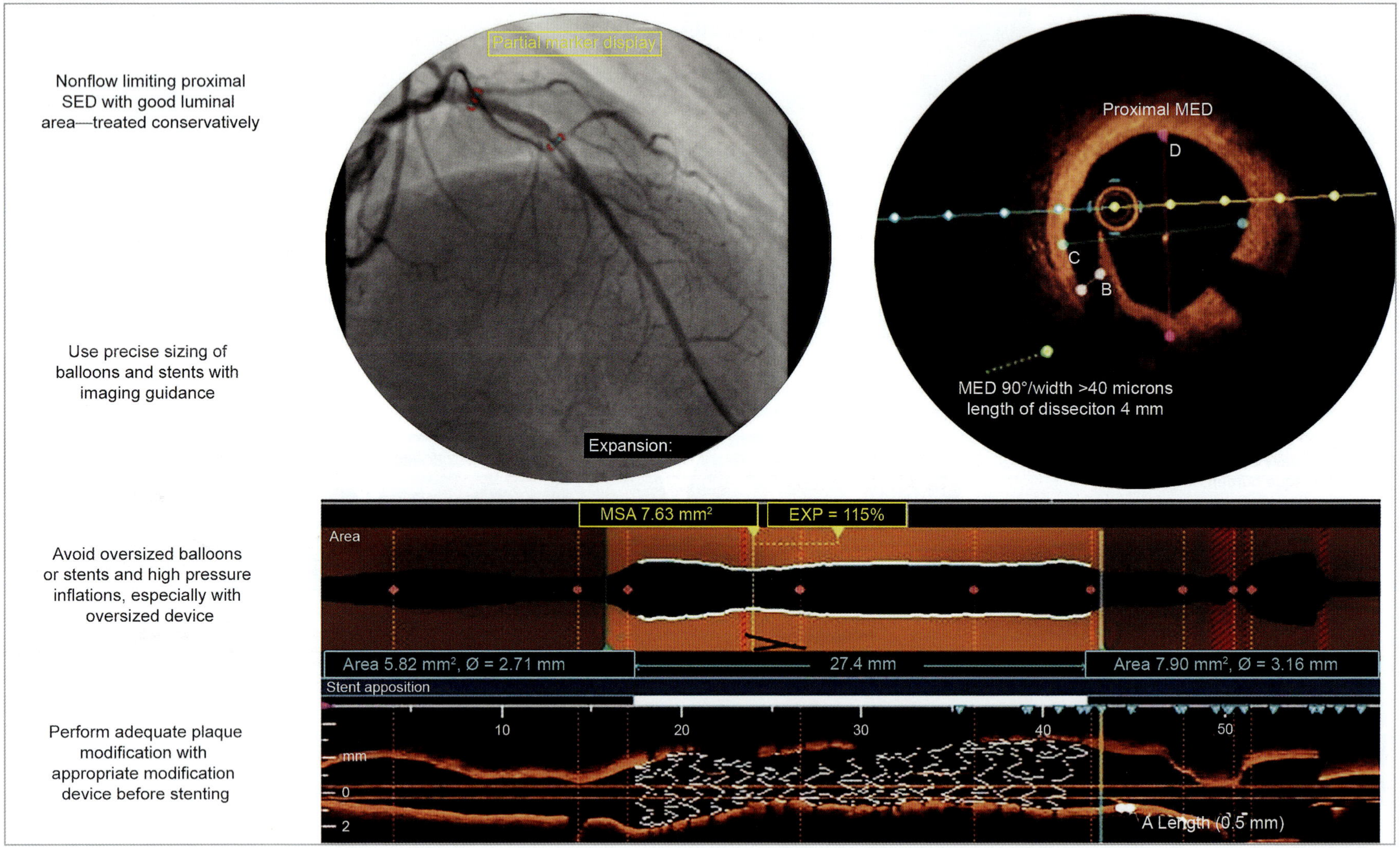

Fig. 2: Case example of proximal edge dissection. (MED: medial edge dissection; MSA: minimal stent area; SED: stent edge dissection)

Risk of PCI increases with advanced age/Long standing risk factors/CKD/CVA/PVD/COPD/High Hb A1c/Calcified lesions/MVD/LMCA/Bifurcation lesions/LV Dysfunction.

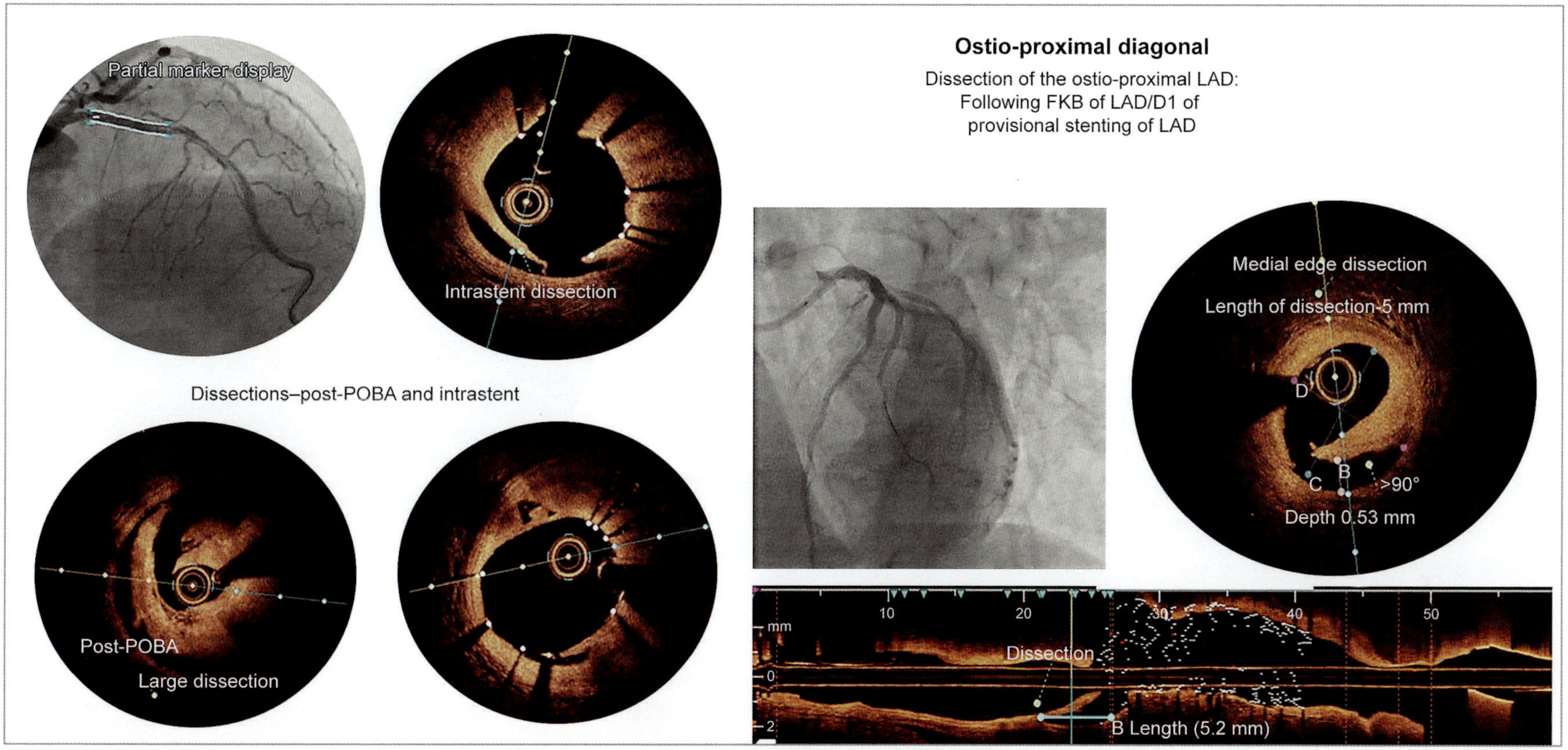

Fig. 3: Case example of proximal edge dissection. (FKB: final kissing balloon; LAD: left anterior descending; POBA: plain old balloon angioplasty)

Morbidity and mortality depends upon the vessel size and its area of myocardial supply.

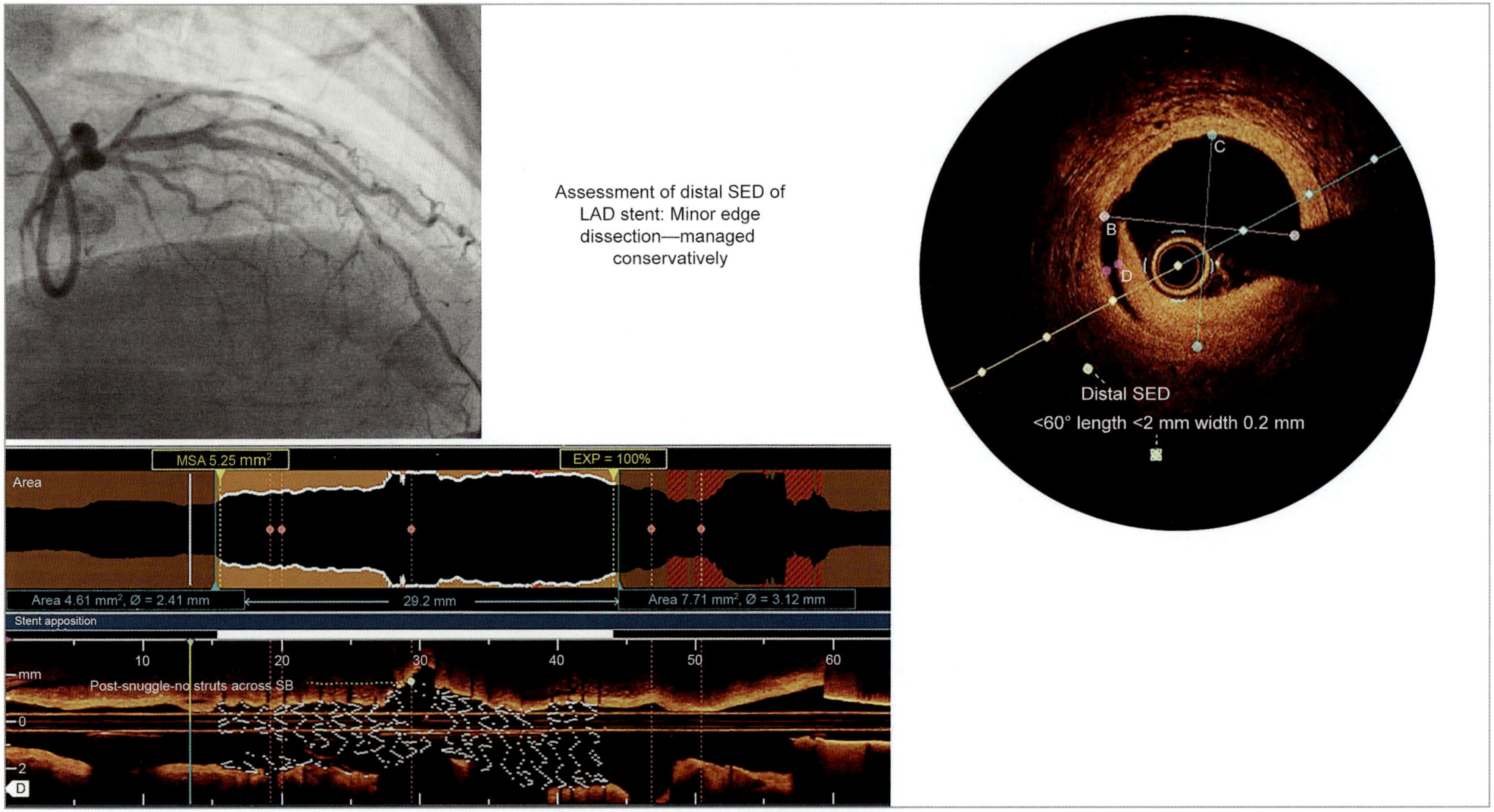

Fig. 4: Case example of distal SED. (LAD: left anterior descending; MSA: minimal stent area; SED: stent edge dissection)

If vulnerable plaques are identified, recommend high dose statins, long-term DAPT. During follow up period special emphasis should be made for optimal control of cardiovascular risk factors with life style modification and appropriate pharmacotherapy to maintain treatment targets for avoiding future progression or regression of atheroma leading to future recurrence of angina or MI.

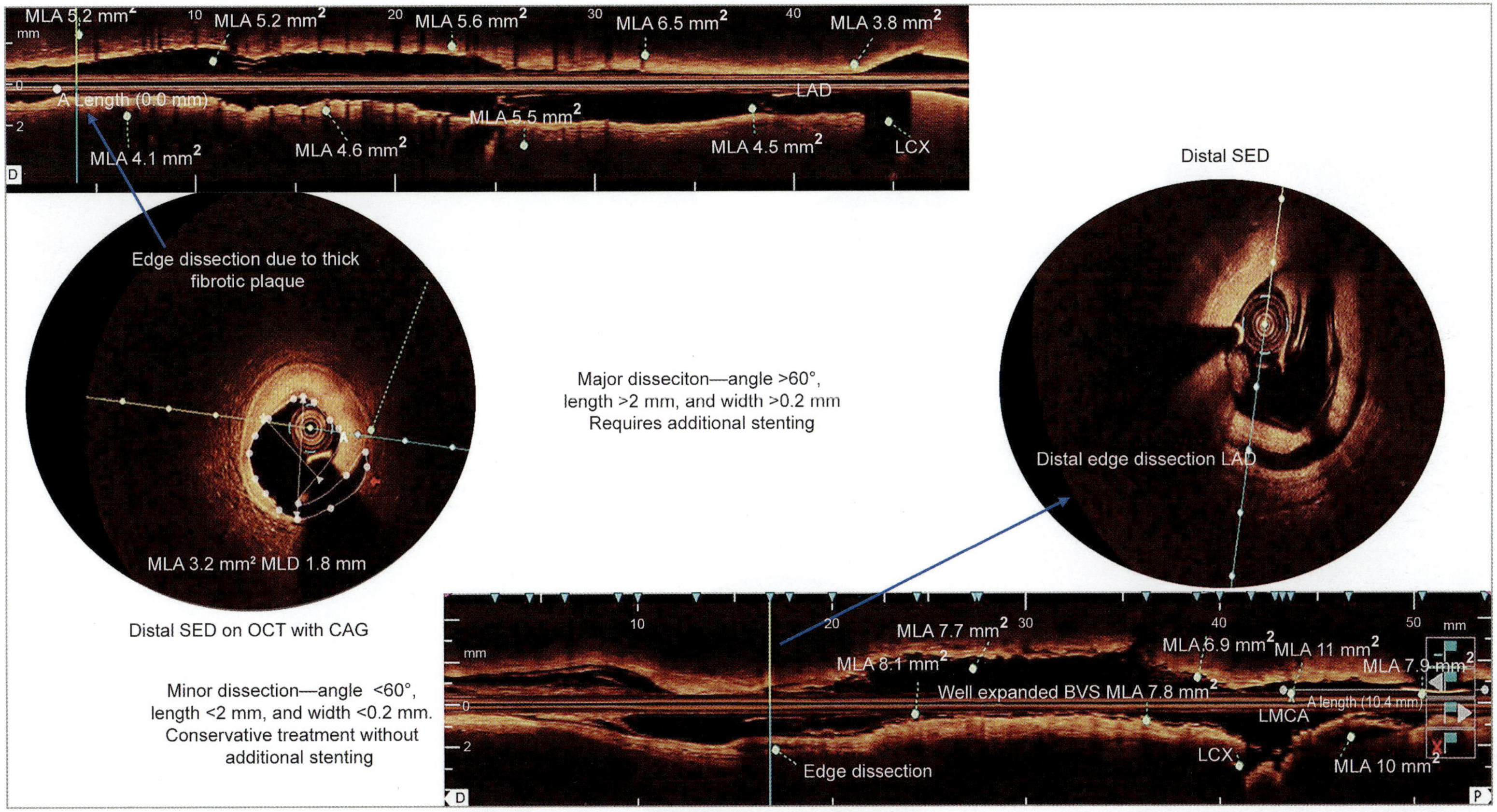

Fig. 5: Case examples of distal edge dissection—major and minor. (CAG: coronary angiogram; LAD: left anterior descending; LCX: left circumflex; LMCA: left main coronary artery; MLA: minimal lumen area; OCT: optical coherence tomography; SED: stent edge dissection)

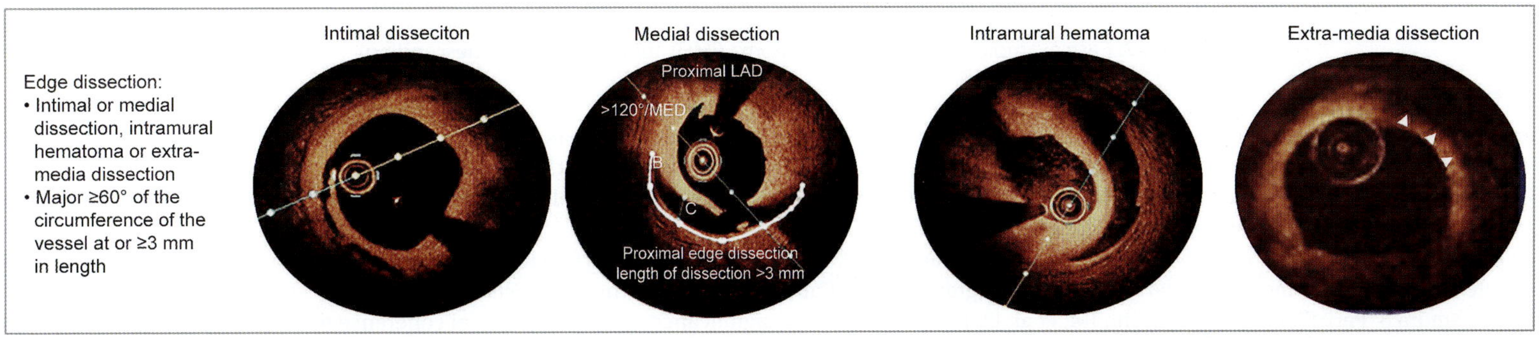

Fig. 6: Spectrum of stent edge dissections by optical coherence tomography (OCT). (LAD: left anterior descending; MED: medial edge dissection)

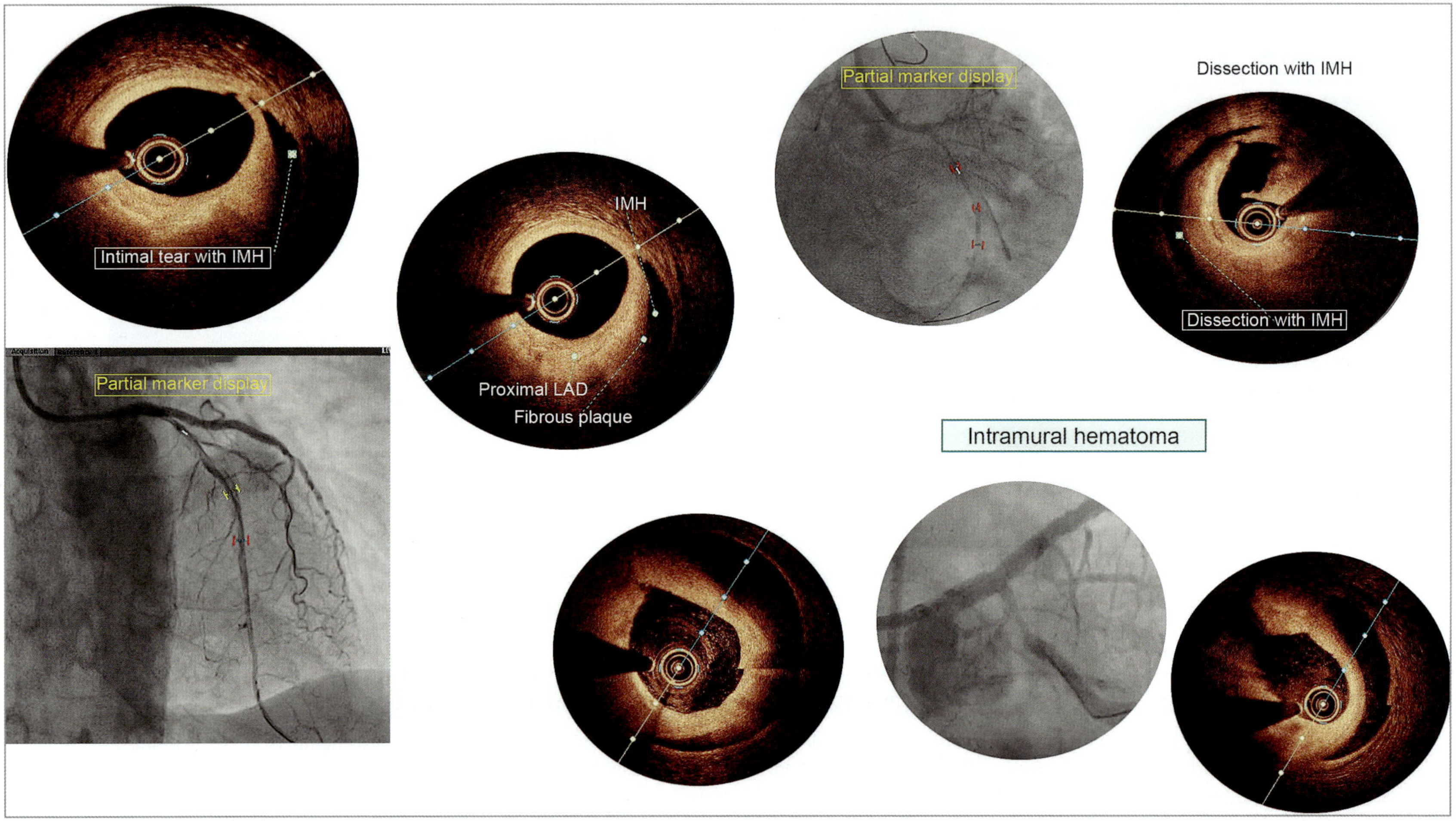

Fig. 7: Case example of intramural hematoma (IMH). (LAD: left anterior descending)

REFERENCES

1. Chamié D, Bezerra HG, Attizzani GF, Yamamoto H, Kanaya T, Stefano GT, et al. Incidence, predictors, morphological characteristics, and clinical outcomes of stent edge dissections detected by optical coherence tomography. JACC Cardiovasc Interv. 2013;6(8):800-13.
2. Gonzalo N, Serruys PW, Okamura T, Shen ZJ, Garcia-Garcia HM, Onuma Y, et al. Relation between plaque type and dissections at the edges after stent implantation: an optical coherence tomography study. Int J Cardiol. 2011;150(2):151-5.
3. Bouki KP, Sakkali E, Toutouzas K, Vlad D, Barmperis D, Phychari S, et al. Impact of coronary artery stent edge dissections on long-term clinical outcome in patients with acute coronary syndrome: An optical coherence tomography study. Catheter Cardiovasc Interv. 2015;86(2):237-46.
4. Soeda T, Uemura S, Park SJ, Jang Y, Lee S, Cho JM, et al. Incidence and clinical significance of poststent optical coherence tomography findings: one-year follow-up study from a multicenter registry. Circulation. 2015;132(11):1020-9.

CASE 1

CLINICAL HISTORY

A 55-year-old female, a known diabetic (uncontrolled) and hypertensive, with stable ischemic heart disease, with recent onset of unstable angina (USA) (episodes of rest angina positive) of 4 days' duration. Electrocardiogram (ECG)—normal sinus rhythm (NSR) within normal limits, two-dimensional (2D) echo—no regional wall motion abnormality (RWMA), good left ventricular (LV) function with ejection fraction (EF) 60%, troponin I positive. *O/I*: Hemoglobin (Hb) 9.8 g/dL, random blood sugar (RBS) 342 mg/dL, serum creatinine (S Cr) 1.03 mg/dL, estimated glomerular filtration rate (eGFR) 61 mL/min, angiogram done outside which revealed triple vessel disease (TVD) with diffuse disease of proximal-to-distal left anterior descending (LAD), tight lesion of left circumflex (LCX) ostium, large obtuse marginal (OM) branch, distal total occlusion of LCX, mid-right coronary artery (RCA) lesion.

PROCEDURE

Left main coronary artery (LMCA) engaged with Judkin's left (JL) 3.5–7 Fr guiding catheter, lesion crossed with 0.014" Sion Blue wire. LCX crossed with 0.014" BMW wire. LAD predilatation done with 2.0 × 15 mm Tazuna. Prestenting OCT to LAD was done which showed long-segment fibrocalcified plaque in proximal–mid LAD **(Figs. 8 and 9)**. Then mid-to-distal LAD stenting done with 2.25 × 28 mm Xience Xpedition stent.

Left circumflex lesion predilatation done with 2.0 × 15 mm Tazuna balloon. "V" stenting done in LAD and LCX. LAD stenting done with 2.75 × 23 mm Xience Xpedition stent. LCX stenting done with 2.0 × 30 mm Resolute Onyx stent. Postdilatation done to LAD with 2.75 × 15 mm noncompliant (NC) Trek at 16 atm and LCX 1.5 × 10 mm at 18 atm and 2.25 × 10 mm Tazuna at 16 atm. Kissing balloon dilatation done with 2.75 × 15 mm NC Trek at 16 atm in LAD and 2.25 × 10 mm Tazuna at 16 atm in LCX. Plain old balloon angioplasty (POBA) to distal LAD with 1.5 × 10 mm Tazuna. Check angio showed well patent LAD and LCX stents without any dissection of LMCA and distal edge of LAD and LCX stents. However, poststenting OCT **(Figs. 10 and 11)** showed significant proximal edge dissection in distal LMCA with angle > 60°, >5 mm length, and width 0.74 mm requiring LMCA–LAD stenting with 3.5 × 18 mm Xience Xpedition stent with crushing of proximal struts of the LCX stent. OCT revealed myocardial bridging of LAD distal to the stent. POT done with 4.0 × 08 mm NC Trek at 14 atm. LCX wire recrossed through stent struts using Fielder FC wire opened with 1.25 × 10 mm Tazuna. First kissing balloon dilatation done with 3.0 × 12 mm NC Trek at 16 atm in LAD and 2.25 × 12 mm Tazuna at 16 atm in LCX. Second kissing balloon dilatation done with 3.0 × 2 mm NC Trek at 16 atm in LAD and 2.5 × 12 mm NC Trek at 16 atm in LCX. Proximal and mid-LAD postdilatation done with 3.5 × 12 mm NC Trek at 16 atm. The final result was good; thrombolysis in myocardial infarction (TIMI-III) flow was achieved.

Femoral artery (FA) sheath check angio showed total occlusion of right (Rt) common FA (CFA) with no antegrade flow of superficial FA (SFA) and popliteal artery, filling of only profunda femoris. Rt brachial approach, Rt iliac angiogram was performed, tried to cross occluded CFA with Terumo, 014 BMW wire but could not cross. Finally, femoral sheath was removed, manual pressure was applied to control bleeding at groin puncture site. After relieving manual pressure at groin site, recheck angio of Rt limb arterial system showed good antegrade flow of CFA, SFA, popliteal, and distal leg vessels, with relief of ischemic symptoms of right leg. Hence, surgical repair of CFA and SFA was differed. Patient developed severe anemia due to groin hematoma

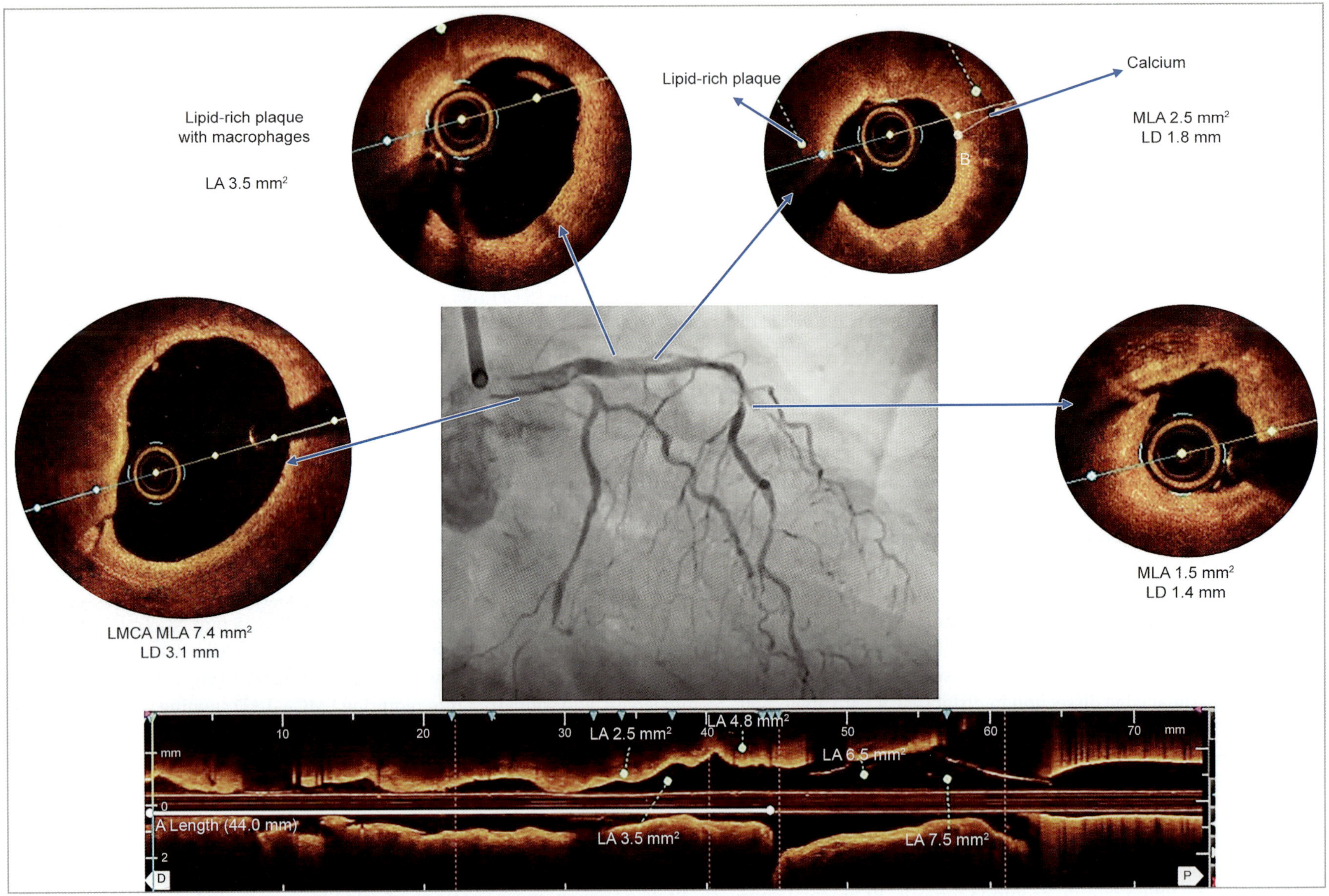

Fig. 8: Minimal lumen diameter (MLD) assessment of proximal and mid LAD. (LA: lumen area; LAD: left anterior descending; LD: lumen diameter; LMCA: left main coronary artery; MLA: minimal lumen area; OCT: optical coherence tomography)

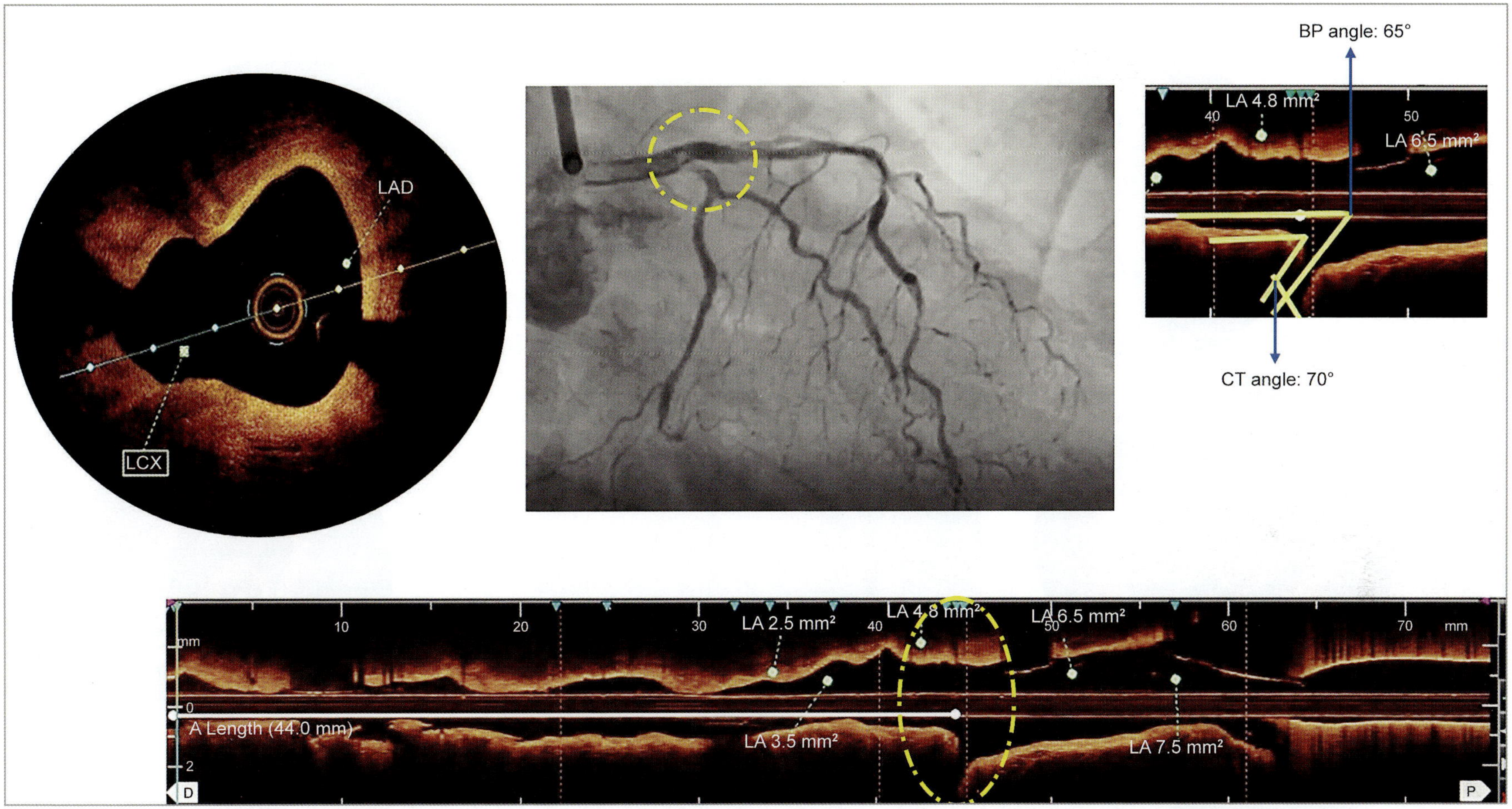

Fig. 9: Assessment of bifurcation and length of the LAD stent. (LA: lumen area; LAD: left anterior descending; LCX: left circumflex)

Bifurcation lesions	Assessment of MLA, plaque burden and extent of plaque length of MV/MB/SB
	CT angle/BP-CT length (spiky carina, eye-brow sign)

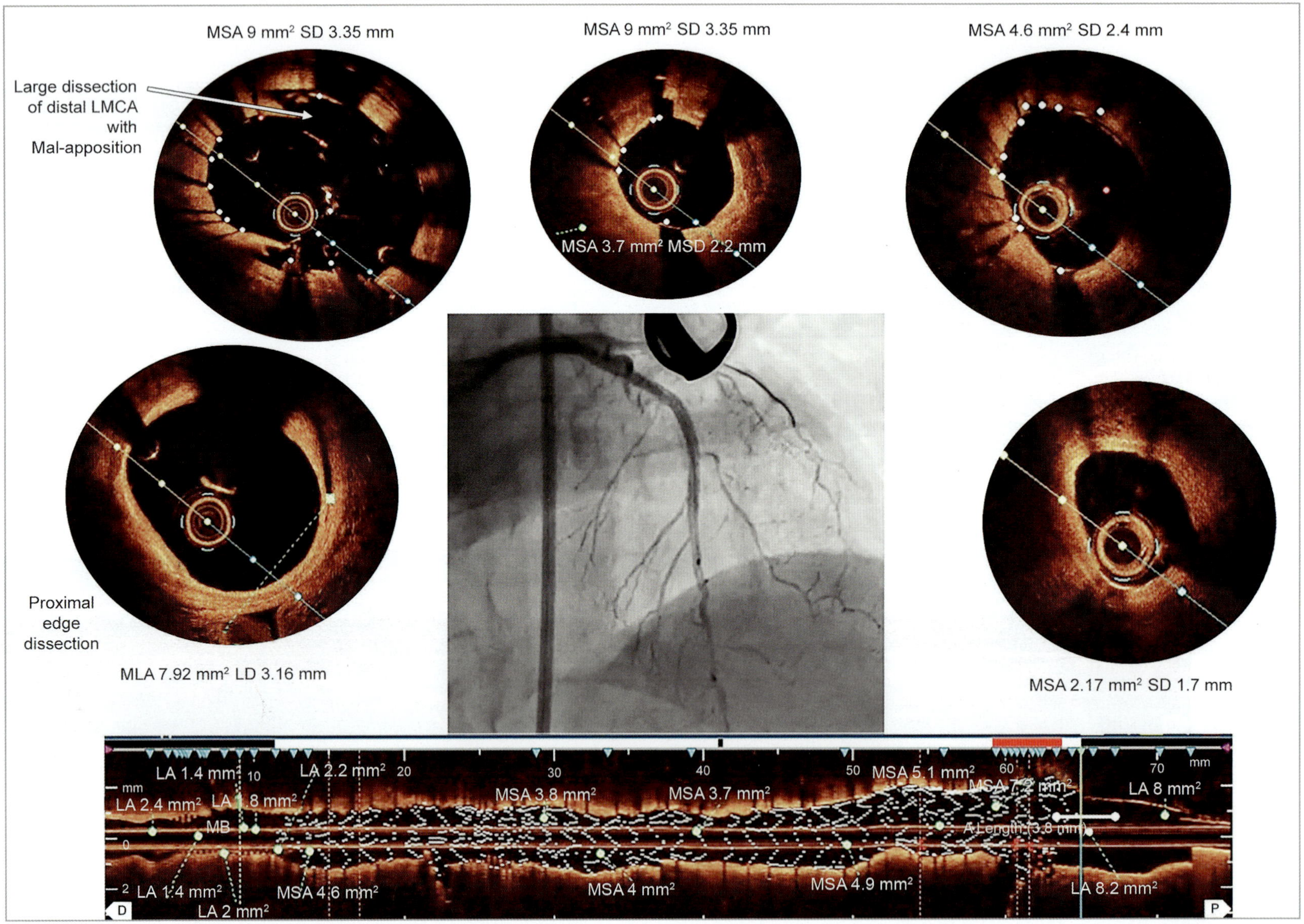

Fig. 10: Proximal edge dissection of LMCA following V-stenting of LAD and LCX—Managed with extension of stent from LAD to LM after crushing LCX stent proximal portion in LMCA. (LD: lumen diameter; LM: left main; MLA: minimal lumen area; MSA: minimal stent area; OCT: optical coherence tomography)

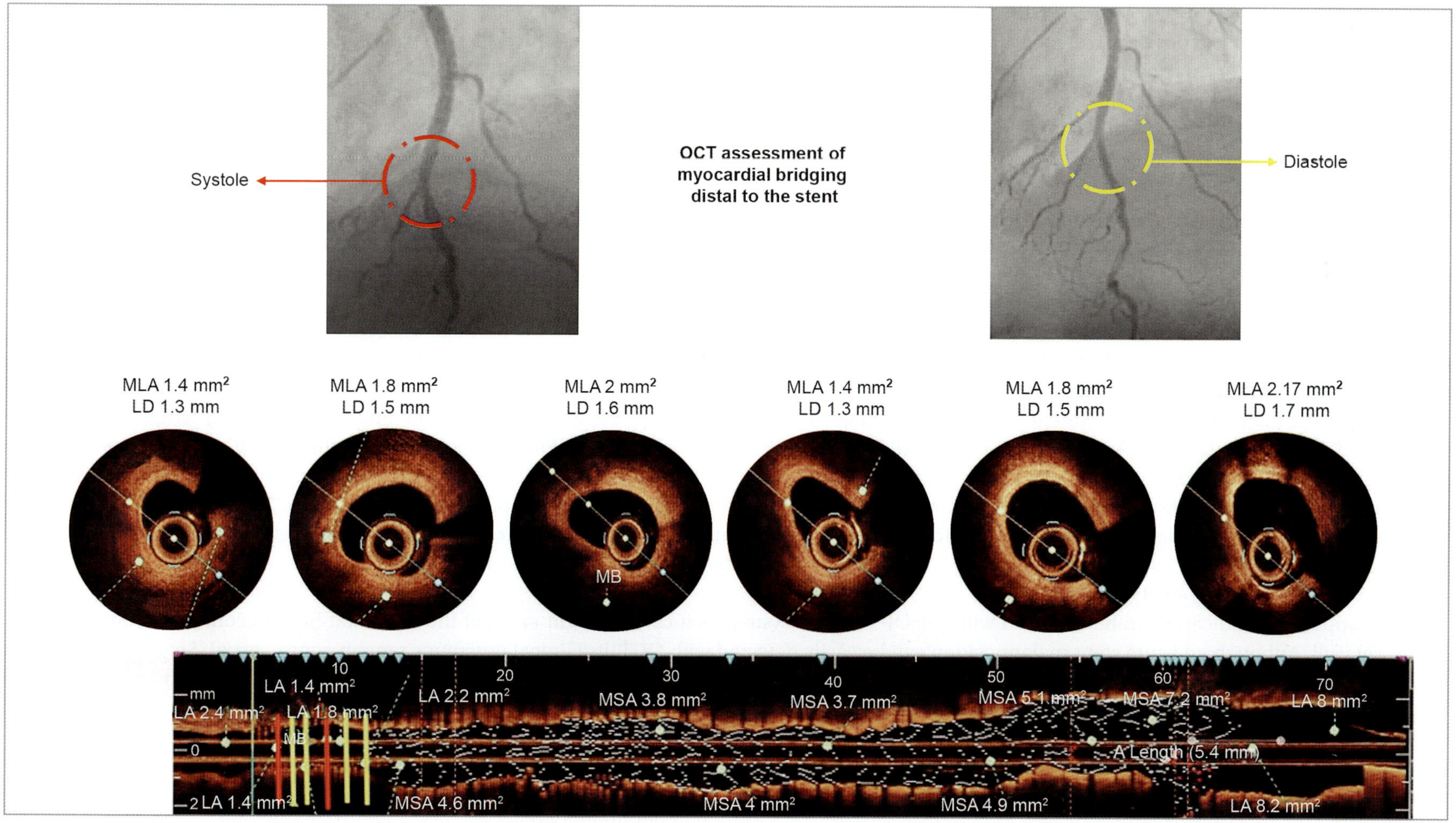

Fig. 11: OCT assessment of myocardial bridging distal to the stent. (LD: lumen diameter; MLA: minimal lumen area; MSA: minimal stent area; OCT: optical coherence tomography)

SGLT-2i and ARNI should be considered for STEMI patients with heart failure and reduced ejection fraction unless contraindicated or not tolerated well.

and FA access bleed which was corrected with 4 units of blood transfusion. Patient became stable for a period of 12 hours without any CV symptoms, shifted toward next day, but developed angina 48 hours later for which recheck angio was done, which showed well-patent stents with good antegrade flow without any thrombus or dissection. Patient was discharged on 3rd postprocedure day in a stable status.

However, OCT has several advantages for percutaneous coronary intervention (PCI) optimization. First, OCT provides more detailed features (such as the presence of thrombi, plaque erosions, and the cap thickness) of the vascular wall that intravascular ultrasound (IVUS) cannot detect. Thus, OCT is a better choice for detecting vulnerable plaque. Second, the pullback speed of OCT is faster than that of IVUS. In addition, OCT provides an automated analysis of the minimal and maximal diameters and lumen dimension of the entire area. Moreover, OCT can automatically point to the position of the minimal lumen area (MLA) in the lesion. Third, OCT can provide a more accurate assessment of the interaction with the vessel wall and stent [e.g., stent apposition, stent coverage, tissue protrusions (TPs), and edge dissections] due to its superior axial and lateral resolution power. However, IVUS overestimated the lumen area compared to OCT (relative reference 10%), suggesting that OCT might be more accurate for assessing coronary lesions than IVUS or coronary angiogram (CAG). The plaque composition may guide the implementation of a preparation strategy.

Stent edge dissections can usually be detected by OCT. However, they may not be detected by CAG. Edge dissection is defined as a linear rim of tissue adjacent to a stent edge (<5 mm) with a width of ≥200 μm. Different factors can affect the edge dissection, including the dissection depth/location/length, dissection flap angle, and residual lumen area at the dissection site.

In ILUMIEN III, edge dissections were defined as being major by OCT when they extend in an arc of >60° and were >3 mm in length based on the ADAPT-DES (Assessment of Dual Antiplatelet Therapy with Drug-Eluting Stents) registry data. Edge dissections at the distal stent edge as viewed by OCT, but not the proximal stent edge, were revealed to be an independent predictor of a MACE in the CLI-OPCI study. Overall, additional intervention may not be needed unless there is an extensive edge dissection with or without a flow limitation. Stent malapposition refers to the lack of contact of the stent struts with the vessel wall of ≥200 μm as viewed by OCT. Underexpansion and stent malapposition can coexist and can also occur independently. Moreover, malapposition can appear in different stages (acute, postprocedural, or late stage) possibly due to the underlying vascular process of inflammation and/or positive remodeling of the vessel wall.

A malapposition indicator can be accessed with the OPTIS-OCT system as it can highlight areas of the stent that have become disconnected from the vessel wall. Although an acute stent malapposition can be easily detected with OCT, its clinical outcomes remain controversial. Several studies have reported that an acute stent malapposition is not associated with adverse clinical outcomes, whereas a high frequency of malappositions has been observed in patients with acute and late-stent thromboses. Thus, when a malapposition is >500 μm, (particularly when it is continuous with a length of >1 mm) and the malapposition exhibits an underexpansion that can deteriorate into a turbulent flow, and when a malapposition occurs in the proximal stented segments that may make the reentry in the vessel difficult, an additional procedure might be needed. Nevertheless, several studies have addressed that stent malappositions of <200 μm may be acceptable for stent.

CHAPTER 6

Geographic Miss

INTRODUCTION

Coronary atherosclerosis is a diffuse process and in a majority of patients not visible angiographically. An intravascular ultrasound (IVUS) study observed significant plaque burden (PB) in the angiographically normal-appearing reference segments. Reference segment PB and lumen area have been associated with increased incidence of stent failure. In the ADAPT-DES (Assessment of Dual Antiplatelet Therapy with Drug-Eluting Stents) study, a proximal reference segment PB of >60% was associated with early-stent thrombosis.[1] Similarly, in the HORIZONS-AMI (Harmonizing Outcomes with Revascularization and Stents in Acute Myocardial Infarction) IVUS substudy, residual edge stenosis (a reference segment PB of ≥70% and a lumen area of <4 mm^2) was associated with early-stent thrombosis. In the CLI-OPCI (the Centro per la Lotta contro l'Infarto-Optimisation of Percutaneous Coronary Intervention) II study, the reference lumen area of <4.5 mm^2 in the presence of large plaque was an important predictor of major adverse cardiovascular events (MACE). In another optical coherence tomography (OCT) study, the presence of lipid-rich plaque (area >185 mm^2) and small mean lumen area (MLA) (<4.1 mm^2) predicted edge restenosis at 9–12-month follow-up. In the IVUS studies evaluating edge restenosis, the reference segment PB that predicted edge restenosis varied from 47% to 57% between different stent types. Further, reference segment injury from inappropriate stent sizing or areas of balloon injury left covered has also been associated with increased incidence of adverse events. The current consensus document recommends stent positioning in reference segments with <50% PB (IVUS) and absence of lipid-rich plaque (OCT).[2] The newer IVUS and OCT systems provide intravascular imaging (IVI) angiography coregistration function that minimizes operator errors in accurately identifying landing zones and may reduce the incidence of geographic miss **(Fig. 1)**.

OCT-MEASURED PLAQUE-FREE WALL ANGLE IS INDICATIVE FOR PLAQUE BURDEN: OVERCOMING THE MAIN LIMITATION OF OCT?

Clinical application of plaque-free wall optical coherence tomography (PFWOCT) angle detection. When a PFWOCT of ≥220° is detected in 78% of the cases, this indicates the presence of a PB <40%, forming an optimal stent landing zone **(Fig. 2)**.

The optimized cutoff value to predict optimal stent landing zone (PB <40%) is ≥220° PFWOCT. Determining an optimal stent-landing zone is critical for the prevention of future stent-related adverse events. An optimal stent-landing zone is a region without lipids and a PB <40%. In contrast to IVUS, OCT is capable of detecting lipids, but the limited penetration depth hampers PB measurements. OCT can however reliably detect the healthy vessel wall. A measurement of the PFW angle provides a reliable estimate of the PB, without the need to fully visualize the outer wall of the vessel.

Geographical miss (GM)—failure to complete cover of previously injured vessel or failure to complete coverage of the atherosclerotic plaque. GM was linked to an increased risk for target vessel revascularization (TVR) and myocardial infarction (MI) at 1 year.

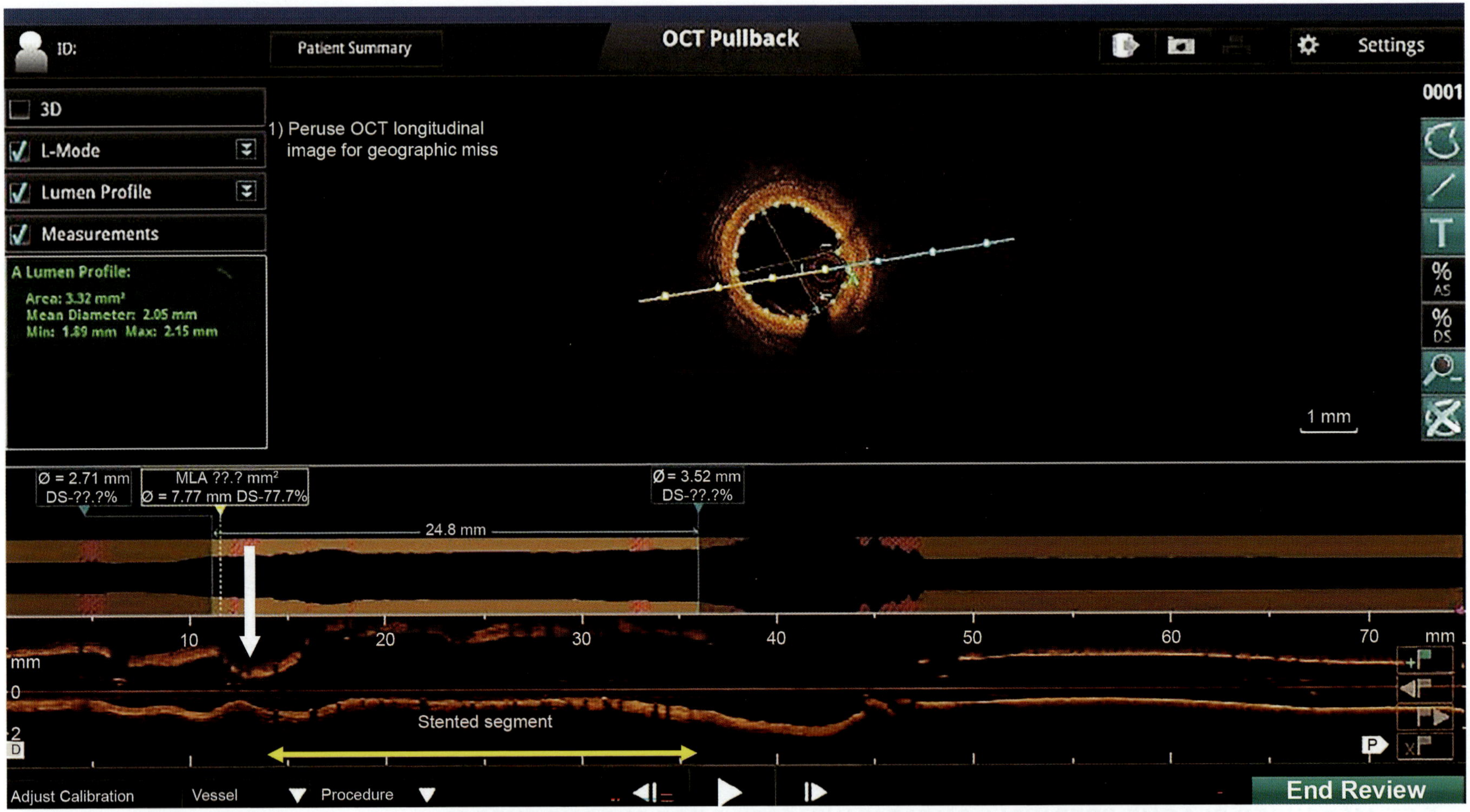

Fig. 1: Ruling out of geographic miss. (OCT: optical coherence tomography)

Patients with acute STEMI advised to control LDL-C <70 mg/dL, and a lower target of LDL-C <55 mg/dL can be considered in STEMI patients.

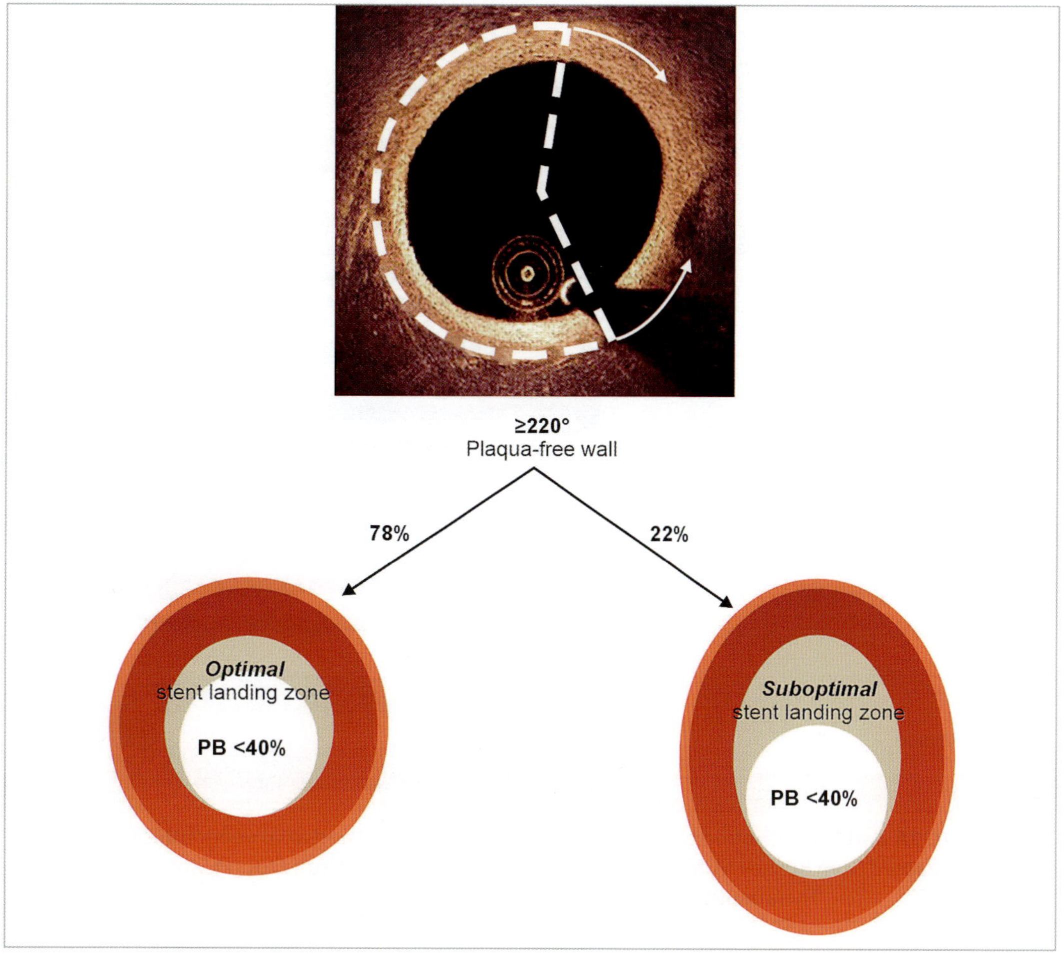

Fig. 2: Clinical application of PFWOCT angle detection. (PB: plaque burden; PFWOCT: plaque-free wall optical coherence tomography)
Source: Adapted from Hoogendoorn A, Gnanadesigan M, Zahnd G, van Ditzhuijzen NS, Schuurbiers JC, van Soest G, et al. OCT-measured plaque-free wall angle is indicative for plaque burden: overcoming the main limitation of OCT? Int J Cardiovasc Imaging. 2016;32(10):1477-81.

Optimal control of hypertension with regular home and occasional office and ambulatory BP monitoring, stressing the need for long term compliance of drug therapy with an aim to maintain BP target—<130/80 mm Hg, preferably with long acting β blocker, ACE inhibitors or ARBs, CCBs is strongly recommended to reduce risk further.

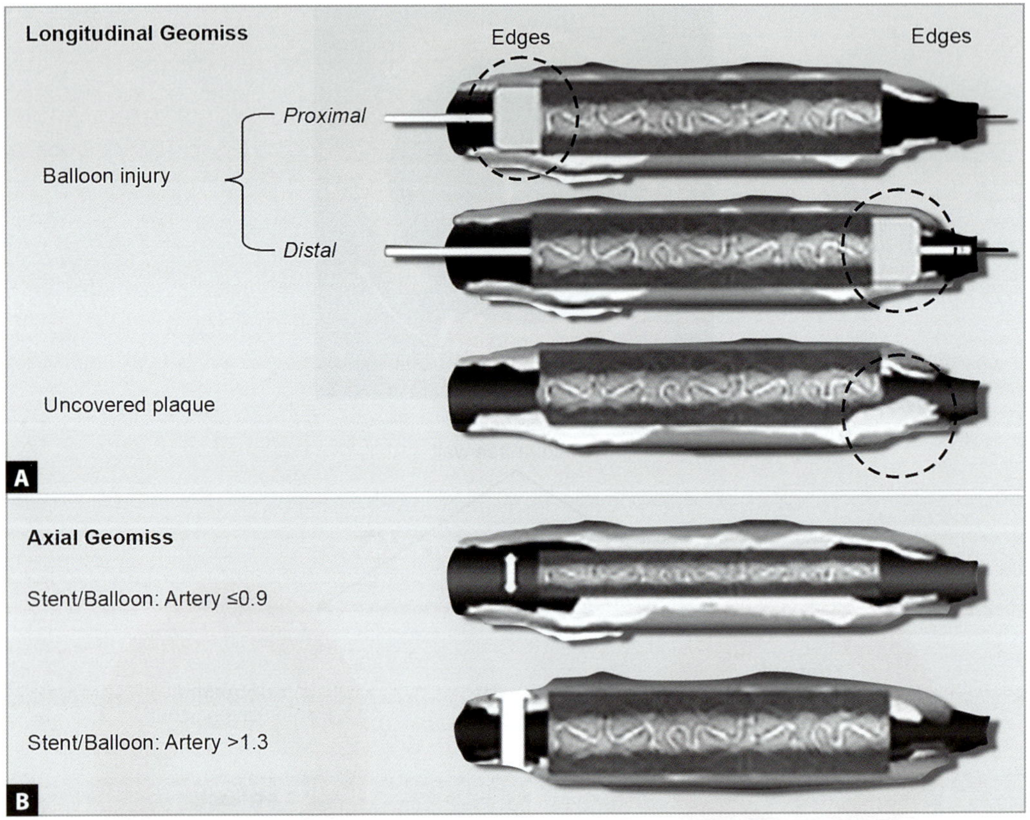

Figs. 3A and B: Description of the mechanisms of longitudinal and axial geographic miss.
Source: Adapted from Boshev M, Magdalena O. In-Stent Restenosis in Drug-Eluting Stents: Issues and Therapeutic Approach. J Cardiol Curr Res. 2016;6(3):00206.

Longitudinal GM refers to an injured or diseased segment not fully covered by drug-eluting stent (DES).

Axial GM refers to an undersized or oversized balloon.

Description of the mechanisms of longitudinal and axial GM as shown in **Figures 3A and B**.

REFERENCES

1. Maehara A, Mintz G, Witzenbichler B, Metzger DC, Rinaldi M, Mazzaferri E, et al. TCT-20 IVUS predictors of stent thrombosis: results from the prospective, multicenter ADAPT-DES study. J Am Coll Cardiol. 2012;60(17 Supplement):B6.
2. Choi SY, Witzenbichler B, Maehara A, Lansky AJ, Guagliumi G, Brodie B, et al. Intravascular ultrasound findings of early stent thrombosis after primary percutaneous intervention in acute myocardial infarction: a Harmonizing Outcomes with Revascularization and Stents in Acute Myocardial Infarction (HORIZONS-AMI) substudy. Circ Cardiovasc Interv. 2011;4(3):239-47.

CASE 1

PCI of ramus and LAD—geographical miss. (LAD: left anterior descending; PCI: percutaneous coronary intervention).

CLINICAL HISTORY

A 46-year old male, a known hypertensive, presented with anterior non-ST-elevation MI (NSTEMI) and chest pain associated with shortness of breath. Electrocardiogram (ECG)—ST depression in anterior leads, two-dimensional (2D) echo—no regional wall motion abnormality (RWMA), normal left ventricular (LV) function, and ejection fraction (EF) 60%.

Investigations: Hemoglobin (Hb) 13.8 g/dL, serum creatinine (S Cr) 0.6 mg/dL, and blood urea 23 mg/dL.

Coronary angiography-left main coronary artery (CAG-LMCA)—normal, left anterior descending (LAD)—proximal 60–70% lesion, ramus—proximal total occlusion, left circumflex (LCX) continuing as major obtuse marginal (OM), right coronary artery (RCA)—proximal 60–70% lesion, posterior descending artery (PDA) and posterior left ventricular branch (PLVB)—normal **(Figs. 4A to D)**.

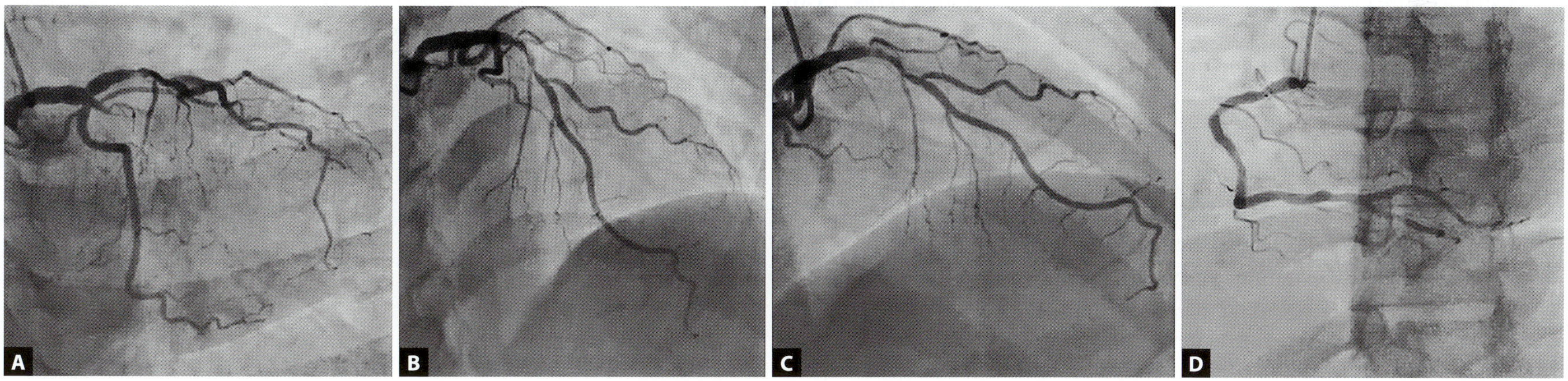

Figs. 4A to D: Coronary angiogram.

PROCEDURE

Percutaneous Coronary Intervention of Ramus

Route—right femoral artery (RFA), using 6 Fr EBU 3.5 guiding catheter, lesion was crossed with 0.014″ Sion Blue wire, predilated with 2.0 × 10 mm Tazuna balloon.

Pre-OCT showed long-segment fibrolipid plaque, tight narrowing of proximal ramus with MLA 2.0 mm^2, mean lumen diameter (MLD) 1.6 mm, distal ramus with MLA 3.8 mm^2, MLD 2.2 mm, LMCA with MLA 16.6 mm^2, MLD 4.6 mm **(Fig. 5)** and post-plain old balloon angioplasty- (POBA)-OCT image showed dissection and distally migrated thrombus **(Fig. 6)**.

Proximal ramus stenting was done with 2.5 × 22 mm Orsiro stent **(Fig. 7)**.

Poststent OCT—distal to ramus stent, there was a GM with lipid-rich plaque (about 9 mm length) **(Figs. 8 and 9)** which was covered with 2.5 × 10 mm Resolute Onyx stent to prevent future in-stent restenosis (ISR) and MACE **(Fig. 10)**.

Postprocedure angio view showed well-implanted stents with thrombolysis in MI-III (TIMI-III) flow without any dissection **(Fig. 11)**.

Percutaneous Coronary Intervention of Left Anterior Descending

Route—RFA, 6 Fr EBU 3.5 guiding catheter, LAD lesion crossed with 0.014″ Sion Blue wire and D1 lesion crossed with 0.014″ Powerturn wire. Predilatation done with 2.0 × 12 mm Mini Trek balloon. Stenting done with 3.0 × 44 mm Vivo ISAR stent. Postdilatation done with 3.5 × 15 mm noncompliant (NC) Trek balloon **(Figs. 12A to D)**.

Postprocedure OCT showed malapposition in proximal stent **(Figs. 13 and 14)**.

Postdilatation done with 3.5 × 15 mm NC Trek balloon. Postprocedure angio view showed well-implanted stents with TIMI-III flow without any dissection. Patient was discharged on third postprocedure day in a stable status.

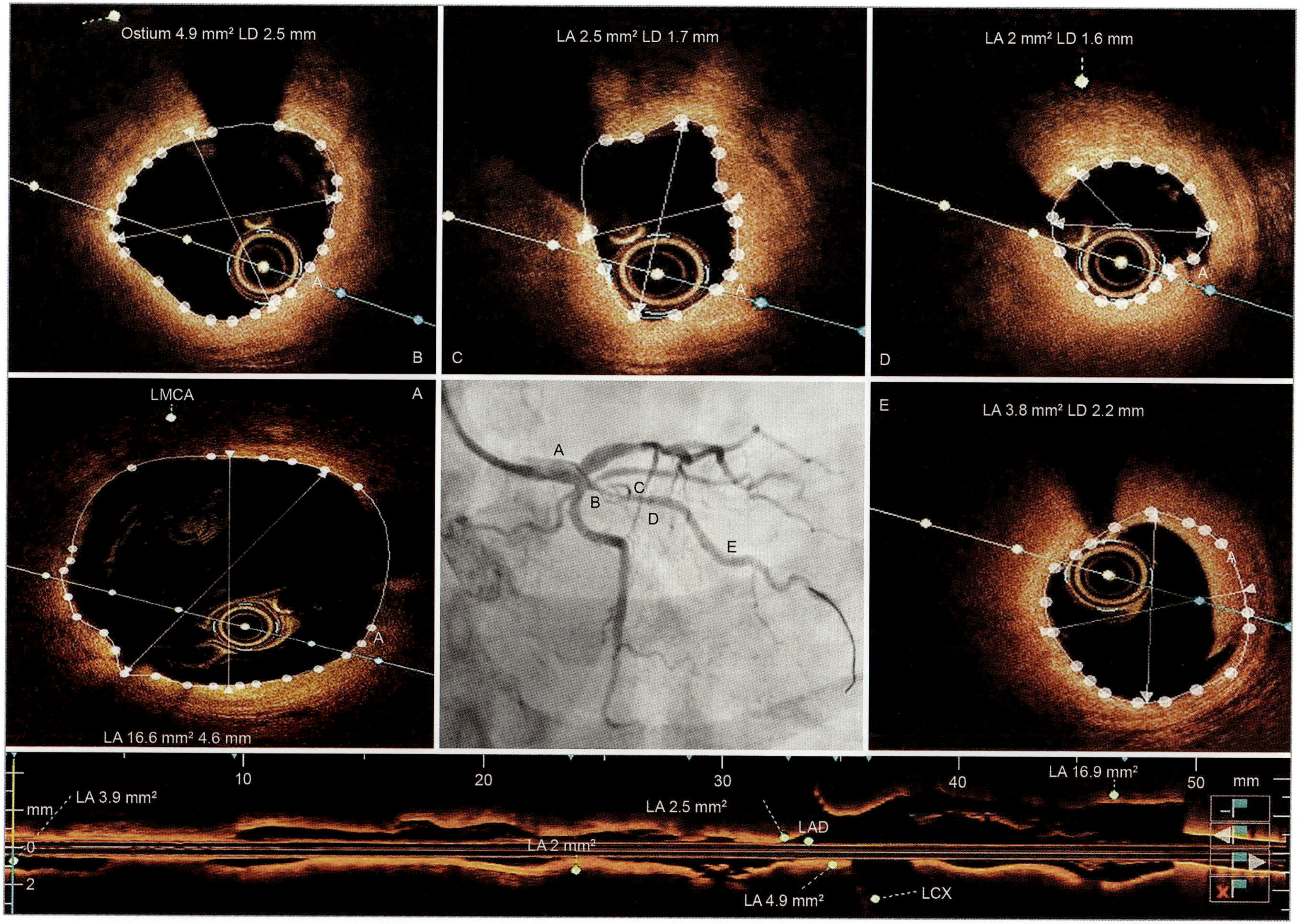

Fig. 5: MLD assessment of ramus-fibrous plaque. (LA: lumen area; LCX: left circumflex; LD: lumen diameter; OCT: optical coherence tomography)

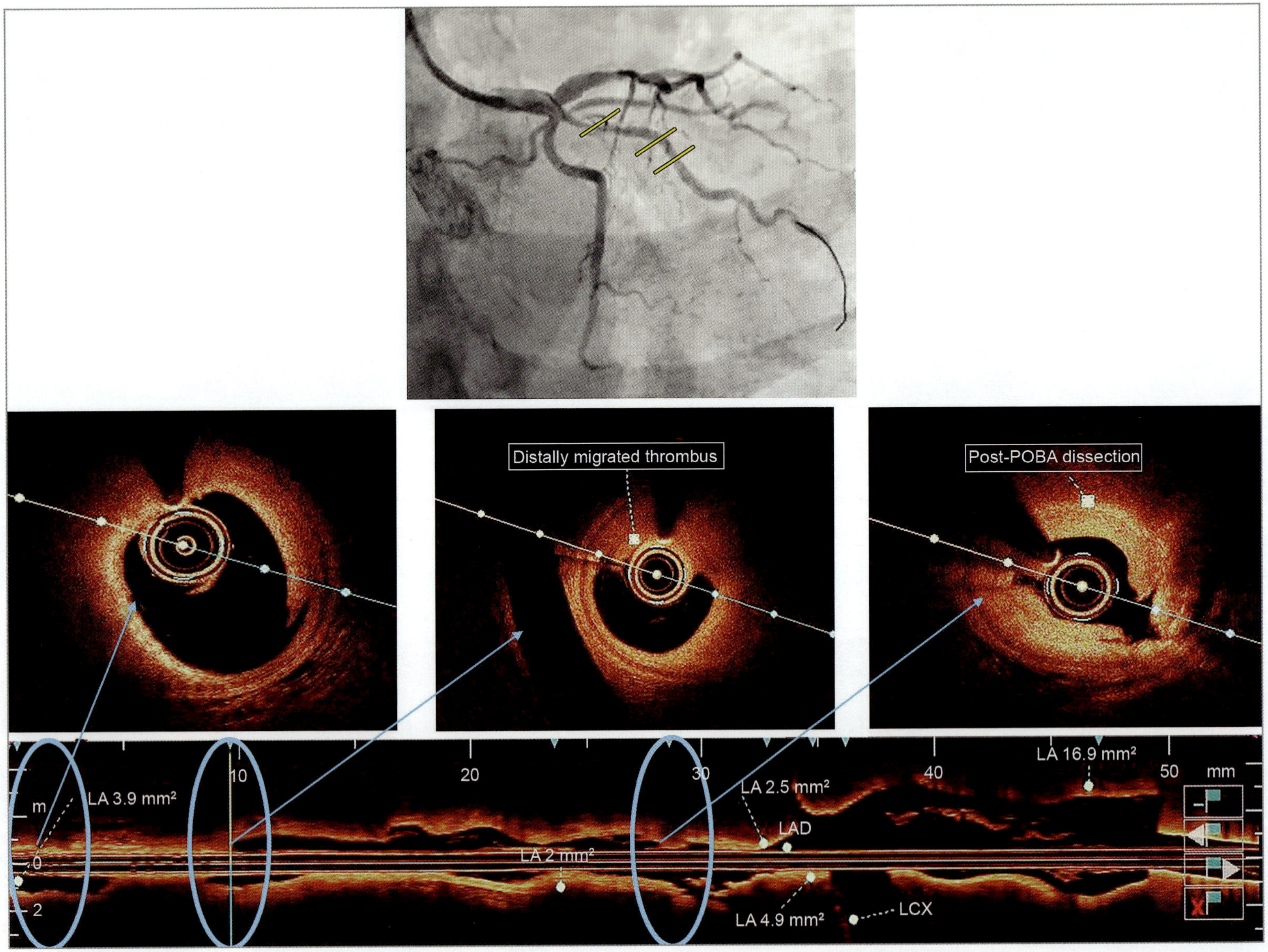

Fig. 6: Assessment of plaque morphology of ramus. (LA: lumen area; LAD: left anterior descending; LCX: left circumflex; POBA: plain old balloon angioplasty)

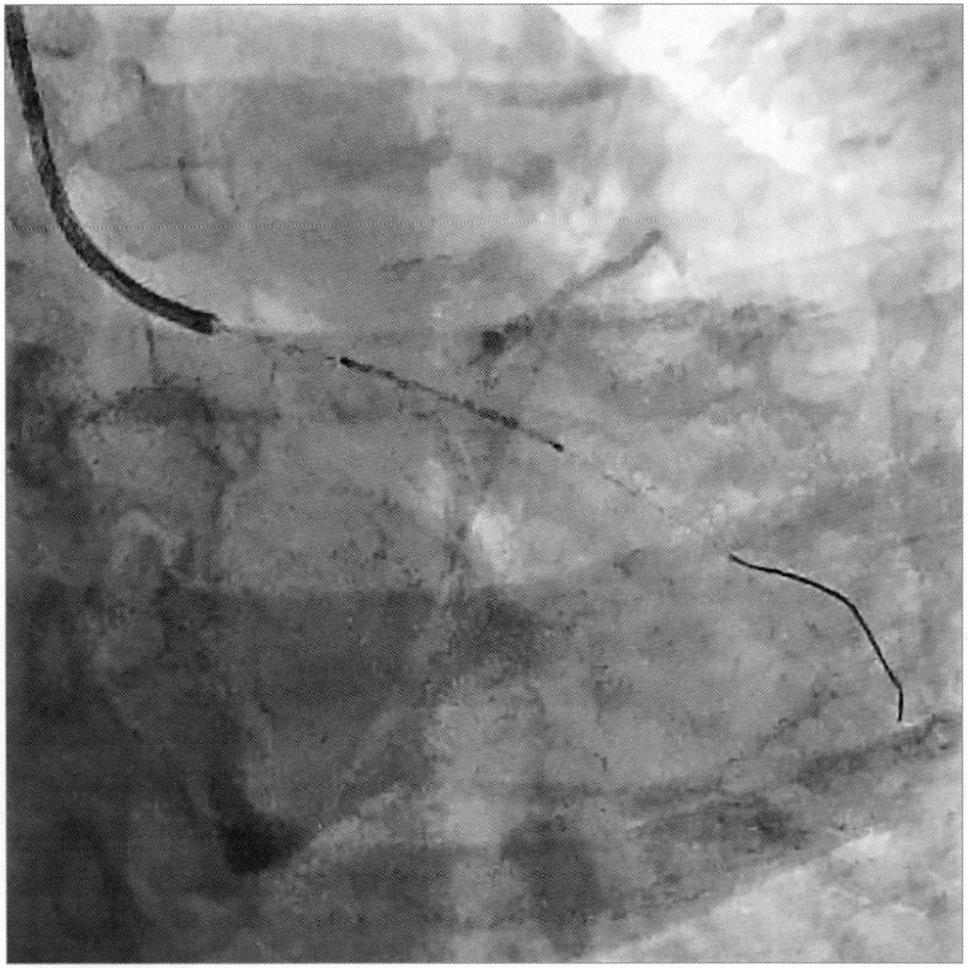

Fig. 7: Coronary angioplasty of ramus.

Adequate LDL-C control should achieved by statin plus non-statin therapies, including ezetimibe, Bempodoic acid, PCSK9i or Inclisiran with full consideration of clinical benefit vs side effects, patient's tolerance, long term drug compliance and cost effectiveness of treatment.

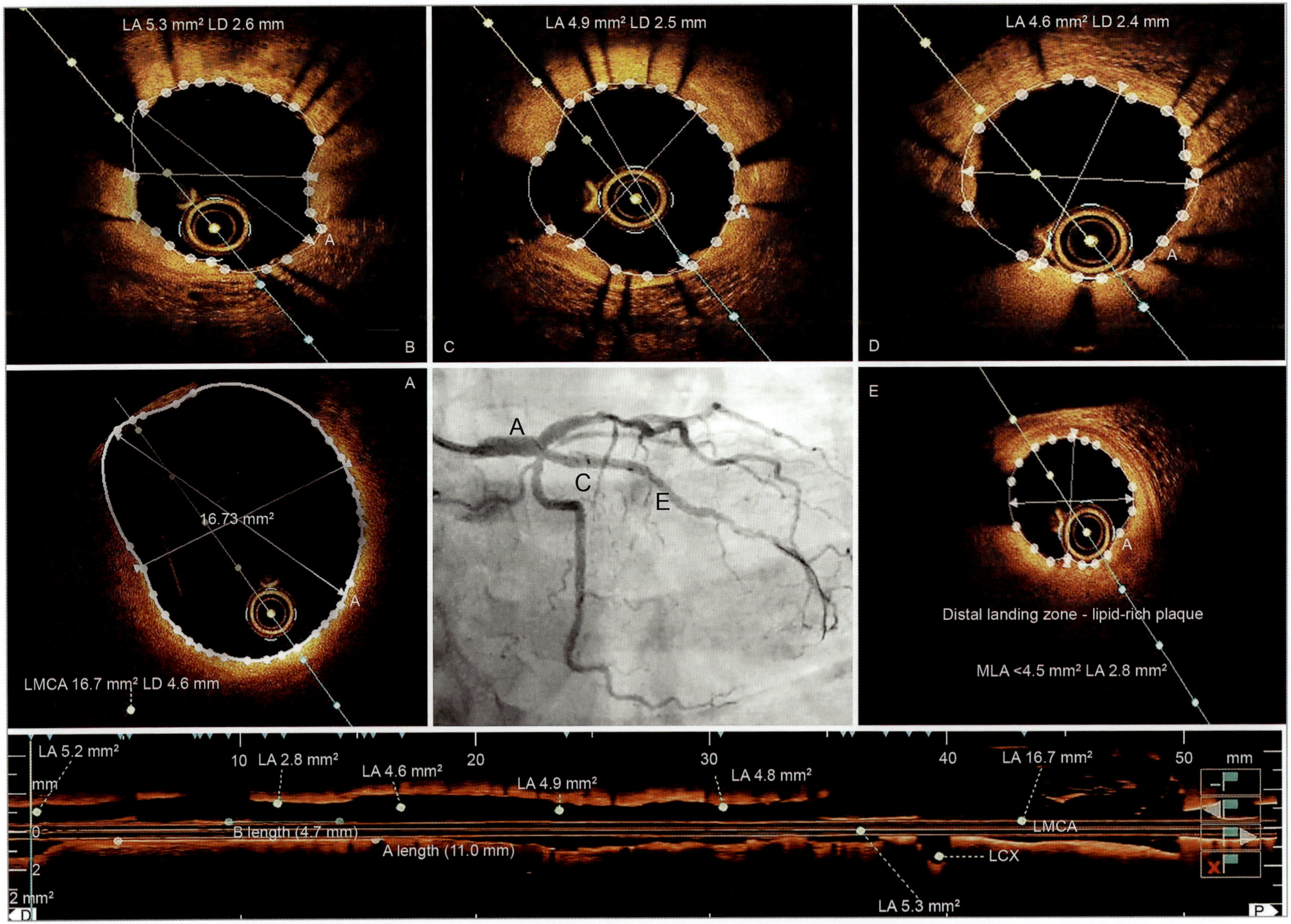

Fig. 8: Post ramus stenting—MAX assessment showed poor landing zone. (LA: lumen area; LCX: left circumflex; LD: lumen diameter; LMCA: left main coronary artery; MLA: mean lumen area; OCT: optical coherence tomography)

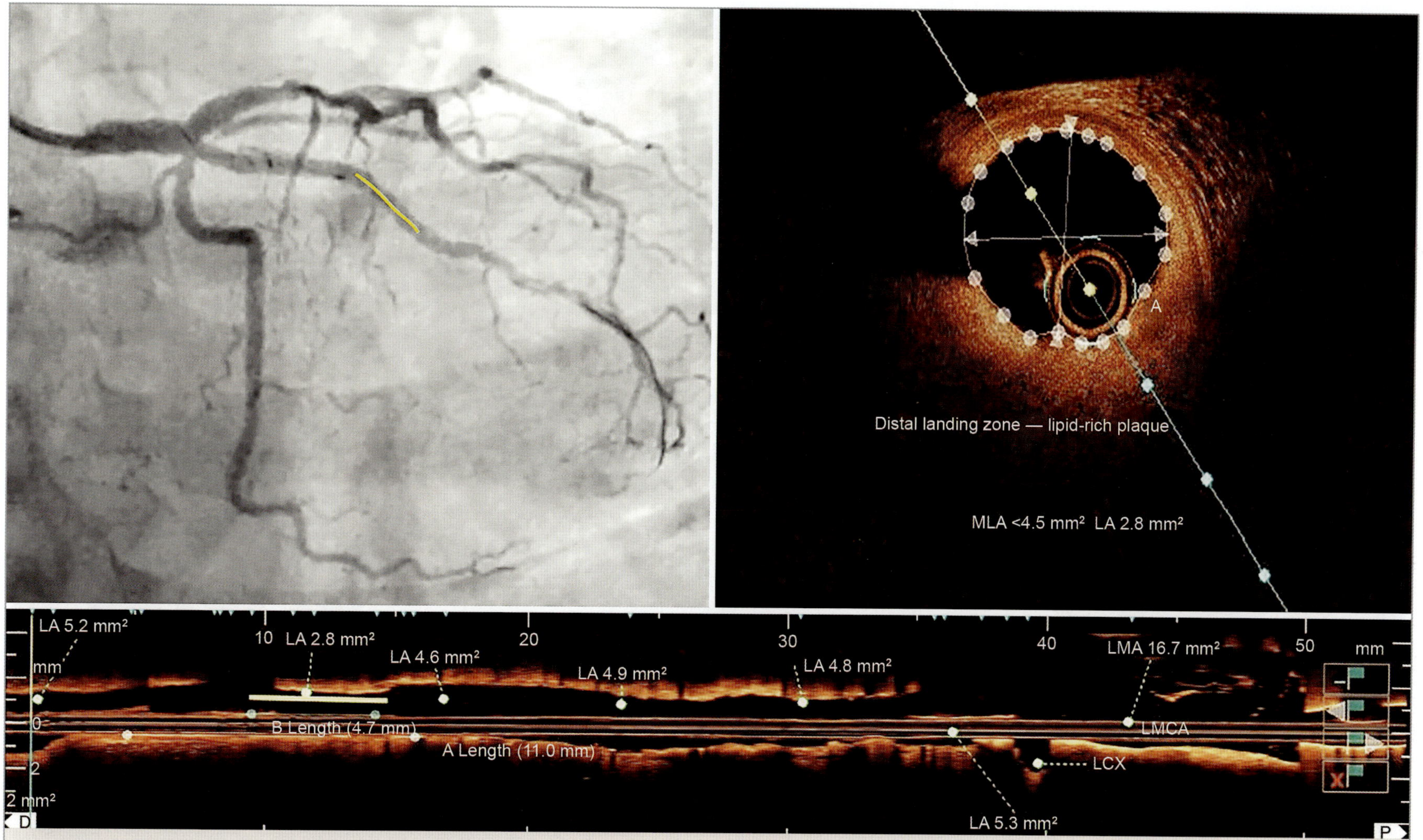

Poststent OCT - Distal landing zone (Geographical miss) of RAMUS stent, 8–9 mm lesion with lipid-rich plaque, covered with 2.5 x 12 mm Resolute Onyx stent to prevent future ISR and MACE.

Fig. 9: Geographical miss at distal landing zone covered with additional stent. (ISR: in-stent restenosis; LA: lumen area; LCX: left circumflex; LMA: left marginal artery; LMCA: left main coronary artery; MACE: major adverse cardiovascular event; MLA: mean lumen area; OCT: optical coherence tomography)

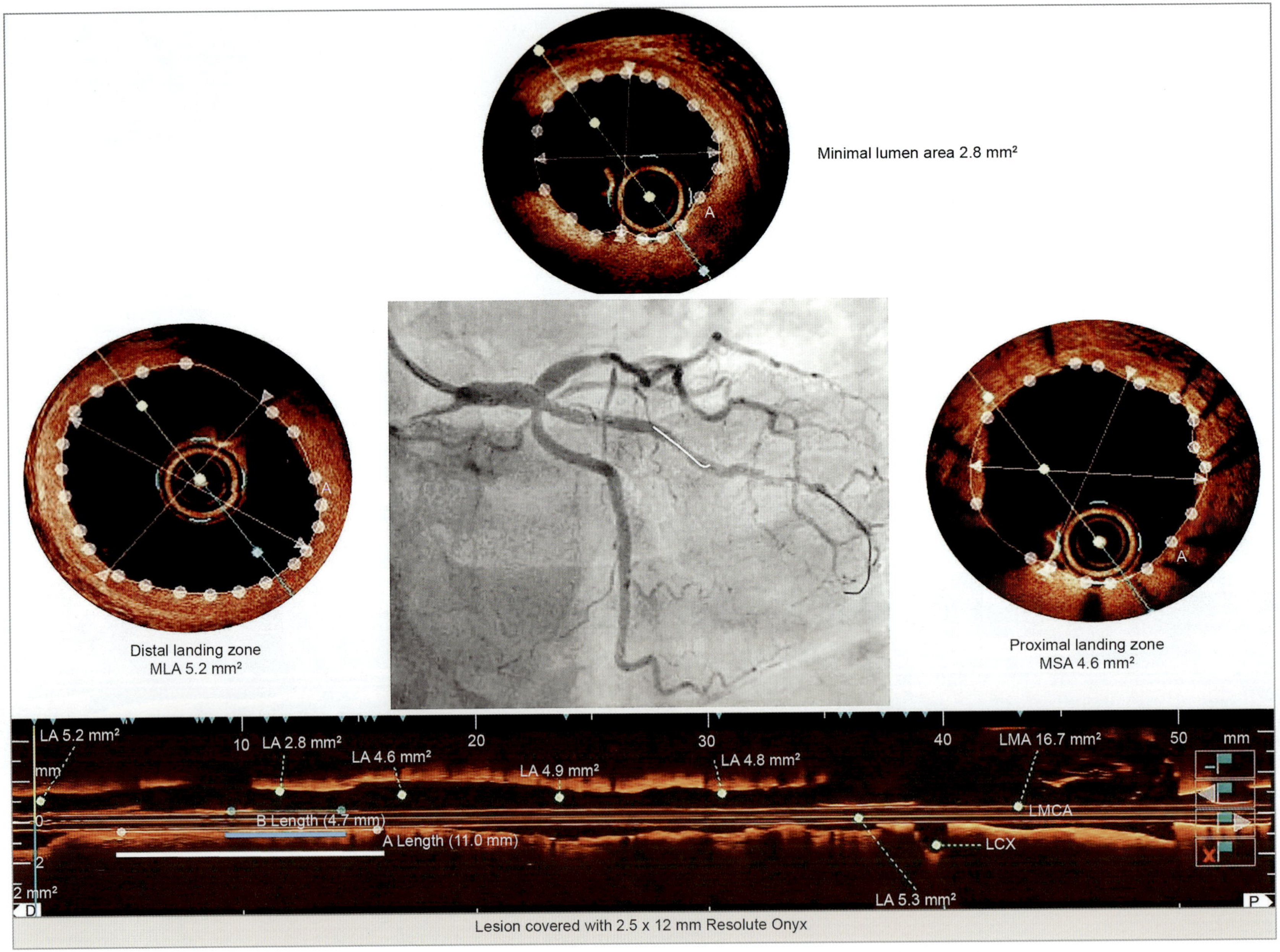

Fig. 10: Correction of geographical miss. (LA: lumen area; LCX: left circumflex; LMA: left marginal artery; LMCA: left main coronary artery; MLA: mean lumen area; MSA: mean stent area)

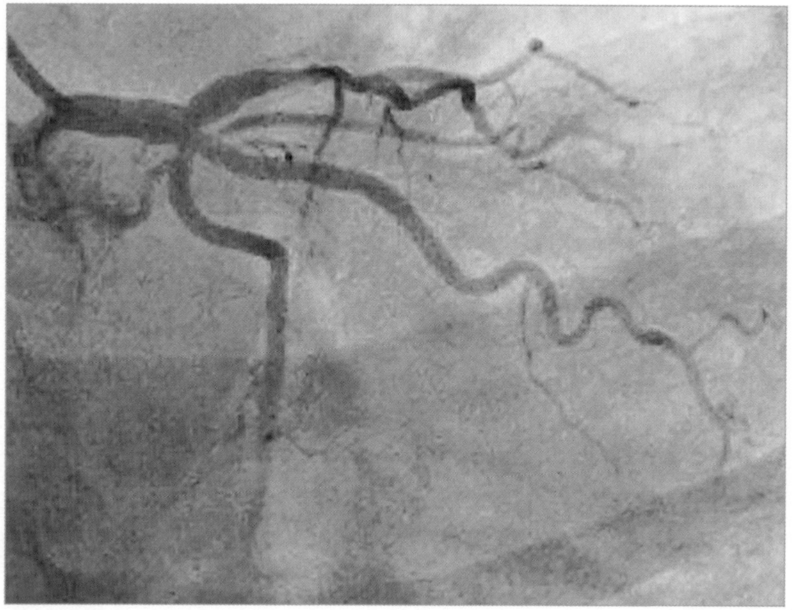

Fig. 11: Final result.

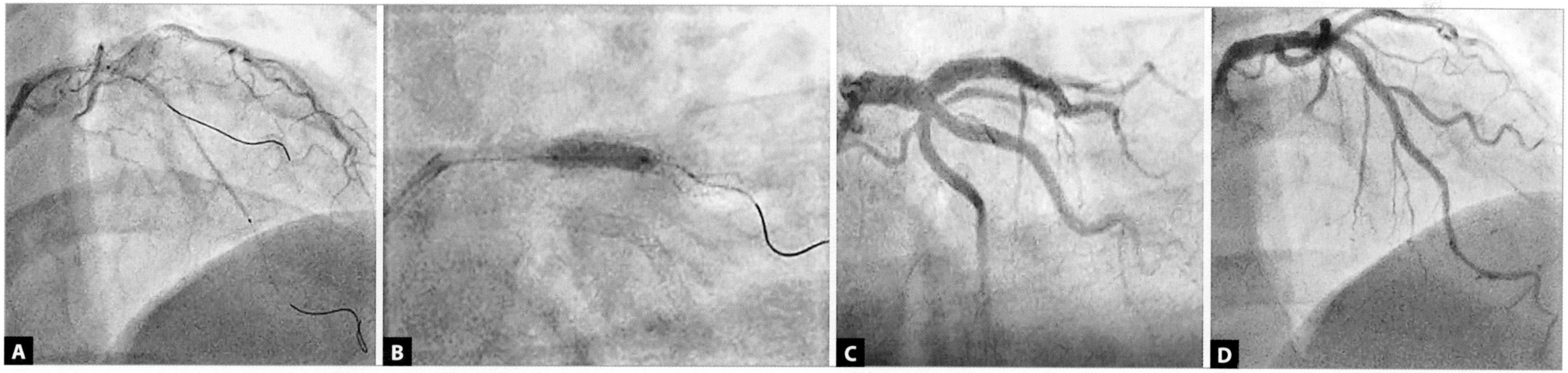

Figs. 12A to D: Coronary angioplasty of left anterior descending (LAD).

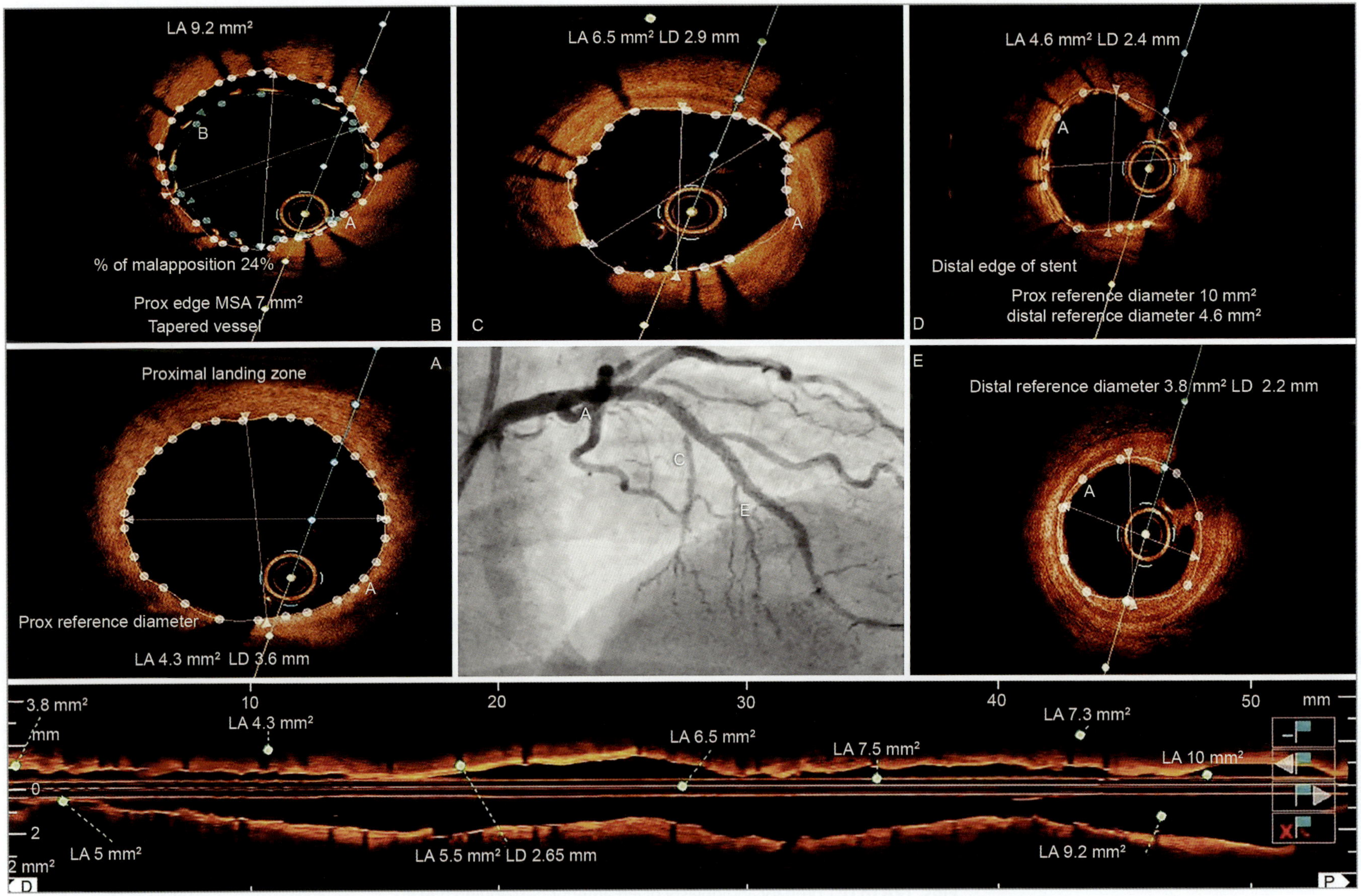

Fig. 13: Poststenting OCT assessment of LAD - MAX assessment of ramus after additional distal stenting. (LA: lumen area; LAD: left anterior descending; LD: lumen diameter; MSA: mean stent area; OCT: optical coherence tomography; Prox: proximal)

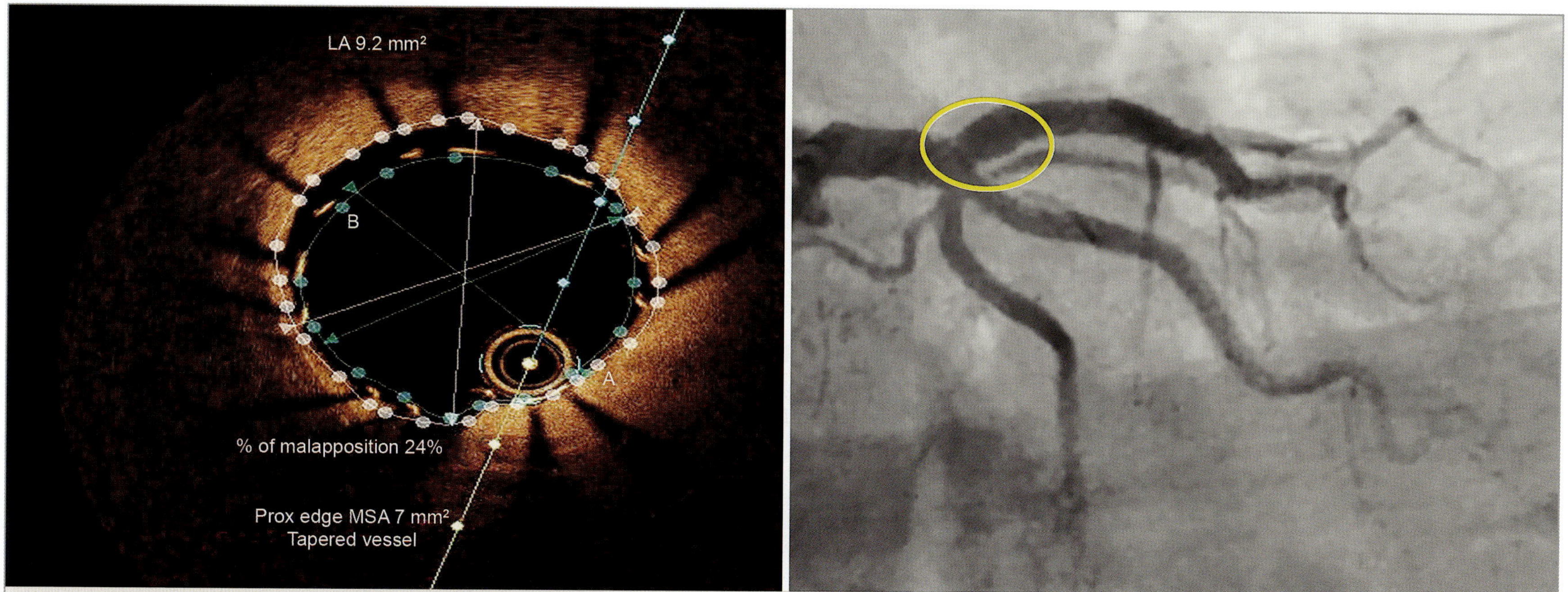

Poststent OCT showed malapposition of the proximal stent (%–24%), corrected with 3.5 x 15 mm NC trek balloon

Fig. 14: Poststent OCT assessment showed malapposition of the proximal stent which was corrected with NC balloon. (LA: lumen area; MSA: mean stent area; NC: noncompliant; OCT: optical coherence tomography)

IVI helps in assessing plaque burden, type of plaque, and vulnerability to rupture, functional significance of the lesion, reference segments, stent size, landing zones, and helps in optimizing DES implantation.

CASE 2

PCI of LAD—assessment of poststenting borderline lesion of proximal landing zone. (PCI: percutaneous coronary intervention; LAD: left anterior descending)

CLINICAL HISTORY

A 74-year old male, a known hypertensive, diabetic, and having bronchial asthma, presented with anterior NSTEMI and chest pain associated with shortness of breath. ECG—ST depression in anterior leads. 2D Echo—mild hypokinesia of LV apex, normal LV function, and EF 62%.

Coronary angiography-LMCA—normal, LAD—proximal 50% lesion, mid 90% lesion, LCX—normal, RCA—distal 30–40% lesion, PDA and PLVB—normal, right ventricular (RV) branch 60–70% lesion **(Figs. 15A and B)**.

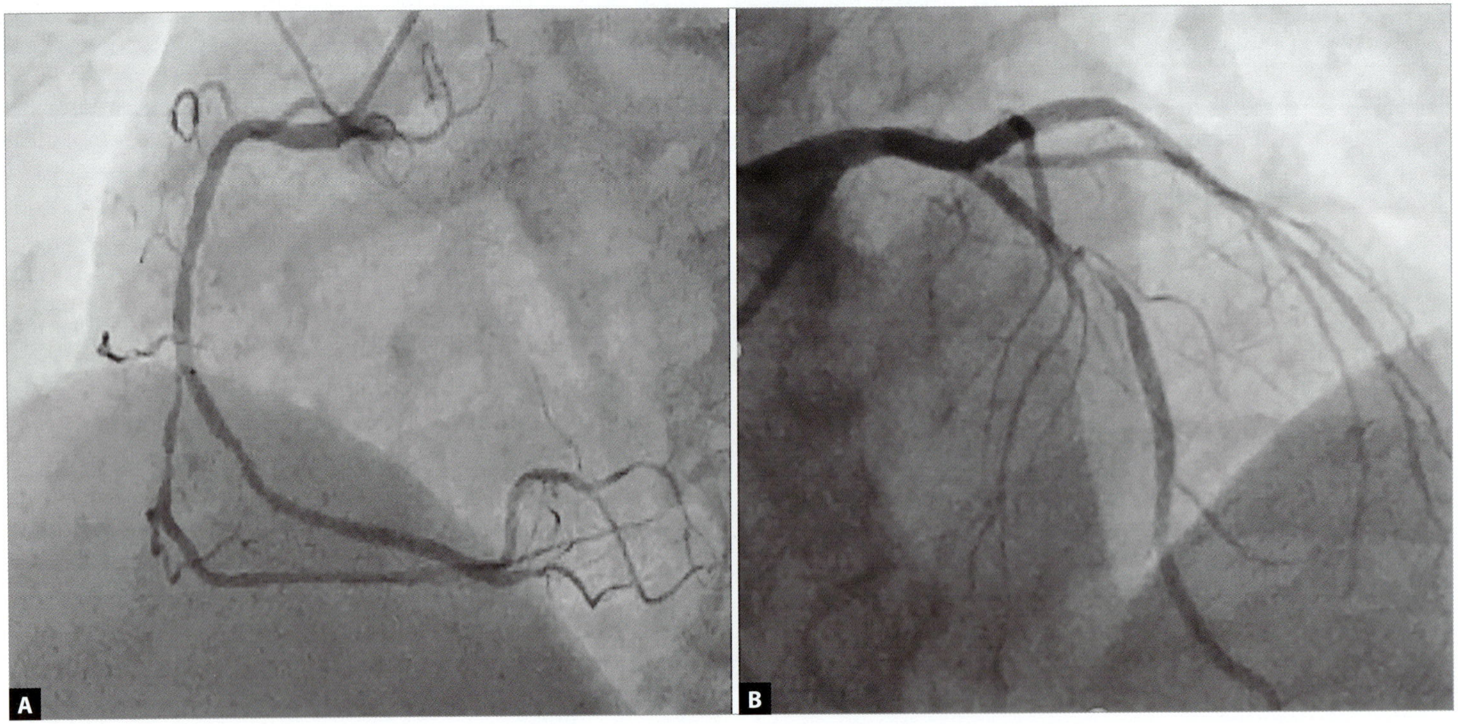

Figs. 15A and B: Coronary angiogram.

PROCEDURE

Route—right radial access (RRA), 6 Fr EBU 3.5 guiding catheter, LAD lesion crossed with 0.014″ Runthrough wire and D1 lesion crossed with Powerturn wire. Predilatation of LAD with 2.0 × 15 mm Tazuna balloon. Mid-LAD stenting with 3.5 × 28 mm Xience Xpedition stent. Postdilatation with 3.0 × 12 mm NC Trek balloon. Poststenting angio showed 50% lesion of proximal LAD.

Post-mid LAD stenting angio showed 50% lesion of proximal LAD. OCT assessment showed thin-cap fibroatheroma (TCFA) with PB of 61% in proximal landing zone; hence, proximal LAD stenting extending from ostium of LAD with overlap of mid-LAD stent was done with 3.5 × 18 mm Xience Xpedition stent, length of the uncovered proximal LAD segment 14.7 mm, distal landing zone of proximal LAD stent—external elastic luminal diameter (ELD) 3.43 × 3.56 mm **(Figs. 16 and 17)**.

Poststenting OCT—well-apposed and well-expanded stent struts without any residual stenosis/edge dissections/thrombosis **(Fig. 18)**.

Postprocedure angio view showed well-implanted stents with TIMI-III flow without any dissection. Patient was discharged on third postprocedure day in a stable status.

Selection of landing zones prior to stent implantation is very important to get best long-term outcomes. If stent edges land in diseased segments with PB >50% is associated with increased ISR due to edge restenosis. Avoid landing zones, especially disease segments with lipid-rich plaques (TCFA-containing plaques), to decrease incidents of future restenosis. Landing zones with calcium >71% and fibrous PB >50% are associated with increased with edge dissection which may contribute to increase in stent thrombosis and ISR.

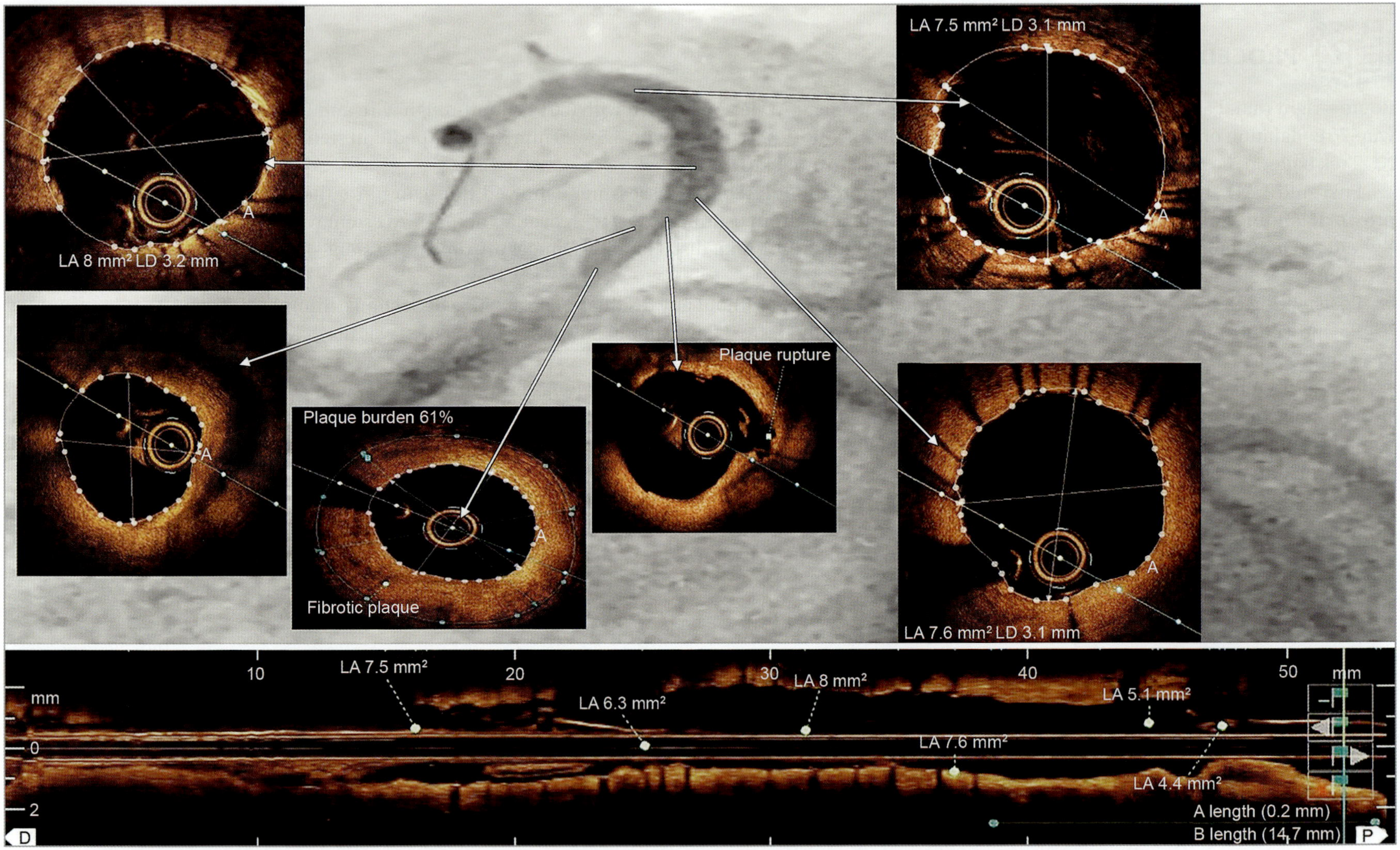

Fig. 16: Poststenting OCT showed more plaque burden proximal to stent. (LA: lumen area; LD: lumen diameter; OCT: optical coherence tomography)

All diabetics should be recommended to control HbA1c <7% in, and The target of HbA1c could be individualized according to patient's condition (<6.5% to <8%). Metformin is recommended as the first-line therapy, and preferable to start early add-on therapy includes SGLT-2i and GLP-1 RA due to well proven cardiovascular beneficial efficacy and safety as evident in recent studies.

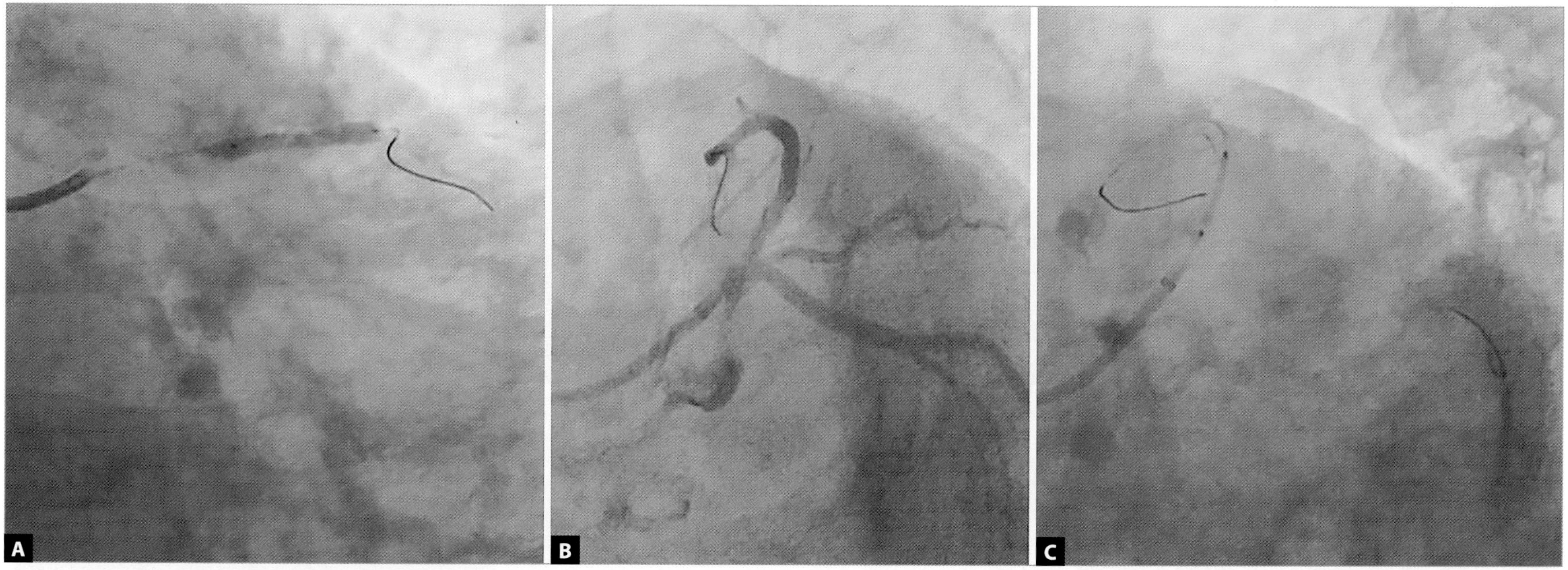

Figs. 17A to C: Coronary angioplasty: (A) Mid-left anterior descending (LAD) stenting done with 3.5 × 28 mm Xience Xpedition stent; (B) poststenting check angio; and (C) proximal LAD stenting done with 3.5 × 18 mm Xience Xpedition stent.

OCT catheter kinking → Slowly remove device or wire and OCT device together totally.

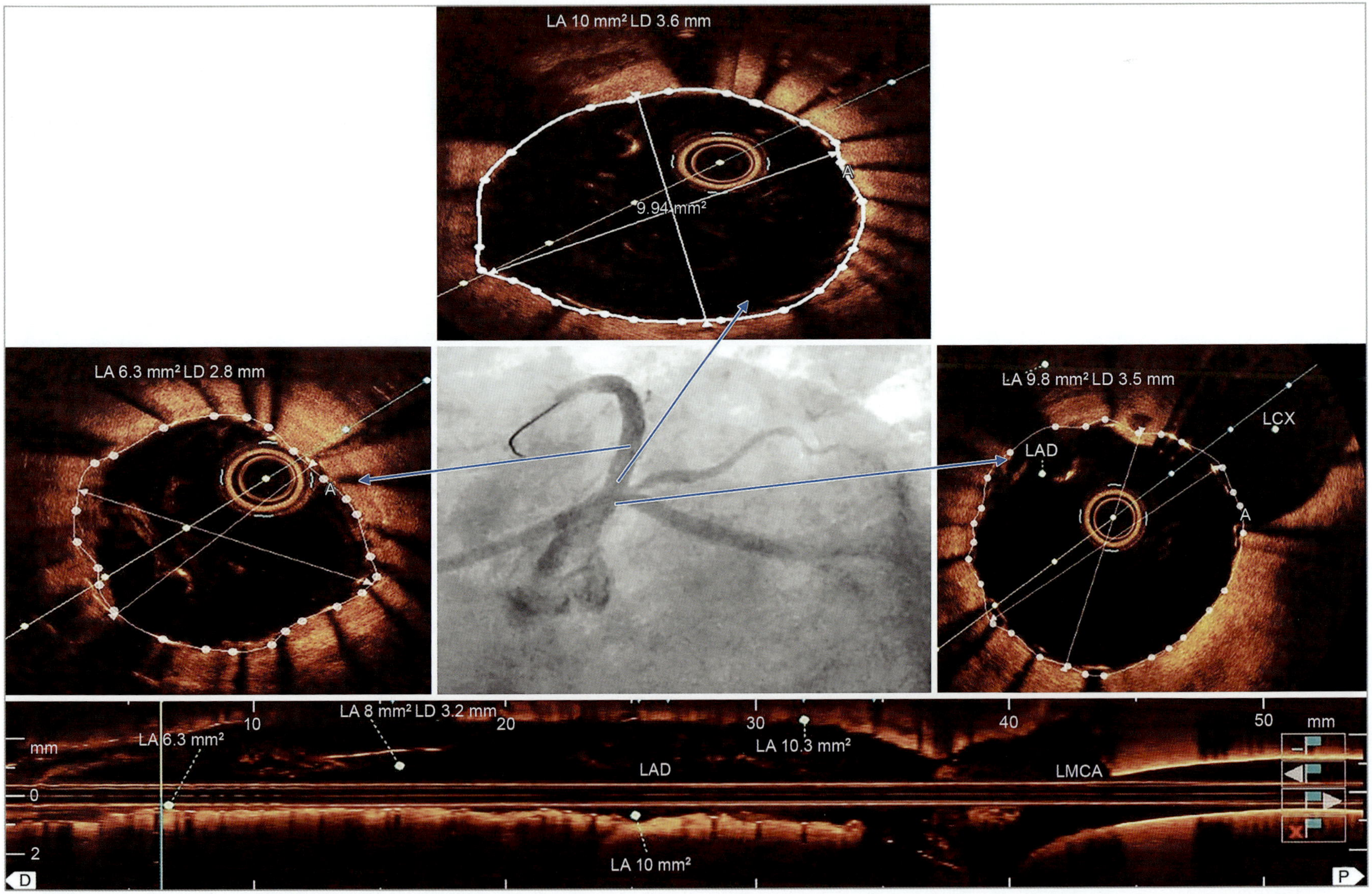

Fig. 18: Poststenting OCT assessment for any medial edge dissections, expansion and apposition of stent struts. (LA: lumen area; LAD: left anterior descending; LCX: left circumflex; LD: lumen diameter; LMCA: left main coronary artery; OCT: optical coherence tomography)

CHAPTER 7

ST-elevation Myocardial Infarction: Acute Coronary Syndrome

ABSTRACT

Acute coronary syndromes (ACS) are associated with high morbidity and mortality, develop from acute thrombus formation secondary to plaque rupture (55–60% of cases) or plaque erosion (30–35%) or eruptive calcium nodule (2–7%). About 17–20% cases of acute coronary syndromes are due to other etiologies such as subocclusive stenosis, recanalized thrombus, spontaneous coronary dissection, coronary embolism, and coronary spasm. Optical coherence tomography (OCT) is useful in assessing morphological features of plaques to differentiate various subsets of ACS thereby guides in the appropriate management decisions.

INTRODUCTION

Optical coherence tomography (OCT) is very useful for acute coronary syndrome (ACS) patients with acute onset of angina and SOB, mainly to assess plaque morphology and etiology of ACS nature. ACS is mainly due to plaque rupture, plaque erosion, eruptive calcific nodule with thrombus, spontaneous coronary artery dissection (SCAD), recanalized thrombus, etc. it is useful to detect the site of lesion, assessing the mean luminal areas, quantification of thrombus, and helpful in differentiating white thrombus and red thrombus. Management of ACS depends upon underlying etiology **(Box 1, Flowcharts 1 and 2, and Figs. 1A and B and Fig. 2A)**.[1]

PATHOLOGY OF CULPRIT LESIONS IN ACUTE CORONARY SYNDROME (FIGS. 1 AND 2A)

Plaque rupture- of ST-elevation myocardial infarction (STEMI) is seen as a presence of fibrous-cap discontinuity with underlying cavity with large lipid-rich plaque with thin-cap fibroatheroma (TCFA). These are associated with a greater extent of cap disruption and a smaller minimal lumen area compared with non-STEMI patients with ruptured plaques. Patients of STEMI is more often associated with "proximal-type" of rupture of the fibrous cap, contrary to "distal-type" of ruptures of non-STEMI patients.

Plaque erosion: Plaque erosion (PE) is visible as evidence of thrombi with an irregular luminal surface. The characteristic of OCT features of erosions is a thick intima without cap rupture and a small or absent lipid core. If the lipid core is present, it does not communicate with luminal thrombi.[2]

BOX 1: OCT for ACS.

- Detects and quantifies thrombus at the culprit site.
- Defines plaque morphology in ACS and guides the appropriate therapy.
- Very useful in ambiguous or borderline lesions to diagnose rare causes such as SCAD, recanalized thrombus, MINOCA and embolism, etc.

(ACS: acute coronary syndrome; MINOCA: myocardial infarction with nonobstructive coronary arteries; OCT: optical coherence tomography; SCAD: spontaneous coronary artery dissection)

Flowchart 1: Unstable plaque morphology by optical coherence tomography (OCT).

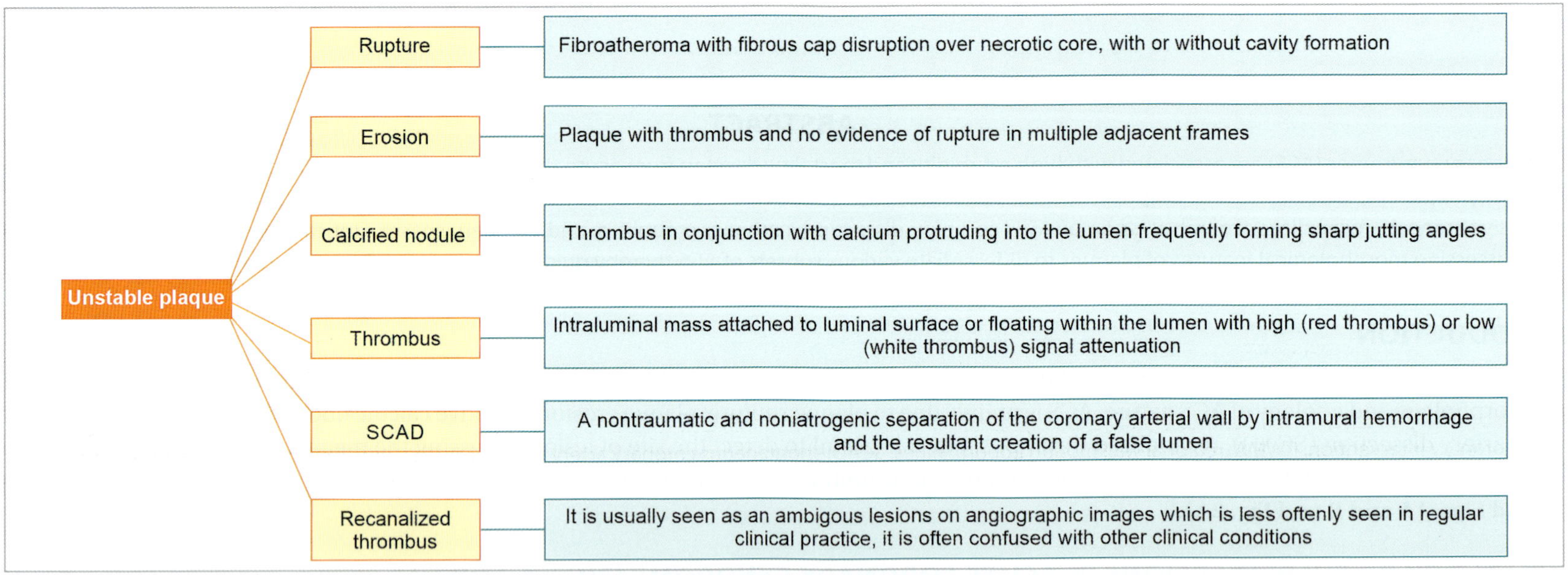

(SCAD: spontaneous coronary artery dissection)

Calcified nodule: OCT shows it as a protrusion of a signal—poor or heterogeneous region with a sharply delineated border. These are more often present with non-STEMI and seen in more often patients with advanced age, chronic kidney disease (CKD), longstanding uncontrolled diabetes, and postcoronary artery bypass grafting (CABG) status.[3,4]

Plaque rupture releases prothrombogenic substrates leading to recurrent local thrombosis and distal embolization, decreases coronary microcirculation, and these are usually associated with worse outcomes after stenting and higher frequency of distal embolization. Patients of PE are associated with less severe obstruction, a less superficial necrotic core, and a smaller plaque burden. However, thrombus in PE is generally due to apoptosis or denudation of superficial endothelial cells and is rich in platelets **(Fig. 2B)**.

Flowchart 2: A treatment algorithm to guide the use of intravascular OCT imaging in patients presenting with acute coronary syndromes.

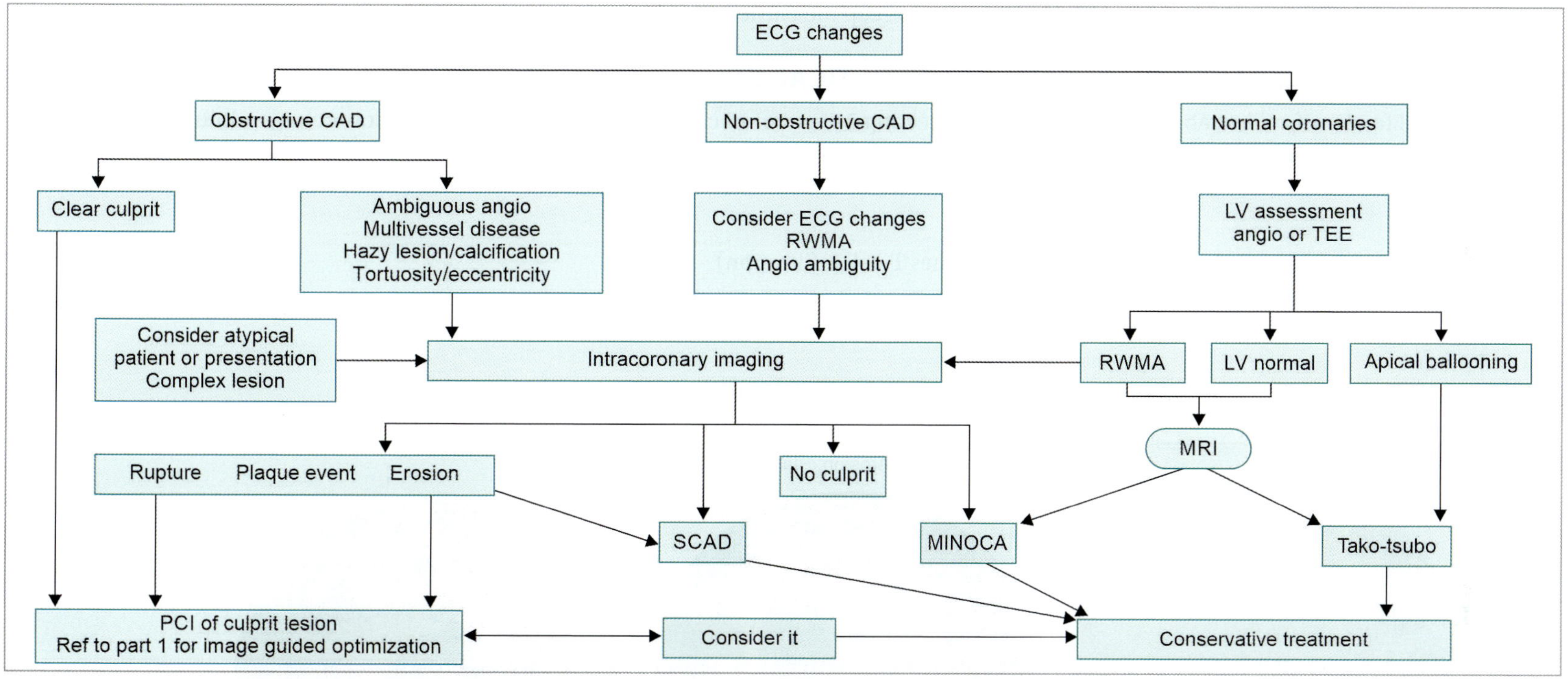

(CAD: coronary artery disease; LV: left ventricular; MINOCA: myocardial infarction with nonobstructive coronary arteries; OCT: optical coherence tomography; PCI: percutaneous coronary intervention; RWMA: regional wall motion abnormalities; SCAD: spontaneous coronary artery dissection; TEE: transesophageal echocardiography)

THROMBUS EVALUATION

OCT assessment of red thrombus is more accurate, and it can be differentiated from platelet-rich white thrombus. It is defined as intraluminal tissue >0.25 mm in diameter and either high backscattering with high attenuation (red-cell-rich thrombus) less back scattering with homogeneous low attenuation (platelet-rich thrombus) or a mixture of both. Thrombus can be quantified by sum up of the total number of quadrants of lumen containing thrombus. The maximum thrombus area is calculated by tracing the outline of the thrombus if the outline is visible or subtracting the minimum area within the thrombus from the adjacent reference lumen area not having thrombus if the outline of thrombus is not visible.

Thrombus burden can be measured quantitatively by planimetry and semi-quantitatively by the OCT thrombus score **(Figs. 3A to F)**. OCT can differentiate between red and white thrombi with high sensitivity (90%) and specificity (80%) (Kume et al.), and mixed thrombus shows intermediate features of both white and red thrombus. Sometimes, it is difficult to differentiate between in-stent plaque prolapse, thrombus protrusion, and acute stent thrombosis by OCT.[5]

Thin-cap fibroatheroma (TCFA) ***(Figs. 4A and B)****:* A fibrous cap is identified as a signal-rich homogenous region overlying a lipid core, which is characterized by a signal—poor region. TCFA is defined as a plaque with a fibrous cap measuring <65 µm.

DETECTION OF VULNERABLE PLAQUE IN VIVO BY OPTICAL COHERENCE TOMOGRAPHY

OCT is the best tool to identify vulnerable plaque **(Fig. 5)** by detecting 7–8 out of 10 criteria except for glistening yellow color, endothelial dysfunction, and intraplaque hemorrhage (**Tables 1 and 2 and Box 2**).

Major Criteria

- Active inflammation (monocyte/macrophage and sometimes T-cell infiltration)
- Thin cap with large lipid core
- Endothelial denudation with superficial platelet aggregation
- Fissured plaque
- Stenosis >90%.

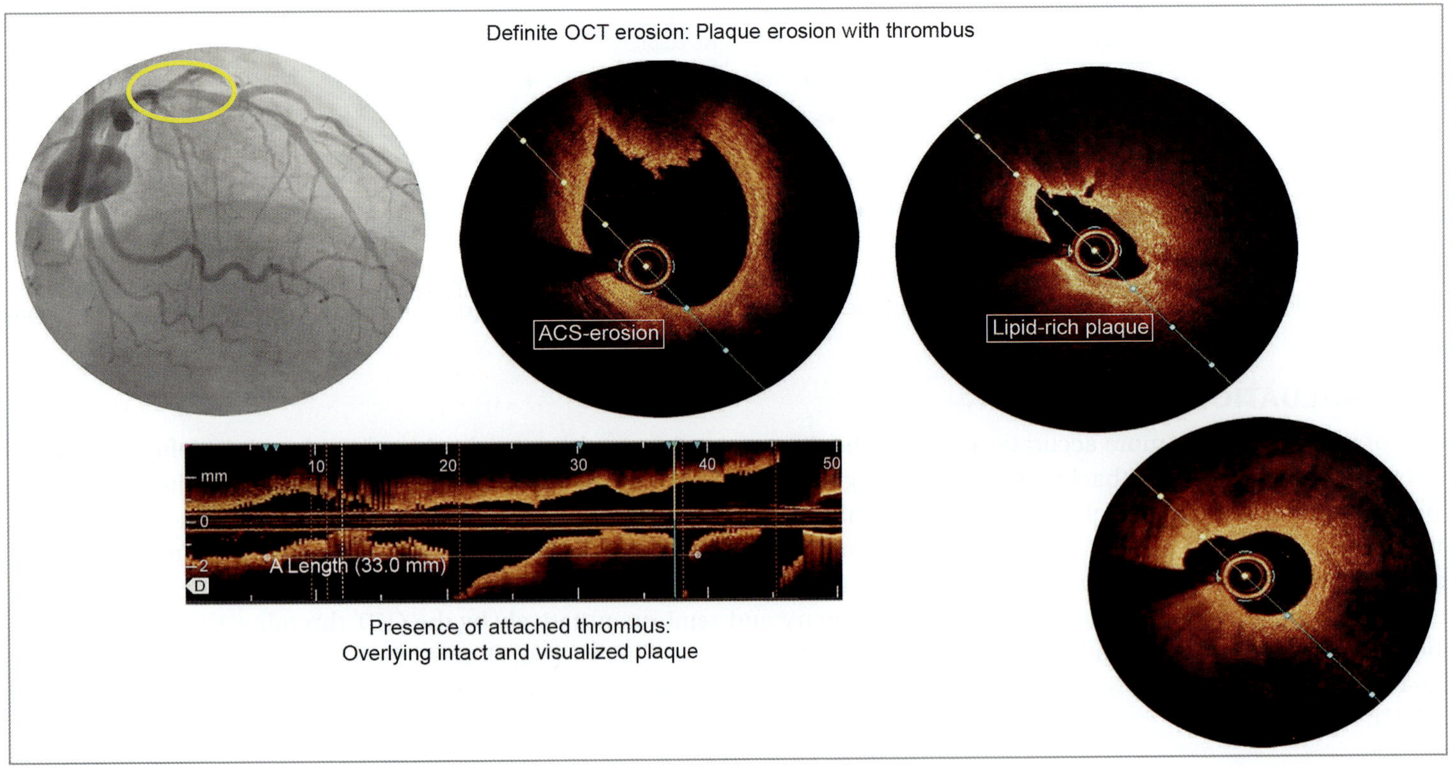

Fig. 1A

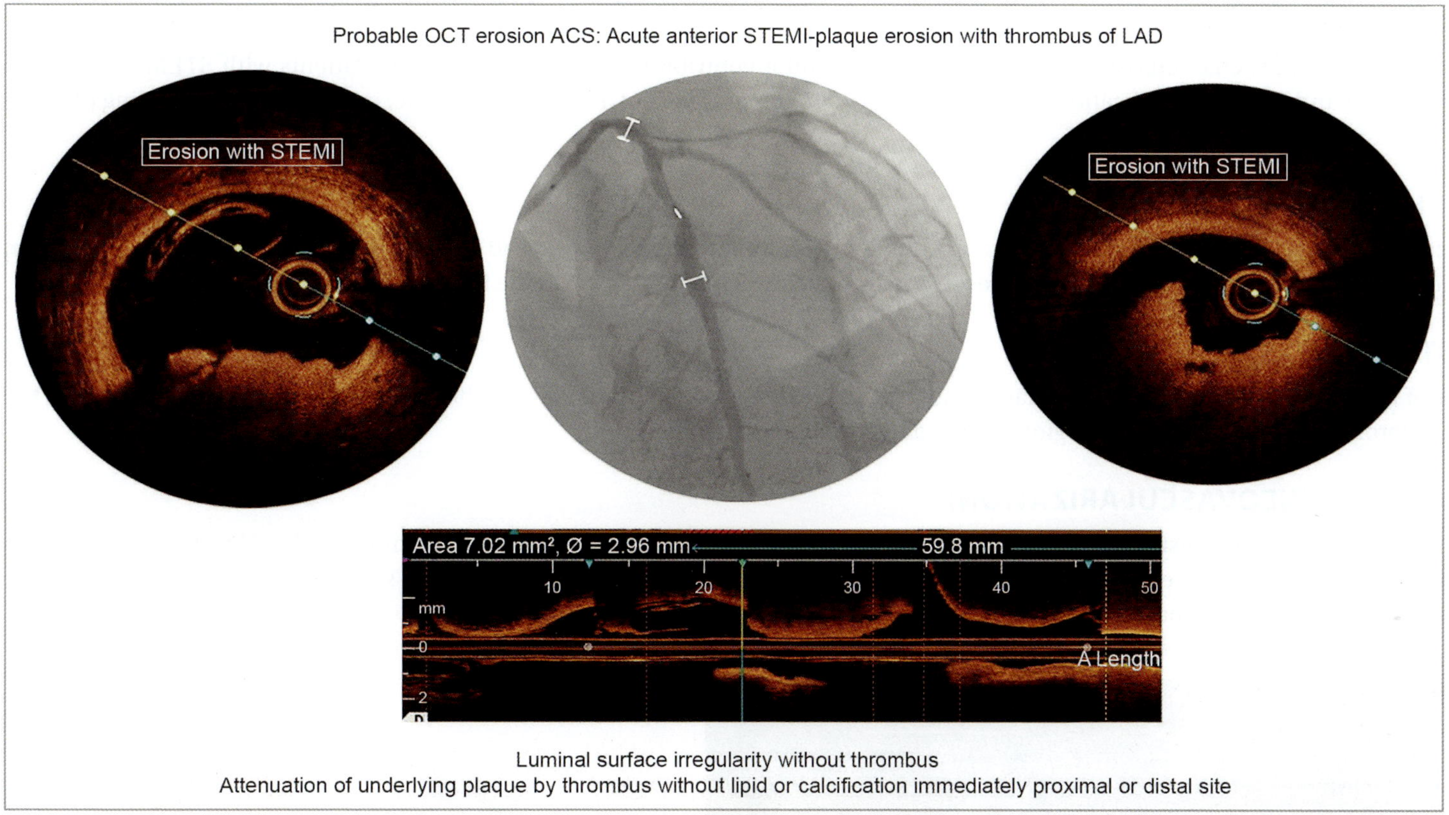

Fig. 1B

Figs. 1A and B: (A) Definite OCT erosion: Plaque erosion with thrombus; (B) Probable OCT erosion ACS: Acute anterior STEMI-plaque erosion with thrombus of LAD. (ACS: acute coronary syndrome; LAD: left anterior descending; OCT: optical coherence tomography; STEMI: ST-elevation myocardial infarction)

Minor Criteria

- Superficial calcified nodule
- Glistening yellow
- Intraplaque hemorrhage
- Endothelial dysfunction
- Outward (positive) remodeling.

SPOTTY CALCIFICATION

A small amount of calcium is characteristic of vulnerable plaque, and it contributes to plaque instability. Patients with STEMI with PR are more often associated with small and discrete calcifications within an arc of <90°, the presence of a fibro-fatty plaque, and positive remodeling of the culprit arterial segment.[6]

MACROPHAGE INFILTRATION

On OCT, macrophages are seen as signal rich, distinct, or confluent punctuate regions that exceed the intensity of background speckle noise, and positive correlation between histological and OCT data with respect to the density of macrophages on the fibrous cap of the plaque was observed.

CHOLESTEROL CRYSTAL

Phagocytosis of cholesterol crystals by macrophages causes and advances an inflammation in the atherosclerotic plaques **(Figs. 6A to H)**. OCT can visualize cholesterol crystals as a thin linear region of high density without attenuation.

VASA VASORUM (NEOVASCULARIZATION)

Vasa vasorum is seen as a sharply distinct tiny black holes (50–100 µm), signal-free voids located on the intimal side of lipid-rich plaques with TCFA, and is usually seen in at least three successive cross-sections **(Figs. 6A to H)**. Microchannels are located as small black holes in the outer plaque near the adventitia and in the thickened intima.

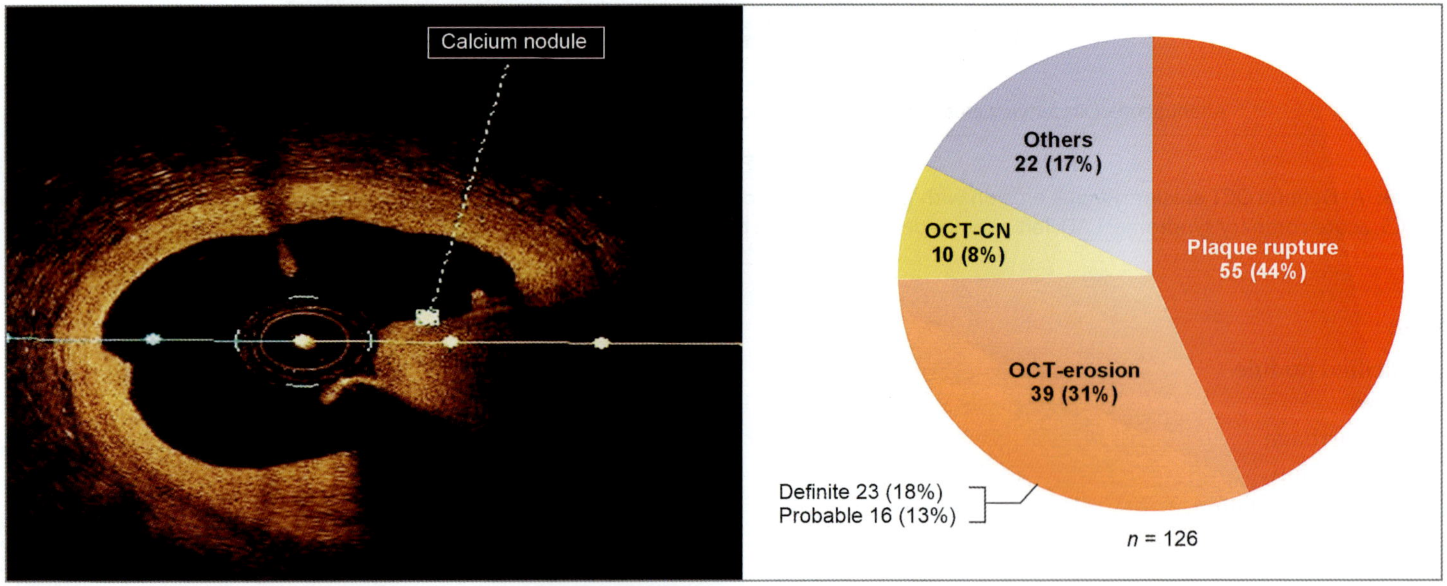

Fig. 2A: Unstable Plaque morphology by OCT.

Rupture	Erosion
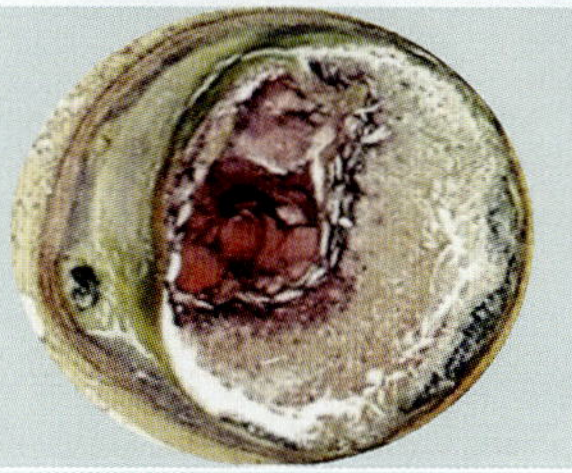 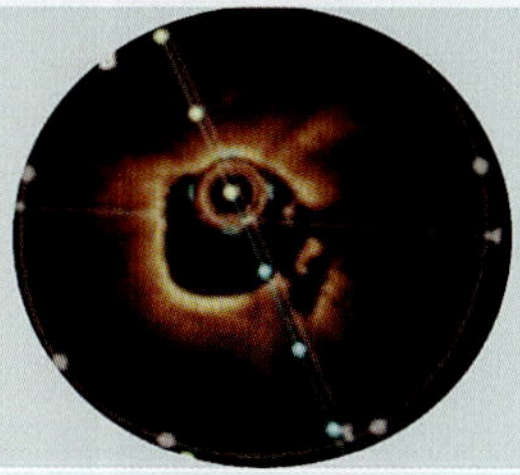	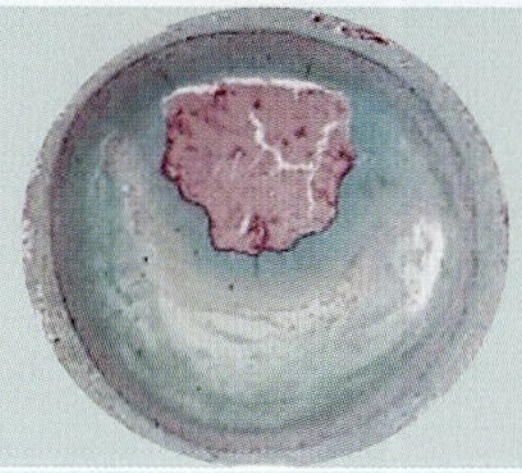 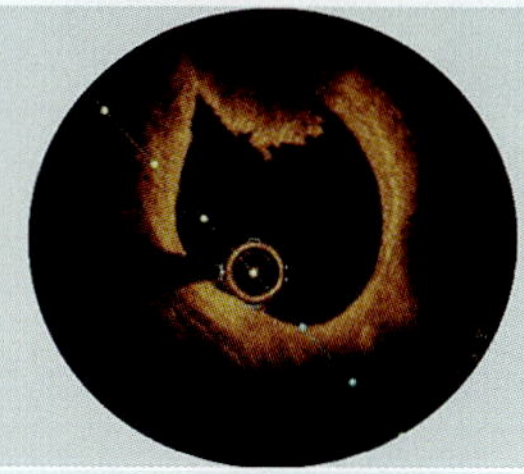
Ruptured thin fibrous cap with empty cavity	Deficiency of endothelium
Smooth muscle cells apoptosis	Endothelial cell apoptosis
Thin fibrous cap	Thick fibrous cap
Large lipid-rich plaque	Less plaque burden
More inflammation	Less inflammation
Majority presents with acute STEMI	Majority presents with NSTEMI and USA
More often in male	More often in female
Majority requires PCI with stenting	Majority can be treated with medical management without intervention

Fig. 2B: Difference between plaque erosion and plaque rupture. (PCI: percutaneous coronary intervention; NSTEMI: non-ST-elevation myocardial infarction)

Vasa vasorum promotes growth of the plaque by increasing blood flow, thereby supplying lipids, inflammatory cells, and cytokines into the plaque, and is frequently associated with positive remodeling and elevated high-sensitive CRP levels. Sometimes, it may cause intraplaque hemorrhage with sudden increase in plaque size and rupture of the plaque, manifest as ACS and sudden death depending upon the acute luminal compromise with reduction in the forward flow of culprit vessel.

Large lipid-rich plaques with TCFA are more often associated with high incidence of slow flow/no reflow, decreased (TIMI) flow, and myocardial blush grade. TCFA is a predictor for type IV (periprocedural) MI and increases the chances of medial edge dissection by six-fold. The presence of ruptured plaque should prompt for an aspiration procedure, followed by implantation of drug eluting stents and an aggressive medical therapy (in particular statins and antiplatelet therapy) and thrombus aspiration may not be useful for patients with plaques containing intact fibrous caps. Plaques with TCFA are seen in about 72% in acute myocardial infarction (AMI), 50% in unstable angina pectoris (UAP), and 20% in SAP. The frequency of OCT-detected plaque

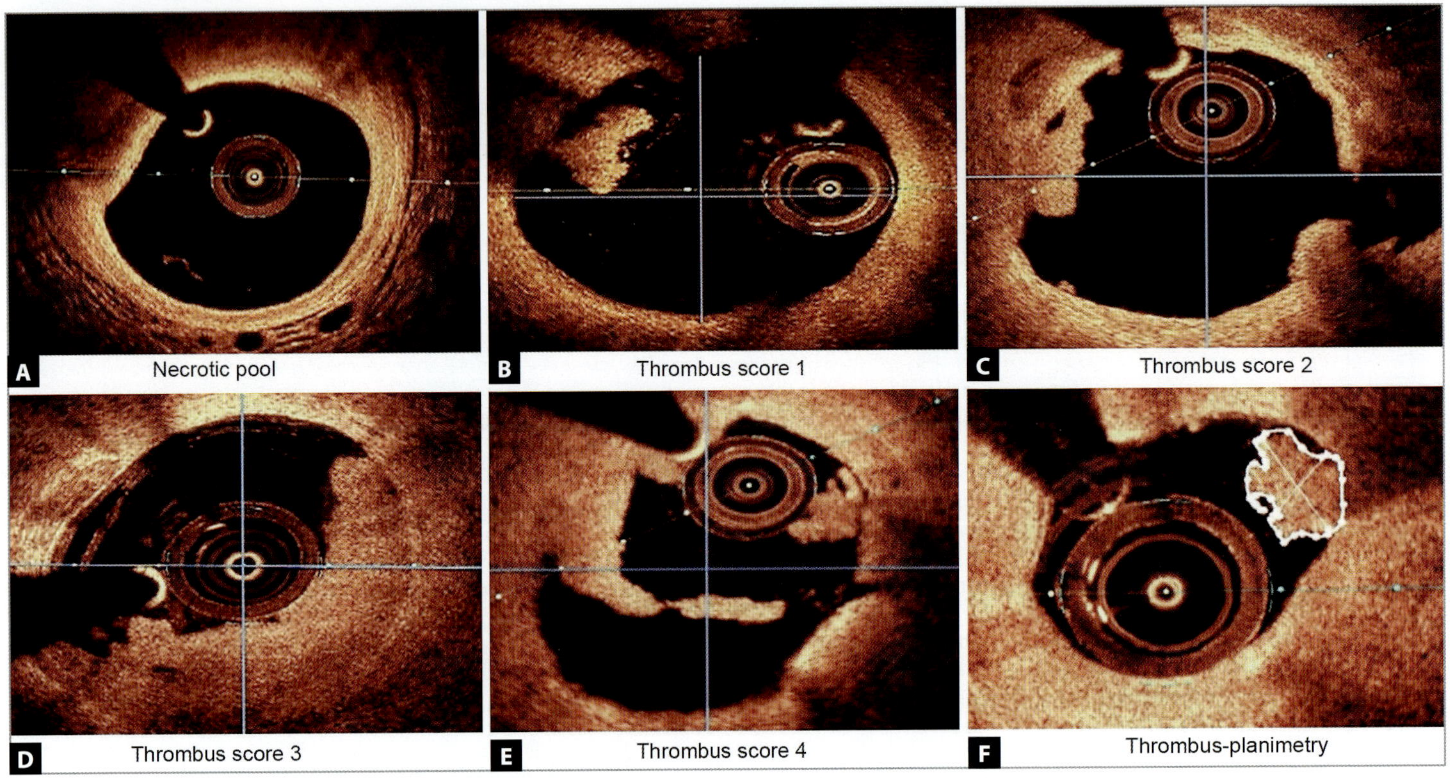

Figs. 3A to F: Thrombus evaluation.

rupture, erosion, and thrombus is similar to that of the pathological reports. ACS may be due to single or multiple culprit large lipid plaques with TCFA and sometimes associated with many nonculprit lesions of culprit or nonculprit vessels which may progress rapidly contributing to increased MACE during follow-up, and is more frequently noticed in diabetic patients.

NEOATHEROSCLEROSIS AND THE VULNERABLE PLAQUE

Neoatherosclerosis with neointimal rupture is one of the most common causes of late and very late drug-eluting stent thrombosis. Neointimal rupture occurs in regions with high-necrotic core content and thin fibrous cap as same as vulnerable plaques of native atherosclerosis. Similarly, it shows high

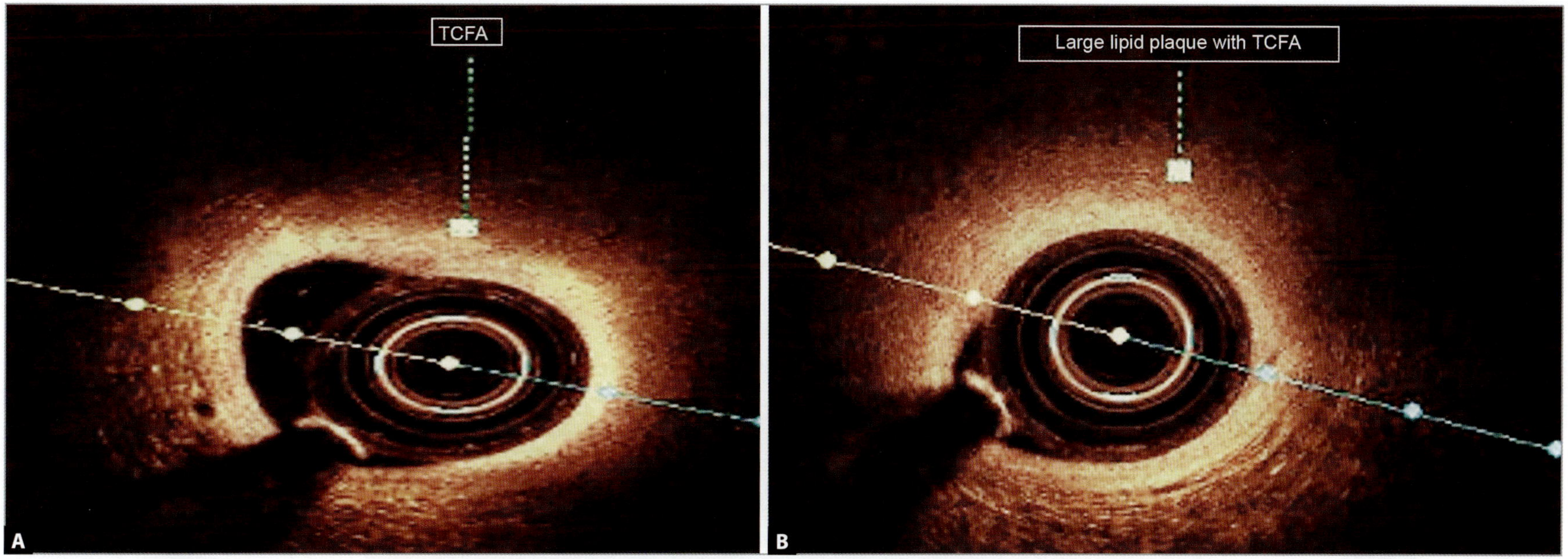

Figs. 4A and B: Thin-cap fibroatheroma (TCFA).

incidence of macrophage infiltration and vasa vasorum. Lipid-rich plaque or coronary thrombus causes OCT signal attenuation, which interferes with visualization of deep layers of coronary artery wall especially in segments with positive remodeling.[8]

OCT can be used safely in patients with STEMI. However, in the case of complete vessel occlusion (TIMI 0–1 flow), restoration of vessel patency with thrombectomy needs to be obtained before the OCT pulls back to ensure adequate clearing of the vessel lumen during contrast injection so that adequate images can be obtained.[9,10]

OCT runs of longitudinal view and three-dimensional (3D) reconstruction with angio co-registration is useful in assessing quantification of thrombus and relationship between the thrombus and the location of the major side branches to select the appropriate stent size and the length with IC nitroglycerine or nicorandil injections.

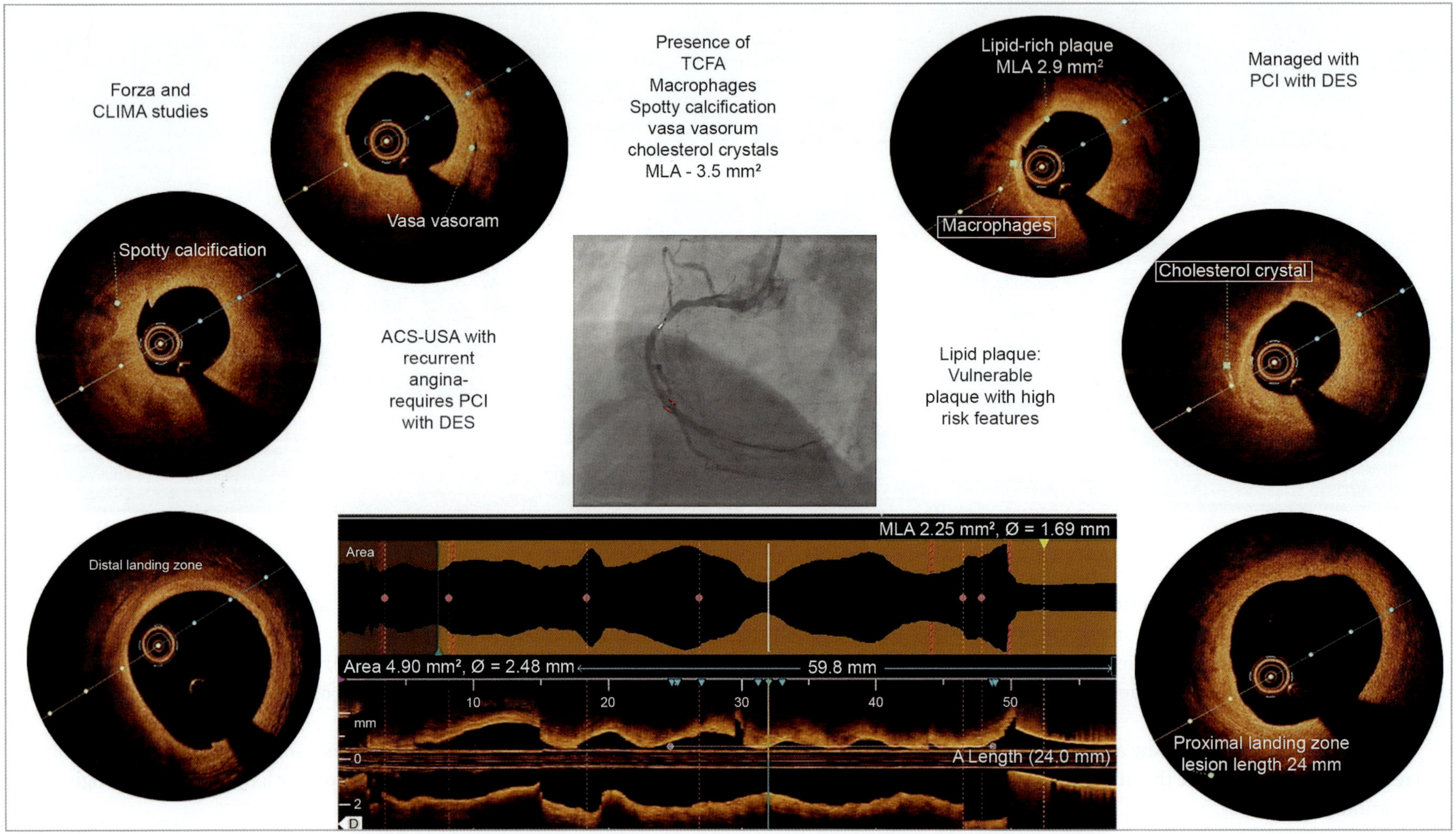

Fig. 5: Detection of vulnerable plaque by OCT imaging. (ACS: acute coronary syndrome; DES: drug eluting stent; MLA: minimal lumen area; PCI: percutaneous coronary intervention; TCFA: thin-cap fibroatheroma)

TABLE 1: Comparison of OCT with IVUS for identification of vulnerable plaques in ACS.

Plaque morphology	***OCT***	***IVUS***
Plaque rupture	3	2
Fibrous cap	3	0
Necrotic core	2	0±1
Thrombus	3	1
Spotty calcification	3	2
Calcified nodule	3	1
Intimal vasculature	1	0
Macrophages	1	0
Remodeling	1	3
Plaque burden	1	3

(0: not visible; 1: less visible; 2: visible; 3: more visible). (ACS: acute coronary syndrome; IVUS: intravascular ultrasound; OCT: optical coherence tomography)

TABLE 2: Studies showing criteria for detecting high-risk vulnerable plaques with event rates.

Study	***Modality***	***Variables***	***Endpoint***	***Follow-up***	***PPV***	***NPV***
PROSPECT (*n* = 697)	IVUS and VH-IVUS	PB >70% and MLA <4 mm^2 and VH-IVUS TCFA	MACE (CD, cardiac arrest, MI, re-hospitalization due to AP)	3 years	17%	98%
ATHEROREMO IVUS (*n* = 581)	IVUS and VH-IVUS	PB >70% and MLA <4 mm^2 and VH-IVUS TCFA	MACE (non-CL related or indeterminate death, ACS, unplanned revascularization)	1 year	23%	93%
PREDICTION (*n* = 506)	IVUS and ESS	PB >58% and low ESS <1.0Pa	PCI	1 year	41%	92%
CLIMA (*n* = 1,003) **(Figs. 6A to H)**	OCT	MLA <3.5 mm^2 and TCFA and lipid arc >180° and macrophage	MACE (CD and TV-MI)	1 year	19%	97%

(ACS: acute coronary syndrome; AP: angiina pectoris; ESS: endothelial shear stress; IVUS: intravascular ultrasound; MACE: ; MLA: minimal lumen area; NPV: negative predictive value; OCT: optical coherence tomography; PB: plaque burden; PPV: positive predictive value; TCFA: thin-cap fibroatheroma; VH-IVUS: virtual histology intravascular ultrasound)

BOX 2: Role of imaging in vulnerable plaque detection and risk stratification.

- Large lipid plaque (>60–70%) indicates proneness for plaque rupture and associated with higher incidence of MACE.
- OCT identifies high-risk vulnerable plaques and is also superior to CTCA in predicting future adverse events.
- Identification of high-risk plaque is helpful to differentiate high-risk patients who would benefit from an aggressive therapy for plaque regression.

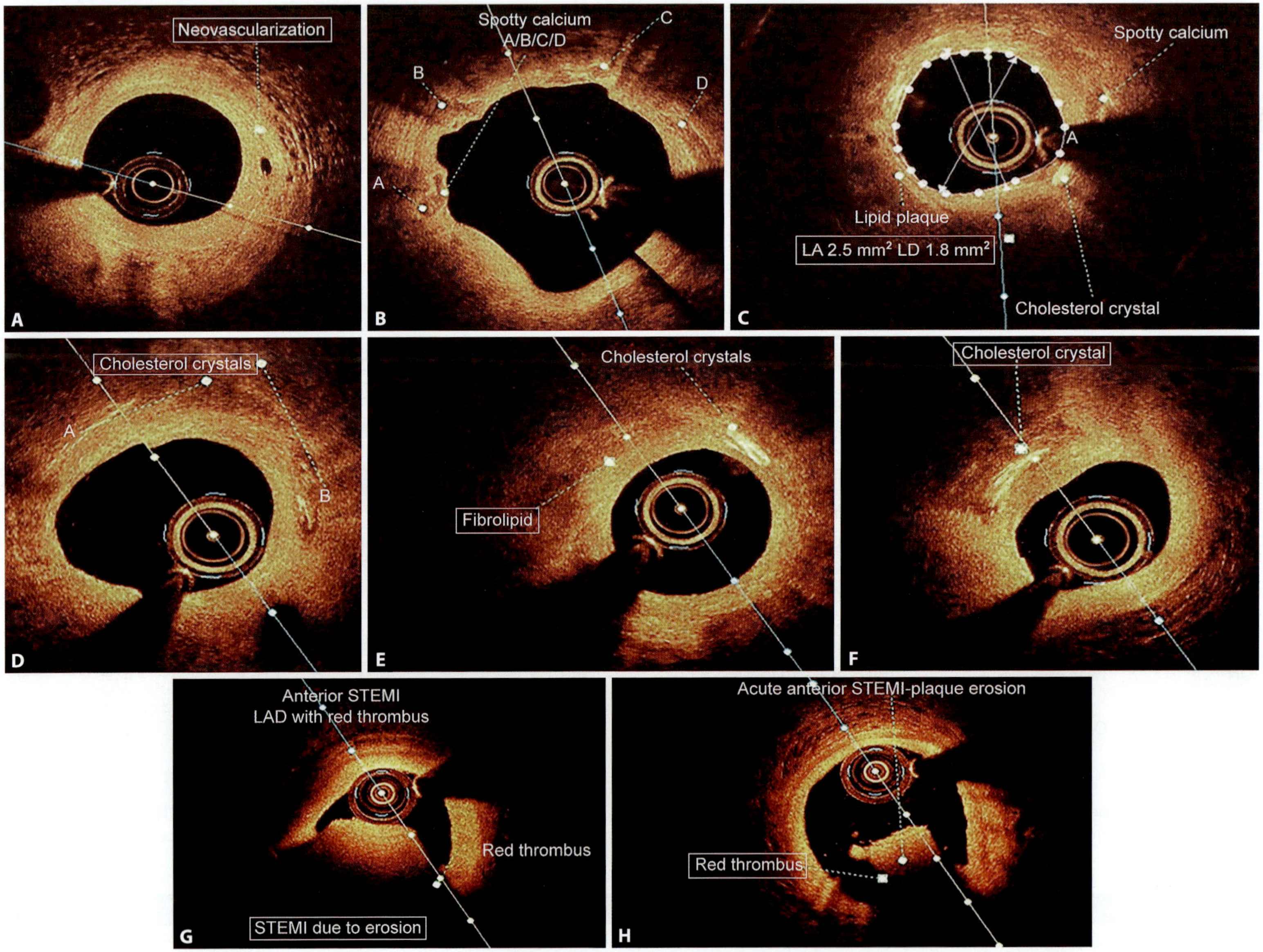

Figs. 6A to H: Phagocytosis of cholesterol crystals by macrophages.

REFERENCES

1. Toutouzas K, Karanasos A, Tousoulis D. Optical coherence tomography for the detection of the vulnerable plaque. Eur Cardiol Rev. 2016;11(2):90.
2. Kubo T, Ino Y, Tanimoto T, Kitabata H, Tanaka A, Akasaka T. Optical Coherence Tomography Imaging in Acute Coronary Syndromes. Cardiol Res Pract. 2011;2011:312978.
3. Akasaka T, Kubo T, Mizukoshi M, Tanaka A, Kitabata H, Tanimoto T, et al. Pathophysiology of acute coronary syndrome assessed by optical coherence tomography. J Cardiol. 2010;56(1):8-14.
4. Mintz GS. Intravascular imaging of coronary calcification and its clinical implications. JACC: Cardiovascular Imaging. 2015;8(4):461-71.
5. Kume T, Akasaka T, Kawamoto T, Ogasawara Y, Watanabe N, Toyota E, et al. Assessment of coronary arterial thrombus by optical coherence tomography. Am J Cardiol. 2006;97(12):1713-7.
6. Hasegawa T, Shimada K. Optical Coherence Tomography for the Assessment of Coronary Plaque Vulnerability. Coron Artery Dis: Assess Surg Prevent. 2015:99.
7. Iannaccone M, Vadalà P, D'ascenzo F, Montefusco A, Moretti C, D'amico M, et al. Clinical perspective of optical coherence tomography and intravascular ultrasound in STEMI patients. J Thorac Dis. 2016;8(5):754.
8. Kitabata H, Akasaka T. Recent developments in intracoronary optical coherence tomography imaging. Imag Med. 2011;3(3):299.
9. Kitabata H, Tanaka A, Kubo T, Takarada S, Kashiwagi M, Tsujioka H, et al. Relation of microchannel structure identified by optical coherence tomography to plaque vulnerability in patients with coronary artery disease. Am J Cardiol. 2010;105(12):1673-8.
10. Johnson TW, Räber L, Di Mario C, Bourantas C, Jia H, Mattesini A, et al. Clinical use of intracoronary imaging. Part 2: acute coronary syndromes, ambiguous coronary angiography findings, and guiding interventional decision-making: an expert consensus document of the European Association of Percutaneous Cardiovascular Interventions: Endorsed by the Chinese Society of Cardiology, the Hong Kong Society of Transcatheter Endocardiovascular Therapeutics (HKSTENT) and the Cardiac Society of Australia and New Zealand. Eur Heart J. 2019;40(31):2566-84.

CASE 1

PCI with stenting LMCA and mid LAD—Ambiguous lesion.

CLINICAL HISTORY

A 74-year-old female (no comorbidities), presented with complaints of chest pain associated with grade II SOB on and off. ECG–ACS–evolved AWMI. 2D Echo–RWMA in LAD territory with mild LV dysfunction–EF-47%.

Investigations: Hb-10.4 g/dL, RBS-96 mg/dL, Serum Cr-1.01 mg/dL, eGFR-55 mL/min, and NT-proBNP-480 pg/mL.

CAG showed ostial LMCA 70–80% lesion, distal LAD 70% lesion, normal LCX and RCA.

LMCA engaged with EBU 3.5–6 Fr guiding catheter, LAD lesion crossed with 0.014" Run through wire and 0.014" BMW wire placed in LCX. Prestenting OCT was done which significant plaque in ostial LAD-LM diameter found to be fibrolipid plaque **(Figs. 7A to C)**.

PROCEDURE

Distal LAD stenting was done with 2.5 × 23 mm Xience Xpedition stent. Then, LMCA stenting is done with 4.0 × 18 mm Xience Xpedition stent. LAD wire recrossed and POT was done with 4.5 × 08 mm NC Trek balloon. Poststenting OCT showed well-expanded stent struts with no edge dissection in LM to LAD stent, underexpansion in distal LAD stent suggestive of postdilatation which was done with 2.75 × 12 mm NC Trek balloon **(Figs. 8 and 9)**. The final result was good with TIMI III flow with no complications.

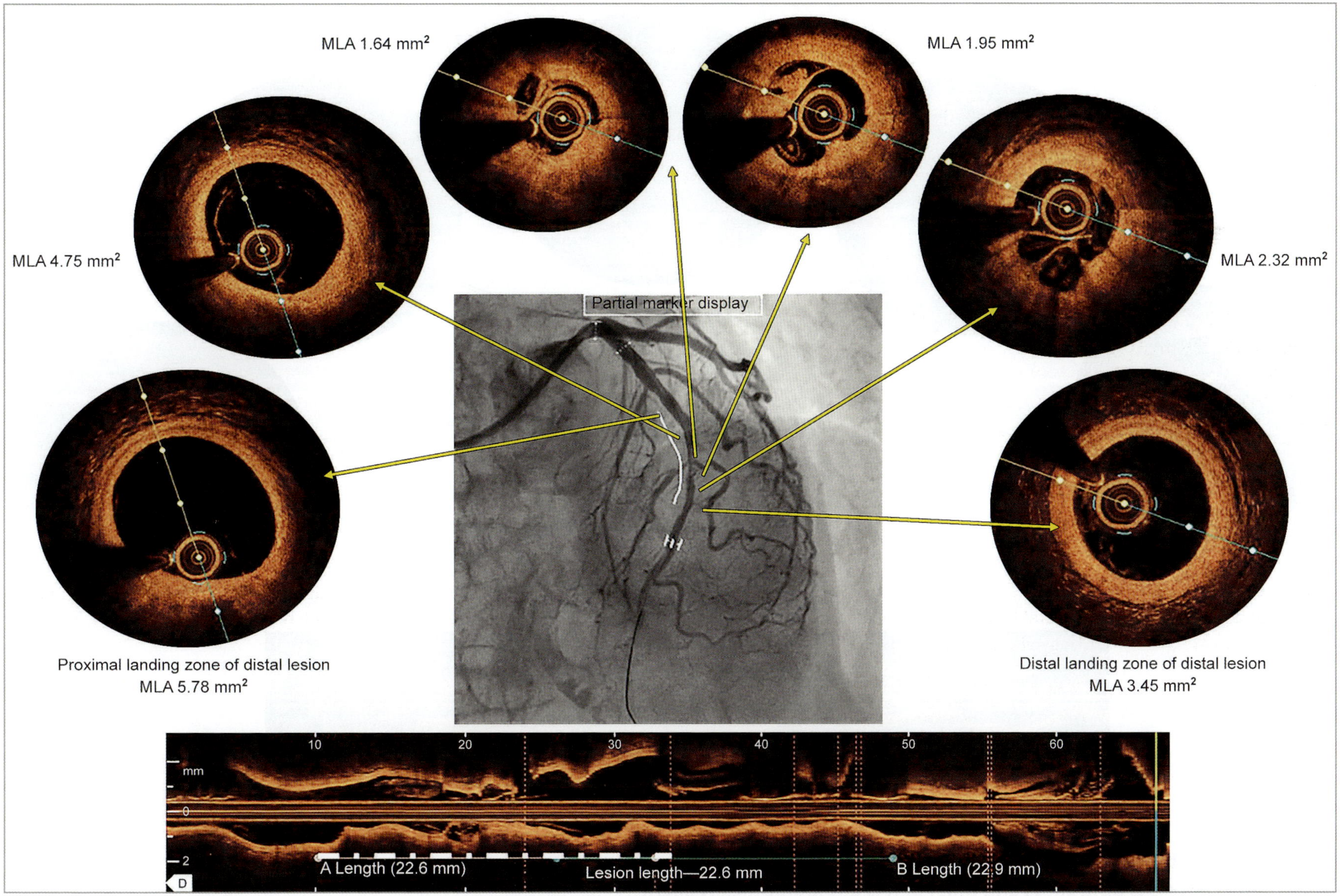

MLA 1.64 mm²
MLA 1.95 mm²
MLA 4.75 mm²
MLA 2.32 mm²
Partial marker display
Proximal landing zone of distal lesion
MLA 5.78 mm²
Distal landing zone of distal lesion
MLA 3.45 mm²
mm
A Length (22.6 mm)
Lesion length—22.6 mm
B Length (22.9 mm)
D

Fig. 7A

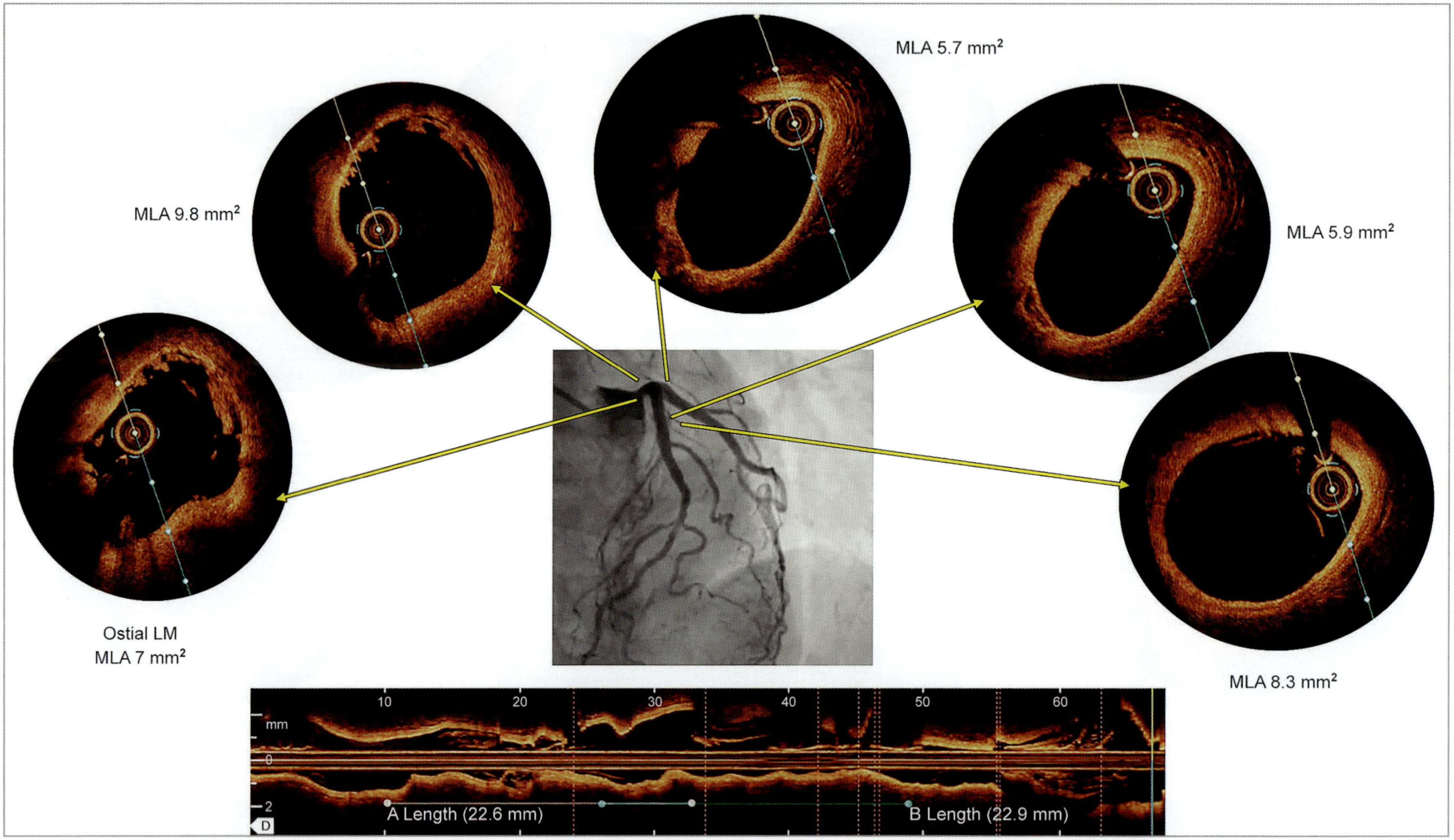

Fig. 7B

Early imaging observations regarding angiography during PCI:

- **Atherosclerosis is ubiquotos and most of it is angiographically silent**
- **The angiogram is often misleading in assessing vessel size.**

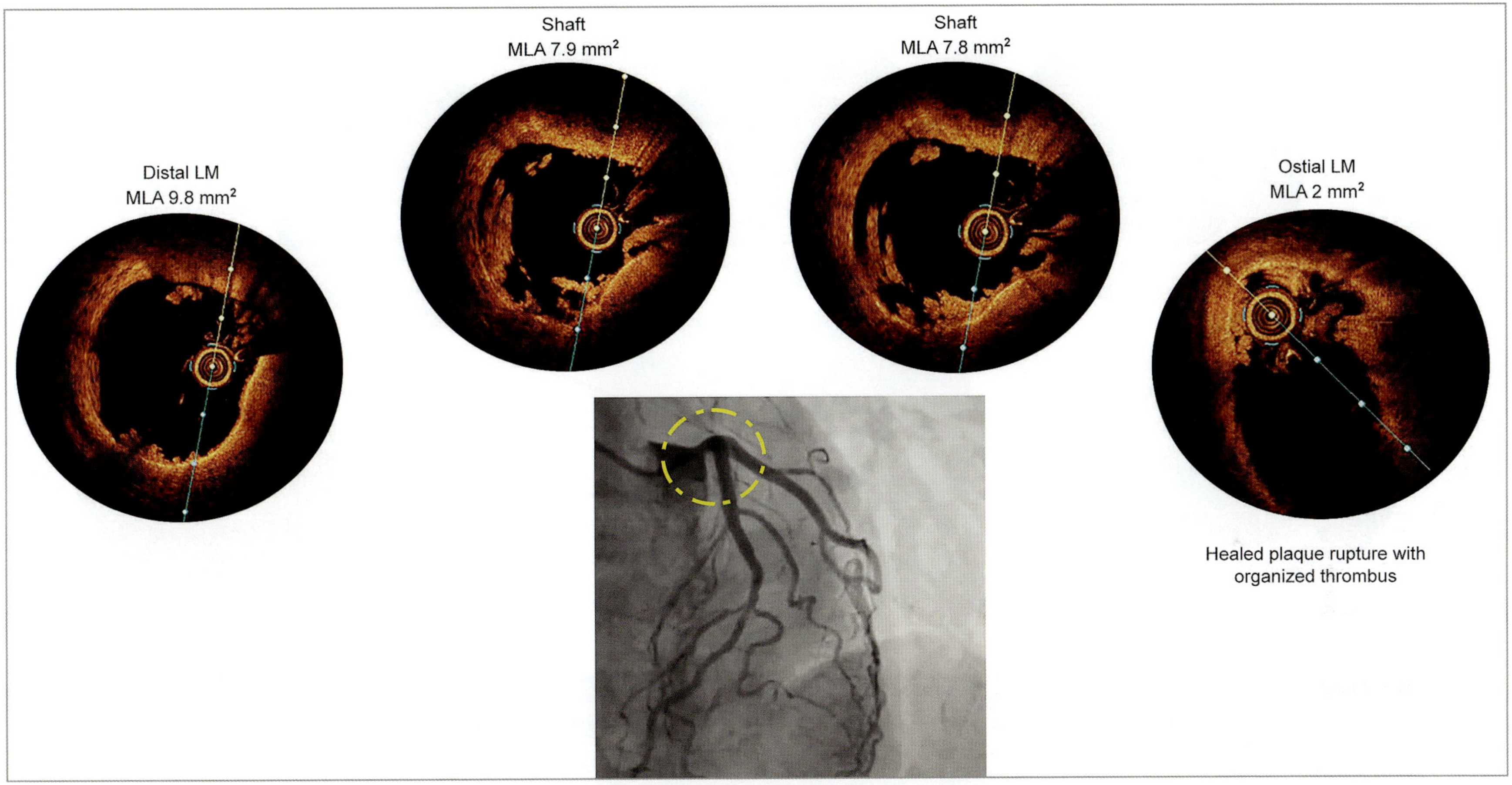

Fig. 7C

Figs. 7A to C: (A) MLD assessment of mid and distal LAD junction showing fibrous plaque with recanalized thrombus; (B) Assessment of ostial LMCA - partially recanalized thrombus at the ostium of LM; (C) Healed plaque rupture with organized thrombus of ostio-proximal LMCA. (LM: left main; MLA: minimal lumen area)

Early imaging observations regarding angiography during PCI:
- **The angiogram is often misleading in assessing the calcification**
- **A good angiographic result is not a guarantee of a good anatomic result.**

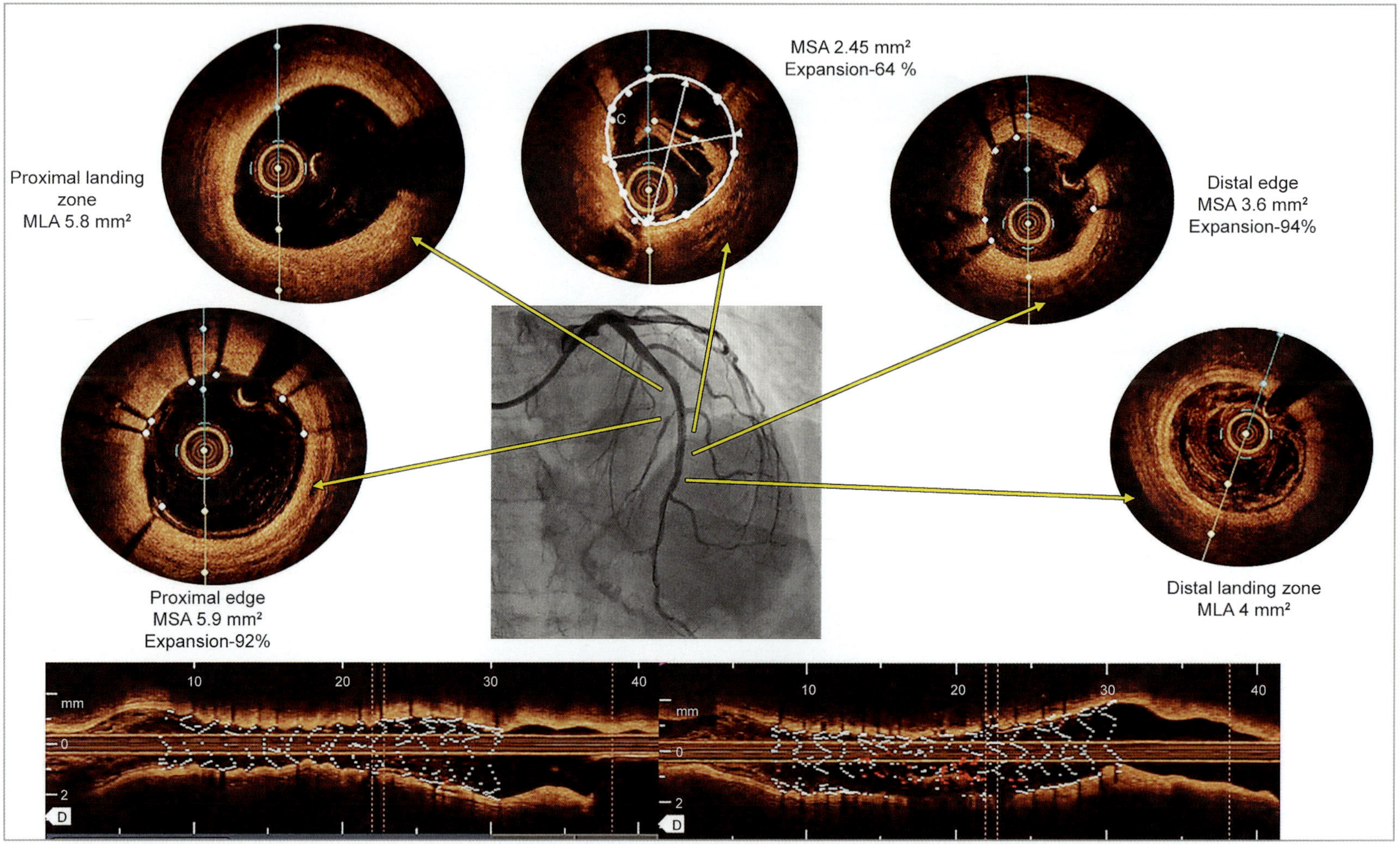

Fig. 8: MAX assessment of LAD stent - under-expansion of the stent. (MLA: minimal lumen area; MSA: minimal stent area)

Correct the MAX criteria and repeat the OCT to confirm the fulfilment of MAX criteria before finishing the procedure.

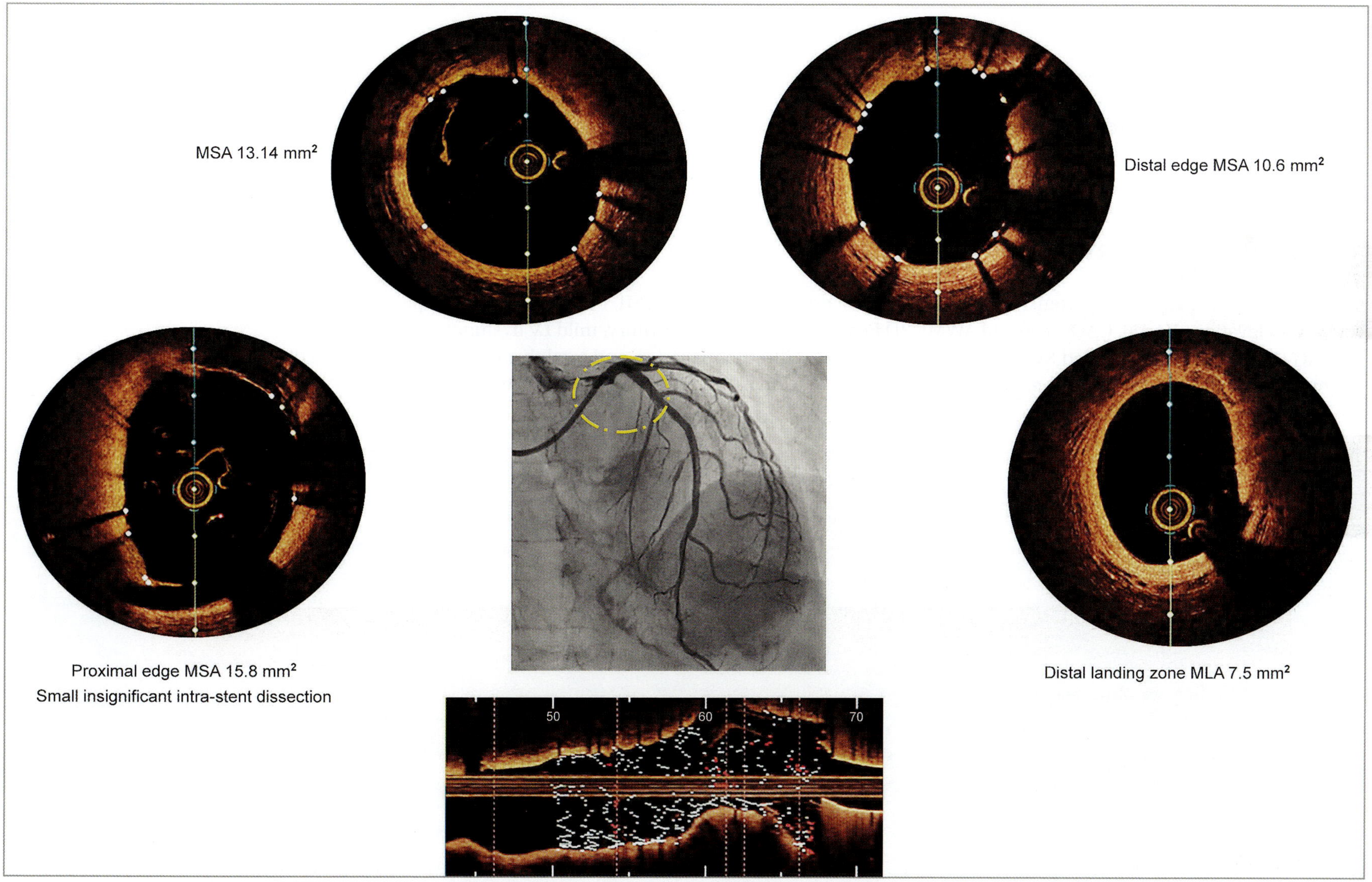

Fig. 9: MAX assessment of LM stent–well expanded and apposed with no medial edge dissections. (MLA: minimal lumen area; MSA: minimal stent area)

CASE 2

ACS-anterior STEMI due to TCFA with plaque rupture of LAD (Red thrombus).

CLINICAL HISTORY

A 47-year-old male, known hypertensive, presented with acute anterior wall STEMI, complaints of chest pain radiating to left arm for 2 days. ECG—QS V3–V6, ST elevations V4–V6, CAD—evolved AWMI, 2D Echo—RWMA in LAD territory, mild LV dysfunction with EF: 42%.

CAG **(Figs. 10A to C)** revealed SVD with proximal LAD 70% thrombotic lesion and total thrombotic occlusion of D1. Investigations: Hb—14.7 g/dL, troponin I—3.70 ng/dL, RBS—134 mg/dL, serum creatinine—0.67 mg/dL, and eGFR—114 mL/min.

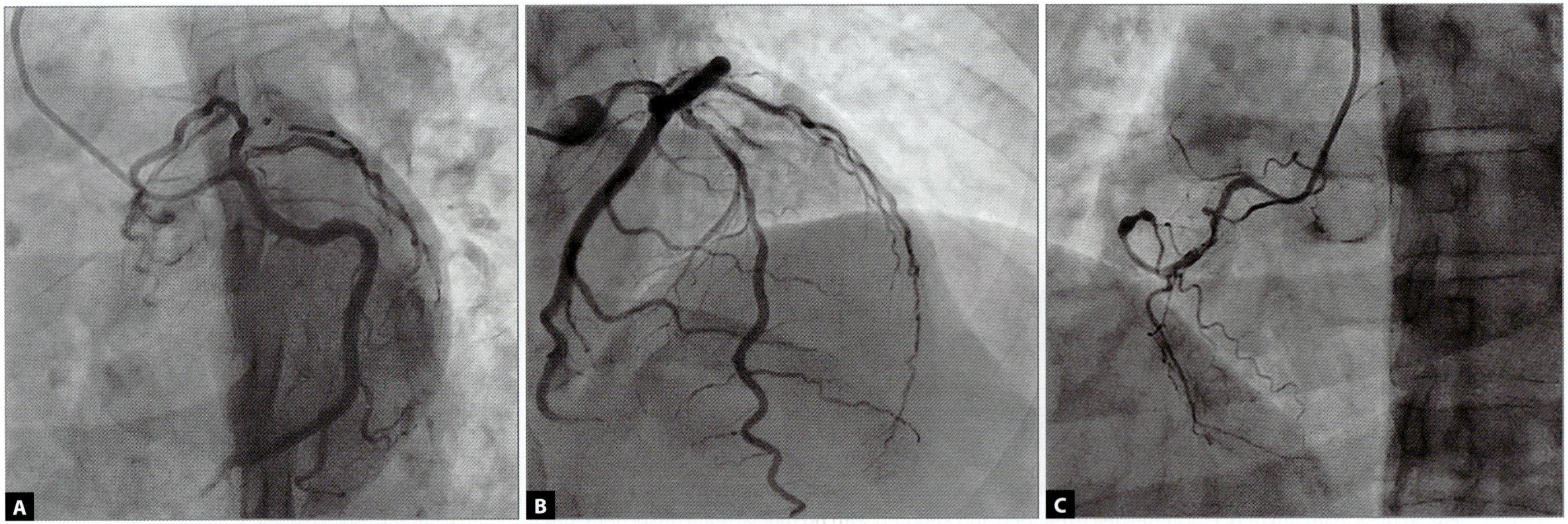

Figs. 10A to C: Coronary angiogram showing LCX, LAD and RCA.

PROCEDURE

LMCA engaged with EBU 3.5–6 Fr guiding catheter, angiogram revealed proximal LAD 70% thrombotic lesion, total occlusion of D1. 0.014″ BMW wire was placed in LAD, D1 wired with 0.014″ Turn track wire.

Presenting OCT showed lipid rich plaque, TCFA with plaque rupture and red thrombus **(Figs. 11A to C)**.

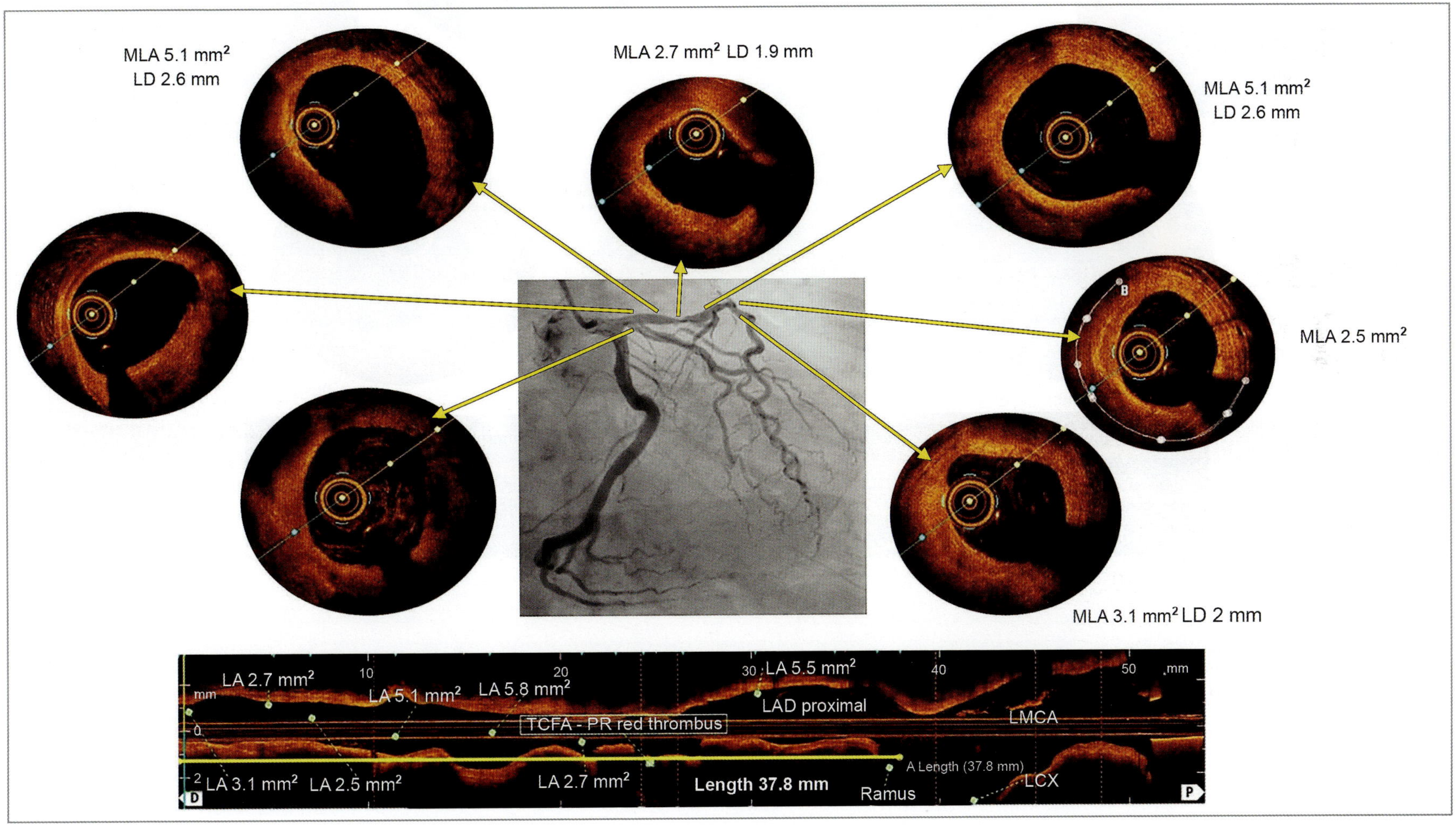

Fig. 11A

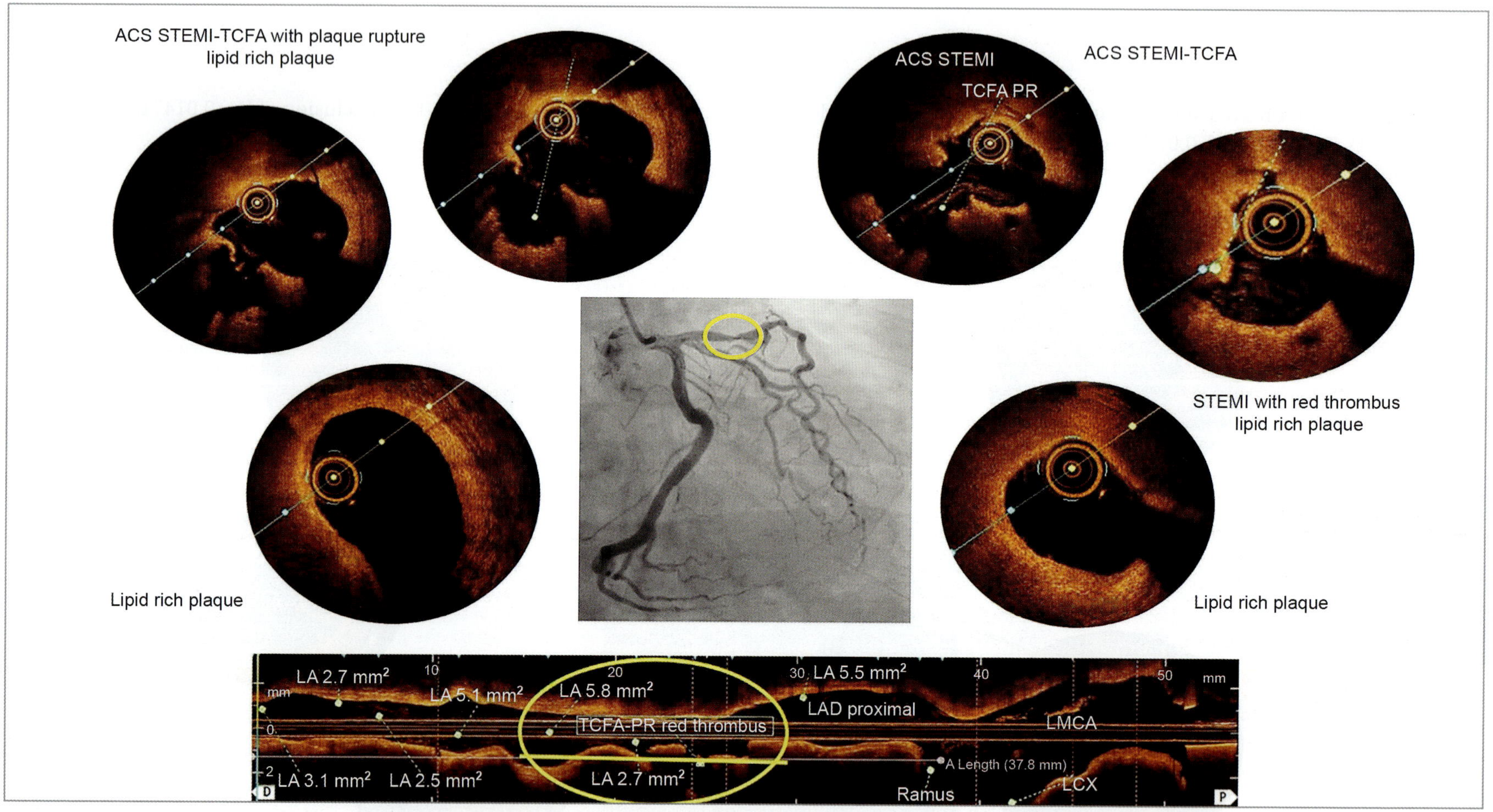

Fig. 11B

Target Vessel Failure (TVF) according to pre-specified optimal IVUS criteria from IVUS-ACS study showed 7.3% (n = 1752) in angio guided PCI, 7.1% (n = 1392) in sub-optimal IVUS guided PCI and 3.2% (n = 351) in optimal IVUS guided PCI at 1 year follow-up.

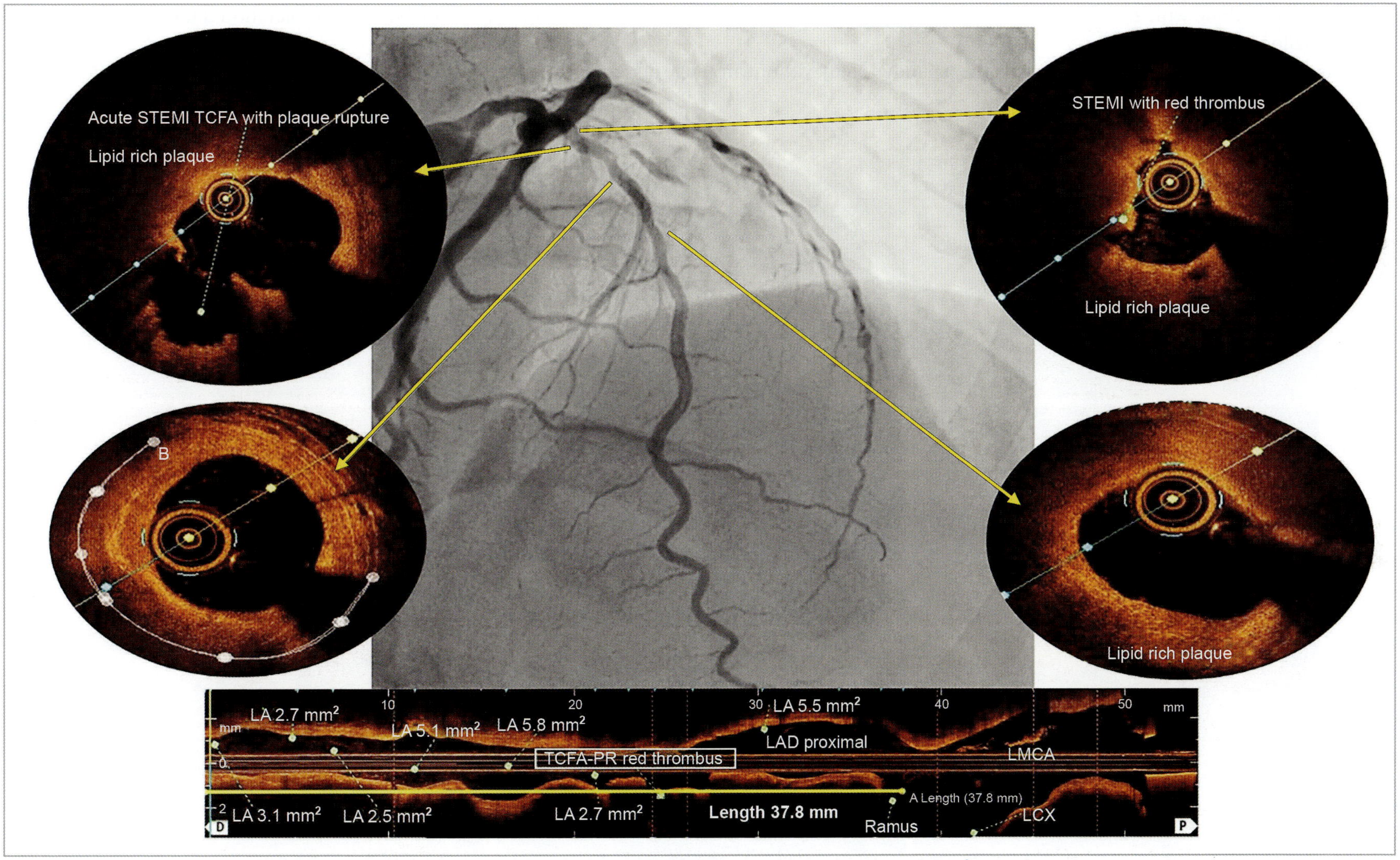

Fig. 11C

Figs. 11A to C: (A) MLD assessment of proximal LAD; (B) Anterior wall STEMI due to–plaque rupture with Red thrombus of proximal LAD; (C) Acute STEMI plaque morphology in LAD segment.

Predilatation done with 2.0 × 10 mm Tazuna balloon, stenting done with 2.75 × 48 mm Xience Xpedition stent. Postdilatation done with 3.0 × 15 mm NC Trek balloon **(Fig. 12)**.

Poststenting OCT showed well-apposed and expanded stent without any edge dissection **(Figs. 13A and B)**. The final result was good with TIMI III flow with no complications.

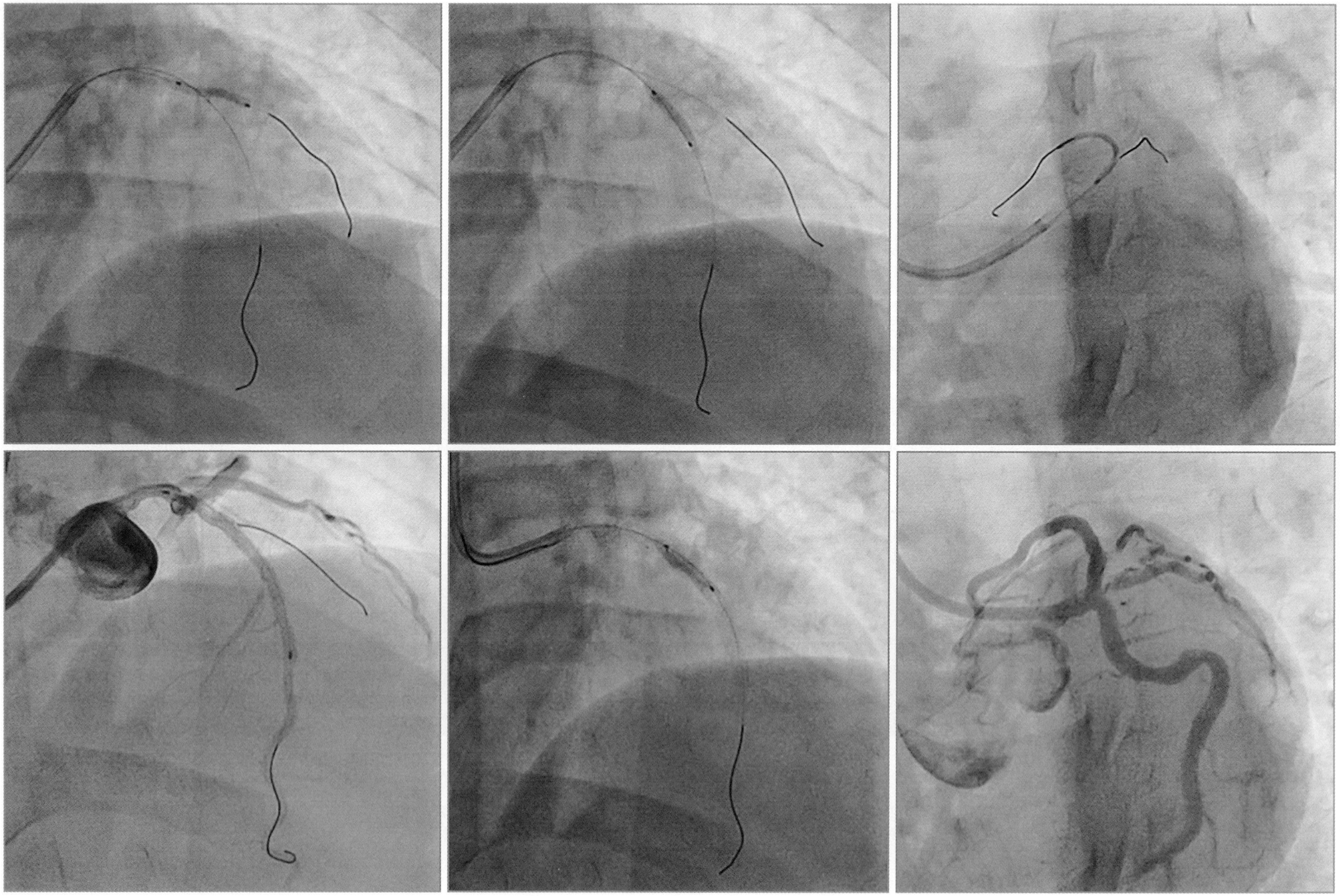

Fig. 12: Coronary angioplasty of LAD showing pre dilatation of D1 and LAD, Stenting of LAD, post dilatation and final result.

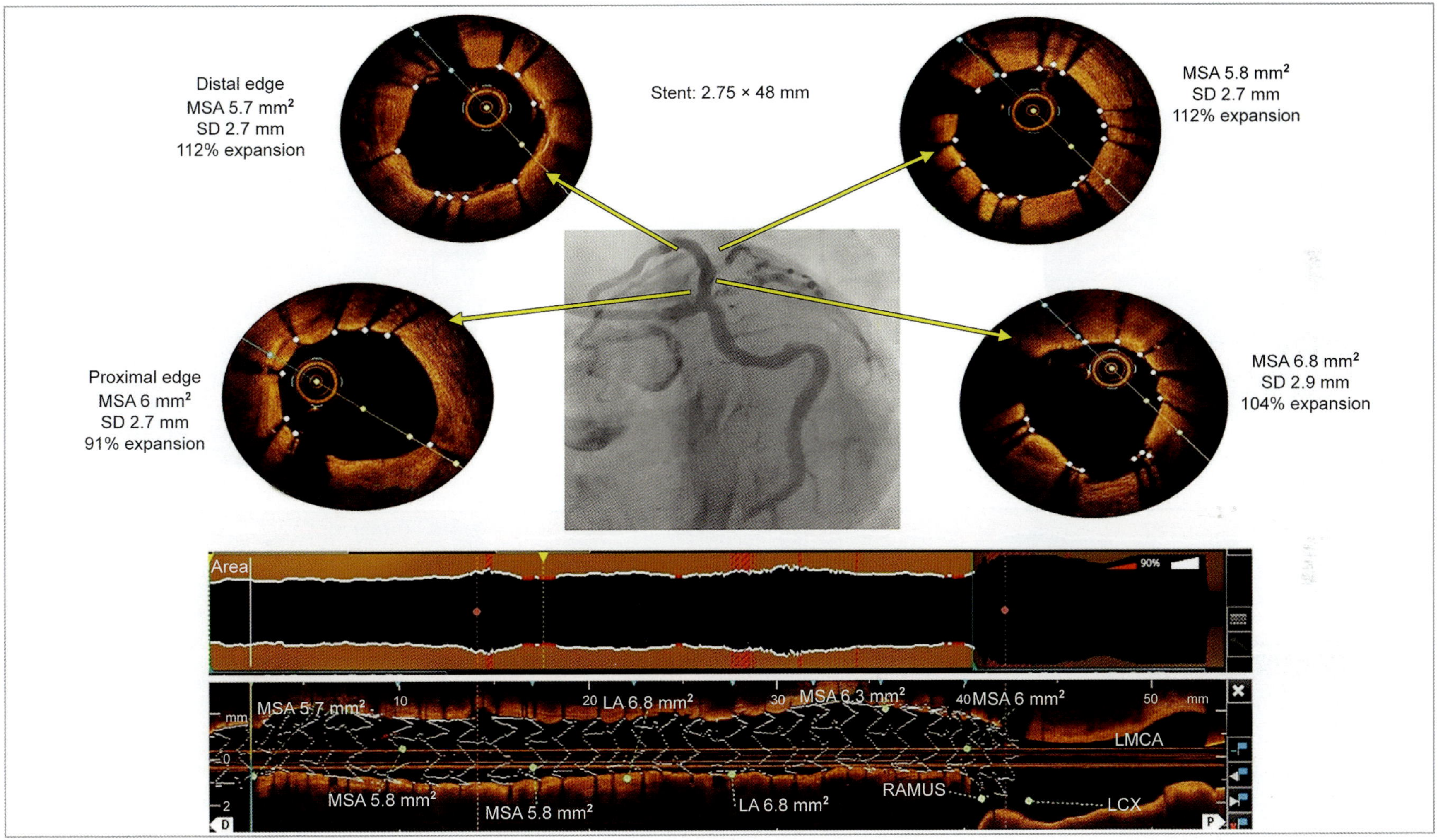

Fig. 13A

Very late events (beyond a year) were similar between BMS and 2nd generation DES-Approximately 1–2%/year, and By Five years, TLF/TVF with Contemporary DES occurs in nearly 1 in 7 patients.

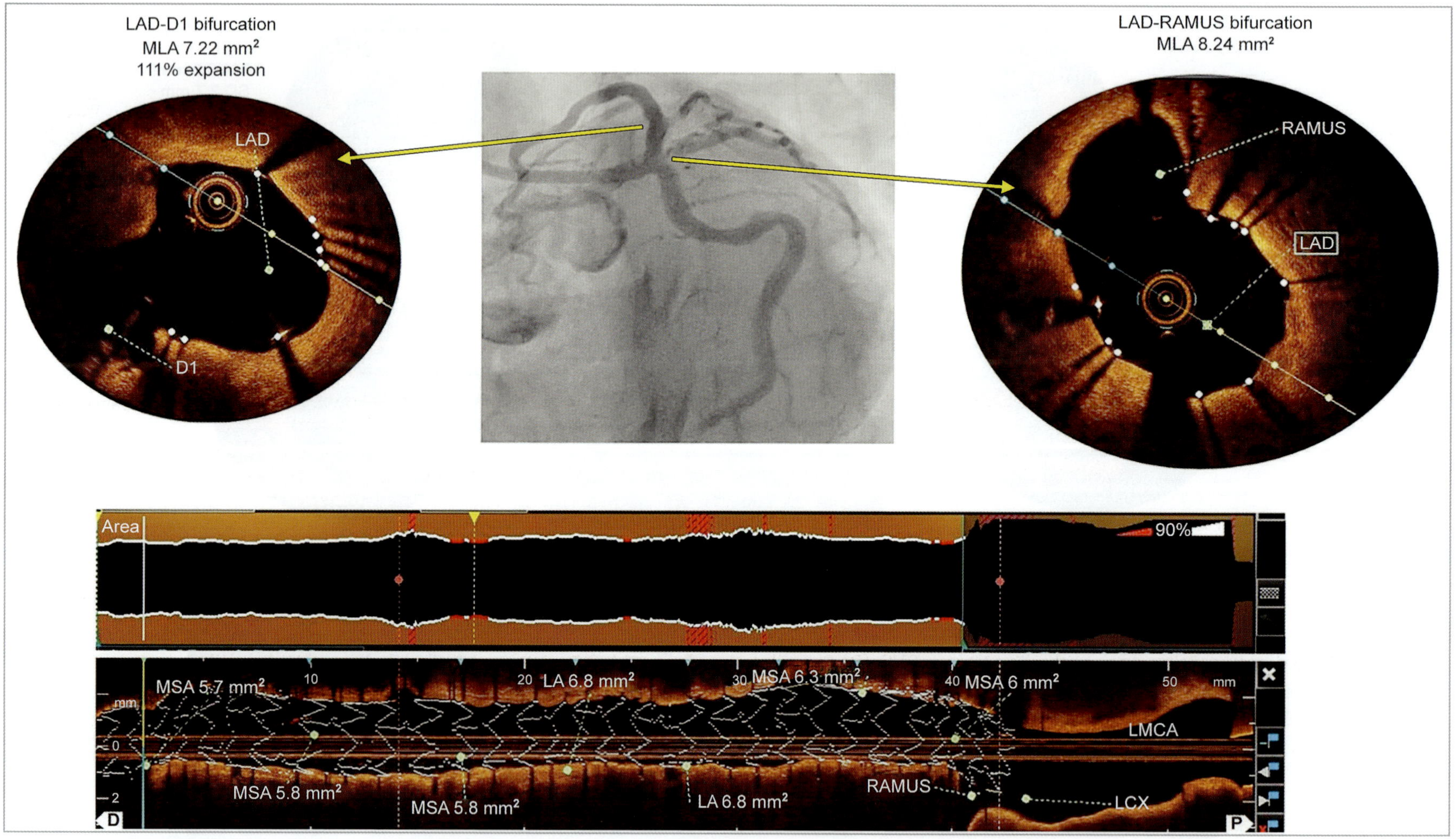

Fig. 13B

Figs. 13A and B: (A) Post LAD stenting OCT assessment for MAX; (B) OCT showing LAD-Ramus and LAD-D1 bifurcation sites.

Post dilate the mal-apposed portion of the stent with appropriately sized semi-compliant balloon at low pressure and reconfirm correction with repeat Imaging.

CASE 3

BVS Stenting of LAD—Anterior STEMI due to plaque rupture.

CLINICAL HISTORY

A 42-year-old male known diabetic with strong family history of CAD presented with acute anterior wall myocardial infarction, STEMI (W/P-2 hours), and chest pain associated with profuse sweating. ECG-ST-elevation in anterolateral leads **(Fig. 14)**. 2D echo-IVS, apex, and anterior wall hypokinetic but with preserved thickness, severe LV dysfunction, EF—36%. He was treated with thrombolytic therapy (IV. Tenecteplase—60 mg) in peripheral hospital, shifted for unrelieved chest pain with persistent ST elevations. CAG—Right transradial approach, LMCA—Normal, LAD—Mid 90% lesion with thrombus **(Fig. 15)**, and LCX and RCA were normal.

PROCEDURE

PCI of LAD performed through RRA-route, using 6 Fr XB 3.0 guiding catheter, LAD lesion was crossed with 0.014" Sion Blue wire. Preprocedure OCT showed LAD plaque rupture thrombus containing lesion leading to acute anterior STEMI, proximal landing zone—10.5 mm^2, MLD—3.65 mm, distal landing zone MLA—5.4 mm^2, MLD—2.6 mm **(Fig. 16A)**, and STEMI due to plaque rupture **(Fig. 16B)**.

(A) Mid-LAD direct stenting done with 3.5 × 18 mm BVS; (B) Postdilatation done with 3.5 × 12 mm NC Trek balloon; (C) Postdilatation—4.0 × 08 mm NC Trek Balloons; (D) Final result **(Figs. 17A to D)**.

Post-OCT showed well-apposed and well-expanded stent struts without any edge dissections **(Fig. 18)** with post-OCT showed distal portion of the BVS MLA—7.7 mm^2, mid-portion of the BVS MLA—10.1 mm^2, MLD—3.59 mm, proximal portion of the BVS MLA—12 mm^2. Postprocedure angio view showed well-implanted stents with TIMI-III flow without any dissection.

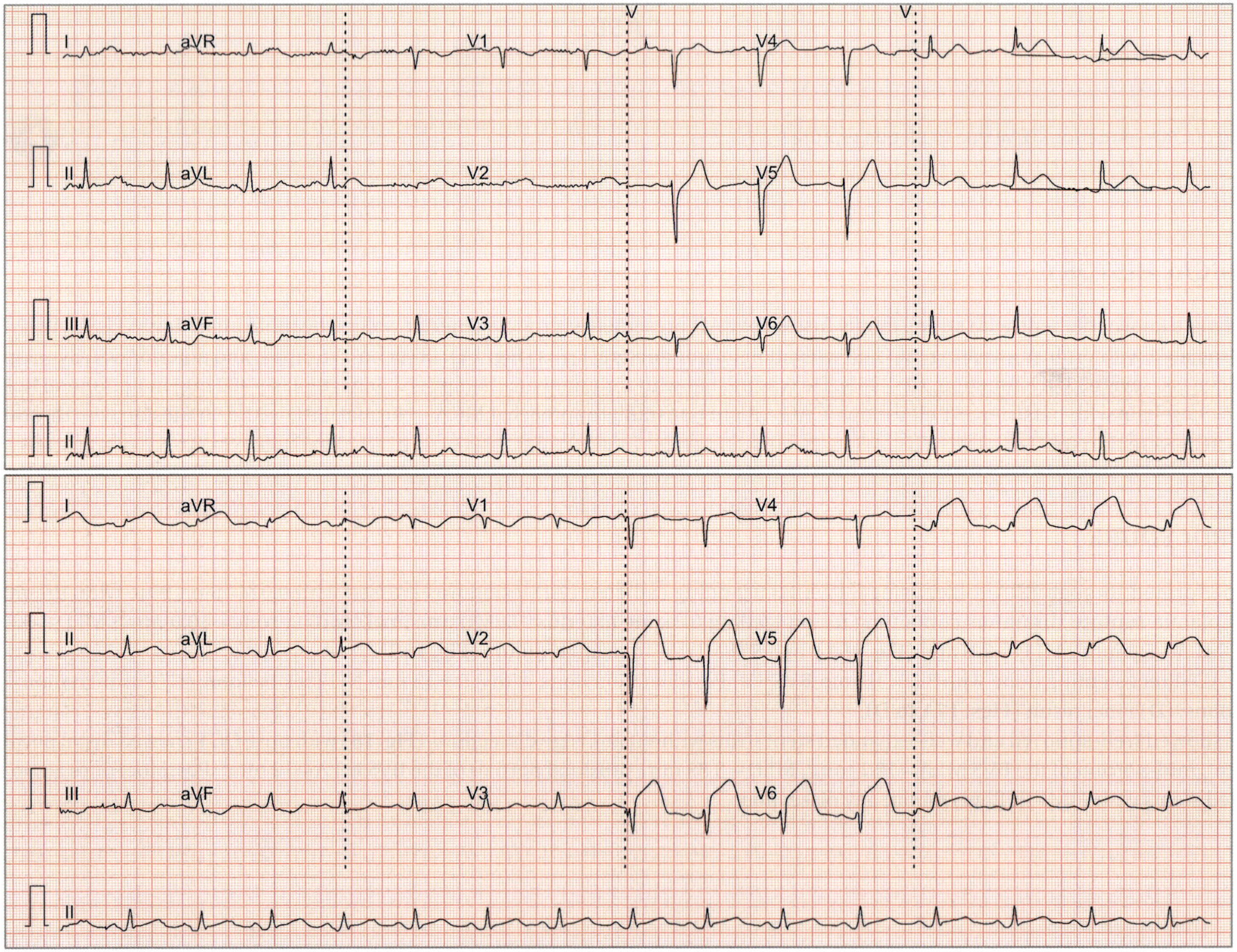

Fig. 14: ECG–showing ST-elevation.

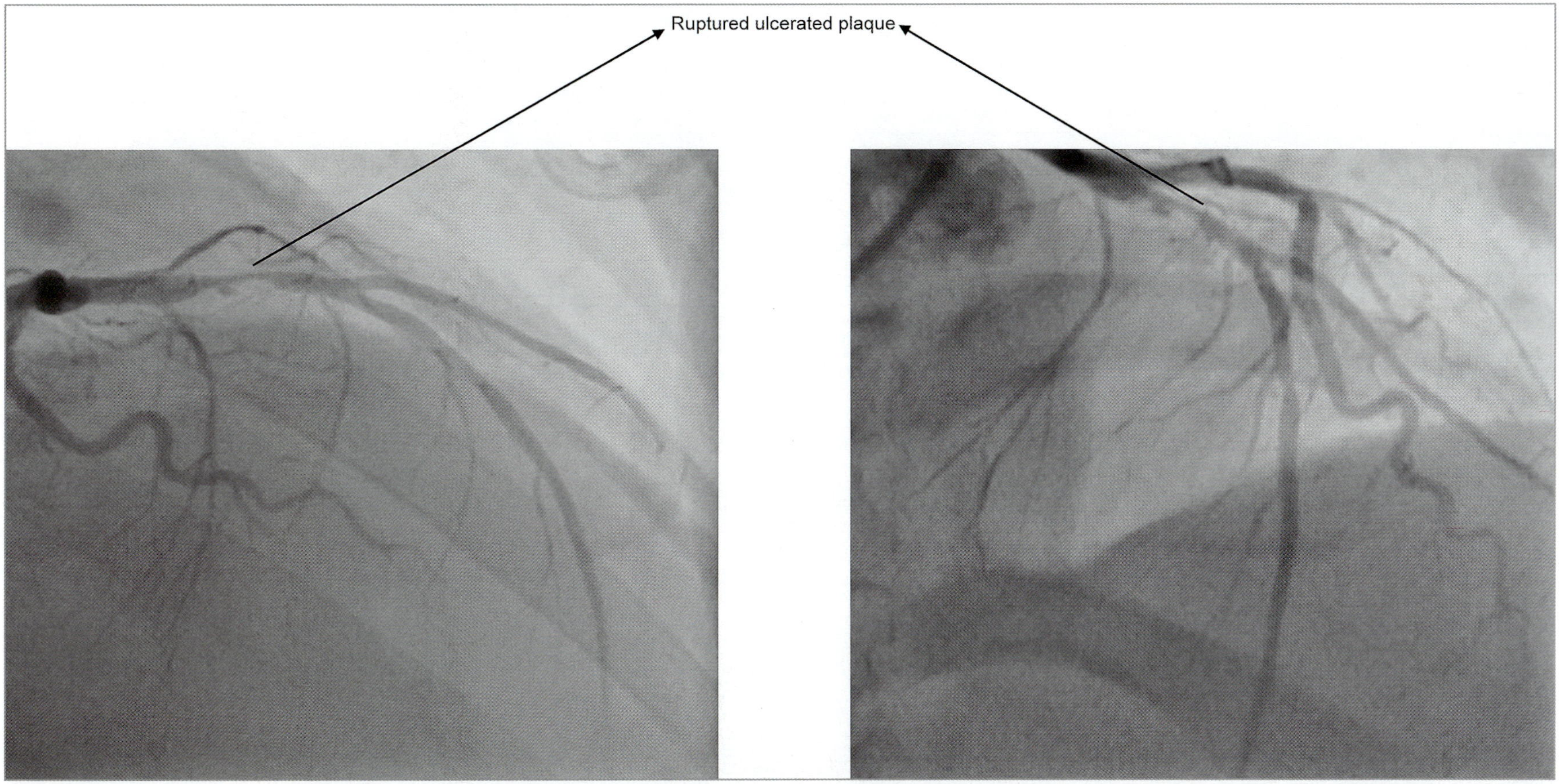

Fig. 15: Coronary angiogram of LAD showing ruptured plaque.

CB/Scoring Balloons- Produces Controlled Dissections with less inflammation and better MLA gain, less chances of IMH, and No melon seed effect with thick fibrotic lesions, and very useful for dilating Ostial fibrotic and mild to moderate fibrotic plaques.

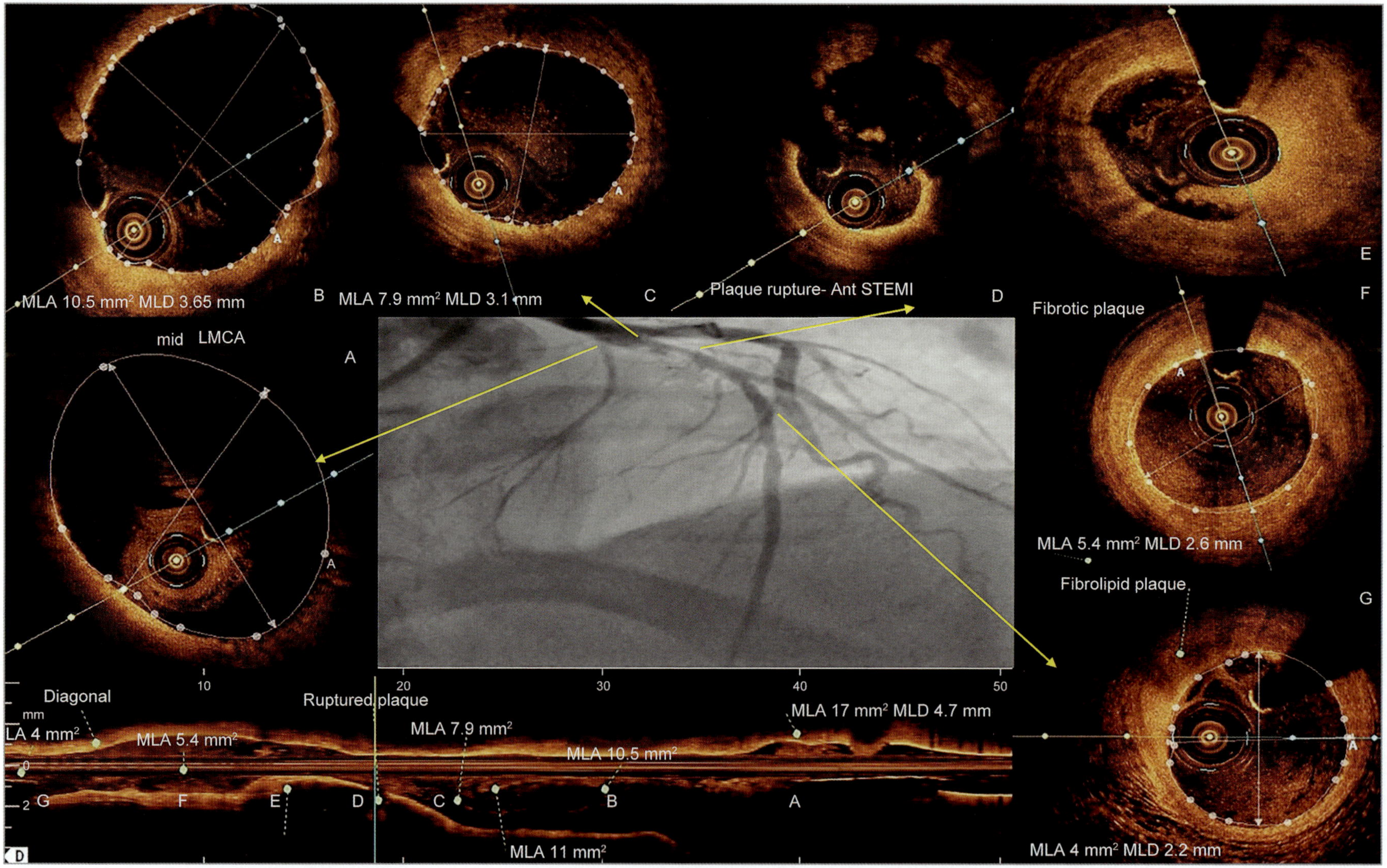
MLA 10.5 mm² MLD 3.65 mm
B
MLA 7.9 mm² MLD 3.1 mm
C
Plaque rupture- Ant STEMI
D
E
F
Fibrotic plaque
mid LMCA
A
MLA 5.4 mm² MLD 2.6 mm
Fibrolipid plaque
G
Diagonal
mm
LA 4 mm²
MLA 5.4 mm²
Ruptured plaque
MLA 7.9 mm²
MLA 10.5 mm²
MLA 17 mm² MLD 4.7 mm
MLA 11 mm²
MLA 4 mm² MLD 2.2 mm
10
20
30
40
50

Fig. 16A

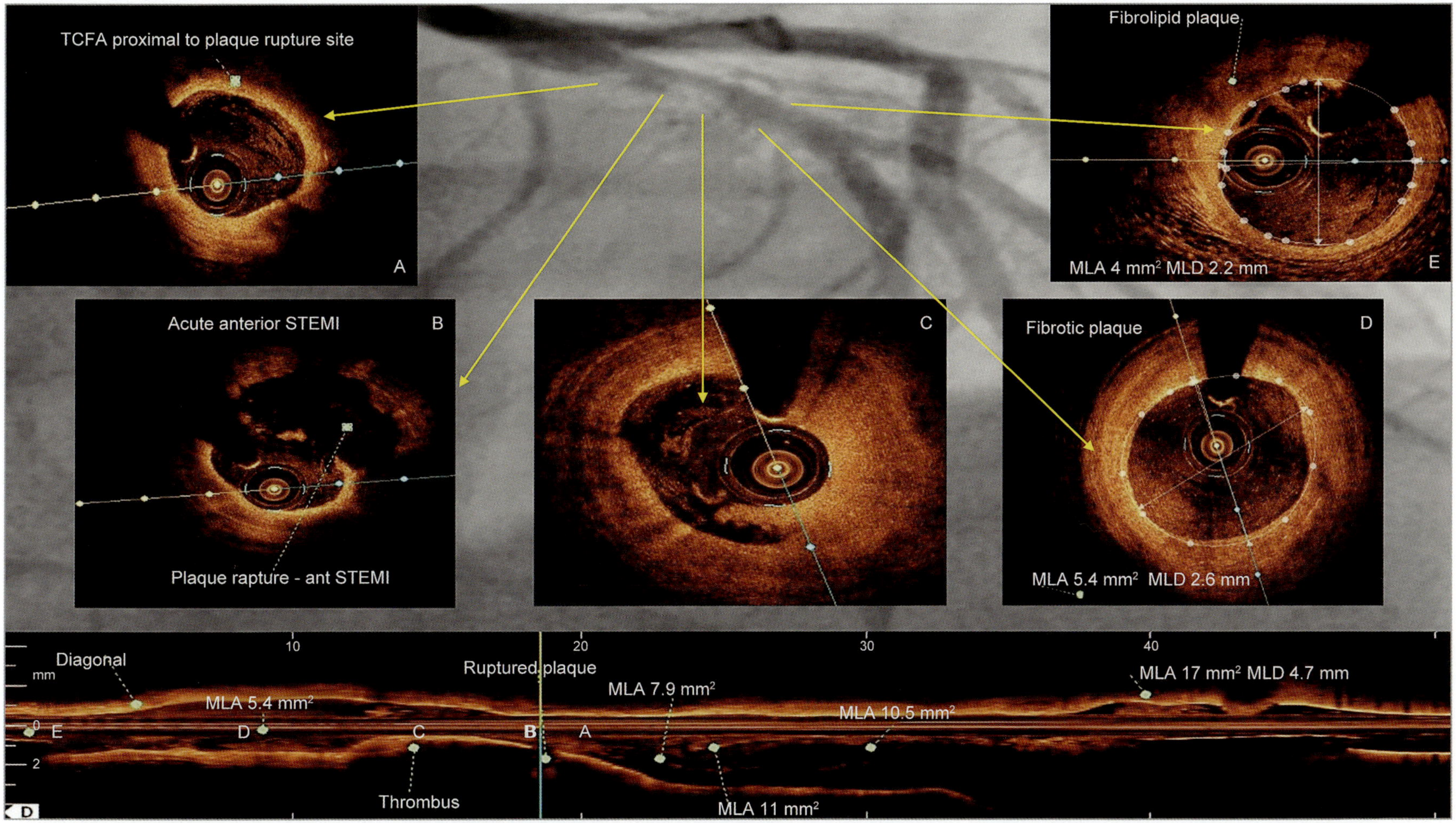

Fig. 16B

Figs. 16A and B: (A) Prestenting OCT assessment of LAD for length and diameter; (B) OCT assessment showing plaque morphology.

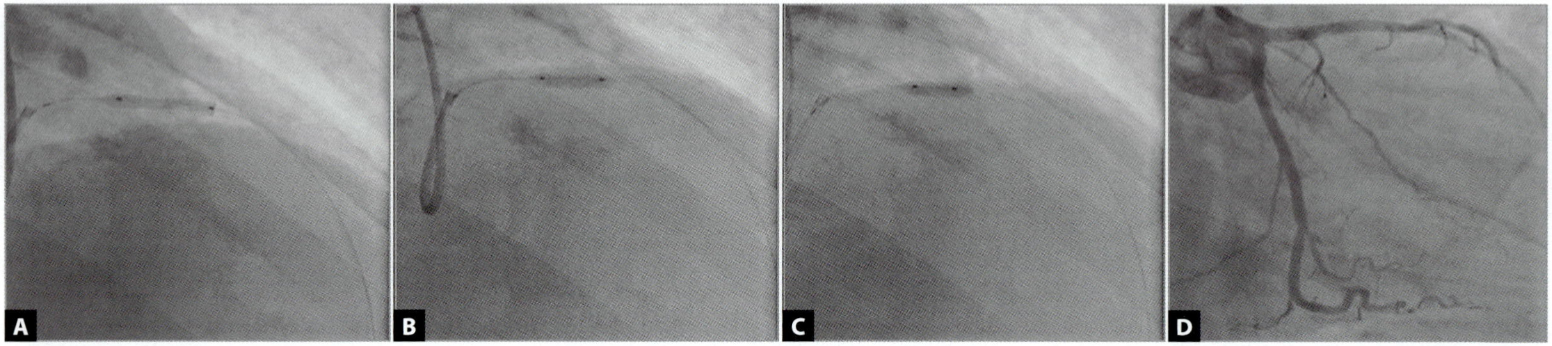

Figs. 17A to D: Coronary angioplasty of LAD.

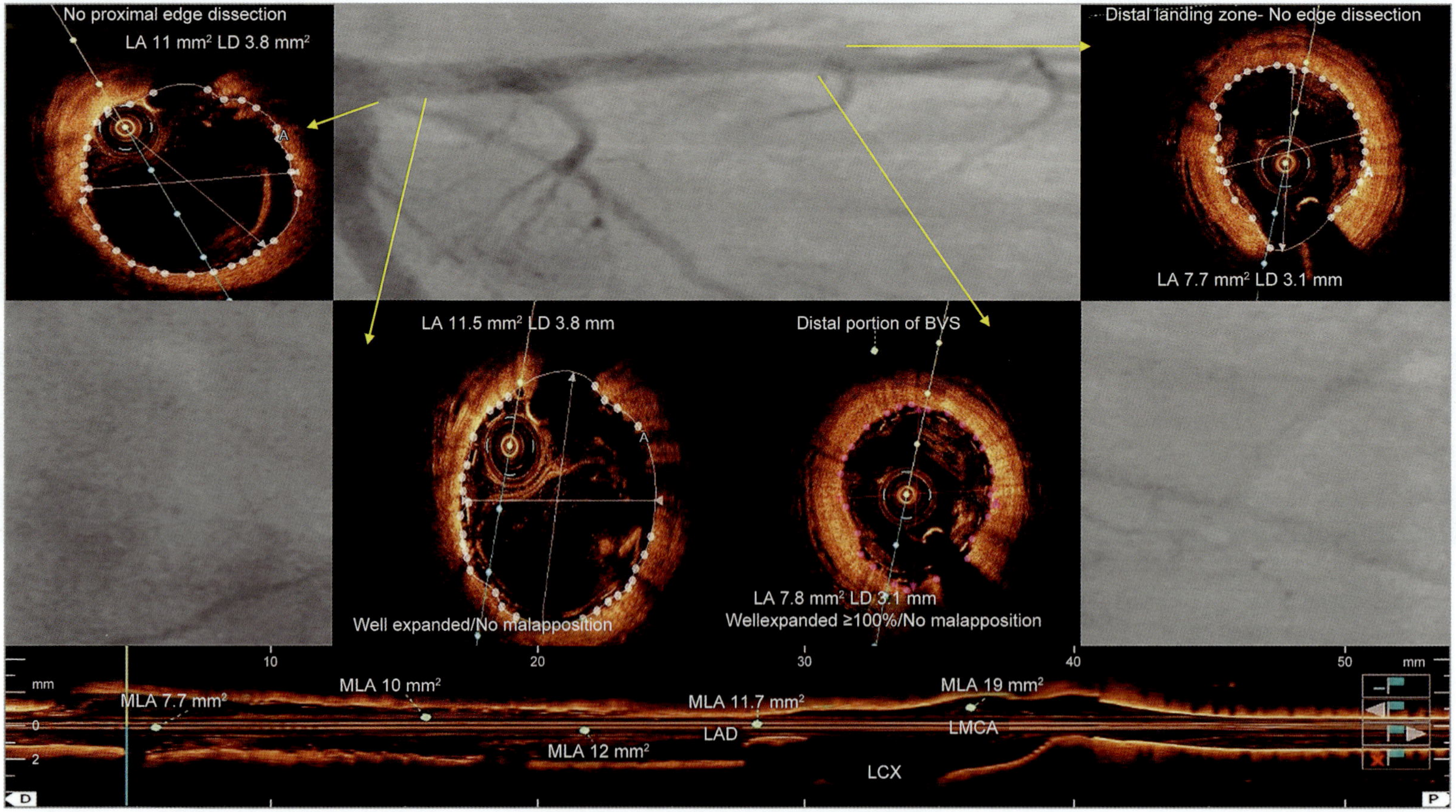

Fig. 18: Poststent OCT assessment for MAX.

CASE 4

STEMI—Plaque erosion with thrombus.

CLINICAL HISTORY

A 42-year-old male presented with evolved AWMI, chest pain associated with SOB, and sweating of 4 hours' duration. ECG-ST-elevation in anterolateral leads, 2D echo—hypokinetic distal IVS, apical and anterior wall, moderate LV systolic dysfunction, EF—40%.

Investigations: RBS—140 mg/dL, blood urea—29 mg/dL, serum creatinine—0.63 mg/dL, eGFR—122. CAG-LMCA—Normal, LAD—Proximal 90% thrombotic lesion, LCX and RCA—Normal **(Fig. 19)**.

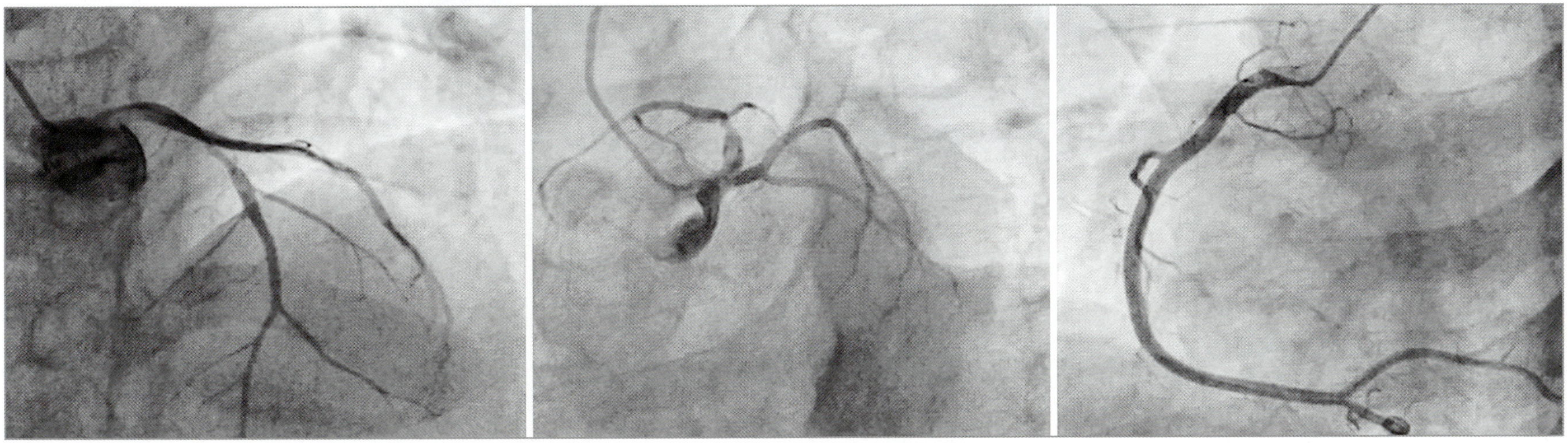

Fig. 19: Coronary angiogram showing LAD, LCX & RCA.

PROCEDURE

Route—RFA, using 6 Fr XB 3.5 guiding catheter, LAD lesion was crossed with 0.014″ Sion Blue wire and LCX crossed with 0.014″ BMW wire.

Pre-OCT showed thrombus and large lipid plaque with critical narrowing with MLA—2.6 mm^2, MLD—1.8 mm, thrombus (Red) burden 20% with MLA—11.1 mm^2, MLD—3.75 mm, total length of the lesion—30.1 mm in proximal LAD **(Fig. 20A)** with thrombus and erosion **(Fig. 20B)**.

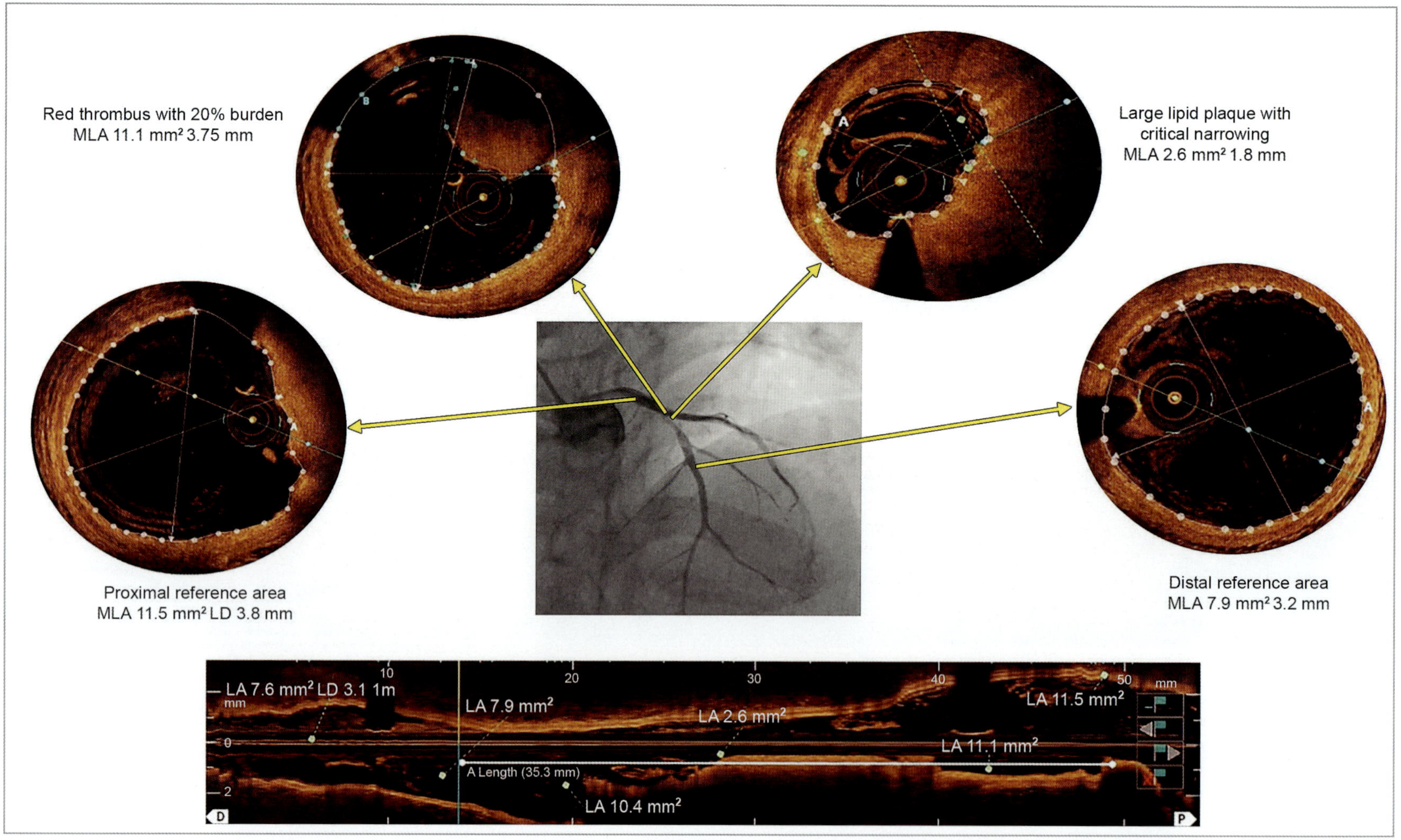

Fig. 20A

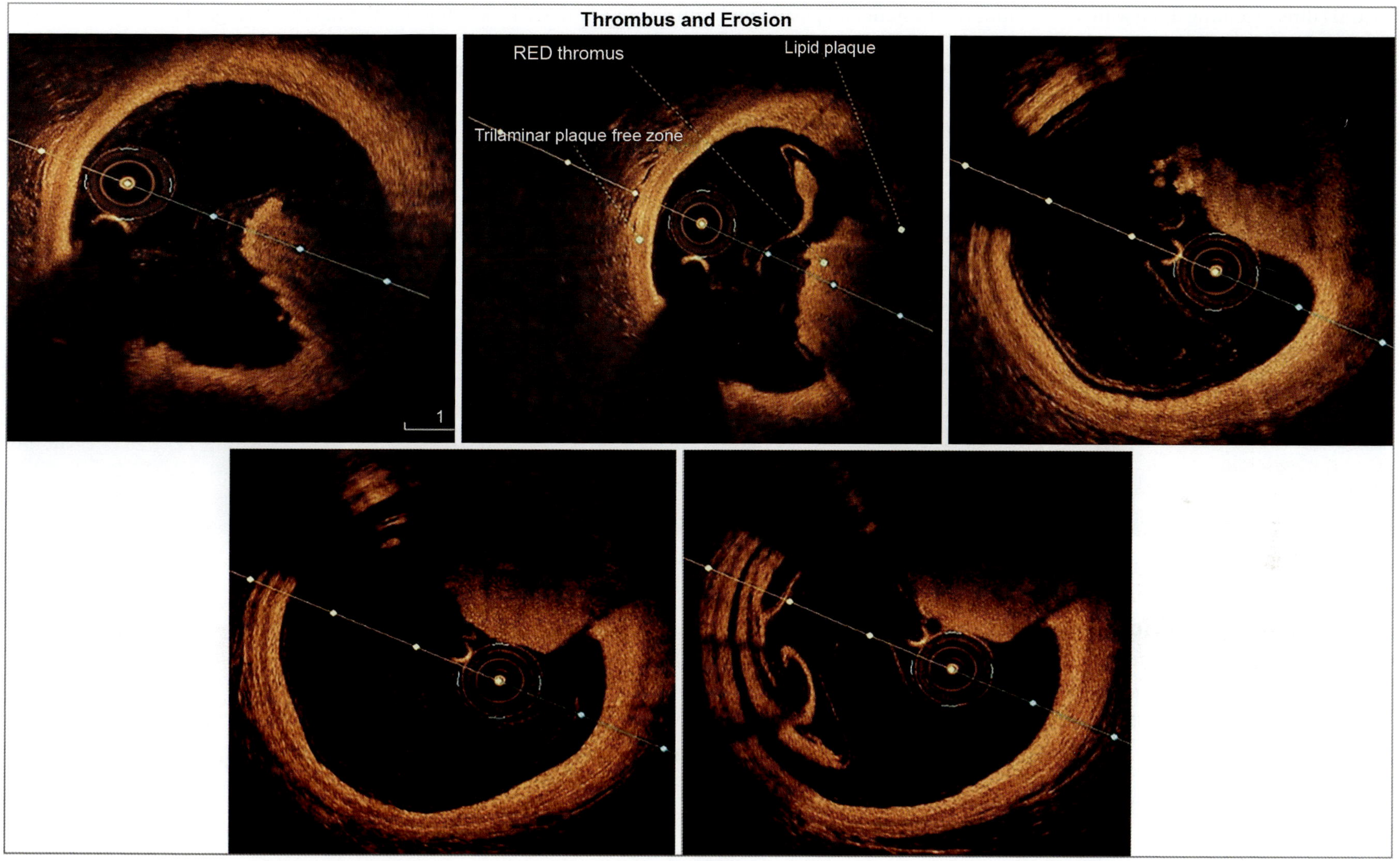

Fig. 20B

Figs. 20A and B: (A) Acute STEMI due to plaque erosion; (B) OCT assessment for plaque morphology.

LAD direct stenting done with 3.5 × 35 mm Orsiro stent and postdilated with 4.0 × 12 mm NC Trek balloon with final result **(Fig. 21)**.

Post-OCT showed proximal landing zone MLA—12 mm^2, MLD—3.9 mm, mid-portion of the stent MLA—7.93 mm^2, MLD—3.2 mm, distal landing zone MLA—7.9 mm^2, MLD—3.2 mm with ostium of the LAD well-apposed and expanded stent struts, no edge dissection with mild tissue prolapse **(Figs. 22A and B)**.

Postprocedure angio view showed well-implanted stents with TIMI-III flow without any dissection.

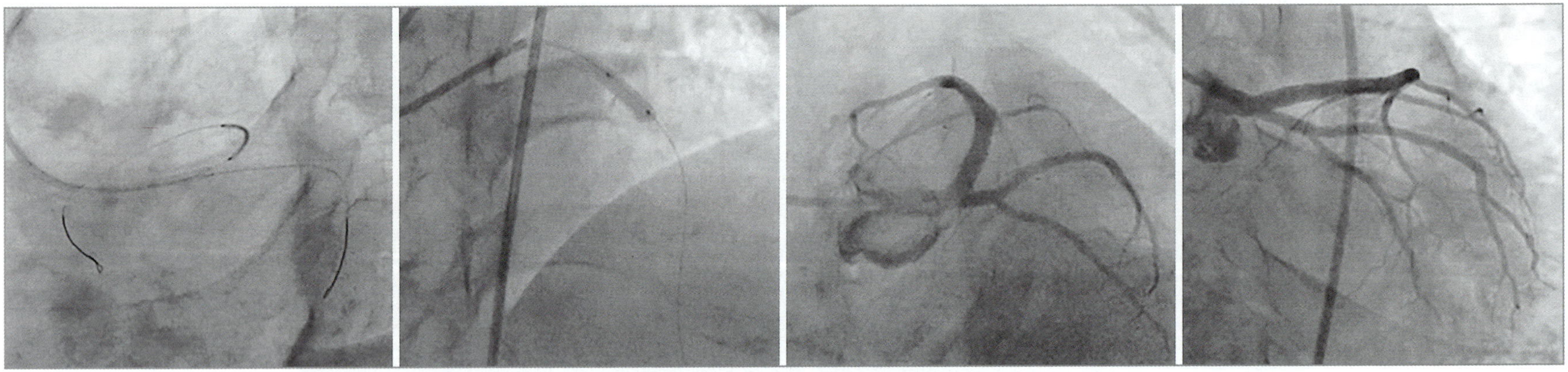

Fig. 21: Coronary angioplasty of LAD.

Coronary Balloon Performance

- *Non-Complaint:*
  - Expand uniformly even in areas of low resistance
  - Exert pressure against focal points of resistance
  - More durable
  - Less flexible
  - Higher crossing/recrossing profile.

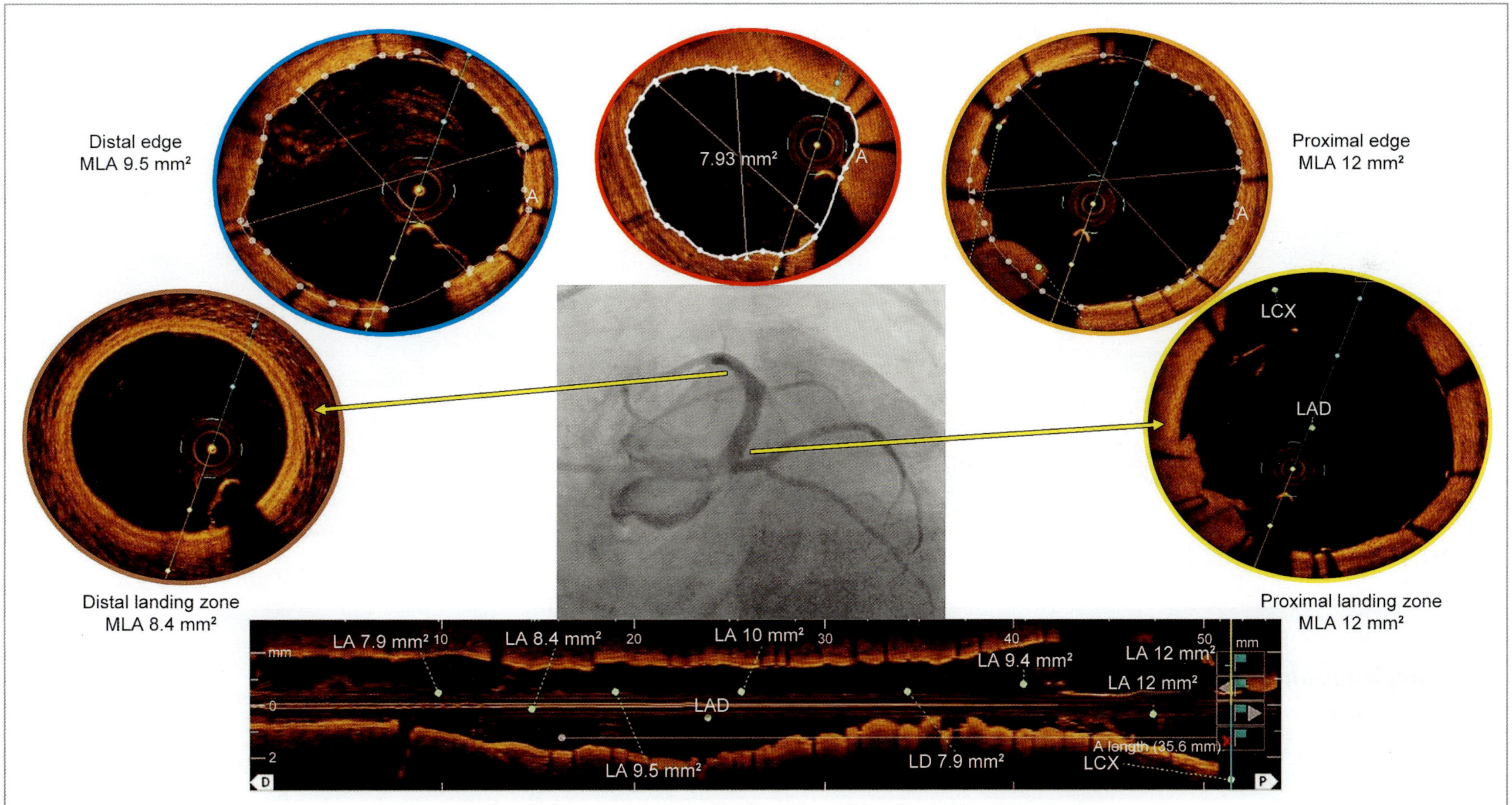

Final result with >100% expansion no edge dissection, mild malapposition /tissue prolapse

Fig. 22A

Patients with Acute STEMI advised to control LDL-C <70 mg/dL, and a lower target of LDL-C <55 mg/dL can be considered in STEMI patients.

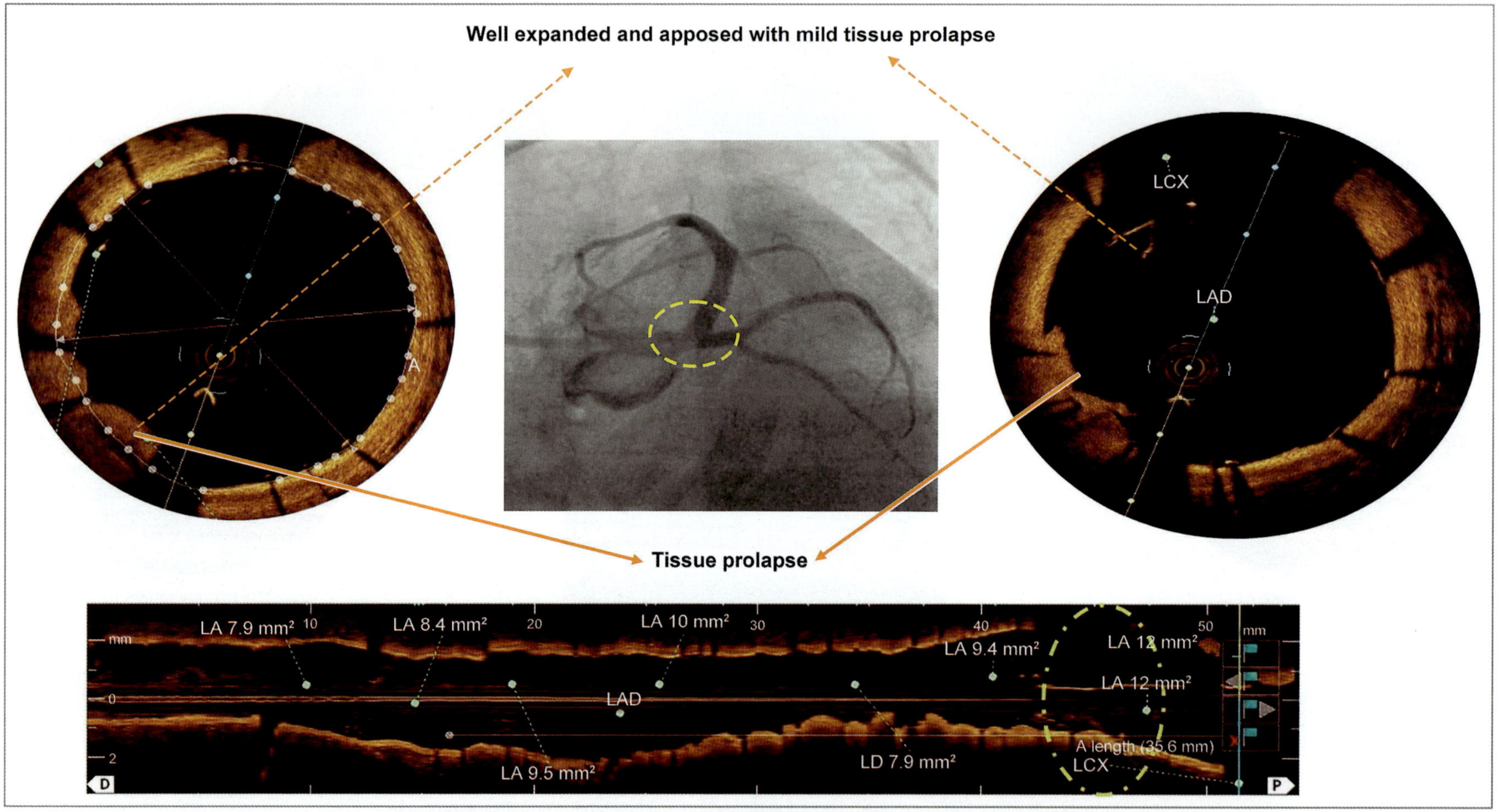

Fig. 22B

Figs. 22A and B: (A) Poststent OCT assessment for MAX; (B) Poststent OCT showing tissue prolapse.

Adequate LDL-C control should achieved by statin plus non-statin therapies, including ezetimibe, Bempedoic acid, PCSK9i or Inclisiran with full consideration of clinical benefit vs side effects , patient's tolerance , long term drug compliance and cost effectiveness of treatment.

CASE 5

PCI of LAD—ACS with plaque rupture.

CLINICAL HISTORY

A 67-year-old male known hypertensive, diabetic presented with CAD—unstable angina, recent onset of chest pain associated with burning sensation and shortness of breath on exertion. 2D echo—No RWMA, normal LV function, EF—62%.

Investigations: RBS—106 mg/dL; blood urea—36 mg/dL; serum creatinine:—1.2 mg/dL; eGFR—62 mL/min. CAG-LMCA—Normal, LAD—Proximal 70–80% long segment lesion, LCX—Normal, RCA—Normal, PDA—70% lesion, PLVB—Normal **(Fig. 23)**.

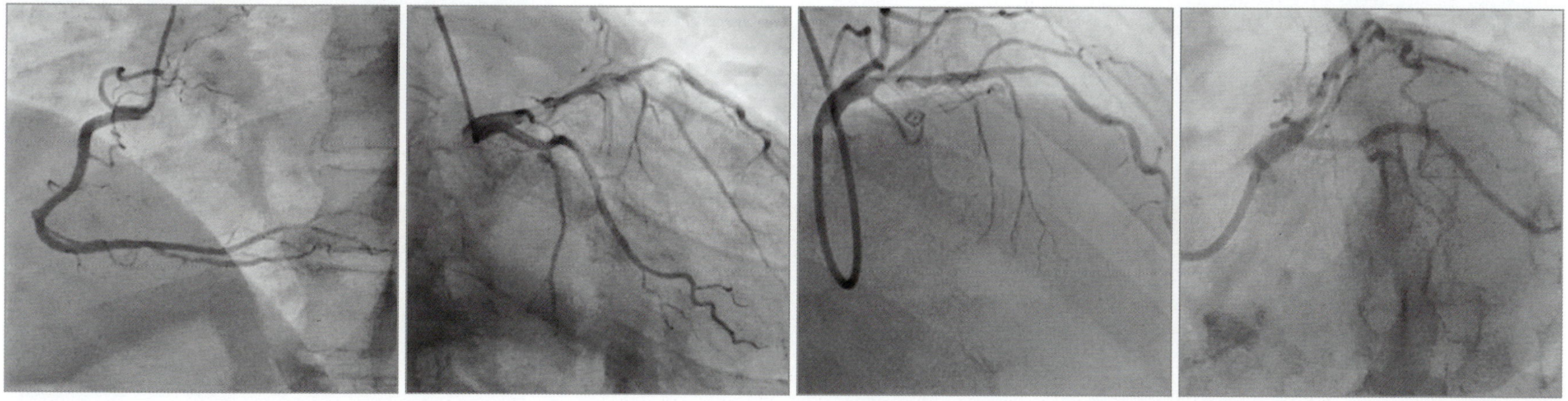

Fig. 23: Coronary angiogram showing RCA, LCX & LAD.

PROCEDURE

Route—RRA, 6 Fr EBU 3.5 guiding catheter, LAD lesion was crossed with 0.014″ Sion Blue wire, predilated with 2.0 × 10 mm Tazuna balloon.

Pre-OCT distal to proximal LAD showed thick fibrotic plaque with distal landing zone MLA—2.49 mm^2, MLD—1.7 mm, mid-LAD tight lesion MLA—1.9 mm^2, lesion length—7.6 mm, diffuse disease and ruptured plaque in proximal LAD, distal LMCA fibrolipid plaque MLA—6.1 mm^2, MLD—2.7 mm, proximal LAD MLA—1.9 mm^2, MLD—1.5 mm, lesion length—15 mm **(Figs. 24A to D)**.

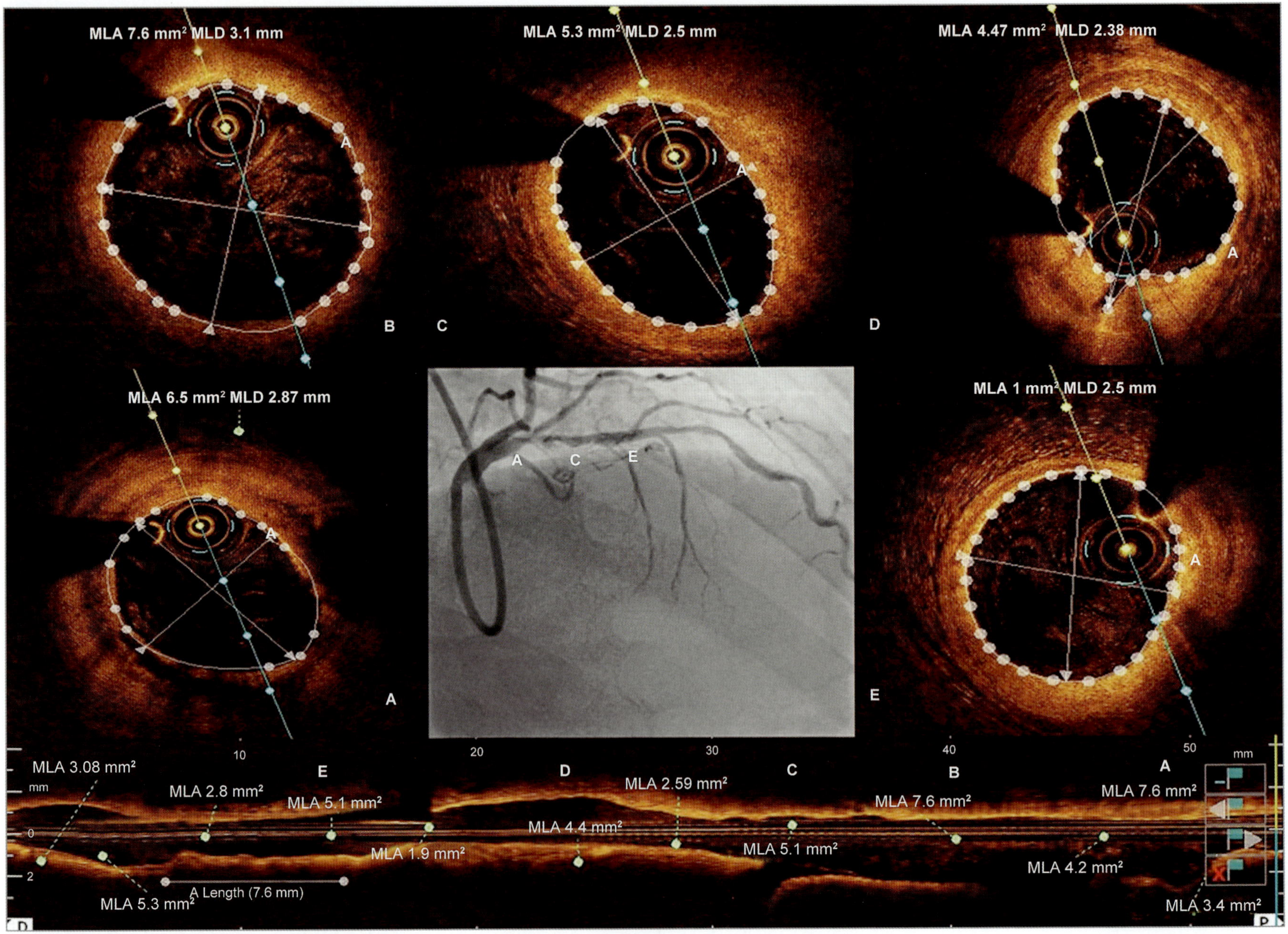
MLA 7.6 mm² MLD 3.1 mm
MLA 5.3 mm² MLD 2.5 mm
MLA 4.47 mm² MLD 2.38 mm
MLA 6.5 mm² MLD 2.87 mm
MLA 1 mm² MLD 2.5 mm
A
B
C
D
E
MLA 3.08 mm²
MLA 2.8 mm²
MLA 5.1 mm²
MLA 1.9 mm²
MLA 4.4 mm²
MLA 2.59 mm²
MLA 5.1 mm²
MLA 7.6 mm²
MLA 4.2 mm²
MLA 7.6 mm²
MLA 3.4 mm²
MLA 5.3 mm²
A Length (7.6 mm)

Fig. 24A

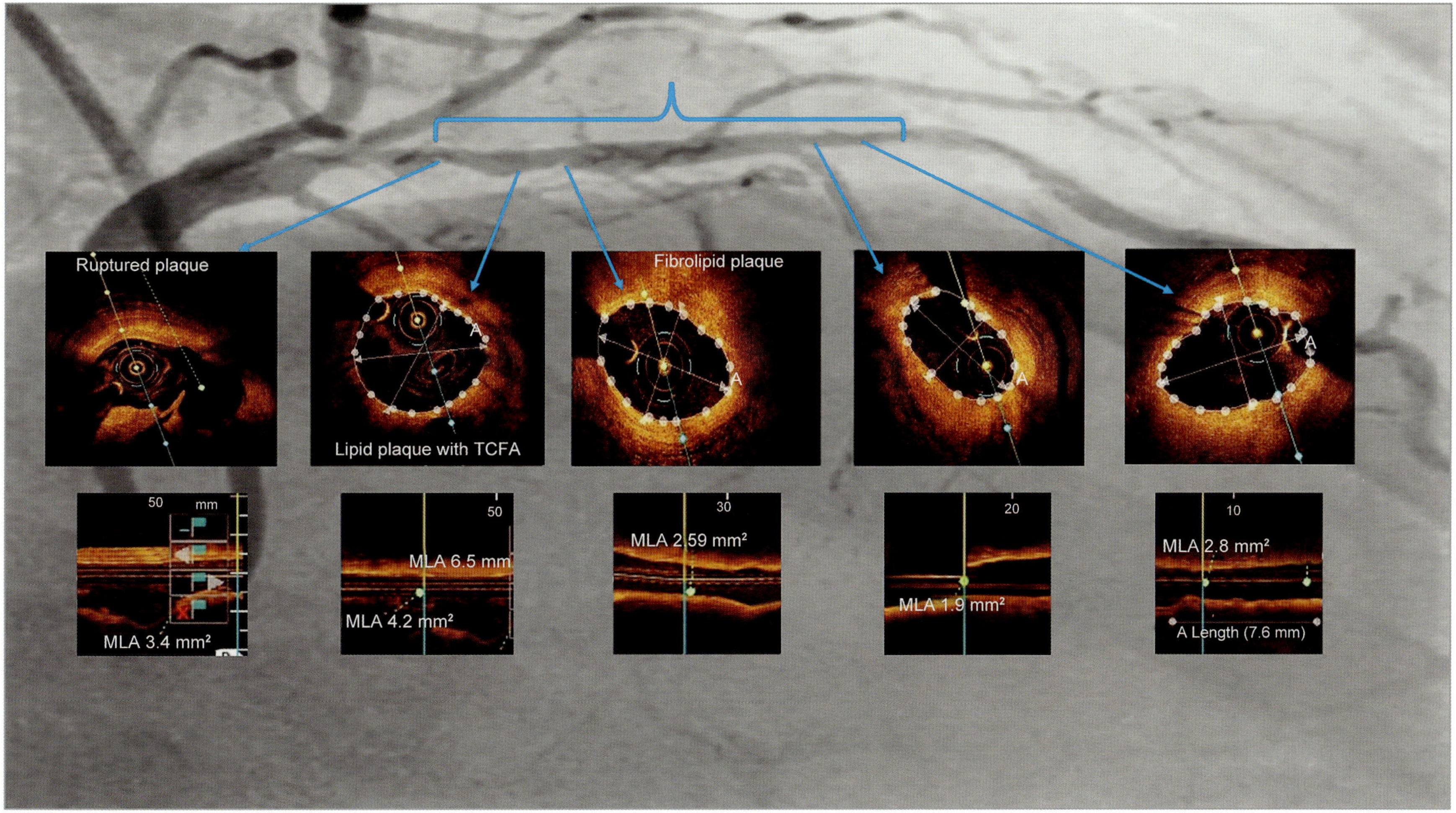
Ruptured plaque
Lipid plaque with TCFA
Fibrolipid plaque
MLA 3.4 mm²
MLA 6.5 mm
MLA 4.2 mm²
MLA 2.59 mm²
MLA 1.9 mm²
MLA 2.8 mm²
A Length (7.6 mm)

Fig. 24B

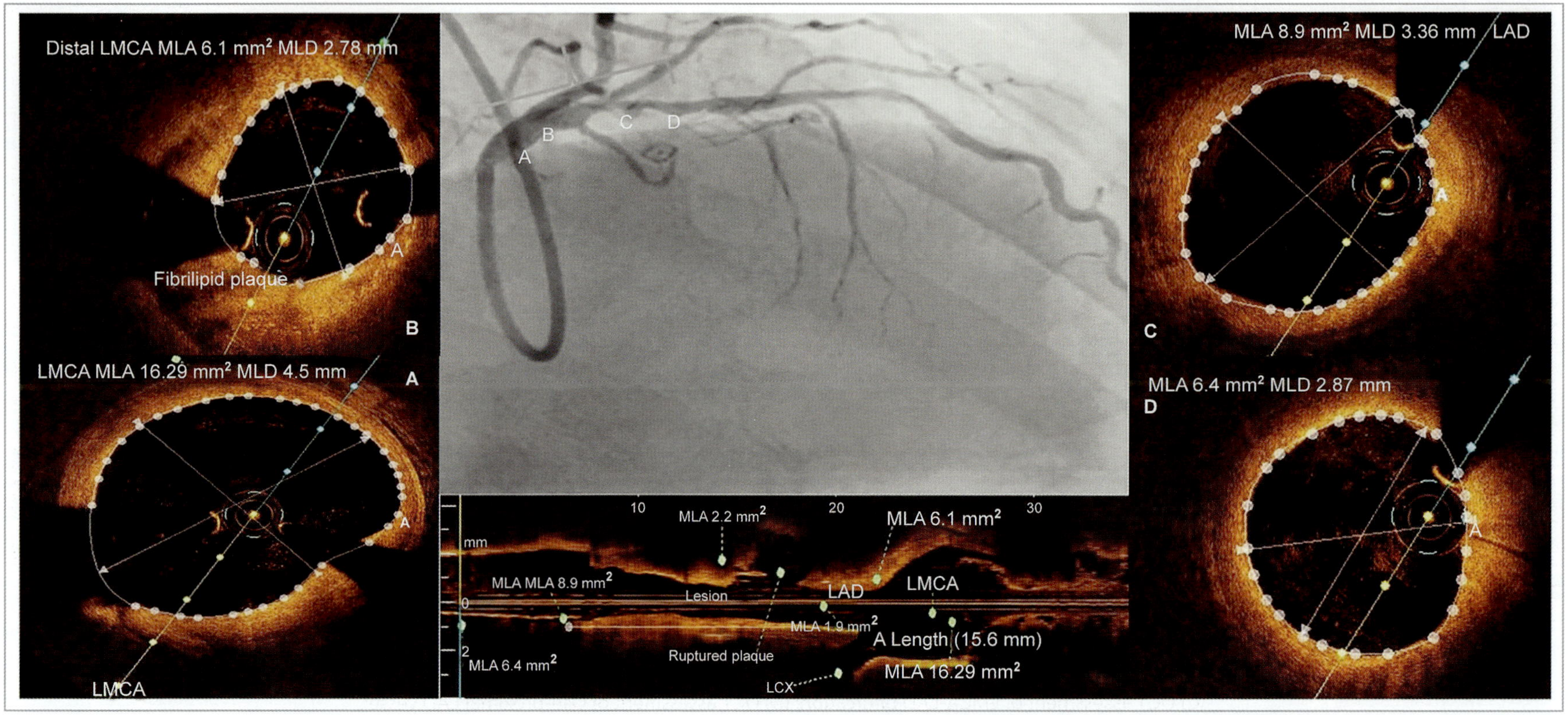

Fig. 24C

Coronary Balloon Performance

- *Semi Complaint:*
  - Expand more as pressure increases
  - Expand preferentially in areas of least resistance
  - Longitudinal growth
  - More flexible
  - Lower crossing/recrossing profile.

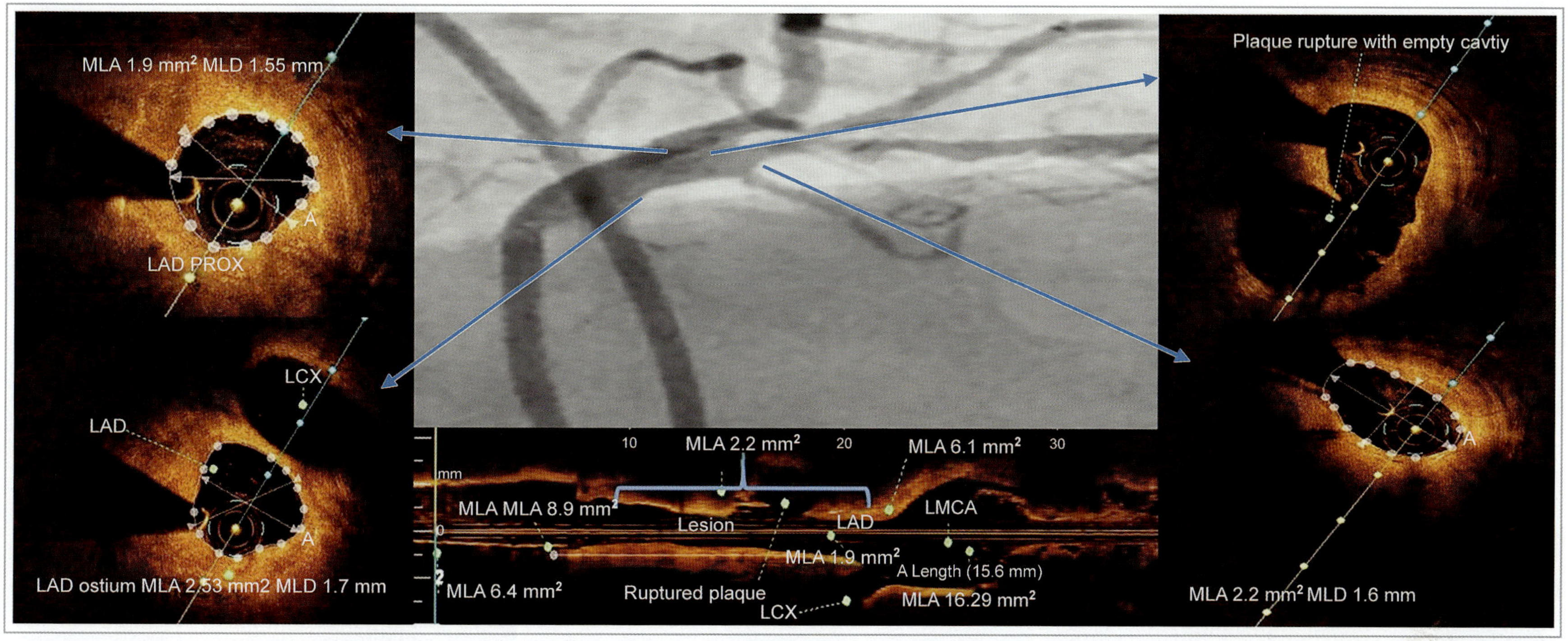

Fig. 24D

Figs. 24A to D: (A) Pre stent OCT assessment of LAD for length and diameter; (B) OCT assessment for plaque morphology; (C) OCT assessment of LMCA-LAD bifurcation; (D) OCT assessment of Osti-proximal LAD vessel.

Predilatation done with 2.0 × 10 mm Tazuna balloon, mid-LAD stenting done with 3.0 × 30 mm Orsiro stent, proximal LAD overlapping stenting done with 3.5 × 30 mm Orsiro stent, postdilatation done with 4.0 × 08 mm NC Trek balloon, with final result **(Fig. 25)**.

Poststenting OCT was done which showed well-apposed and well-expanded stent struts, without any edge dissections with distal edge of stent MLA—5.75 mm^2, MLD—2.7 mm, proximal LAD MLA—5.69 mm^2 **(Fig. 26)**. Postprocedure angio view showed well-implanted stents with TIMI-III flow without any dissection.

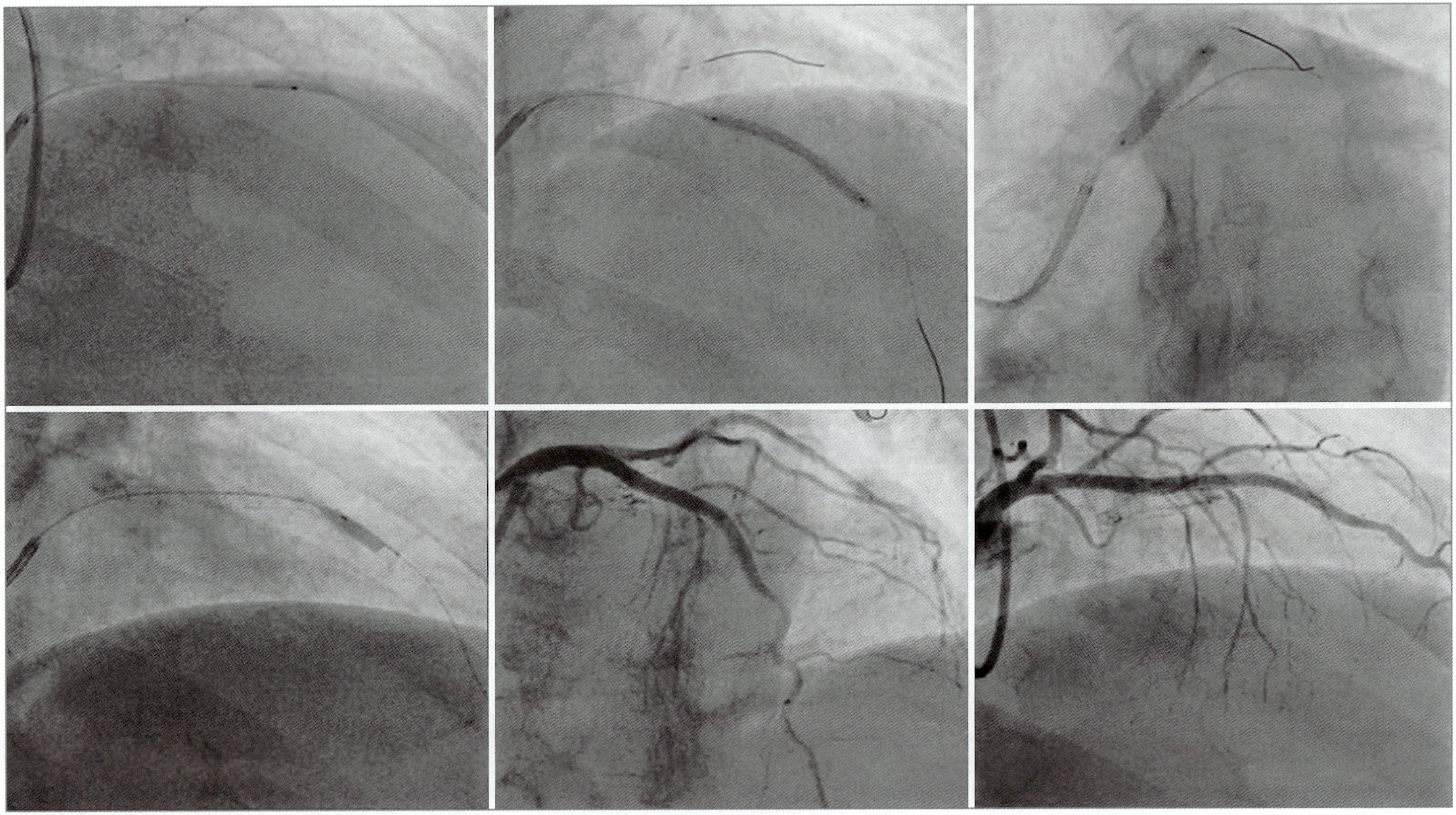

Fig. 25: Coronary Angioplasty.

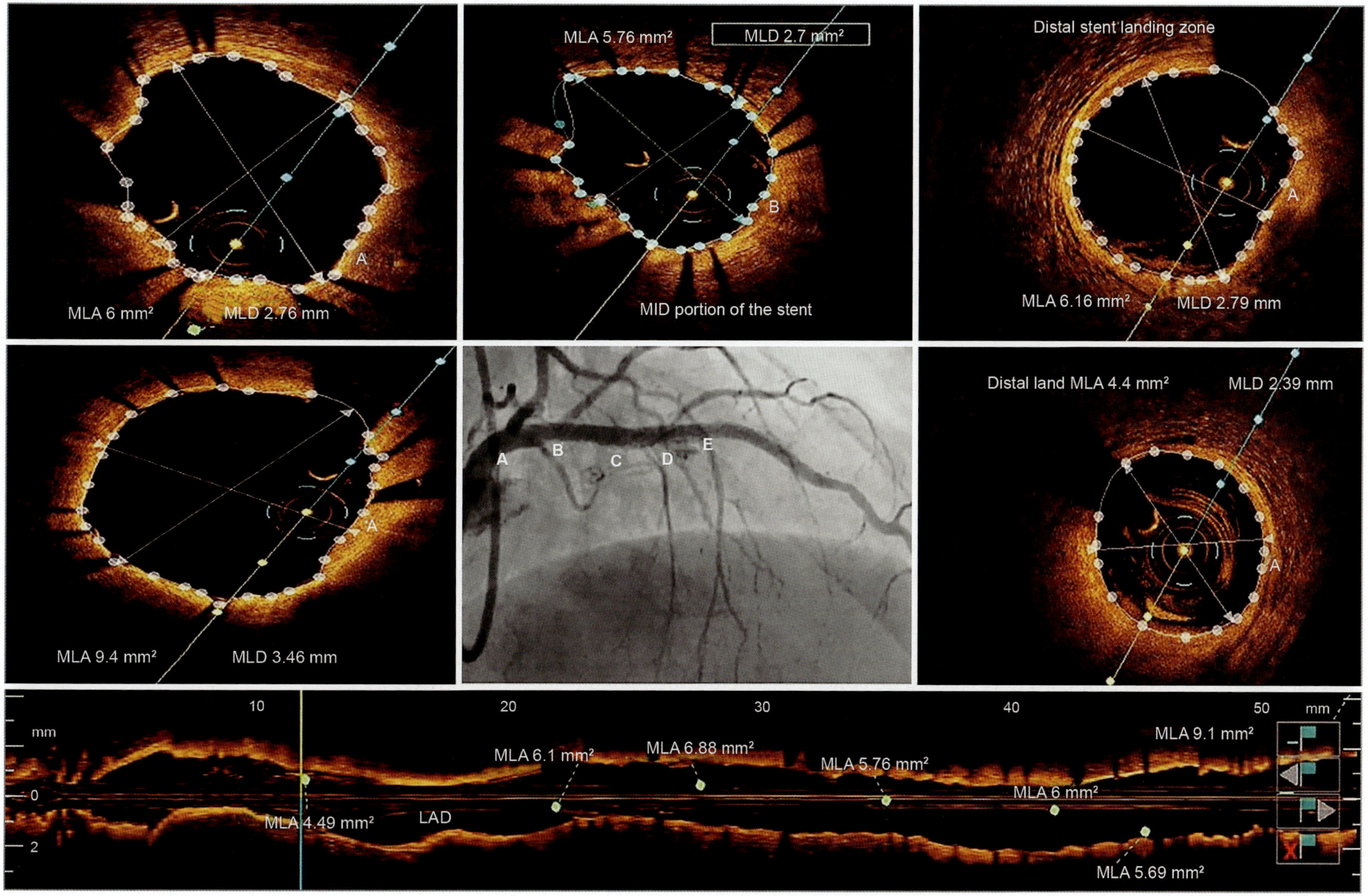

Fig. 26: Post LAD stenting OCT assessment for MAX.

CASE 6

OCT Assessment of calcium during PCI (ACS due to CN).

CLINICAL HISTORY

A 53-year-old male presented with CAD-old MI, known hypertensive, diabetic associated with chest pain, past history of CABG in 2017, 2D echo-No RWMA, normal LV function, EF—64%.

CAG-LMCA—Normal, LAD—Proximal 60–70% lesion, mid-total occlusion, D1—Proximal 80–90% lesion, LCX—proximal 70% lesion of OM1 branch, RCA—Proximal 90% lesion, Mid-80% lesion, PDA—70–80% lesion, graft angiogram-LIMA to LAD, D1, OM2—patent grafts, SVG to RCA-occluded graft **(Fig. 27)**.

PROCEDURE

Route—RRA, 6 Fr JR 3.5 guiding catheter, RCA lesion was crossed with 0.014″ power turn wire. Predilatation was done with 1.5 × 10 mm Tazuna balloon. Stenting attempted with guide liner support but could not cross the lesion in view of heavy calcification. Hence, further procedure abandoned.

After 1 month patient admitted for PCI of RCA, route—RFA, using 6 Fr JR 3.5 guiding catheter, check angiogram revealed RCA—Proximal to mid-long segment 90% stenosis, which was crossed with 0.014″ Sion Blue wire using microcatheter support, rotablation of RCA done with 1.5 mm Burr with TPI support.

Post-rota-OCT analysis **(Figs. 28A to C)** showed superficial calcium with thrombus and fibrocalcific plaque.

Mid-RCA stenting was done with 3.0 × 34 mm Resolute Onyx stent. Proximal RCA stenting was done with 3.5 × 34 mm Resolute Onyx stent. Ostial RCA stenting was done with 4.0 × 08 mm Resolute Onyx stent. Mid-RCA postdilatation was done with 3.5 × 15 mm Pantera balloon **(Fig. 29)**.

Poststenting OCT was done which showed well-apposed and well-expanded stent struts without any edge dissections **(Figs. 30A to C)**. Postprocedure angio view showed well-implanted stents with TIMI-III flow without any dissection.

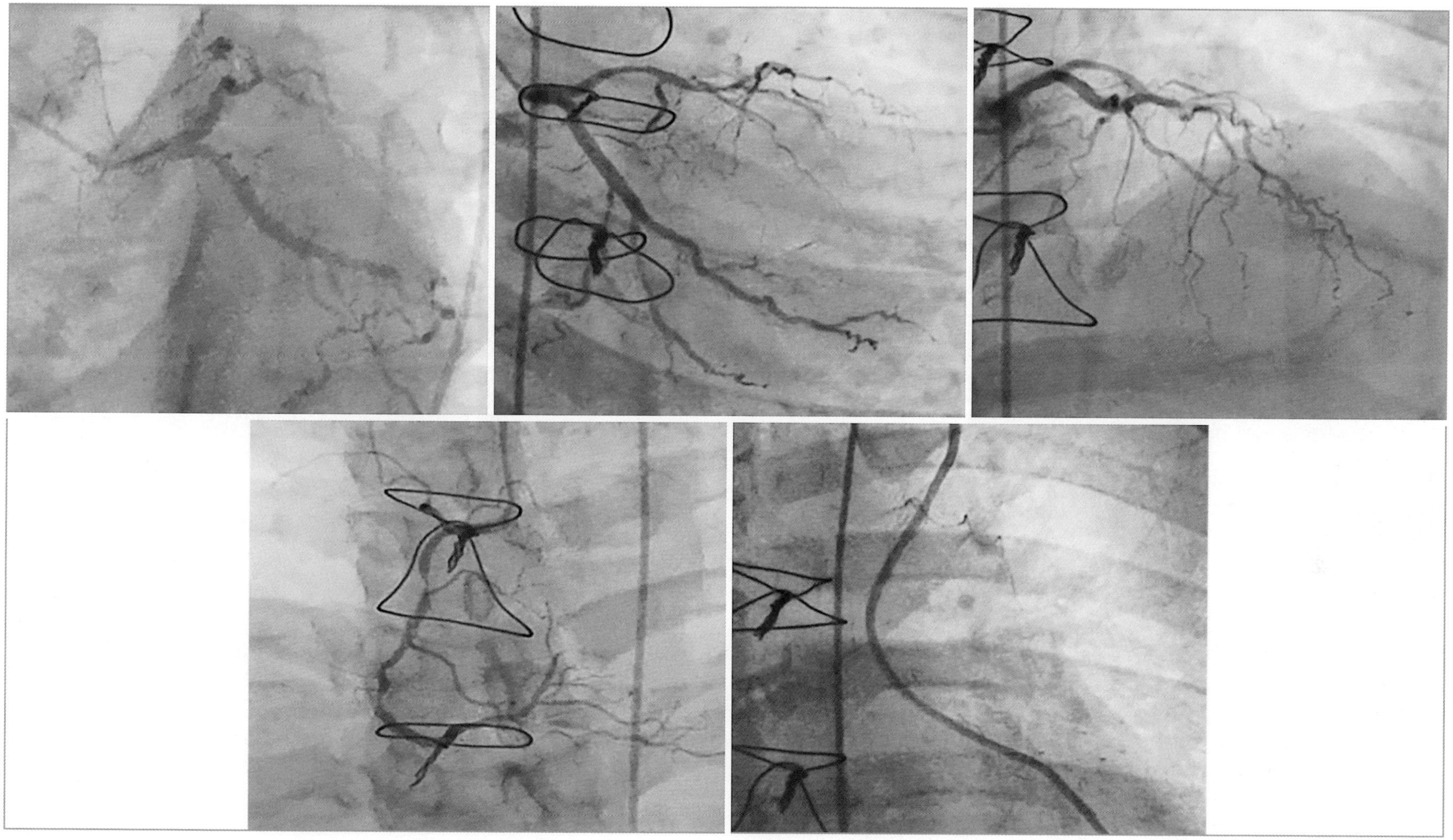

Fig. 27: Coronary angiogram followed by graft angio.

All patients with PCI should be implimented with standard DAPT therapy, and special emphasis should be made for optimal control of cardiovascular risk factors with life style modification.

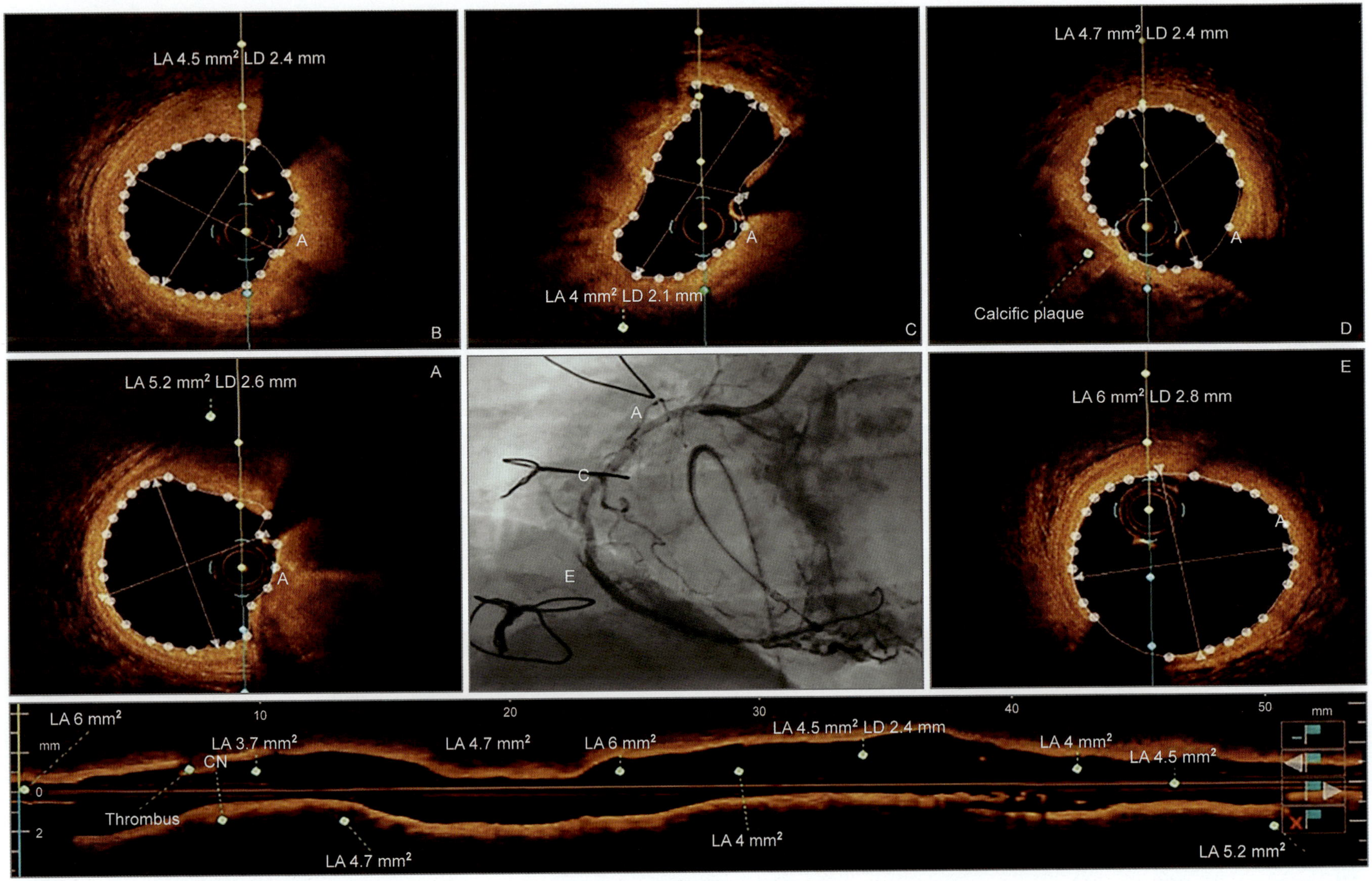

LA 4.5 mm² LD 2.4 mm
A
B
LA 4 mm² LD 2.1 mm
A
C
LA 4.7 mm² LD 2.4 mm
A
Calcific plaque
D
LA 5.2 mm² LD 2.6 mm
A
A
C
E
LA 6 mm² LD 2.8 mm
A
E
LA 6 mm²
mm
0
2
10
20
30
40
50
mm
LA 3.7 mm²
CN
Thrombus
LA 4.7 mm²
LA 4.7 mm²
LA 6 mm²
LA 4.5 mm² LD 2.4 mm
LA 4 mm²
LA 4 mm²
LA 4.5 mm²
LA 5.2 mm²

Fig. 28A

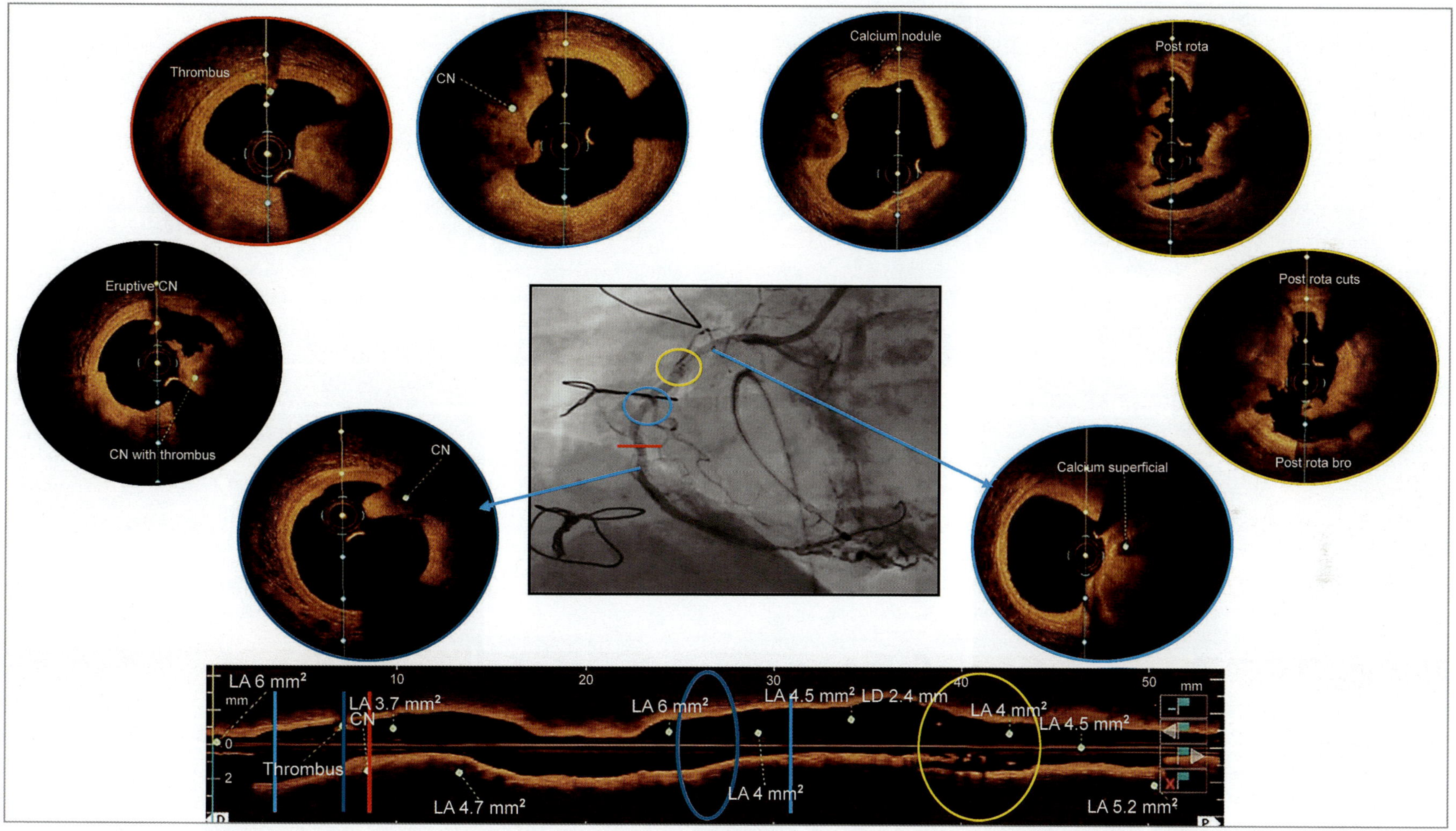

Fig. 28B

Patients with vulnerable plaques on OCT imaging need high dose statins with or without other lipid therapeutic drugs combination to maintain LDL levels in the optimal range.

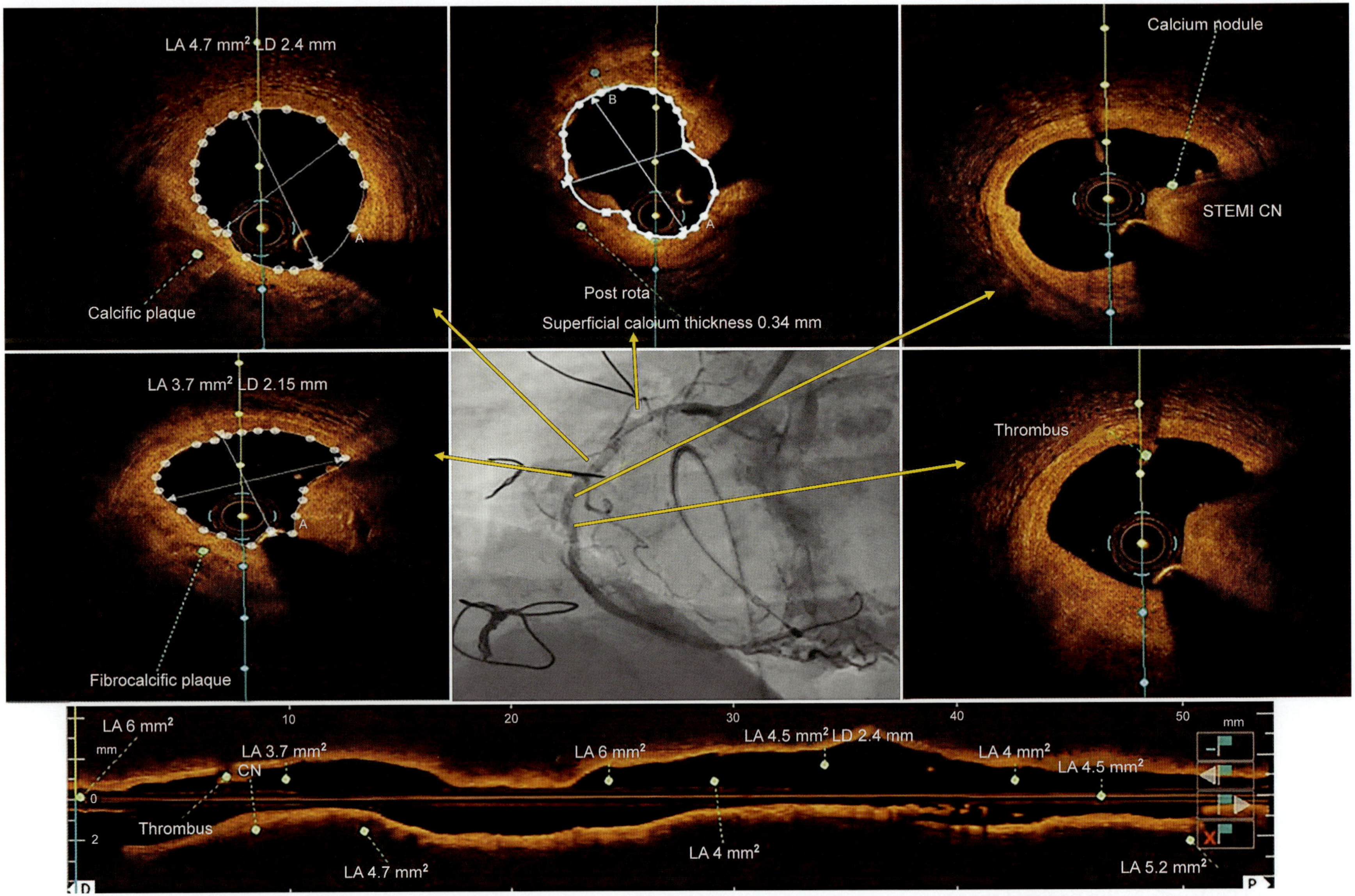

Fig. 28C

Figs. 28A to C: (A) Post ROTA OCT assessment for length and diameter; (B) Post ROTA OCT assessment for ROTA cuts and plaque morphology; (C) Post ROTA OCT assessment for sizing of the devise.

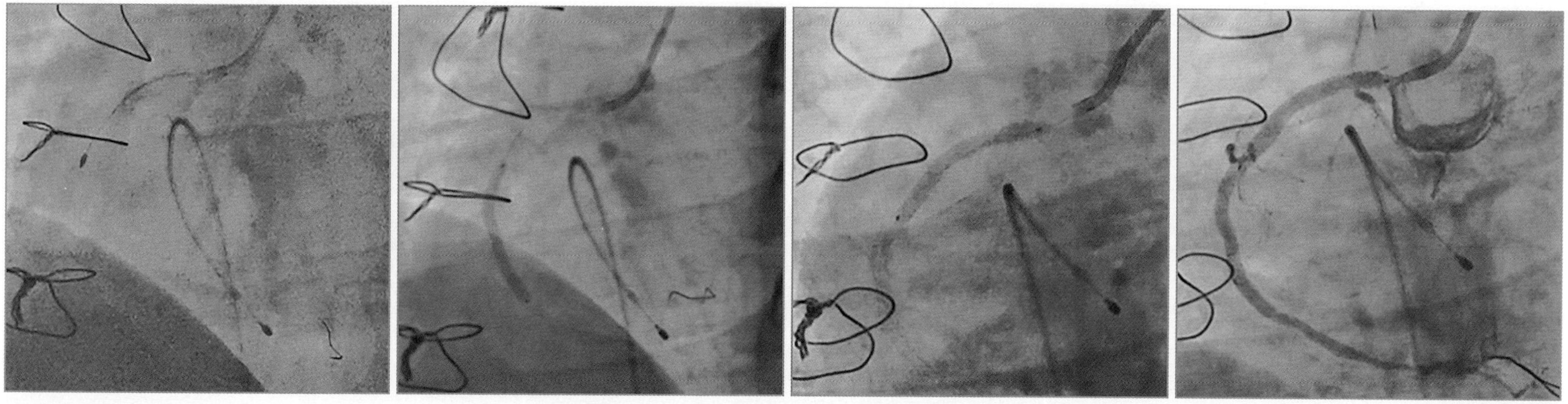

Fig. 29: Rotablation followed by coronary angioplasty.

Basic principles of operating Rota include use of single 1.5 mm burr (appropriate in >90% of the cases) with burr-to-artery ratio of 0.6, rotational speed of about 140,000 to 180,000 rpm, gradual burr advancement with a slow pecking motion, 15 to 20 sec of short ablative runs guided by fluoroscopy, acoustic and tactile inputs, and avoid significant deceleration in rotational speed >5000 rpm to reduce complications like burr entrapment/burr stall/burr detachment, and finish the procedure with 1or 2 final polishing runs.

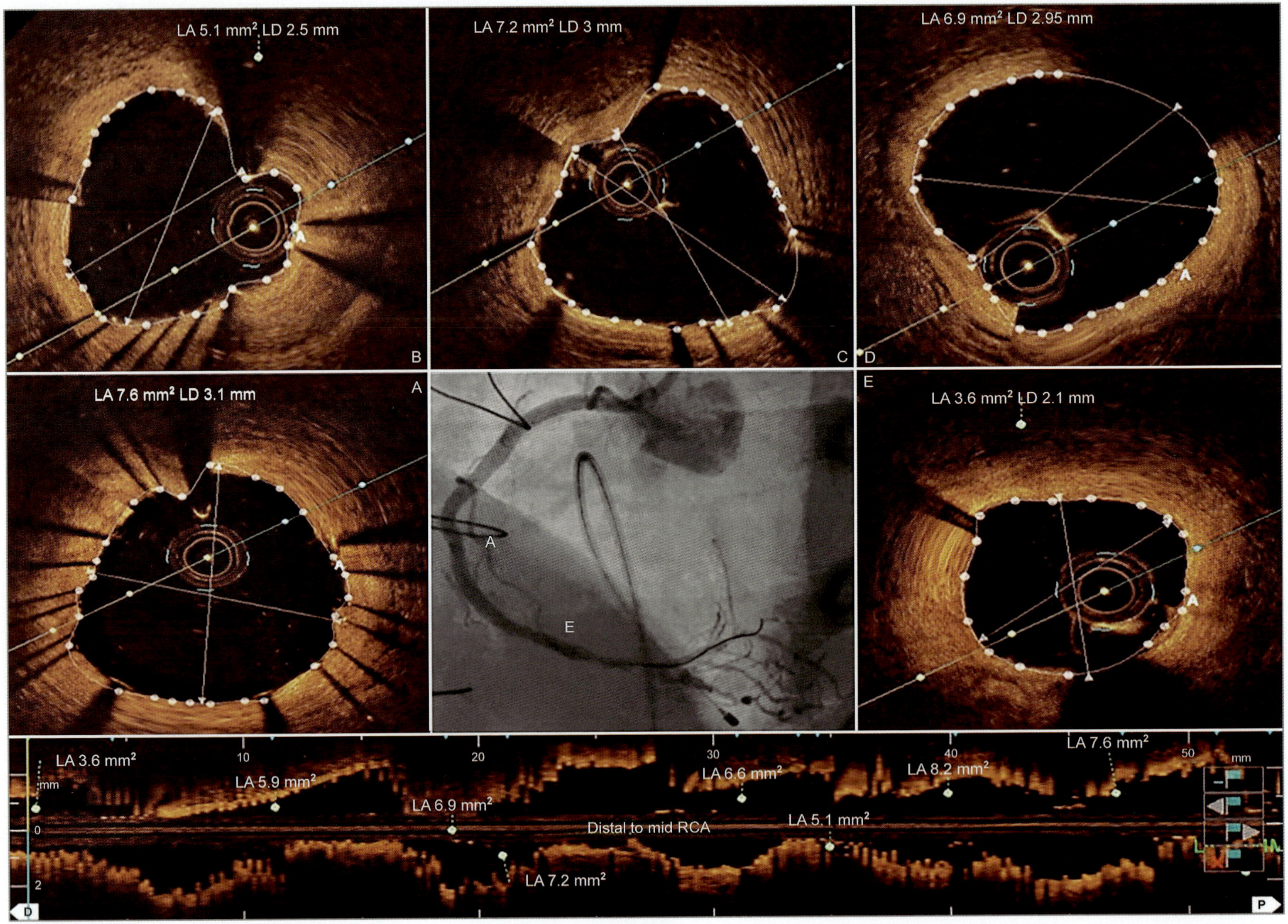
LA 5.1 mm² LD 2.5 mm
B
LA 7.2 mm² LD 3 mm
C
LA 6.9 mm² LD 2.95 mm
D
LA 7.6 mm² LD 3.1 mm
A
E
LA 3.6 mm² LD 2.1 mm
LA 3.6 mm²
LA 5.9 mm²
LA 6.9 mm²
LA 7.2 mm²
Distal to mid RCA
LA 6.6 mm²
LA 5.1 mm²
LA 8.2 mm²
LA 7.6 mm²
D
P

Fig. 30A

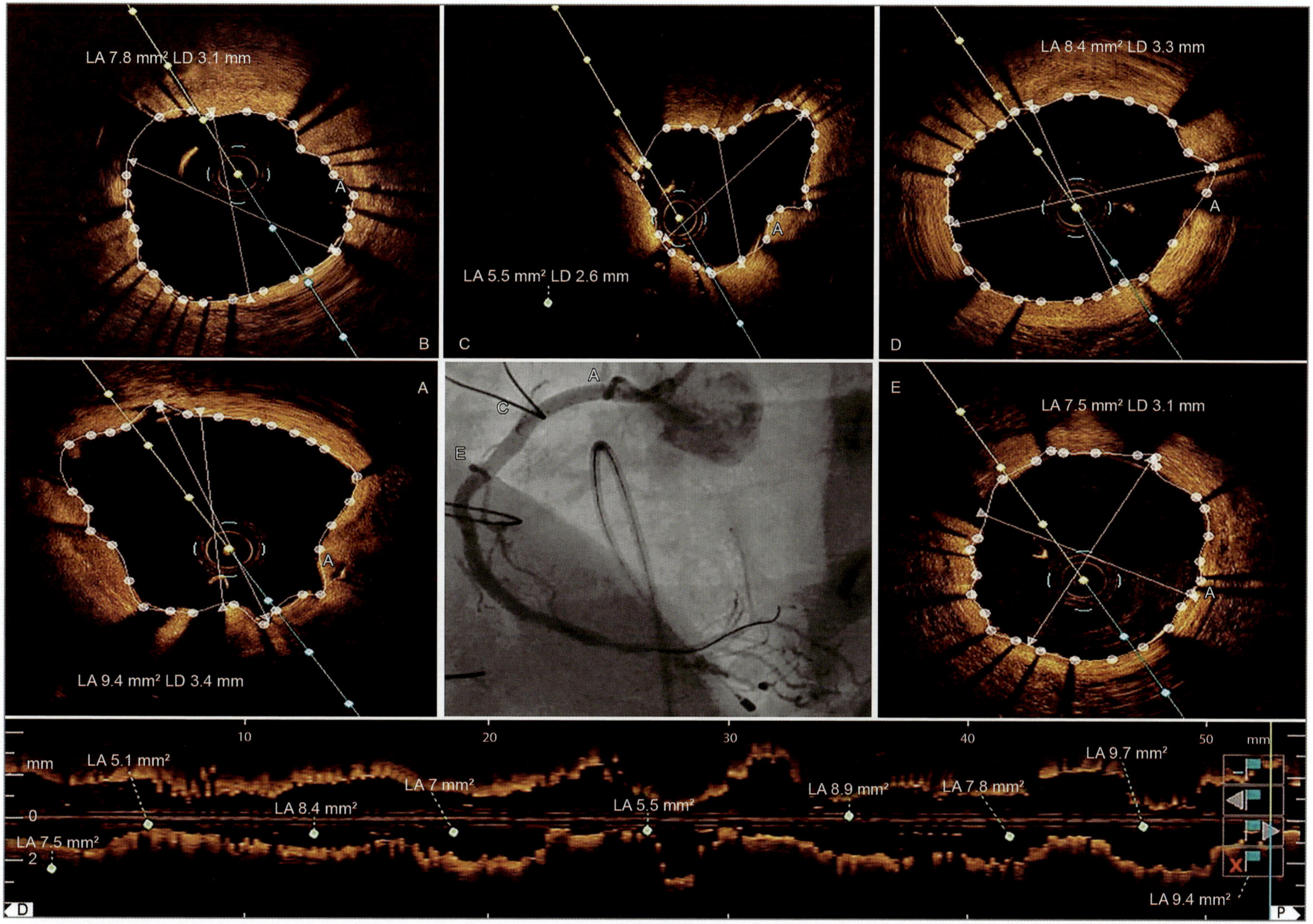
LA 7.8 mm² LD 3.1 mm
B
LA 5.5 mm² LD 2.6 mm
C
LA 8.4 mm² LD 3.3 mm
D
A
LA 9.4 mm² LD 3.4 mm
E
LA 7.5 mm² LD 3.1 mm
mm
LA 5.1 mm²
LA 8.4 mm²
LA 7 mm²
LA 5.5 mm²
LA 8.9 mm²
LA 7.8 mm²
LA 9.7 mm²
LA 7.5 mm²
LA 9.4 mm²
D
P

Fig. 30B

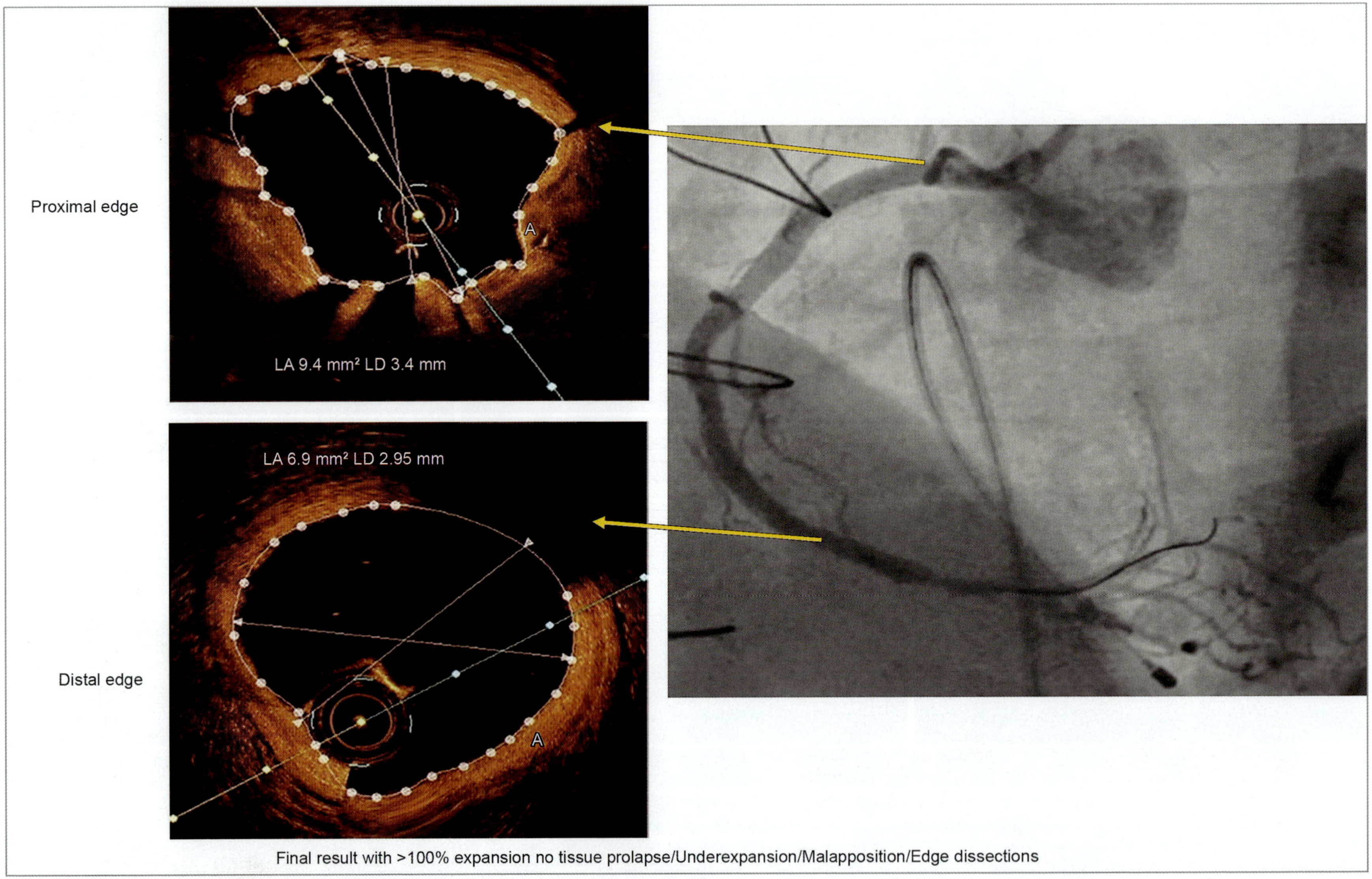

Fig. 30C

Figs. 30A to C: (A) Post distal RCA stenting OCT assessment for MAX; (B) Post Proximal RCA stenting OCT assessment for MAX; (C) Post RCA stenting OCT showing no medial edge dissection with good apposition and expansion of the stents.

CASE 7

PCI of LAD in ACS-TP and slow flow.

CLINICAL HISTORY

A 60-year-old male presented with ACS-NON-STEMI, known as hypertensive, diabetic associated with shortness of breath. 2D echo-hypokinetic distal IVS, apex, anterior wall, mild LV systolic dysfunction, EF—47%.

Investigations: Hb—8.8 g/dL, serum creatinine—0.8 mg/dL, blood urea—13 mg/dL, eGFR—93 mL/min, troponin I—0.30 ng/mL, CAG-LMCA—Normal, LAD—Proximal 80–90% lesion, mid 30–40% lesion, LCX and RCA—Normal **(Fig. 31)**.

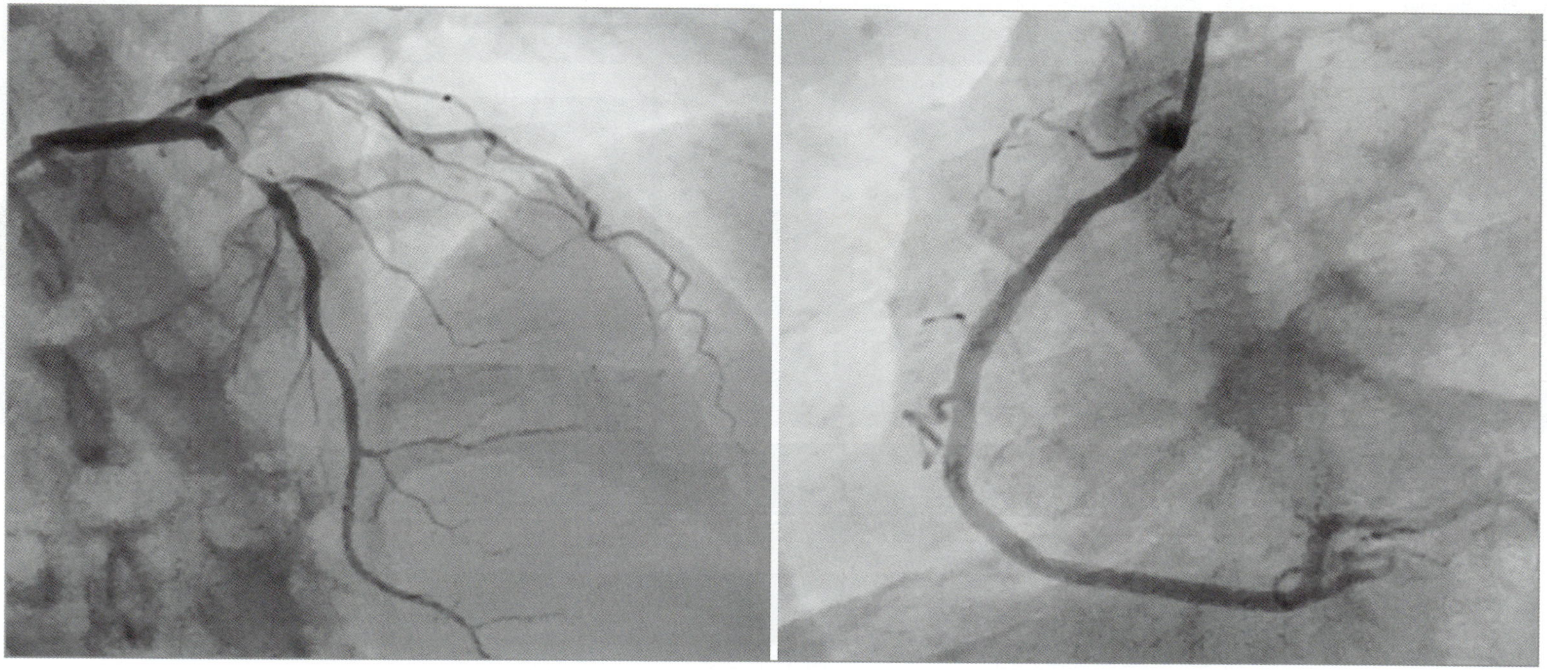

Fig. 31: Coronary angiogram showing LAD, LCX and RCA.

PROCEDURE

RRA—Route, 6 Fr XB 3.5 guiding catheter, angiogram revealed proximal 80–90% lesion which was crossed with run through wire. Predilatation with 1.5 × 10 mm Tazuna balloon.

Pre-OCT showed diffuse long-segment disease, lipid plaque with TCFA which indicated the possibility of slow flow/no flow **(Fig. 32)**.

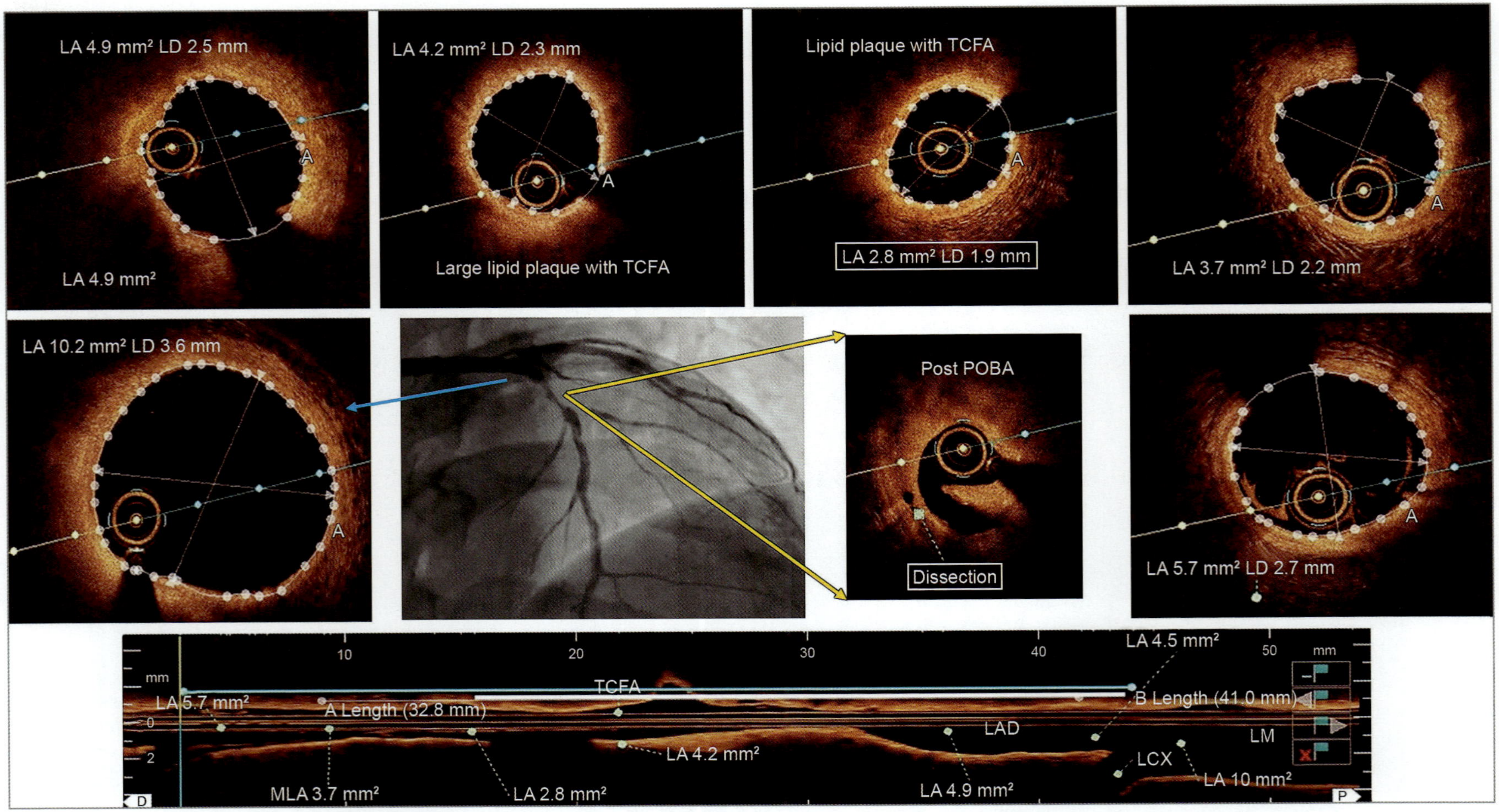

Fig. 32: Prestenting OCT assessment for post POBA dissection, plaque morphology, length and diameter.

Proximal LAD stenting with 3.0 × 34 mm resolute Onyx. Poststenting check angiogram showed slow flow due to diffuse long-segment disease, large lipid plaque with TCFA treated with IV-NTG 200 μg/Nikoran 2 mg, IC GP IIb/IIIa 10 mL (eptifibatide) **(Fig. 33)**.

Post-OCT showed well-expanded and well-apposed stent struts with no edge dissection/underexpansion with visible tissue prolapse due to ACS–NSTEMI **(Figs. 34A and B)**. Postdilatation with 3.5 × 12 mm NC Trek balloon. Postprocedure angio view showed well-implanted stents with TIMI-III flow without any dissection.

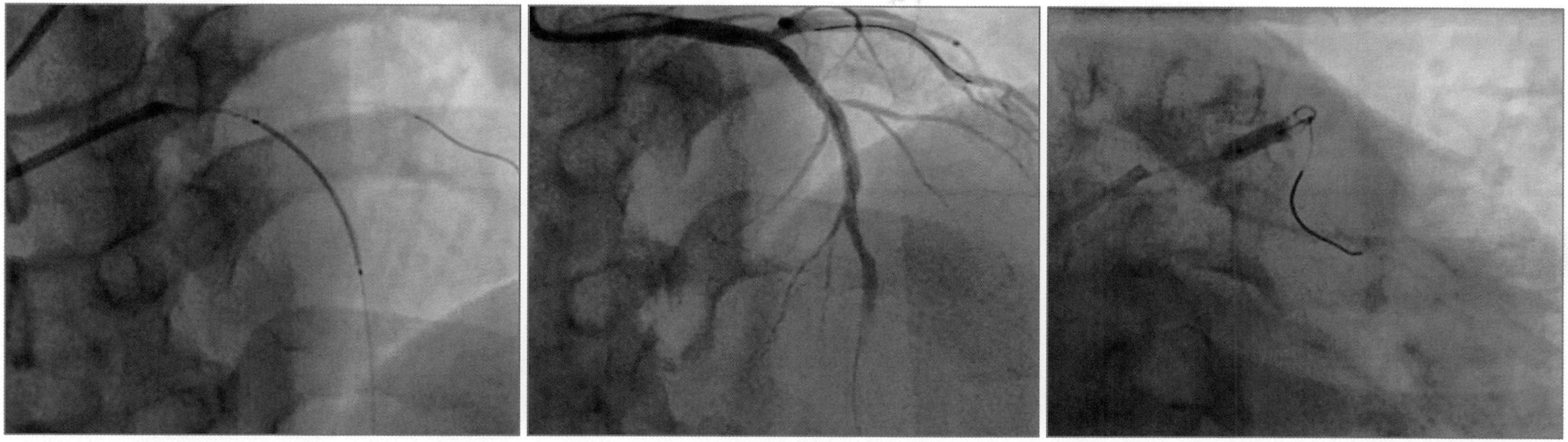

Fig. 33: LAD stenting followed by post dilatation.

Image guided PCI associated with decreased incidence of stent thrombosis and MACE rate which is evident in recently published Meta-analysis, ADAPT-DES , ULTIMATE , IVUS-XPL, OCTOBER, and OCT-IVUS studies.

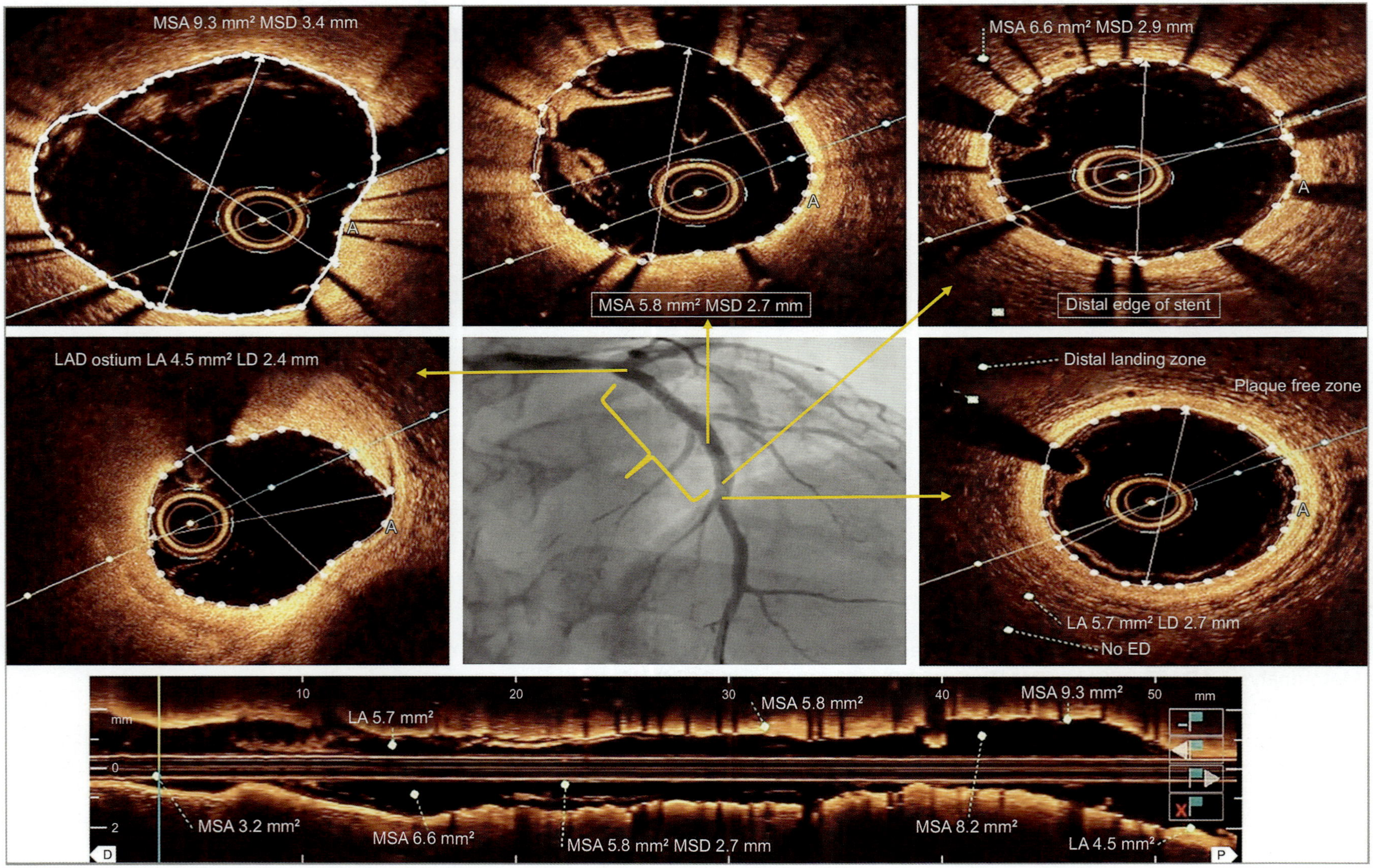
MSA 9.3 mm² MSD 3.4 mm
MSA 5.8 mm² MSD 2.7 mm
MSA 6.6 mm² MSD 2.9 mm
Distal edge of stent
LAD ostium LA 4.5 mm² LD 2.4 mm
Distal landing zone
Plaque free zone
LA 5.7 mm² LD 2.7 mm
No ED
A
10
20
30
40
50
mm
LA 5.7 mm²
MSA 5.8 mm²
MSA 9.3 mm²
MSA 3.2 mm²
MSA 6.6 mm²
MSA 5.8 mm² MSD 2.7 mm
MSA 8.2 mm²
LA 4.5 mm²
D
P

Fig. 34A

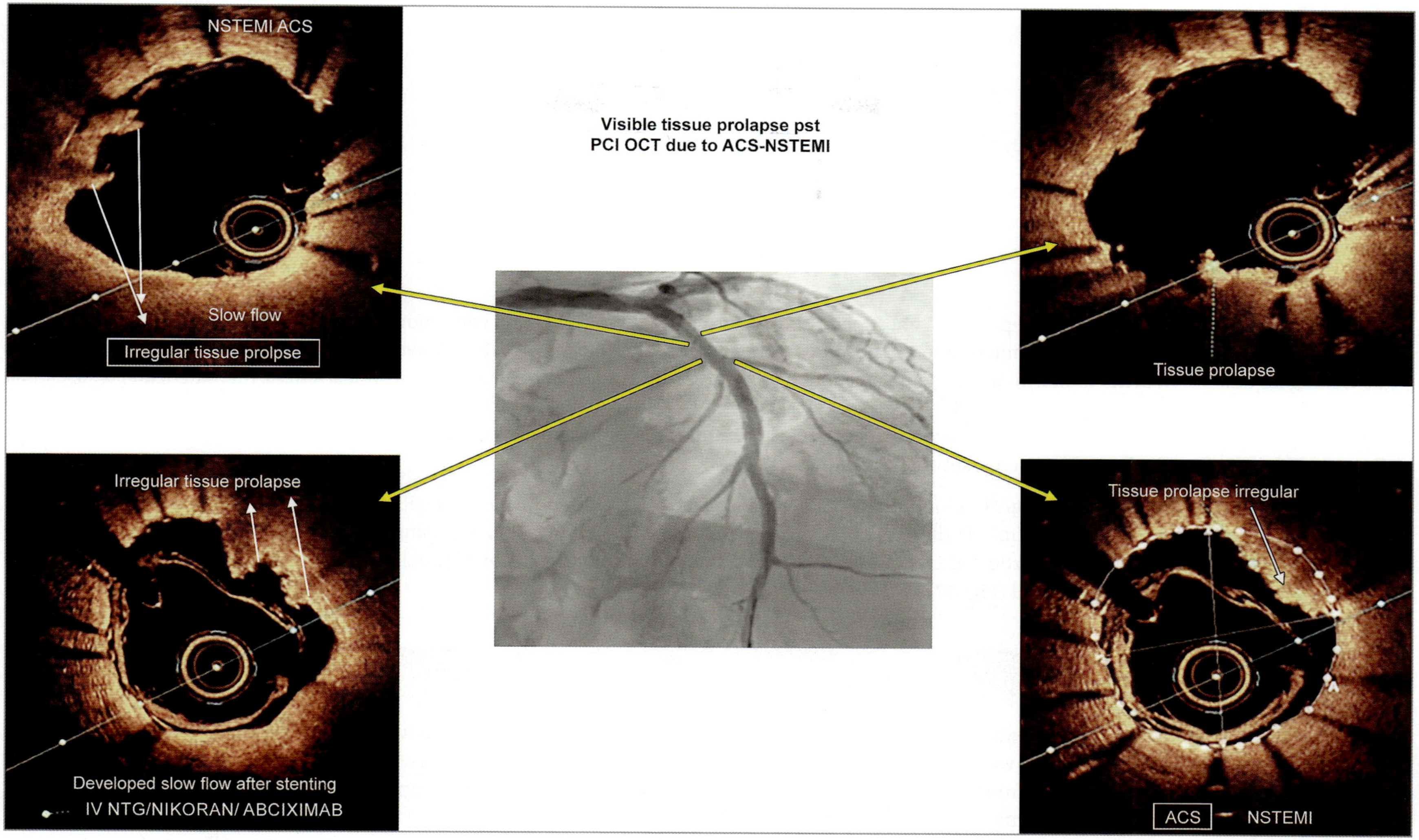

Fig. 34B

Figs. 34A and B: (A) Poststenting OCT assessment for MAX; (B) OCT assessment for Poststenting Slow-flow due to tissue prolapse which was corrected by adequate post dilatation.

CASE 8

Primary PCI with ECMO support—STEMI with cardiogenic shock.

CLINICAL HISTORY

A 32-year-old female presented with one episode of chest pain, shortness of breath, and sweating early morning on the day of admission. Patient was accompanying her father-in-law to get admitted into the hospital who had been suffering from COPD. Patient suddenly collapsed outside the causality while waiting for admission of her father-in-law. Patient had sudden onset of seizure and collapse, decreased responsiveness, intubated, and resuscitated at emergency room. (CPR was carried out for 30 minutes as per ACLS and DC shock delivered for VT/VF 5 Shocks). ECG—Anterior wall myocardial infraction with wide QRS complexes **(Fig. 35)**. 2D echo-akinetic apical IVS, and apical anterior wall, hypokinesia of mid IVS, anterolateral wall RWMA with well-preserved thickness of infarcted segments, severe LV dysfunction, EF—30%.

Investigations: CRP—66 mg/L, Hb—11.5 g/dL, blood urea—17 mg/dL, serum creatinine—0.7 mg/dL, eGFR—102 mL/min, Troponin-I—>24 ng/mL, RBS—310 mg/dL, NT-Pro-BNP—3,962 pg/mL, D-dimer—1,653 ng/mL. Under ECMO support **(Fig. 36)** using right femoral vein and left femoral artery sites, angio was done through RFA, which showed LMCA—normal, LAD—total thrombotic occlusion of proximal LAD, LCX—normal, RCA—Proximal to mid-30% stenosis. PDA and PLVB—Normal **(Fig. 37)**.

PROCEDURE

RFA—Route, using 7 Fr EBU 3.5 guiding catheter, angiogram revealed LAD—Proximal total thrombotic occlusion. LAD lesion was crossed with 0.014 × 190 cm" BMW wire. Predilatation was done with 2.5 × 15 mm Tazuna balloon. OCT was done to assess the cause of acute MI in young female, which showed long-segment of fibrotic plaque extending from proximal to distal LAD **(Figs. 38A and B)**. Proximal LAD stenting was done with 3.0 × 26 mm Resolute Onyx stent **(Fig. 39)**. Post-OCT showed long-segment of fibrotic plaque distal to stent **(Figs. 40A and B)**. Mid-LAD stenting was done with 2.75 × 38 mm Resolute Onyx stent. Postdilatation was done with 3.0 × 12 mm NC Trek balloon **(Fig. 41)**. Post-OCT showed fibrotic plaque distal to stent **(Figs. 42A and B)**. Distal LAD stenting was done with 2.5 × 15 mm Resolute Onyx stent. Postprocedure angio view showed well-implanted stents with TIMI-III flow without any dissection **(Fig. 43)**. Post-OCT showed well-apposed and expanded stent without any dissection and no under expansion **(Fig. 44)**.

Patient developed repeated episodes of VT during first 48 hours which were treated with IV-cordarone, $MgSO_4$ infusions, and DC shocks. Repeat check angio was performed on second day due to re-elevation of ST-segment in anterior leads to rule out any stent thrombosis which revealed patent stents, no ST with good antegrade flow. Patient was maintained on high inotropic, and ECMO support for 4 days.

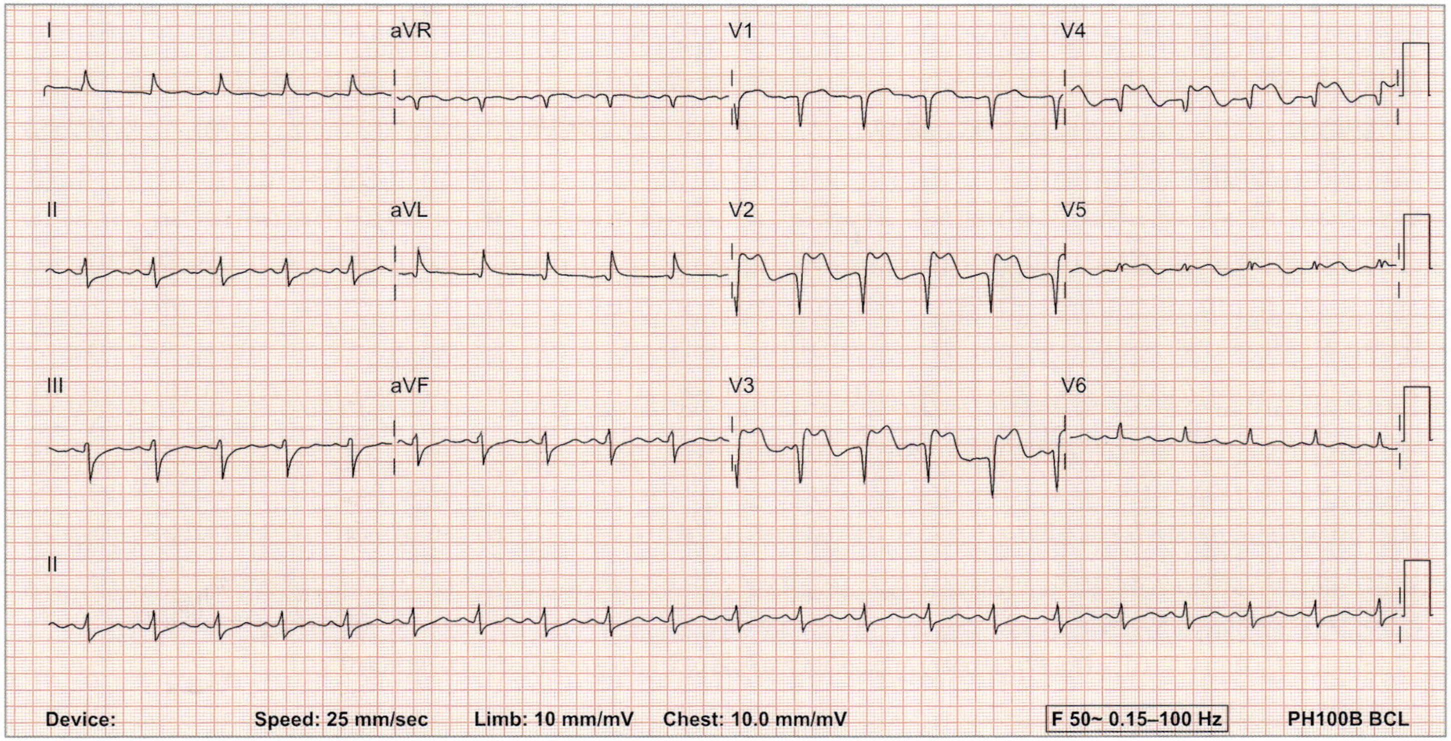

Fig. 35: ECG—showing ST-elevation.

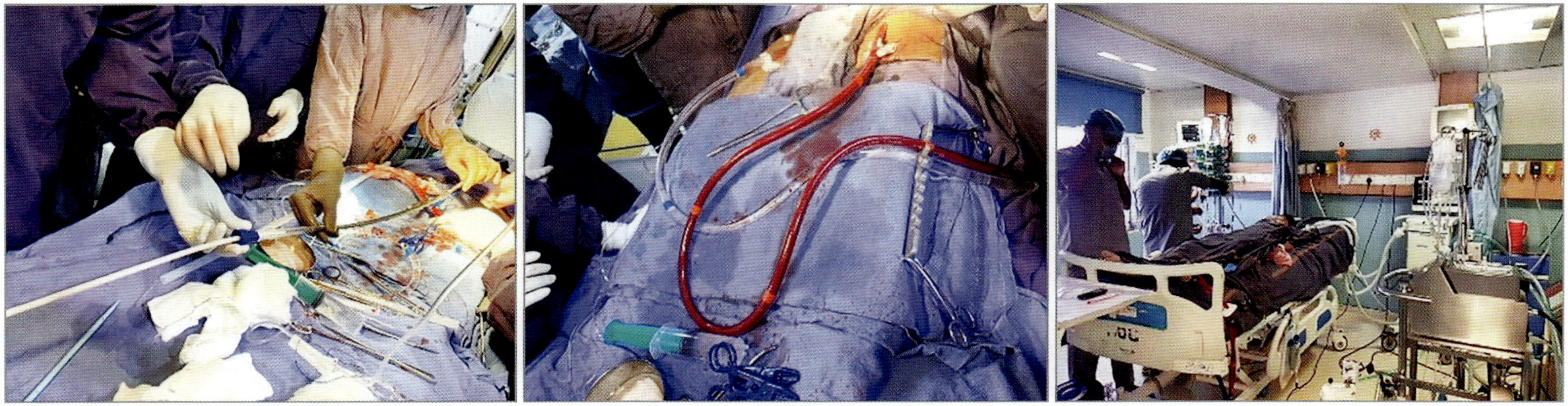

Fig. 36: ECMO support.

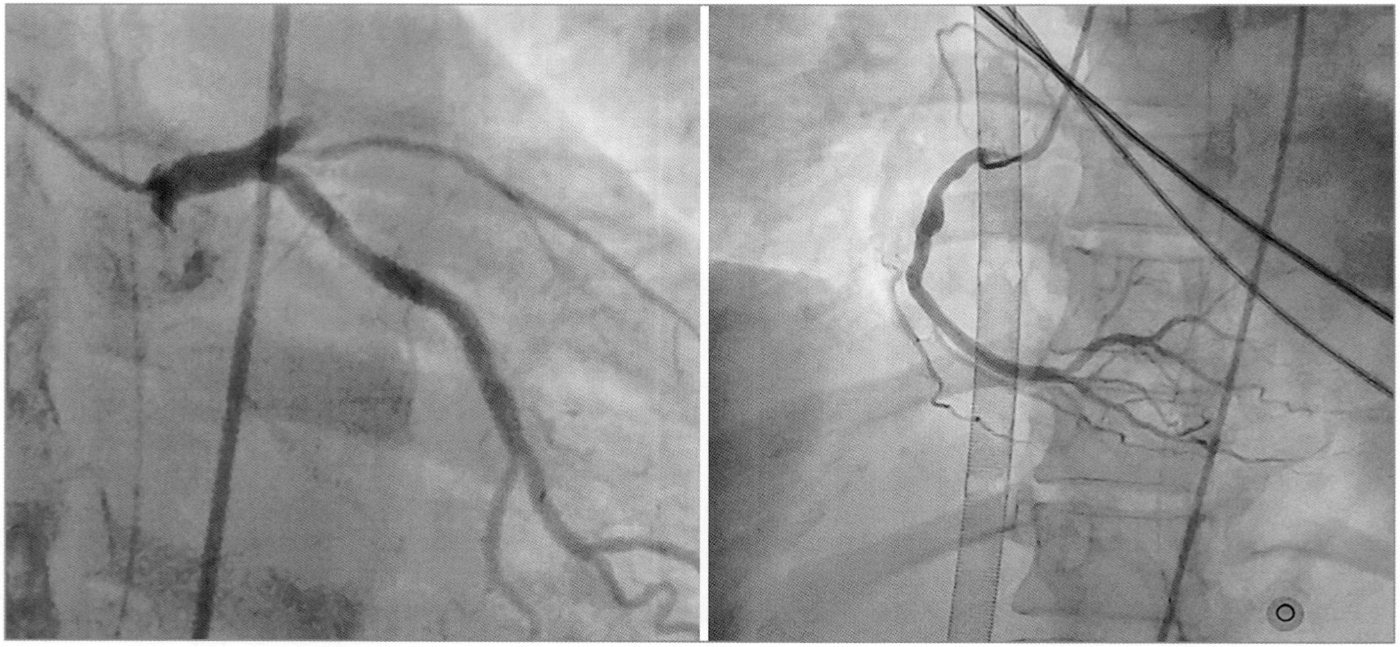

Fig. 37: Coronary Angiogram showing LCX, totally occluded LAD and RCA.

Patient developed right upper limb venous thrombosis leading to right upper arms swelling, treated with IV-heparin, and NOACS. Patient developed right leg massive hematoma due to oozing from perivenous sheath of ECMO resulting in elevated bilirubin, significant fall of Hb (5.5 gm%) requiring multiple blood transfusions. ECMO support was weaned off from 3 L to 1 L, finally removed on 4th day with repair of arterial and venous insertion sites at the groins. Patient was discharged on 12th postprocedure day in a stable status with relief of right upper limb edema.

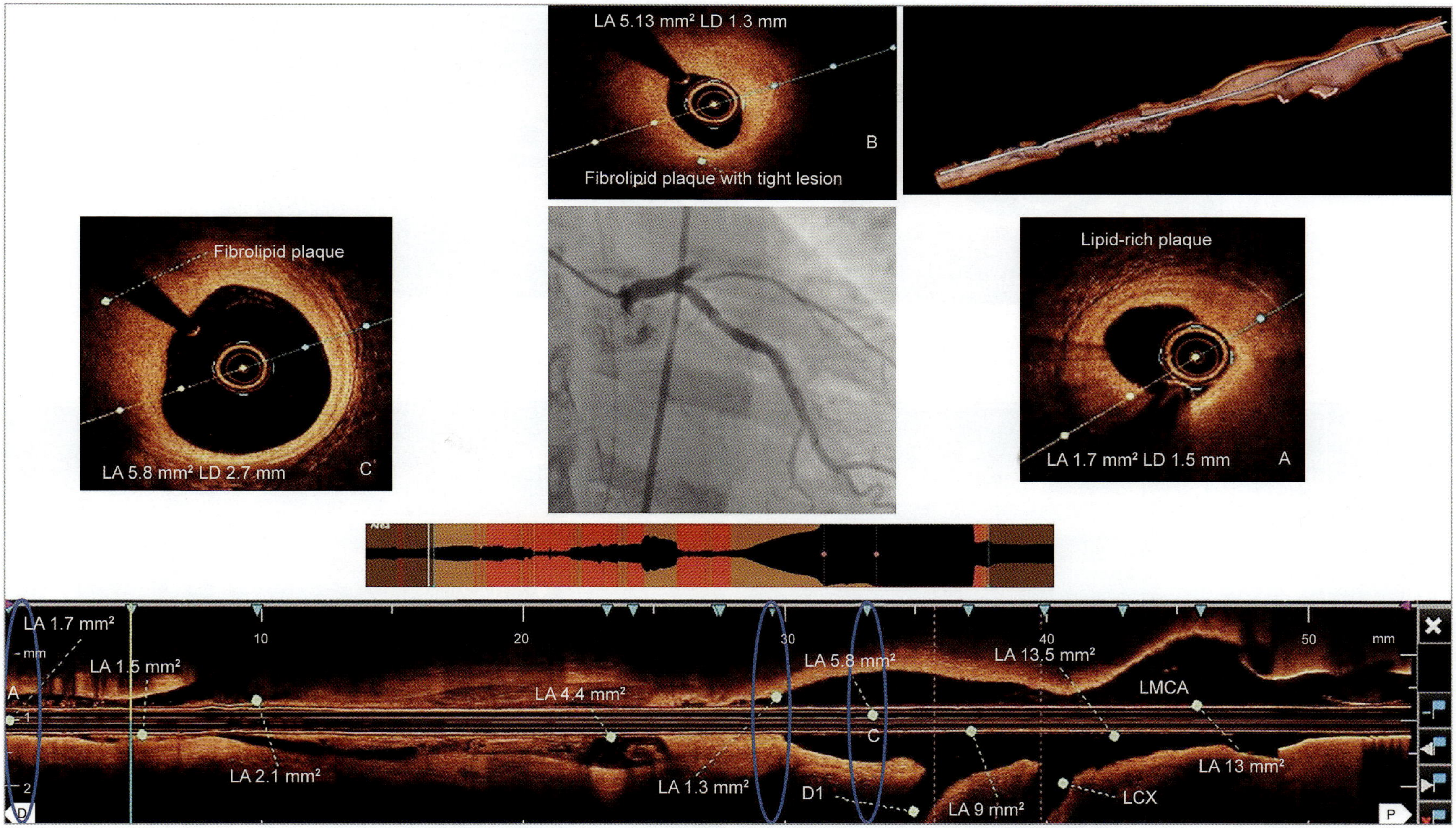

Fig. 38A

Before the MCS initiation, assess the ability of MCS to provide hemodynamic or circulatory support in terms of only LV or RV support vs. Biventricular support and effect on CPO and PAPI, coronary perfusion, and myocardial protection ability of MCS to off load the ventricle.

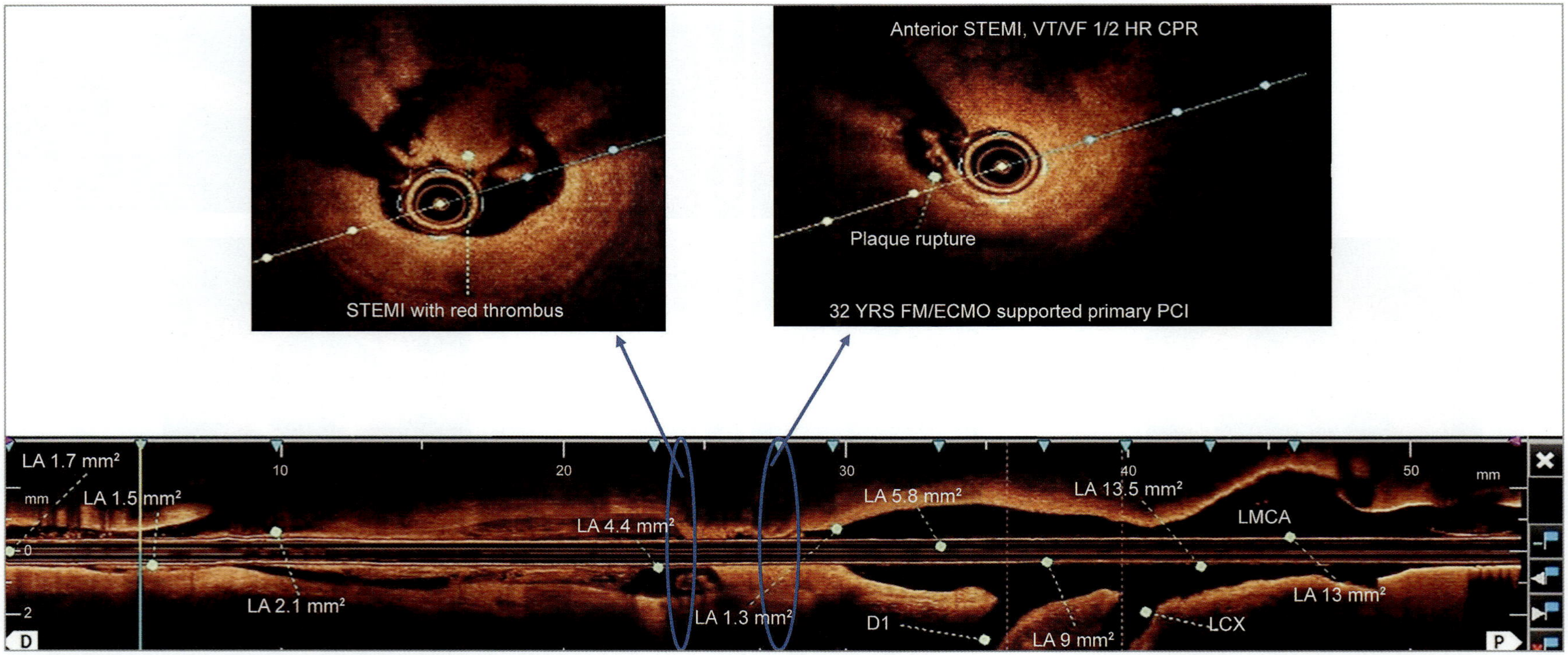

Fig. 38B

Figs. 38A and B: (A) Pre stenting OCT assessment showing Length and diameter of the vessel; (B) Pre stenting OCT assessment showing morphology.

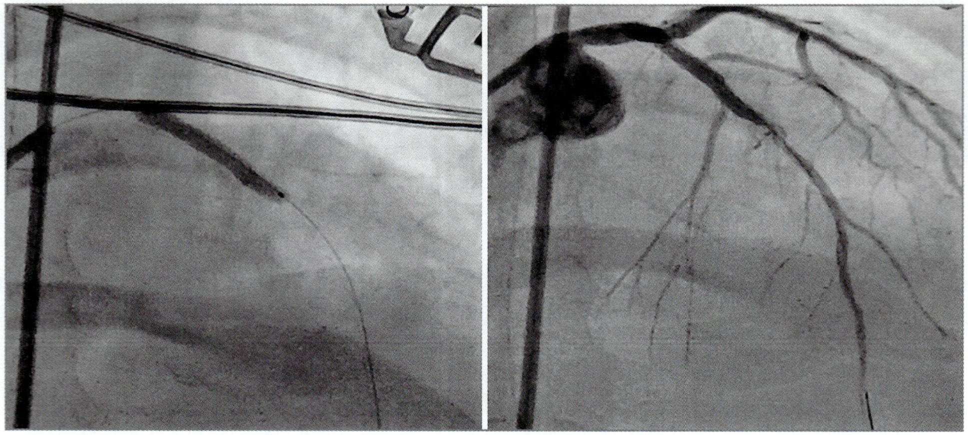

Fig. 39: Proximal LAD angioplasty.

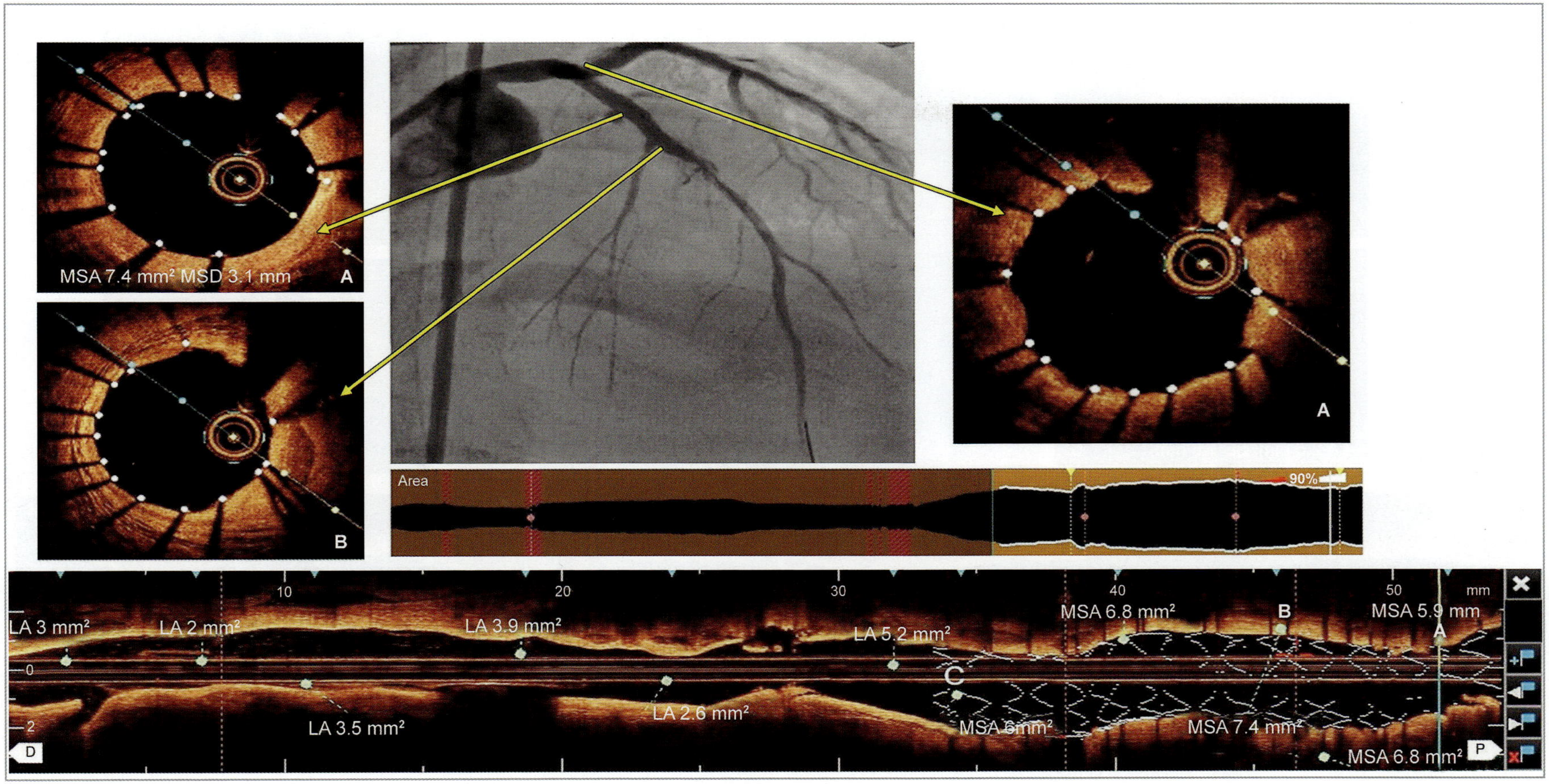

Fig. 40A

Prior to the commencement of the MCS, it is also essential to rule out absolute contraindications which include irreversible cardiac failure with a lack of an exit strategy (i.e., heart transplantation or durable mechanical circulatory support) and concomitant irreversible non-cardiac multi-organ failure or other terminal illnesses.

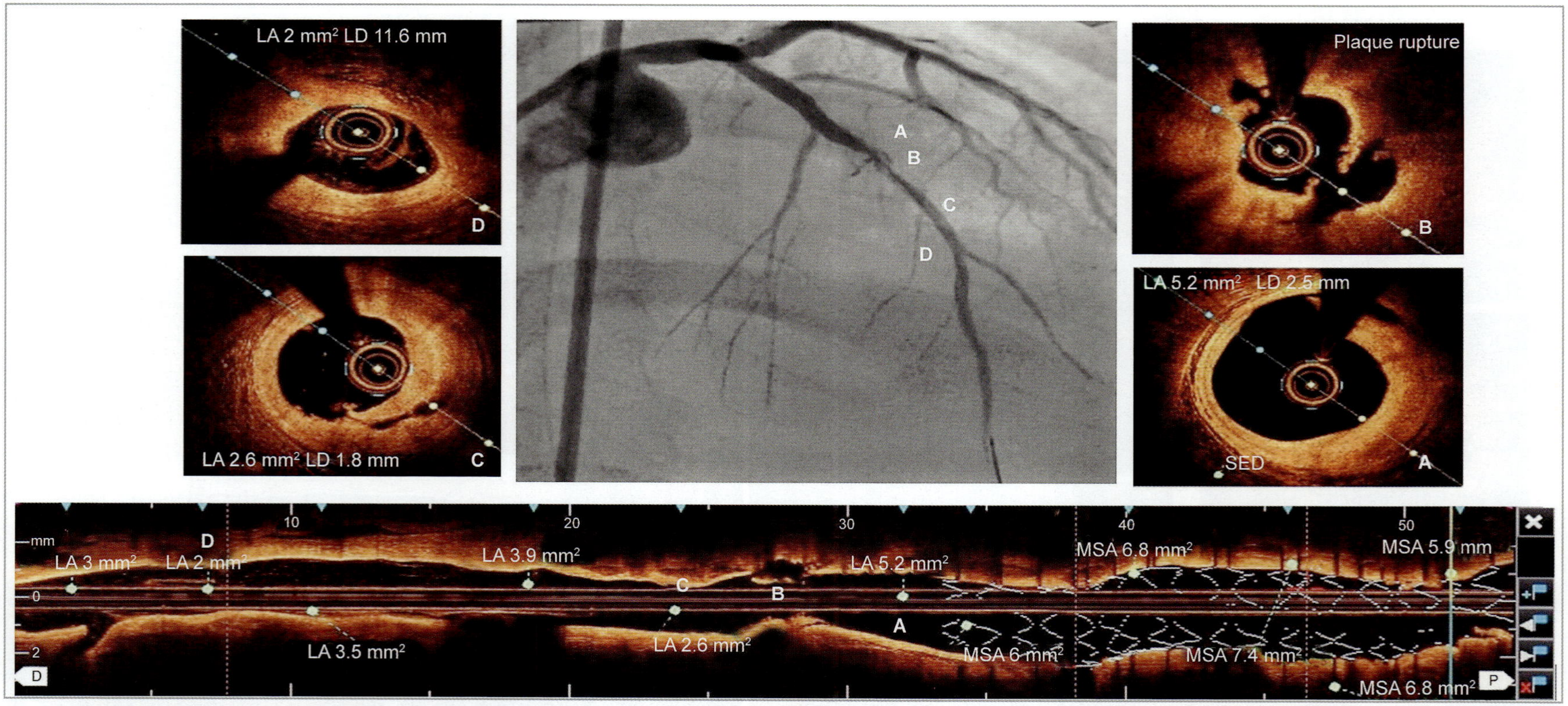

Fig. 40B

Figs. 40A and B: (A) Post proximal LAD stenting assessment for MAX; (B) Pre stenting mid LAD OCT assessment for plaque morphology.

MCS for High-risk PCI- MCS may be considered to patients who are surgically unsuitable or high risk due to associated co-morbidities, Complex coronary disease of LM, MVD, and severely calcified lesions requiring plaque modification devices, severe LV dysfunction-EF <25%, Systolic BP, 100 mm Hg, and LVEDP >25 mm Hg.

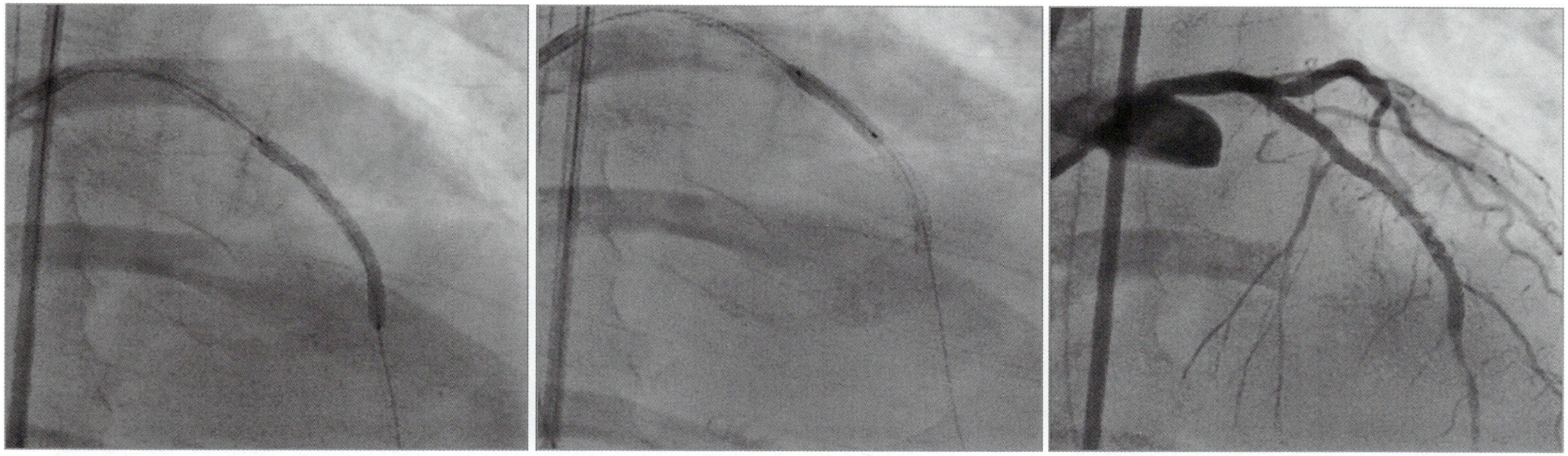

Fig. 41: Angioplasty of mid LAD – stenting, post dilatation and check angio.

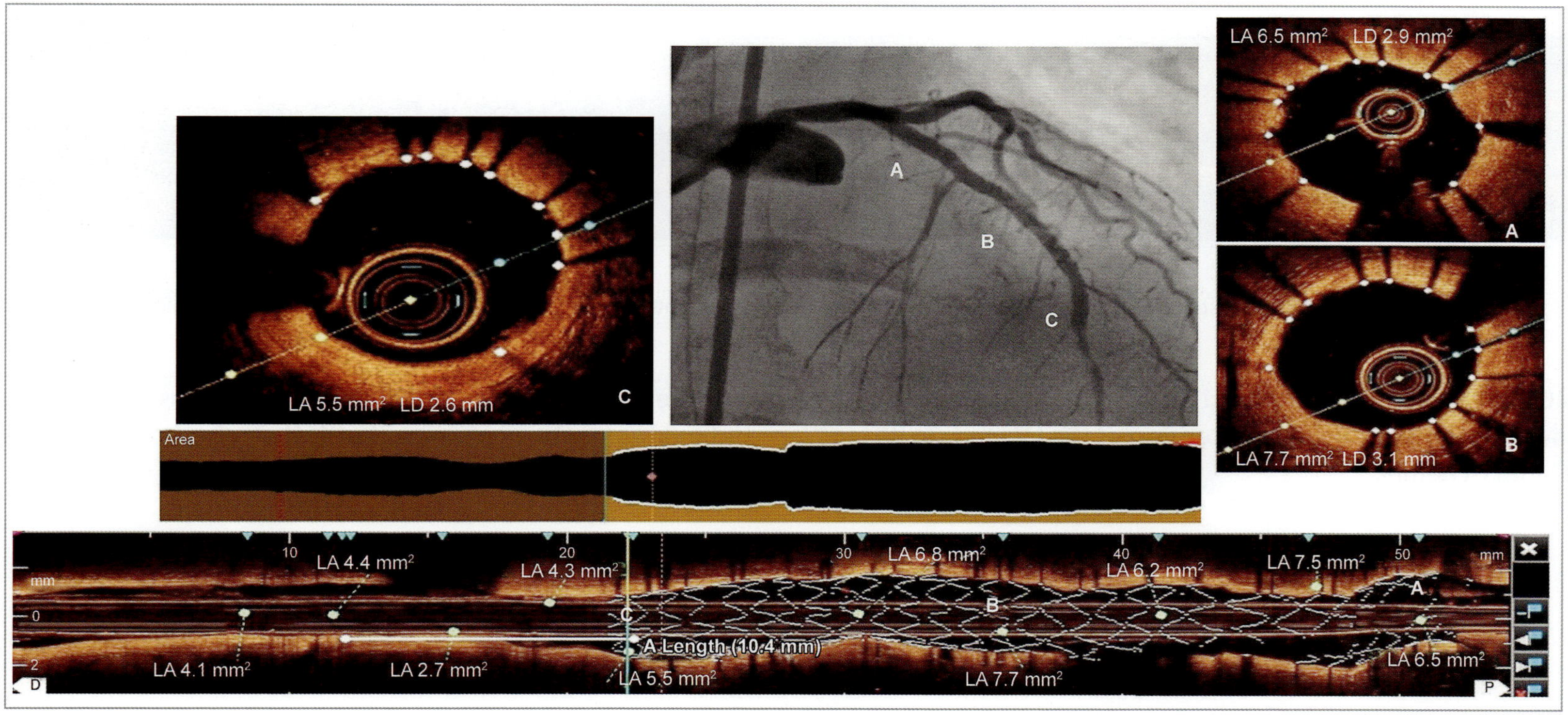

Fig. 42A

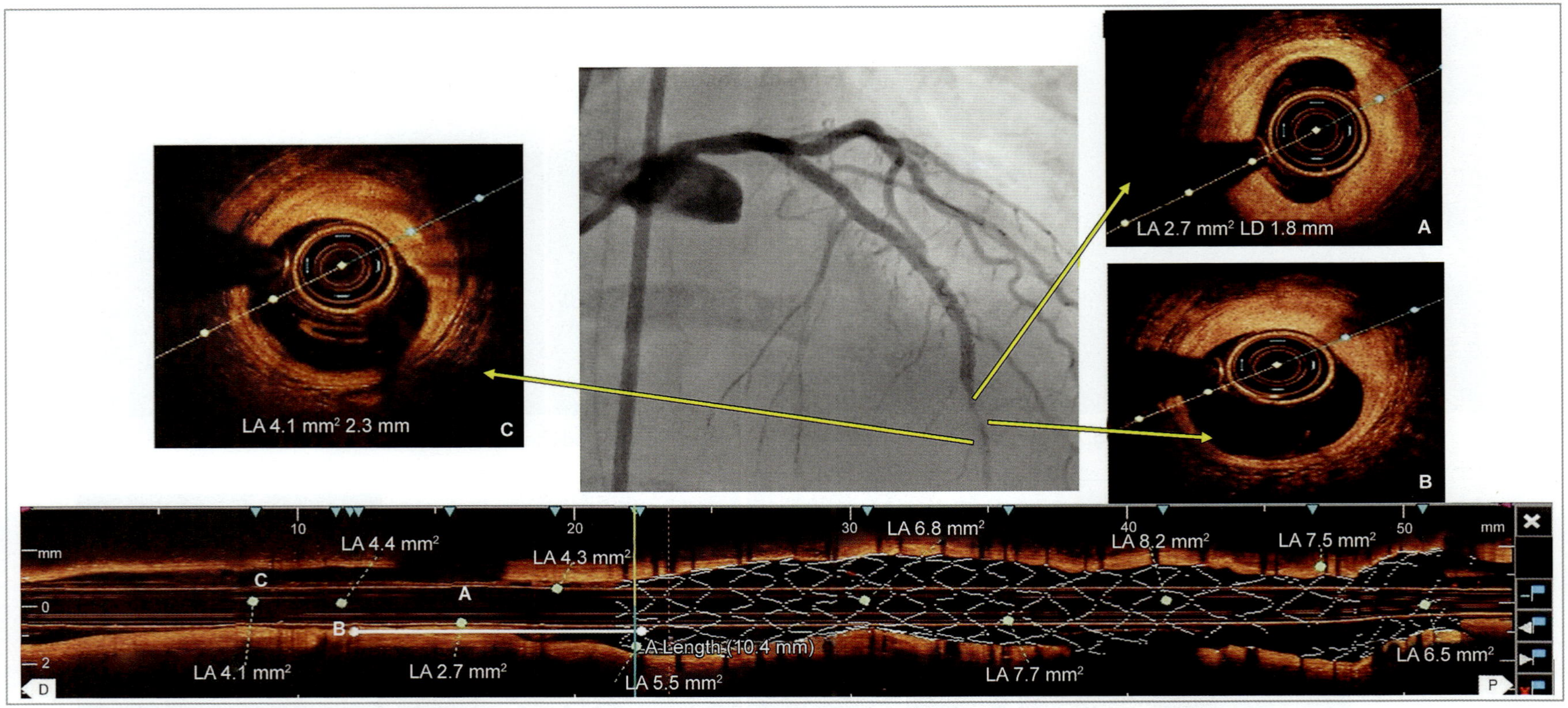

Fig. 42B

Figs. 42A and B: (A) Post mid LAD stenting OCT assessment for MAX; (B) Pre stenting distal LAD OCT assessment for plaque morphology.

ECMO provides biventricular and pulmonary support and carries some of the disadvantageous like dual vessel access with large sized cannulas, non pulsatile flow, distension of the LV limiting its recovery and pulmonary haemorrhage, Aortic thrombus, cerebral hypoxia, and Limb ischemia.

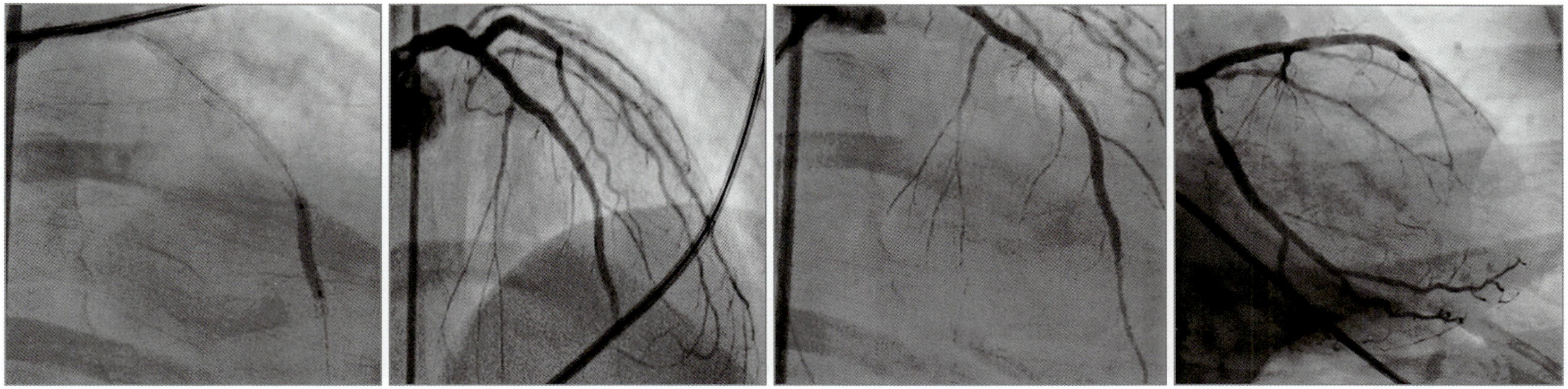

Fig. 43: Distal LAD angioplasty and final result.

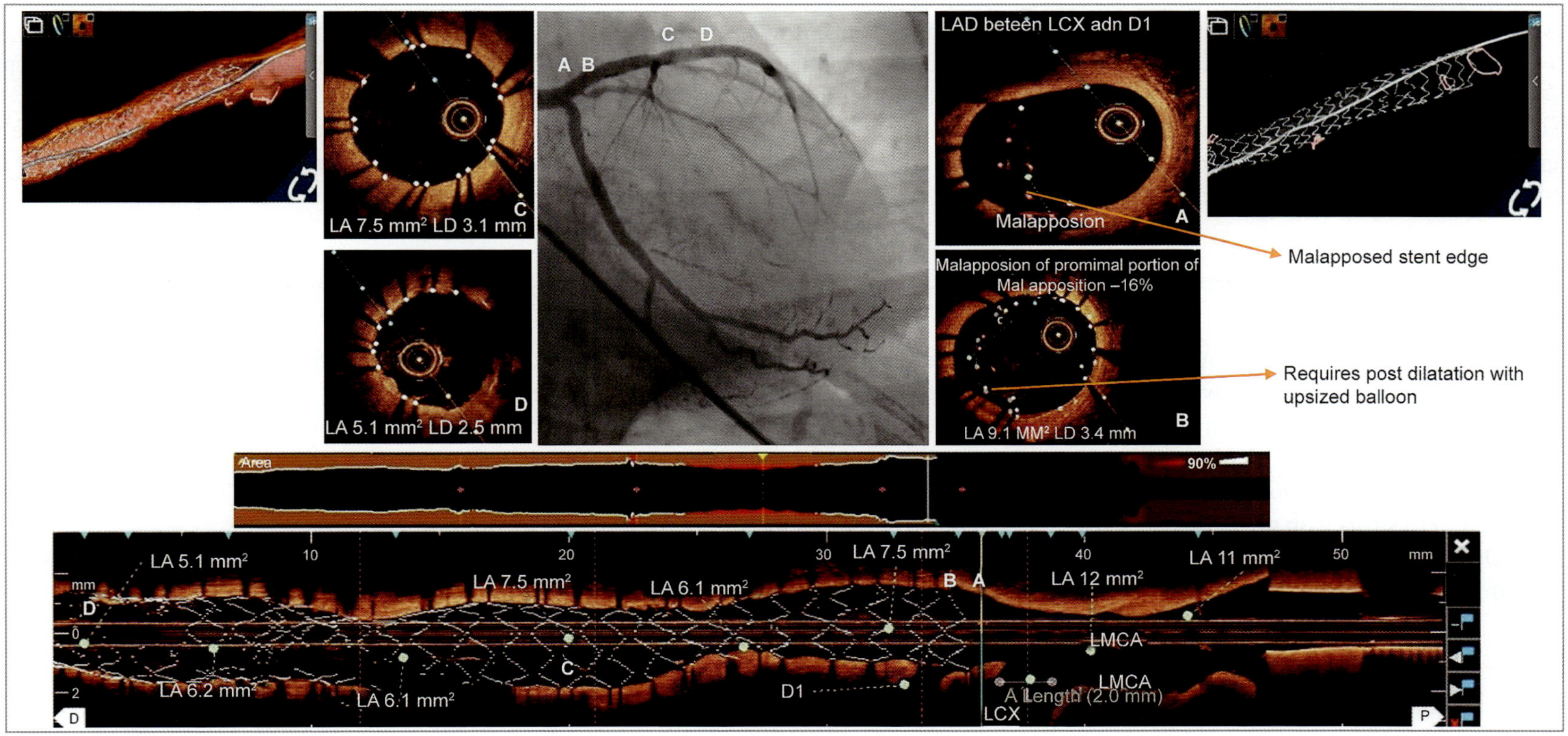

Fig. 44: Post LAD stenting OCT assessment for MAX.

CASE 9

PCI with direct stenting of thrombus containing lesion of LAD due to plaque erosion.

CLINICAL HISTORY

A 48-Year-old male, with a past history of Bariatric surgery, and Lung sarcoidosis under remission with medical management presented with H/o retrosternal chest pain associated with SOB of 1 week duration. ECG - T inversions in Anterior leads, 2D Echo-RWMA of Anterior wall and anterior septum, Good LV function with EF:58%.

Investigations: Hb-13.7 g/dL, RBS-119 mg/dL, serum Cr-1.05 mg/dL, eGFR-80 mL/min, Trop I-33.1 ng/L.

CAG—Rt radial approach with Tiger catheter showed critical thrombus containing lesion of proximal and mid LAD junction. In view of ongoing chest pain with NSTEMI emergency PCI of LAD was planned after giving loading doses of Aspirin and Ticagrelor.

LCA was engaged through RRA with XBU 3.0–6 Fr guiding catheter, LAD was crossed with Run through wire. Prestenting OCT showed large red thrombus containing lesion with areas of fibrotic plaque and lipid rich plaque with TCFA and no evident plaque rupture. As the OCT showed Lipid rich plaque with TCFA, we opted for direct stenting of LAD without any other plaque preparation strategy.

PROCEDURE

LAD stenting was done with Xience Alpine 3.5 × 33 mm stent, and it was post dilatated with NC Trek 4.0 × 15 mm balloon.

Post LAD stenting OCT showed well expanded and apposed stent struts with no medial edge dissections.

Distal to the stent showed 15 mm length lipid rich plaque which was managed with additional stenting by overlapping the distal edge of the proximal stent using Xience Alpine 3.0 × 18 mm stent.

High pressure post dilatations of proximal stent was performed again with NC Trek 4.0 × 15 mm balloon. Post LAD stenting OCT showed well expanded and apposed stent struts with no medial edge dissections. Final result was good with TIMI III flow with no complications.

Final OCT run for MAX assessment—showed smooth type of Tissue prolapse (<10% of MSA with good MSA), well expanded, and apposed stent struts without any MED.

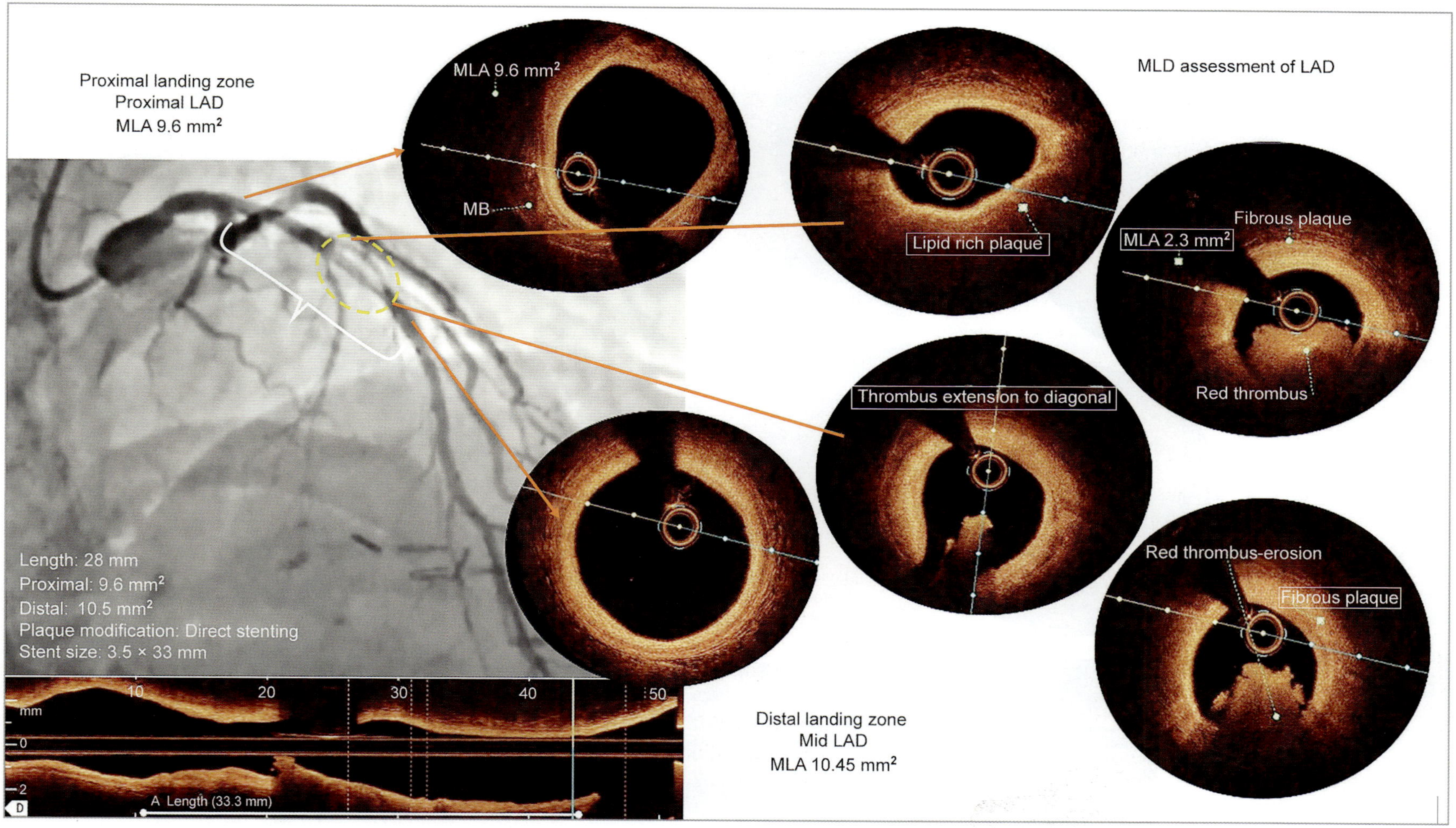

Fig. 45: Prestenting OCT assessment showing MLD for selection of the stent size. (M: morphology; L: length; D: daiameter)

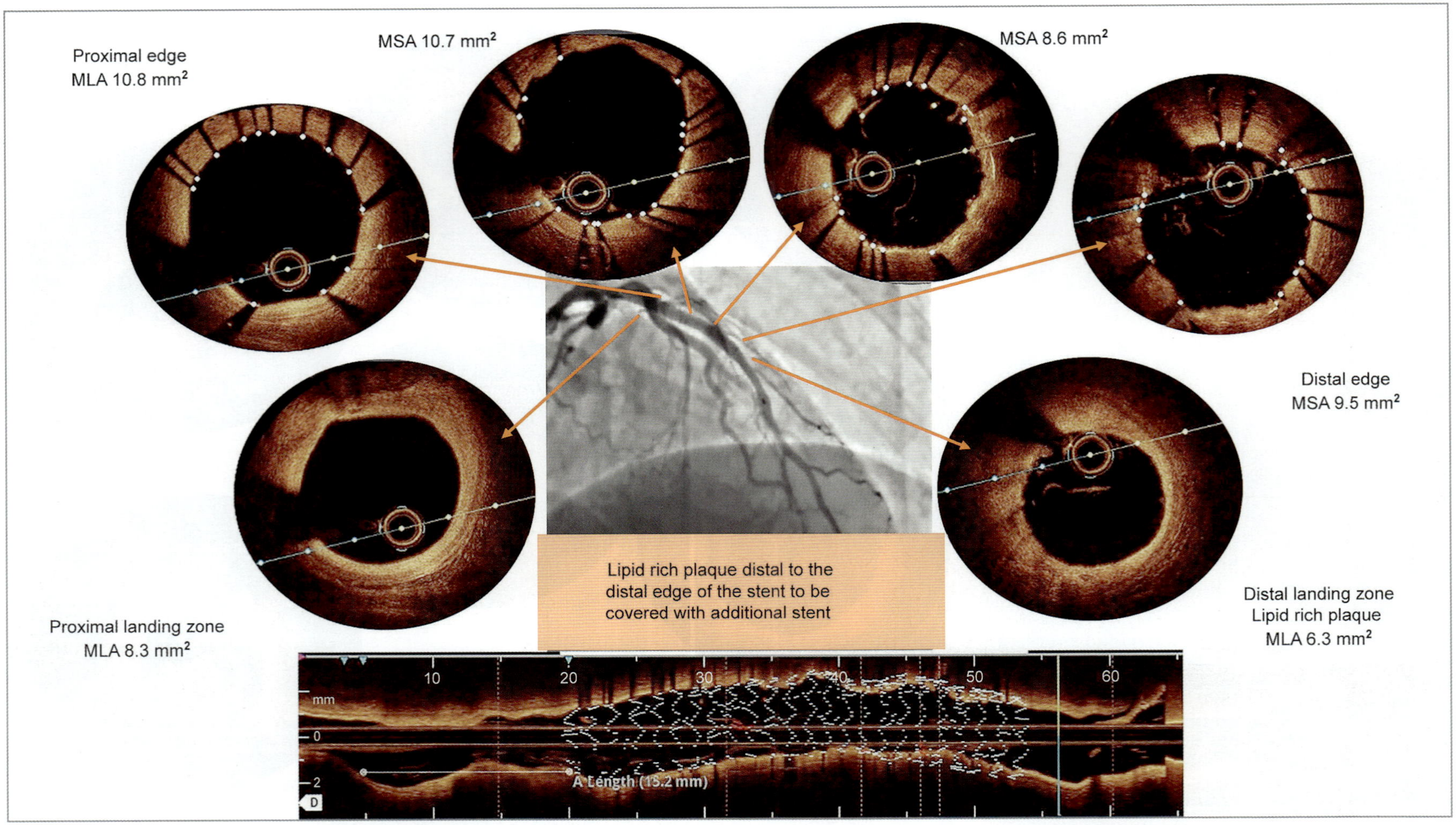

Fig. 46: Poststenting OCT shoing well expanded and well apposed stent struts with no edge dissections and found lipid rich plaque distal to the stent.

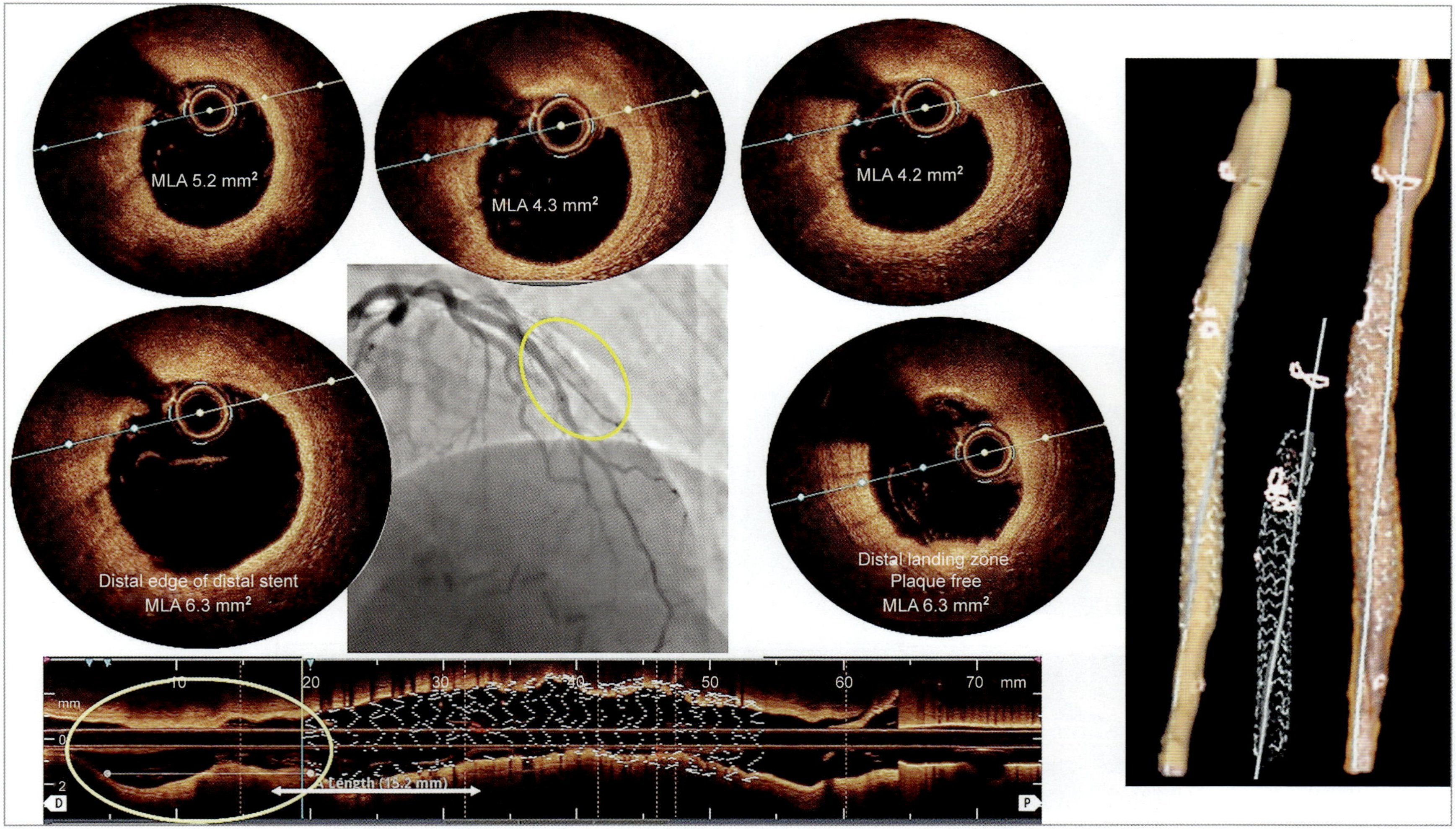

Fig. 47: OCT showing lipid rich plaque distal to the stent requires additional stent.

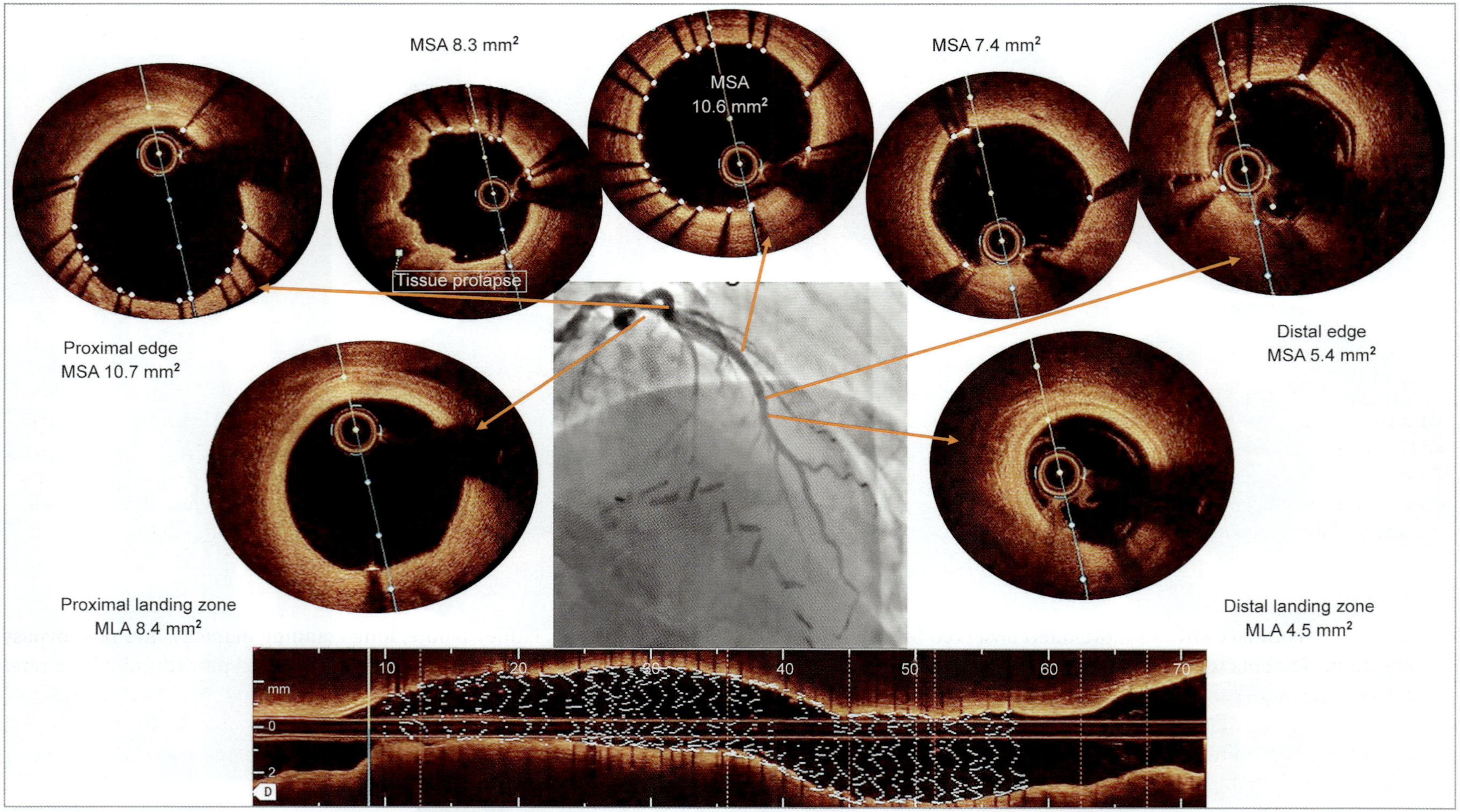

Fig. 48: Final OCT showing well expanded and apposed stent struts with no medial edge dissections.

CHAPTER 8

Assessment of Calcium and Plaque Modification

ABSTRACT

Coronary calcification is observed in 15–20% cases of coronary artery disease and its prevalence increases with age and associated comorbidities, most often seen in lesions with tortuosity and angulation. PCI of calcified lesions are usually associated with high incidence of complications due to undilatable nature which might lead to underexpansion, dislodgement of stent, dissection, perforation, and stent thrombosis. Angiographic assessment of severity of calcium is not very accurate, it detects only in 45–50% of patients with calcium and poor in detecting lesions with mild-to-moderate calcium compared to those with severe calcium. OCT can assess calcium severity more reliably in measuring depth, length, and circumferential extent of calcium plaque which helps in estimating calcium expansion index and also useful in assessing effectiveness of plaque modification prior to PCI and optimization of DES implantation by implementing MLD-MAX algorithm.

INTRODUCTION

Calcification of coronary arteries more often observed in patients with advanced age, chronic kidney failure, long-standing diabetes, and post-bypass surgery status. Patients with calcified coronary arteries carry high mortality and morbidity particularly in terms of increased procedural failure rate, periprocedural complications and recurrence of disease after interventional procedures or bypass surgery. ADAPT-DES reported incidence of moderate (26.1%) to severe (5.8%) calcium in 30.8% of STEMI and NSTEMI PCI patients. Calcium is usually noticed in 50% among people in the age group of 40–49 years and 80% among people in the age group of 60–69 years. As per the results of HORIZONS-AMI and ACUITY CORONARY CALCIUM there was a significant increase in the MACE rate at 1 year follow-up in patients with the severe calcium.[1,2]

CORONARY ANGIOGRAPHIC ASSESSMENT OF CALCIUM

Angiographic assessment of severity of calcium may not be reliable in making proper clinical decisions because of its limited planar resolution and two-dimensional images of three-dimensional vascular structure. PCI of severely calcified lesions are prone for underexpansion, dislodgement of stent, dissection, perforation, and stent thrombosis and stenting without adequate plaque modification is associated with stent underexpansion which is a major predictor of restenosis and stent thrombosis.[3] Proper and adequate plaque modification shortens procedure time, improves acute and long-term outcomes.[4]

Although the diagnostic accuracy of CAG is poor in detecting mild-to-moderate calcium compared to severe calcific lesions, enough attention should be paid to assess severity of calcium **(Table 1)** to decide any need for proper plaque modification strategy to avoid procedure-related problems prior to planning of revascularization strategies **(Box 1)**.

IVUS FOR ASSESSMENT OF CALCIUM

Calcium is a powerful reflector of ultrasound and the leading edge of calcific plaque shown as a hyperechoic area that is brighter than the reference adventitia with shadowing. IVUS is associated with high sensitivity (90%) and specificity (100%) for large dense calcific deposits or microcalcification clusters, whereas the majority of small flecks of calcium being below IVUS resolution may not be visible properly or missed in majority of lesions **(Box 2)**.

The IVUS classifies calcium according to the arc and length of the calcium, diameter of the vessel, and presence or absence of calcific nodule. The greater the arc, length or thickness of calcium, the greater the likelihood of stent underexpansion which indicate severity of calcium **(Fig. 1 and Table 2)**.

The IVUS specific scoring system to predict underexpansion and score of >2 suggests plaques modification prior to stenting.

OCT ASSESSMENT OF CALCIUM

The OCT helps in assessing plaque morphology, severity of calcific plaque, choosing appropriate plaque modification devices, adequacy of plaque modification, any need for upscaling of burr size and additional plaque modification devices and optimization of stent implantation by using simple and easy to implement MLD-MAX algorithm while performing PCI of calcific lesions.

TABLE 1: ACC/AHA classification of coronary calcification.

Type A lesion	*None:* No radiopacity
	Mild: Faint radiopacities noted during cardiac cycles
Type B lesion	*Moderate:* Dense radiopacities noted during cardiac cycle before contrast injection
	Severe: Dense radiopacities noted on both sides of the arterial wall (tram track) without cardiac motion before contrast injection

BOX 1: Clinical problems relevant to of PCI of calcified coronary arteries.

- Associated with a greater number of complications and procedure failures if no proper plaque modification.
- Associated with greater number of dissections resulting in abrupt closure and thrombosis.
- Might result in poor expansion which may require high pressure inflations leading to perforation and pericardial tamponade.
- Prolonged procedure time leading to bleeding complications, increased radiation exposure, and CIN due to increase in contrast load.
- Requires more plaque modification devices, balloons, and other adjunctive devices.

BOX 2: Limitations of IVUS in assessing calcium.

- Detects only the leading edge of a calcific deposit, not its thickness.
- Cannot detect a deep calcific deposit behind a superficial calcific deposit due to dense shadow behind the bright leading edge of the calcium.
- Poor penetration of calcific plaque by IVUS results in shadow behind bright white arc which makes improper judgement in measuring thickness of severe calcific plaque.
- Superficial calcium that is concordant to the maximum plaque thickness may represent a thicker calcific deposit compared with deeper lesion calcium.

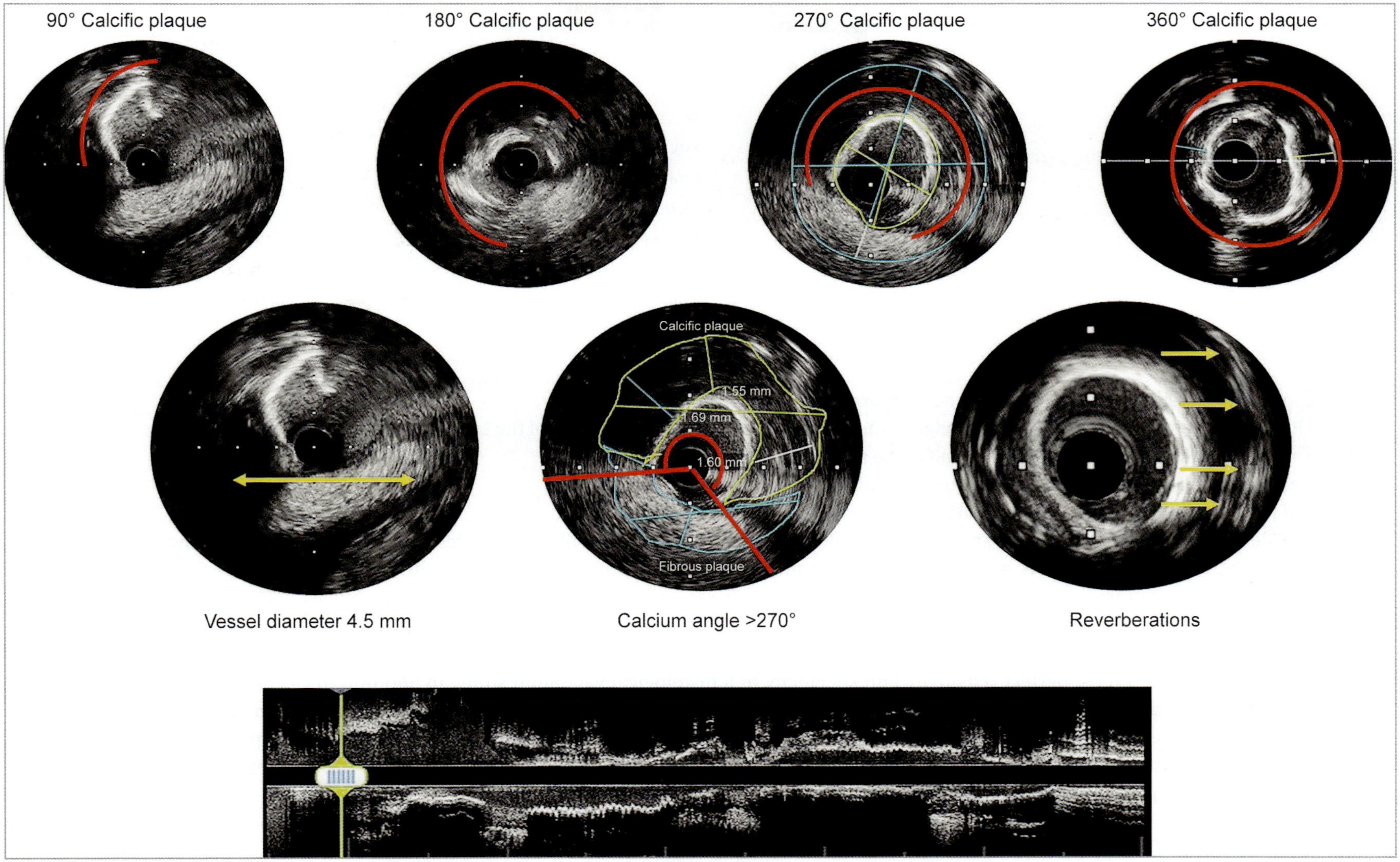

Fig. 1: IVUS analysis on calcium.

TABLE 2: IVUS score.

IVUS characteristic	*Parameter*	*Score*
Ca^+ arc	<360°	0
	360°	1
Length of >270° Ca^+	≤5 mm	0
	>5 mm	1
Diameter	>3.5 mm	0
	≤3.5 mm	1
Calcific nodule	Absent	0
	Present	1

Calcific plaques are classified into four types based on morphological appearance:

1. Superficial dense calcified plates—a leading edge of the calcified plate located within half of the superficial intima side.
2. Deep intimal calcifications—located within half of the adventitial side.
3. Scattered microcalcification—small purple dots accumulating within the intima.
4. Calcified nodules—calcification that protruded into the lumen.

The OCT detects calcification with 90% sensitivity and 100% specificity, it[3] classifies fibrocalcific lesions as mild (0–180° arc), moderate (180°–270° arc), and severe (>270° arc) calcification. Intravascular imaging should be considered in PCI of vessels with moderate-to-severe fluoroscopic coronary calcification. The use of rotational or orbital atherectomy or IVL is strongly recommended in vessels with calcium angles >270° and thicker than 500 µm.

The OCT predicts underexpansion when calcium length >5 mm, arc >180°, and thickness >0.5 mm **(Fig. 2)**.

The IVUS is sensitive for the detection of CAC, but due to reflection of acoustic waves, cannot measure depth. Compared to IVUS, OCT is superior in diagnosing calcium with almost perfect sensitivity and specificity in a histological validation study. In addition to calcium arc and length, OCT can assess its thickness, area, and volume, because it can penetrate calcified plaques. Sometimes, superficial lipid accumulation can mask underlying deep calcification due to relatively poor depth penetration of OCT, and calcium is often confused with lipid or necrotic core (the signal-poor regions of calcium are sharply delineated vs. the signal poor regions of lipid or a necrotic core have poorly defined or diffuse borders). IVUS scores over OCT for patients with ostial LM and RCA, unstable hemodynamic status, severe LV dysfunction, CKD, and allergic to contrast.

VARIETY OF CALCIUM MORPHOLOGY (FIGS. 3A AND B)

The OCT can identify various morphological types of calcium such as superficial calcium, deep calcium, and calcium nodule **(Box 3)**. It also identifies distribution of calcium in relation to vessel circumference—eccentric versus concentric distribution, circumferential versus horseshoe, or semilunar distribution and thickness of calcium at various levels of vessel circumference and length. During follow-up period of PCI patients, recurrence of ISR may be due to neoatherosclerosis with calcific plaque or underexpansion of stent due to severe calcium which are very well identified by OCT imaging.

The PCI of diffusely calcified coronaries require adequate proper plaque modification and adequate stent expansion to cover entire diseased segment by landing in landing zones with no plaque or minimal plaque burden without leaving any clinically significant edge dissections and malapposition,

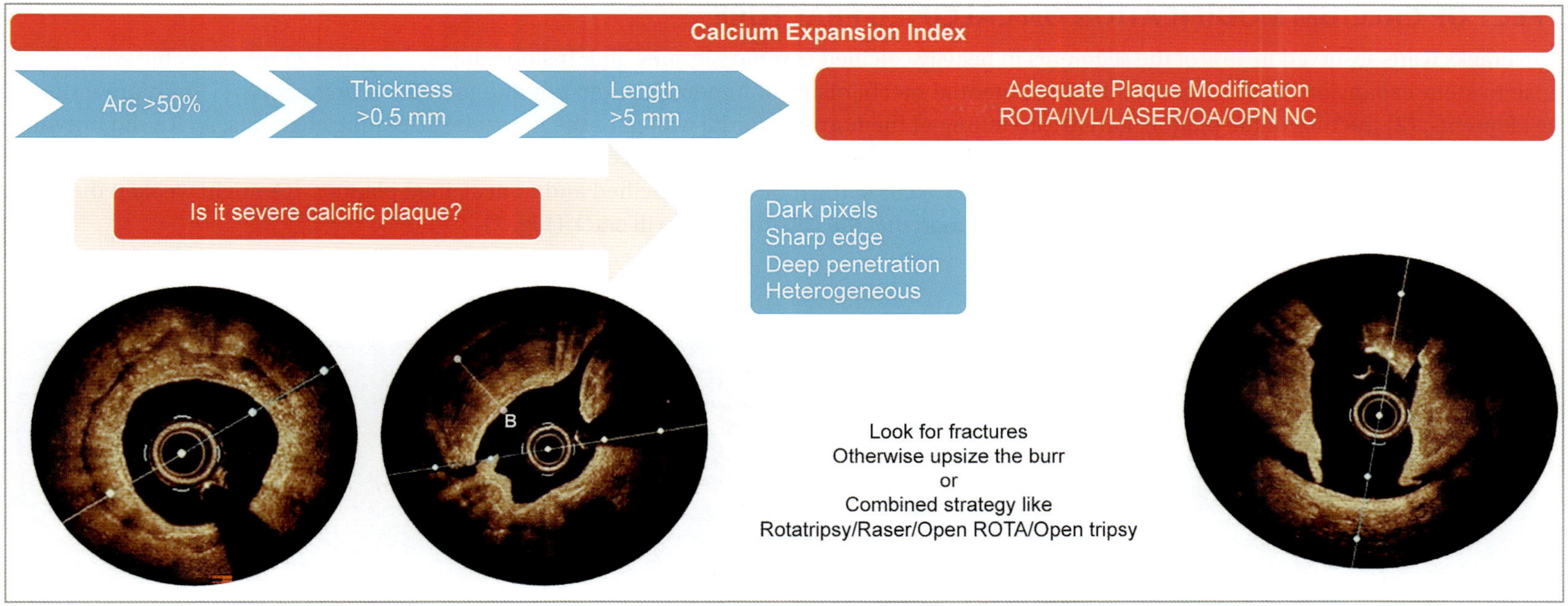

Fig. 2: Calcium expansion index.

otherwise it may lead to increase in MACE rates. PCI of calcified coronaries is a challenging procedure, needs adequate guide support, supportive wires, plaque modification, guide extension catheters, etc. **(Table 3)**.

PLAQUE MODIFICATION OF CALCIFIC PLAQUE DURING PCI

Rotational atherectomy/OA/IVL/ELCA/cutting or scoring balloon are frequently used in calcified vessels as adjunctive plaque modification devices to modify calcific plaque. Superficial calcium close to the lumen is more difficult to expand than deeper calcium limiting expansion of the stent. Devices like cutting or scoring balloons improve vessel compliance through incisions at the edges between calcified and noncalcified components results in greater stent expansion through controlled dissection. Sometimes resistant lesions may require high-pressure balloon inflations, thereby greatly increasing the risk of vessel injury and rupture[3] **(Figs. 4 and 5)**. The super high-pressure balloon OPN NC balloon is a twin layered NC balloon that allows balloon inflations up to 35–40 atm to handle more resistant fibrocalcific lesions compared to maximum inflation of 18–20 atm of conventional NC balloons.

Upsizing of ROTA burr may not be needed to achieve optimal stent expansion in lesions with minimal calcium thickness <0.67 mm, and further use of an oversized burr can be detrimental. In contrast, if the minimal calcium thickness is >0.67 mm after RA, the burr size can be upsized to promote formation of calcium crack[5] **(Fig. 6)**.

EFFECT OF CALCIUM MODIFICATION ON CALCIFIED FRACTURE

Calcium cracks were observed in 49% of the segments in heavily calcified coronary lesions after balloon angioplasty and were associated with a favorable response to stent expansion. Waller described three potential mechanisms of lumen enlargement due to balloon angioplasty: (1) Compression of soft plaque elements; (2) fracture of the plaque; and (3) stretching of the normal arterial wall or of the more elastic plaque elements. As RA did not influence the soft or elastic plaque components, fracture of the plaque or stretching of normal segments is considered the key mechanism for lumen enlargement in heavily calcified coronary lesions. The dissections typically occur at the junction of calcified and noncalcified plaques. RA might weaken the structural integrity by ablating calcium and thereby increase the likelihood that the calcium itself will crack **(Fig. 7)**.

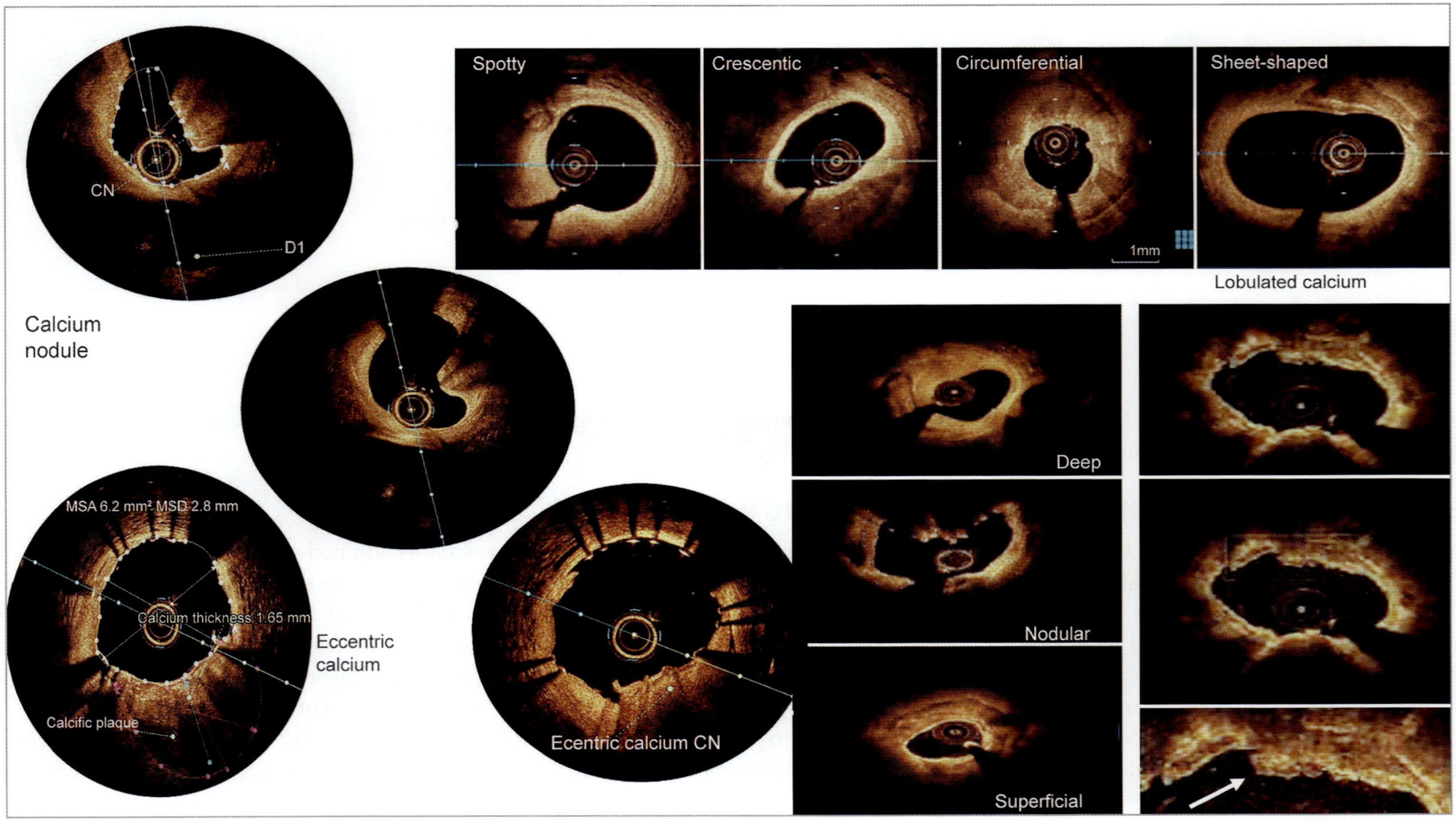

Fig. 3A

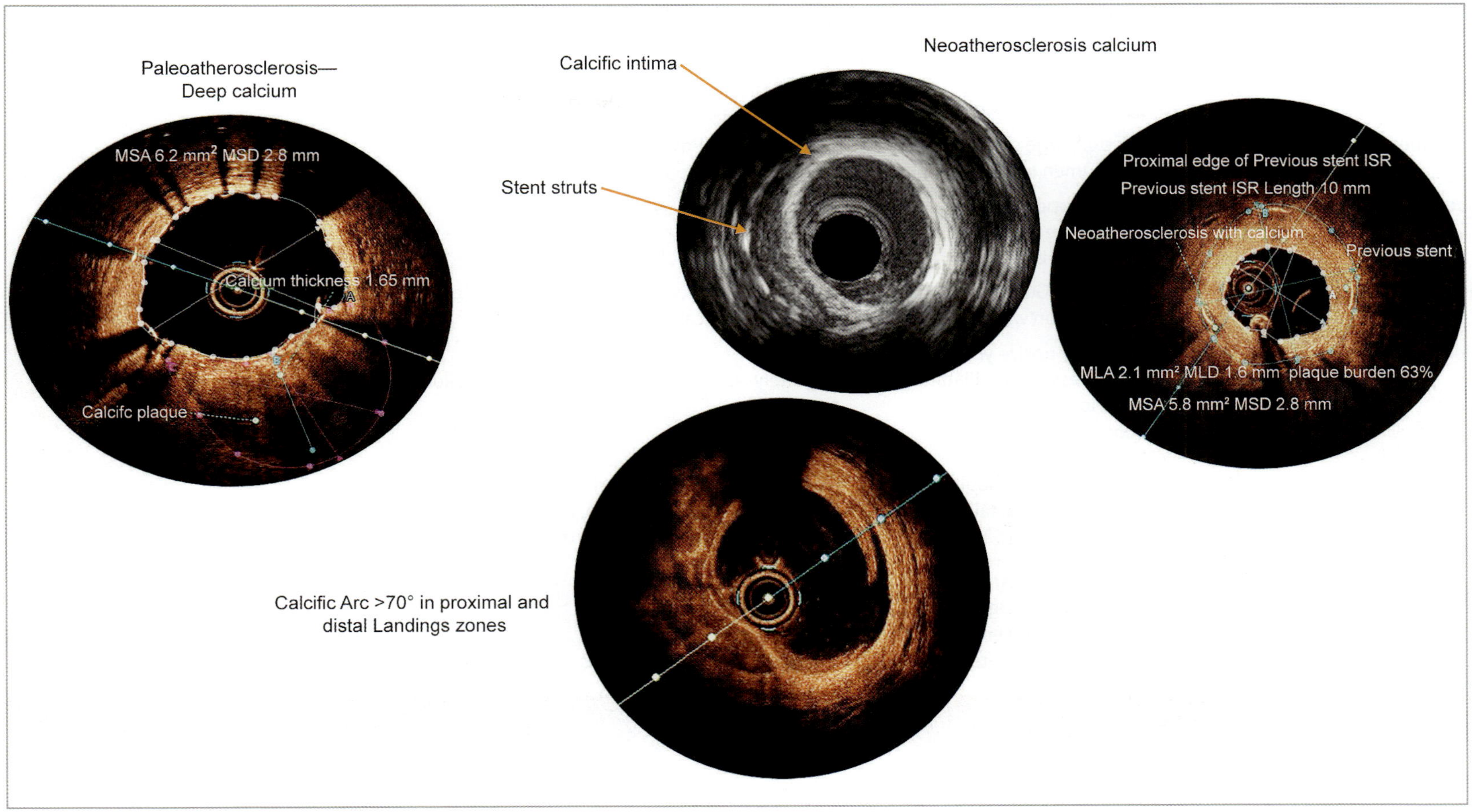

Fig. 3B

Figs. 3A and B: (A) Assessment of calcification by OCT; (B) Assessment of calcium during follow-up of PCI.

BOX 3: OCT for calcific coronaries.

- Assessment of plaque morphology, severity of calcium plaque, and expansion index.
- Usefulness of OCT criteria for choosing appropriate debulking devices.
- Assessment of effectiveness of debulking, upscaling of burr, and any need for additional adjunctive modification devices.
- Optimization of DES implantation with MLD-MAX algorithm

<table>
<tr><th colspan="3">TABLE 3: PCI of diffusely calcified coronaries.</th></tr>
<tr><td>Good guide catheter support (shape and size)</td><td colspan="2">• Ideally 7/8 Fr
• EBU/XB
• Left Amplatz for right coronary</td></tr>
<tr><td>Microcatheter</td><td colspan="2">• For exchange of guidewires and for placement of RotaWire
• Dual lumen catheter for placing guidewires in tortuous/angulated lesions.</td></tr>
<tr><td>Guidewire</td><td colspan="2">• Good supportive wires
• Buddy wire technique
• Anchoring balloons</td></tr>
<tr><td>Guide extension–GuideLiner</td><td colspan="2">• Guidezilla/GuideLiner for placing balloons and stents to facilitate placement even after adequate plaque
• Modification when there is a difficulty in crossing calcified lesions</td></tr>
<tr><td>Lesion preparation</td><td colspan="2">• Gradually upsize your balloons
• High pressure NC dilatation (use adequately-sized balloons (1:1) and check balloon expansion with adequate contrast filling)
• Cutting balloon
• Score flex
• Open NC
• Covered stents should be available (e.g., Papyrus, Graftmaster)
• Rotablation, orbital atherectomy, intravascular lithotripsy, ELCA, and brachytherapy</td></tr>
<tr><td rowspan="2">Imaging</td><td colspan="2">CTCA</td></tr>
<tr><td>IVUS/OCT</td><td>• Arc
• Depth
• Length of calcium plaque
• Determine calcium modification strategy (goal is to develop adequate calcium cracks for adequate expansion).</td></tr>
<tr><td>Physiology</td><td colspan="2">FFR/IFR/RFR</td></tr>
<tr><td>Stents</td><td colspan="2">DES</td></tr>
</table>

The OCT imaging is superior in assessing the effectiveness of modification and debulking method: (1) Ca modification-defined as a round, concave, and polished lumen surface and (2) Ca fracture-defined as complete discontinuity of calcified plaque after stenting. Fujine et al. suggested thickness of calcific plaque <0.54 mm, arc <221° by OCT are predictor of calcific plaque fractures or cracks **(Fig. 8)**.

PREDICTORS FOR FRACTURE THICKNESS <0.24 MM, ARC <225° BY OCT

The primary objective of plaque modification by RA in complex calcified coronary lesions is to cross and adequately dilate stenotic lesions by adjunctive balloon angioplasty and subsequent stent implantation. The OCT showing large calcium angle (>270°) and thickness (>670 µm) predicts nondilatable lesions. OCT predicts calcium fractures if calcium arc >270° and calcium thickness <0.67 mm. OCT evidence of these parameters indicate or defer the use of atherectomy before stent implantation and guide optimization of PCI.[6]

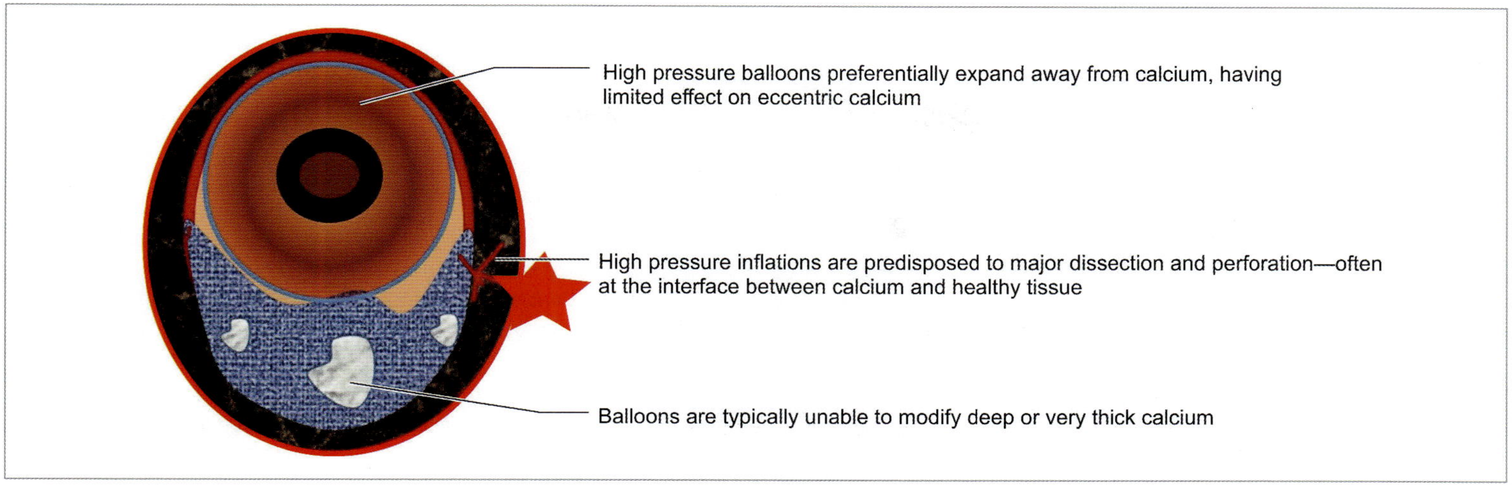

Fig. 4: Balloon-based therapies in calcified lesions.

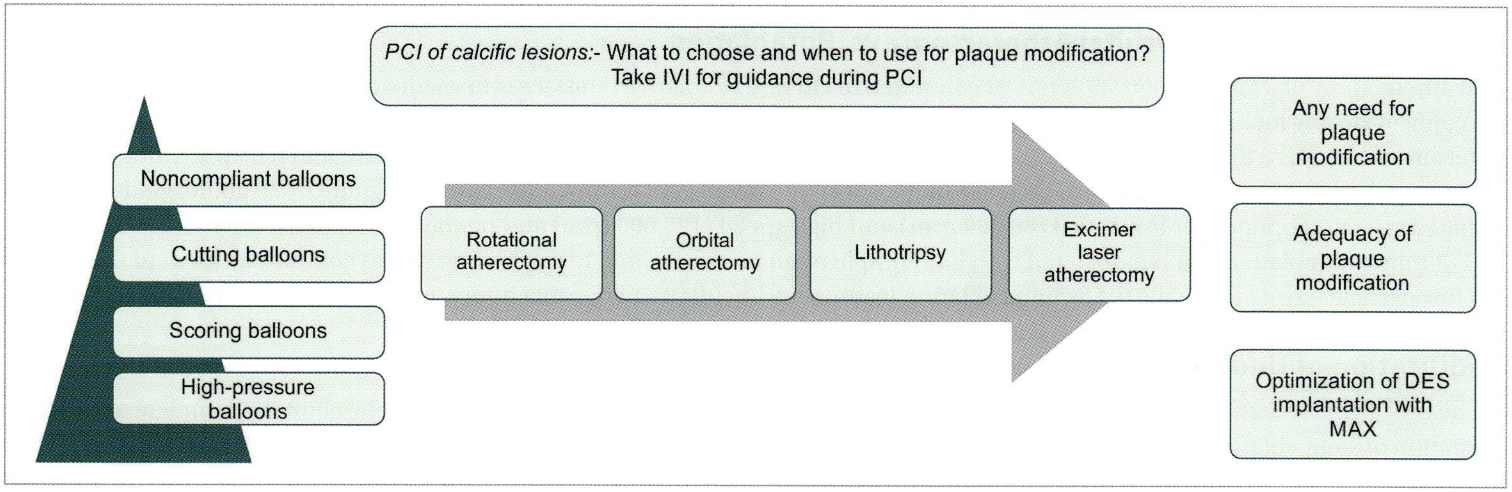

Fig. 5: Selection of plaque modification and optimization of DES based on intravascular imaging.

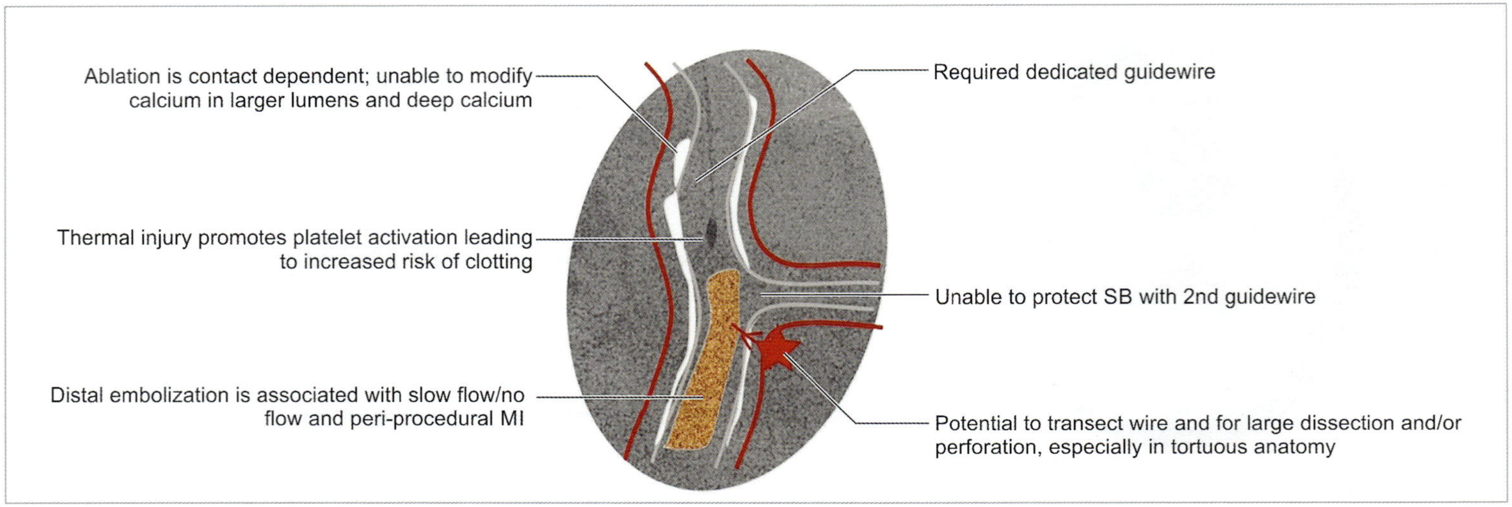

Fig. 6: Rotablation for plaque modification.

Atherectomy Device of Choice: Orbital Atherectomy vs. Rotablation

The rotational atherectomy has more penetration power compared to OA due to ablative interface is immediately at the tip of the diamonds-studded burr, with ablation capacity during forward motion. Rotablator is more useful compared to OA in ostial lesions, chronic total occlusions, and balloon uncrossable lesions. Orbital atherectomy is a diamond-coated 1.25-mm crown which spins (orbits) and ablates during forward and backward motion of device, ease of use, and increase in size of ablation capacity with increase in the speed of crown. OA is compatible with a 6F guide or 7F guide/guide extension pair, it is console has speed selection options for low speed (80,000 rpm) and high speed (120,000 rpm) and operator can move crown in both directions at slowly at a speed of 1–3 mm/s for ablation. OA is associated with low complication rate compared to rotablation due to continuous forward flow of lubricant and generation of low particle size <2 µm while performing ablation leads to low incidence of thermal injury, heart block, and slow flow **(Fig. 8)**.

Plaque Modification of Underexpanded Stent

Debulking of heavy calcific lesions with rotablation of the metallic component of underexpanded stents, thereby allowing complete expansion of lesions. The main limitation of stent ablation is slippage of the burr through the underexpanded stent without ablating the metal and leaving the burr immovable. Burr movement should be more gradual and careful to avoid burr entrapment and burr stall. The slow flow/no flow can happen due to the metallic debris, and stent thrombosis due to more heat generation is also possible **(Figs. 9A and B)**. Stent ablation of an underexpanded stent in a heavily calcified lesion should be carried out by experienced operator only as it is associated with a danger of burr entrapment/burr stall/burr detachment and once the stent ablation is performed, post-OCT evaluation may reveal the complete removal of the stent struts. Stents should be avoided in lesions which are resistant to expand adequately despite using all possible strategies.[7] IVL is the best mode of plaque modification device for underexpanded stent with severe calcification which can break/fracture thick calcific plaque underneath the stent struts. Neoatherosclerosis with severely calcific plaques should be managed like native vessel atherosclerosis with calcific lesions using appropriate modification devices.

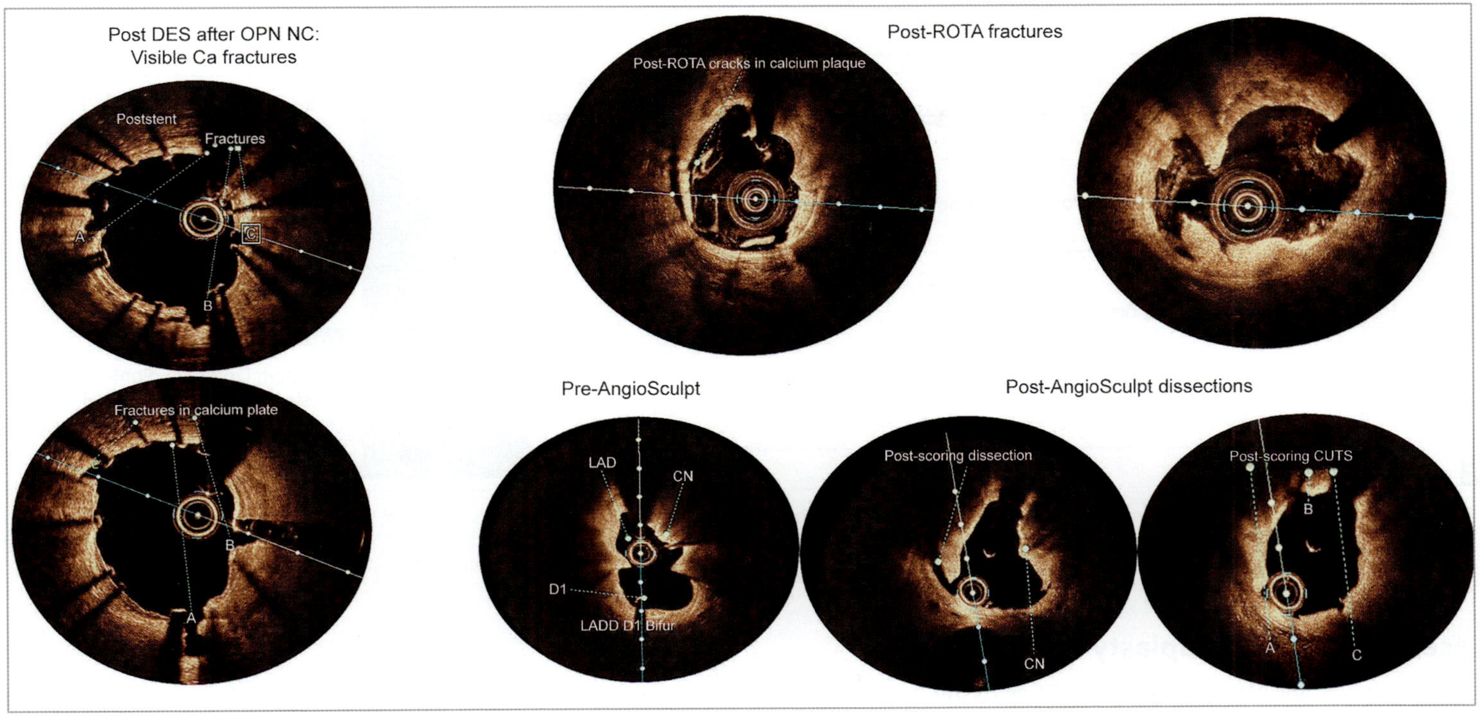

Fig. 7: Postplaque modification–evidence of fractures indicates favorable outcome.

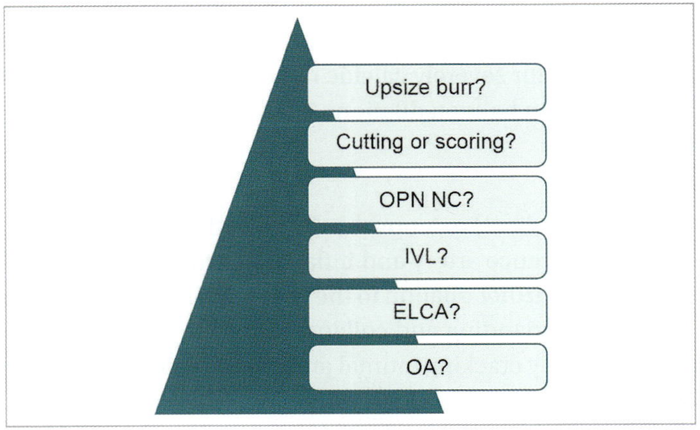

Fig. 8: Atherectomy device of choice for additional plaque modification.

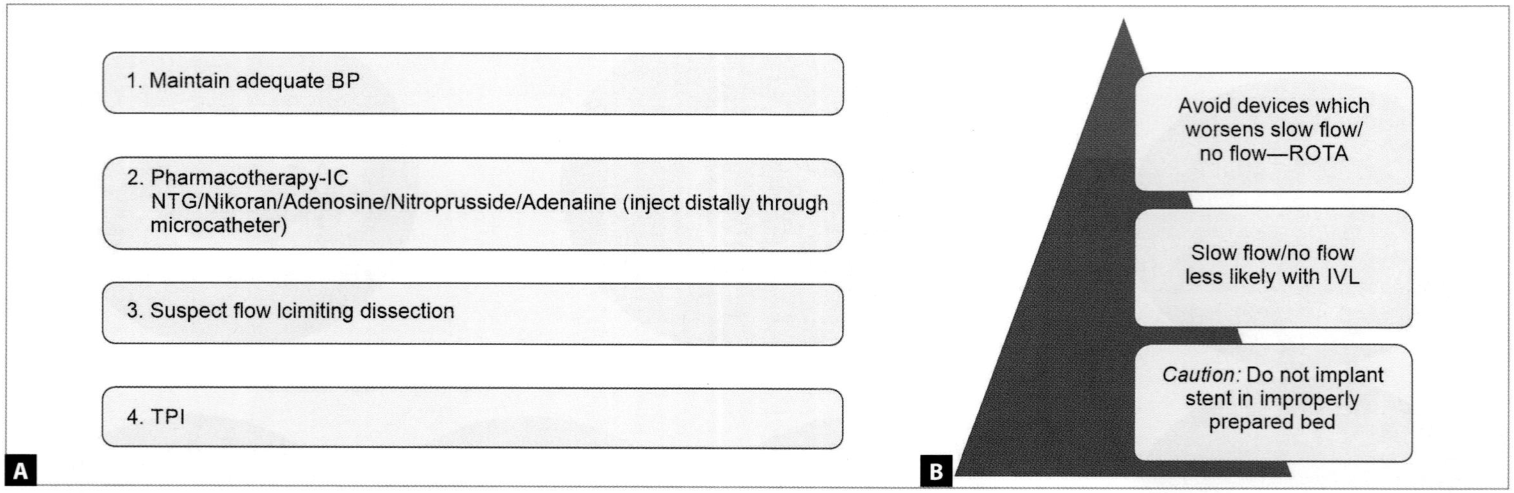

Figs. 9A and B: Slow flow/no flow phenomenon.

Excimer Laser Coronary Angioplasty

Excimer laser coronary angioplasty (ELCA) modifies tissue by three distinct mechanisms: Photochemical, photothermal, and photomechanical effects. The first is a unique laser feature that is capable of breaking down tissue at the molecular level. Photoablation is extremely efficient in fibrotic tissue as well as thrombus but not so much on calcium.[6]

Excimer laser catheters are compatible with standard coronary guidewires, and may also be used to create channel to permit RotaWire with subsequent passage of microcatheter to carry RA ("RASER" technique) or OA to take advantage of the combined benefits of each individual technology. ELCA is currently indicated for the treatment of mild-to-moderate calcific lesions resistant to balloon inflation, saphenous venous grafts and in-stent restenosis. The combined use of RA and ELCA is particularly effective for severely calcific noncrossable and nondilatable lesions. ELCA can also be used in cases of underexpanded stents even after atherectomy and maximum balloon dilation.

Intravascular Lithotripsy

The intravascular lithotripsy (IVL) system (Shockwave Medical) is a novel balloon catheter-based device that utilizes pulsatile mechanical energy to disrupt calcified lesions. IVL balloon is sized 1:1 to the reference artery and inflated to 4 atmospheres, to allow contact with the vessel wall but minimize static barotrauma, and 10 pulses are delivered, followed by further dilation to the nominal pressure of 6 atmospheres. Electrical discharge from the emitters vaporizes the fluid within the balloon, creating a rapidly expanding and collapsing bubble that generates sonic pressure waves which create a localized field effect that travels through soft vascular tissue, selectively cracking intimal and medial calcium within the vessel wall. During ablation both RA and OA generate nanoparticles that may emboli distally and impair microcirculatory function, whereas larger calcium fragments generated by lithotripsy remain in situ. IVL is an operator friendly technique with a short learning curve, and it has potential advantage over the ROTA particularly in high-risk bifurcation

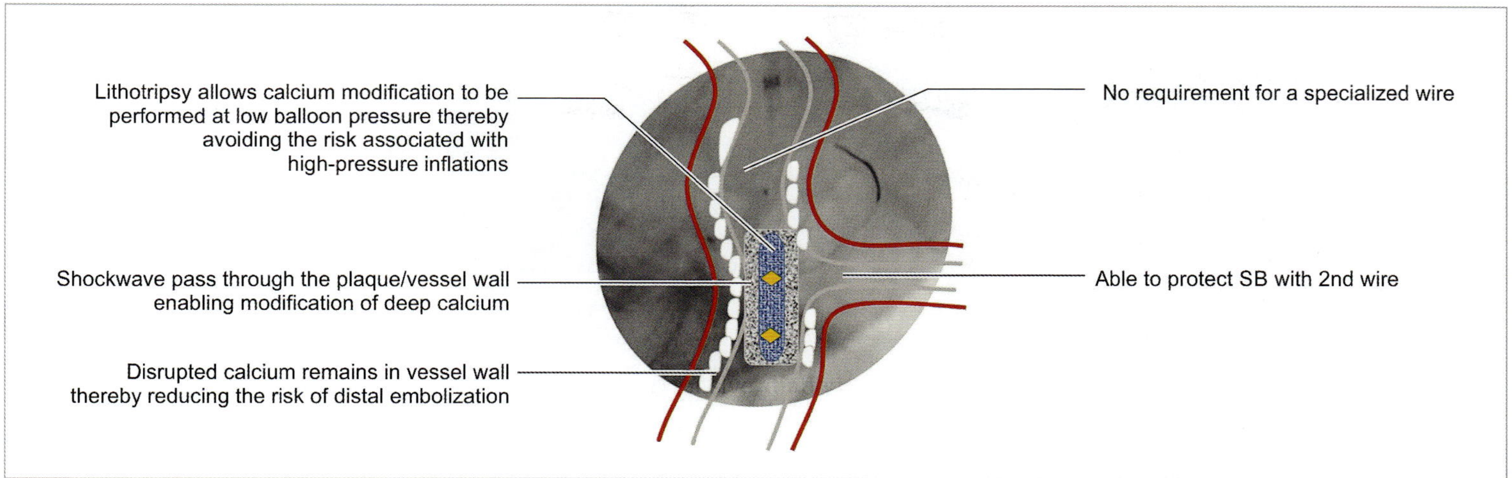

Fig. 10: Intravascular lithotripsy for plaque modification.

lesions with high prediction for SB closure where there is no need to remove the side branch guidewire, and patients with severe LV dysfunction who at risk of high risk of slow flow or no flow **(Figs. 10 and 11)**. Incidence of dissection, perforation, and slow flow is very low with IVL compared to ROTA and OA as evident in DISRUPT I and DISRUPT II studies with high success rate in severe calcified lesions, but it is unsuitable for balloon uncrossable lesions. Sometimes, combination of IVL and ROTA may be useful in patients with severely calcified lesions which is called ROTA-Tripsy when adequate modification is not optimal with either of the device.

OCT AFTER LITHOTRIPSY AND DISRUPT CAD CORONARY OCT

The IVL selectively interact with calcified plaques even in their inner adventitial layer, produces calcium fractures or cracks in 70–75% of calcium plaques but main mechanism responsible for stent expansion is alteration of vessel compliance due to its ability to produce microfracture which were evident in micro-CT and histological studies and it avoids the trauma produced by blades or burrs and their related risk like coronary dissection or perforation.[8]

Salient features of each device is described in **Table 4** to choose the appropriate device for plaque modification strategies based on the clinical situation and operator's experience.

TOP 10 TIPS AND TRICKS FOR PCI OF CALCIFIED VESSELS

Step 1: Decide on the initial strategy: Assess calcium severity based on fluoroscopy, CT-Angio, and intravascular imaging IVUS/OCT.

Step 2: Optimize your support: Proper guide catheter support, GuideLiner/Guidezilla, balloon anchoring, and buddy wire.

Step 3: Gradually upsize your balloons: Use low profile CTO balloons if unable to cross such as Nick Nano, Acrostat 1.0 mm × 5 mm/1.0 × 10 mm, Tazuna 1.25 mm balloon. Upsize the balloon according to vessel size, not to exceed balloon artery size >1:1.1.

Step 4: Consider using a modified balloon: Scoreflex/cutting balloon/AngioSculpt/Open NC (high pressure inflation up to 35–40 atm).

Step 5: Make sure the balloons have expanded

Step 6: Choose appropriate strategy quickly: Balloon Escalation Strategy (BEST) for uncrossable, undilatable, and failure to cross lesions **(Figs. 12A and B)**.

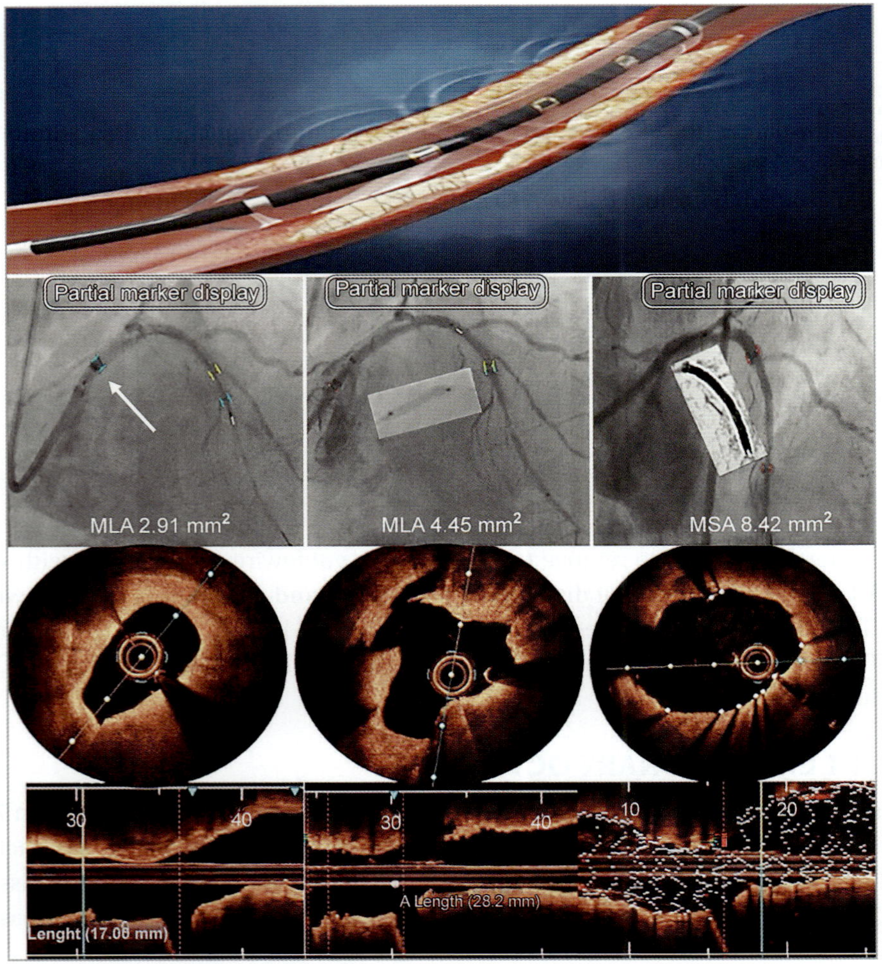

Fig. 11: IVL-induced calcium fractures after plaque modification for optimal stent expansion.

Step 7: Use atherectomy if required: ROTA/orbital atherectomy/IVL/ELCA.

Step 8: Stent advancement (with caution): Avoid pushing forcefully if any resistance, try to use GuideLiner, balloon anchoring, and buddy wire if any difficulty in placing stent.

Step 9: Stent optimization: Using proper NC/OPN NC balloon with image guidance, OCT/IVUS **(Figs. 13A to C)**.

Step 10: Anticipate complications and manage on emergency basis to avoid morbidity and mortality: If there is any perforation, use balloon occlusion proximal to perforation to decrease flow through perforation site, covered stent for sealing perforation site, and coils or subcutaneous fat to occlude perforations of small branches. Plan for emergency pericardiocentesis if any symptoms and signs of pericardial tamponade appear.

While performing OCT evaluation for calcified coronary arteries, algorithmic approach is very useful as mentioned in **Flowchart 1 and Box 4**.

TABLE 4: Angioplasty, atherectomy, and lithotripsy device comparison.

Device	*ROTA*	*OA*	*IVL (balloon-based device at inflation of 4–6 atm)*	*ELCA*	*OPN NC*
Mechanism	Rotational motion in a concentric and forward motion, ablation only during forward motion (central cutting)	Orbital motion centrifugal cutting and ablation during forward and backward motion	Circumferential mechanical energy—formation of microbubbles by producing 40–50 atm pressure with rapid expansion and collapse causes disruption of calcified lesions	Ablation of calcific lesions by catheter based UV light	High pressure NC balloon double layered—can be inflated up to 35–40 atm
Guidewire	RotaWire (Floppy and Extra Support)	ViperWire Advance® guidewire	Standard coronary guidewire	Standard coronary guidewire	Standard coronary guidewire
Concept	Differential cutting	Differential sanding	Electrical energy is delivered to the emitter, initiating the steam bubble, which expand and collapses—creating sonic pressure waves	Thermal creation of microbubbles and modification of plaque	Balloon expansion
Device size selection	1.25, 1.50, 1.75, 2.00, 2.15, 2.25, 2.38, and 2.50 mm (Burr). Majority (90%) of patients requires 1.5 mm burr for plaque modification. Burr can be upsized if no visible fractures and Ca^+ thickness >0.5 mm	*1.25 mm (crown):* Single crown by increasing the speed of burr increases burr capacity	*Balloons (mm):* 2.5–4.0 mm in 12 mm length	*Catheters (mm):* 0.9, 1.4, 1.7, and 2.0	*Balloons (mm):* 1.5–4.5 mm
Ablation speed	Plaque modification usually achieved at low speeds (135,000–180,000 rpm) to reduce risk of complications	Low speed (80,000 rpm) or high speed (120,000 rpm) initial treatment for each lesion must start at low speed	–	–	–
Continuous blood flow during ablation	No	Yes (minimizing the potential for ischemia and thermal trauma)	No	No	No
Flush	Rotablation cocktail with verapamil, nitrates and heparin in saline recommended	No specific recommendation	No specific recommendation	No specific recommendation	No specific recommendation
Particle size	5–10 µm	2 µm	<10 µm	–	–
Complications	No flow, dissection, perforation, burr entrapment, burr stall, AV block	No flow, dissection, perforation, abrupt closure (less compared to ROTA)	Dissection, electric signals similar to pacing spikes, low incidents of slow flow or no flow	Dissection, perforation	Dissection, contained perforation—low incidents of pericardial tamponade

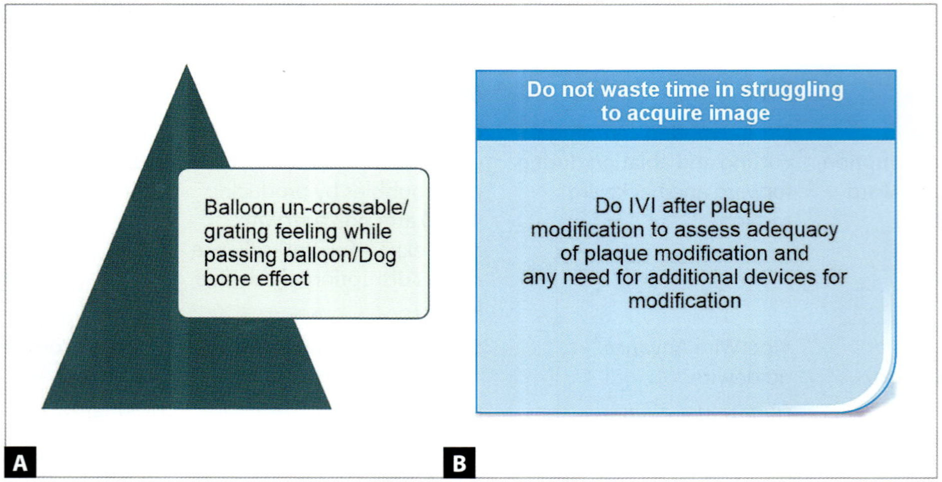

Figs. 12A and B: Strategy for balloon uncrossable lesions.

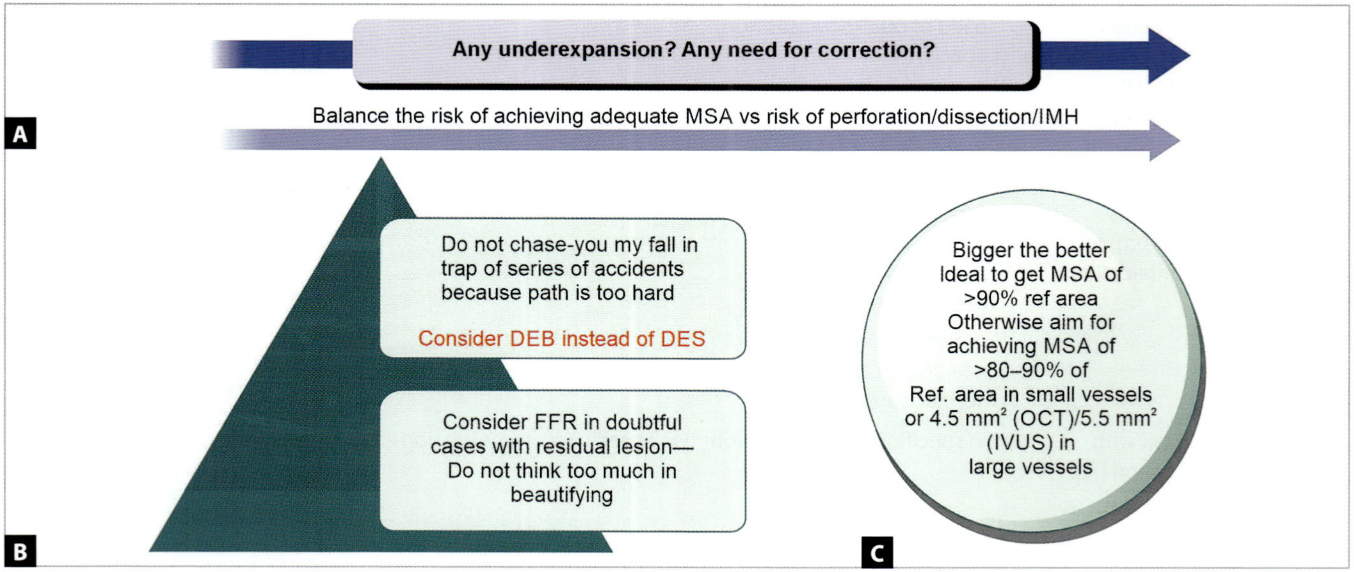

Figs. 13A to C: Adequate optimization of the device.

Flowchart 1: Algorithmic approach to the treatment of heavily calcified coronary lesions.

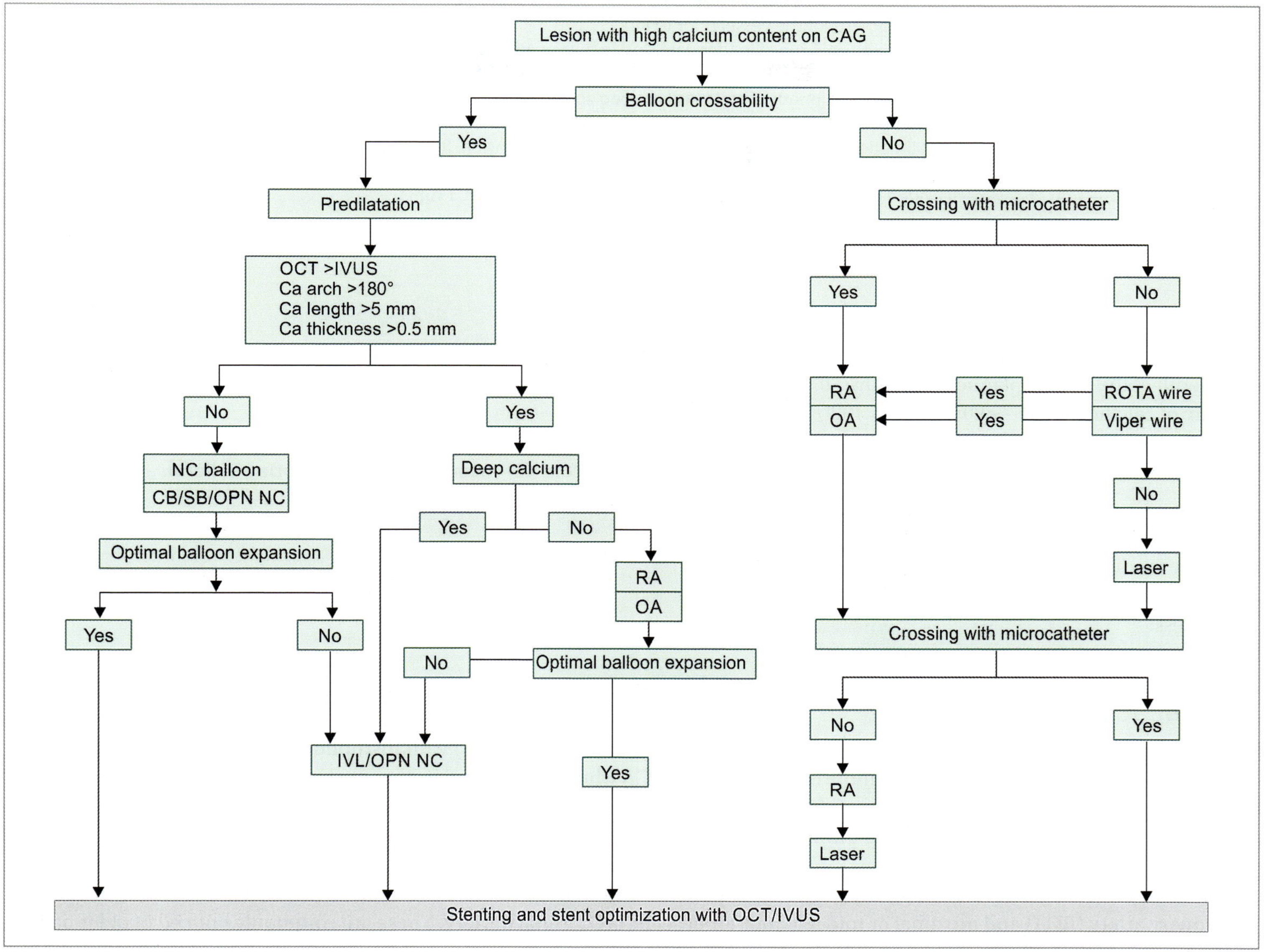

BOX 4: Key points for use of imaging with implantation with DES.

- Use OCT to assess morphology. Lesion length, and diameter of the vessel prior to PCI
- Ensure adequate plaque modification and confirm it with OCT run, if inadequate upsize burr or additional adjunct devices for further modification of plaque before implanting stent.
- Use Angio-coregistration for choosing precise diameter and length of stent and landing zones.
- Avoid mismatch with reference vessel (oversizing leads more frequent MACE and undersizing leads more frequent malapposition and stent thrombosis).
- Use high pressure NC balloon or OPN NC balloon inflations for adequate stent apposition and expansion. It will be effective only when the plaque modification is adequate.
- Assess and implement correction of any medial edge dissection, apposition, and expansion with final OCT run.

SUMMARY

Assessment of calcified vessel by OCT for preprocedure planning:

- Decide plaque morphology—deep calcific plaque/superficial calcific plaque/CN
- Decide the depth of the calcific plaque—<0.5 mm/>0.5 mm
- Decide the arc of calcific plaque—<90°/>90° to <180°/>180°
- Decide the length of the calcific plaque—<5 mm/>5 mm
  If score >2—needs plaque modification by ROTA/orbital atherectomy/IVL. If score <2—needs NC/cutting/scoring balloon.

Calcium Scoring System

Rule of 5 for plaque modification of calcific plaque:

- 50% circumference
- 0.5 mm thickness
- 5 mm length.

Calcium Nodule

Calcified nodule defined as an accumulation of nodular calcification (small calcium deposits) with disruption of fibrous cap on the calcified plate. It is usually formed due to breaks in the calcified sheet, more often in the mid-RCA where mechanical factors, such as a coronary hinge motion might break the calcium sheet. It can contribute to coronary thrombosis (2–7%) and is one of the common causes of ACS presentation in advanced age. Disrupted luminal surface by nodules of dense calcium with overlying thrombus and little or no underlying necrotic core in arteries that are highly calcified, tortuous, and often have a large sheet of calcification.[9,10]

Calcium nodule is observed in 4.2–7% of the culprit lesions of patients presenting with ACS and more often seen in the lesions involving the ostium or mid right coronary artery (RCA) and proximal or mid left anterior descending coronary artery. These are commonly noticed in older patients, females, diabetics, post-coronary bypass graft surgery, and CRF patients. ACS patients with culprit lesions of CN showed lesser lipid-rich plaque, fewer thin-cap fibroatheroma, and plaque ruptures compared with those without a CN. Sometimes, CN resembles a red thrombus on OCT which might result in difficulty in interpreting images leading to improper clinical decisions while performing PCI.[11,12]

Calcium nodule is potentially more amenable to OA due to bidirectional cutting and movement or spin of the crown along the periphery of the vascular lumen compared to unidirectional cutting during forward movement with central probing of the ROTA burr and no need to see wire alignment with CN while performing ablation. Sometimes, to improve stent results more aggressive lesion preparation such as RA in combination with orbital atherectomy or RA with cutting balloon or intravascular lithotripsy might be necessary. However, because of more frequent association of thrombus with unstable features and heterogeneous hardness of CN, distal embolization of CN with slow flow can occur more often during plaque modification. CN can produce wire bias, whereby the guidewire for the debulking device is positioned closer to the soft tissue wall than nodule. The position of the IVUS catheter can indicate likelihood of wire bias, and providing that the bias is suitable for successful rotablation.[13]

Ultreon

The Ultreon Software with an intuitive interface offers physicians a user-friendly on-screen information and step-by-step guidance following MLD-MAX workflow to aid with decision-making; to determine a proper treatment technique pre-PCI, and to ensure optimal stent expansion results post-PCI.

Pre-PCI: Ultreon 1.0 Software uses artificial intelligence (AI) to automatically detect degree and thickness of calcification. Autodetects and highlights calcification arc and max thickness, displays calcification angle and max thickness values throughout the pullback in real-time, and highlights calcification overlays on the vessel with the co-registration view.

Device selection: Automatically detect external elastic lamina (EEL) and lumen to help identify landing zones for accurate stent placement, provides vessel diameter measurements, facilitates measuring lesion length and identification of optimal user-adjusted stent landing zones on a single screen, autodetects and provides measurement of lumen and detectable external elastic lamina (EEL) for quick visualization, and facilitates stent length selection through co-registration.

Postprocedure: It provides side-by-side viewing of live and co-registered Angio to help physicians guide precise stent deployment, helps to ensure complete lesion coverage and avoid stent edges in high-risk morphology, and ensure optimal stent expansion and apposition with instantaneous display of expansion and apposition results.

The Ultreon™ Software with an intuitive interface offers physicians a user-friendly on-screen information and step-by-step guidance following MLD-MAX workflow to aid with decision-making; to determine a proper treatment technique pre-PCI, and to ensure optimal stent expansion results post-PCI.

Ultreon™ 1.0 Software uses artificial intelligence (AI) to automatically detect degree and thickness of calcification.

- Autodetects and highlights calcification arc and max thickness
- Displays calcification angle and max thickness values throughout the pullback in real-time
- Highlights calcification overlays on the vessel with the coregistration view

Sizing

Ultreon™ 1.0 Software uses artificial intelligence (AI) to automatically detect external elastic lamina (EEL) and lumen to help identify landing zones for accurate stent placement.

- Provides vessel diameter measurements
- Facilitates measuring lesion length and identification of optimal user-adjusted stent landing zones on a single screen
- Autodetects and provides measurement of lumen and detectable external elastic lamina (EEL) for quick visualization
- Facilitates stent length selection through coregistration.

Deployment of the stent with Ultreon Software

- Provides side-by-side viewing of live and coregistered Angio to help physicians guide precise stent deployment.
- Helps to ensure complete lesion coverage and avoid stent edges in high-risk morphology.
- Helps to ensure optimal stent expansion and apposition with instantaneous display of expansion and apposition results.

REFERENCES

1. Sharma SK, Vengrenyuk Y, Kini AS. IVUS, OCT, and coronary artery calcification: is there a bone of contention? JACC Cardiovasc Imaging. 2017;10(8):880-2.
2. Saita T, Fujii K, Hao H, Imanaka T, Shibuya M, Fukunaga M, et al. Histopathological validation of optical frequency domain imaging to quantify various types of coronary calcifications. Eur Heart J Cardiovasc Imaging. 2016;18(3):342-9.
3. Shimamura K, Guagliumi G. Optical coherence tomography for online guidance of complex coronary interventions. Circ J. 2016;80:2063-72.
4. Mintz GS. Intravascular imaging of coronary calcification and its clinical implications. JACC Cardiovasc Imaging. 2015;8(4):461-71.
5. Maejima N, Hibi K, Saka K, Akiyama E, Konishi M, Endo M, et al. Relationship between thickness of calcium on optical coherence tomography and crack formation after balloon dilatation in calcified plaque requiring rotational atherectomy. Circ J. 2016;80:1413-9.
6. Mehanna E, Abbott JD, Bezerra HG. Optimizing percutaneous coronary intervention in calcified lesions: Insights from optical coherence tomography of atherectomy. Cir Cardiovasc Interv. 2018;11(5):e006813.
7. Koide M, Inoue K, Matsuo A, Fujita H. Optical coherence tomography findings after longitudinal ablation for an underexpanded stent in a heavily calcified lesion: a case report. BMC Cardiovasc Disord. 2016;16(1):241.
8. Virmani R, Kolodgie FD, Burke AP, Farb A, Schwartz SM. Lessons from sudden coronary death: a comprehensive morphological classification scheme for atherosclerotic lesions. Arterioscler Thromb Vasc Biol. 2000;20(5):1262-75.
9. Lee JB, Mintz GS, Lisauskas JB, Biro SG, Pu J, Sum ST, et al. Histopathologic validation of the intravascular ultrasound diagnosis of calcified coronary artery nodules. Am J Cardiol. 2011;108(11):1547-51.
10. Yahagi K, Davis HR, Arbustini E, Virmani R. Sex differences in coronary artery disease: pathological observations. Atherosclerosis. 2015;239(1):260-7.
11. Lee T, Mintz GS, Matsumura M, Zhang W, Cao Y, Usui E, et al. Prevalence, predictors, and clinical presentation of a calcified nodule as assessed by optical coherence tomography. JACC Cardiovasc Imaging. 2017;10(8):883-91.
12. Sénior JM, Tamayo N, Rodríguez A, Fernández A. Rotational atherectomy for the management of inadequate stent expansion (stent ablation). Revista Colombiana de Cardiología. 2017;24(6):625.
13. Yamamoto K, Natsuaki M, Serikawa T, Okabe M, Yamamoto Y. Nodular calcification in saphenous vein graft successfully treated by percutaneous coronary intervention. Case Rep Cardiol. 2018;2018:5138705.

CASE 1

OCT-guided plaque modification with orbital atherectomy.

CLINICAL HISTORY

A 67-year-old male, known diabetic with positive TMT, admitted for further evaluation of coronary artery disease. 2D echo—no RWMA, normal LV function, EF—60%, O/I: Hb—8.6 g/dL, WBC—15,600, Trop-I—819.77 ng/L, CPK-MB—18.9 U/L, serum creatinine—0.60 mg/dL, eGFR—95 mL/min, RBS—160 mg/dL **(Fig. 14)**.

RCA was engaged with JR 3.5-6 Fr guiding catheter, lesion was crossed with 0.014″ runthrough wire with Guide plus support, predilated with 1.5 × 15 mm Ryurei balloon at 12 atm. Postdilatation OCT run of RCA showed significant fibrotic plaque with calcified lesions **(Fig. 15)**.

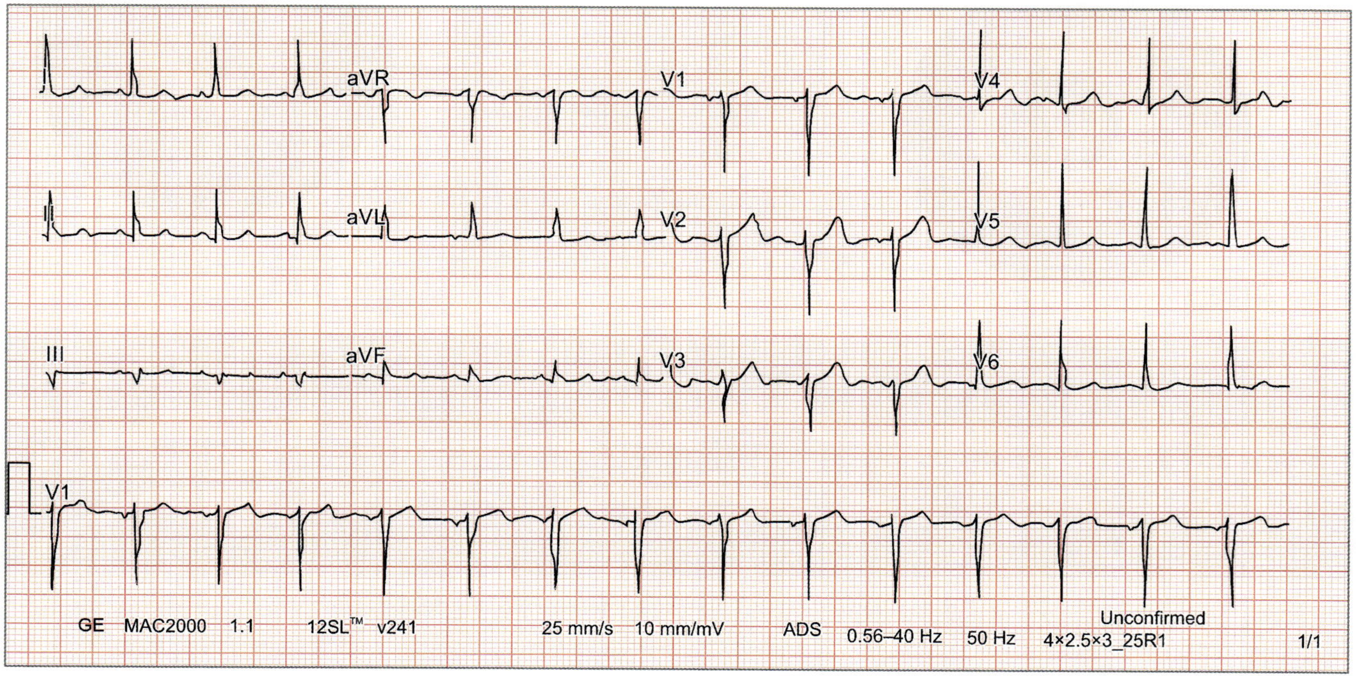

Fig. 14: Electrocardiogram (ECG).

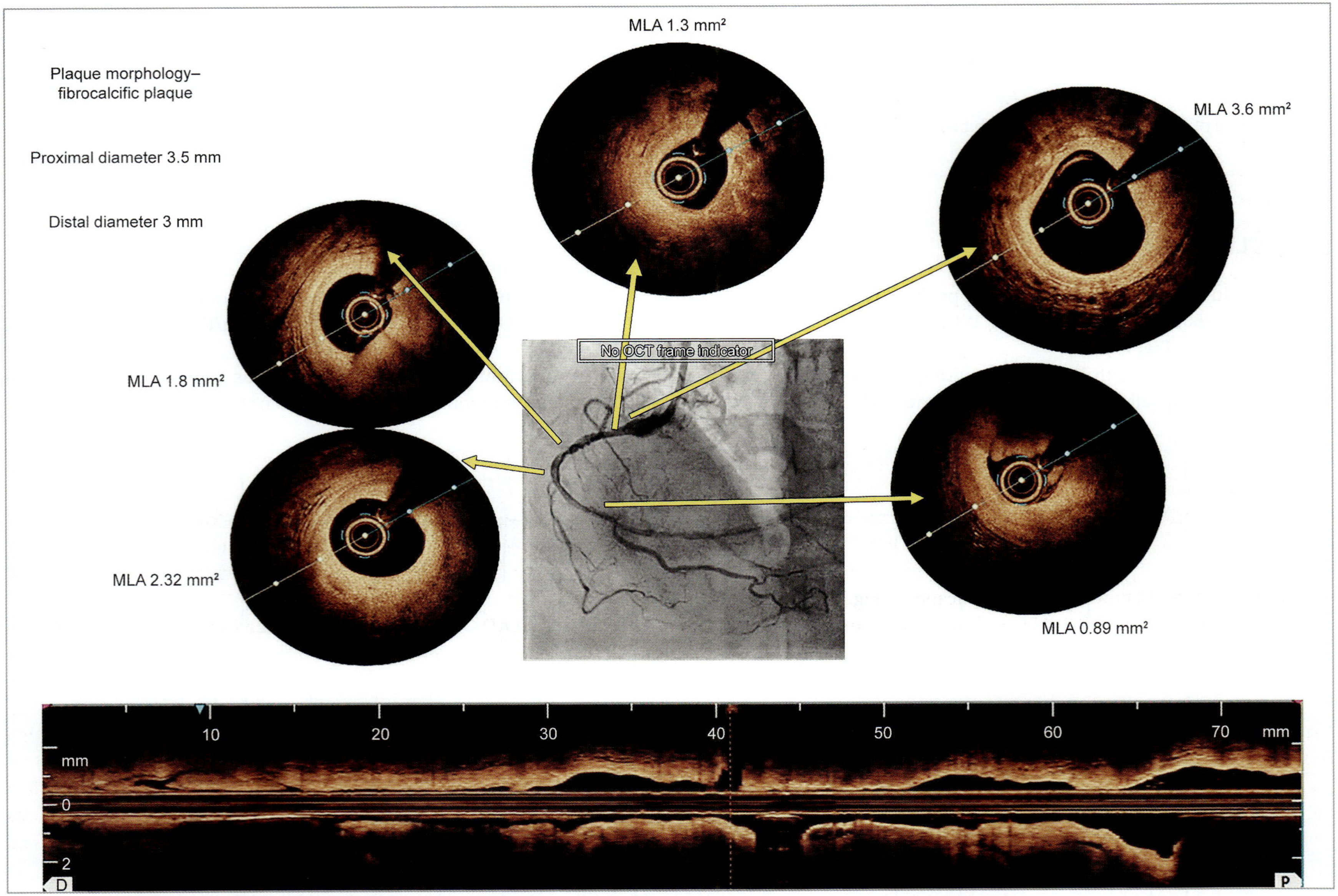

Fig. 15: Prestenting OCT assessment for sizing of the device.

Plaque modification was performed with scoring using 3.0 × 15 mm AngioSculpt balloon through Guide plus II catheter due to difficulty in placing devices.

Balloon Uncrossable Lesion Algorithm

- *Increase support:*
  - Better guide catheter (bigger shape)
  - Guide extension
  - Anchor wire/balloon
- Small balloon
- Balloon-assisted microdissection (BAM)—"grenadoplasty"
- *Add a microcatheter:*
  - Torquable (Corsair Pro and Turnpike)
  - Lower profile (FineCross, Turnpike LP, Corsair Pro, and Caravel)
  - Threaded (Turnpike Spiral and Turnpike Gold)
- Laser
- Atherectomy (free wire with RotaWire)
- *Subintimal techniques:*
  - External crush/subintimal plaque modification
  - Dissection and re-entry

Initially, stenting of distal RCA was done with 3.0 × 48 mm Xience Xpedition at 12 atm inflations, postdilated with 3 × 15 NC balloon inflations. Then, proximal RCA was stented with 3.5 × 48 mm Xience Xpedition stent with 2–3 mm overlap of proximal edge of distal stent. Postdilatations were carried out with 3.0 × 15 mm NC Trek balloon at 16–18 atm. Poststent OCT run showed well expanded and apposed stent struts with no edge dissection. The final result was good with TIMI III flow without complications **(Fig. 16)**.

LCA was engaged with XB 3-7 Fr guiding catheter, and Runthrough wire was placed in the LAD. Then, lesion was predilated with 3.0 × 15 mm NC Trek balloon at 12 atm. Presenting OCT run of proximal LAD showed severe calcific plaque with high calcium expansion index score suggestive of adequate plaque modification prior to stenting **(Fig. 17)**.

Plaque modification with PA was planned due to severely calcific plaque. ViperWire was exchanged with Runthrough wire using FineCross microcatheter. Orbital atherectomy device with 1.25 mm crown was used to ablate calcific plaque of proximal LAD plaque using 80k rpm × 6 cycles and final two polishing runs using crown speed of 120k rpm **(Fig. 18)**.

Post-OCT run showed adequate plaque modification of calcific plaque with evidence of calcium fracture, dissections and increase in the mean luminal areas at various levels of ablated area **(Fig. 19)**. Then, LAD stenting was done with 2.75 × 38 mm Xience Alpine stent at 12–16 atm inflations. Postdilatations were done with 3.0 × 15 mm NC Trek balloon at 16–18 atm. Final OCT run showed well-expanded stent, no malapposition, and medial edge dissection. The final result was good with TIMI III flow without complications.

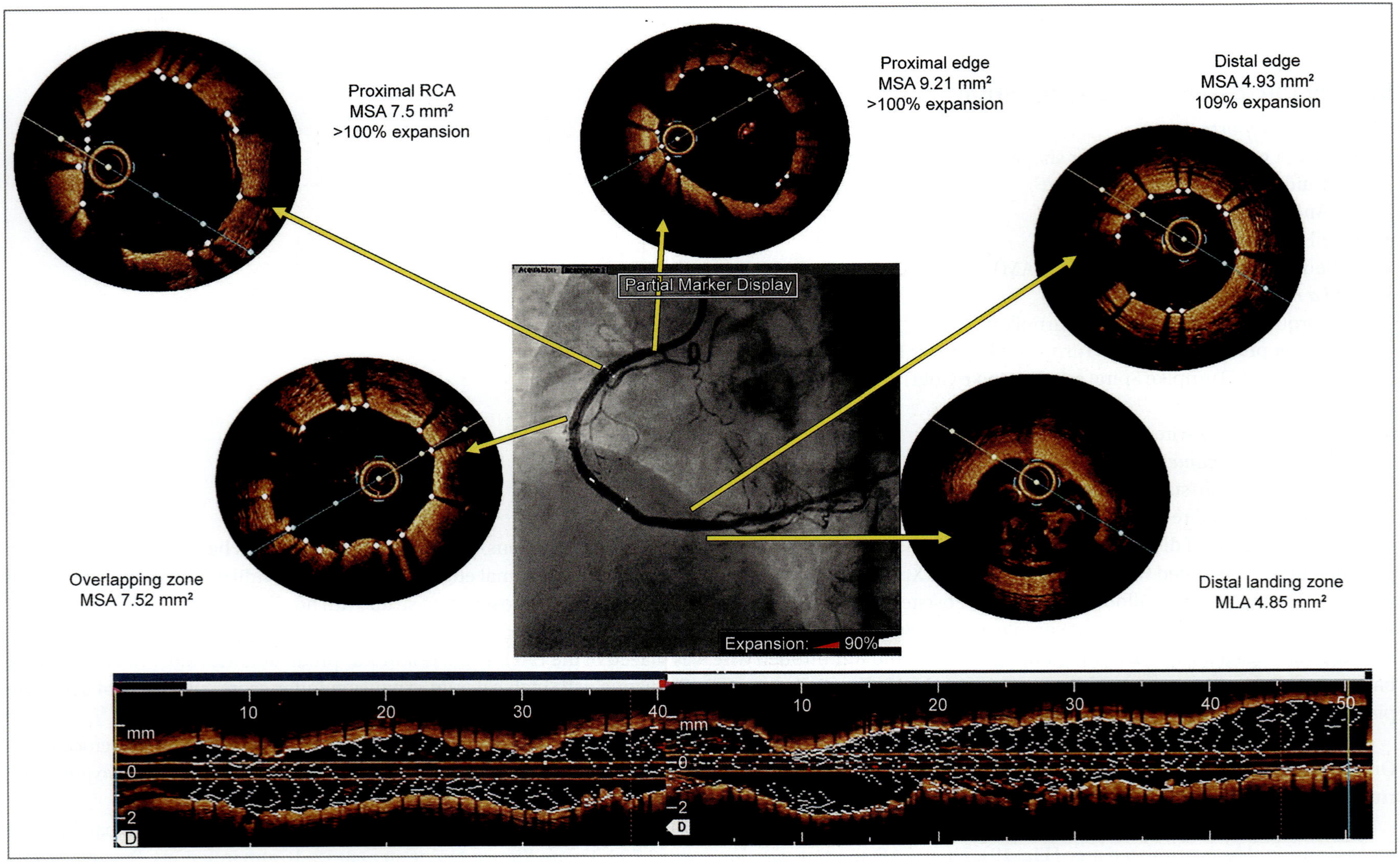

Fig. 16: Post stenting OCT assessment of RCA showing well expanded and apposed stent struts with no medial edge dissections.

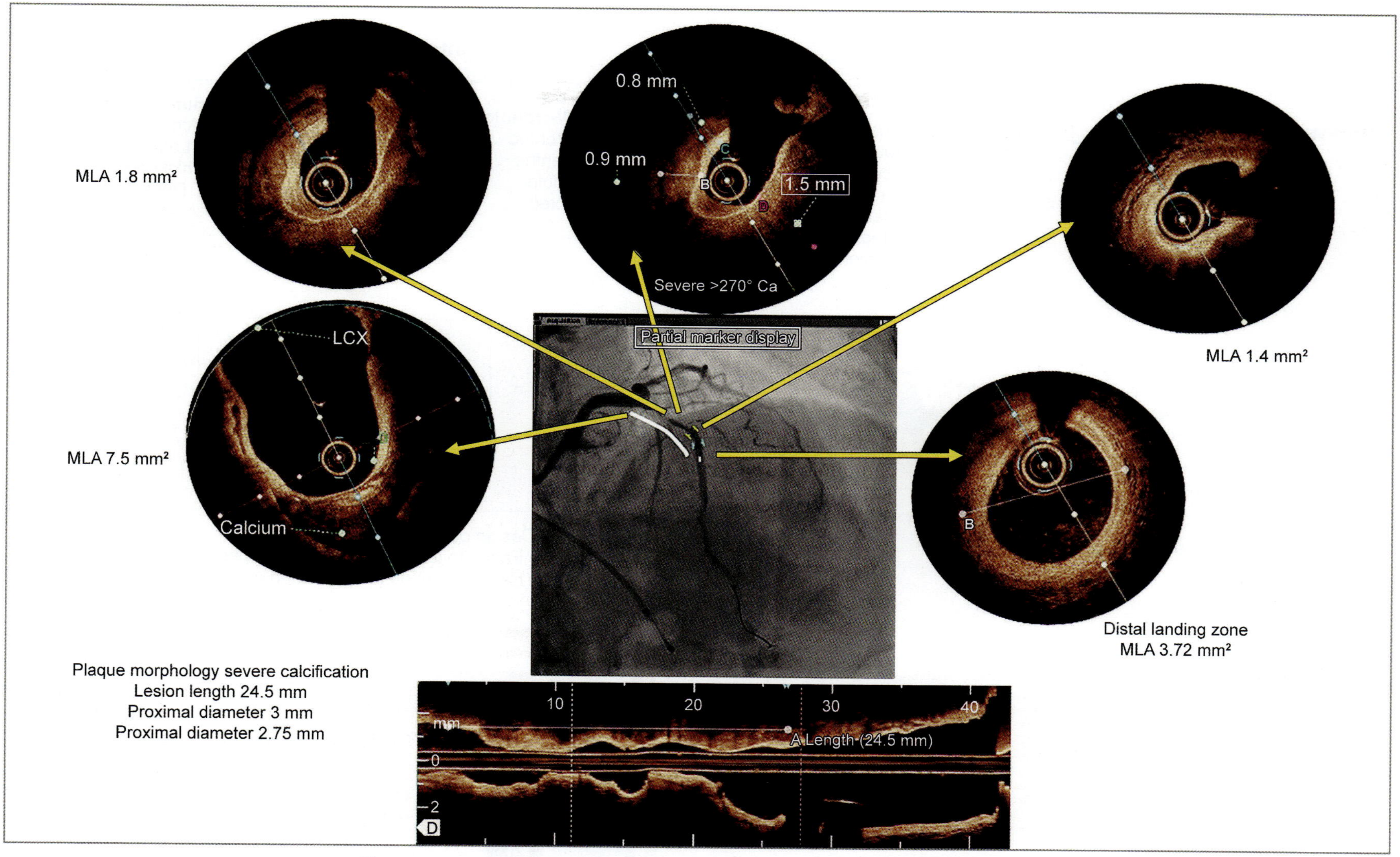

Fig. 17: Presenting OCT assessment for plaque morphology and selection of device.

In vast majority of cases, OA can be performed using radial approach, hence it can reduce significant number of access site related complications and shortens the duration of hospitalization.

OA is more useful for ablating large vessels, lesions with severe superficial calcium, eccentric calcium or CN, and crossable Aorto-ostial lesions with reverse cutting.

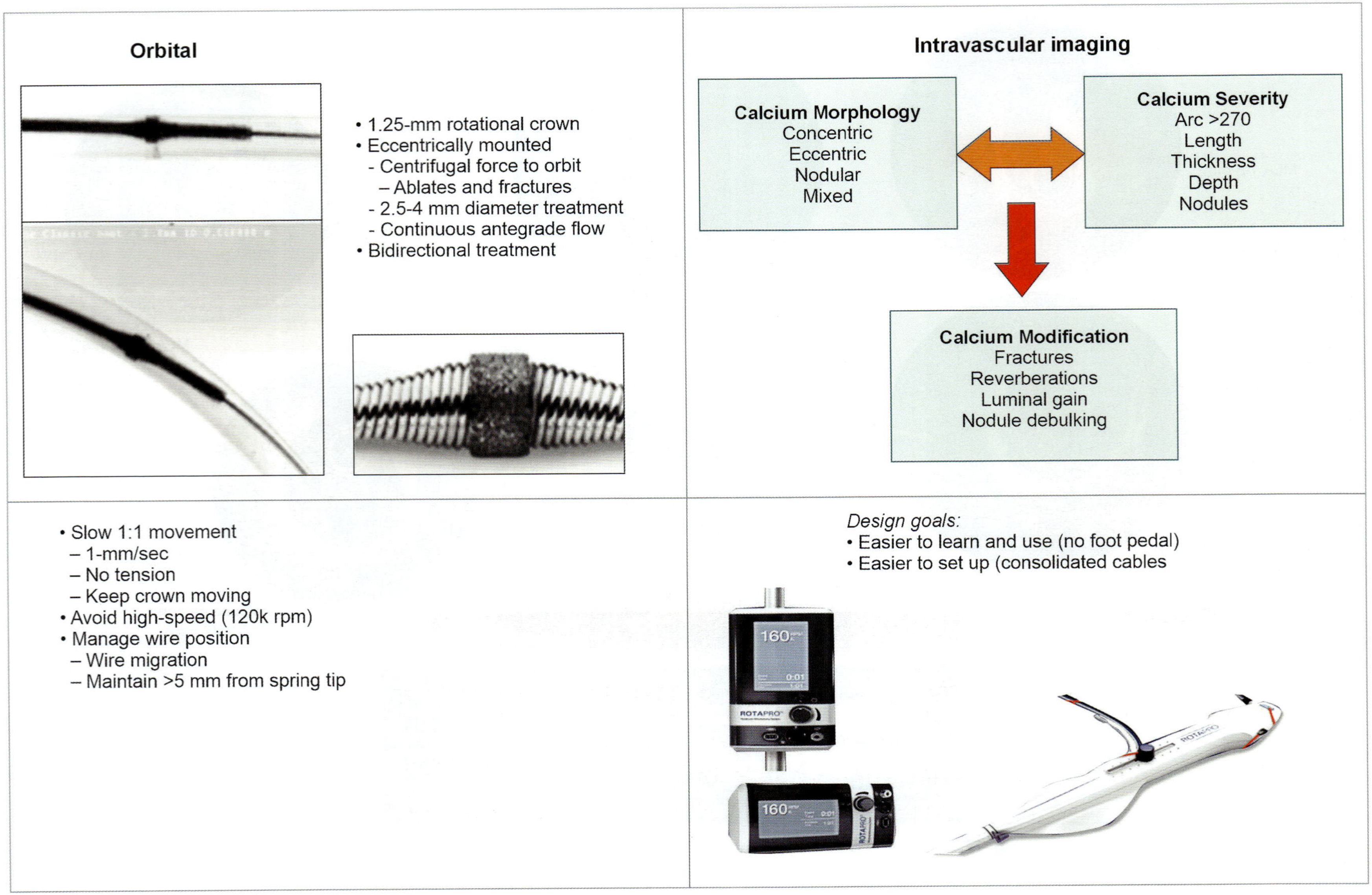

Fig. 18: Description of orbital atherectomy.

Recent edition of OCT with Ultreon software helps in the automatic detection of vessel size and quantification of calcium by using artificial intelligence.

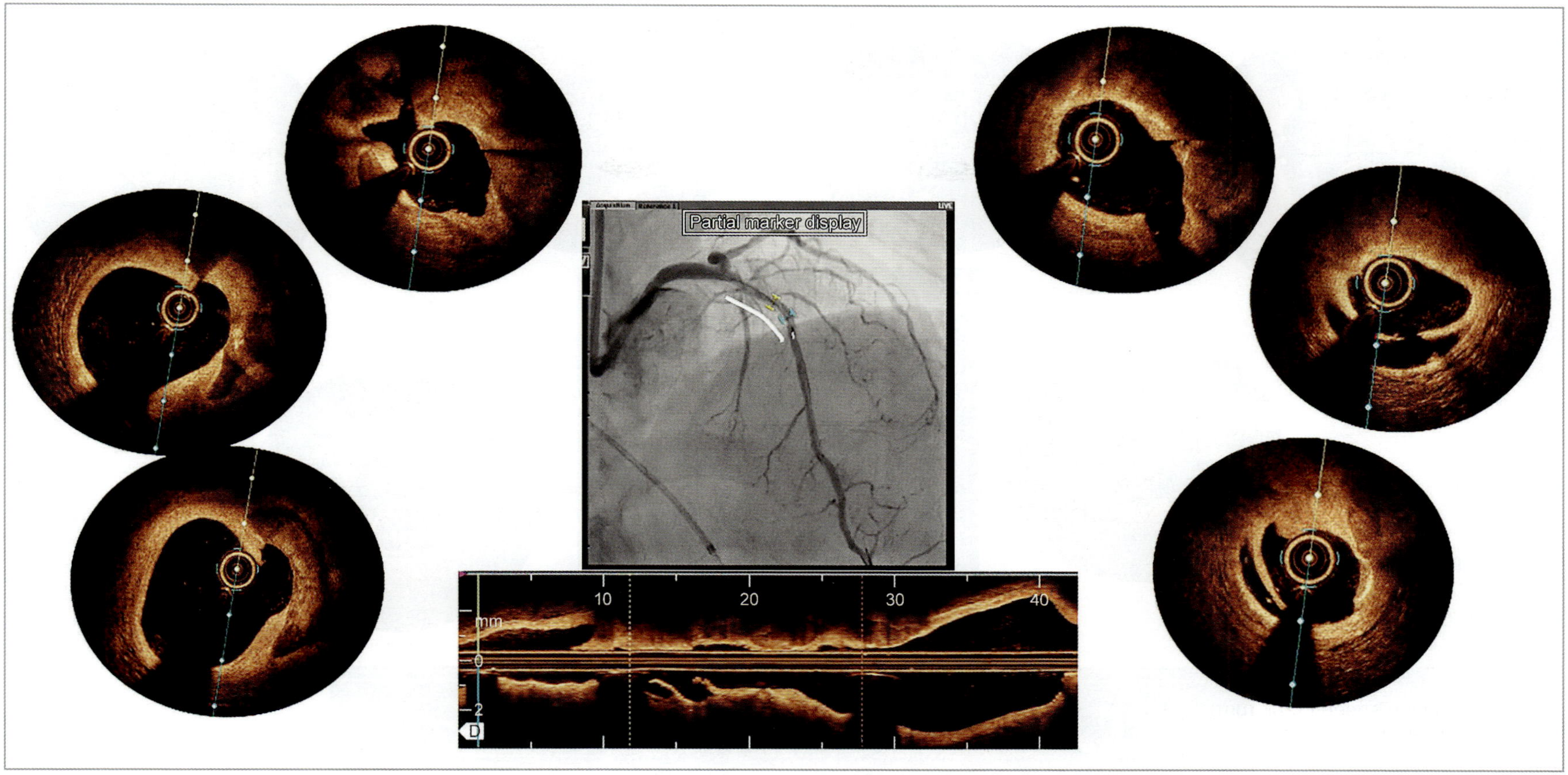

Fig. 19: Postorbital atherectomy showing increased luminal gain, calcium fractures and dissections.

Technical features of Rotablation (RA) and Orbital Atherectomy (OA)

RA	***OA***
Front cutting unidirectional burr	Diamond coated crown, bidirectional
Speed: 140,000–180,000 rpm, avoid deceleration >5,000 rpm	*Speed:* 80,000–1,20,000 rpm, larger ablative arc with higher speed
Burr movement with pecking motion/short ablative runs (<25 sec)	Continuous slow forward and backword crown movement

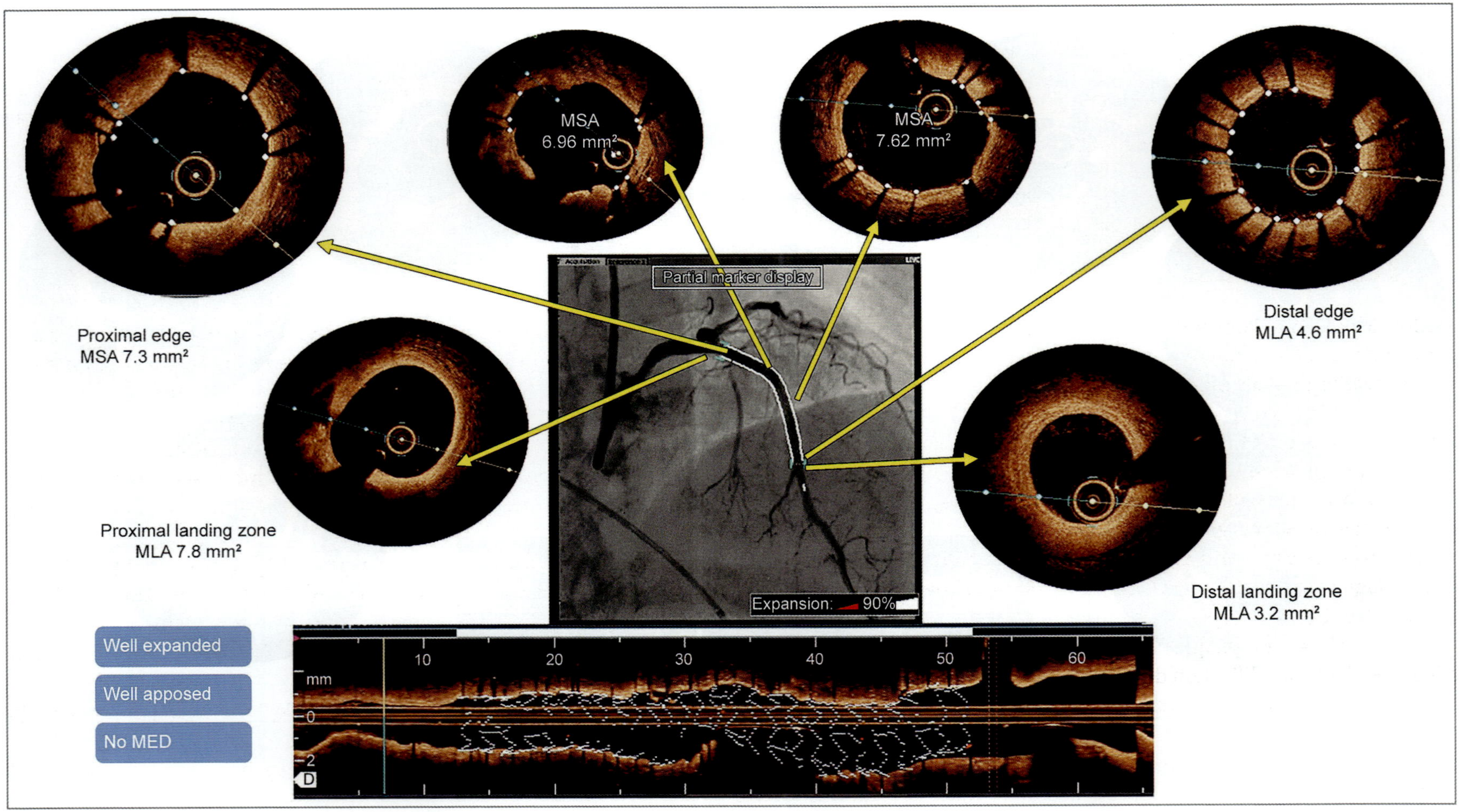

Fig. 20: Poststenting OCT showing expanded and apposed stent struts with no medial edge dissections.

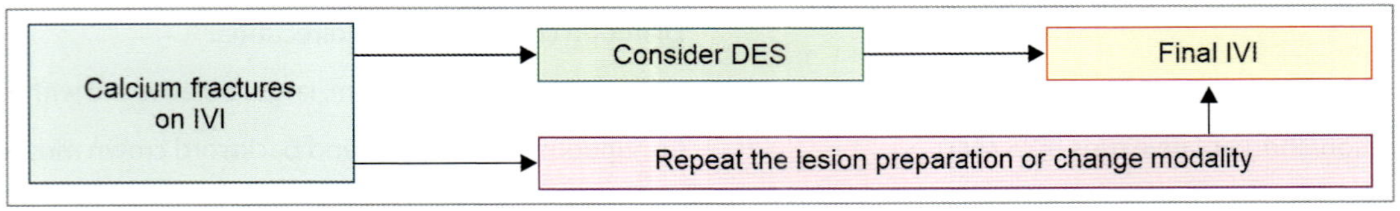

CASE 2

OCT + IVUS-guided IVL plaque modification of LM-LAD.

CLINICAL HISTORY

A 72-year-old male, known diabetic, presented with ACS, acute inferior + RVMI with complaints of giddiness for 5 days associated with sweating and hypotension. ECG—acute IWMI + RVMI, 2D echo—showed RWMA of RCA territory, mild LV dysfunction, EF—48%, O/I: Hb—14.7 g/dL, RBS—211 mg/dL, serum creatinine—0.64 mg/dL, eGFR—99 mL/min.

Coronary Angio revealed two-vessel disease with LAD—proximal 70–80%, distal 70% lesion, LCX—nondominant, normal; RCA—proximal to mid long segment 99% lesion. Planned for PTCA + stent to RCA and staged OCT/IVUS-guided PCI with stenting of LAD with IVL plaque modification.

RCA was engaged with JR 3.5–6 Fr guiding catheter, lesion was crossed with 0.014 × 190 cm″ Sion Blue Wire. Predilatation was carried out with 2.0 × 10 mm Tazuna balloon. Then, stenting of RCA was done with 2.5 × 48 mm Xience Xpedition, postdilatations were done with 2.5 × 12 mm NC Apollo balloon, final result was good with TIMI III flow.

LCA was engaged with EBU 3.5–7 Fr guiding catheter, LAD lesion was crossed with 0.014 × 190 cm″ BMW wire and LCX was wired with 0.014″ Runthrough wire. Prestenting OCT and IVUS runs showed severe calcific lesion with >270° circumferential calcium and total lesion length was 38 mm **(Figs. 21A to D)**.

IVL was chosen for plaque modification and total 80 pulses delivered using 3.0 × 12 mm IVL balloon. Post-IVL runs of OCT and IVUS analysis showed adequate plaque modification done **(Fig. 22)**.

Proximal LAD stenting was done with 3.0 × 38 mm Resolute Onyx stent, postdilatation was done with 3.0 × 15 mm NC Trek. Poststenting OCT and IVUS runs showed lipid rich and fibrocalcific plaque distal to the stent about 18 mm length **(Figs. 23A to C)**.

Which was covered with 2.25 × 18 mm Resolute Onyx Stent with poststent optimization. Poststenting OCT showed well expansion and apposition and no medial edge dissection. Final result was good with TIMI III flow **(Fig. 24)**.

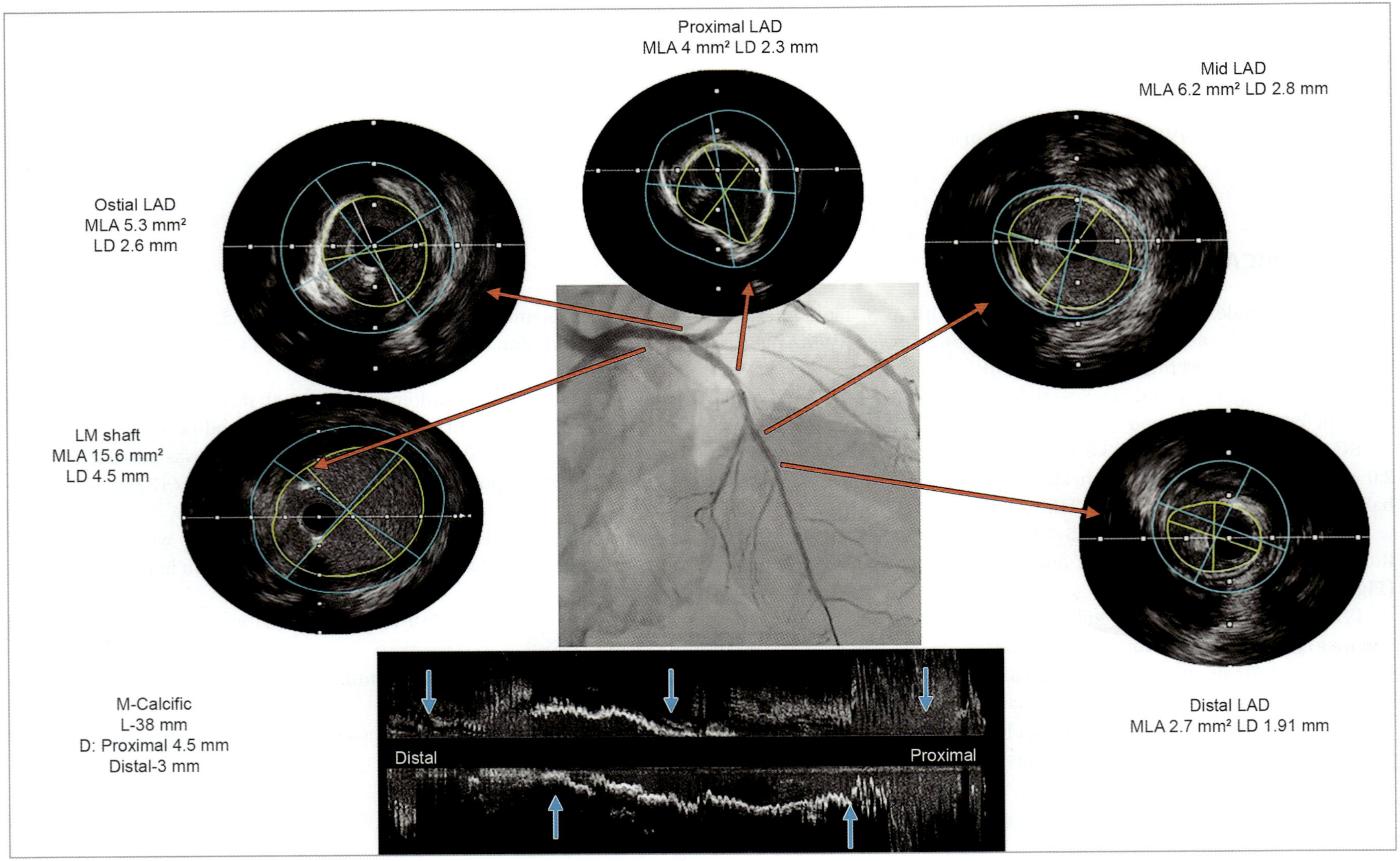
Proximal LAD
MLA 4 mm² LD 2.3 mm
Mid LAD
MLA 6.2 mm² LD 2.8 mm
Ostial LAD
MLA 5.3 mm²
LD 2.6 mm
LM shaft
MLA 15.6 mm²
LD 4.5 mm
M-Calcific
L-38 mm
D: Proximal 4.5 mm
Distal-3 mm
Distal
Proximal
Distal LAD
MLA 2.7 mm² LD 1.91 mm

Fig. 21A

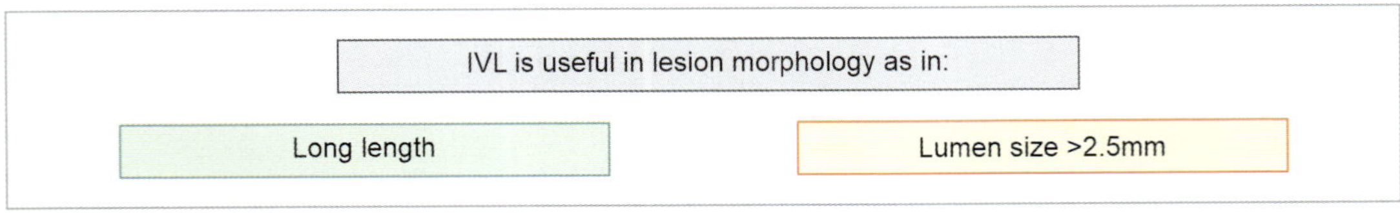
IVL is useful in lesion morphology as in:
Long length
Lumen size >2.5mm

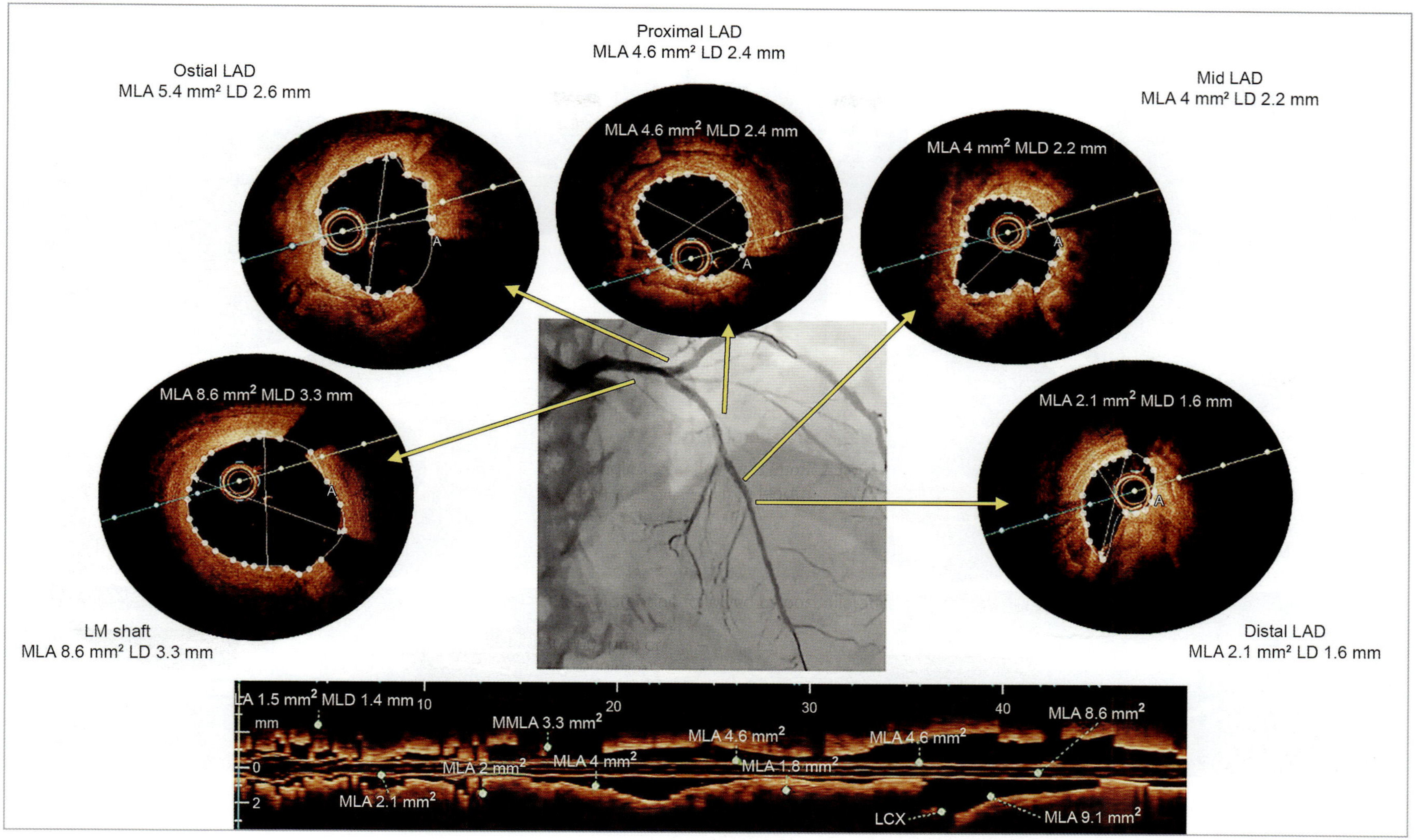

Fig. 21B

IVL is useful in lesion morphology as in:

Tortuosity

Stent failure

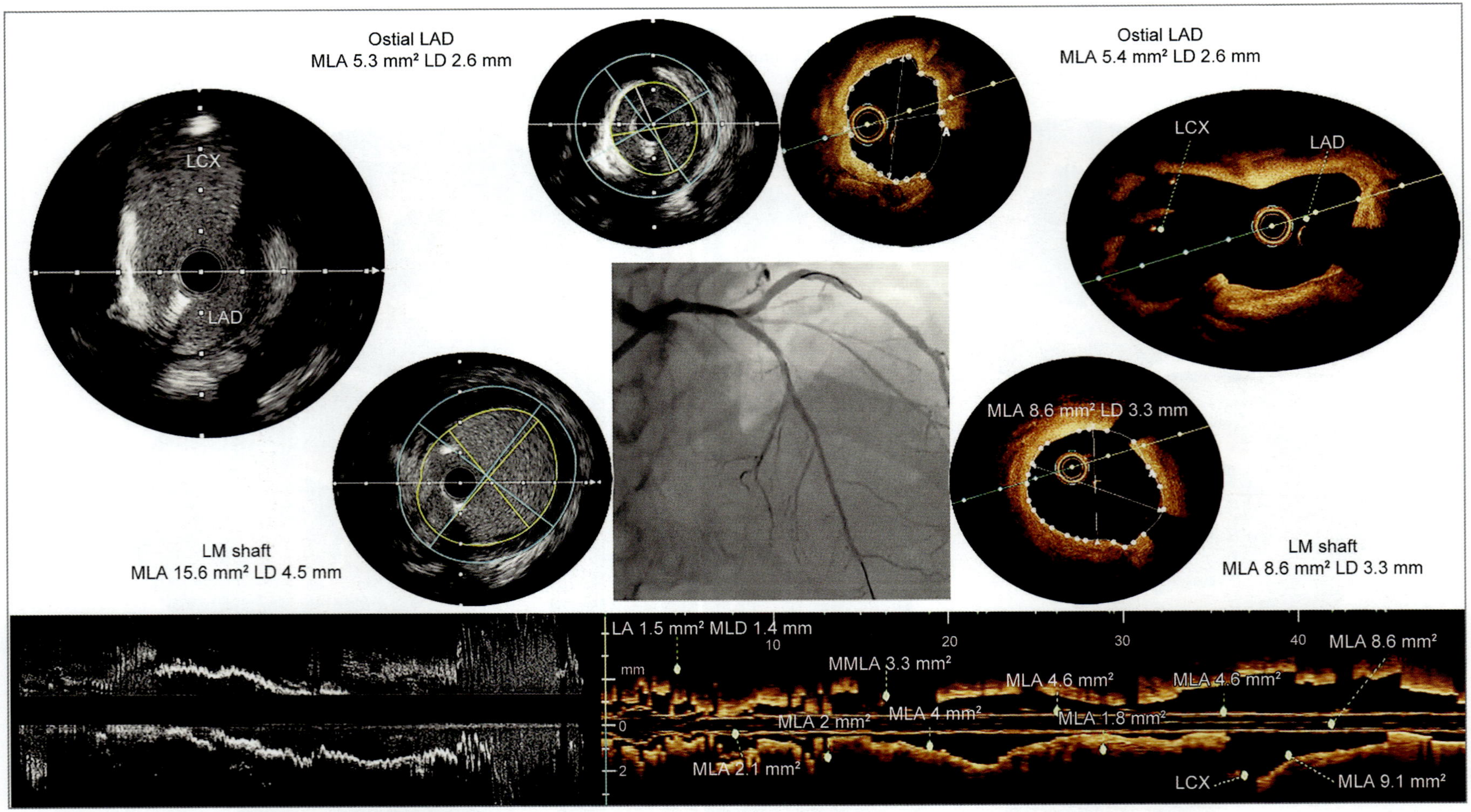

Fig. 21C

IVL is useful in lesion location at:

- Left main
- Ostial RCA
- CTO
- SVG

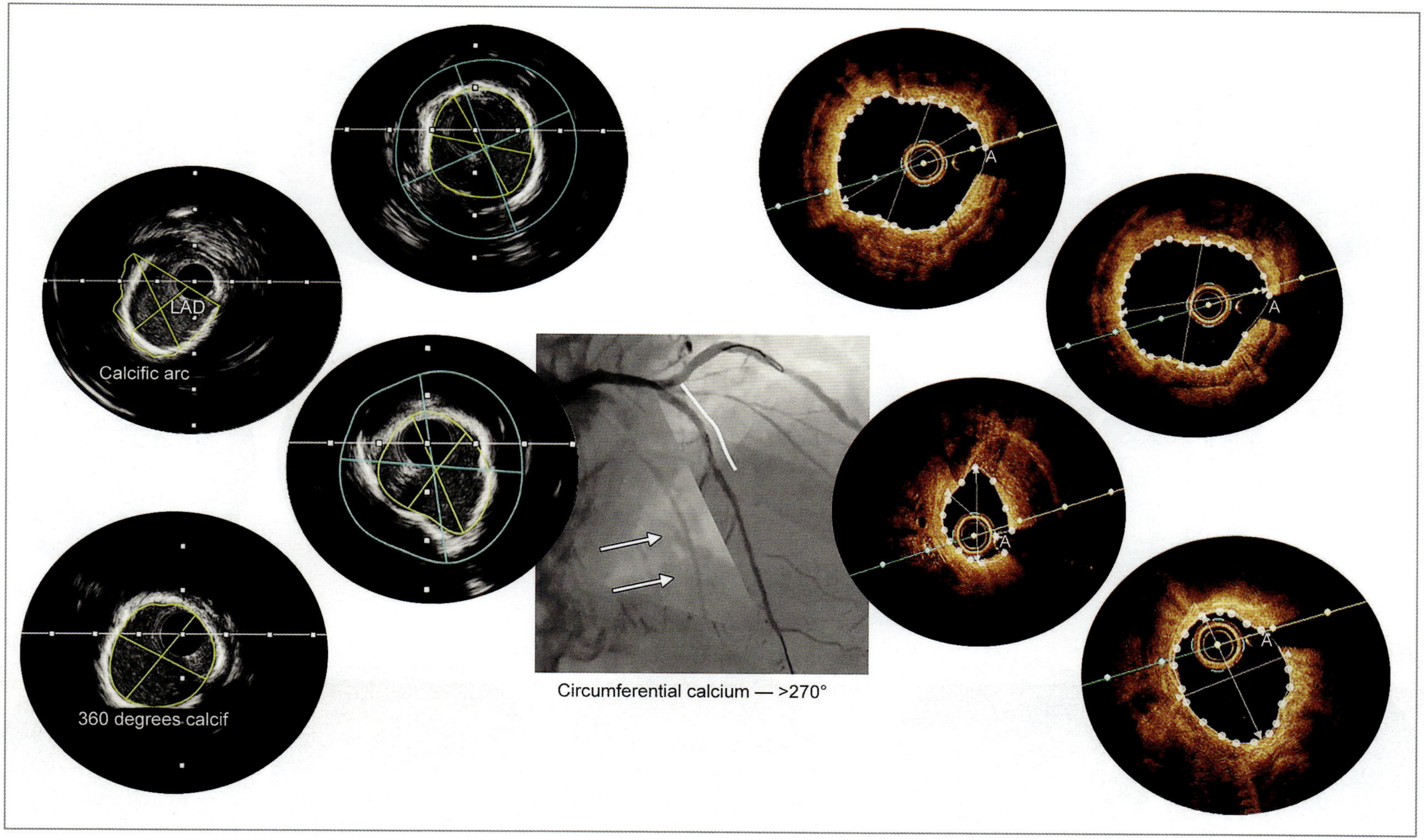

Fig. 21D

Figs. 21A to D: (A) Presenting IVUS assessment for plaque morphology; (B) Presenting OCT assessment for plaque morphology; (C) Presenting IVUS and OCT assessment; (D) IVUS and OCT showing circumferential calcium.

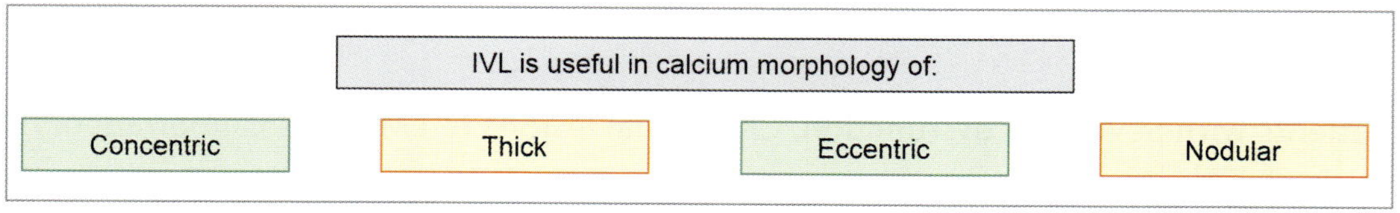

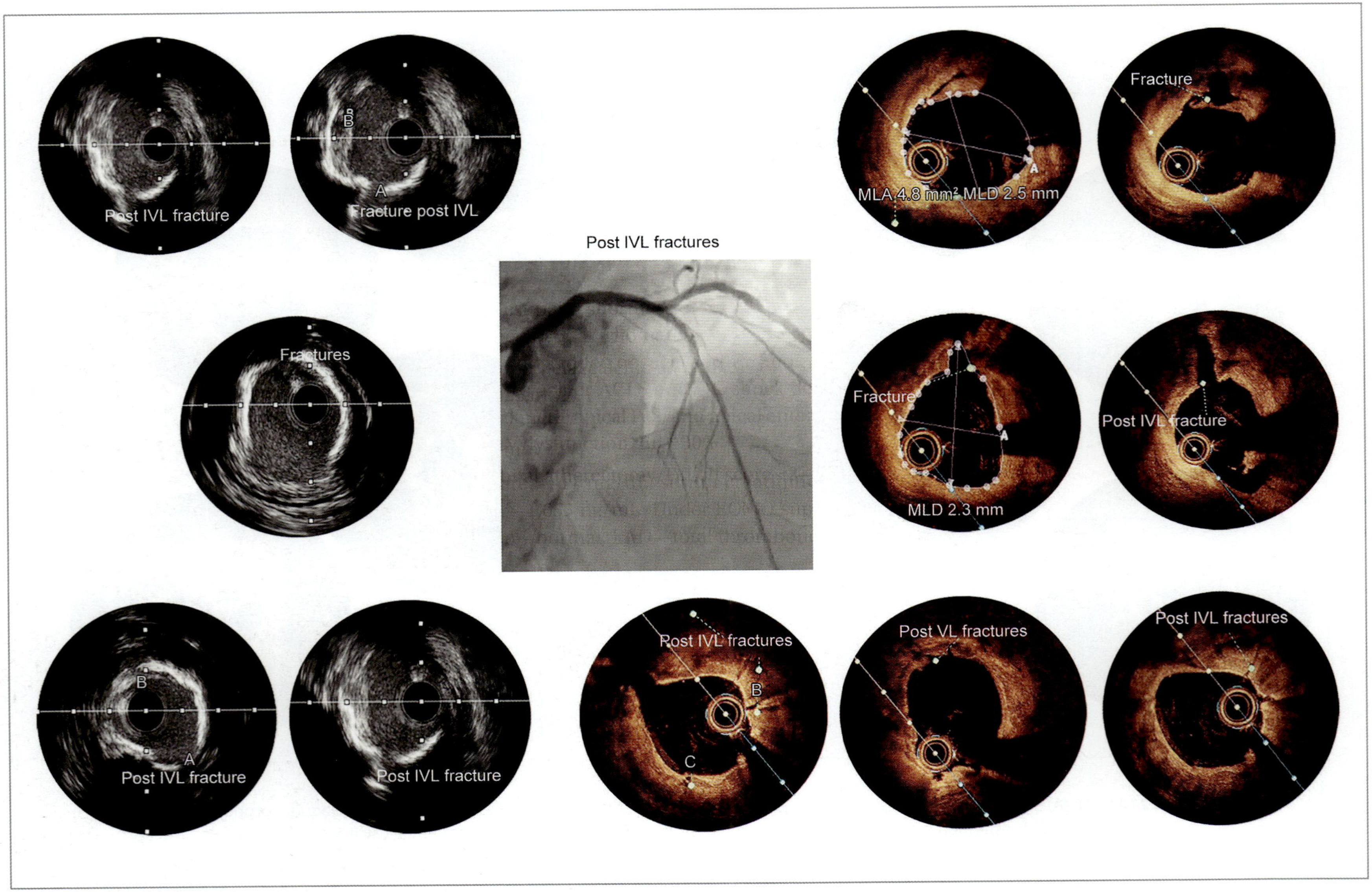

Fig. 22: Postplaque modification IVUS and OCT showing fractures.

IVUS scores over OCT in patients with Severe LV dysfunction, CKD, ostial lesions of LM, large caliber/aneurysmal vessels and unstable hemodynamic status.

Ostial LM PCI

For ostial LM lesions, the specific technique to align the proximal edge of the stent with the LM ostium (ideally 1–2 mm into the aorta) is important to avoid lesion miss.

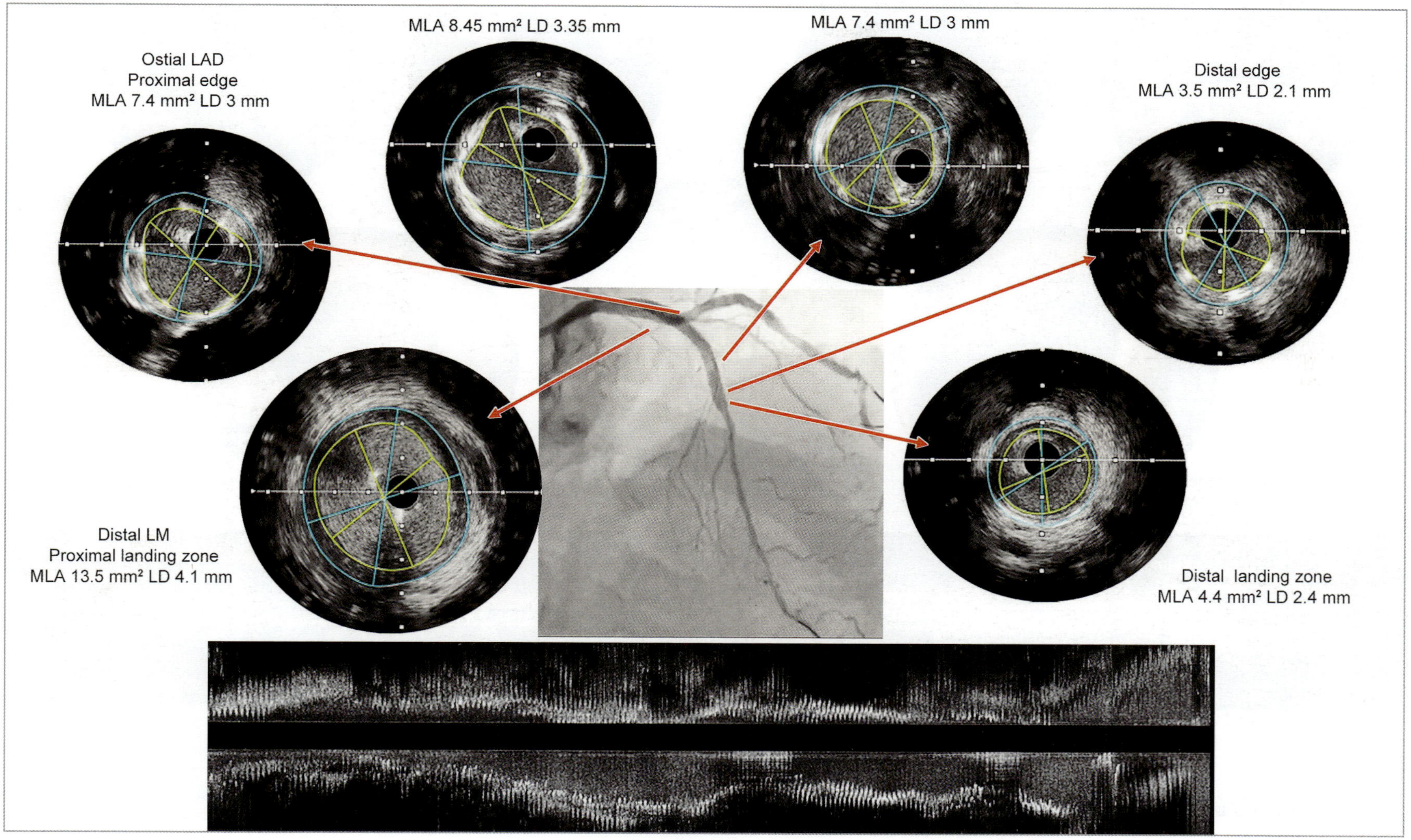

Fig. 23A

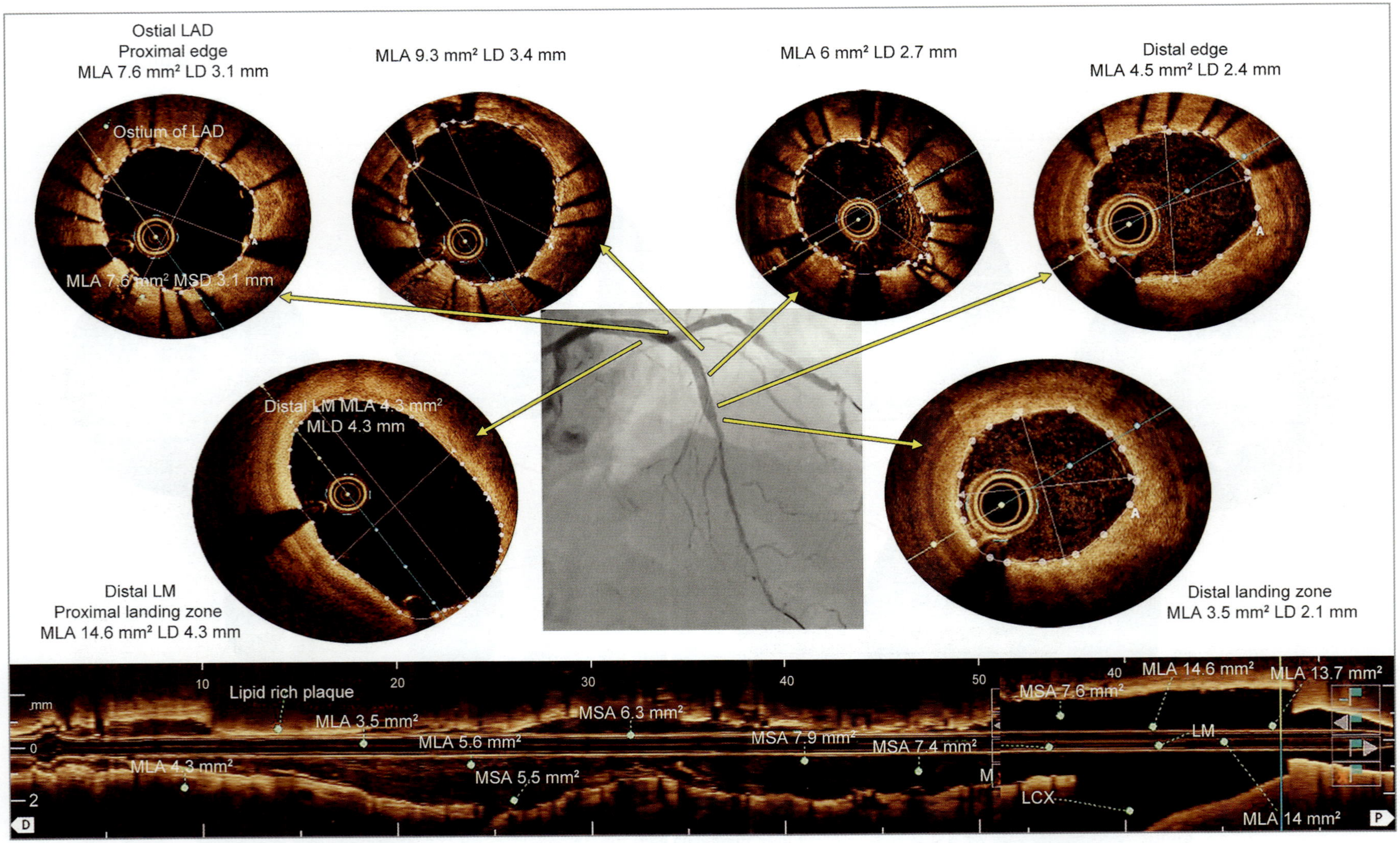

Fig. 23B

When assessing an ostial LMCA or RCA (or SVG) lesion – it is necessary to disengage the guiding catheter.

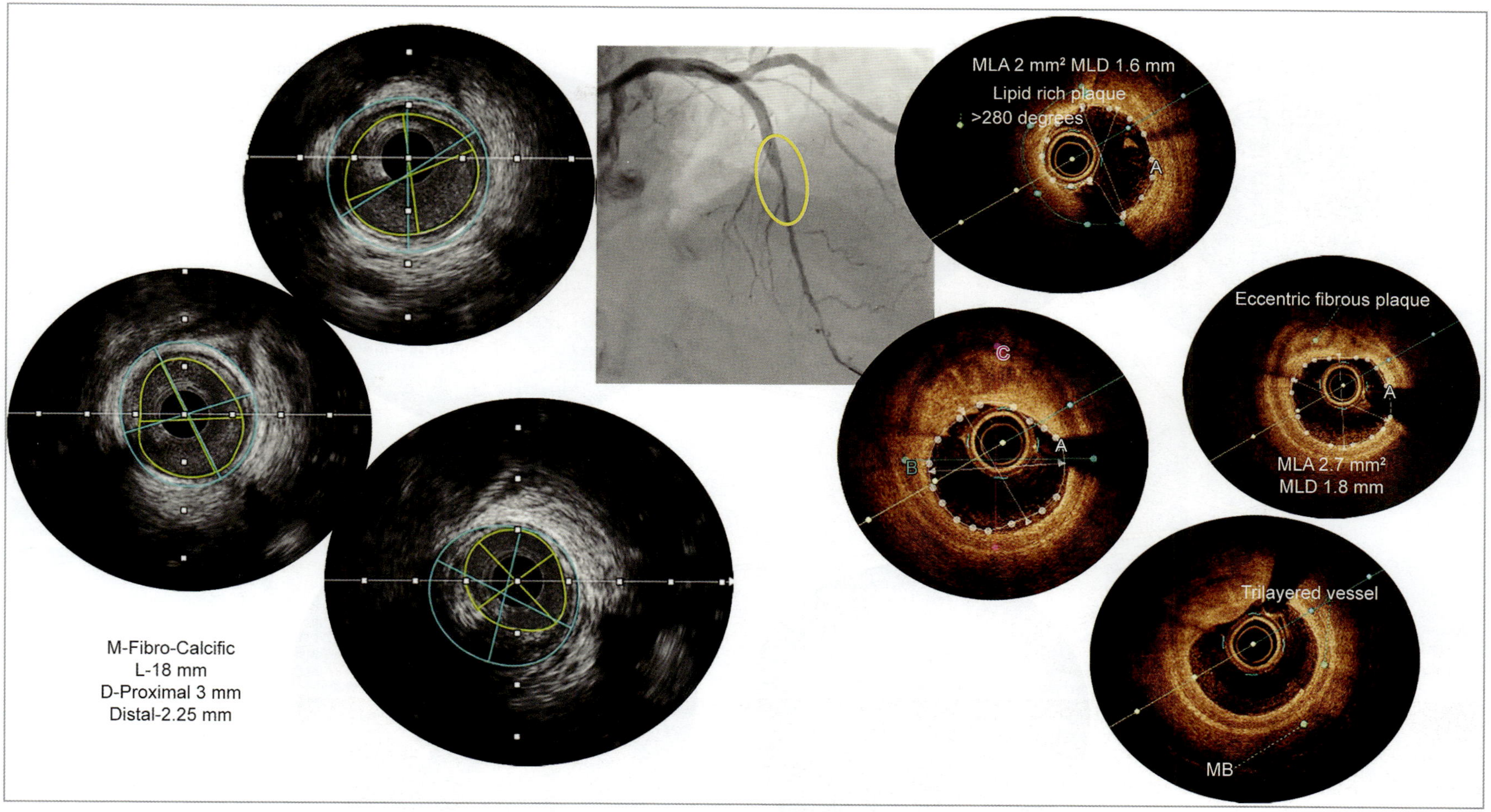

Fig. 23C

Figs. 23A to C: (A) Post-LM-proximal LAD stenting IVUS assessment for MAX; (B) Post-LM-proximal LAD stenting OCT assessment for MAX; (C) Poststenting OCT and IVUS runs showed lipid rich and fibrocalcific plaque distal to the stent about 18 mm length.

Sheath/Guide Compatibility

- Sheaths are measured inner diameter
- Catheters are measured outer diameter
- 8 fr guide catheter is compatible with an 8 fr sheath.
  Generally there us a 2 fr size difference between the inner diameter and outer diameter of both sheaths and guiding catheters.

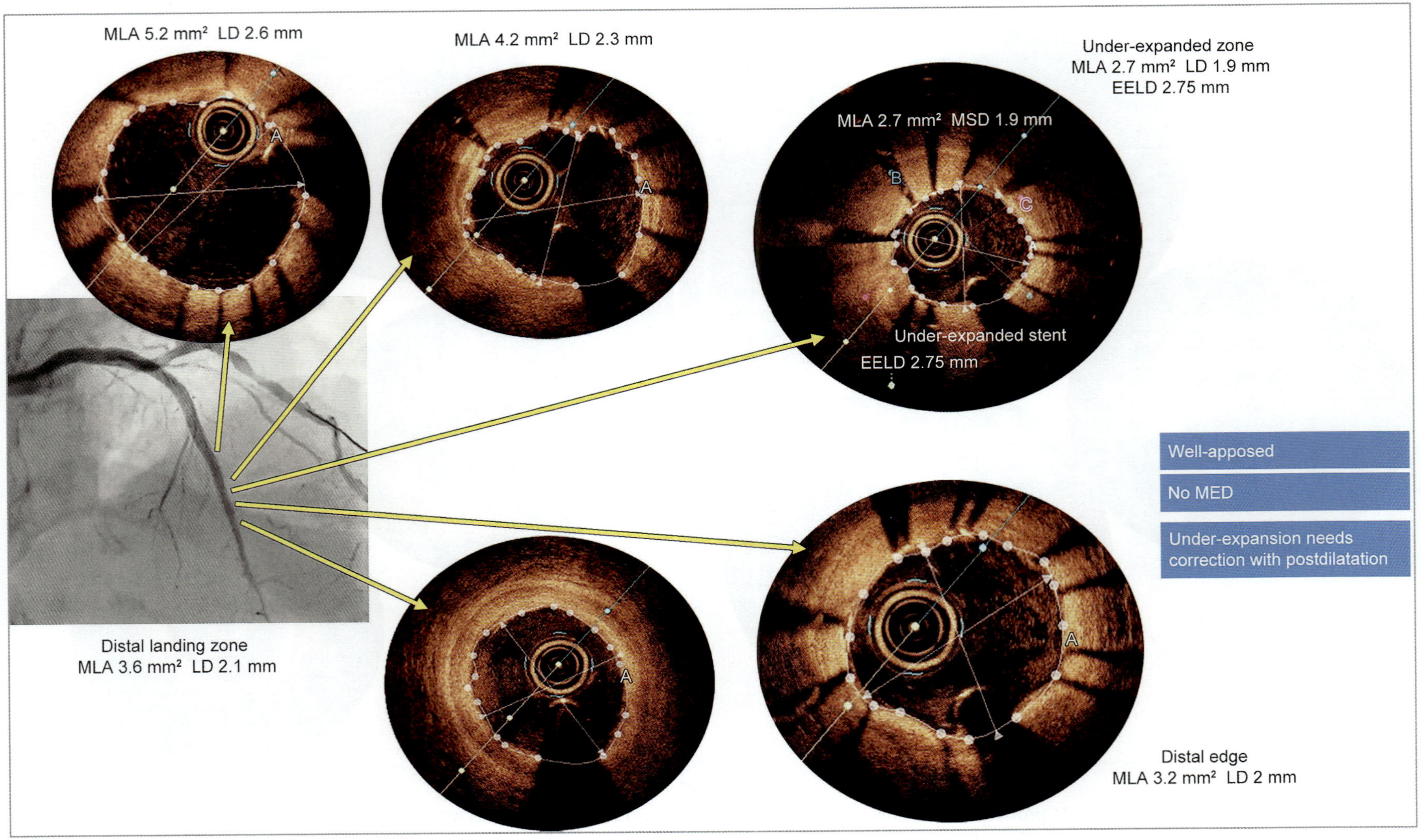

Fig. 24: Postdistal LAD stenting OCT showing well apposed and expanded stent struts.

CASE 3

OCT-guided PCI of LMCA + triple vessel disease—plaque modification using IVL.

CLINICAL HISTORY

A 72-year-old, known DM, HTN, old CVA—right hemiparesis recovered (2018), presented with complaints of giddiness and fall at 8:30 AM yesterday. Height—161 cm, weight—68 kg. CAD: ACS-NSTEMI. ECG showed Q in III, aVF, poor R wave progression, 2D echo showed no RWMA, normal LV function with EF—58% **(Fig. 25)**, CAG done outside (13/09/2021) showed LM + TVD, LMCA—ostial mild disease, followed by distal 60%, LAD—calcific vessel, proximal diffuse disease with maximum of 90% stenosis at D1, D1—ostial 80% stenosis, LCX—mild disease, RCA—50–60% stenosis, PDA—proximal 70% stenosis.

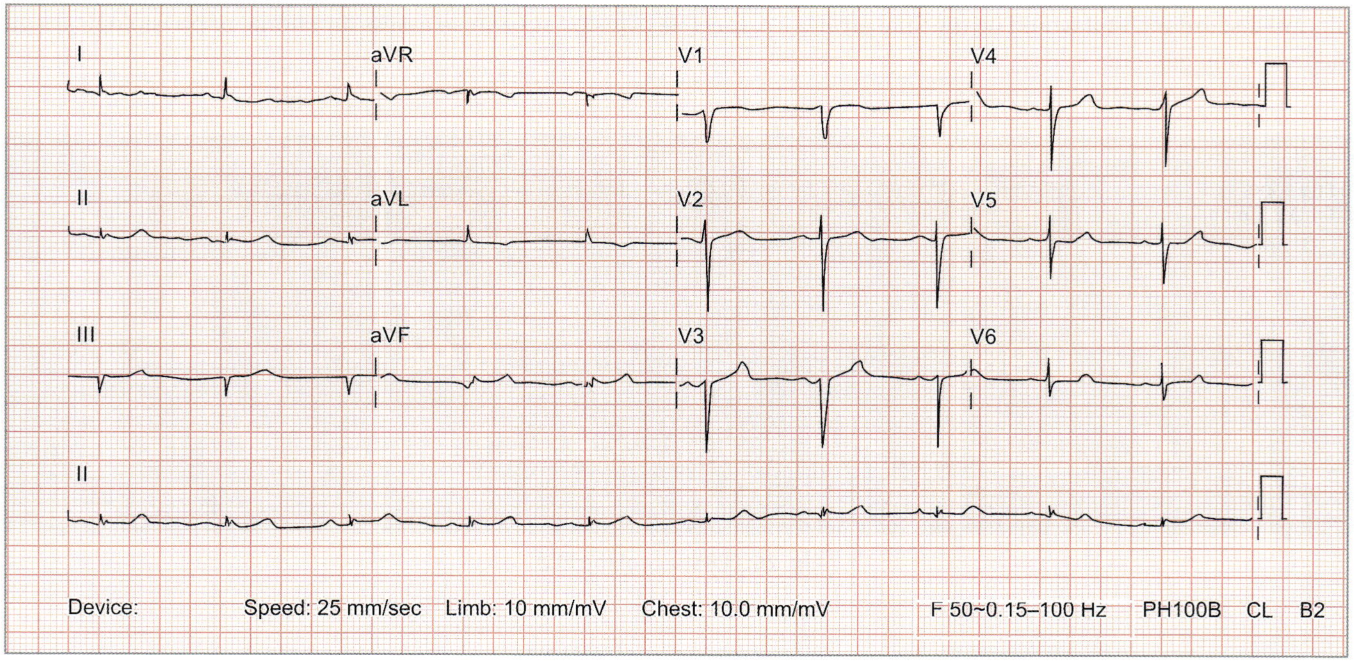

Fig. 25: Electro cardiogram showing Q waves in III, aVF, poor R wave progression.

Investigations: Hb—15.5 g/dL, RBS—212 → 188 mg/dL, serum creatinine—1.18 → 0.84 mg/dL, GFR—87 mL/min, Trop T—18.66 ng/L (pg/mL). SYNTAX score—38, EURO score II—1.29%.

FFR Study of the RCA

RCA engaged with JR 3.5-6 Fr, guiding catheter, RCA lesion crossed with PressureWire (0.014′ PressureWire "CERTUS"), FFR performed after injection NTG followed by intracoronary administration of injection adenosine @140 μg/kg/min **(Fig. 26)**.

LMCA engaged with EBU 3.5-6 Fr guiding catheter, LAD lesion crossed with 0.014″ BMW wire. D1 crossed with Runthrough wire. LCX crossed with 0.014 Sion Blue Wire. LAD predilatation done with 2.5 × 15 mm Tazuna balloon. Presenting OCT was done which showed fibrocalcific lesion 270° **(Figs. 27A and B)**.

IVL using GuideLiner support with 3.0 × 12 mm IVL × 8 cycles from mid LAD to LMCA **(Fig. 28)**.

Proximal to mid LAD 2.5 × 28 mm Xience Xpedition stent deployed at 12 atm. Postdilatation done with 3.0 × 15 mm NC balloon at 16 atm. Distal LAD predilatation done with 3.0 × 15 mm balloon at 4–6 atm. DEB done to distal LAD with 2.25 × 25 mm MagicTouch balloon at 6 atm twice for 1 minute each. OCT showed well-expanded stent with no edge dissection **(Fig. 29)**.

LMCA-LAD stenting done with 3.5 × 28 mm Xience Xpedition stent deployed at 16 atm. Ostial flaring done with stent balloon at 16 atm. POT done to LMCA with 4.5 × 12 mm NC balloon at 12 atm. LAD postdilatation done with 3.0 × 15 mm NC balloon at 12 atm. Poststenting OCT was done which showed well-expanded stent struts with no edge dissection. The final result was good with TIMI III flow with no complications **(Fig. 30)**.

As per the consensus statement of the SCAI, instead of relying solely on angiographic criteria of severity when there is no stress test present, or the stress test/anatomy results are discordant, FFR would be the final arbiter irrespective of lesion severity to assess functional or physiological significance of lesion to decide PCI vs medical management.

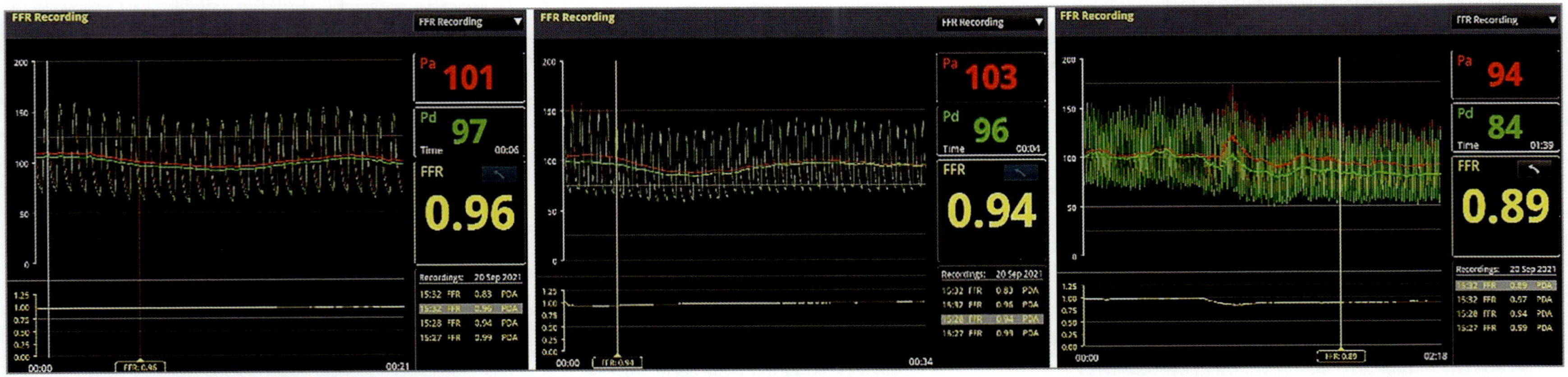

Fig. 26: FFR study of the RCA.

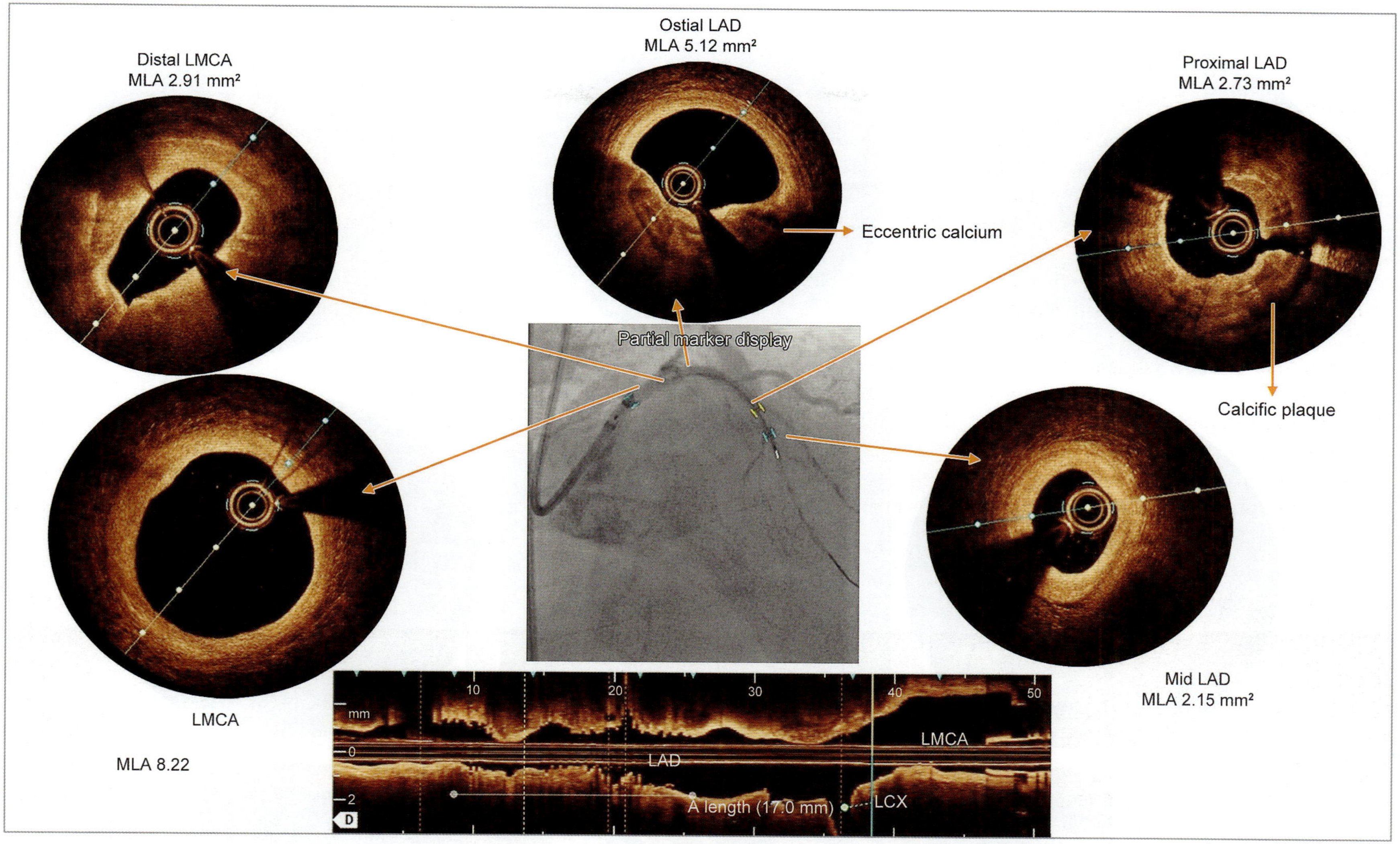
Ostial LAD
MLA 5.12 mm²
Distal LMCA
MLA 2.91 mm²
Proximal LAD
MLA 2.73 mm²
Eccentric calcium
Partial marker display
Calcific plaque
LMCA
MLA 8.22
Mid LAD
MLA 2.15 mm²
mm
10
20
30
40
50
0
2
LMCA
LAD
A length (17.0 mm)
LCX
D

Fig. 27A

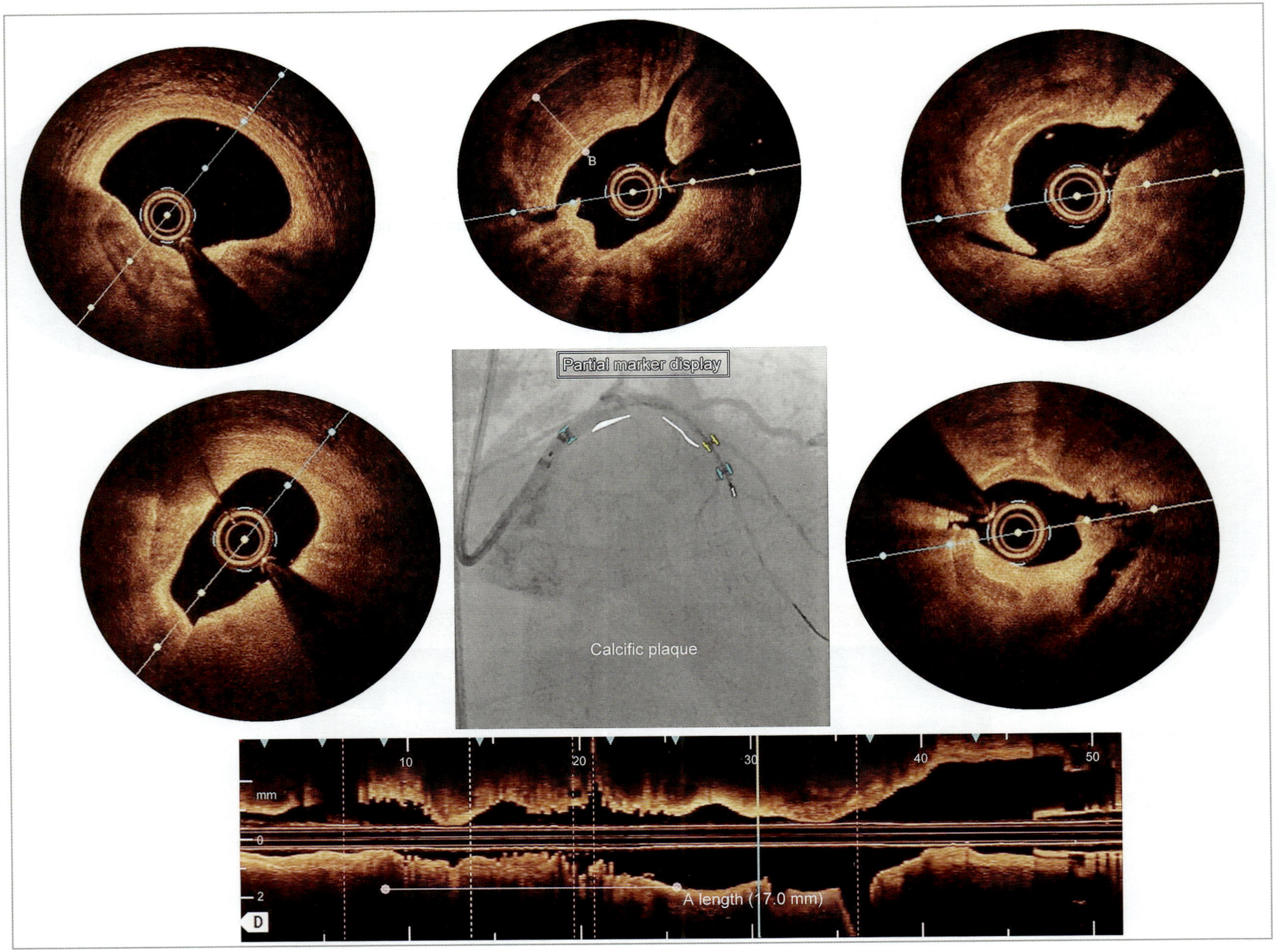

Fig. 27B

Figs. 27A and B: (A) Presenting OCT assessment for device selection; (B) Presenting OCT showing severe calcific plaque.

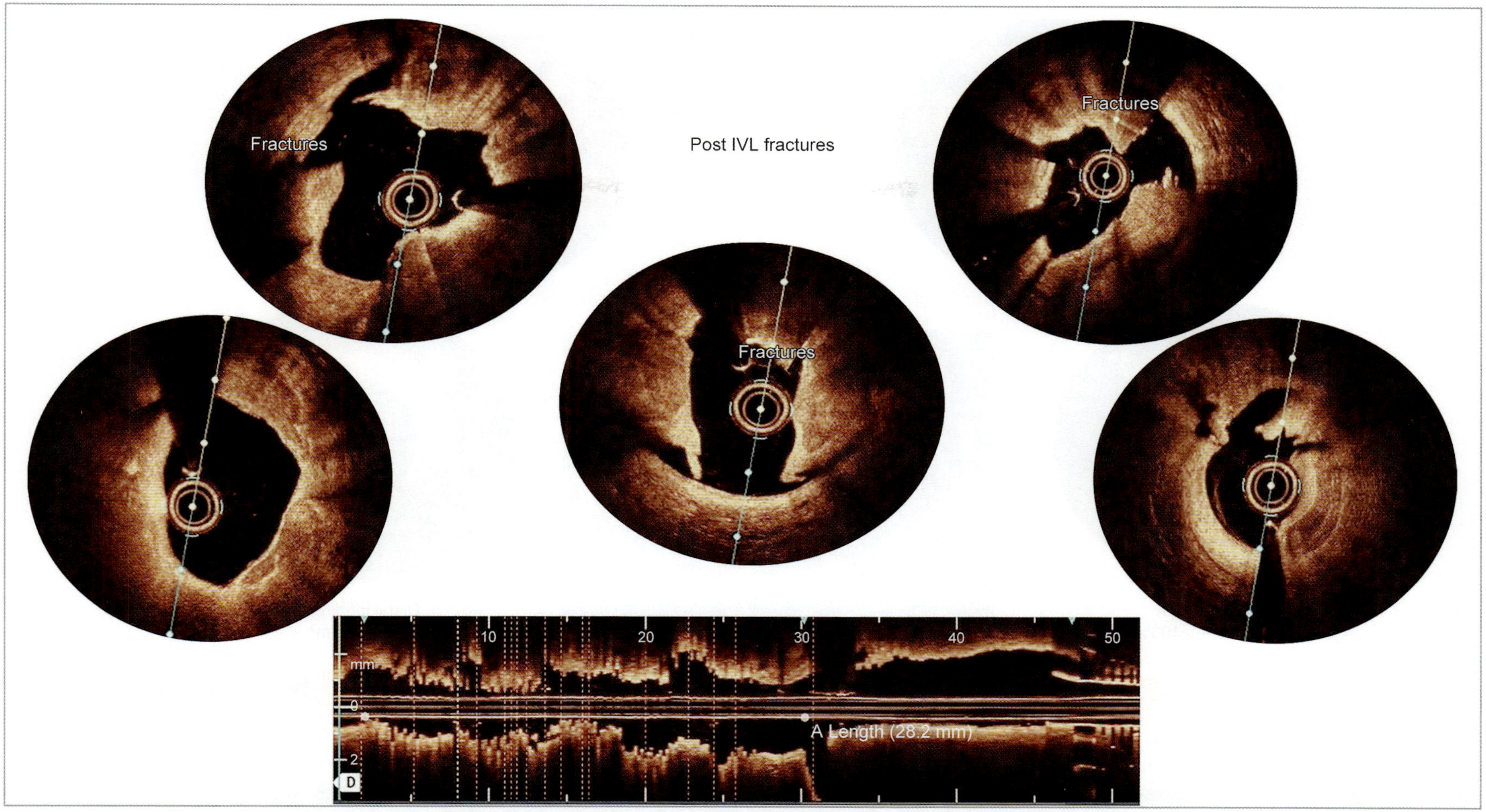

Fig. 28: Postplaque modification OCT assessment showing fractures.

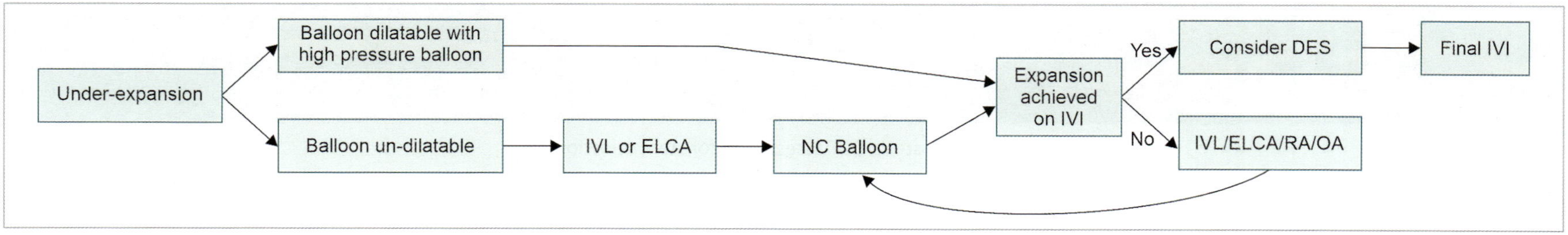

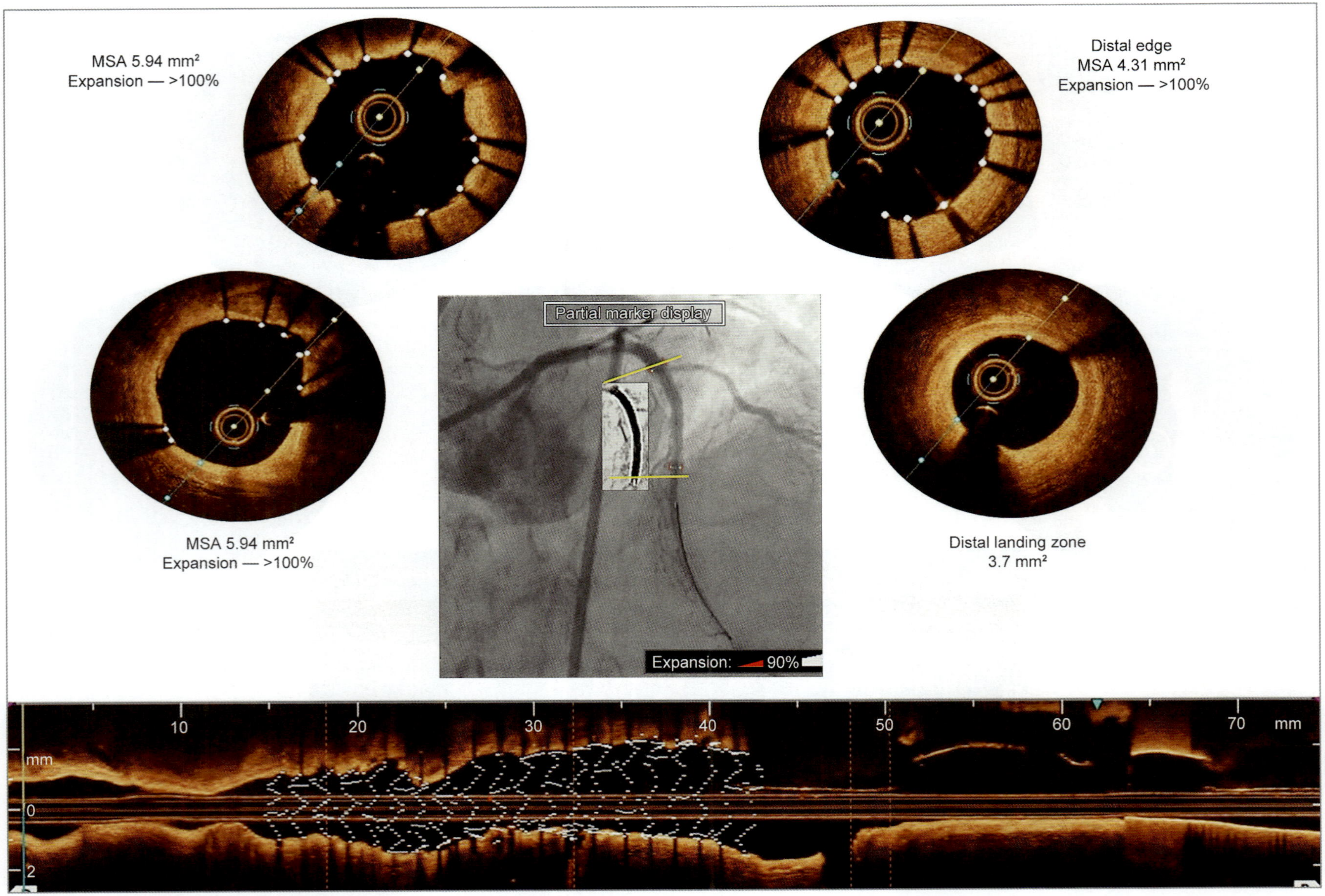

Fig. 29: Post-IVL OCT assessment for stent selection.

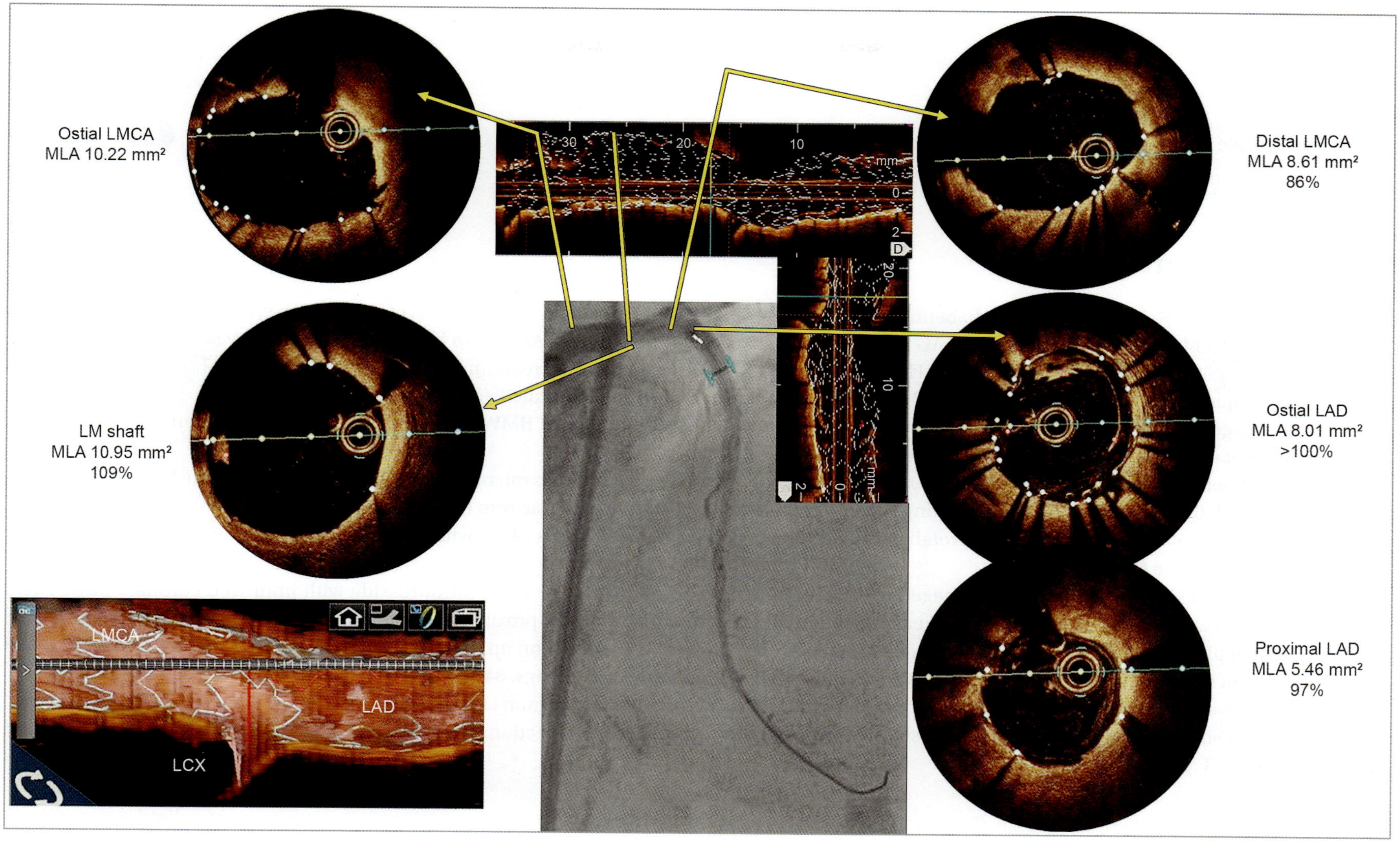

Fig. 30: Poststenting LM-LAD and LCX OCT showing well expanded and apposed stent struts.

CASE 4

Oct guided plaque modification with ROTA-Tripsy PCI with stenting of severe calcified LAD.

CLINICAL HISTORY

A 67-year-old male, known hypertensive and diabetic, presented with complaints of chest pain and shortness of breath on exertion, CAD—evolved AWMI, 2D echo showed mild LV dysfunction, EF: 48%, CAG was done, and failed attempt of PCI of LAD due to balloon uncrossable severely calcific LAD lesion in another tertiary care hospital on 04.08.2022, O/I: Hb—13.5 g/dL, RBS—225 mg/dL, serum creatinine—0.89 mg/dL, eGFR—96 mL/min. Procedure was planned with plaque modification using ROTA and OCT-guided PCI with stenting of severely calcified LAD **(Fig. 31)**.

LCA was engaged with EBU 3.5–7 Fr guiding catheter, LAD lesion was crossed with 0.014″ BMW wire, and tried to cross the lesion with 2.0 × 10 mm Ryurei balloon but could not cross even with multiple negotiations.

In view of balloon uncrossable lesion, RotaWire exchanged with BMW by keeping Finecross microcatheter at the tightest site of the lesion. Rotablation was carried out with 6 runs followed by final polishing runs using 1.5 mm ROTA burr with 1.6 lac rpm **(Figs. 32A to C)**.

Due to inadequate plaque modification with rotablation, additional plaque modification was done with 3.0 × 12 mm IVL balloon, and delivered 8 cycles of 10 pulses per each cycle **(Figs. 33A to C)**.

Patient developed slow flow which was managed with intracoronary injection NTG, injection nitroprusside with improved coronary flow. Then, distal LAD stenting was done with 2.75 × 33 mm Xience Alpine stent deployed at 12 atm and proximal LAD stenting was done with 3.5 × 48 mm Xience Xpedition stent deployed at 12 atm. Postdilatations were done with 3.0 × 12 mm NC Trek balloon up to 16 atm. Poststenting OCT was done which showed underexpansion of stent, which was optimized with 3.5 × 15 mm NC Trek balloon at 12 atm **(Figs. 34A to D)**.

Post-OCT showing underexpansion, which was corrected with postdilatation with 3.0 × 15 mm OPN NC balloon at 35–40 atm.

Final OCT run showed well expanded and apposed stent struts without medial edge dissection. The final result was good with TIMI III flow without any complications **(Fig. 35)**.

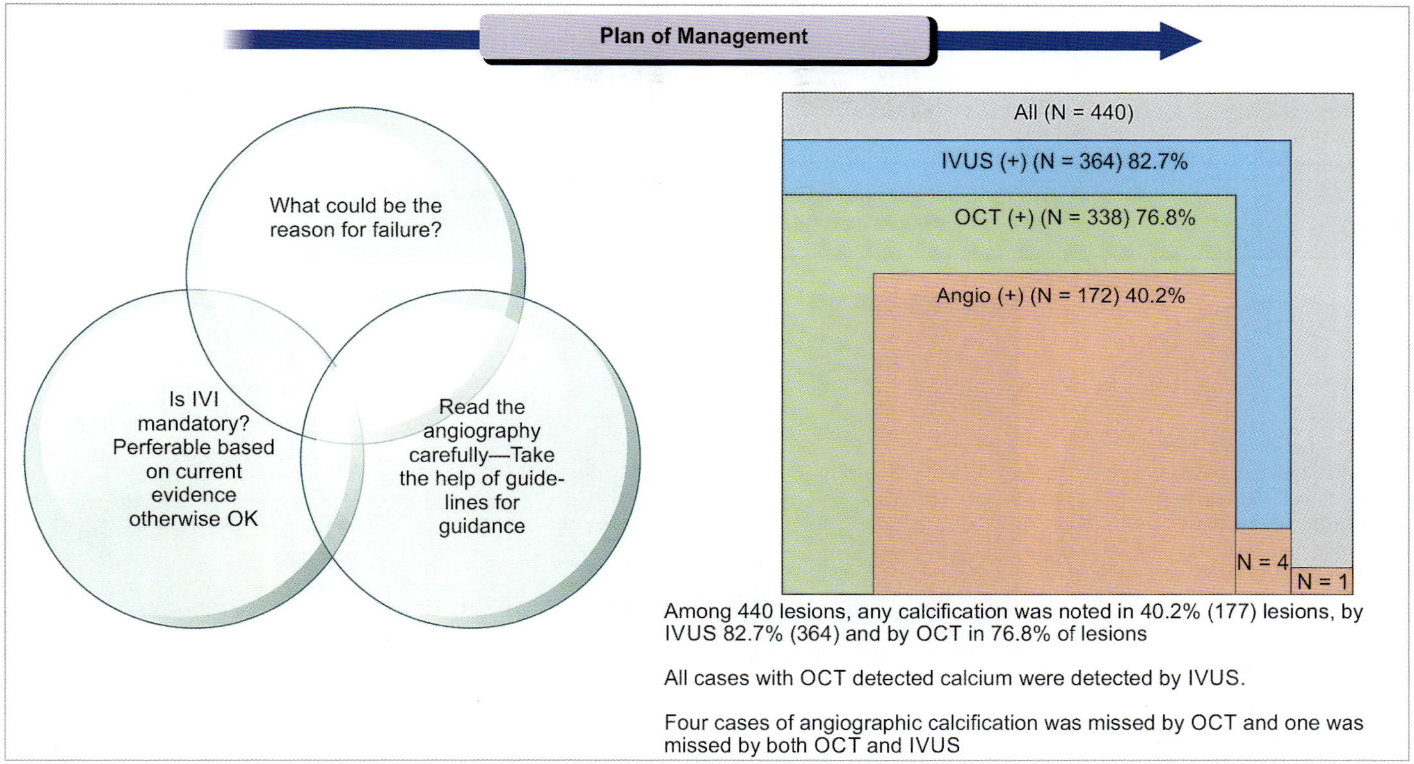

Fig. 31: Plan of management.

Recommendations for use of intravascular imaging.		
COR	***LOE***	***Recommendations***
2a	B-R	In patients undergoing coronary stent implantation, IVUS can be useful for procedural guidance, particularly in cases of LM or complex coronary artery stenting, to reduce ischemic events
2a	B-R	In patients undergoing coronary stent implantation. OCT is reasonable alternative to IVUS for procedural guidance, except in ostial LM disease

Lawton JS, Tamis-Holland JE, Bangalore S, Bates ER, Beckie TM, Bischoff JM, Bittl JA, Cohen MG, DiMaio JM, Don CW, Fremes SE. 2021 ACC/AHA/SCAI guideline for coronary artery revascularization: executive summary: a report of the American College of Cardiology/American Heart Association Joint Committee on Clinical Practice Guidelines. Circulation. 2022 Jan 18;145(3):e4-17.

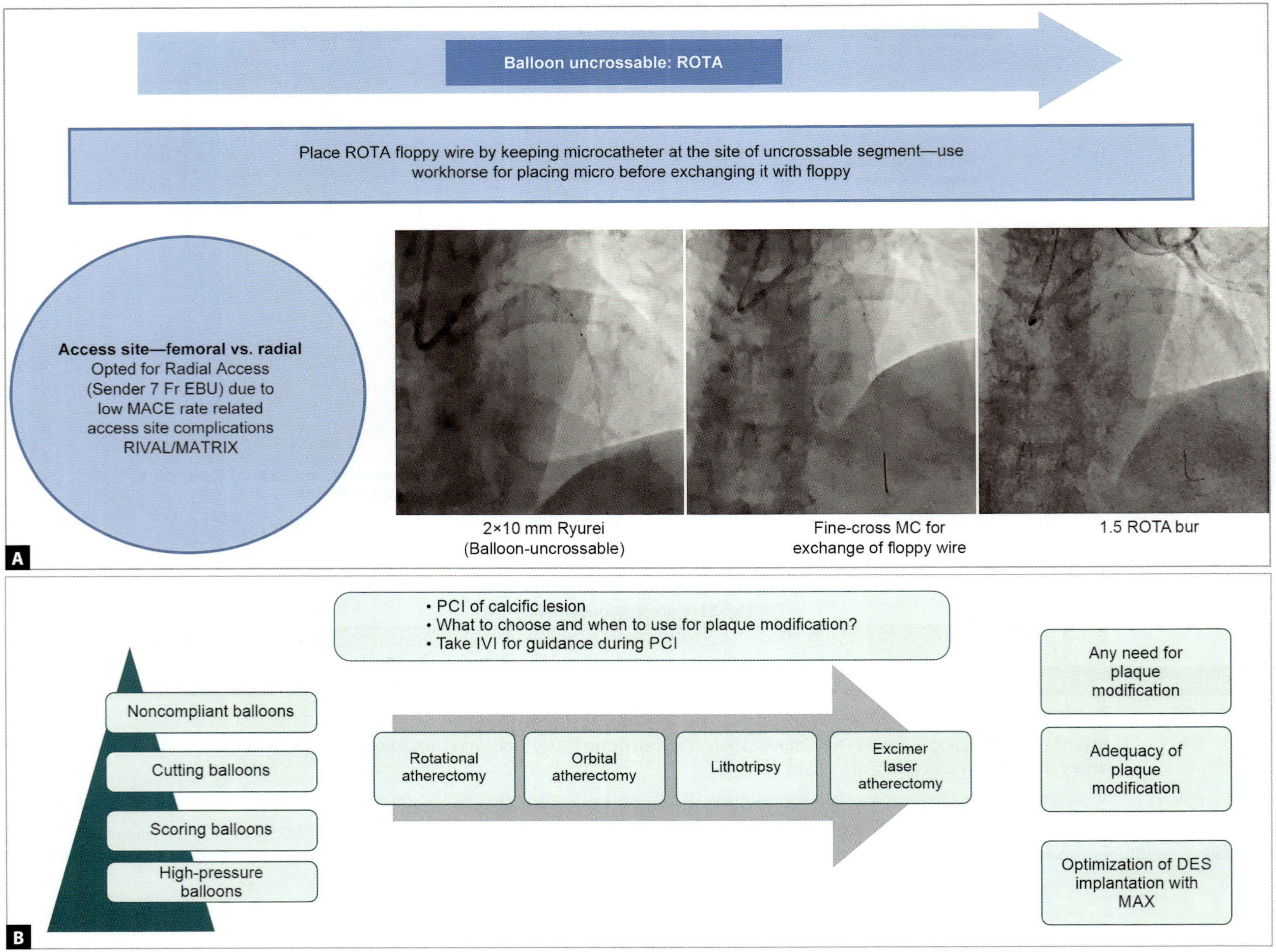

Figs. 32A and B

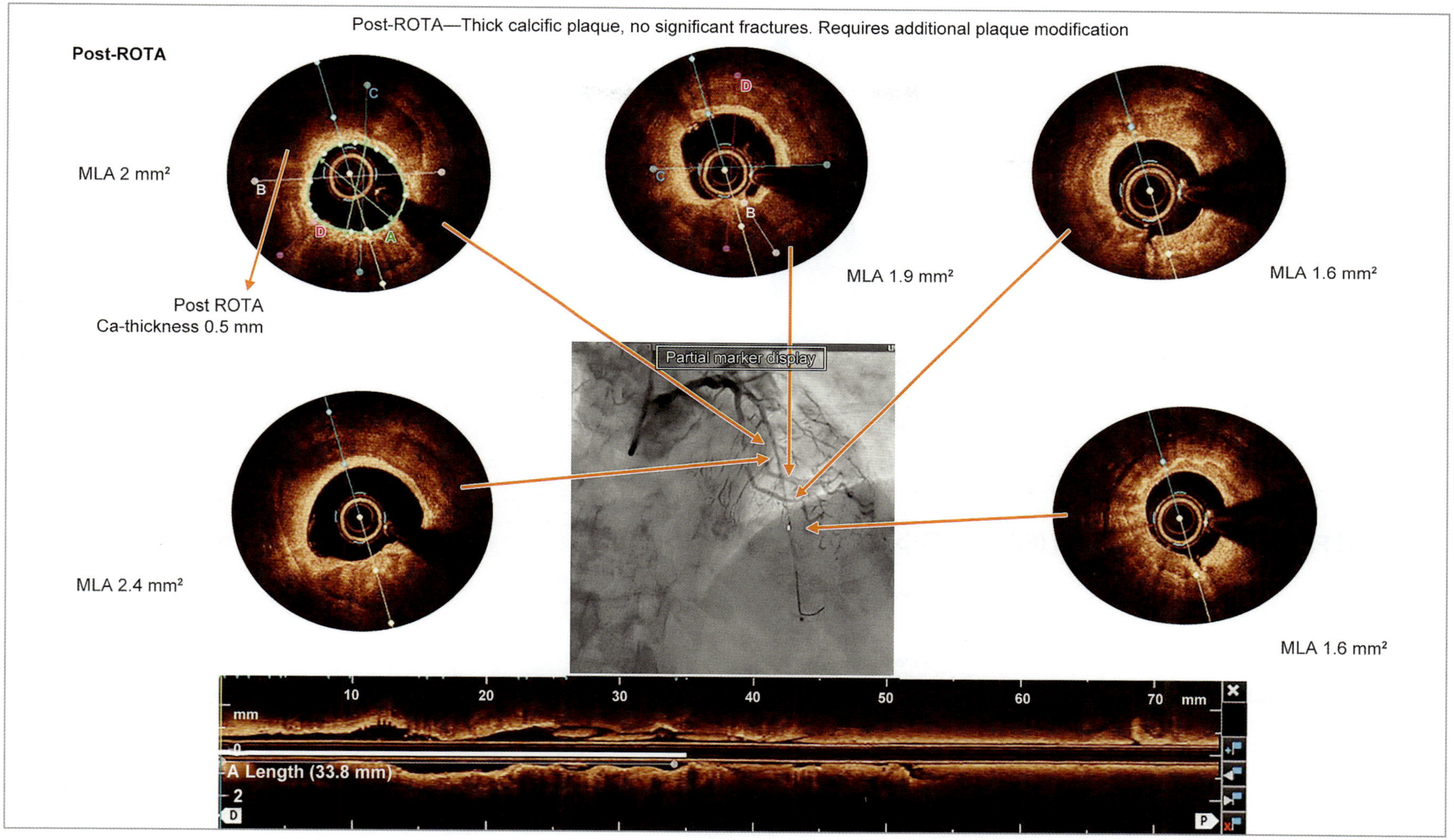

Fig. 32C

Figs. 32A to C: (A) Rotablation for balloon uncrossable lesion; (B) Imaging for proper selection of plaque modification device and optimization DES implantation; (C) Post-ROTA OCT assessment for adequate plaque modification.

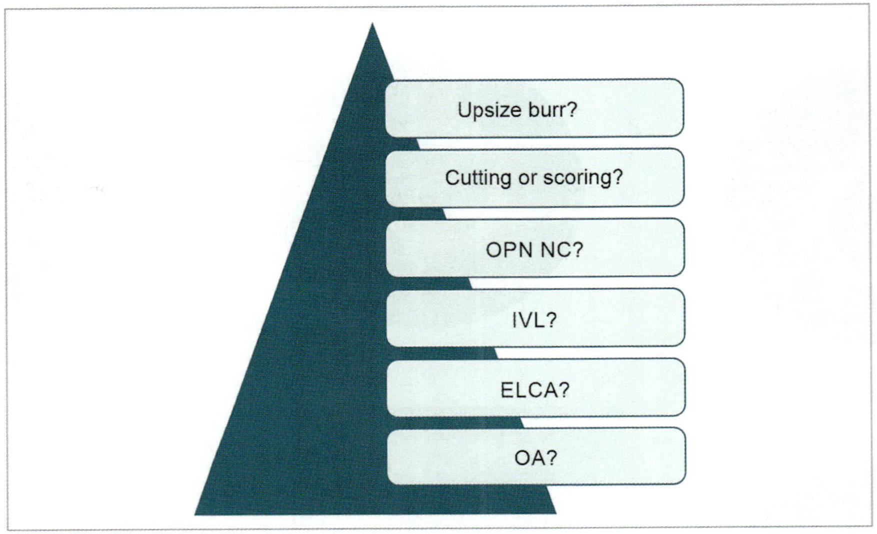

Fig. 33A

Technical Features of Rotablation (RA) and Orbital Atherectomy (OA)

Feature	***RA***	***OA***
Device	Rotablator	Diamondback 360
Available sizes	1.25, 1.5, 1.75, 2.0, 2.25, 2.38 and 2.5	1.25 mm
Guid Catheter compatibility	<1.75 mm burrs; 6Fr guide	6 Fr guide

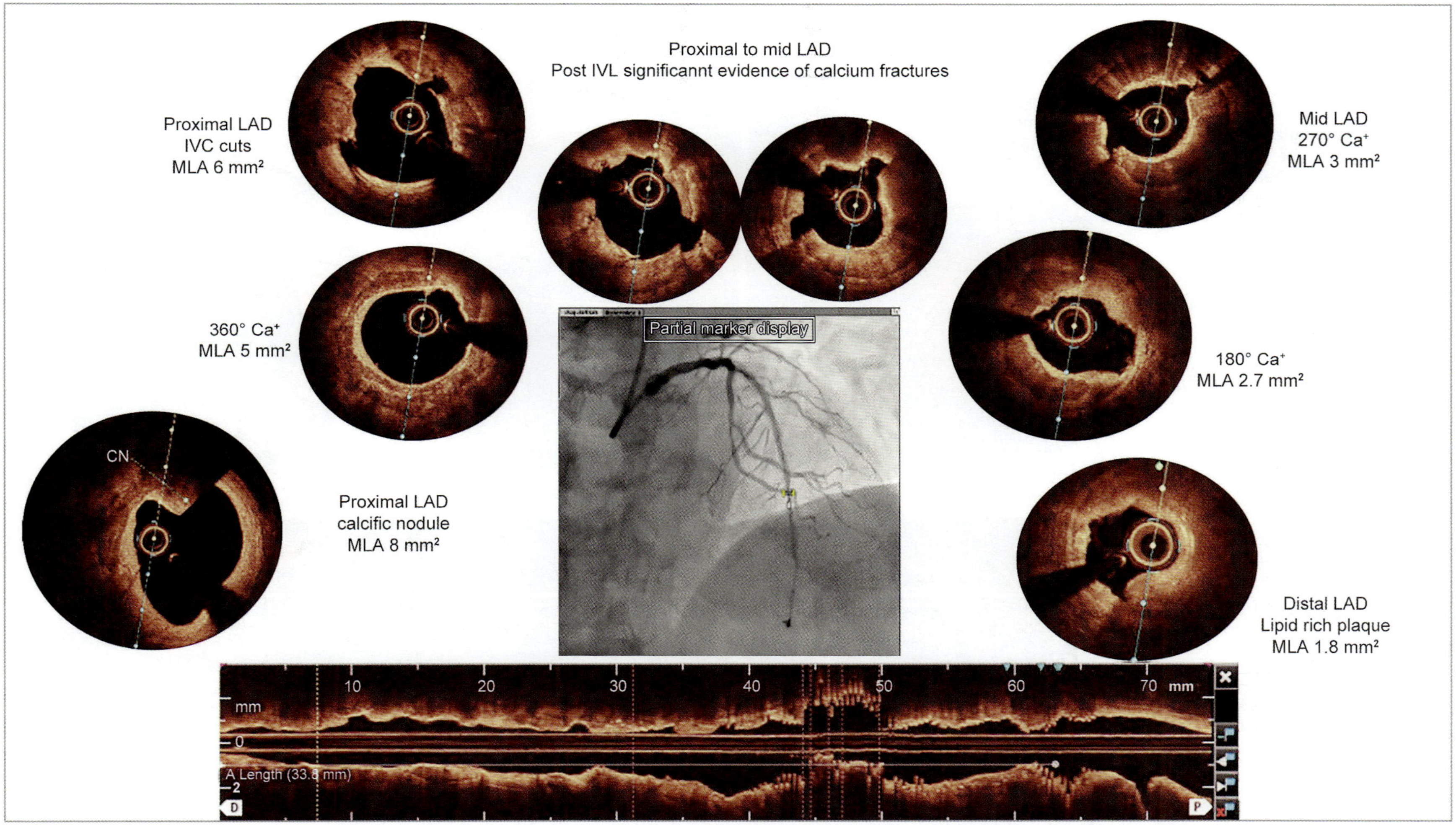

Fig. 33B

For every 1 mmol/L increase in LDL-C, risk of MI is 30% higher.

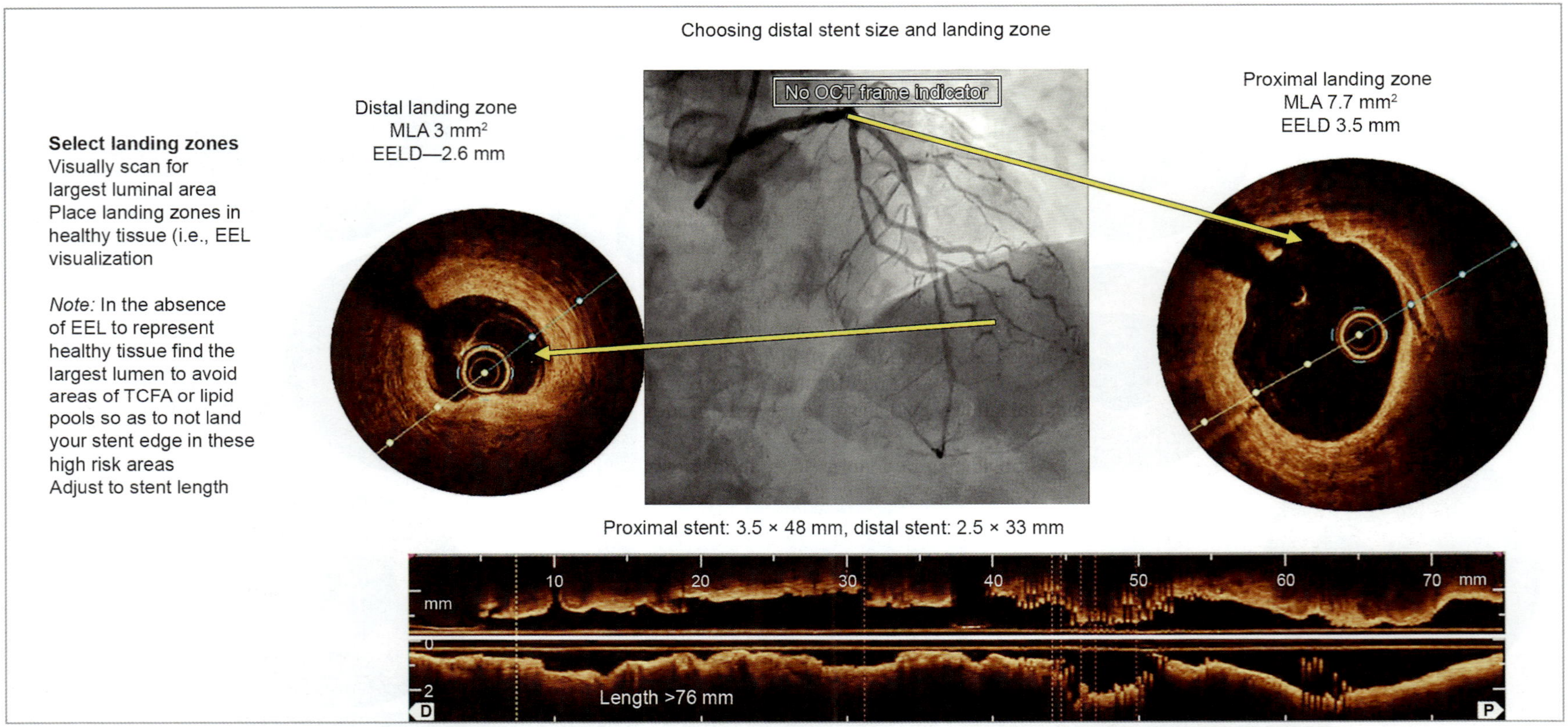

Fig. 33C

Figs. 33A to C: (A) Plan for inadequate plaque modification–requires combined strategy; (B) Post-ROTA and IVL OCT assessment for calcium fractures—evidence of adequate plaque modification (presence of fractures and gain in MLA); (C) Post-IVL OCT assessment for selection of the stent.

MCS for High-risk PCI- MCS may be considered to patients who are surgically unsuitable or high risk due to associated co-morbidities, Complex coronary disease of LM, MVD, and severely calcified lesions requiring plaque modification devices, severe LV dysfunction-EF <25%, Systolic BP, 100 mm Hg, and LVEDP >25 mm Hg.

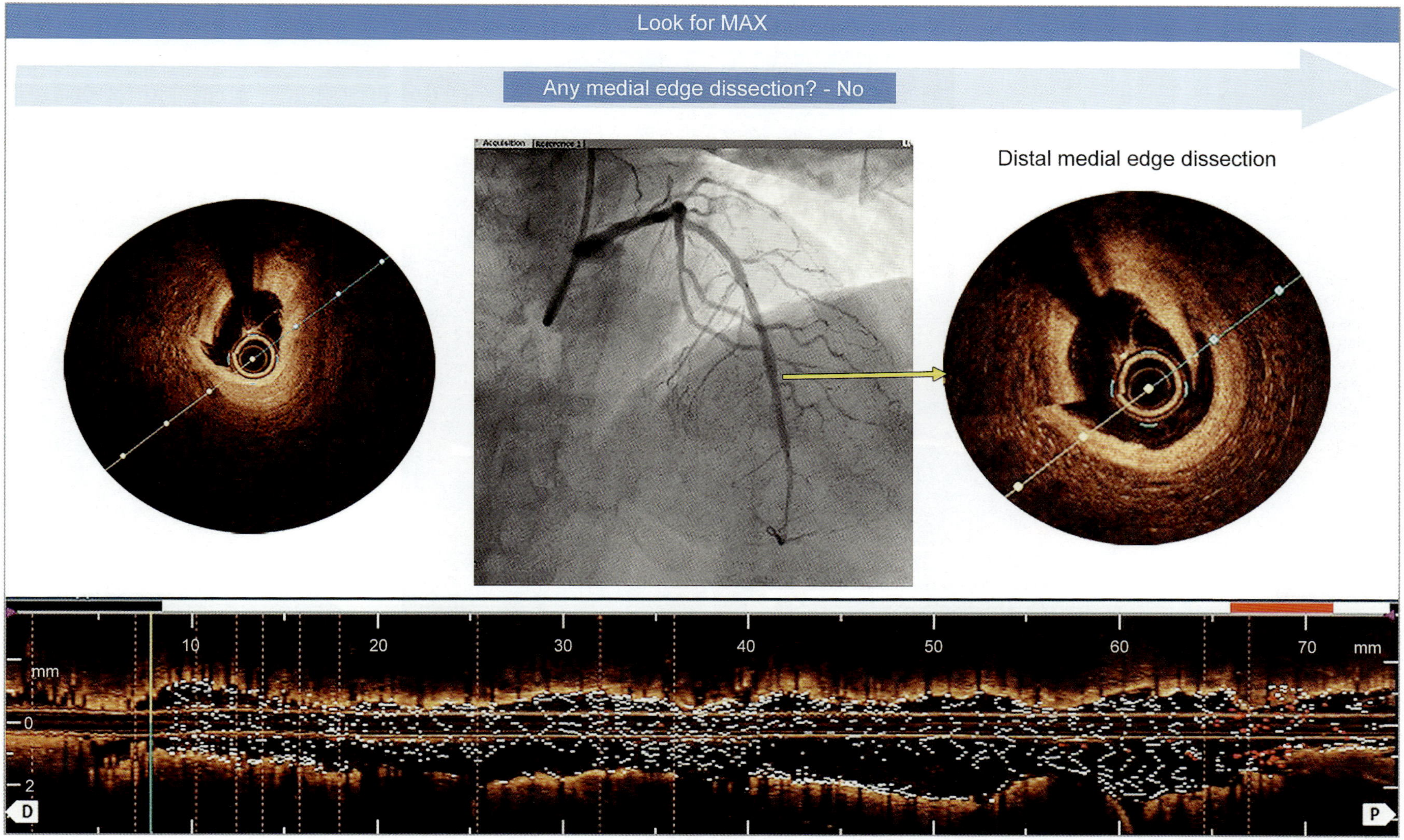

Fig. 34A

Physiology (FFR/IFR) allows an accurate estimation of the severity of LM lesions.

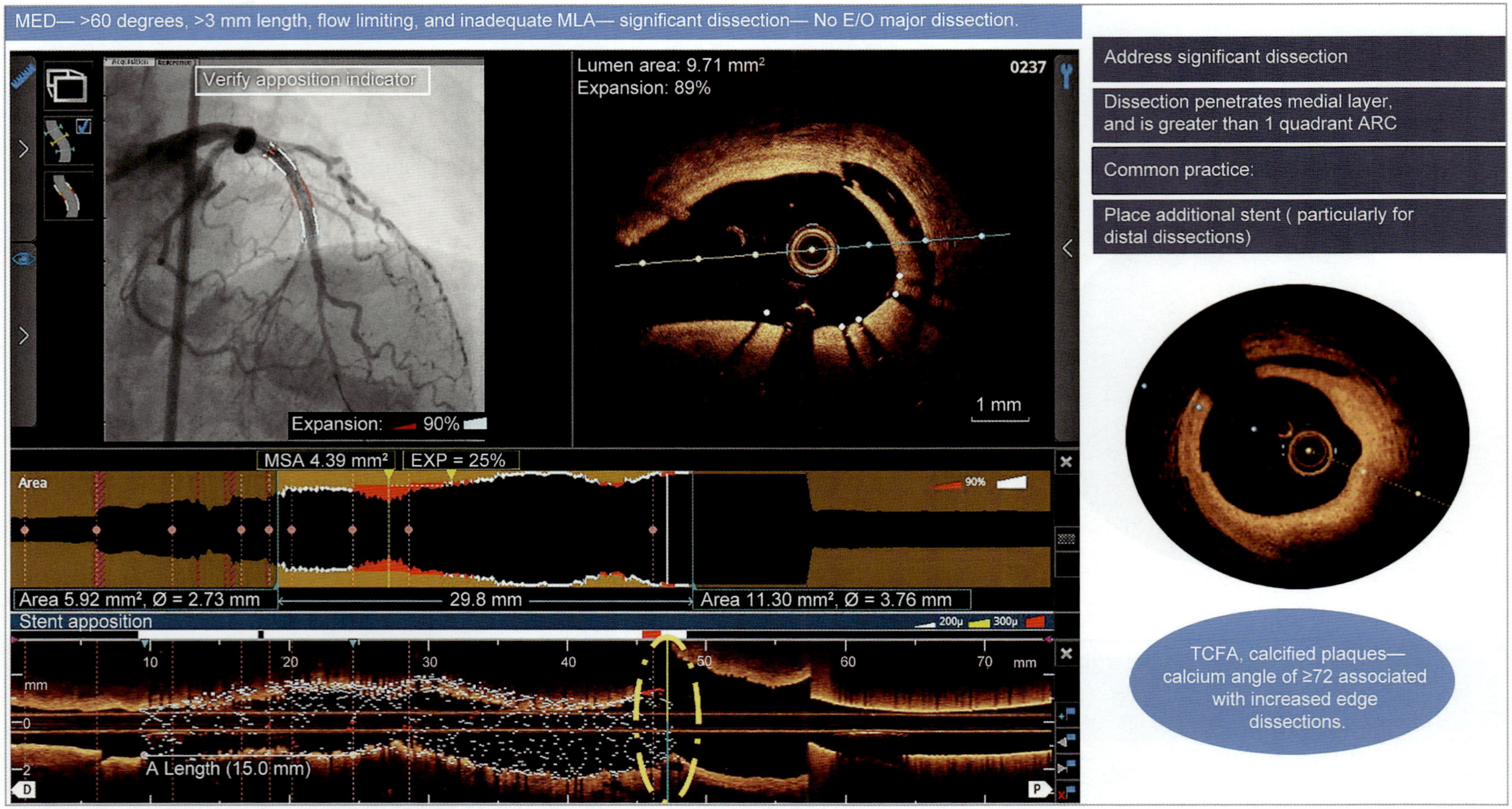

Fig. 34B

IVUS and OCT imaging is key to plan and optimize PCI procedures in LM.

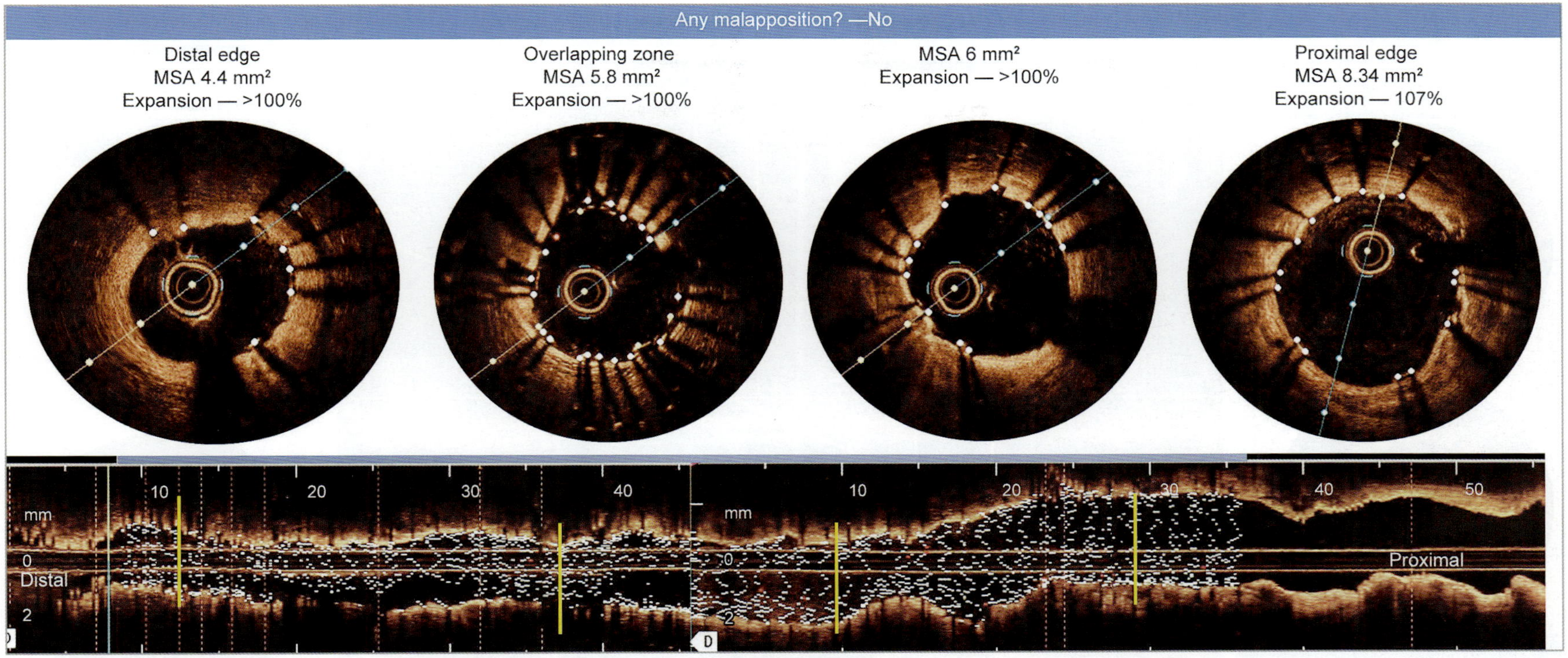

Fig. 34C

If the wire entrapped within the lesion, don't pull it:

- Advance the microcatheter & pull en masse
- Advance a balloon over the wire, inflate to dislodge the wire and then pull
- Pass a guide extension with balloon, pull en masse
- Snare it
- Cut with bioptome or atherectomy. Stent to pin to the vessel wall.

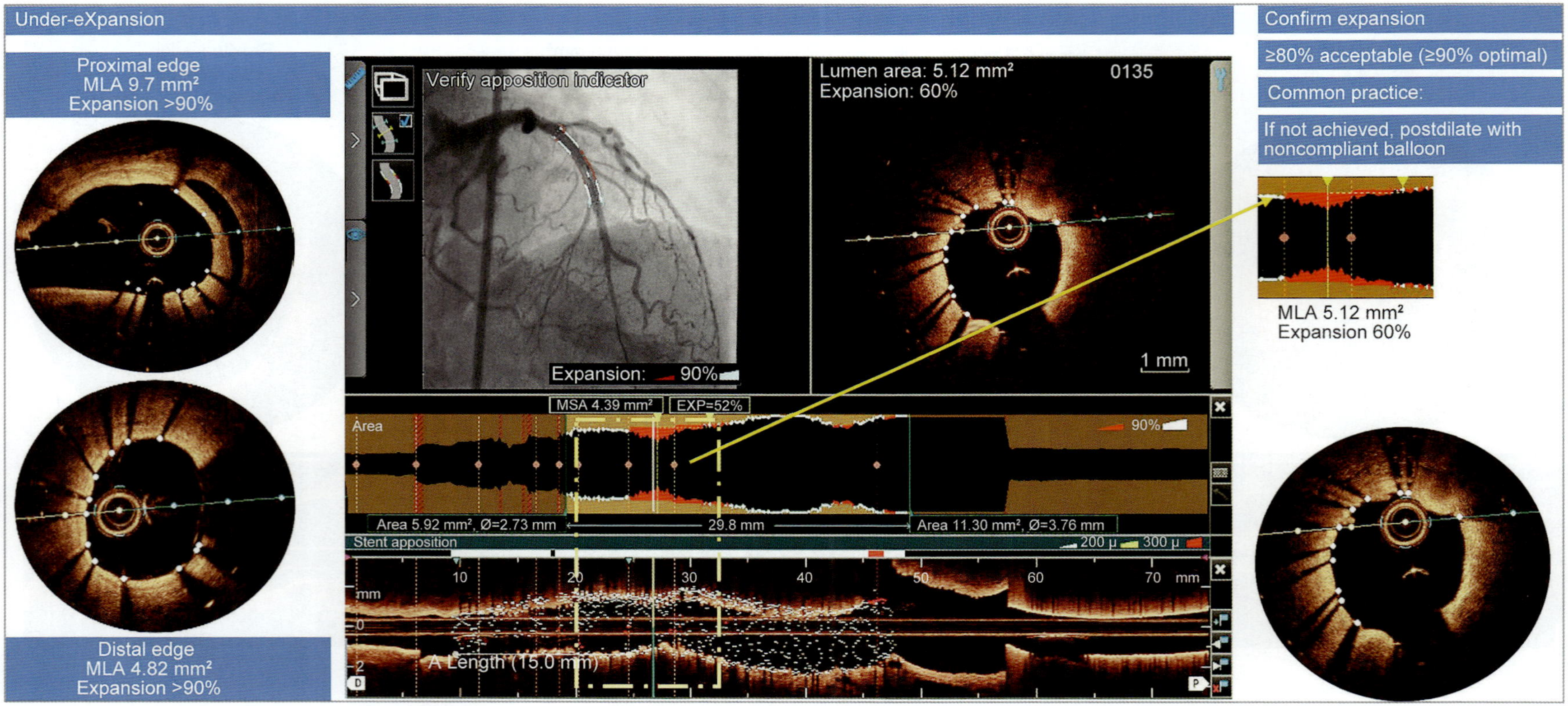

Fig. 34D

Figs. 34A to D: (A) Poststenting OCT showing distal edge dissection; (B) Poststenting OCT showing proximal and distal edge dissection (case example); (C) Poststenting OCT showing no malapposition; (D) Poststenting OCT showing under-expansion to be corrected with additional balloon (case example).

Most patients with LM+ MVD lesions have additional stenoses, the influence of downstream stenoses on measured FFR value should always be considered.

Use 1.25 mm burr for long tortuous lesions and if unable to cross the lesion with 1.5 mm burr, then upsize the burr or other modification devices for further modification.

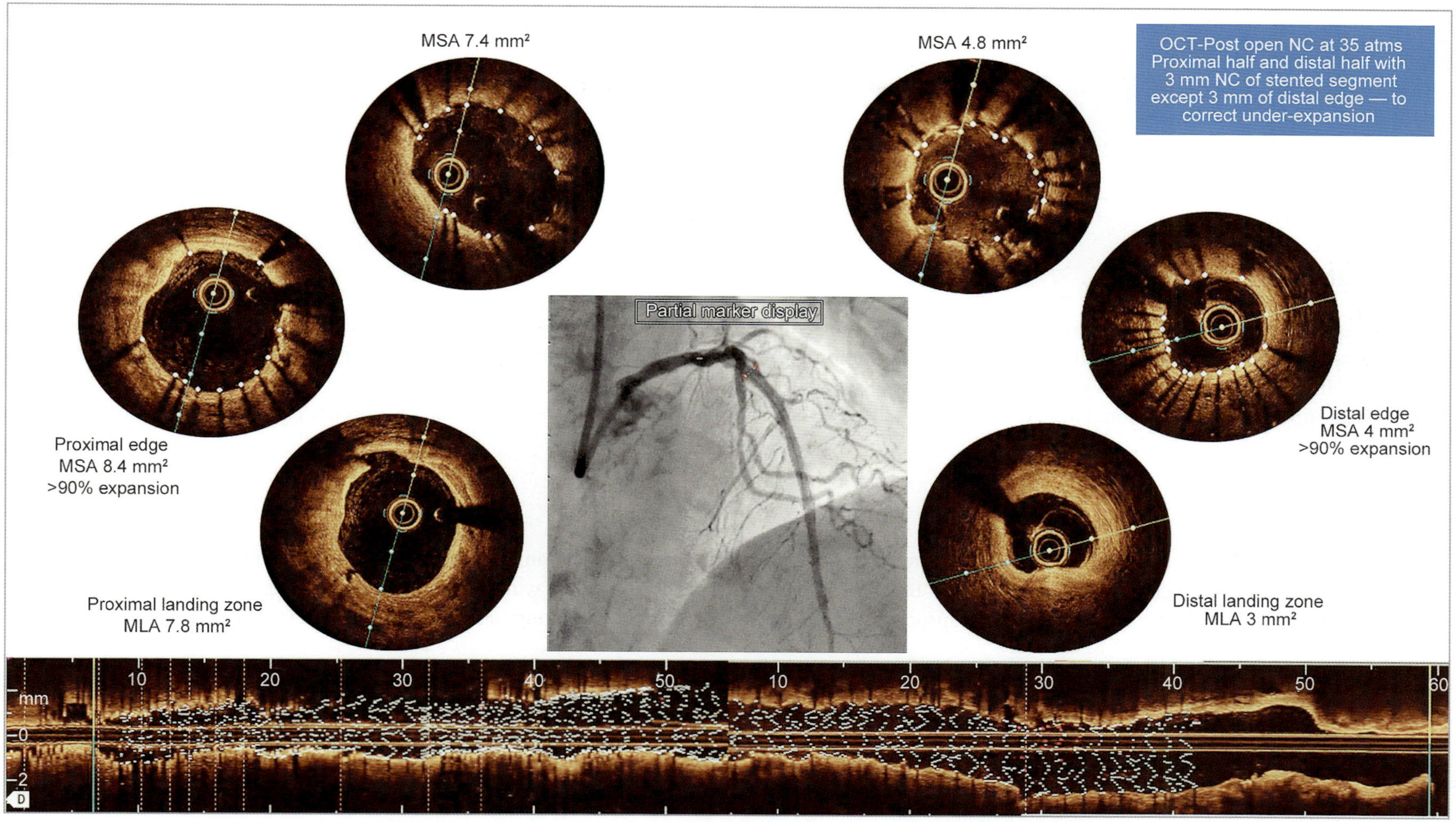

Fig. 35: Poststenting OCT showing well expanded and apposed stent struts with no medial edge dissections.

Tandem Lesions-Initially perform lesion with max gradient, repeat FFR and if +ve perform 2nd stenting. Diffuse long lesions- initially do stenting of segment with max step-up, and repeat FFR.

CASE 5

PCI of severely calcified RCA balloon uncrossable lesion.

CLINICAL HISTORY

A 77-year-old female known hypertensive, history of fall at home resulting in left intertrochanteric fracture and discontinued tablet Ecosprin for 3 days. Patient developed episodes of classical angina of 1 week duration. Past history of left hemiparesis in 2013. ECG—evolved inferior wall MI, 2D echo—hypokinetic basal inferior wall, mild LV systolic dysfunction, EF—50%.

CAG-LMCA—normal, LAD—proximal mild disease, LCX—distal 80–90% calcified lesion, RCA—mid 90% calcified lesion, PDA and PLVB—normal.

PROCEDURE

Route—right femoral artery, using 6 Fr JR 3.5 guiding catheter, RCA was crossed with 0.014 Sion Blue Wire. 2.25 × 12 mm Mini Trek balloon could not cross the lesion even with microcatheter support. Sion Blue Wire exchanged with ROTA floppy wire using microcatheter support. Rotablation was done with 5 runs of 1.5 mm ROTA burr at 150,000 rpm. Preprocedure IVUS showed proximal to mid long segment 90% calcified lesion. Predilatation done with 2.25 ×12 mm NC Trek balloon.

Post-ROTA OCT Analysis

Pre-OCT showed 270° deep calcium with MLA—4.9 mm^2, MLD—2.5 mm, thickness of calcium >500 µm, lipid plaque with TCFA MLA—3.3 mm^2, MLD—2 mm **(Figs. 36A and B)**.

Stenting done with 3.0 × 40 mm Orsiro stent. Postdilatation done with 3.0 × 12 mm and 3.5 × 12 mm NC Trek balloons.

CAG-RCA—mid 90% calcified lesion, PDA and PLVB—normal, Sion Blue Wire exchanged with ROTA floppy wire using microcatheter support. Rotablation was done using 1.5 mm ROTA bur at 150,000 rpm, 5 runs, predilatation done with 2.25 × 12 mm NC Trek balloon, RCA stenting done with 3.0 × 40 mm Orsiro stent, postdilatation done with 3.0 × 12 mm and 3.5 × 12 mm NC Trek balloon, final result **(Figs. 37A to F)**.

Post-ROTA stenting OCT analysis: Asymmetrical stent expansion due to thick calcific plaque.

Post-OCT showed distal landing zone with MLA—6.6 mm^2, MLD—2.9 mm, midportion of the stent with MLA—4.7 mm^2, MLD—2.4 mm, and proximal landing zone with MLA—8.5 mm^2, MLD—3.3 mm **(Fig. 38)**.

OCT showed well-apposed stent struts, no residual stenosis and no thrombosis. Postprocedure Angio view showed well-implanted stents with TIMI-III flow without any dissection. Patient was discharged on third postprocedure in a stable status.

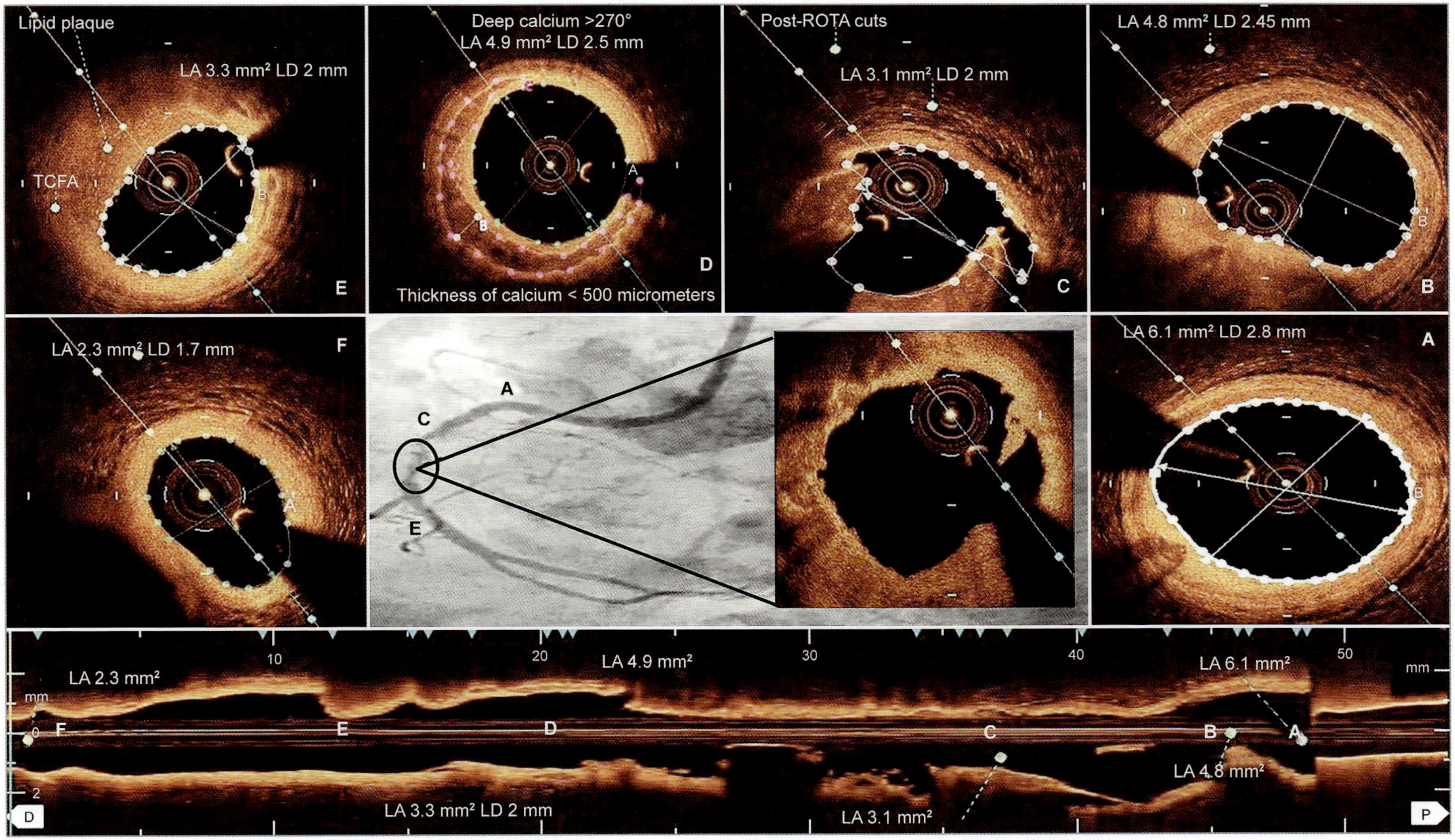

Lipid plaque
LA 3.3 mm² LD 2 mm
TCFA
E
Deep calcium >270°
LA 4.9 mm² LD 2.5 mm
D
Thickness of calcium < 500 micrometers
Post-ROTA cuts
LA 3.1 mm² LD 2 mm
C
LA 4.8 mm² LD 2.45 mm
B
LA 2.3 mm² LD 1.7 mm
F
A
C
E
LA 6.1 mm² LD 2.8 mm
A
10
20
30
40
50
mm
LA 2.3 mm²
LA 4.9 mm²
LA 6.1 mm²
F
E
D
C
B
A
LA 4.8 mm²
LA 3.3 mm² LD 2 mm
LA 3.1 mm²
D
P

Fig. 36A

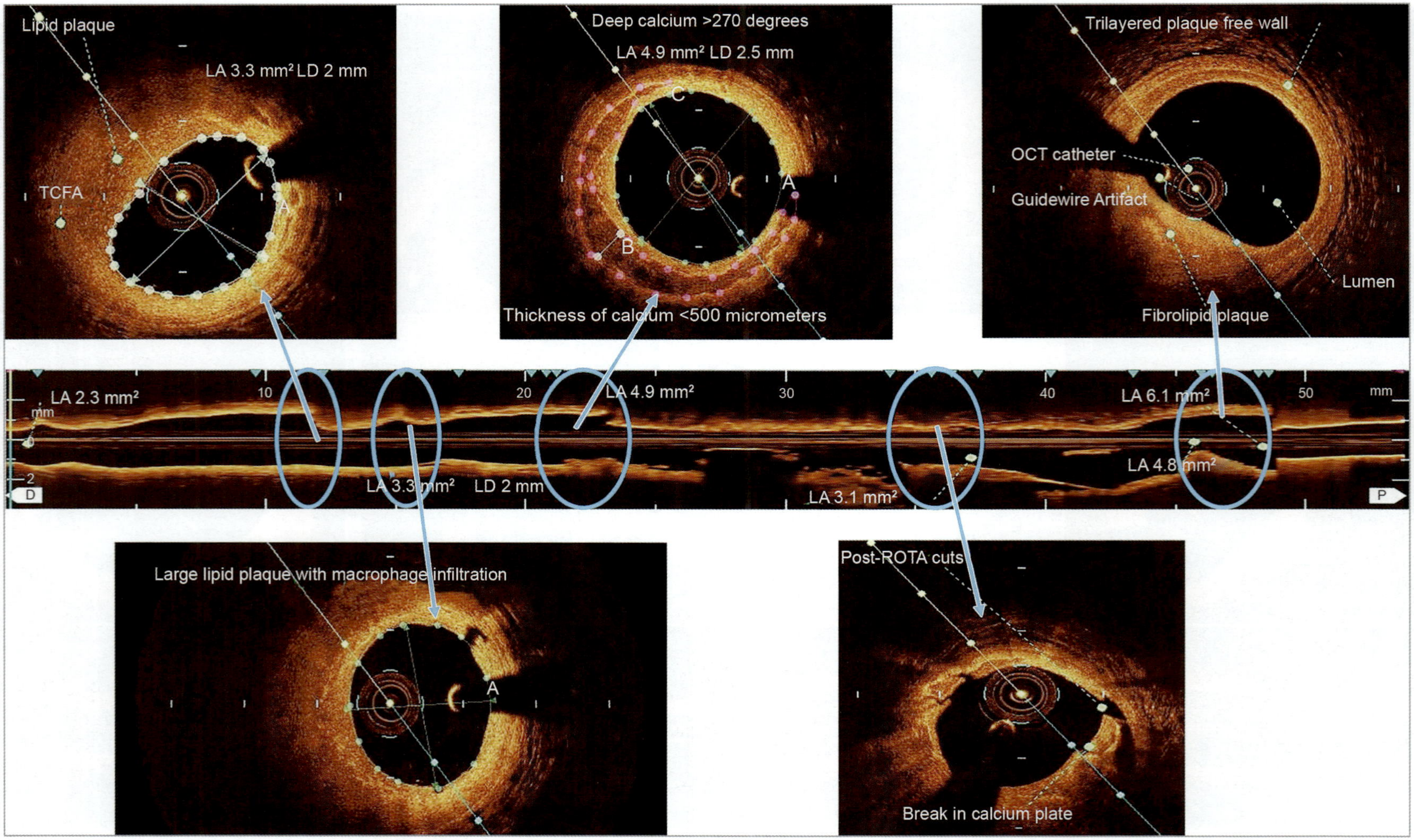

Fig. 36B

Figs. 36A and B: (A) Prestenting OCT assessment for device selection; (B) Prestenting OCT assessment for plaque morphology.

Thick calcific plaque can lead to irregular and inadequate expansion of stent. Sometimes patients may require upsized bur for adequate modification of plaque to debulk calcium plaque. These lesions can also be managed with additional usage of intravascular lithotripsy (IVL)-ROTA-Tripsy or high-pressure OPN NC balloon inflation at 40–50 atm to get adequate expansion and apposition, otherwise these may lead to stent thrombosis and ISR.

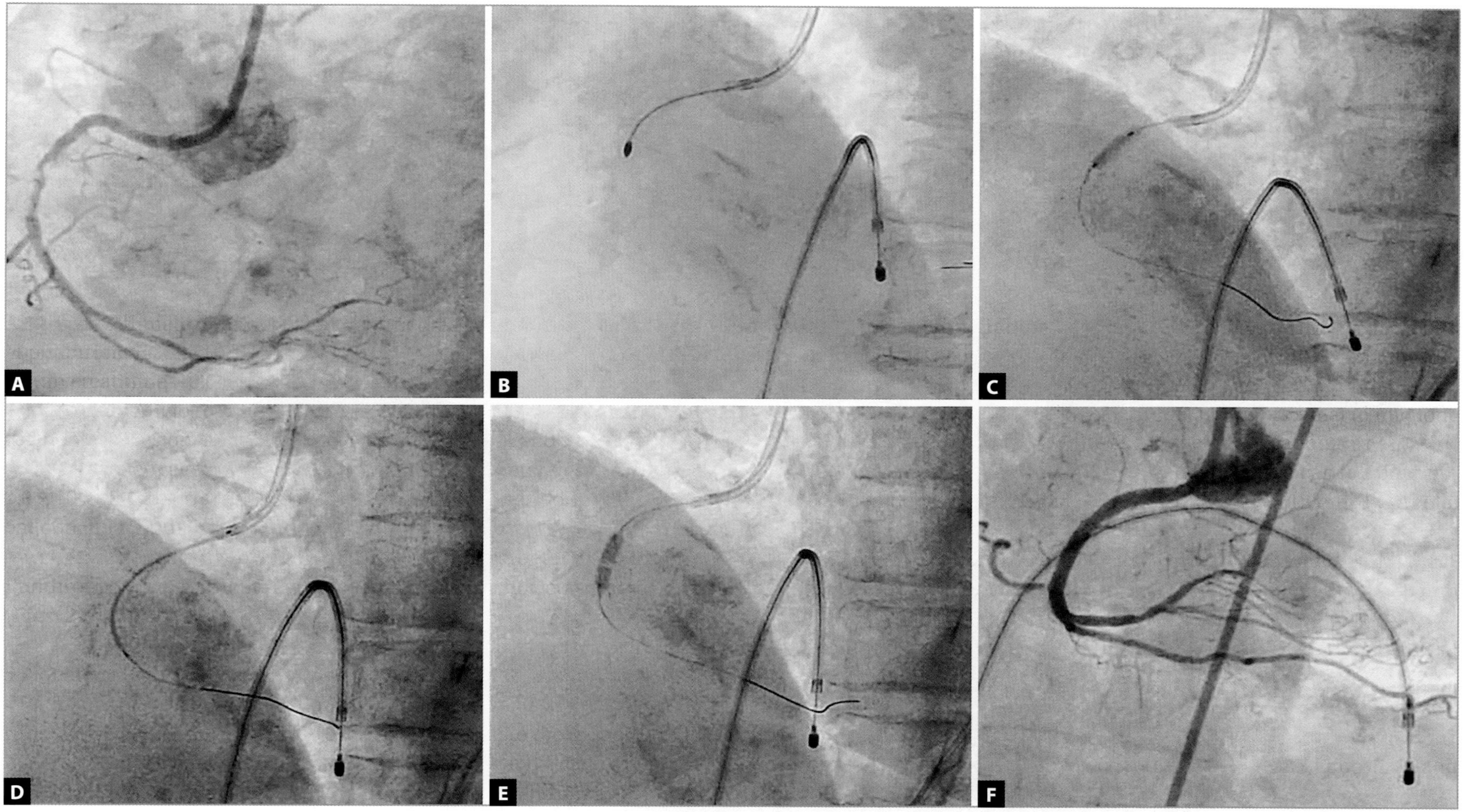

Figs. 37A to F: Plaque modification of RCA followed by stenting and postdilatation. (A) Check angio; (B) Rotablation; (C) Predilatation; (D) Stenting; (E) Postdilatation; (F) Final result.

Use 1.25 mm burr for long tortuous lesions and if unable to cross the lesion with 1.5 mm burr, then upsize the burr or other modification devices for further modification.

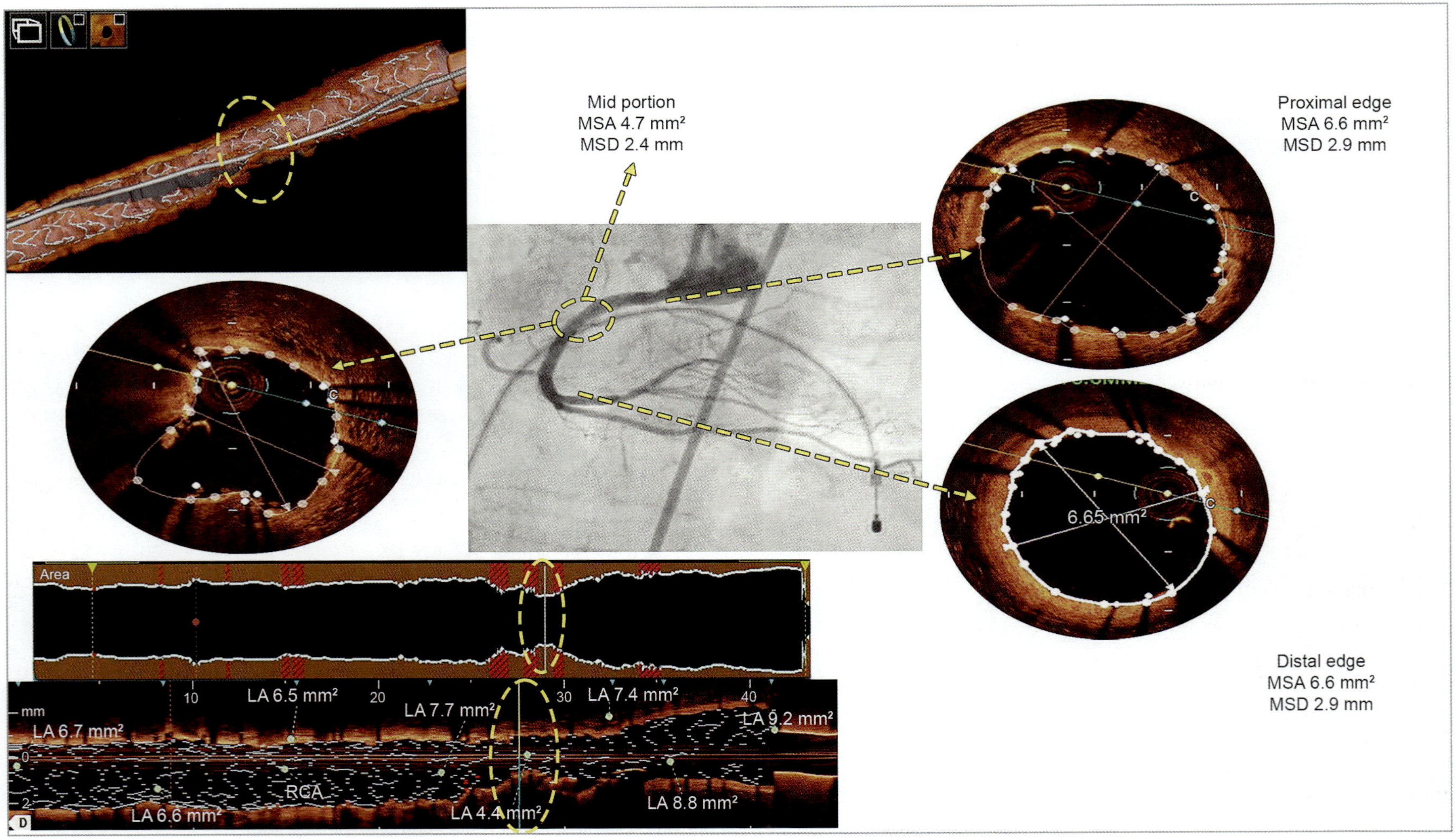

Fig. 38: Poststenting OCT showing well expanded and apposed stent struts.

Basic principles of operating Rota include use of single 1.5 mm burr (appropriate in >90% of the cases) with burr-to -artery ratio of 0.6, rotational speed of about 140,000 to 180,000 rpm, gradual burr advancement with a slow pecking motion, 15 to 20 sec of short ablative runs guided by fluoroscopy, acoustic and tactile inputs, and avoid significant deceleration in rotational speed >5,000 rpm to reduce complications like burr entrapment/burr stall/burr detachment, and finish the procedure with 1or 2 final polishing runs

CASE 6

PCI with DES of diffusely Calcified RCA.

CLINICAL HISTORY

A 65-year-old male known hypertensive, diabetic presented with inferior NSTEMI with recent onset of angina. ECG—ST depression in inferior leads, 2D echo—no RWMA, normal, LV function with EF—64%. TMT +ve for inducible ischemia. Investigations: Hb—10.8 g/dL, RBS—99 mg/dL, serum creatinine—0.89 mg/dL with eGFR 90 mL/min.

CAG-LMCA—normal, LAD-mild disease, D1 70% lesion, LCX—normal, RCA—proximal to mid long segment 80-90% lesion **(Fig. 39)**.

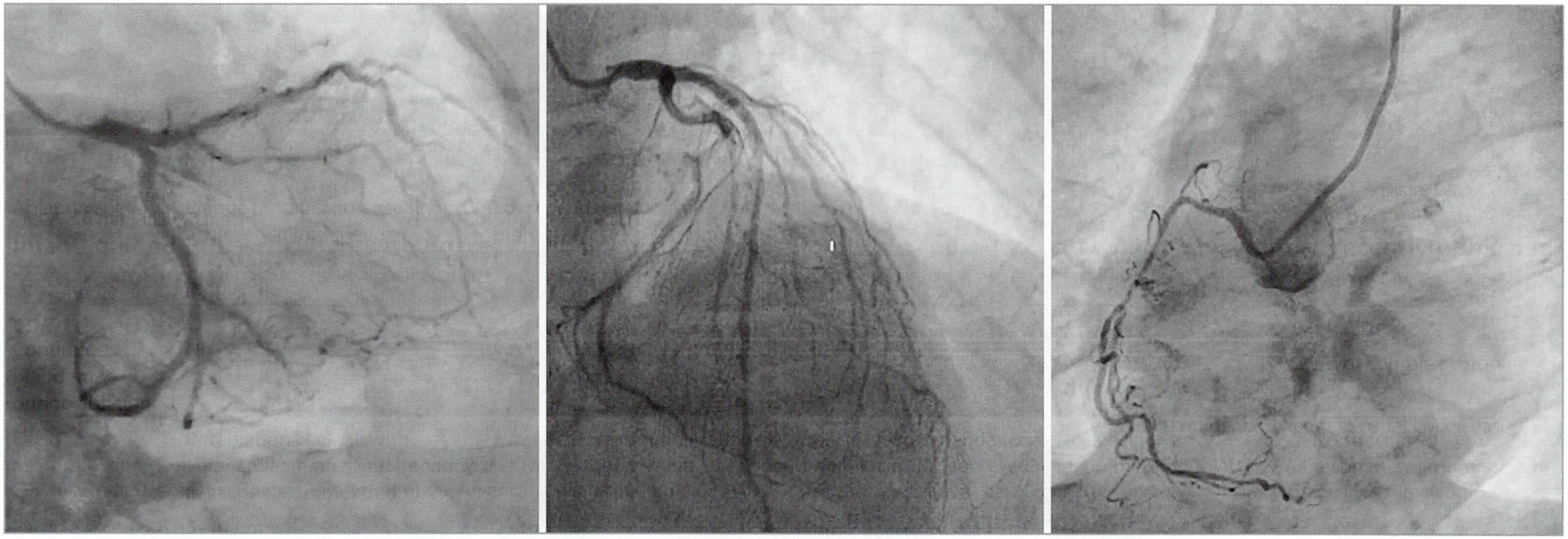

Fig. 39: Coronary angiogram.

PROCEDURE

Route—RFA, using 6 Fr JR 3.5 guiding catheter, RCA was crossed with 0.014″ Power turn wire. Pre-OCT balloon dilatation done with 2.0 × 10 mm Tazuna balloon for smooth passage of OCT catheter.

Pre-OCT assessment distal landing zone-LD—2.2 mm × 2.1 mm with intimal hyperplasia-0.27 mm, proximal landing zone: LD—3.27 mm × 2.9 mm, total lesion length—46 mm, calcium thickness 0.72 mm, ARC <180° with MLA—2.9 mm^2, mid RCA dissected plaque **(Figs. 40A and B)**.

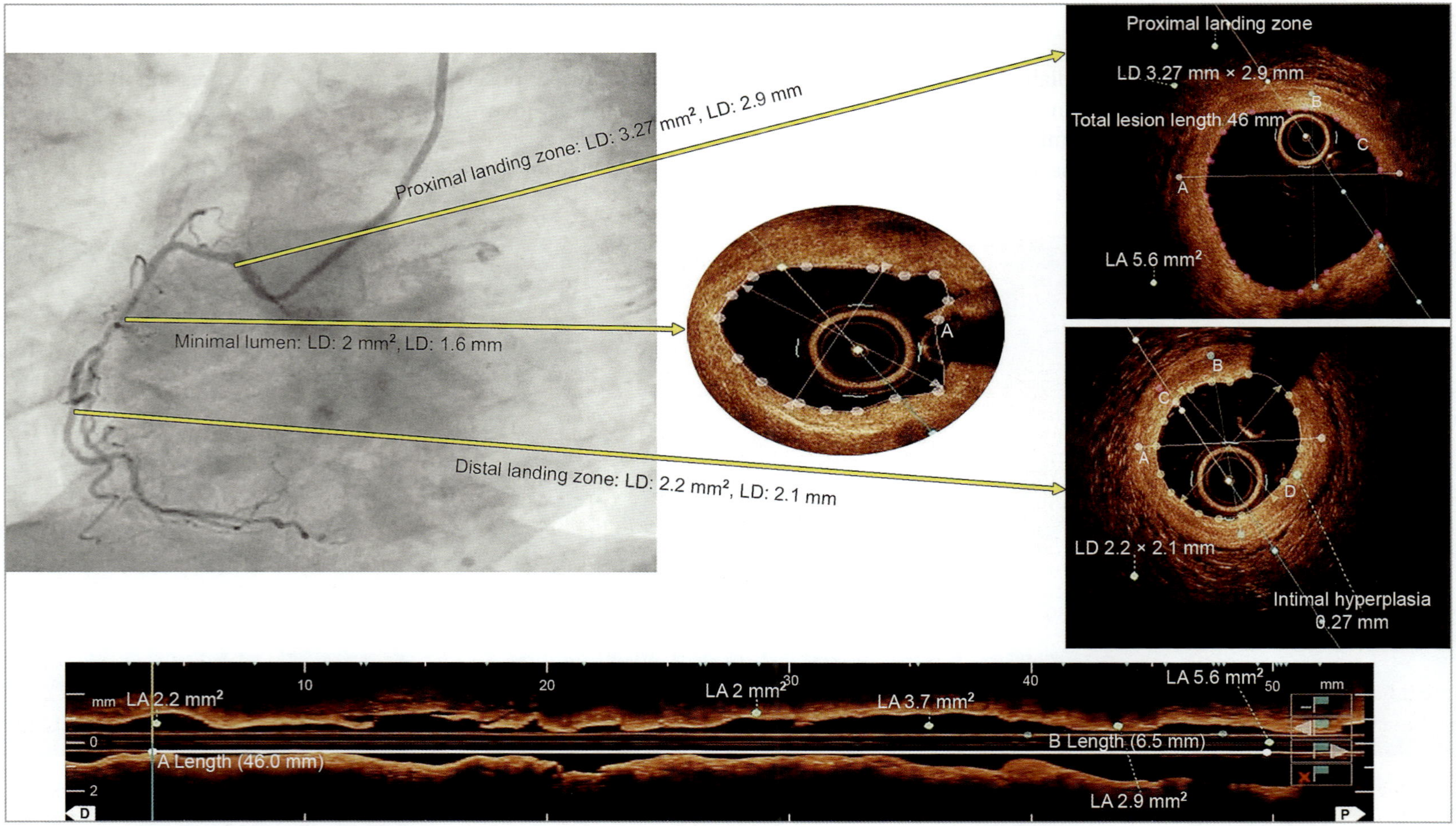

Fig. 40A

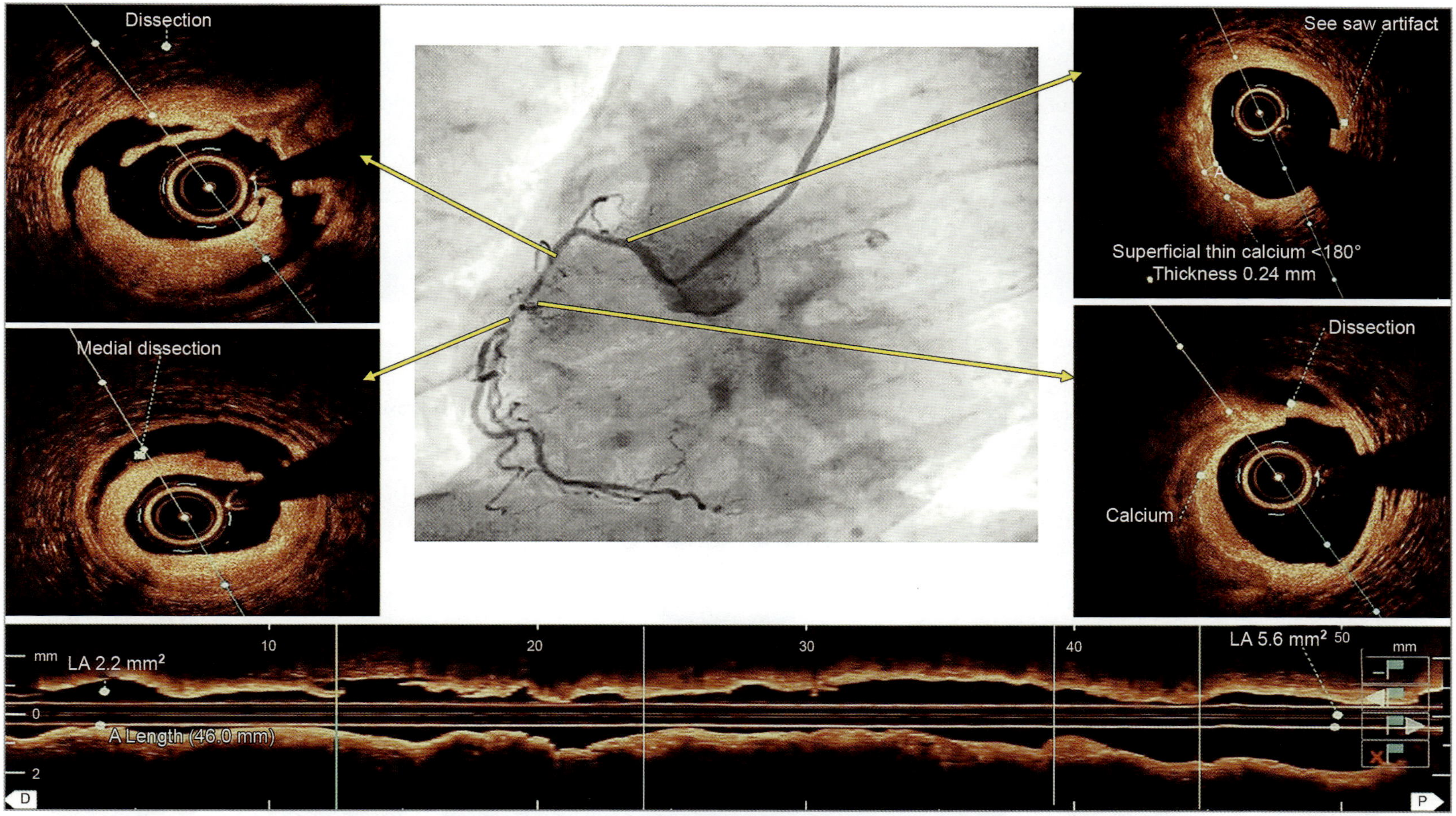

Fig. 40B

Figs. 40A and B: (A) Presenting OCT assessment for the selection of the stent size; (B) Presenting OCT assessment for plaque morphology.

Mid to distal RCA stenting done with 2.25 × 26 mm Resolute Onyx stent. Proximal RCA stenting done with 2.75 × 26 mm Resolute Onyx stent. Postdilatation done with 3.0 × 12 mm NC Apollo balloon **(Fig. 41)**. Post-OCT showed well-apposed stent, no underexpansion, no tissue prolapses and edge dissection **(Figs. 42A and B)**. Postprocedure Angio view showed well-implanted stents with TIMI-III flow without any dissection. Patient was discharged on third postprocedure in a stable status.

OCT helps in choosing precise devise length to cover entire diseased segment particularly in diffuse long segment lesions, and choosing landing zones with disease free or with minimal plaque burden. Distal stent diameter should be selected according to distal reference mean lumen area or EEL derived diameter, proximal portions of the stent expansion should be done according to the mean reference luminal diameter or EEL-derived diameter by appropriately sized NC balloon.

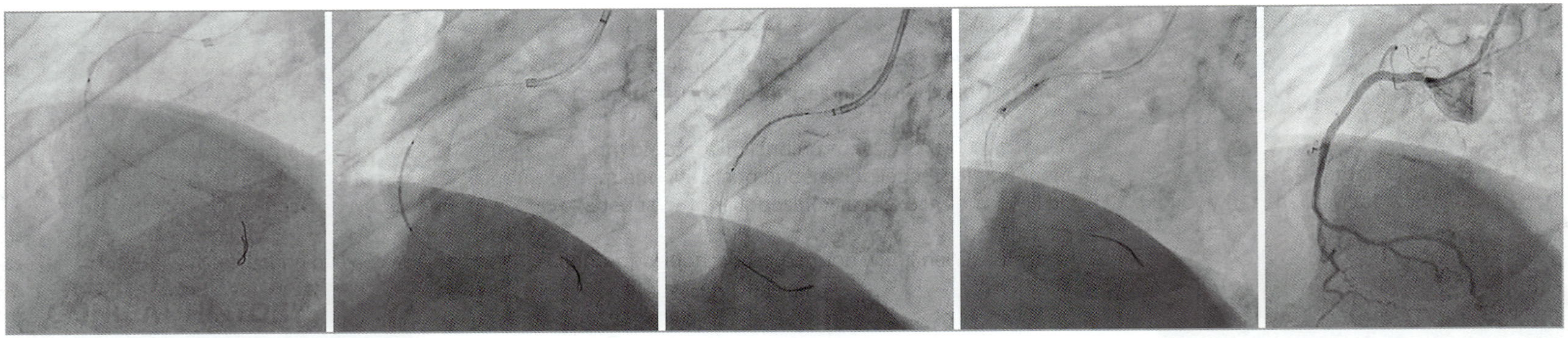

Fig. 41: Coronary angioplasty stenting of RCA.

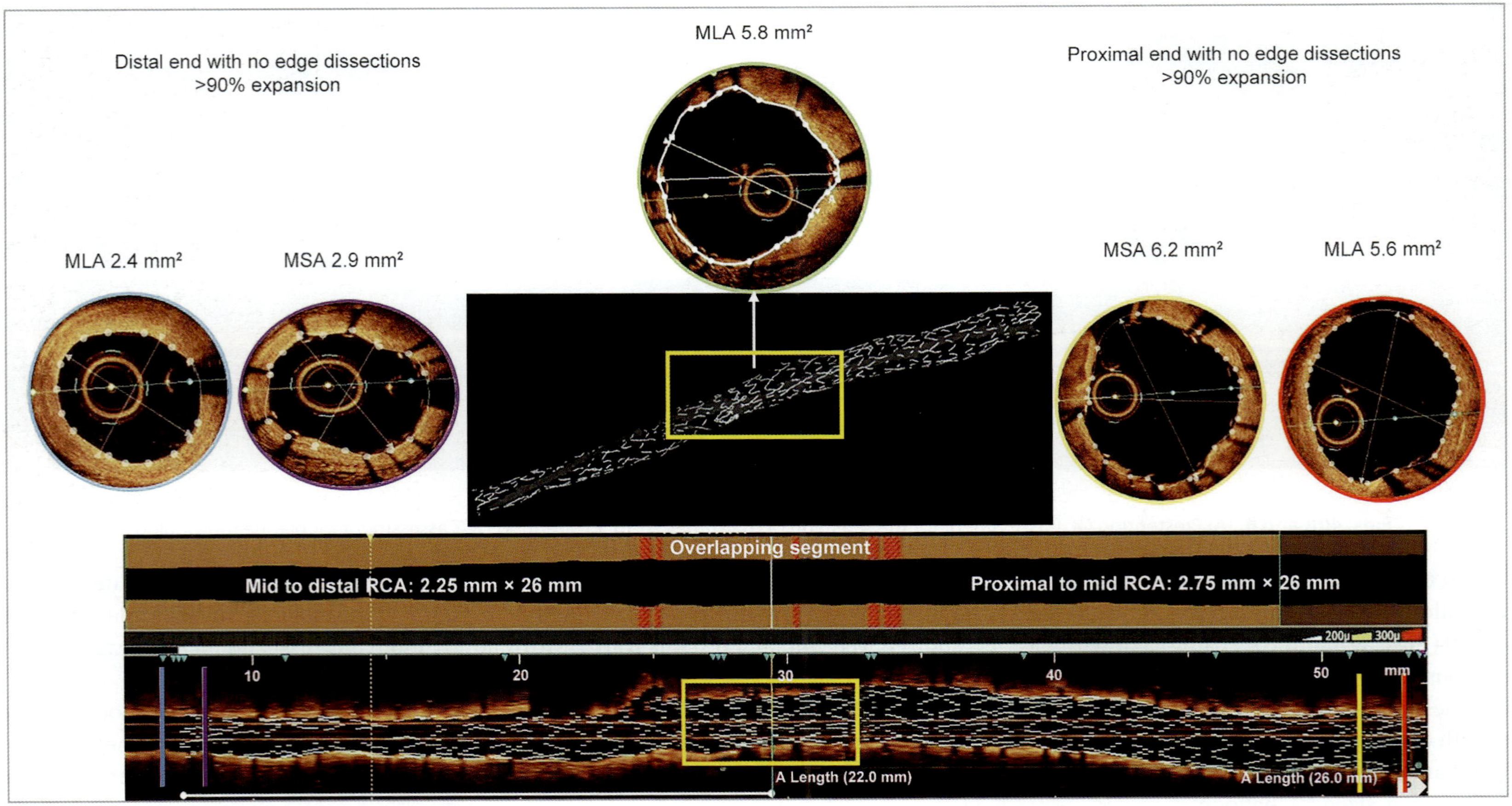

Fig. 42A

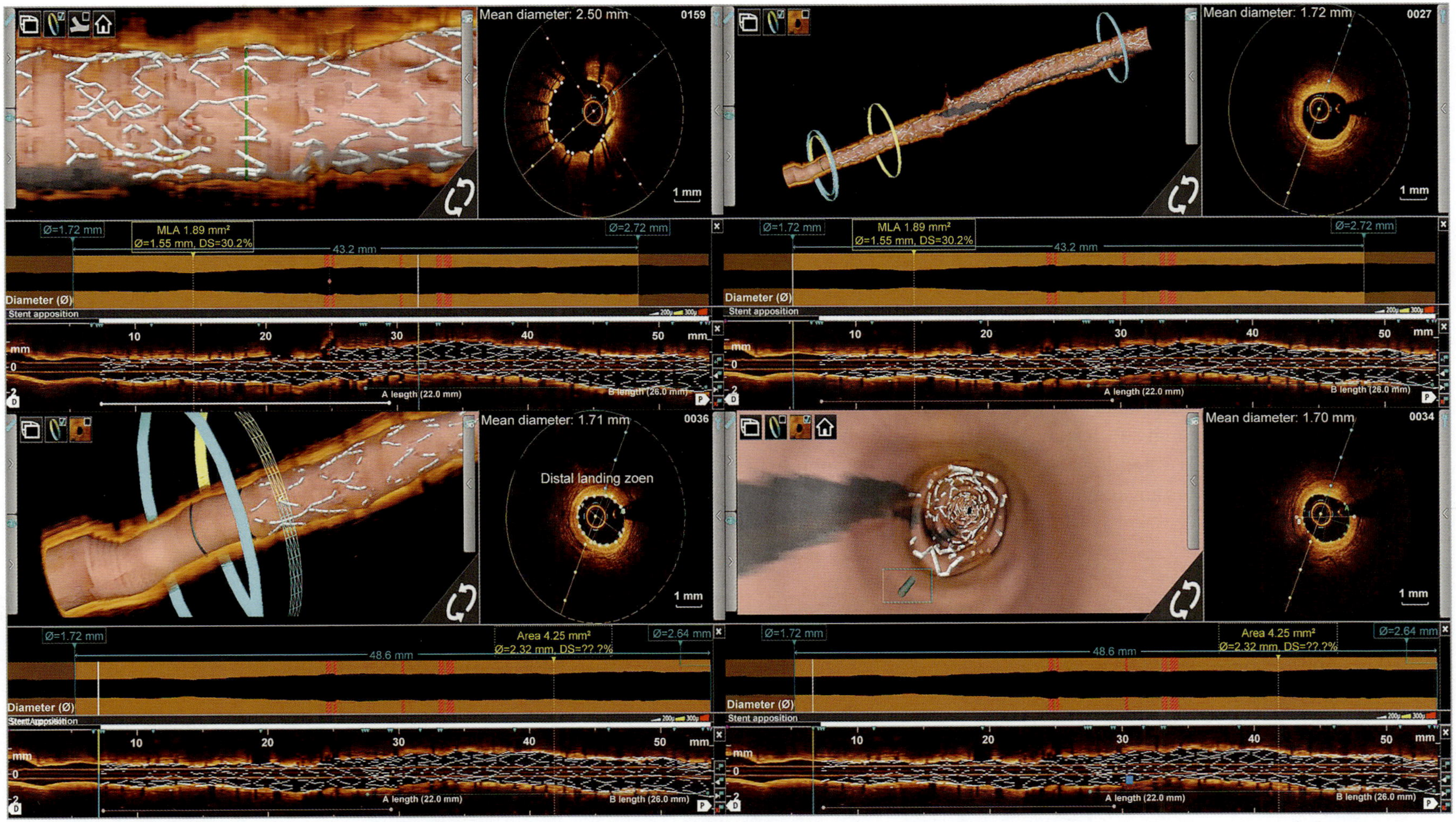

Fig. 42B

Figs. 42A and B: (A) Poststenting OCT showing well expanded and apposed stent struts; (B) Poststent 3D OCT view.

CASE 7

OCT-guided PCI of calcified LAD.

CLINICAL HISTORY

A 78-year-old male known hypertensive, diabetic presented with history of effort angina class II to III for 1 month duration with recent worsening of angina with rest episodes. CAD-unstable angina. Past history of PCI of RCA and proximal LCX with DES in 2000. 2D echo—no RWMA, good LV function, EF—61%. Thallium study showed negative for inducible ischemia with good LV function, hence advised medical management. In view of persistent angina, CAG was done which showed LAD proximal to mid long 90% segment severely calcified lesion (visible Ca lines on both sides of vessel walls of proximal LAD and proximal LCX), OM1—proximal 80% lesion, RCA CTO—ISR with severe calcific lesion **(Fig. 43)**.

Initial plan was to do ROTA stenting of LAD in view of angiographic evidence of severe calcium. Preprocedure intracoronary imaging was done to assess calcium severity and to assess any need for plaque modification with rotablation.

PROCEDURE

Route—RFA, 7 Fr EBU 3.5 guiding catheter, temporary pacing was inserted through right femoral vein, LAD lesion was crossed with 0.014 Sion Blue, predilated with 1.5 × 10 mm Tazuna balloon.

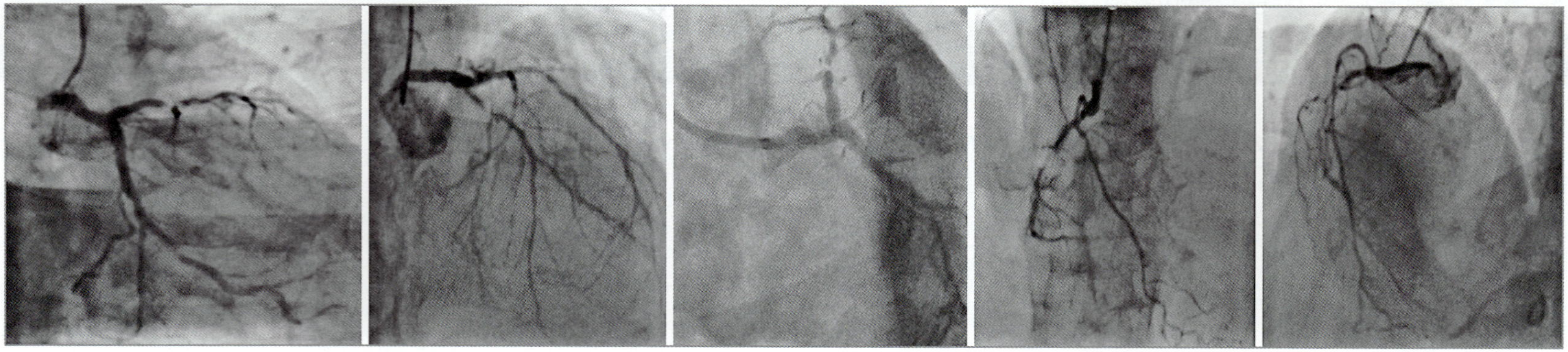

Fig. 43: Coronary angiogram.

Pre-OCT showed long segment calcific lesion extending from proximal to mid LAD. Calcium arc <180°, length <5 mm with more of deep calcium, thick fibrotic plaque at the area of tight stenosis, hence ROTA was deferred **(Figs. 44A to C)**.

Predilatation done with 2.75 × 12 mm Tazuna balloon **(Fig. 45)**. LAD stenting with 3 × 33 mm Xience Xpedition, postdilatation with 3 × 15 mm NC Trek **(Fig. 46)**. Poststenting OCT showed malapposition of proximal LAD **(Figs. 47A and B)**. Postdilatation done with 3.5 × 14 mm NC Trek balloon. Postprocedure Angio views showed well implanted stents with TIMI-III flow without any dissection.

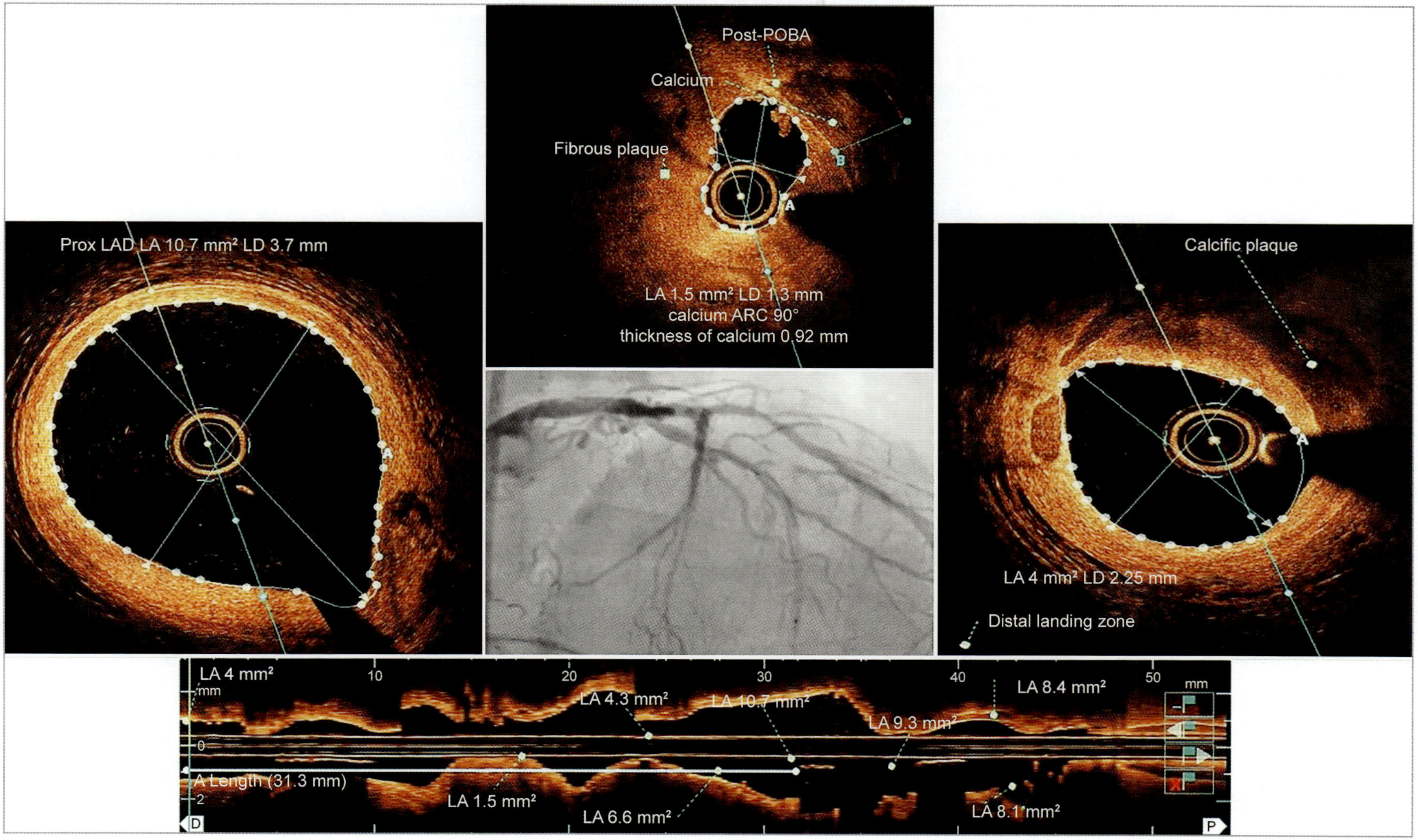

Fig. 44A

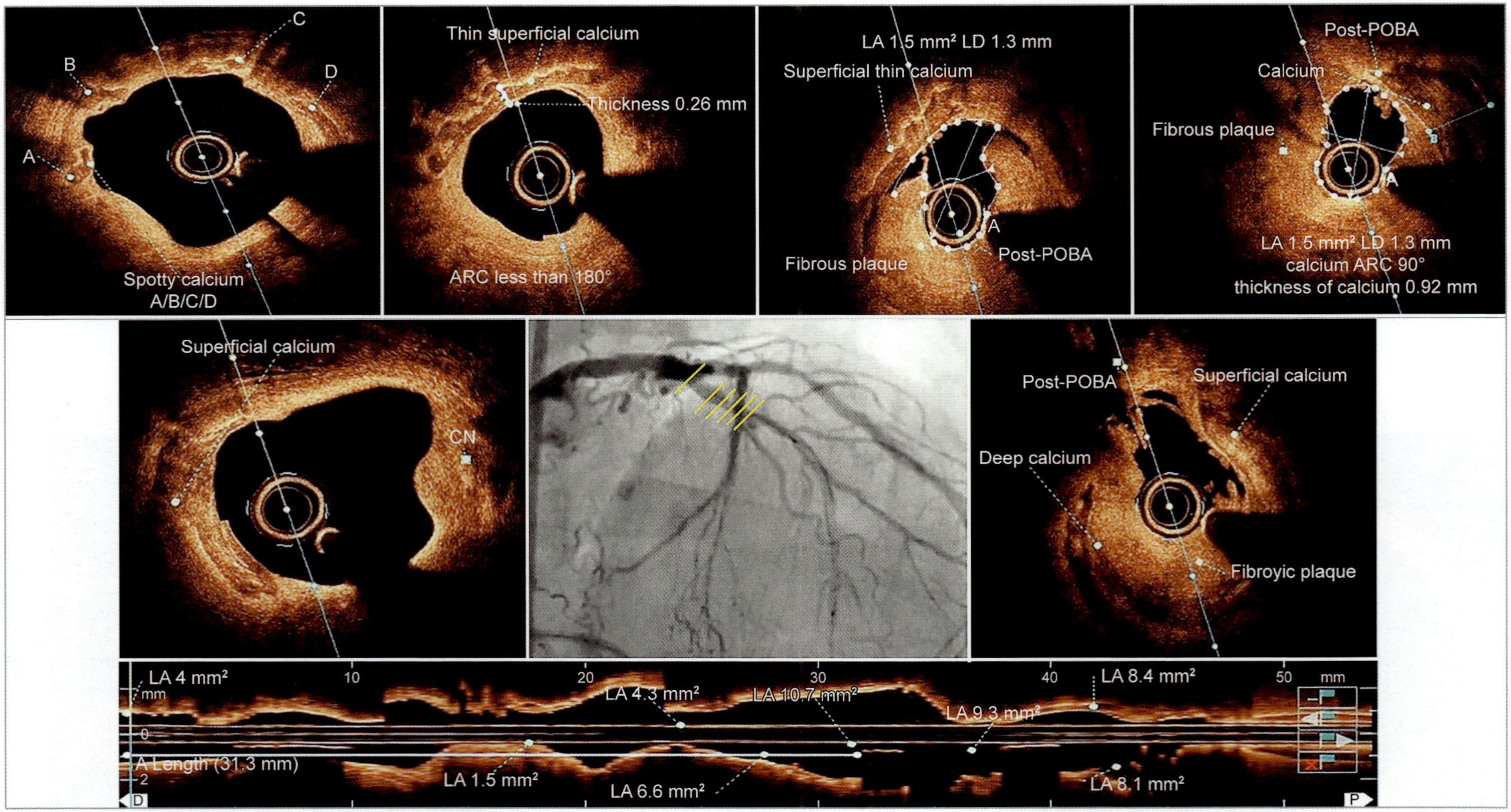
C
B
D
A
Spotty calcium
A/B/C/D
Thin superficial calcium
Thickness 0.26 mm
ARC less than 180°
LA 1.5 mm² LD 1.3 mm
Superficial thin calcium
A
Fibrous plaque
Post-POBA
Post-POBA
Calcium
Fibrous plaque
A
LA 1.5 mm² LD 1.3 mm
calcium ARC 90°
thickness of calcium 0.92 mm
Superficial calcium
CN
Post-POBA
Superficial calcium
Deep calcium
Fibroyic plaque
LA 4 mm²
LA 4.3 mm²
LA 10.7 mm²
LA 9.3 mm²
LA 8.4 mm²
A Length (31.3 mm)
LA 1.5 mm²
LA 6.6 mm²
LA 8.1 mm²

Fig. 44B

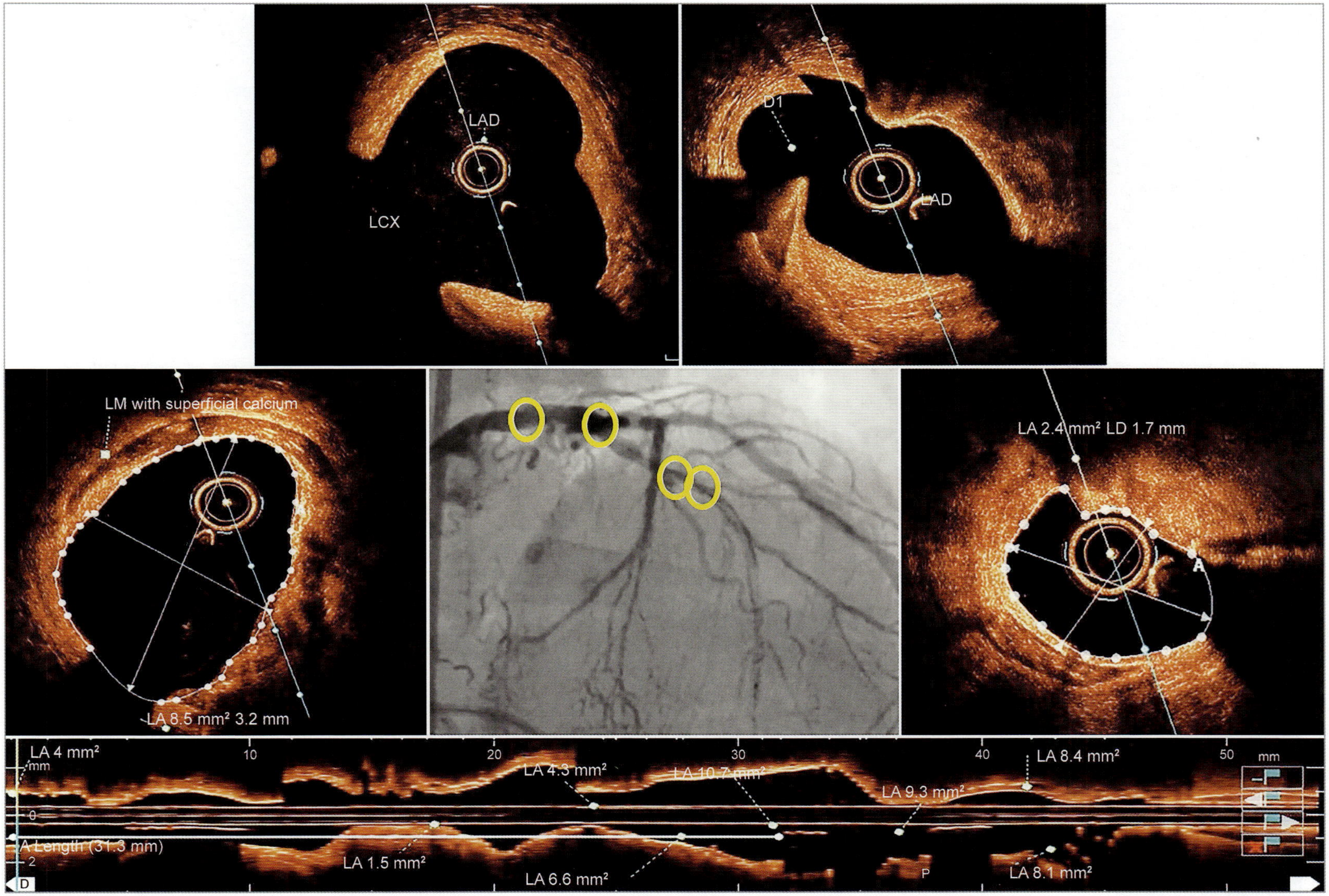

Fig. 44C

Figs. 44A to C: (A) Prestent OCT assessment for device selection; (B) Prestent OCT assessment showing fibrocalcific plaque; (C) OCT showing LM and LAD bifurcation zones.

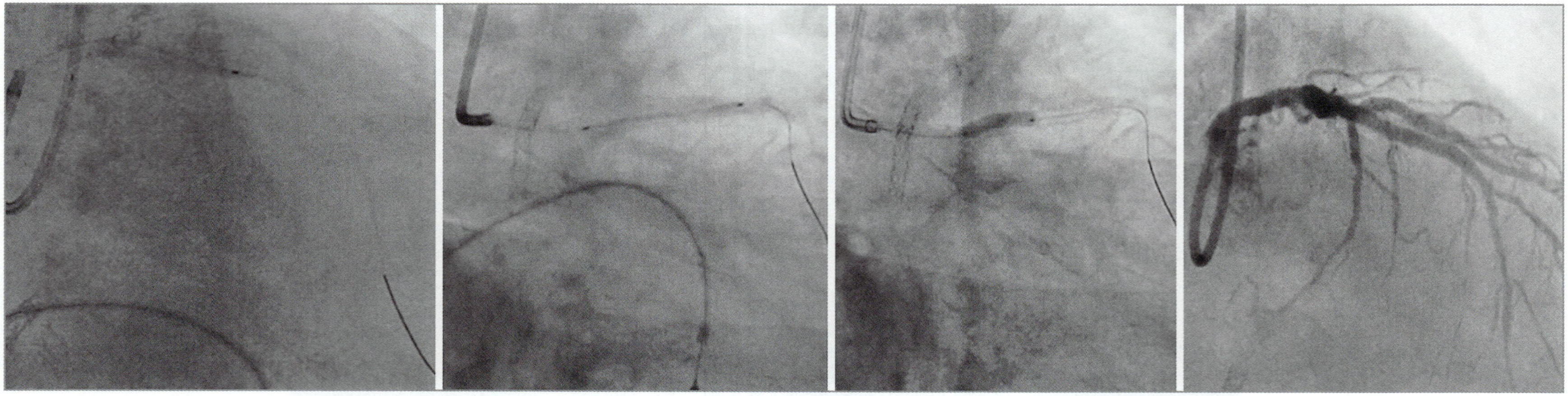

Fig. 45: Coronary angioplasty of LAD.

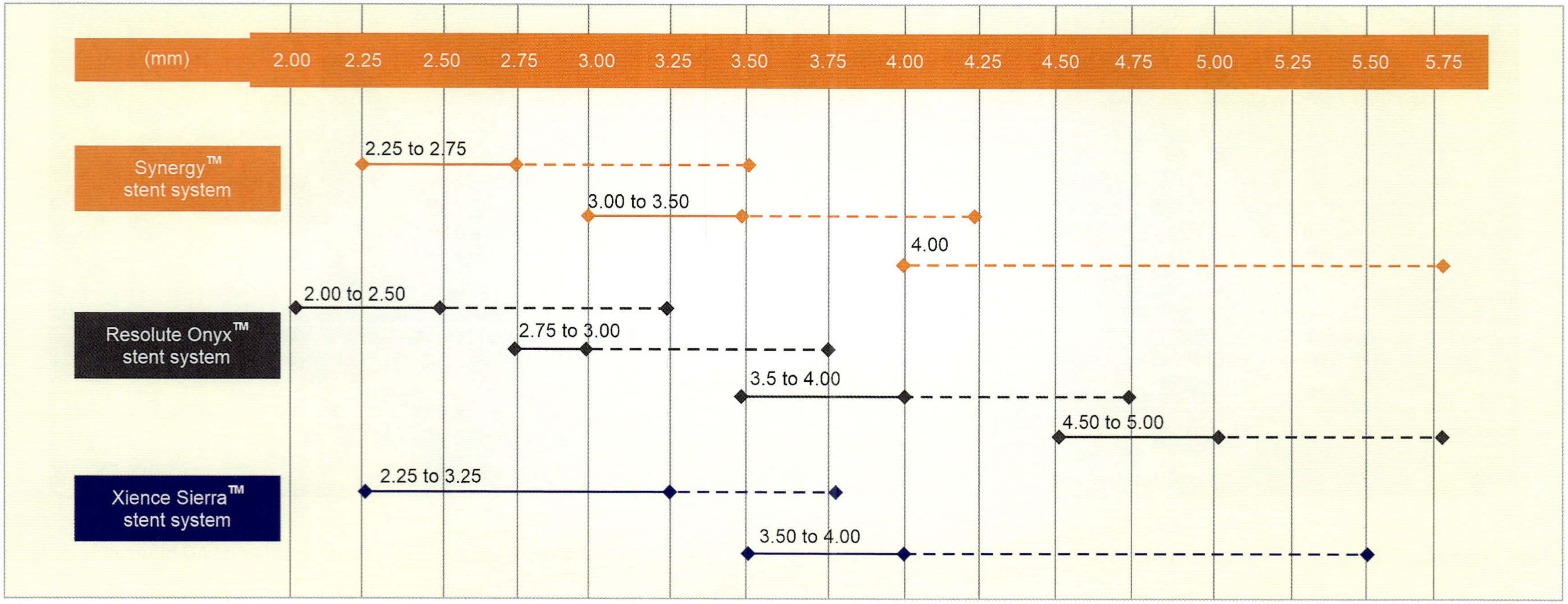

Fig 46: Stent expansion capability–1.
Source: https://www.bostonscientific.com/en-US/products/stents—coronary/synergy-megatron.html

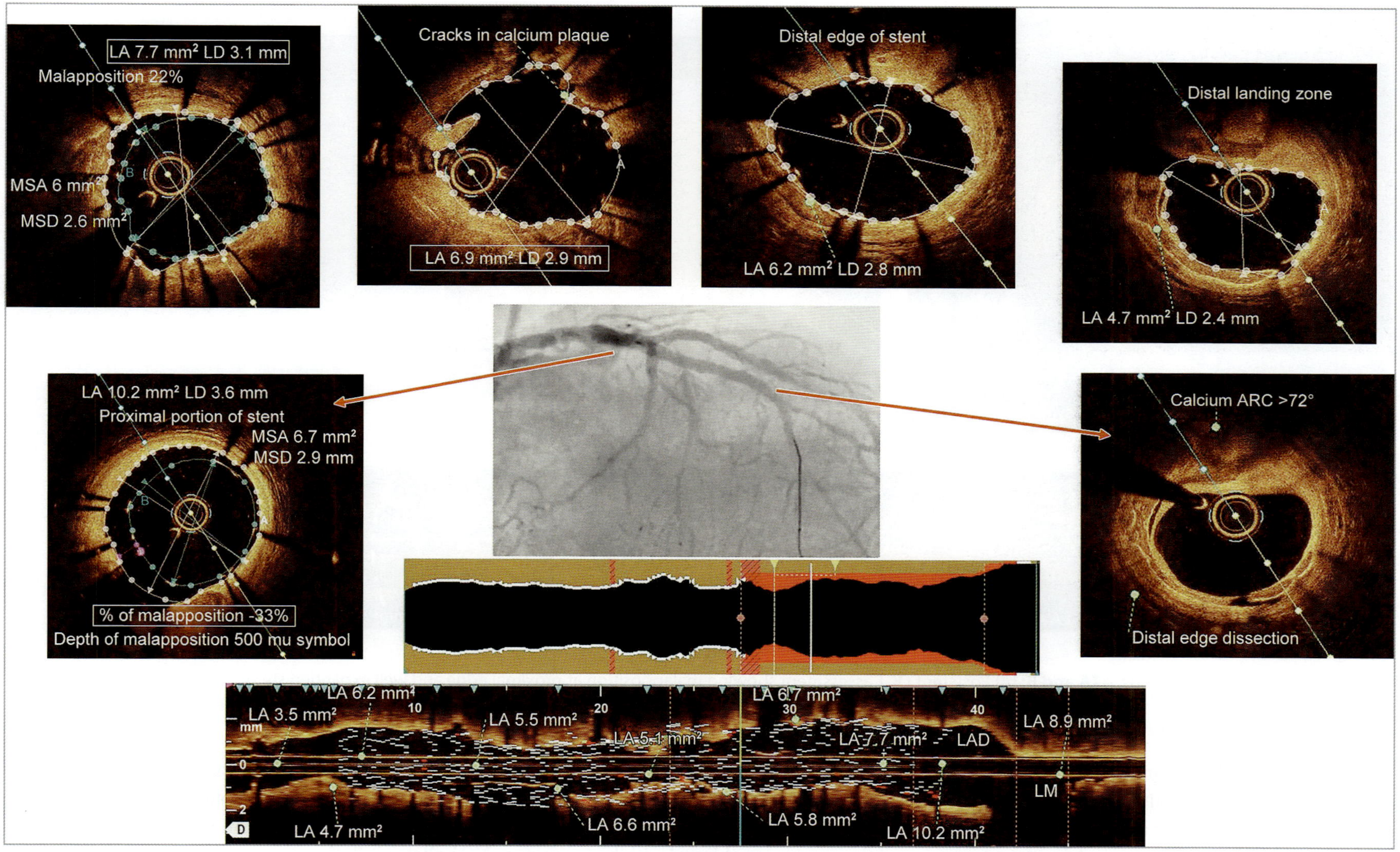

LA 7.7 mm² LD 3.1 mm
Malapposition 22%
MSA 6 mm²
MSD 2.6 mm²
Cracks in calcium plaque
LA 6.9 mm² LD 2.9 mm
Distal edge of stent
LA 6.2 mm² LD 2.8 mm
Distal landing zone
LA 4.7 mm² LD 2.4 mm
LA 10.2 mm² LD 3.6 mm
Proximal portion of stent
MSA 6.7 mm²
MSD 2.9 mm
% of malapposition -33%
Depth of malapposition 500 mu symbol
Calcium ARC >72°
Distal edge dissection
LA 6.2 mm²
LA 3.5 mm²
LA 5.5 mm²
LA 5.1 mm²
LA 6.7 mm²
LA 7.7 mm²
LAD
LA 8.9 mm²
LM
LA 4.7 mm²
LA 6.6 mm²
LA 5.8 mm²
LA 10.2 mm²

Fig. 47A

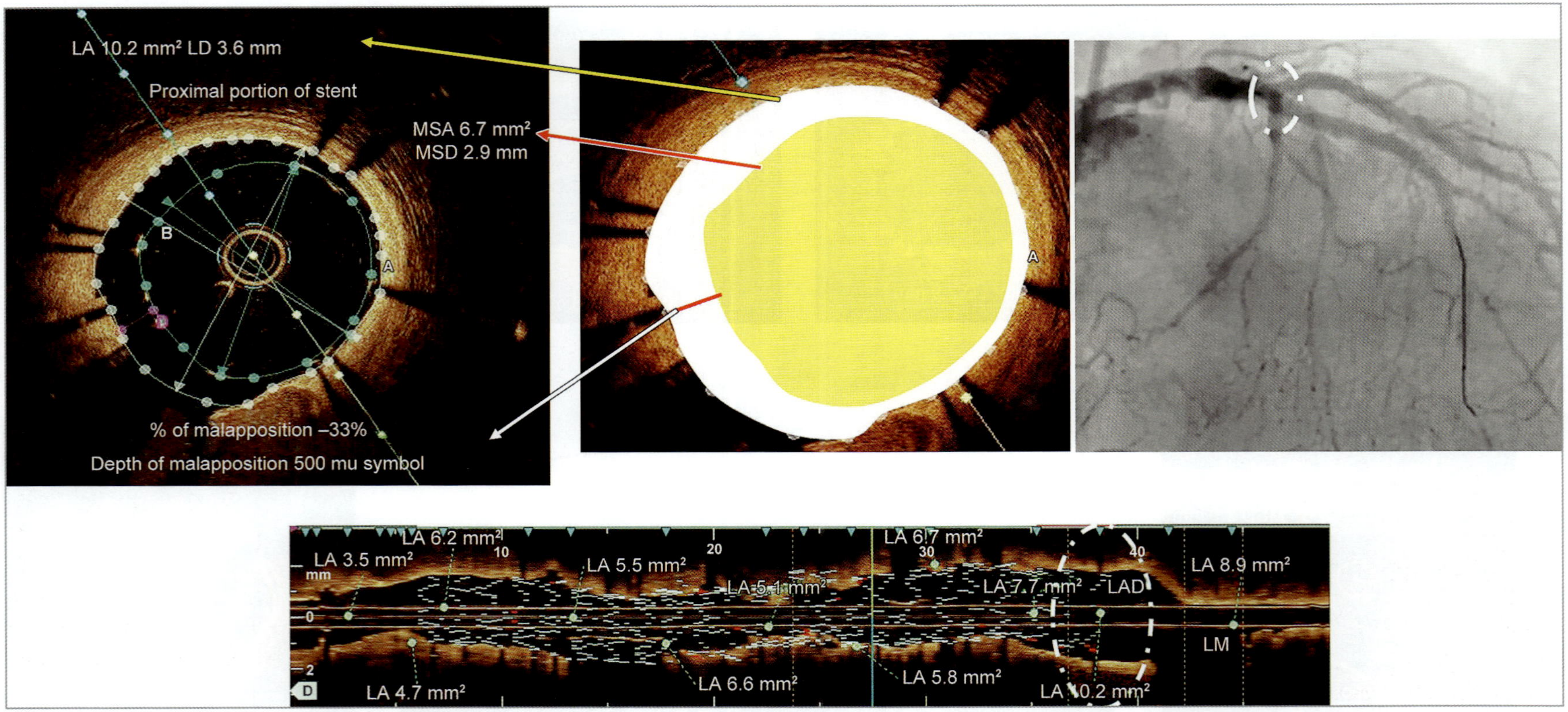

Fig. 47B

Figs. 47A and B: (A) Poststent OCT assessment showing malapposition at proximal edge and well expanded stent; (B) OCT assessment of malapposition which was corrected with upsized NC balloon.

Angiographic detection of calcium is associated with low sensitivity (45–50%) whereas OCT and IVUS is associated with sensitivity of 75–80% in identifying significantly calcified lesions. IVI assess the severity assessment and differentiating various types of coronary calcium such as superficial, deep calcium, and CN. Despite angiographic evidence of severe calcium, OCT guided us in avoiding ROTA for plaque modification which showed more of fibrotic tissue with deep calcium. Adequate expansion of the stent was achieved with high pressure NC balloon inflation.

CASE 8

PCI of diffusely calcified LAD.

CLINICAL HISTORY

A 69-year-old male known hypertensive, diabetic presented with anterior wall STEMI, associated with chest heaviness and shortness of breath. ECG—ST elevations in anterior leads. 2D echo—RWMA of anterior wall with mild LV dysfunction and EF—45%. *Investigations*: RBS—231 mg/dL, blood urea—26 mg/dL, serum creatinine—0.86 mg/dL, eGFR—88.

CAG-LMCA—mild distal disease, LAD—proximal to mid long segment severely calcified lesion, D1—50-60% lesion, LCX—normal, RCA—mild disease **(Fig. 48)**.

PROCEDURE

Route—RFA, 6 Fr XB 3.5 guiding catheter, LAD crossed with 0.014 Sion Blue Wire, 0.014 Versaturn wire placed in LCX. Preprocedure FFR to LCX showed negative (0.93). Pre-IVUS to LAD showed proximal to distal near about 270° calcium. ROTA floppy wire exchanged with microcatheter and 6 runs of 10–15 seconds rotablation at a speed of 1.5 lac rpm by using 1.5 mm ROTA burr **(Figs. 49A to D)**.

Post-ROTA OCT showed thick calcific plaque with thickness >1 mm in multiple areas, and no visible fractures despite plaque modification with multiple ROTA runs which indicates inadequate plaque modification requiring upsized ROTA bur or additional plaque modification with IVL or ELCA or high pressure OPN NC balloon. On the day of procedure there was no availability of 1.75 mm/2 mm burr, and IVL, hence we proceeded with DES implantation with an option of high pressure NC balloon inflation, and if needed OPN NC postdilatations at 45-50 atm **(Fig. 50)**.

Pre-OCT showed distal LMCA with MLA—11.1 mm^2, MLD—3.75 mm, ostial LAD with MLA—5.5 mm^2, MLD—2.6 mm, mid LAD with MLA—3.2 mm^2, MLD—2 mm and distal LAD with MLA—2.4 mm^2, MLD—1.7 mm.

Post-ROTA OCT showed dissection, >1 mm thick, >270° calcific plaque—no fractures, fibrous plaque with deep calcific plaque **(Fig. 50)**.

Distal LAD stenting done with 2.5 × 38 mm Promus Premier stent. LMCA to proximal LAD stenting done with 3.5 × 38 mm Promus Premier stent. LM POT was done with 4.0 × 8 mm NC and LAD postdilatation done with 3.0 × 10 mm OPN NC balloon to correct the underexpansion of the LAD stent. LMCA POT done with 4.5 × 8 mm NC Trek balloon to correct the malapposition of the LM stent at the ostio-proximal site.

Rotablation of LAD done with 1.5 mm burr, stenting done with 2.5 × 38 mm Promus Premier stent with GuideLiner support, LMCA—proximal LAD was stented with 3.5 × 38 mm Promus Premier stent with GuideLiner support **(Fig. 51)**, poststenting check Angio-persistent waist in distal portion of the proximal stent, postdilatation done with 3.0 × 10 mm OPN NC balloon, LMCA POT done with 4.5 × 8 mm NC Trek balloon. In view of inadequate plaque modification with ROTA resulted in underexpansion of distal portion of LAD stent which was postdilated with 3 mm NC high pressure inflation at 22 atm.

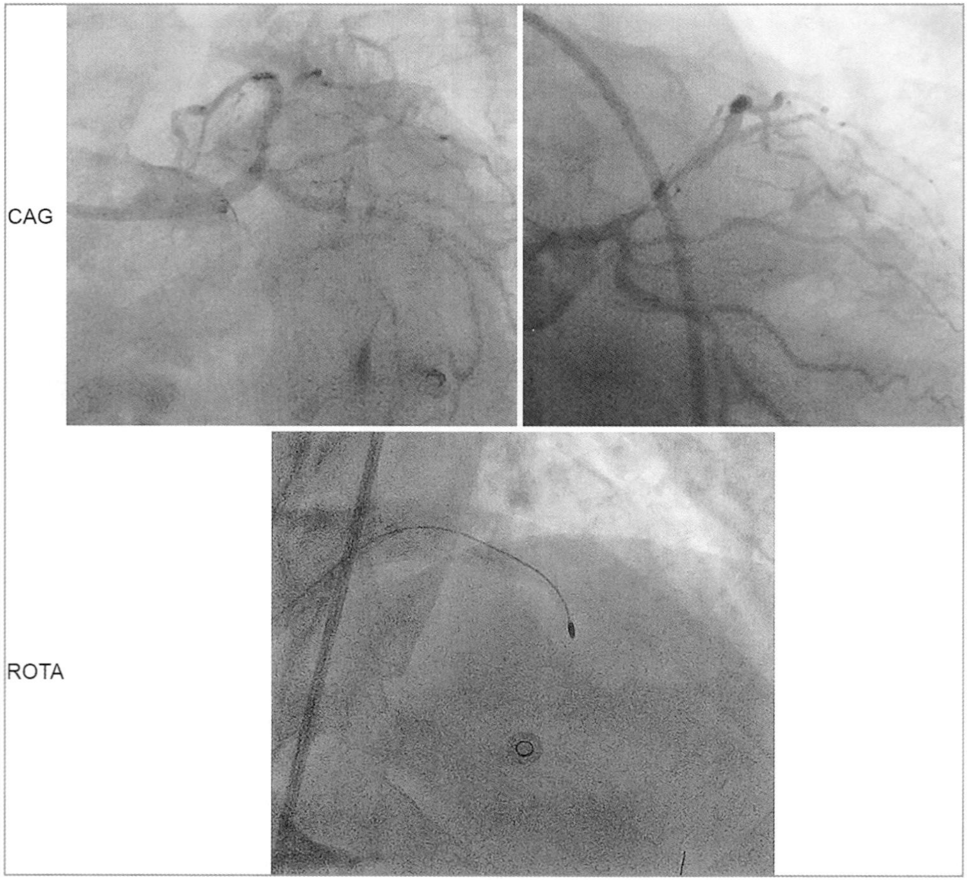

Fig. 48: Coronary angiogram and rotablation.

Despite high pressure underexpanded stent segment was not yielding with NC at 22 atm, hence opted for high pressure OPN NC balloon inflation at 45 atm which resulted in adequate expansion **(Figs. 52A to C)**.

Post-OCT Analysis

Post-OCT showed distal landing zone with MLA—5.3 mm^2, MLD—2.6 mm, mid portion of the stent with MLA—8.5 mm^2, MLD—3.3 mm, LMCA with MLA—11.5 mm^2, MLD—3.8 mm, post-OCT showed underexpansions due to calcium plaque with MLA—4.2 mm^2, MLD—2.3 mm, arc >180° and MLA—3.5 mm^2, arc >270°. Post-OCT showed malapposition near LMCA ostium with MLA—17 mm^2, MLD—4.7 mm, mean diameter 4.68 mm **(Figs. 52A to C)**.

OCT also revealed LMCA significant malapposition which was rectified with 4.5 mm NC balloon. Postprocedure Angio view showed well-implanted stents with TIMI-III flow without any dissection. Patient was discharged on third postprocedure in a stable status.

Postprocedure side branch (LCX) FFR study showed negative, hence LCX stenting avoided **(Fig. 53)**. Postprocedure Angio view showed well-implanted stents with TIMI-III flow without any dissection. Patient was discharged on third postprocedure in a stable status.

Preprocedural OCT showed severe circumferential calcium with expansion index of 4, decision of plaque modification with ROTA was made using 1.5 burr. Despite adequate rotablation with multiple runs post-ROTA OCT did not reveal any calcium fractures and thickness of calcium was >1 mm in multiple areas suggesting inadequate rotablation. In such circumstances, better to upsize the burr, otherwise underexpansion of the stent is expected.

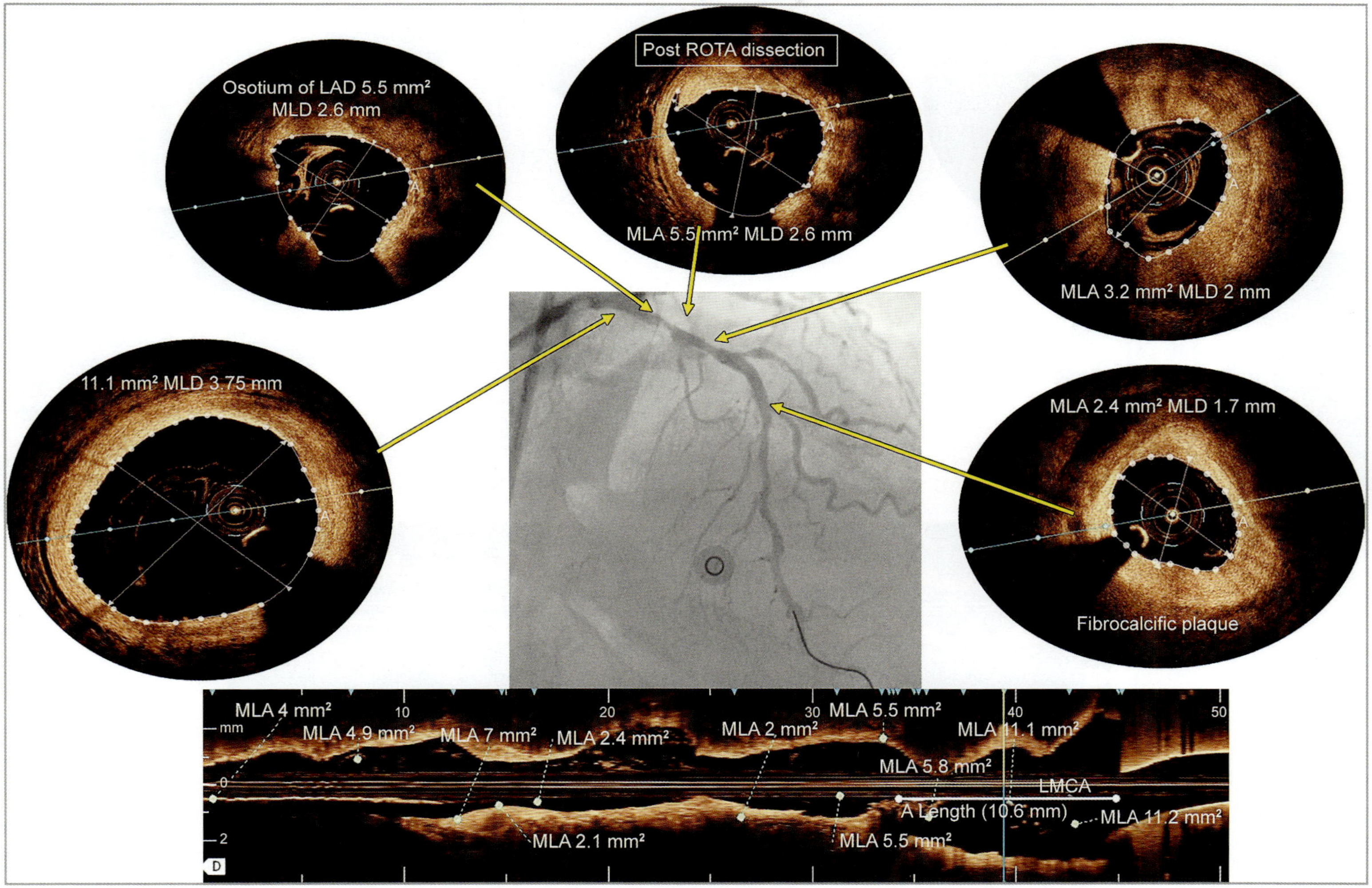

Fig. 49A

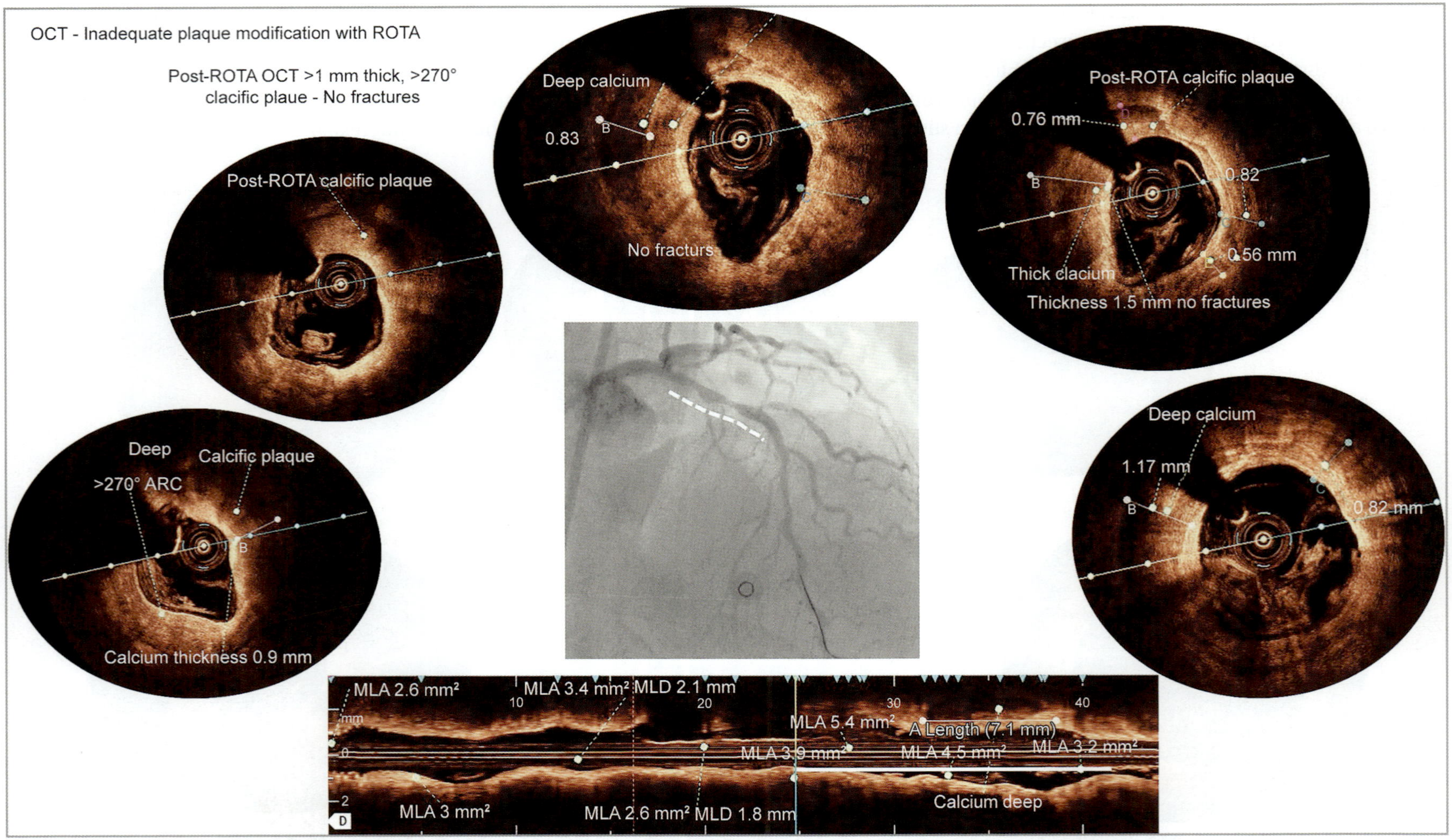
OCT - Inadequate plaque modification with ROTA
Post-ROTA OCT >1 mm thick, >270°
clacific plaue - No fractures
Deep calcium
0.83
No fracturs
Post-ROTA calcific plaque
0.76 mm
0.82
0.56 mm
Thick clacium
Thickness 1.5 mm no fractures
Post-ROTA calcific plaque
Deep
Calcific plaque
>270° ARC
Calcium thickness 0.9 mm
Deep calcium
1.17 mm
0.82 mm
MLA 2.6 mm²
MLA 3.4 mm² MLD 2.1 mm
MLA 5.4 mm²
A Length (7.1 mm)
MLA 3.9 mm²
MLA 4.5 mm²
MLA 3.2 mm²
MLA 3 mm²
MLA 2.6 mm² MLD 1.8 mm
Calcium deep

Fig. 49B

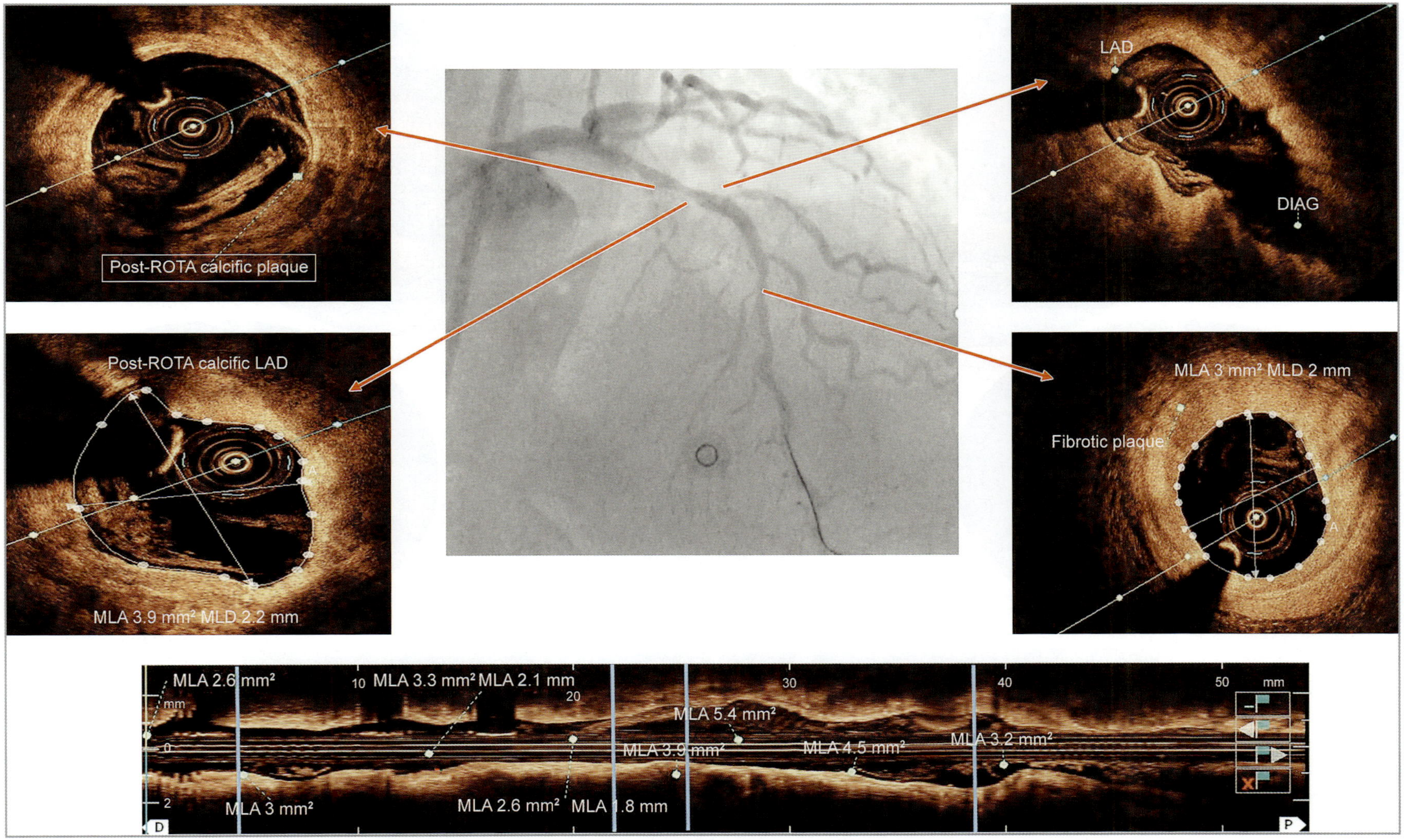
Post-ROTA calcific plaque
LAD
DIAG
Post-ROTA calcific LAD
MLA 3.9 mm² MLD 2.2 mm
MLA 3 mm² MLD 2 mm
Fibrotic plaque
MLA 2.6 mm²
MLA 3.3 mm² MLA 2.1 mm
MLA 5.4 mm²
MLA 3.9 mm²
MLA 4.5 mm²
MLA 3.2 mm²
MLA 3 mm²
MLA 2.6 mm² MLA 1.8 mm

Fig. 49C

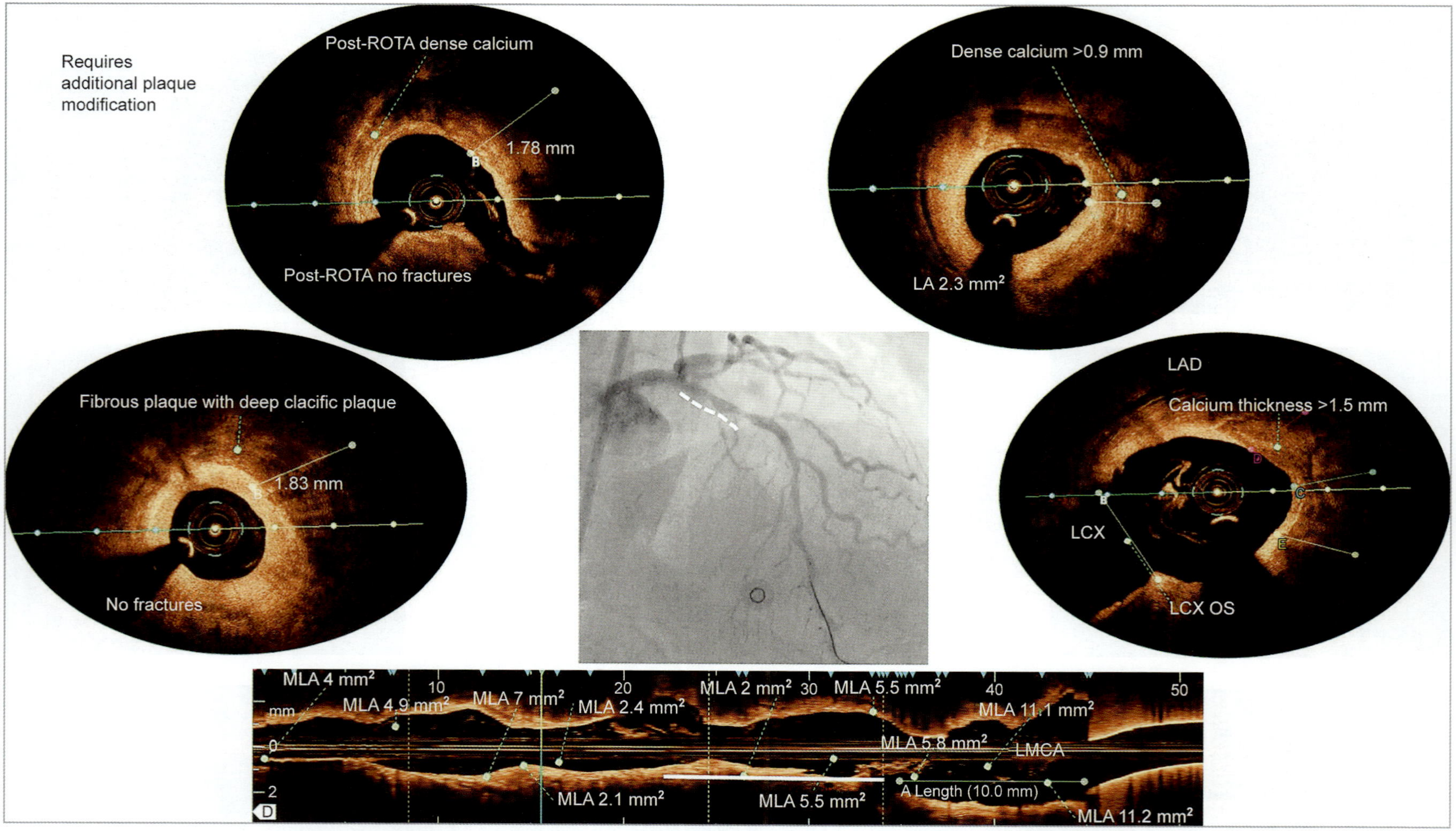

Fig. 49D

Figs. 49A to D: Presenting OCT assessment. (A) For devise selection; (B to D) Calcium assessment.

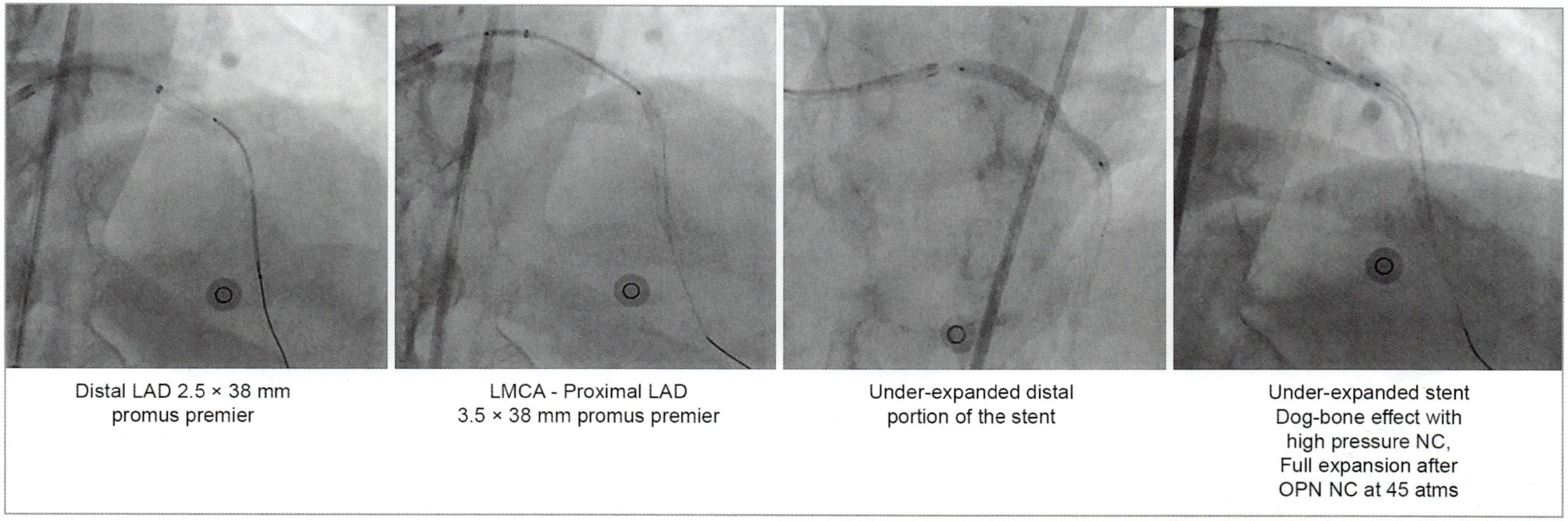

Fig. 50: Coronary angioplasty. Underexpansion even after plaque modification with ROTA. Corrected with OPN NC balloon.

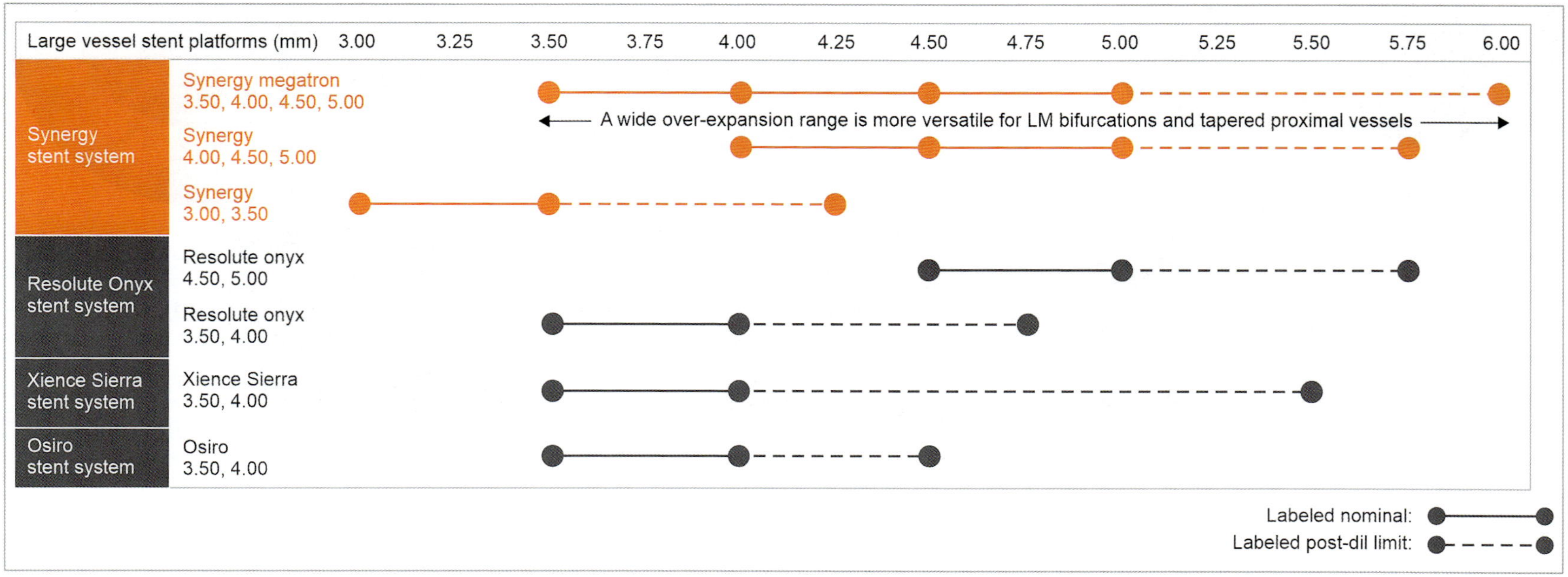

Fig. 51: Stent expansion capability–2.
Source: https://www.bostonscientific.com/en-US/products/stents—coronary/synergy-megatron.html.

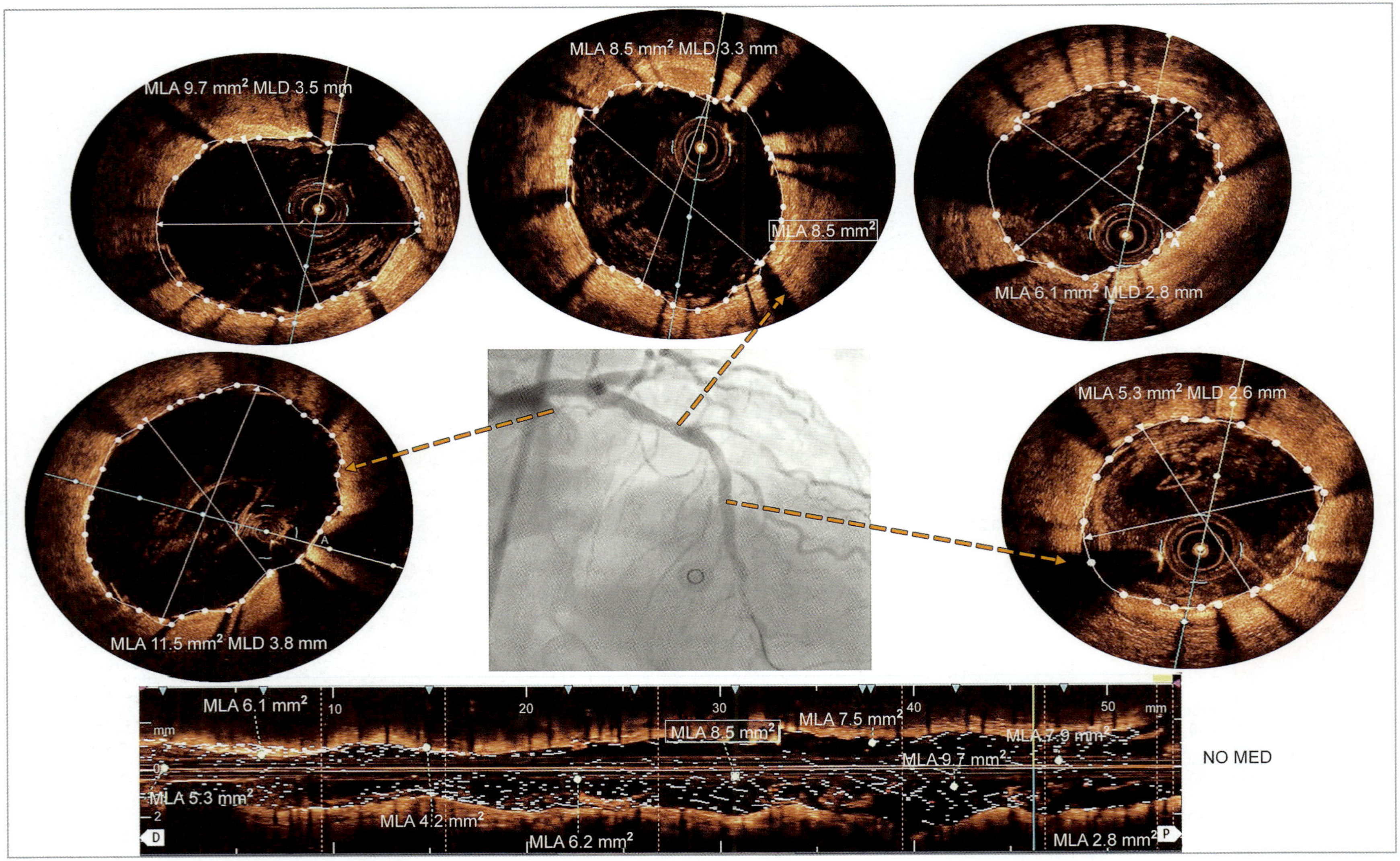
MLA 9.7 mm² MLD 3.5 mm
MLA 8.5 mm² MLD 3.3 mm
MLA 8.5 mm²
MLA 6.1 mm² MLD 2.8 mm
MLA 11.5 mm² MLD 3.8 mm
MLA 5.3 mm² MLD 2.6 mm
MLA 6.1 mm²
MLA 8.5 mm²
MLA 7.5 mm²
MLA 7.9 mm²
MLA 9.7 mm²
MLA 5.3 mm²
MLA 4.2 mm²
MLA 6.2 mm²
MLA 2.8 mm²
10
20
30
40
50
mm
D
P
NO MED

Fig. 52A

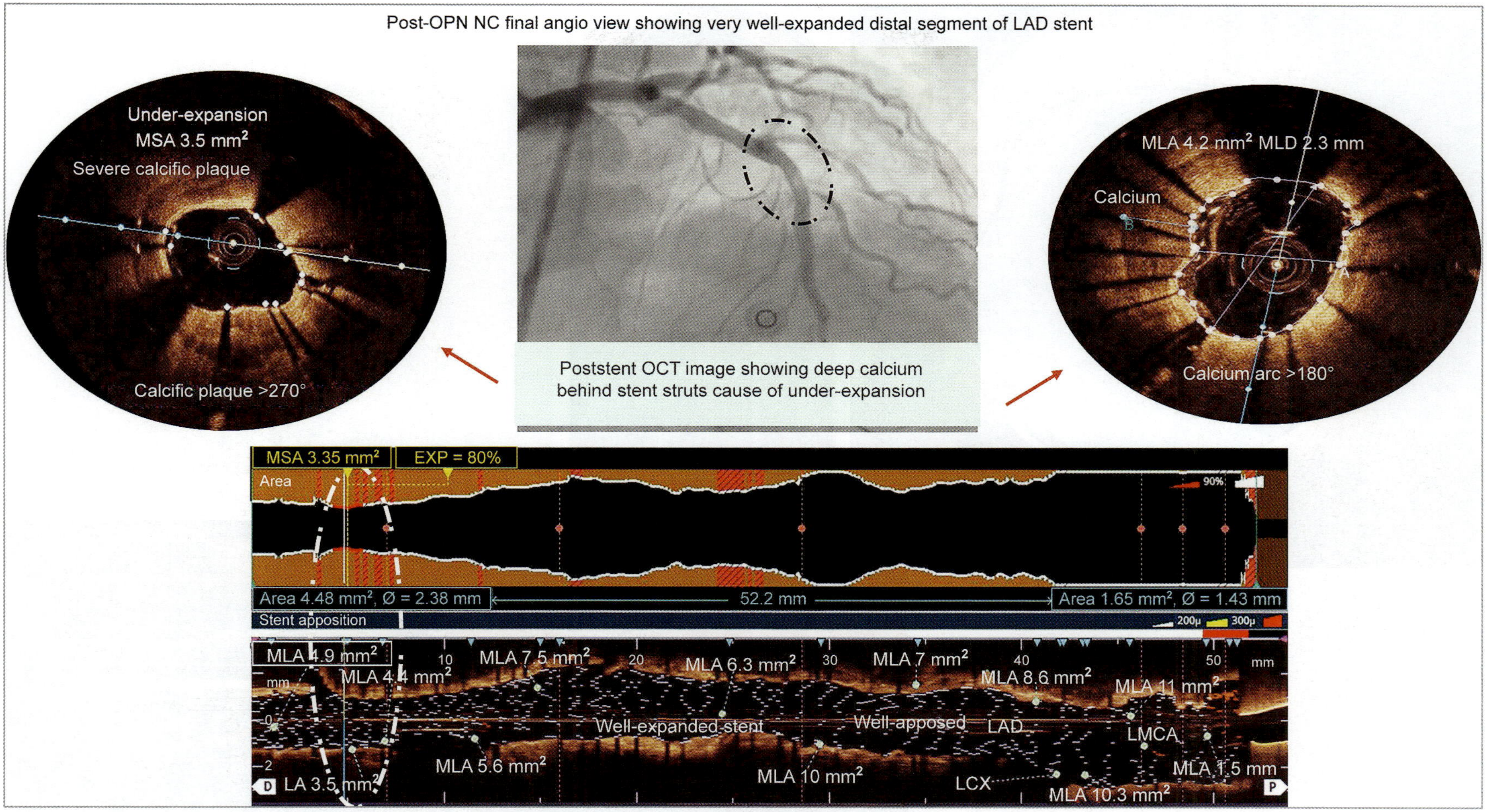
Post-OPN NC final angio view showing very well-expanded distal segment of LAD stent
Under-expansion
MSA 3.5 mm²
Severe calcific plaque
Calcific plaque >270°
Poststent OCT image showing deep calcium behind stent struts cause of under-expansion
MLA 4.2 mm² MLD 2.3 mm
Calcium
Calcium arc >180°
MSA 3.35 mm²
EXP = 80%
Area
Area 4.48 mm², Ø = 2.38 mm
52.2 mm
Area 1.65 mm², Ø = 1.43 mm
Stent apposition
MLA 4.9 mm²
MLA 4.4 mm²
MLA 7.5 mm²
MLA 6.3 mm²
MLA 7 mm²
MLA 8.6 mm²
MLA 11 mm²
Well-expanded stent
Well-apposed
LAD
LMCA
MLA 5.6 mm²
MLA 10 mm²
LCX
MLA 1.5 mm
LA 3.5 mm²
MLA 10.3 mm²

Fig. 52B

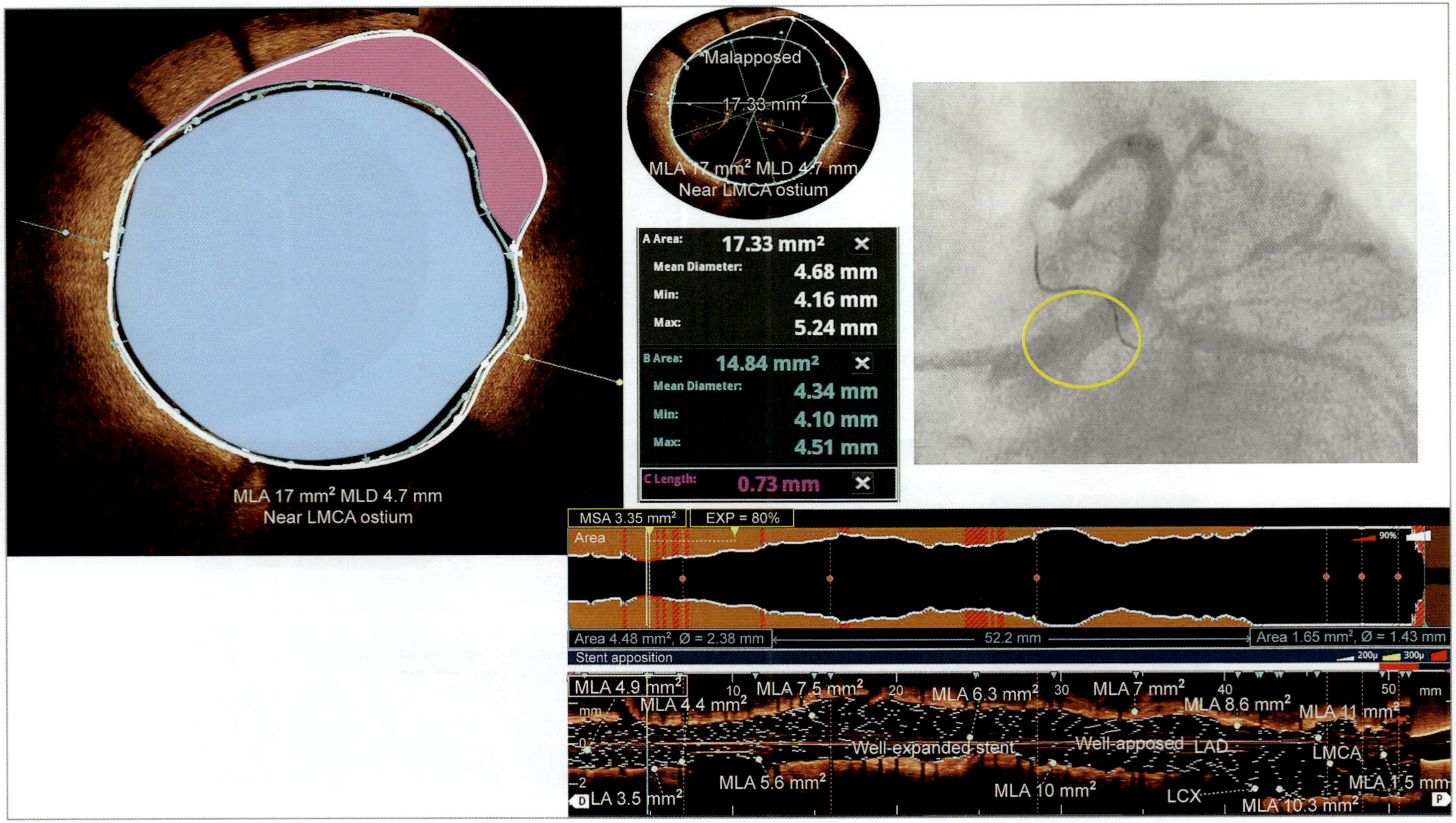

Fig. 52C

Figs. 52A to C: Poststenting OCT assessment. (A) For any for medial edge dissections; (B) Detection of underexpansion; (C) Detection of malapposition at proximal edge.

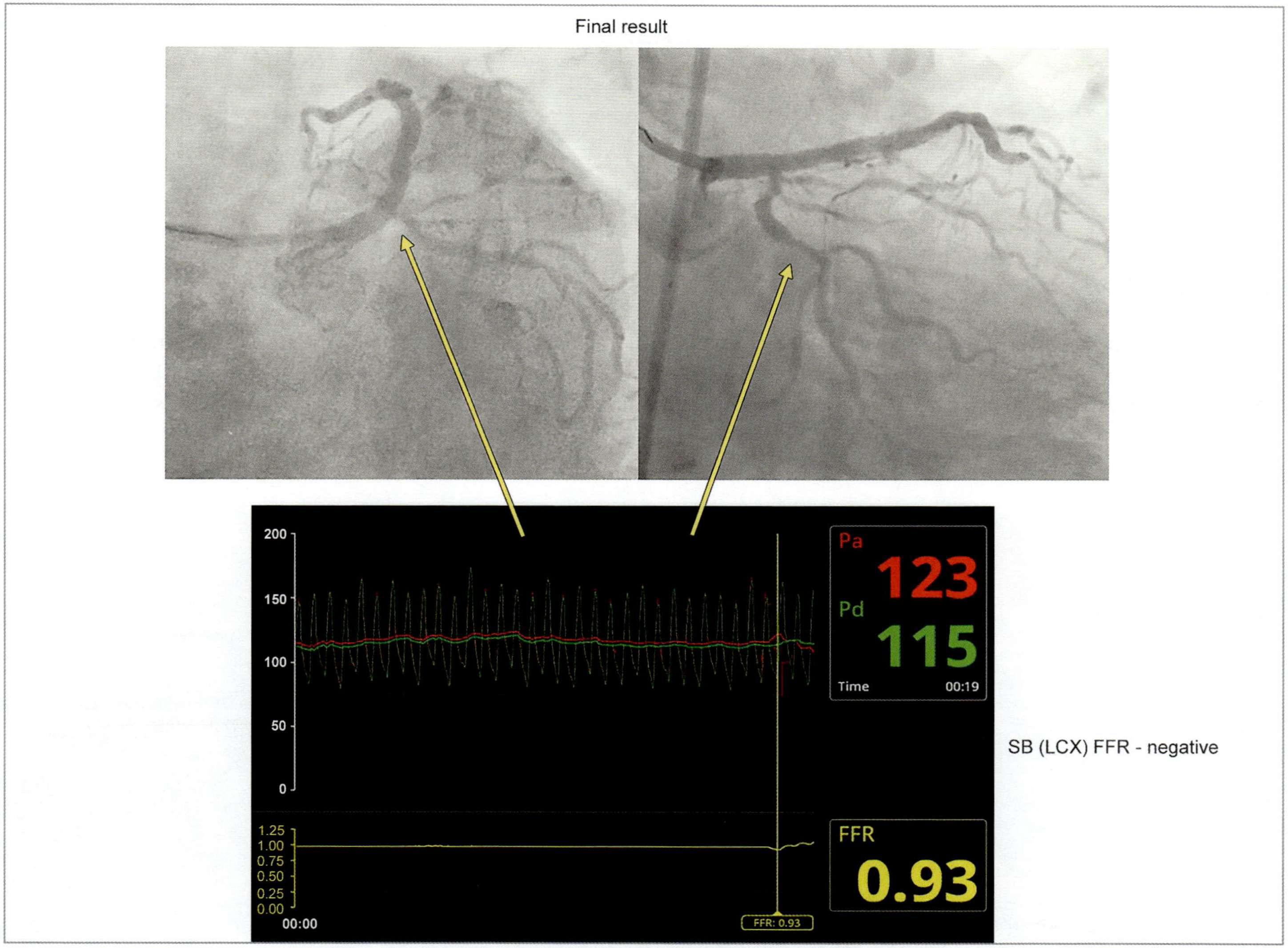

Fig. 53: FFR to study to side branch (LCX) and final result.

The presence of a critical stenosis at one branch can divert flow more to the other branch and influence FFR value (branch steal phenomenon).

As long as the stenosis in the LAD or LCx is not very tight (FFR <0.60), it hardly influences the FFR value of the LM.

CASE 9

Assessment of calcium.

CLINICAL HISTORY

A 71-year-old male known hypertensive, diabetic presented with chest discomfort. Past history of CAG-DVD with PCI of LAD in 2019 (3.0 × 34 mm Resolute Onyx) and admitted for PCI of RCA. ECG—normal, 2D echo no RWMA, good LV function with EF 62%, TMT revealed positive for inducible ischemia. *Investigations*: Hb—12.6 g/dL, RBS—205 mg/dL, HbA1C—6.4%, serum creatinine—0.8 mg/dL with eGFR—89 mL/min. CAG showed severe calcified RCA **(Fig. 54)**.

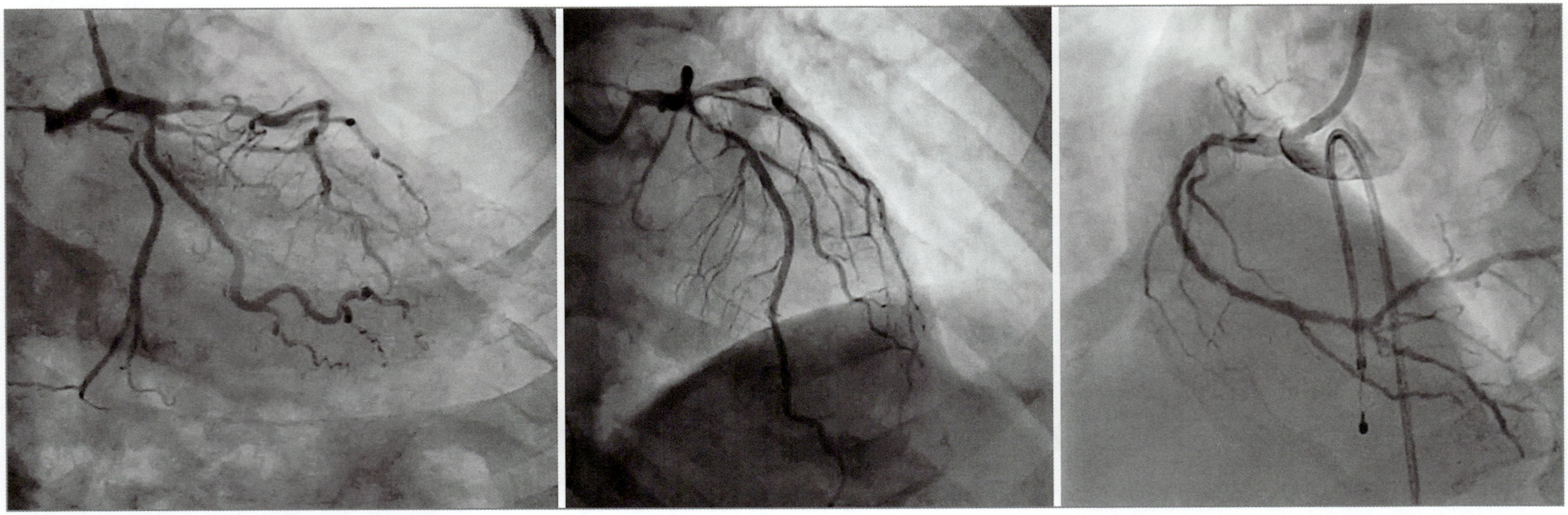

Fig. 54: Coronary angiogram.

PROCEDURE

Route—right radial approach using JR 3.5–7 Fr guiding catheter, TPI through right femoral vein approach, lesion crossed with 0.014" Turntrac wire, then exchanged with Sion Blue Wire. Later Sion Blue Wire exchanged with RotaWire using microcatheter support. Rotablation done with 1.5 mm burr at 160,000 rpm (5 runs). Predilatation done with 2.5 × 18 mm NC Trek balloon **(Flowchart 2)**.

Post-ROTA OCT study showed multiple fractures of calcium plaque and calcium nodule **(Figs. 55A and B)**.

Predilatation done with 3.0 × 15 mm NC Trek balloon. Mid RCA stenting done with 3.0 × 30 mm Resolute Onyx stent, proximal RCA stenting done with 3.5 × 38 mm Resolute Onyx stent with GuideLiner support. Postdilatation done with 3.5 × 12 mm NC Trek balloon **(Fig. 57)**.

Post-OCT showed well-expanded stent struts **(Fig. 56A)** and fibrotic calcified lesion in distal RCA to PLVB **(Fig. 56B)**.

Distal RCA to PLVB predilatation done with 2.0 × 18 mm Tazuna balloon. Distal RCA stenting done with 2.25 × 30 mm Resolute Onyx stent. Postprocedure Angio view showed well-implanted stents with TIMI-III flow without any dissection. Patient was discharged on third postprocedure day in a stable status.

Rotablation done with 1.5 mm burr at 160,000 rpm (5 runs), predilatation done with 2.5 × 18 mm NC Trek balloon, Mid RCA stenting done with 3.0 × 30 mm Resolute Onyx stent, proximal RCA stenting done with 3.5 × 38 mm Resolute Onyx stent, check Angio, distal RCA to PLVB predilatation done with 2.0 × 18 mm Tazuna balloon, distal RCA stenting done with 2.25 × 30 mm Resolute Onyx stent, final result **(Fig. 57)**.

PCI of calcified coronary artery throws many challenges despite usage of rotablation for plaque modification. Patient required Guidezilla support for placing stents in RCA, postproximal to mid RCA stent OCT image showed diffuse long lesion of distal RCA extending to PLV requiring additional distal stent to cover disease segment of distal RCA. OCT run reveals position and size of the Guidezilla at the ostium of RCA. Guidezilla/GuideLiner will be very useful in placing OCT catheter in tortuous/vessels with acute angles to get adequate OCT images.

Flowchart 2: Algorithmic approach in case of failure to advance a balloon or stent into the main branch or side branch of a coronary bifurcation.

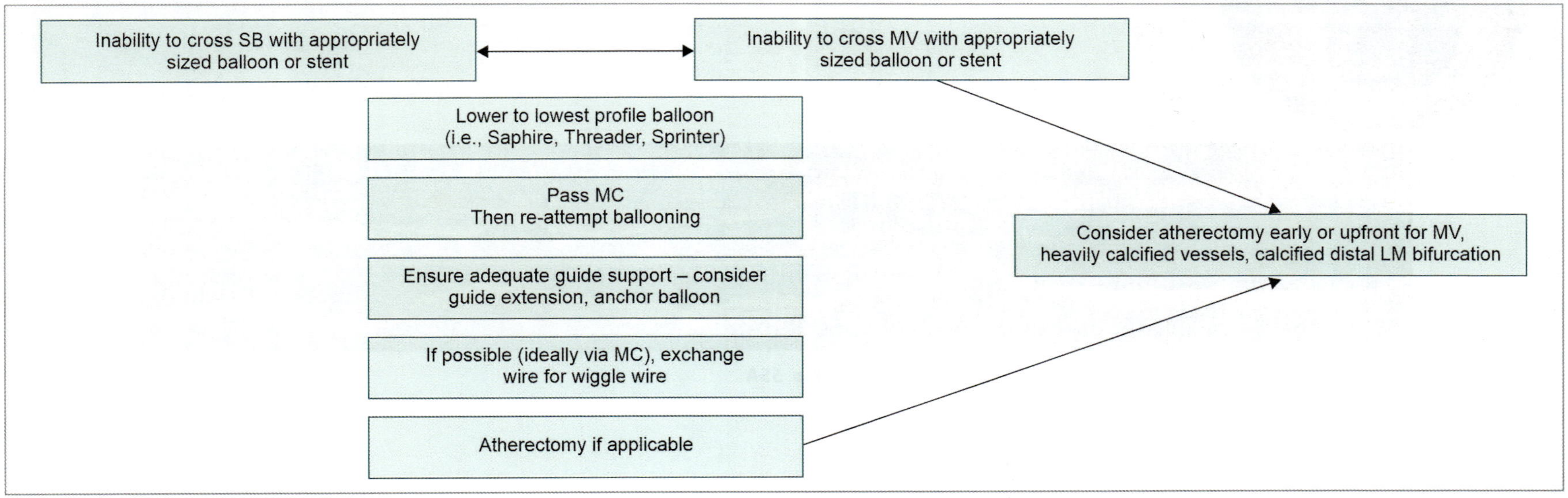

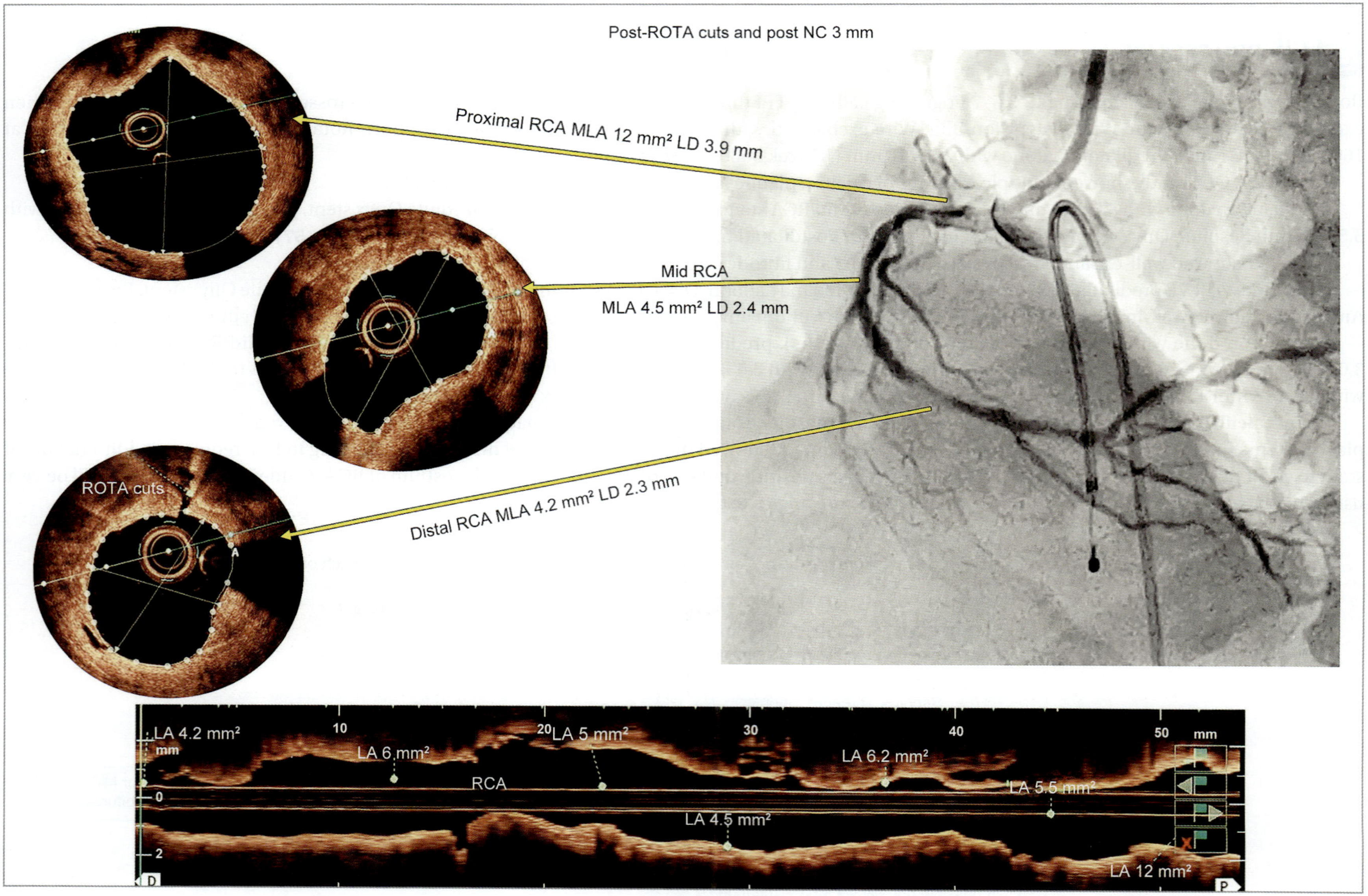
Post-ROTA cuts and post NC 3 mm
Proximal RCA MLA 12 mm² LD 3.9 mm
Mid RCA
MLA 4.5 mm² LD 2.4 mm
ROTA cuts
Distal RCA MLA 4.2 mm² LD 2.3 mm
LA 4.2 mm²
LA 6 mm²
LA 5 mm²
LA 6.2 mm²
LA 5.5 mm²
LA 4.5 mm²
LA 12 mm²
RCA
10
20
30
40
50
mm
0
2
D
P

Fig. 55A

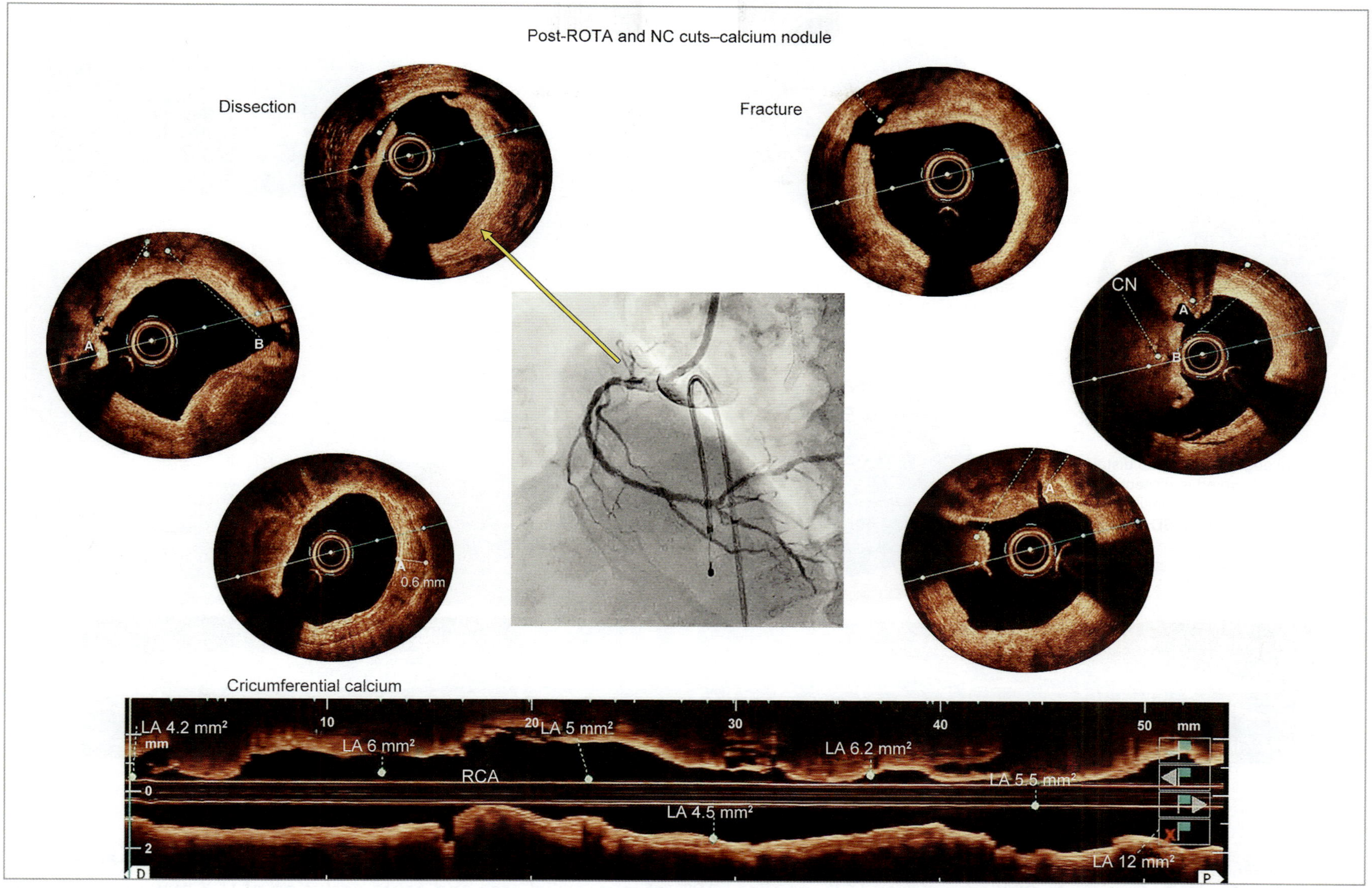

Fig. 55B

Figs. 55A and B: (A) Post-ROTA OCT assessment showing ROTA cuts and measurements for selection of the stent; (B) OCT showing post-ROTA cuts and calcium nodule.

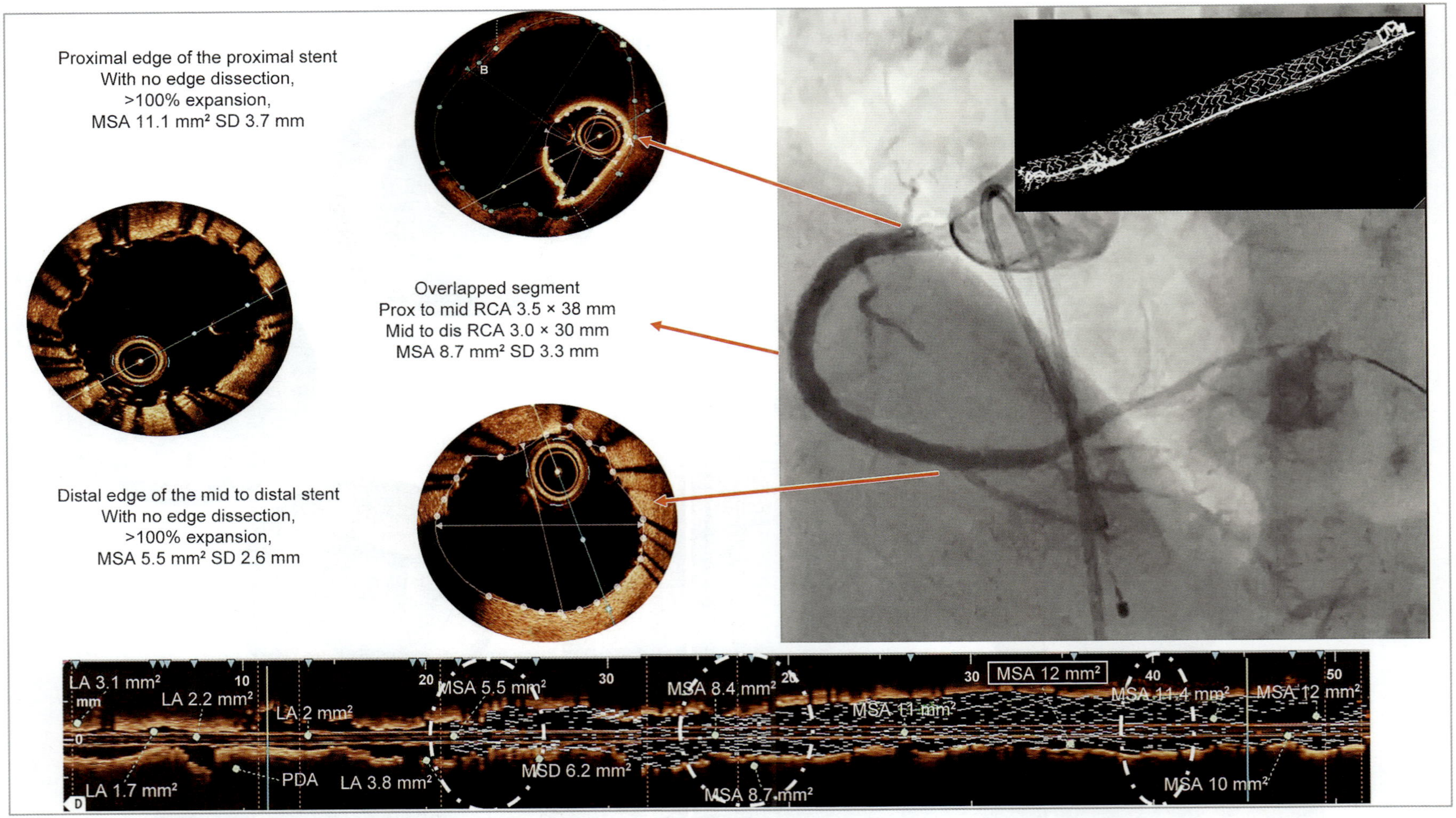

Fig. 56A

In LM cases, the SB is the circumflex artery (LCX) in most instances. It generally has a large diameter and is not always easily accessible, especially after MB stenting. In 90% of patients, LCX supplies >10% of myocardial area and acute occlusion of LCX may lead to acute severe ischemic MR with acute pulmonary oedema contributing to high morbidity and mortalitype text here

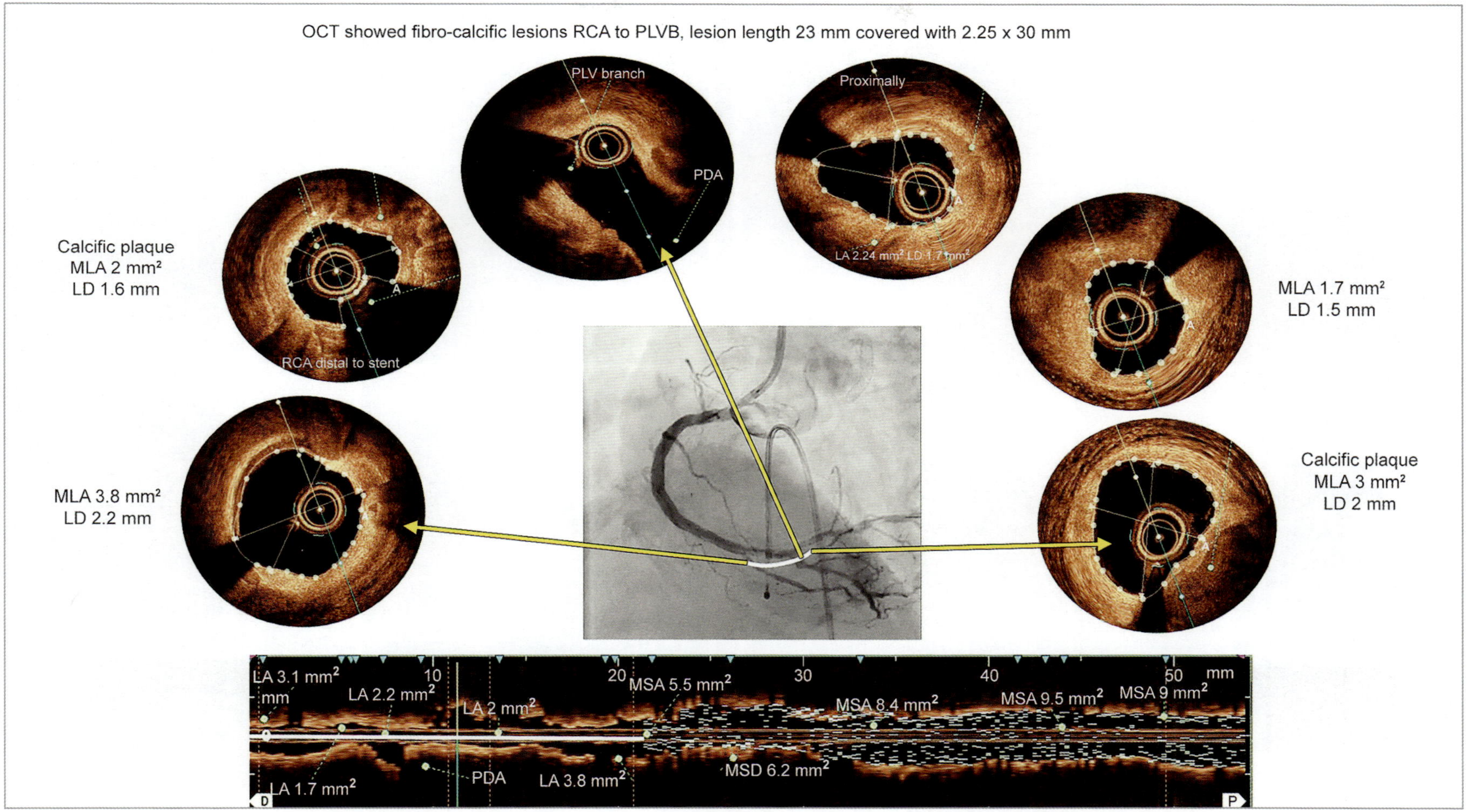

Fig. 56B

Figs. 56A and B: (A) Post-RCA stent OCT assessment showing well expanded and apposed stent struts; (B) OCT showing fibrocalcific lesions at distal RCA and PLVB.

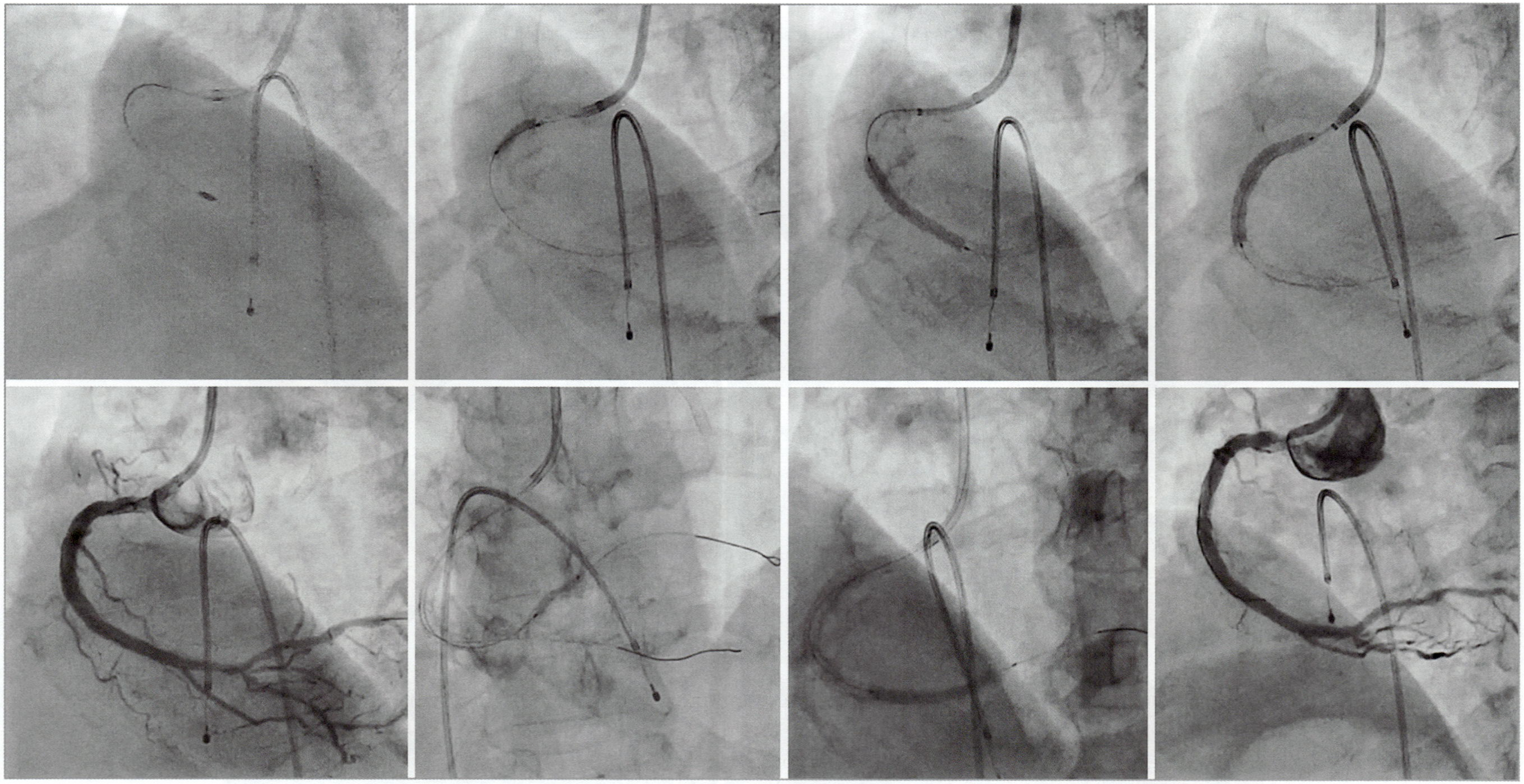

Fig. 57: Coronary angioplasty of RCA and PLVB.

Mechanism of Actions of Rotablation (RA) and Orbital Atherectomy (OA)

RA	*OA*
Diamond-tipped burr spins concentrically on the wire	Eccentrically mounted diamond coated crown uses centrifugal force
Athero-ablation via differential cutting	Athero-ablation via differential sanding
Particle size (5–10 μm)	Particle size (<2 μm)

CASE 10

Poststenting OCT assessment of eccentric calcium of LAD lesion.

CLINICAL HISTORY

A 64-year-old female known diabetic and hypertensive presented with CAD—USA, S/P CAG—TVD, ECG—NSR, no significant ST-T changes, 2D echo—good LV function.

Investigations: Hb—8.2 g/dL (corrected with 3 PRBC units, Post-Hb—11.0 g/dL), Trop I—4.26 ng/mL, serum creatinine—0.65 mg/dL, eGFR—99 mL/min, NT-proBNP—3,672 pg/mL. CAG shows LMCA normal, proximal to mid LAD eccentric calcified lesion, ostio-proximal LCX 90% stenosis, OM1 proximal 70% lesion, RCA—chronic total occlusion **(Fig. 58)**.

LCA engaged with XB 3.5–7 Fr guiding catheter, 0.014″ Runthrough wire placed in OM1 and 0.014″ Versaturn wire placed in LCX and 0.014″ BMW wire placed in LAD. OM predilated with 1.5 × 10 mm and 2.25 × 10 mm Tazuna balloons. Then OM distal stenting was done with 2.25 × 22 mm Resolute Onyx stent. Postdilatation done with 2.5 × 12 mm NC Trek balloon, proximal LCX stented with 3.0 × 15 mm Resolute Onyx and crushed with 3.0 × 12 mm NC balloon placing in LAD **(Fig. 58)**. Predilatation of proximal calcified LAD tried with 2.5 × 10 mm Tazuna which was undilatable (dog bone effect) due to severely calcified lesion, hence predilatations were carried out with 2.5 × 10 mm OPN NC at 45 atm which was ruptured, reattempted with another 2.5 × 15 mm OPN NC at 45 atm that is also ruptured, finally 3.0 × 15 mm OPN NC balloon was used with Guidezilla support to dilate undilatable LAD lesion with adequate dilatation of LMCA and proximal to mid LAD. LMCA to LAD stenting was done with 3.0 × 38 mm Resolute Onyx and POT of LMCA was performed with 4.5 × 8 mm NC balloon and DOT of LAD with 3.5 × 12 mm NC Trek balloon **(Fig. 59)**. LCX struts crossed with Fielder FC wire and opened with 0.85 × 10 mm Nick Nano balloon and 1.5 × 10 mm Tazuna balloon, but failed attempt to cross LCX ostium with 3 mm NC. Failed Reattempt to place NC balloon after performing re-POT of LMCA with 4.5 × 8 mm NC balloon. Multiple attempts were made to cross LCX ostial struts with different wires, exchanged wires to avoid entanglement, able to cross LCX with different wires but unable to cross struts across LCX ostium with 3.0 × 12 mm NC for FKB despite opening side branch ostial struts with 1.5 and 2 mm Tazuna balloons. Poststent OCT was done **(Fig. 60A)** to evaluate the side branch ostial struts and position of SB wire due to difficulty in crossing balloons for FKB despite crossing side branch ostium with wires and dilatations with Nick Nano balloon and 1.5 × 10 mm Tazuna balloons. OCT revealed position of side branch wire in the crushed portion of side branch stent struts which were not allowing 3 mm NC balloon to place across LCX ostium. We decided to choose another strut to cross with another wires using dual lumen Sasuke catheter over the side branch wire which went through the crushed portion of SB stent, then another wire was to cross another strut of SB ostium avoiding wire going through crushed portion of stent struts. Stent struts across the LCX ostium opened with 1.25 × 10 mm, 1.5 × 15 mm, and 2.5 × 15 mm Tazuna balloons. FKB done with 3.0 × 12 mm NC Trek in LCX and 3.5 × 12 mm NC Trek in LAD and LAD DOT with 3.5 × 12 mm NC Trek. Final OCT showed irregular expansion of stent due to eccentric calcium, well-expanded stent struts, well-apposed, without medial dissection at stent edges. OCT also revealed calcific nodules and post-OPN NC calcium fractures **(Fig. 60B)**. Final POT of LMCA was performed with 4.5 × 8 mm NC balloon. The final result was good with TIMI III flow with no complications **(Fig. 61)**.

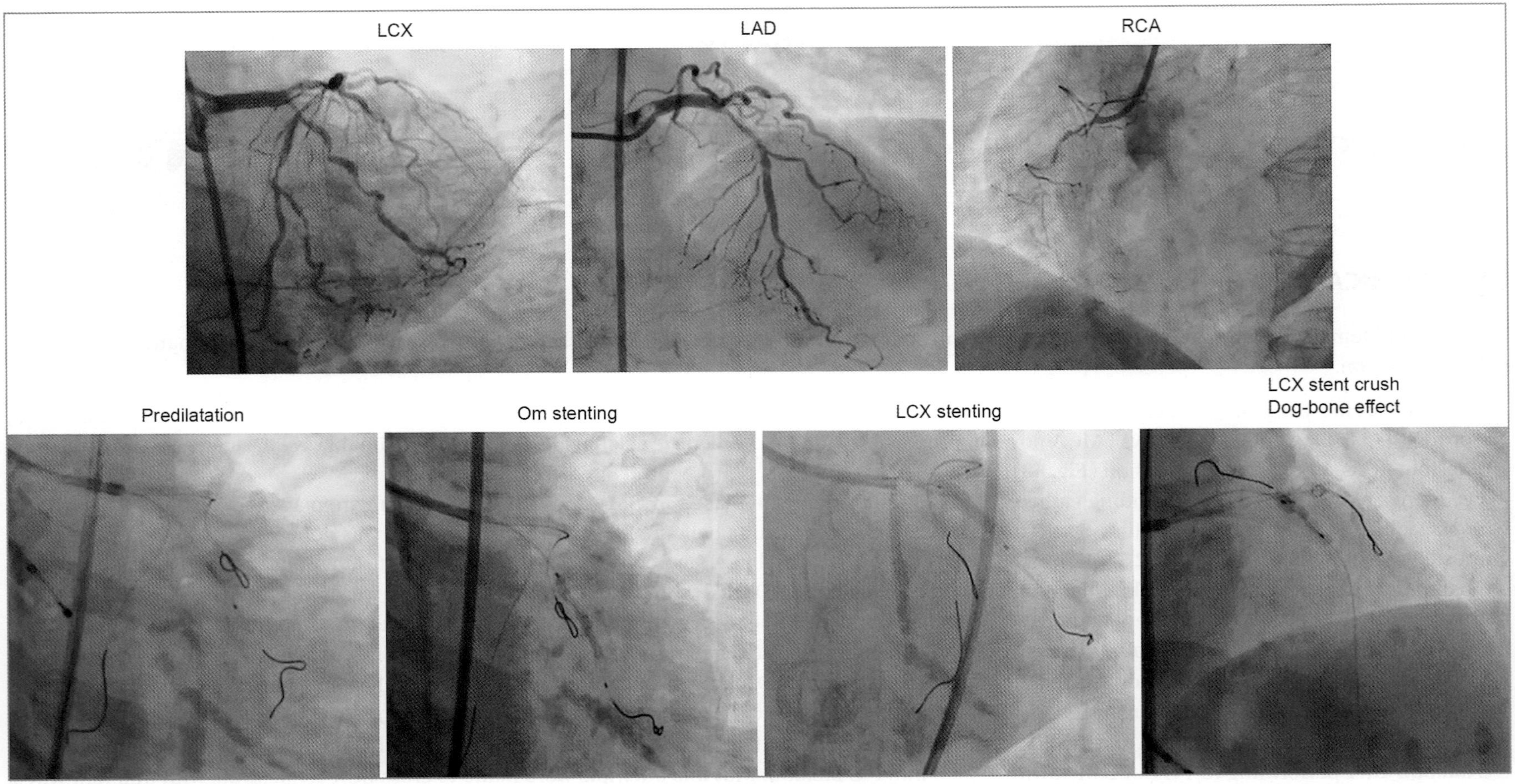

Fig. 58: Coronary angiogram and OM and LCX stenting.

OA is more useful for ablating large vessels, lesions with severe superficial calcium, eccentric calcium or CN, and crossable Aorto-ostial lesions with reverse cutting.

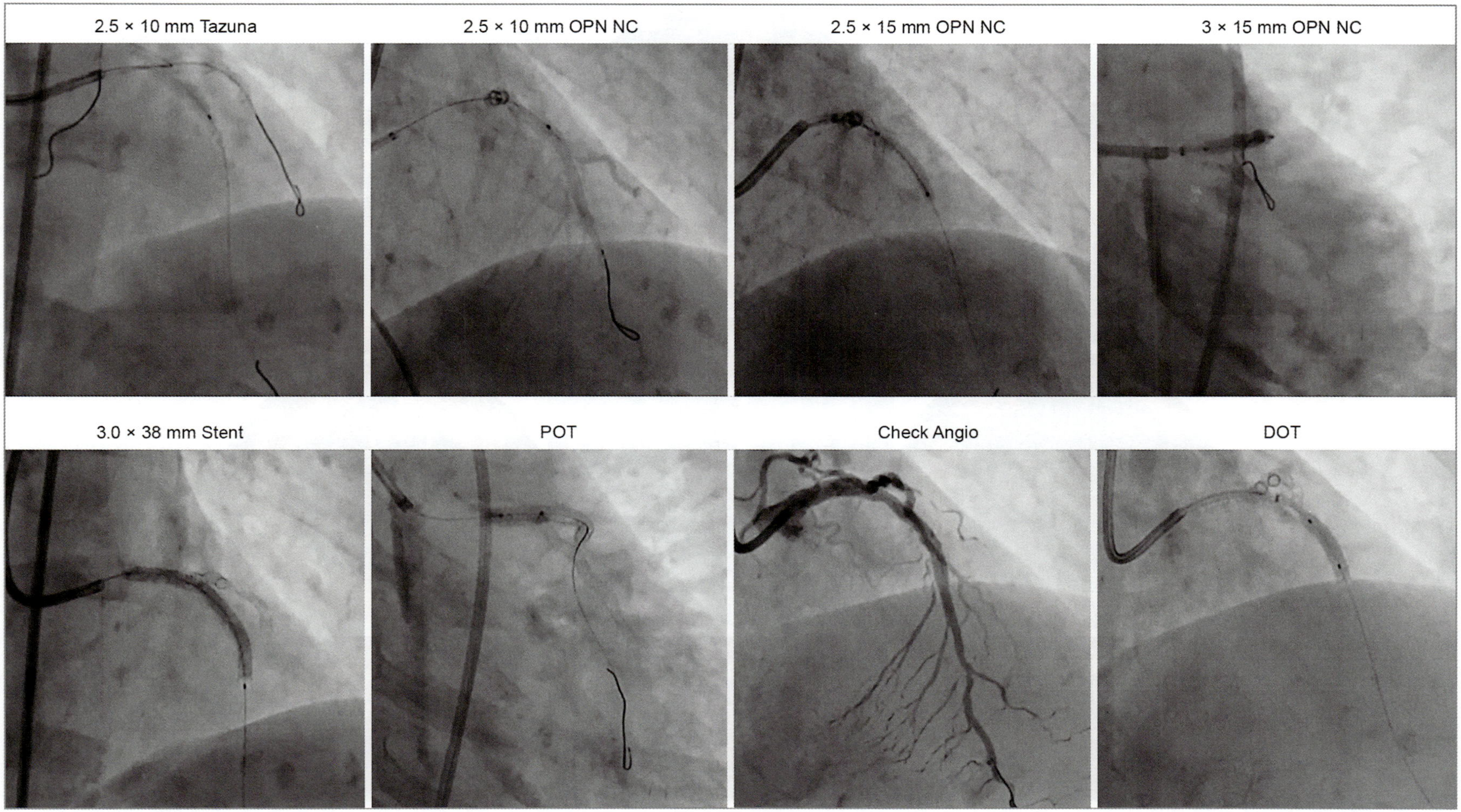

Fig. 59: Coronary angioplasty of LAD lesion.

High pressure OPN NC ballons (super-NC balloon) is a twin -layered balloon with minimal increase of diameter at burst pressure 35 atms (Maximal pressure tested up to 45 ATMs) is suitable to tackle crossable un-dilatable calcified lesions (avoid eccentric calcific or CN lesions to avoid perforation) and under expanded stents. However, it has high profile with poor capability to cross very tight lesions compared to regular NC balloons.

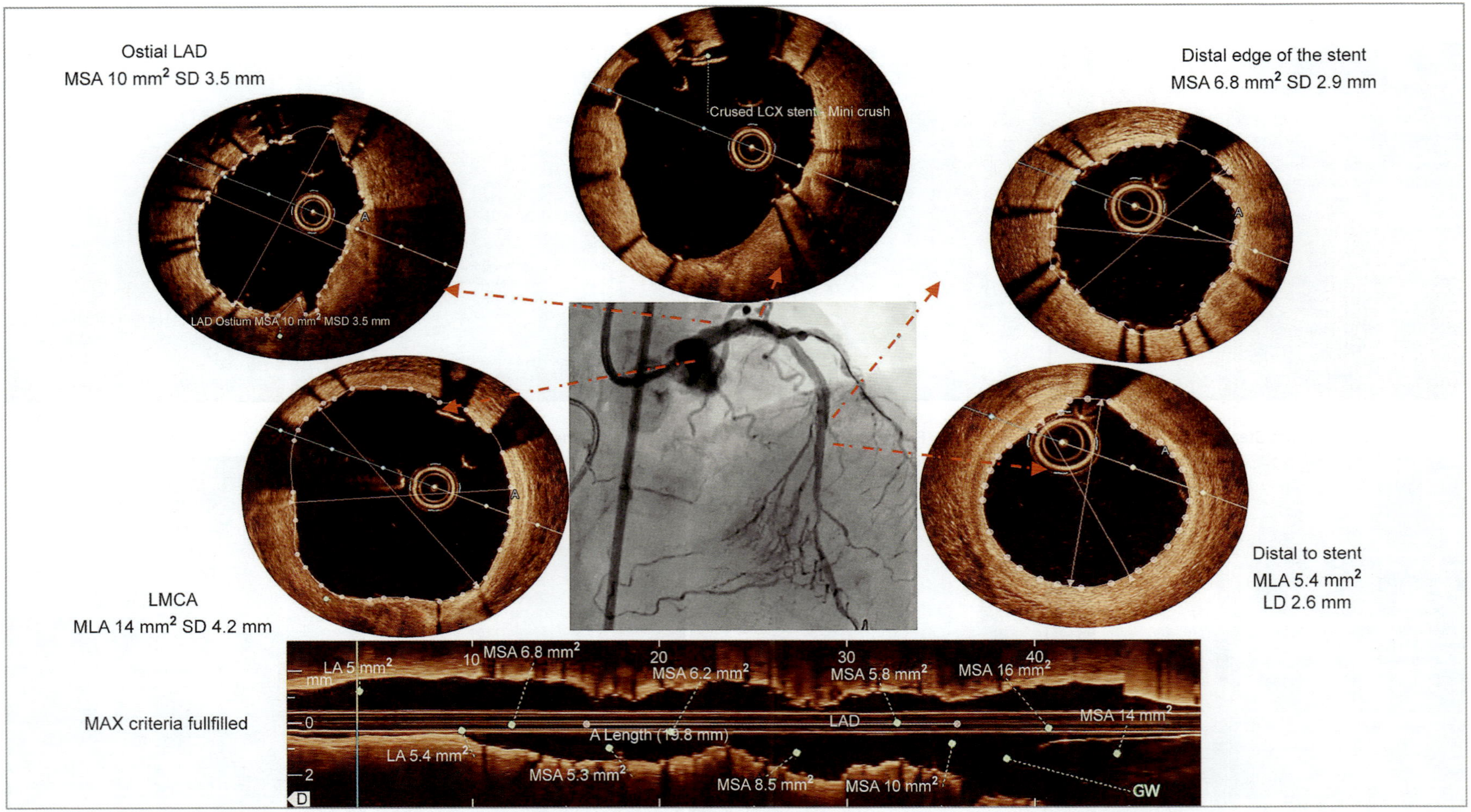
Ostial LAD
MSA 10 mm² SD 3.5 mm
LAD Ostium MSA 10 mm² MSD 3.5 mm
Crused LCX stent - Mini crush
Distal edge of the stent
MSA 6.8 mm² SD 2.9 mm
LMCA
MLA 14 mm² SD 4.2 mm
Distal to stent
MLA 5.4 mm²
LD 2.6 mm
MAX criteria fullfilled
LA 5 mm²
MSA 6.8 mm²
MSA 6.2 mm²
MSA 5.8 mm²
MSA 16 mm²
MSA 14 mm²
LAD
A Length (19.8 mm)
LA 5.4 mm²
MSA 5.3 mm²
MSA 8.5 mm²
MSA 10 mm²
GW

Fig. 60A

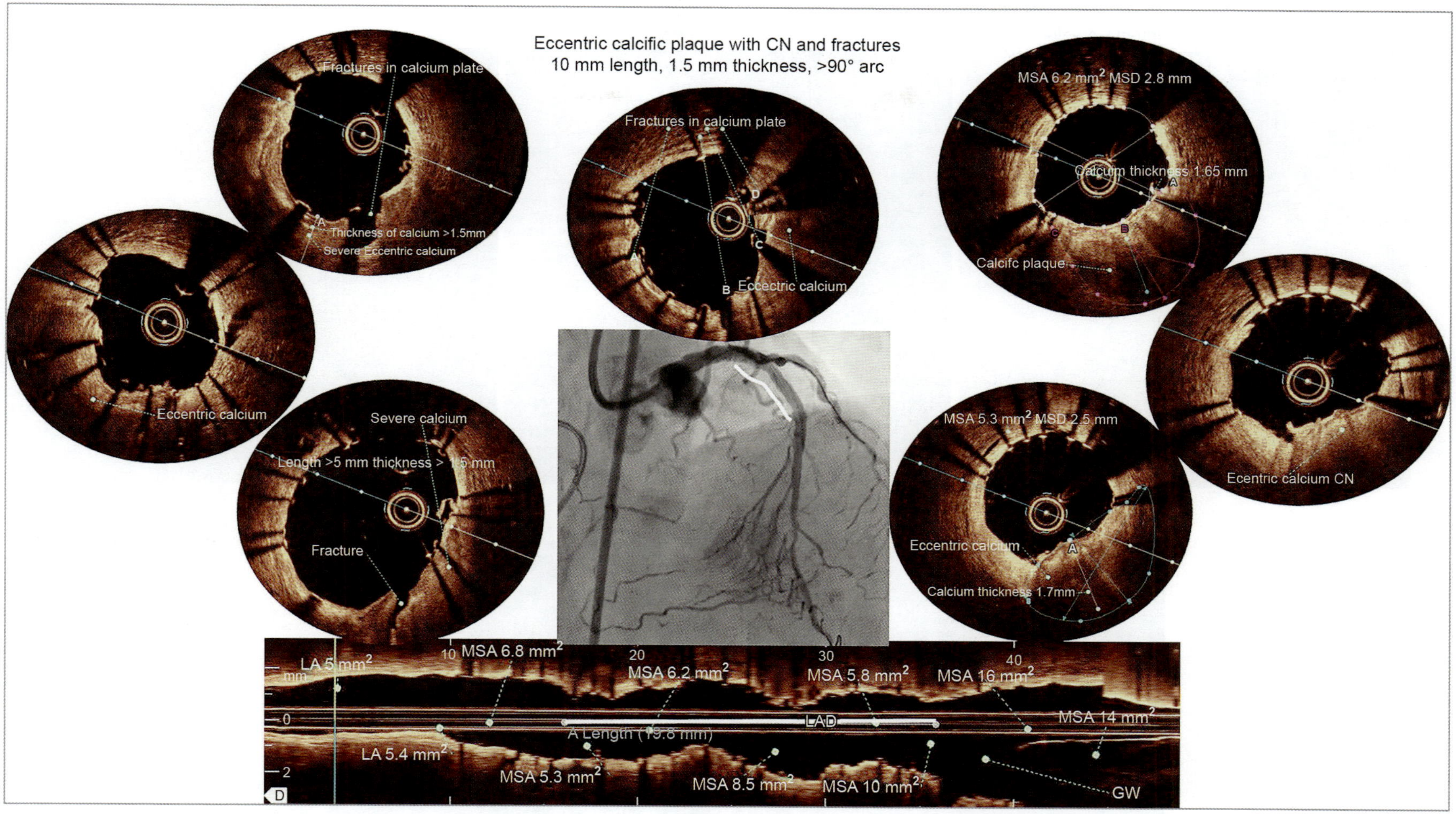

Fig. 60B

Figs. 60A and B: (A) Post-LAD stenting OCT assessment; (B) Morphology of LAD vessel for eccentric calcium which results in irregular stent expansion.

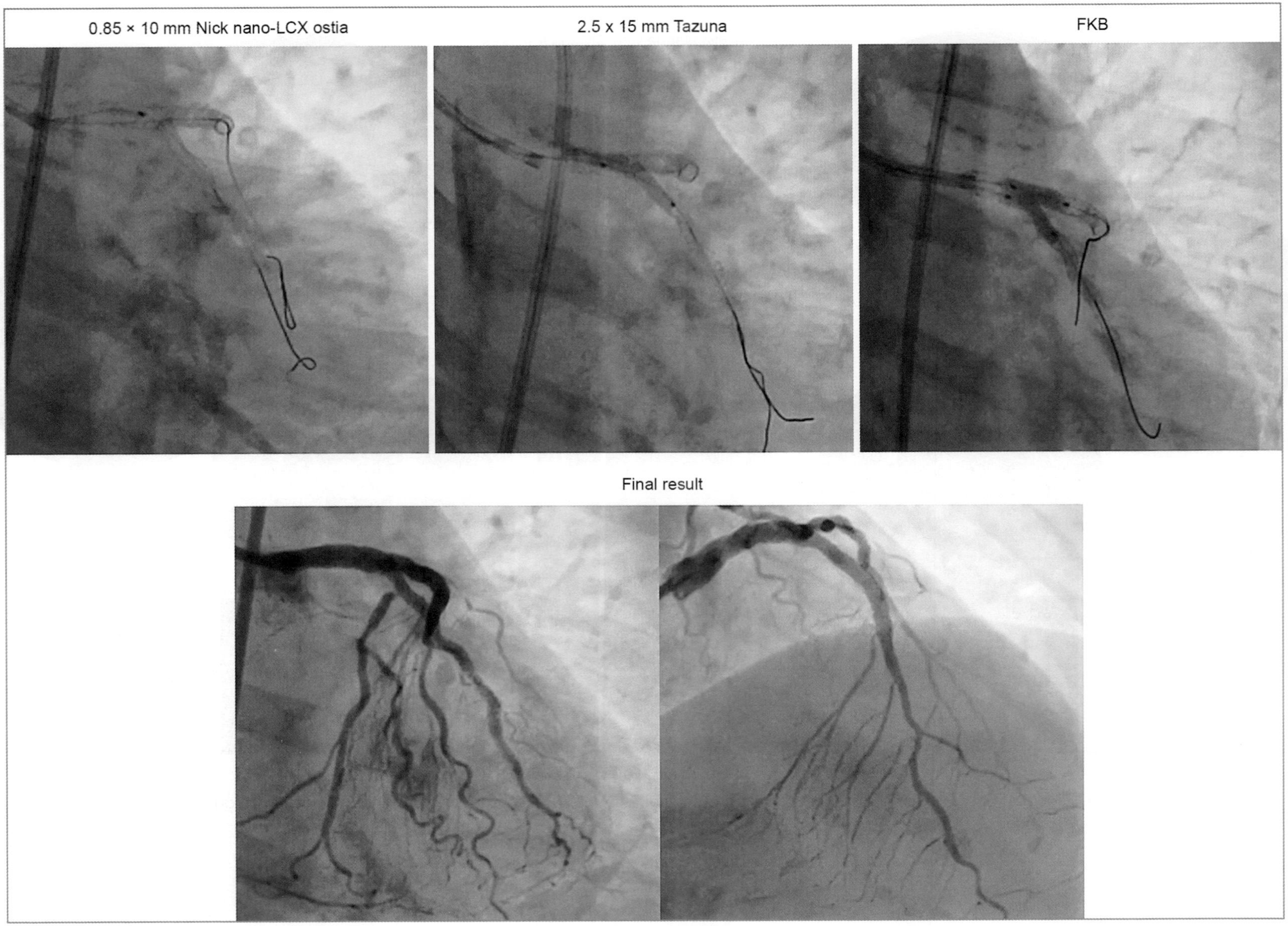

Fig. 61: Final kissing balloon dilatation and final result of LAD, LCX, and OM in a case of thick calcium particularly when deeply located in the intimal and medial layers, atherectomy (Rotational or Orbital) may result in eccentric ablation with no effect on deeper calcium and subsequent suboptimal lesion dilatation associated with potential stent underexpansion.

CASE 11

Calcium nodule—plaque modification with IVL.

CLINICAL HISTORY

A 78-year-old male, known hypertensive, and diabetic with past history of CABG (LIMA-D1, RA to LAD), presented with complaints of angina and breathlessness on minimal exertion on and off for 1 month. CAD—unstable angina, 2D Echo—mild LV dysfunction, EF—40%.

Investigations: Hb—11.3 g/dL, serum creatinine—0.7 mg/dL, eGFR—86 mL/min, Trop I—219 ng/L.

CAG—triple vessel disease with patent grafts to LAD and D1, LMCA: Distal 50–60% lesion (calcified), extending into LCX, LAD: Ostioproximal 95% lesion. LCX: Ostial 70% lesion, calcified. Distal mild disease. RCA: Mid total cutoff after RV branch. Distal vessel filling retrogradely from left system. LIMA—Diagonal graft: Patent. RA—LAD graft: Patent.

LCA engaged with JL 3.5–7 Fr guiding catheter, lesion crossed with 0.014" Run through wire.

PROCEDURE

OCT run was acquired for MLD assessment of LM to proximal LCX segment for choosing appropriate plaque modification strategy and selection of the stent size. OCT showed severe calcification with large calcific nodule of the ostioproximal LCX with extension to LM confluence and distal LM. Plaque modification was planned with AngioSculpt and IVL with guide extension support due to difficulty in placing devices **(Fig. 62)**.

Plaque modification was done with 3.0 × 15 mm AngioSculpt balloon. Lesion further dilatation with 3.0 × 12 mm NC Trek balloon. 4 × 12 mm IVL balloon was used for plaque modification with guideliner support,and total 80 pulses delivered in the LMCA and proximal LCX.

Postplaque modification OCT showed fractures of CN suggestive of adequate plaque modification **(Fig. 63)**.

LMCA-LCX stenting was done with 3.5 × 18 mm Xience Alpine Stent, and POT of LMCA was carried out with 4.5 × 12 mm NC Trek and DOT of LCX was done with 3.5 × 12 mm NC Trek balloon. Final Angio result was good with TIMI III flow and no complications.

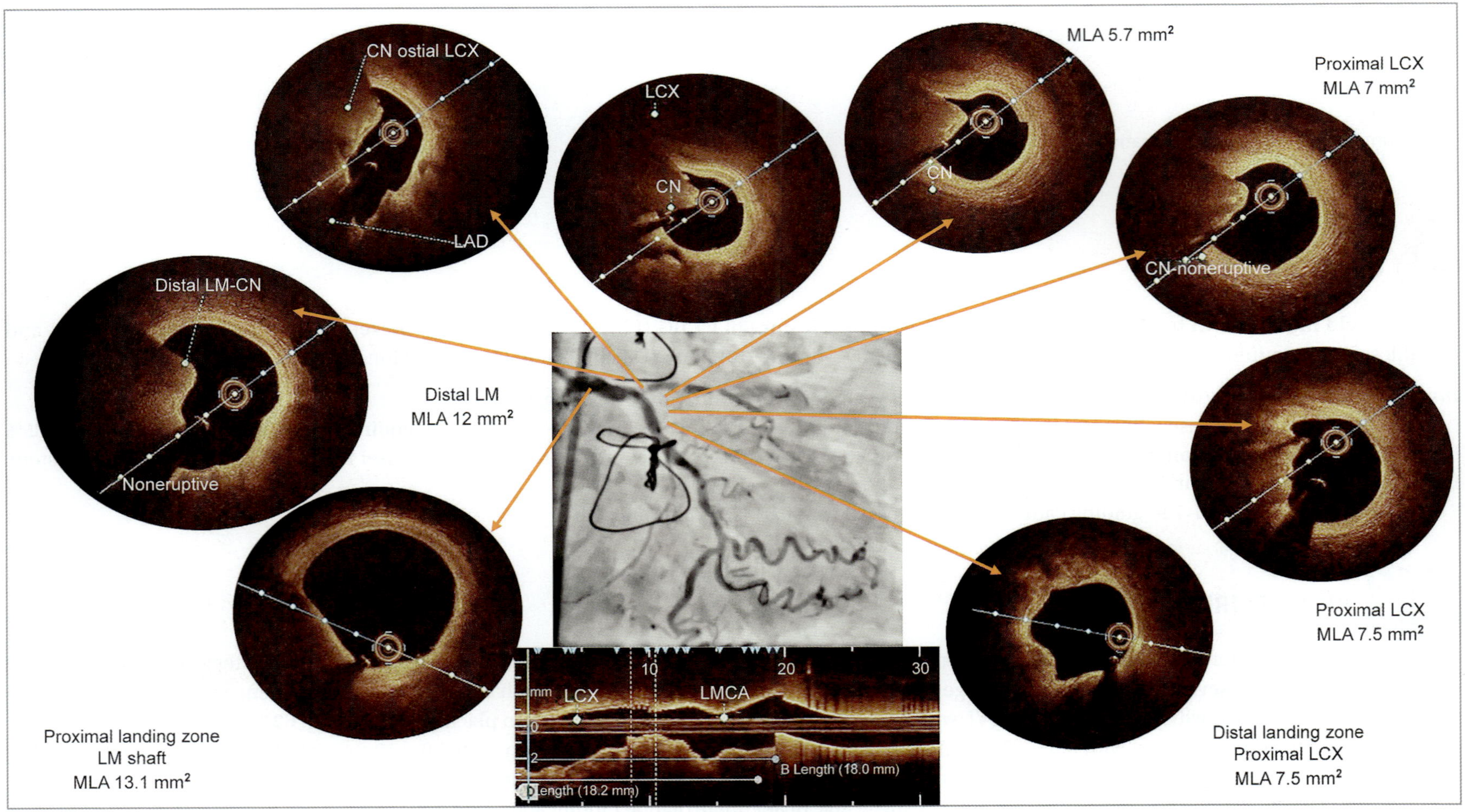

Fig. 62: Presenting IVL showed severe calcification with large calcific nodule of theostio-proximal LCX with extension to LM confluence and distal LM.

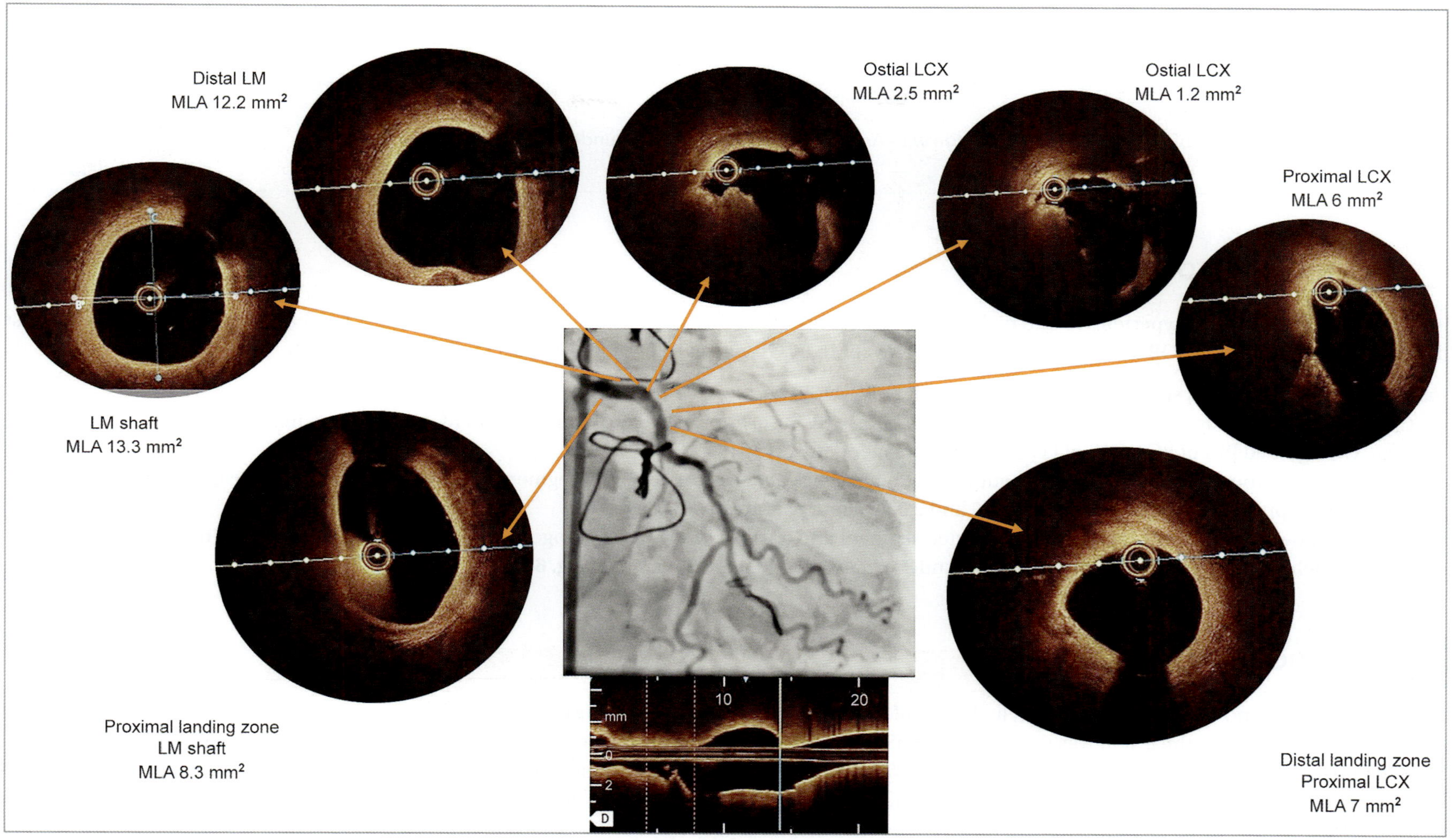

Fig. 63: Post-IVL OCT showing fractures of CN suggestive of adequate plaque modification.

CASE 12

Heterogeneous ISR of CTO of RCA—plaque modification with AngioSculpt and correction of under-expansion with OPN NC.

CLINICAL HISTORY

A 75-year-old male, known hypertensive and diabetic with a past history of PCI + stents to LAD, LCX and RCA (2012 and 2018) presented with c/o chest discomfort associated with SOB for 2 weeks, CAD - ACS - NSTEMI, ECG—normal, 2D Echo—normal LV function, EF—60%.

Investigations: Hb—10 g/dl, serum creatinine—0.9 mg/dL, RBS—157 mg/dL.

CAG—LAD ostioproximal 60–70% stenosis, mid 70% stenosis, LCX—ostioproximal 80% stenosis, and RCA—ostioproximal CTO.

Plan: OCT-guided PCI of RCA. PCI of LCX and LAD on later date.

RCA engaged through RRA with AL 1 - 7 Fr guiding catheter, check angio was taken, CTO segment of RCA was crossed with Fielder XT 0.014" wire with microcatheter support. Predilated with Ryurei 1.25 and 2.0 × 10 mm balloons.

OCT run showed fibrotic narrowing beyond stented segment and areas of Intra-stent homogeneous ISR, heterogeneous neointimal proliferation with calcification behind sent, peri-strut infiltration, and under expansion of the previous stent **(Fig. 64)**.

PROCEDURE

Heterogeneous ISR and under expanded stent at the site of previously overlapped stents **(Figs. 65 and 66)**.

Plaque modification of the lesion was done with AngioSculpt 3.0 × 15 mm scoring balloon, mid RCA stenting was performed with Ultimaster Nagomi 3.0 × 50 mm stent, proximal RCA stented with Ultimaster Nagomi 3.5 × 28 mm stent and postdilatated with NC Trek 3.5 × 20 mm balloon.

Poststent OCT showing well under-expanded, apposed stent struts with no medial edge dissections **(Fig. 67)**.

Under expanded stent segment was not expanded adequately despite usage of plaque modification with AngioSculpt and high pressure NC dilatations therefore it was dilated with OPN NC 3.0 × 15 mm balloon at 35–40 atms with guideliner support which resulted in adequate expansion of the stent.

Final result was good with TIMI III flow with no complications

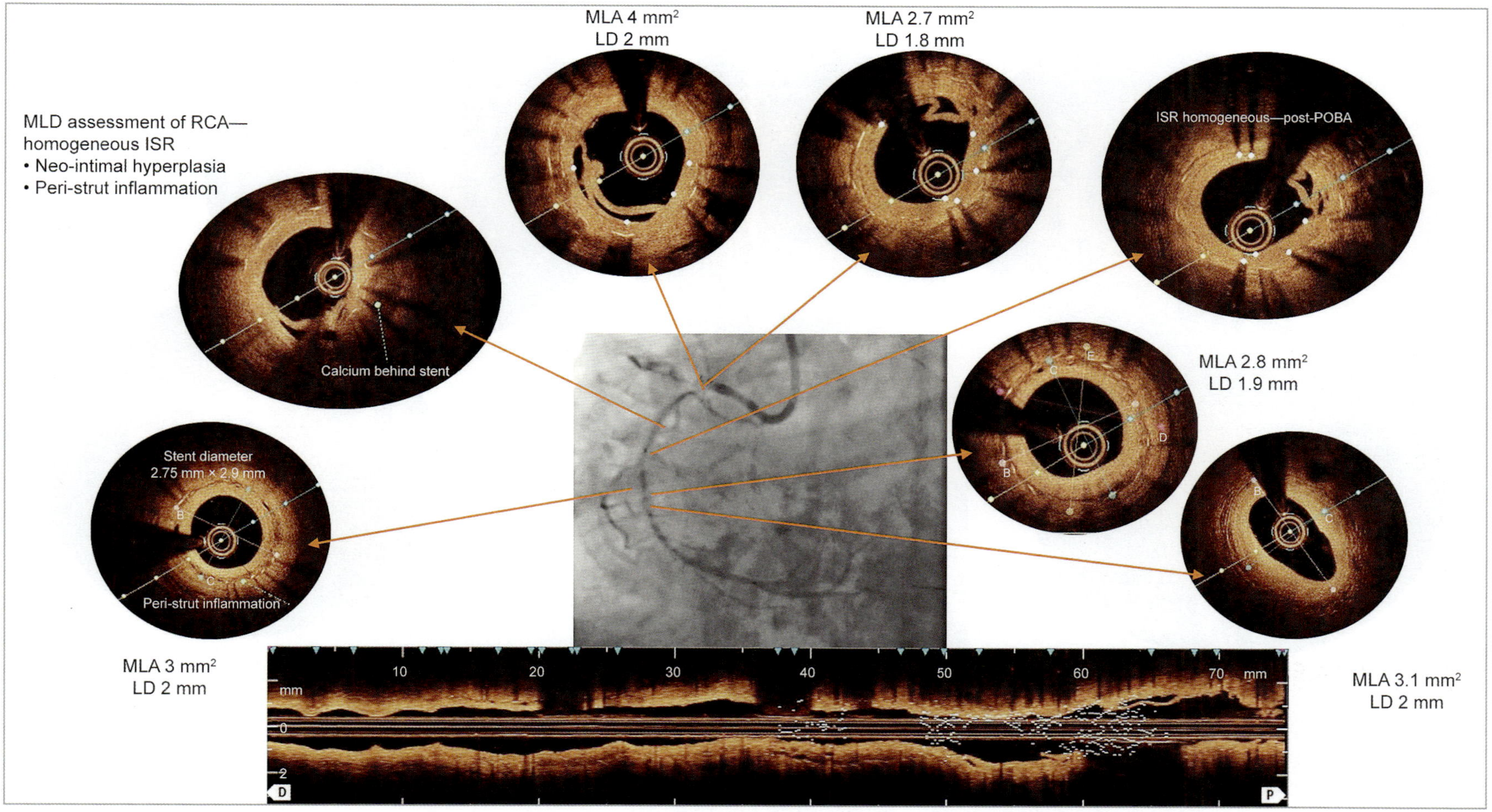

Fig. 64: MLD assement of RCA by OCT.

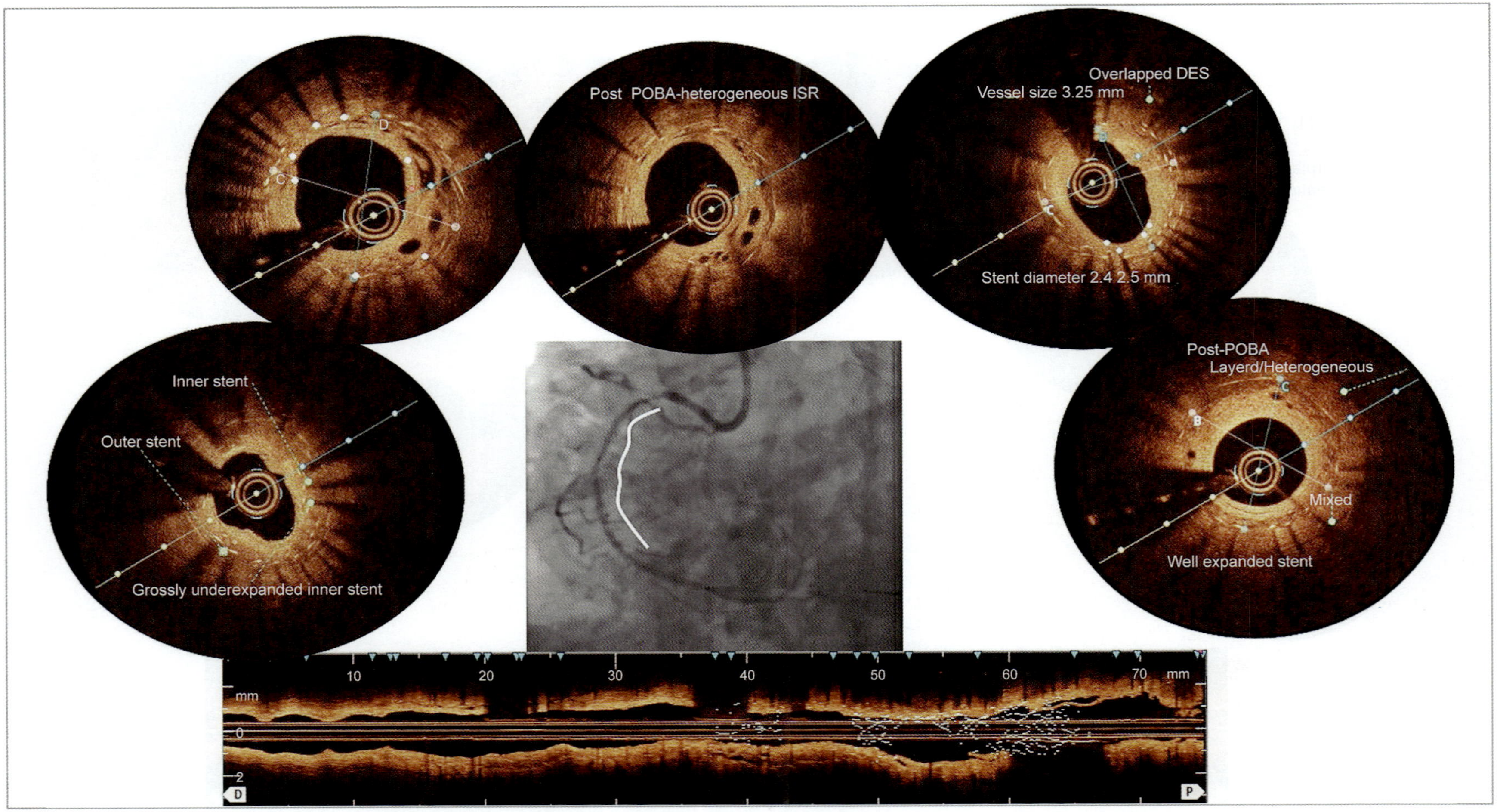

Fig. 65: Post-POBA OCT assessment showing heterogenous ISR.

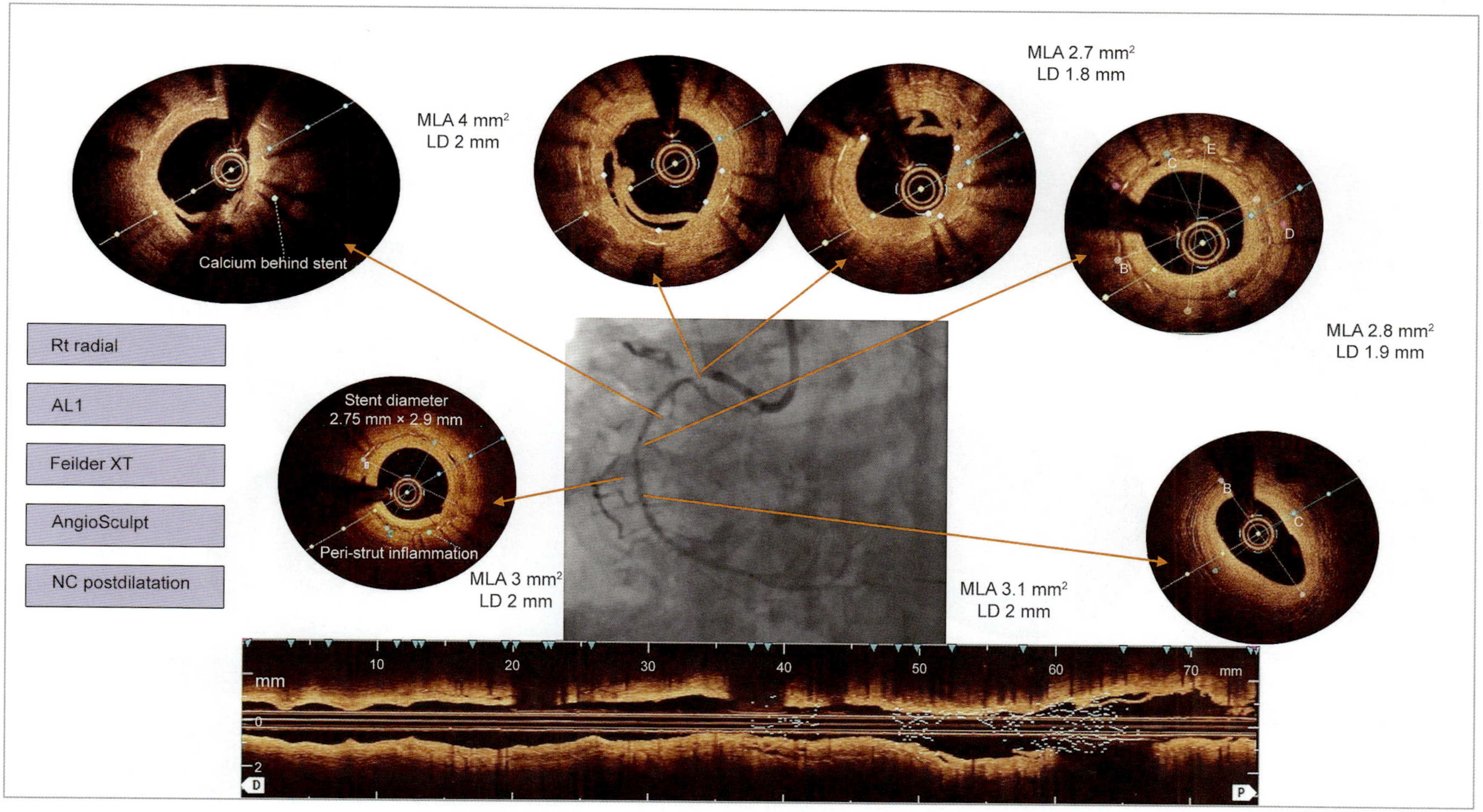

Fig. 66: Presenting OCT of RCA assessment for the selection of stent.

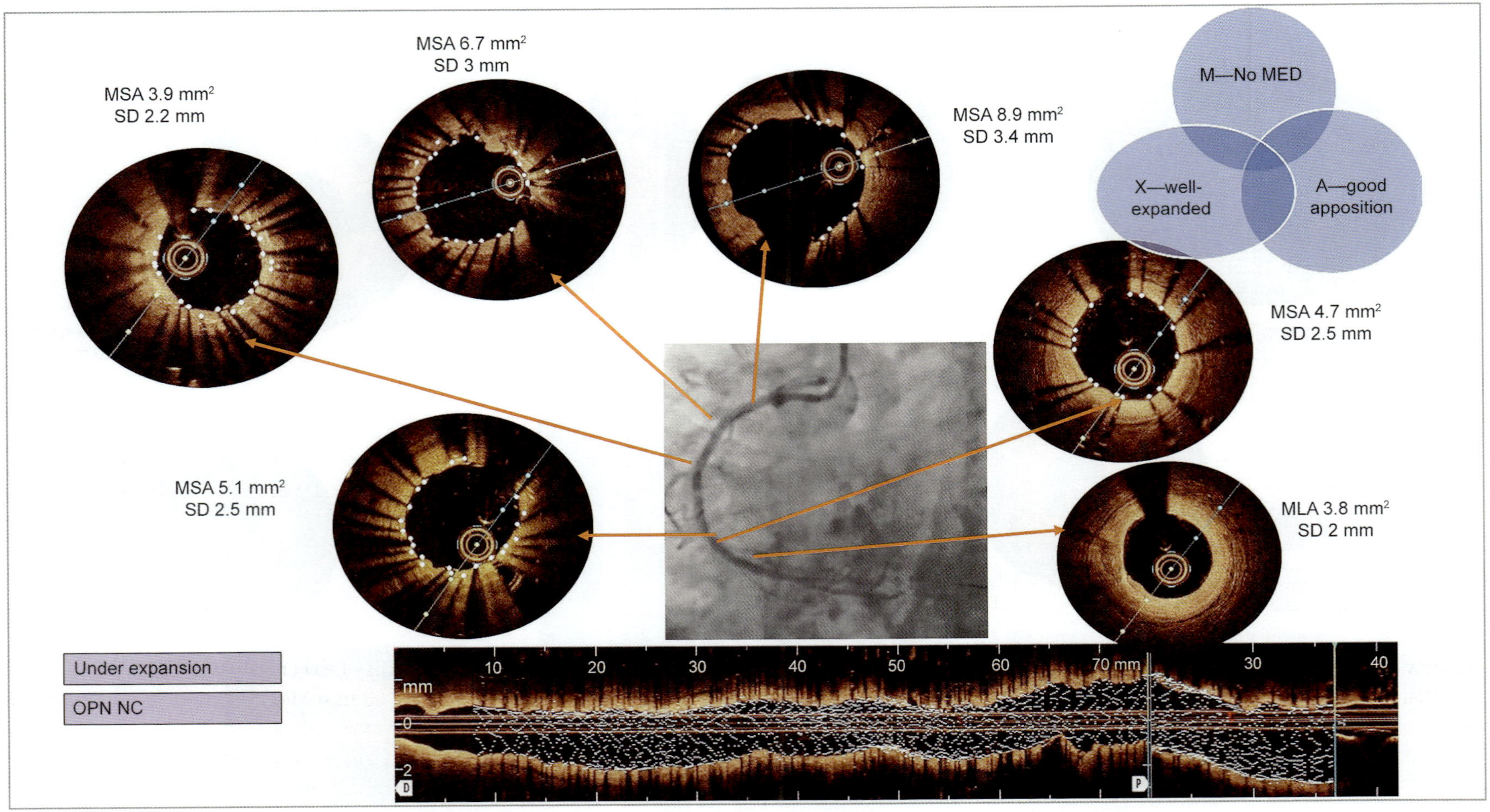

Fig. 67: Poststent of RCA showing under-expansion, well apposed with no medial edge dissection.

CASE 13

ROTA-TRIPSY for severe calcified LAD.

CLINICAL HISTORY

A 67-year-old female, known DM, HTN, S/p CABG (2015), presented with chest pain radiating to back. ECG-NSR, 2D Echo—RWMA in RCA territory, mild LV dysfunction, EF—48%.

Investigations: Hb—12 g/dL, serum creatinine—1.16 mg/dL, eGFR—49.5 mL/min, RBS—143 mg/dL. CAG—native TVD.

LMCA engaged with EBU 3.5-7 Fr guiding catheter, lesion crossed with 0.014″ run through wire. Lesion tried to cross with 2.0 × 15 mm balloon not negotiated. Then tried with 1.25 × 10 mm balloon, not negotiated. Hence wire exchanged with Rota drive wire, 1.25 mm Burr taken and lesion ablated with multiple passes. Post-ROTA OCT was done which showed dense calcification in proximal LAD, fibrotic lesion in mid-LAD and calcification with cuts in distal LAD **(Figs. 68 and 69)**.

PROCEDURE

In view of dense calcification IVL was opted, 3.5 × 12 mm IVL balloon crossed and 120 pulses delivered from LMCA - LAD **(Figs. 70 to 72)**.

Distal dilated with 2.5 × 10 mm wolverin cutting balloon at 10–18 atms. Dista LAD stenting done with 2.5 × 33 mm Xience Alpine Stent deployed at 10 atms. Then overlapping stenting done with 3.5 × 48 mm Xience Alpine Stent deployed at 12 atms with guide extension support. Post dilatation done with 3.0 × 10 mm NC balloon and 3.5 × 10 mm NC balloon at 10 atms. POT done with 5.0 × 08 mm NC Trek balloon at 12 atms. Post-OCT was done which showed well expanded stent struts with no edge dissection. The final result was good with TIMI III flow with no complications **(Figs. 73 and 74)**.

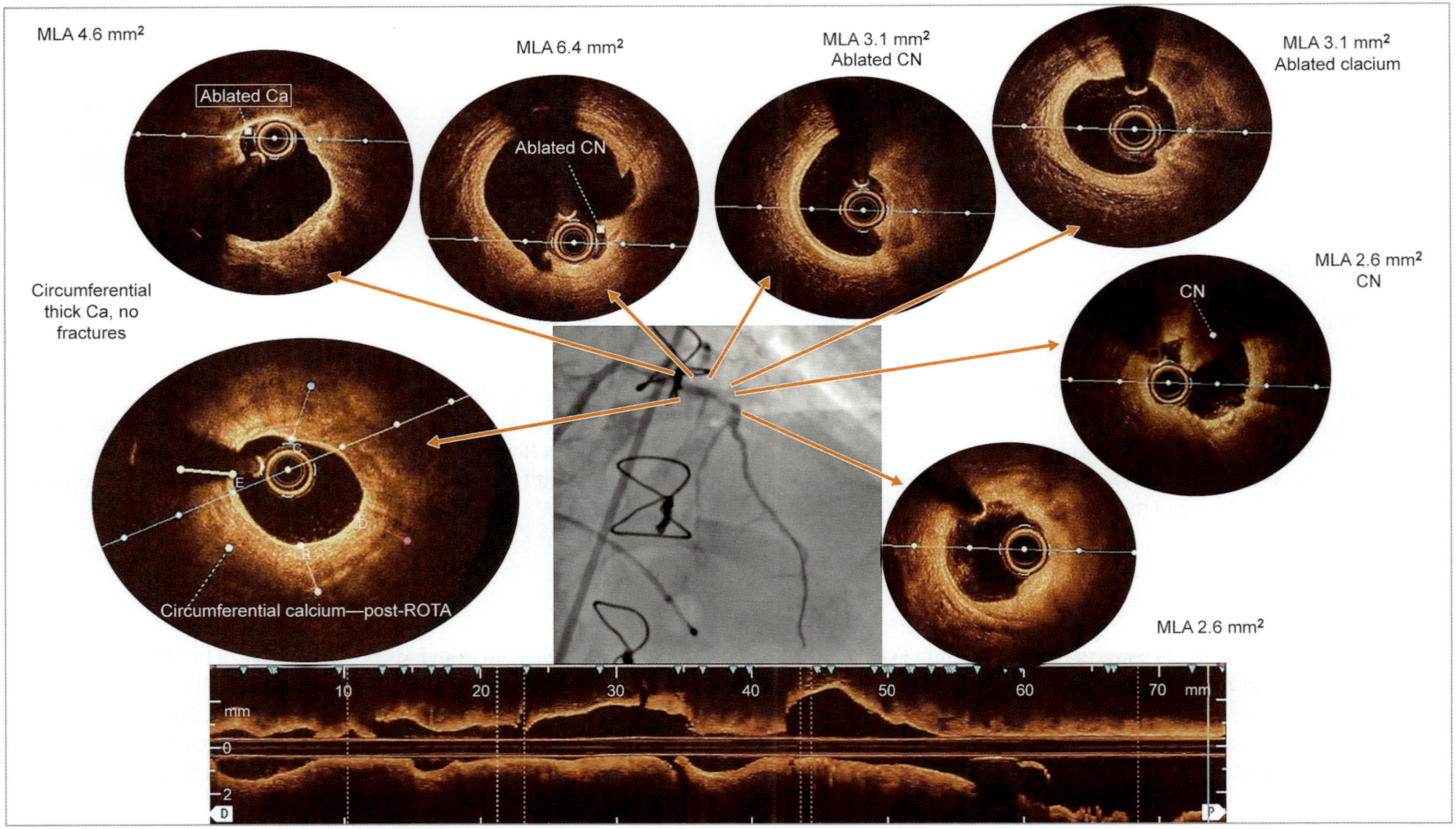

Fig. 68: Prestenting OCT assessment for stent size.

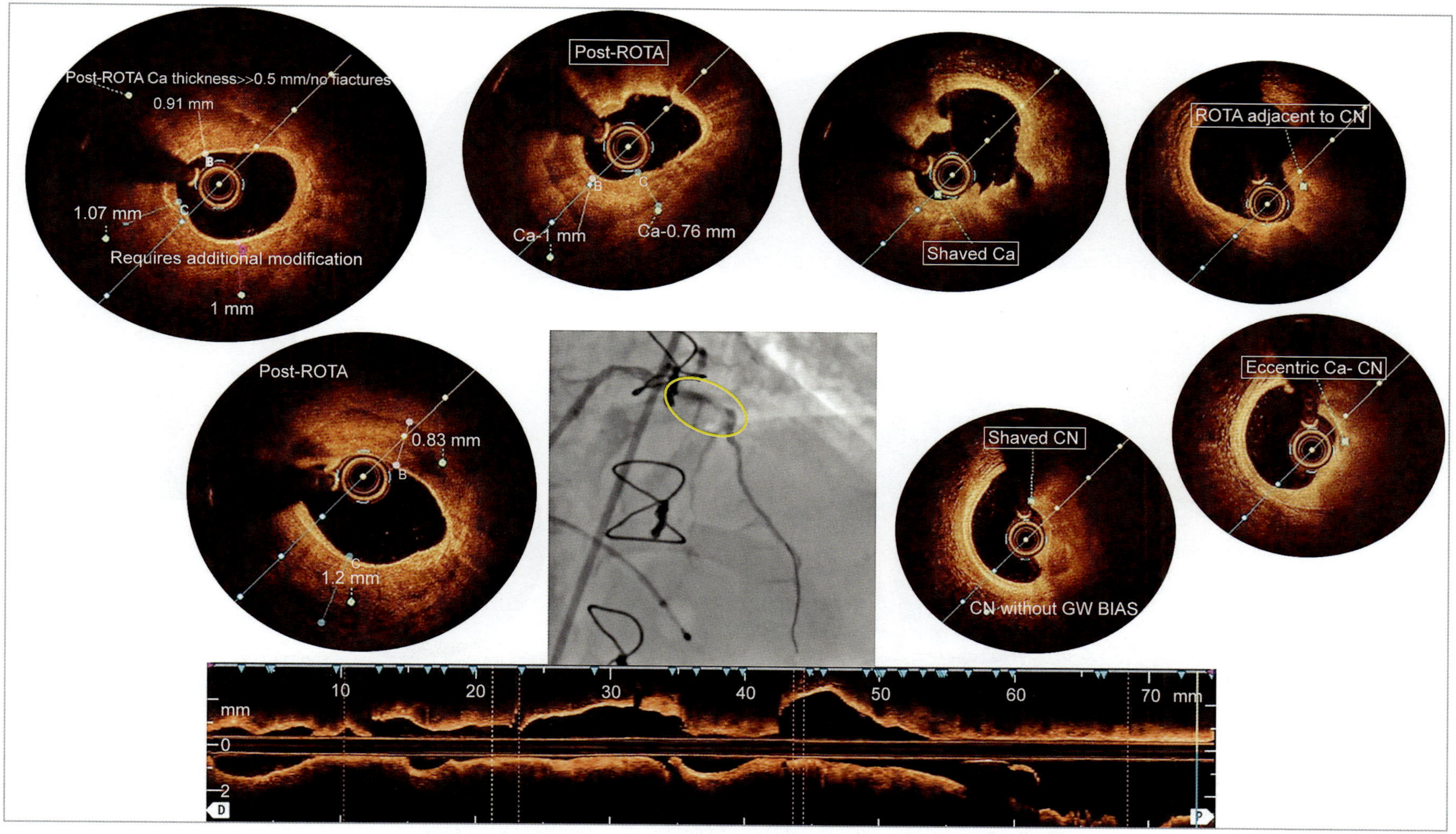

Fig. 69: Prestenting OCT assessment showing circumferential thick calcium—requires IVL for plaque modification.

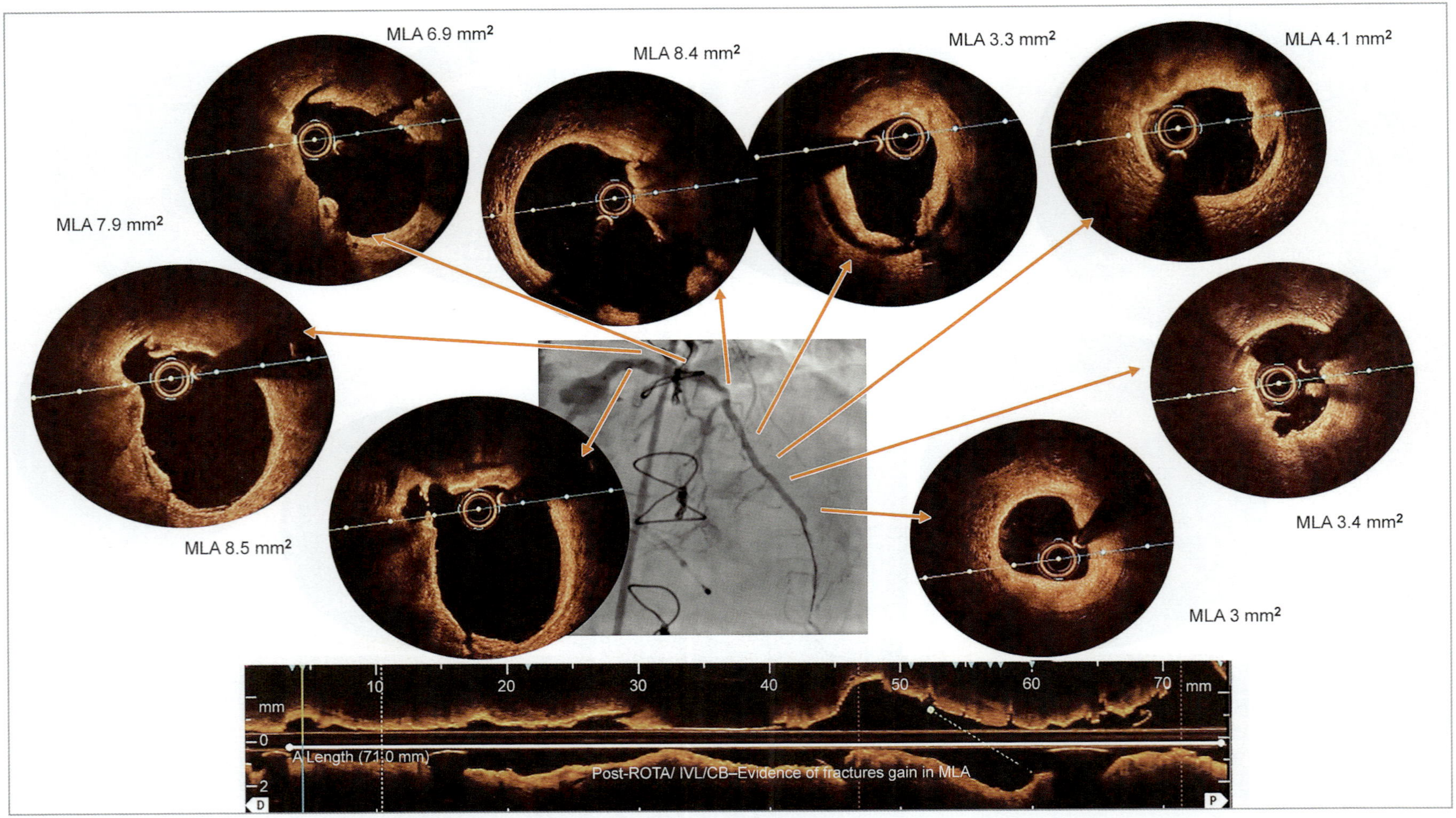

Fig. 70: Post-IVL more effective plaque modification—evidence of more fractures.

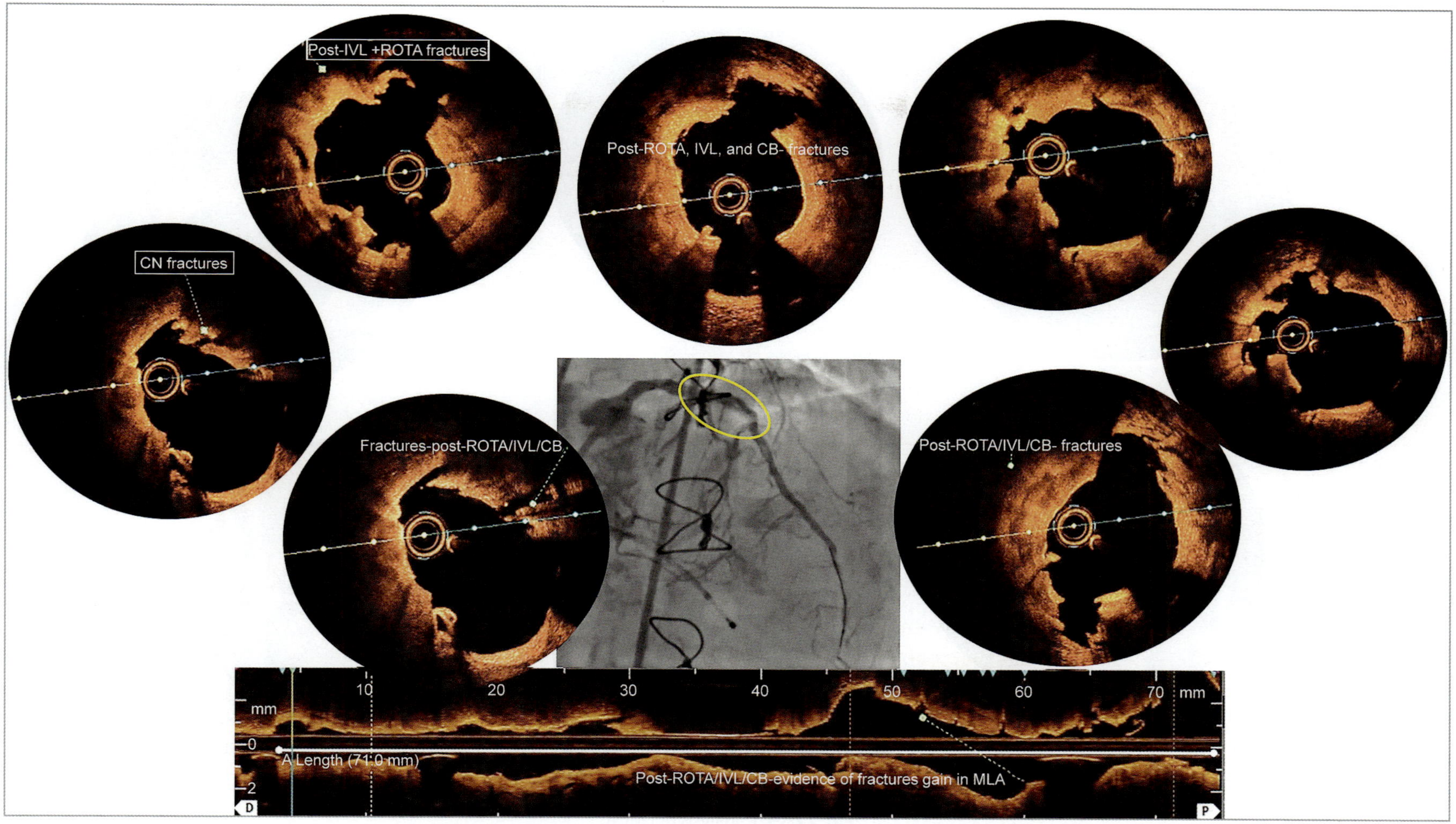

Fig. 71: Post-IVL OCT showing adequate luminal gain and fractures.

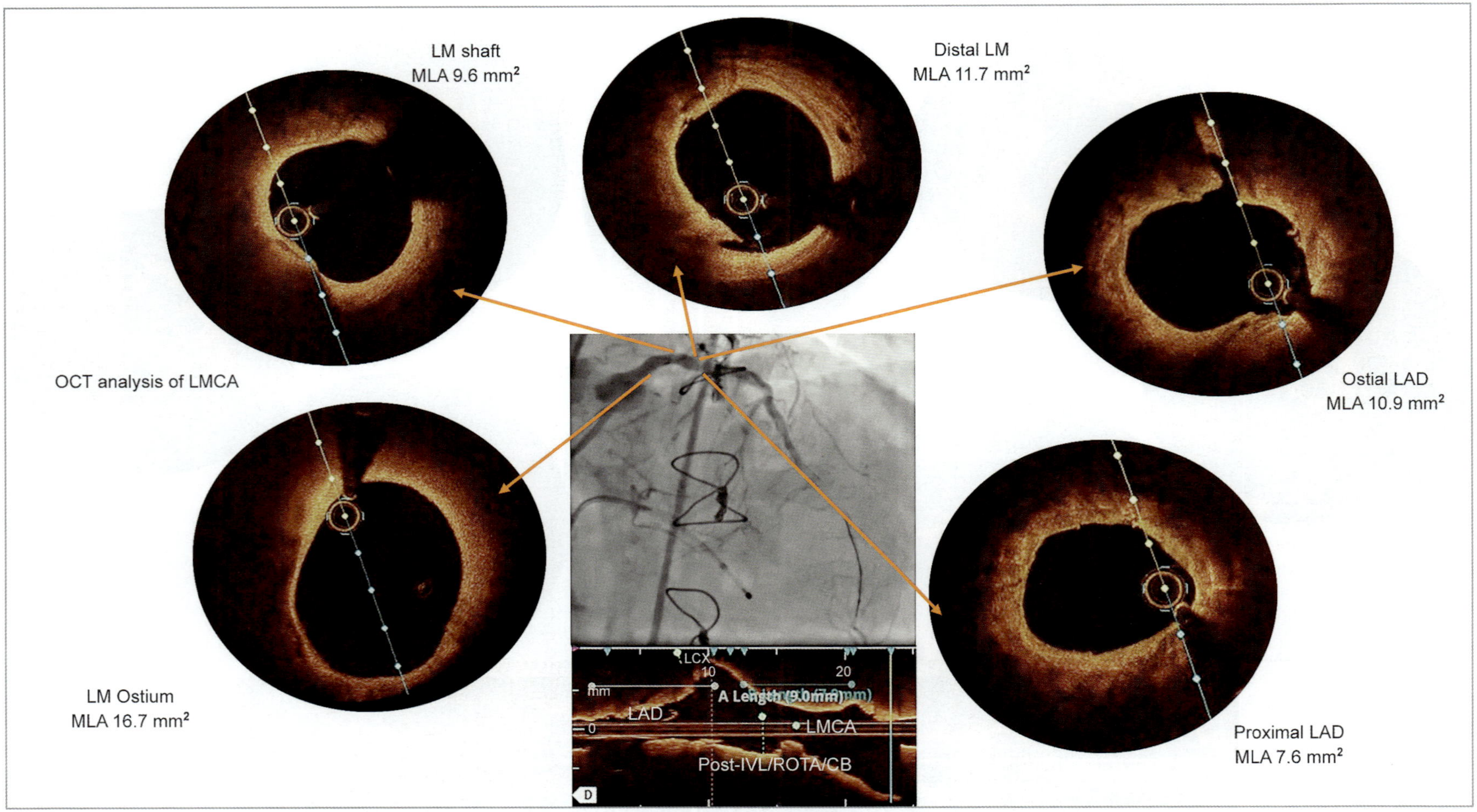

Fig. 72: OCT analysis of LMCA.

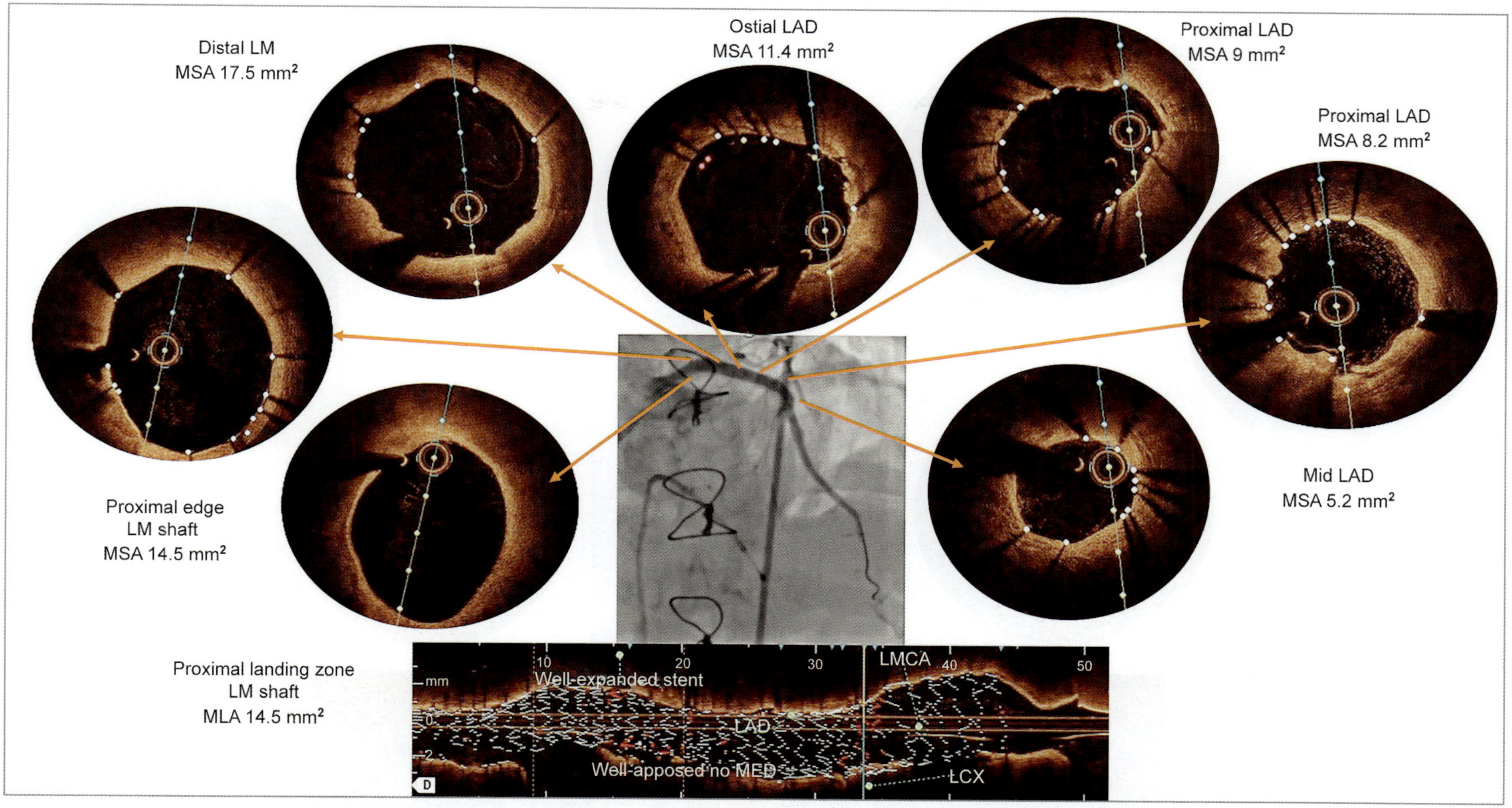

Fig. 73: MAX assessment of LM-LAD showing well expanded and apposed stent struts with no medial dissections.

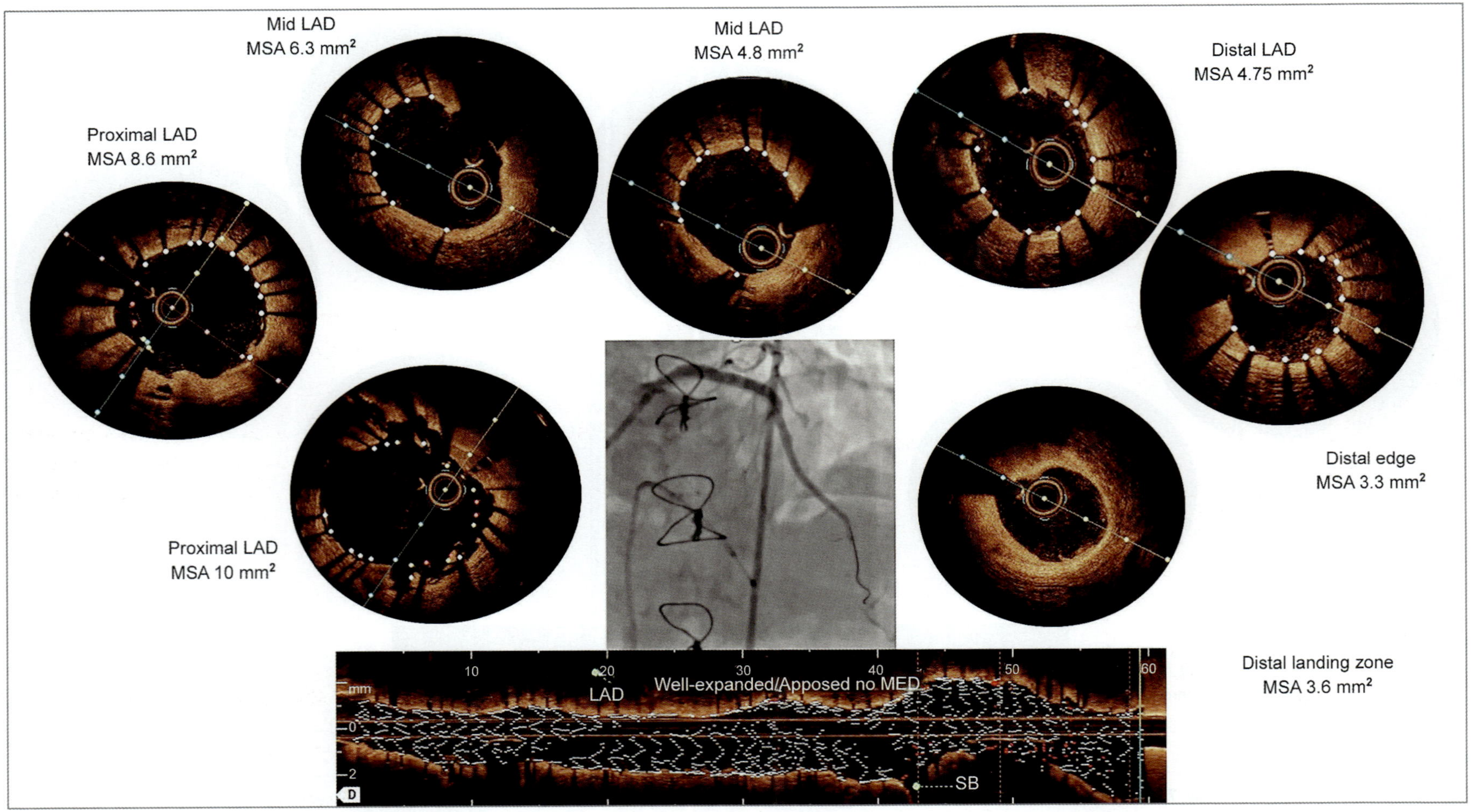

Fig. 74: MAX assessment of LAD showing well expanded and apposed stent struts with no medial dissections.

CASE 14

Plaque modification with IVL severe calcified ostal LAD.

CLINICAL HISTORY

A 60-year-old male, known diabetic, hypertensive presented with CAD—unstable angina for having chest pain 15 days prior to admission with ECG—no significant abnormality, 2D Echo—normal LV function, EF—60%. CAG done outside which revealed single vessel disease with proximal LAD 90% long severe calcific lesion.

O/I: Hb—15 g/dL, creatinine—0.81 mg/dL, TCL—50 mg/dL, TGL—185 mg/dL.

LCA engaged with EBU 3.5-6 Fr guiding catheter, and LAD lesion was crossed with 0.014" run through guidewire. OCT imaging was acquired for MLD assessment of LM, ostioproximal to distal LAD to decide plaque modification strategy, selection of the stent size and choosing proper landing zones. OCT run also showed myocardial bridge segment in the distal LAD, fibrotic plaque and thick eccentric calcific plaque of ostioproximal and mid LAD with MLA of 1.6 mm2 at the narrowest luminal area **(Fig. 75)**.

PROCEDURE

Presenting OCT of LAD revealed myocardial bridging distally **(Fig. 76)**.

Plaque modification was done with IVL shock wave 3.5 × 12 mm C2 plus balloon and 120 pulses delivered from mid LAD to Ostial LAD lesion **(Fig. 77)**. Then it was pre dilated with Wolverine 3.0 ×15 mm cutting balloon at 12 atms. After plaque modification OCT run was acquire to assess the adequacy of plaque modification before stenting which showed adequately modified plaque with evidence of significant fractures of calcific plaque, and gain in the mean luminal area **(Fig. 78)**.

Then LAD stenting was done with Xience Sierra 3.0 × 33 mm Stent at 12 to 16 atms, and it was post dilatated with NC Trek 4.0 × 15 mm balloon at 16–18 atms. Final OCT run was taken for the MAX assessment which revealed well expanded and apposed stent of the most of the stent without MED but with focal segment of under-expansion in the middle of stent 4.8 mmsq **(Figs. 79 and 80)**.

OPN NC balloon 3.0 × 10 mm was used to tackle under expanded stent by post dilating it up to 35 atms. Subsequently OCT run was repeated which revealed well expanded stent, no dissection, and no mal-apposition. The final result was good with TIMI III flow with no complications **(Fig. 81)**.

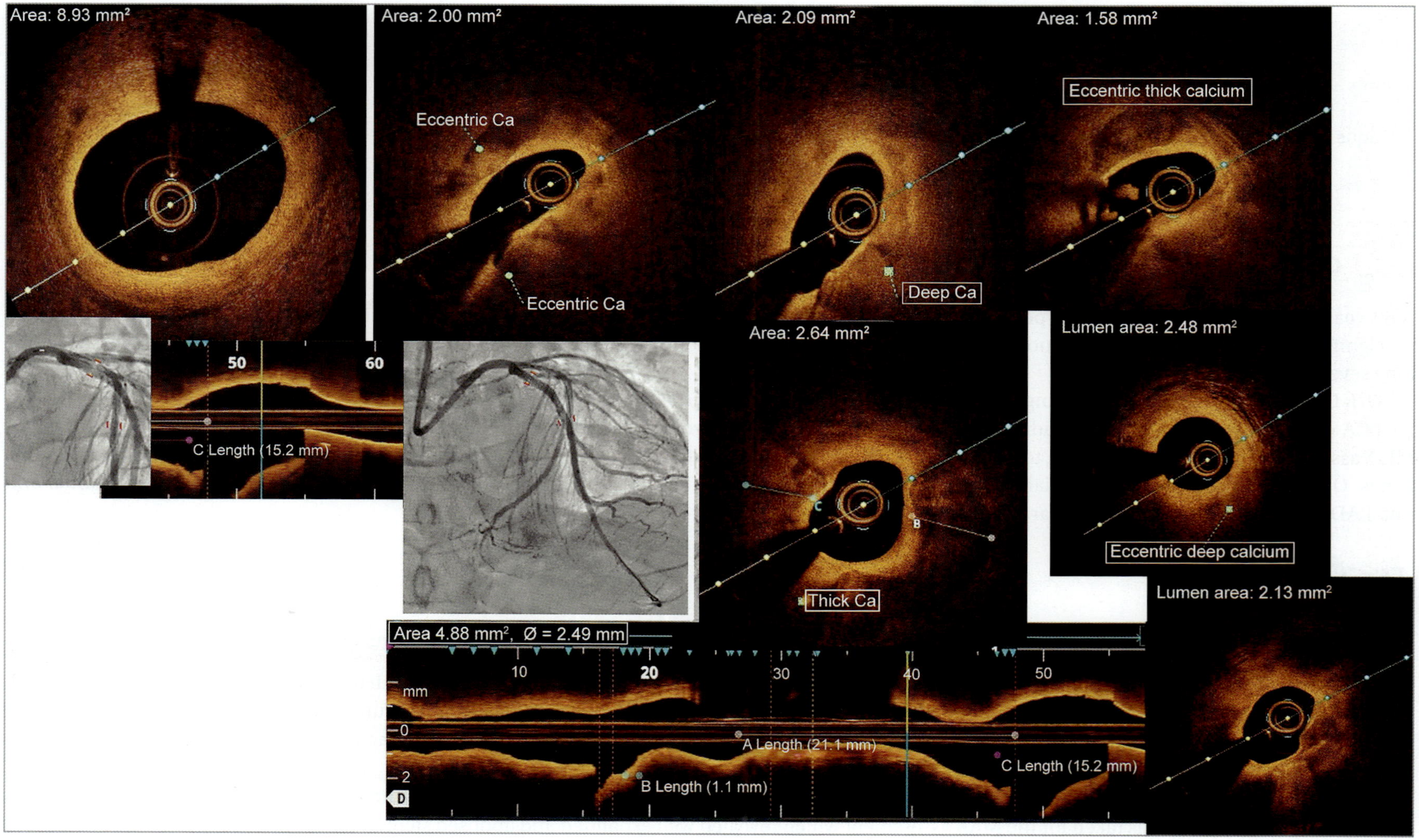

Fig. 75: MLD assessment of LAD for deciding plaque modification strategy.

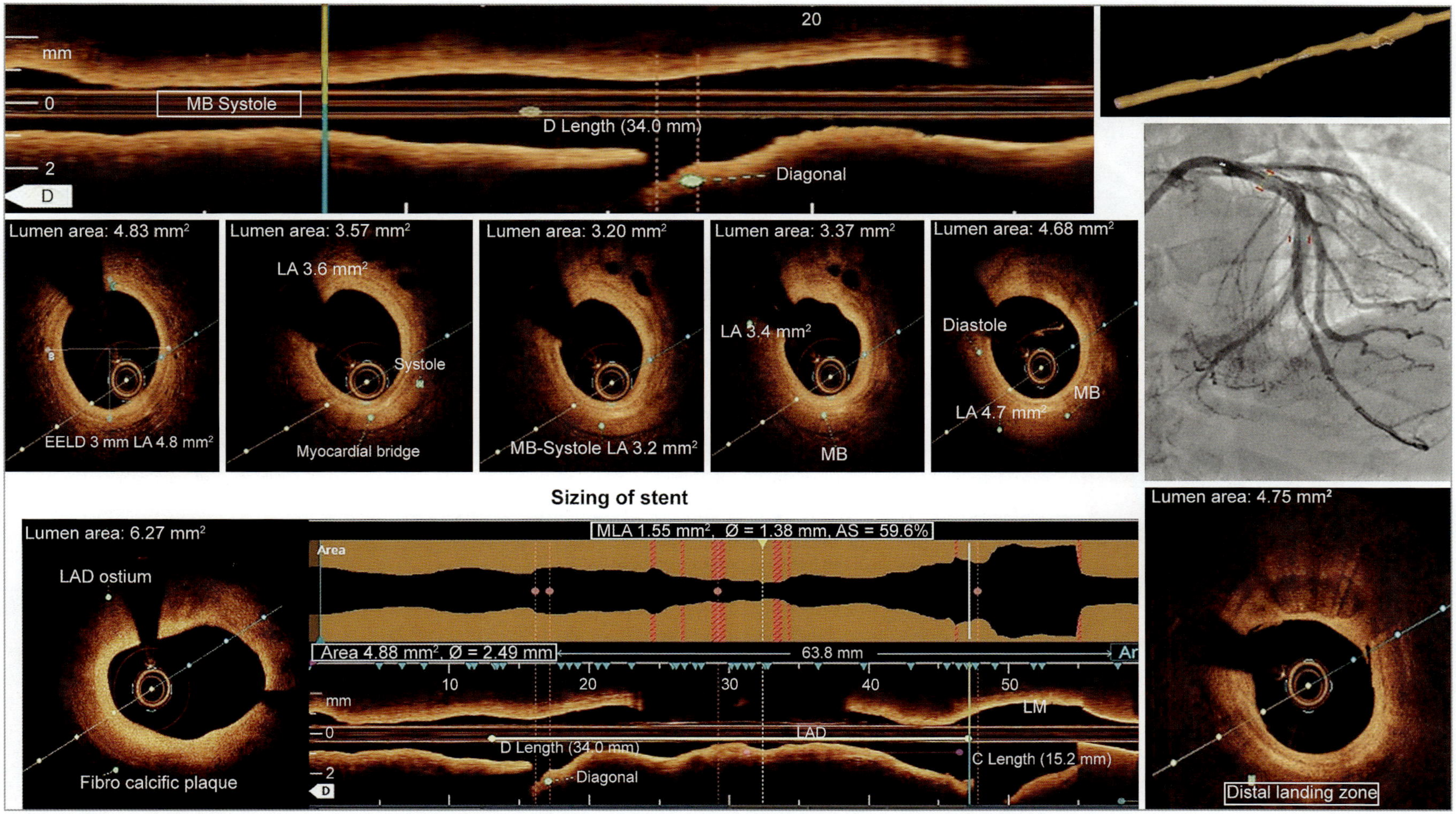

Fig. 76: Myocardial Bridging assessment of distal LAD and sizing of the stent.

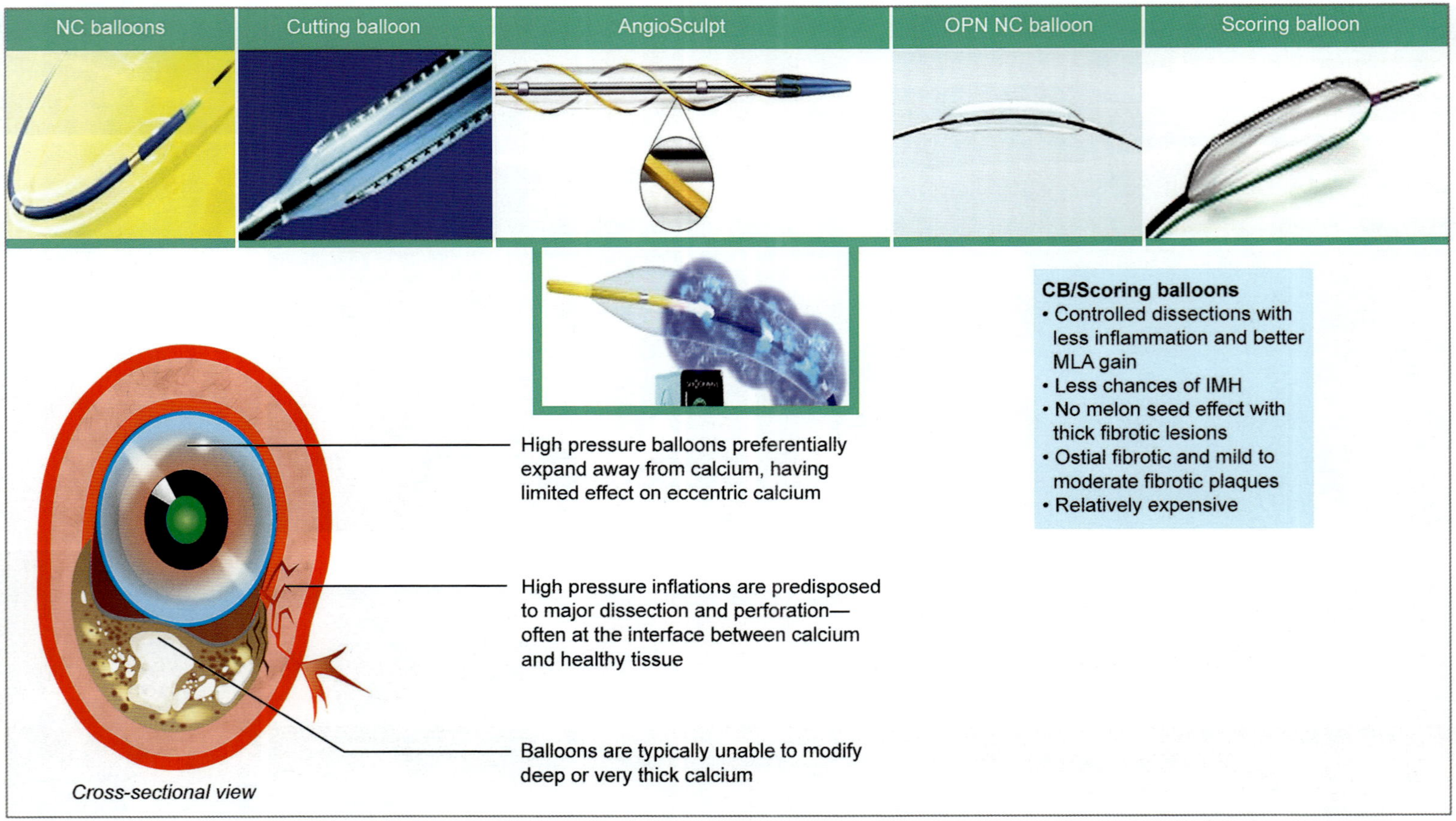

Fig. 77: Limitations of convetional tools in calcium.

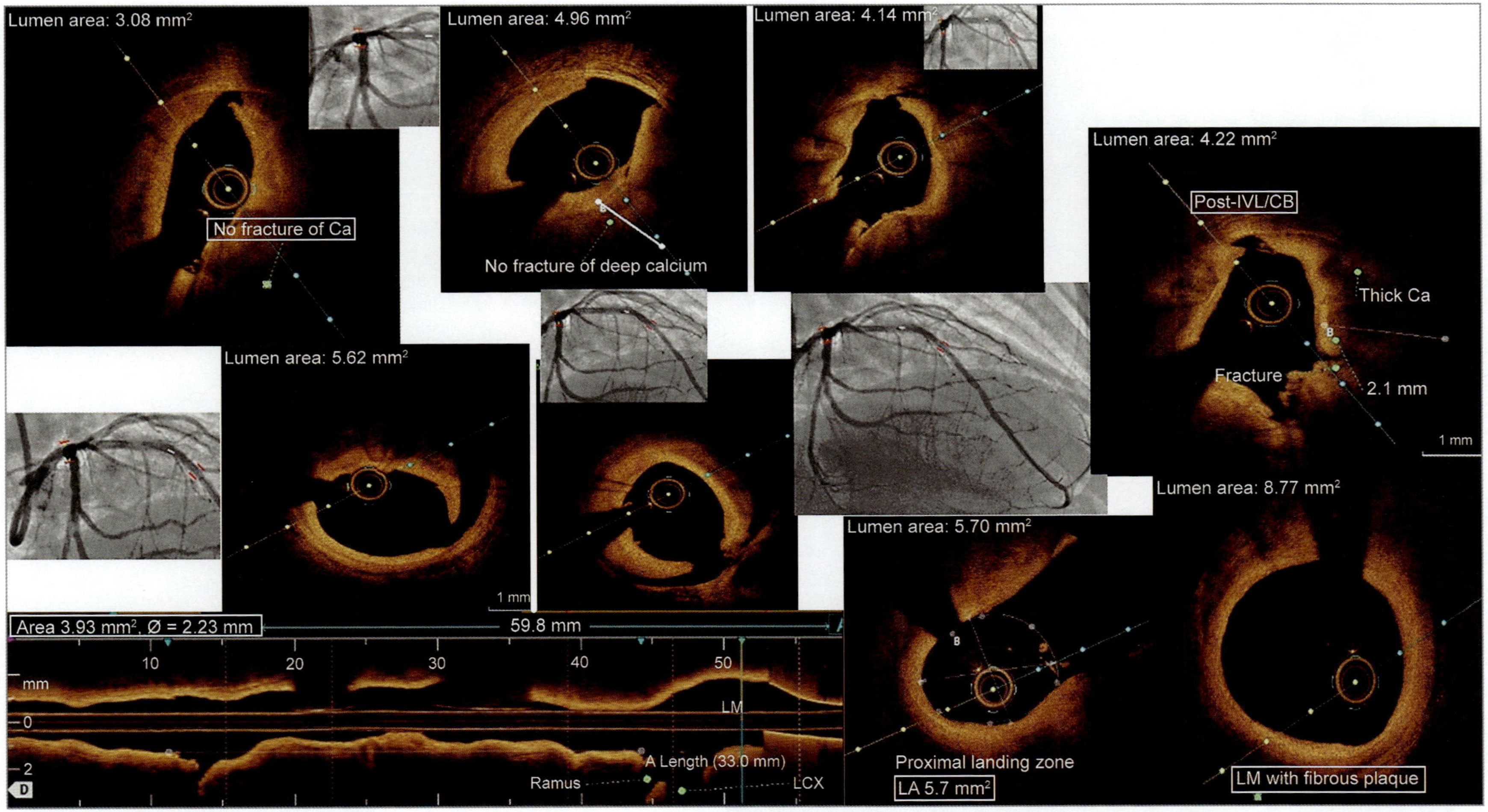

Fig. 78: Assessment of plaque modification post-IVL/CB/4 mm NC.

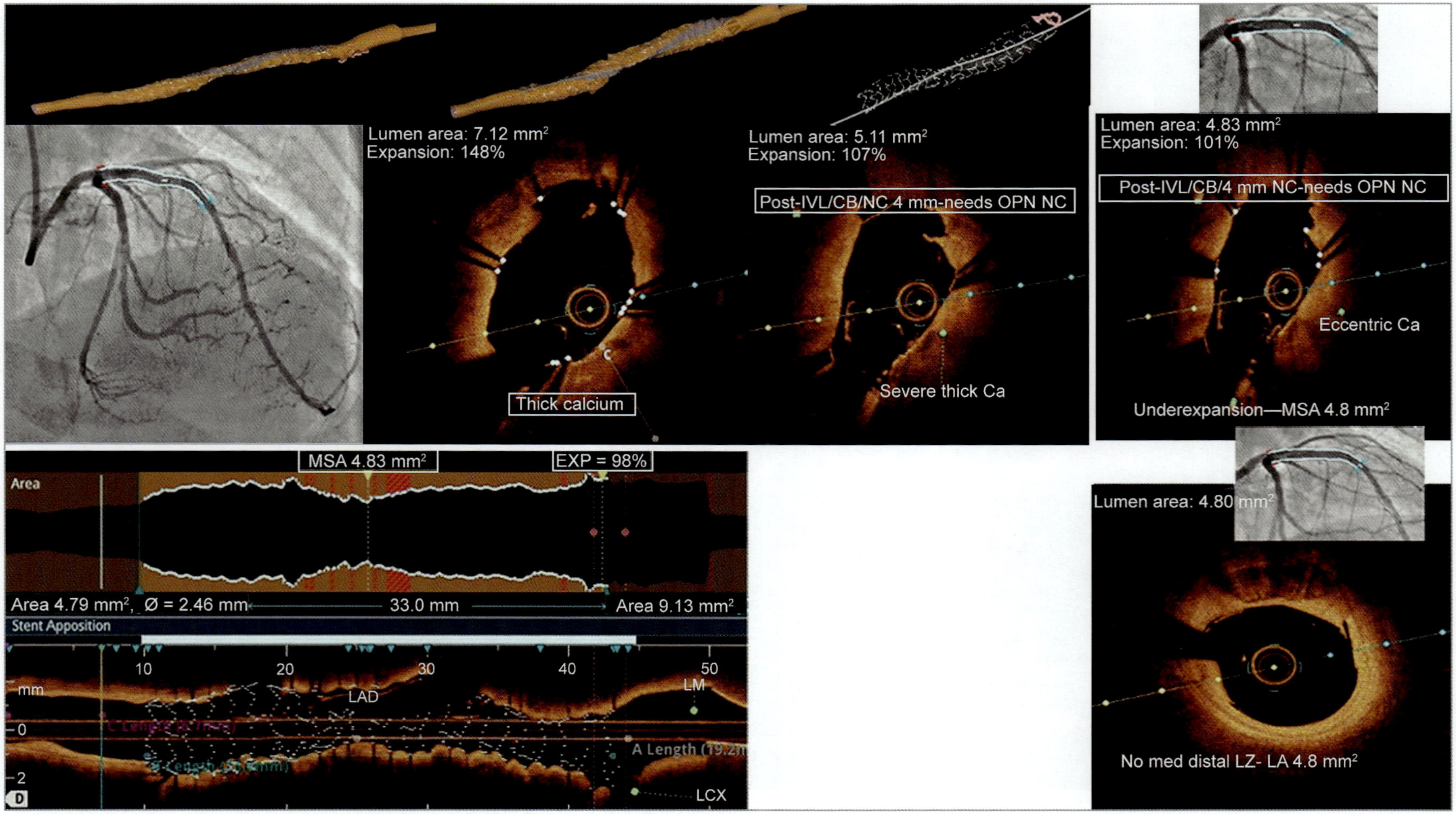

Fig. 79: Assessment of MAX revealed under-expansion needs high pressure balloon dilatations (OPN NC).

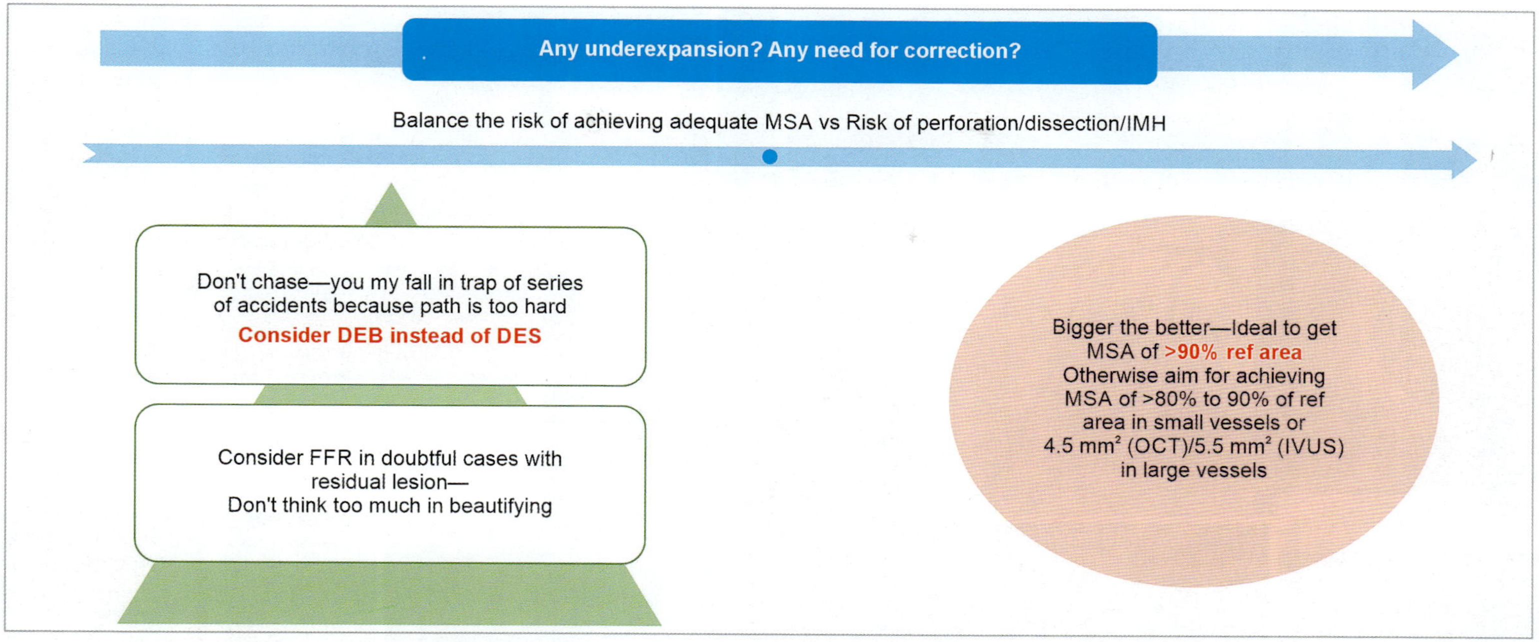

Fig. 80: Balance the risk of achieving MSA vs. risk of perforation/dissection/IMH.

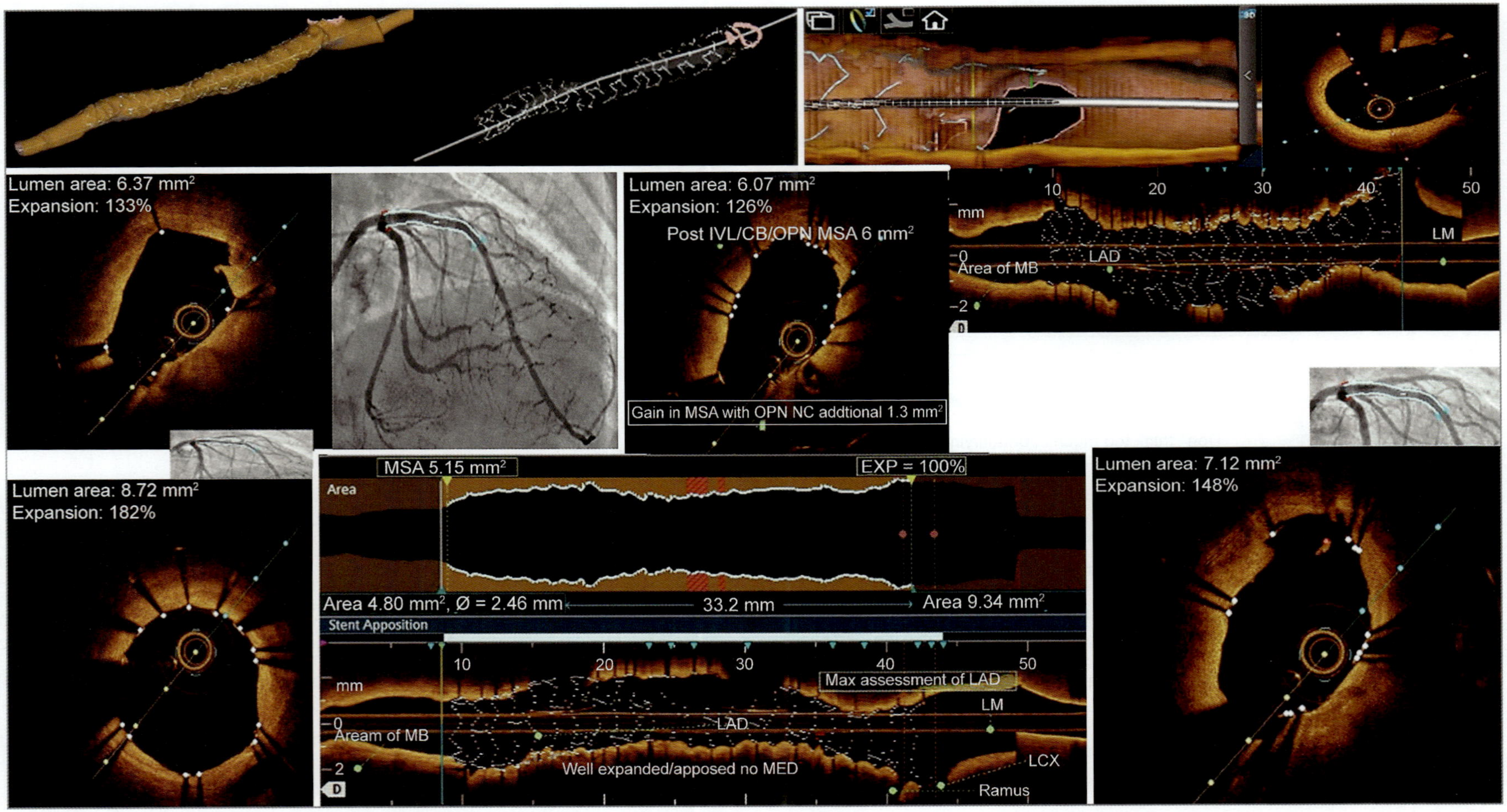

Fig. 81: Assessement of MAX after OPN NC-well expanded apposed and no MED.

CHAPTER 9

Percutaneous Coronary Intervention of Left Main Coronary Artery and Non-left Main Coronary Artery Bifurcation

ABSTRACT

Left main coronary artery (LMCA) is a crucial segment in the coronary tree because it supplies a large majority of the left ventricular myocardium in the setting left dominance; the left main (LM) contributes nearly to its entire blood supply. Current clinical practice guidelines from both the American College of Cardiology/American Heart Association (ACC/AHA) and the European Society of Cardiology (ESC) recommend revascularization for all patients with ≥50% stenosis of the LMCA. Assessment of LMCA disease is sometimes very difficult by angiography due to its ambiguity, particularly in complex bifurcation lesions. Angiography is highly accurate when defining critical or very severely obstructive lesions; its precision declines when contrast-filling defects or intermediate stenosis are involved. Optical coherence tomography (OCT) provides high-resolution images at the cost of limited penetration compared with intravascular ultrasound (IVUS) with an axial spatial resolution of 10–20 µm vs. 100–200 µm, lateral resolution of 20 vs. 200 µm, and penetration depth of 1–2.5 vs. 10 mm, respectively. OCT measurements were proved to be nearer to the actual luminal areas, whereas IVUS measurements were overestimated and were less reproducible in the phantom model. OCT and IVUS are proved to be a valid guidance for optimization of percutaneous coronary intervention (PCI). However, usefulness of OCT in day-to-day practice is very limited in the assessment of LM disease. A novel technique using OCT-guided angiographic coregistration to optimize stent placement in true ostial bifurcation lesion. Both imaging technologies have different distinct features; these are complementary and should be opted carefully for each patient based on pros and cons and clinical indications of each technique. Although experience of OCT usage for assessment of LMCA is very limited, but it is being used by more and more operators throughout the world due to very high-resolution images, especially in patients with distal LMCA disease. We feel this will play a great role in guiding LMCA interventions.

INTRODUCTION

Assessment of left main coronary artery (LMCA) disease is sometimes very difficult by angiography due to its ambiguity, particularly in complex bifurcation lesions. Angiography is highly accurate when defining critical or very severely obstructive lesions; its precision declines when contrast filling defects or intermediate stenosis are involved. Although utility of optical coherence tomography (OCT) usage for assessment of LMCA is very limited, but it is being used by more and more operators throughout the world due to very high-resolution images, especially in patients with distal LMCA disease.

Significant left main (LM) disease is seen in about 4–6% of patients who undergo coronary angiography and untreated LM disease carries >20% mortality rate at 1 year. Current clinical practice guidelines from both the American College of Cardiology/American Heart Association (ACC/AHA) and the European Society of Cardiology (ESC) recommend revascularization for all patients with ≥50% stenosis of the LMCA **(Fig. 1)**. Regardless of symptomatic status or associated ischemic burden, the guidelines recommend LMCA percutaneous coronary intervention (PCI) in patients with stable

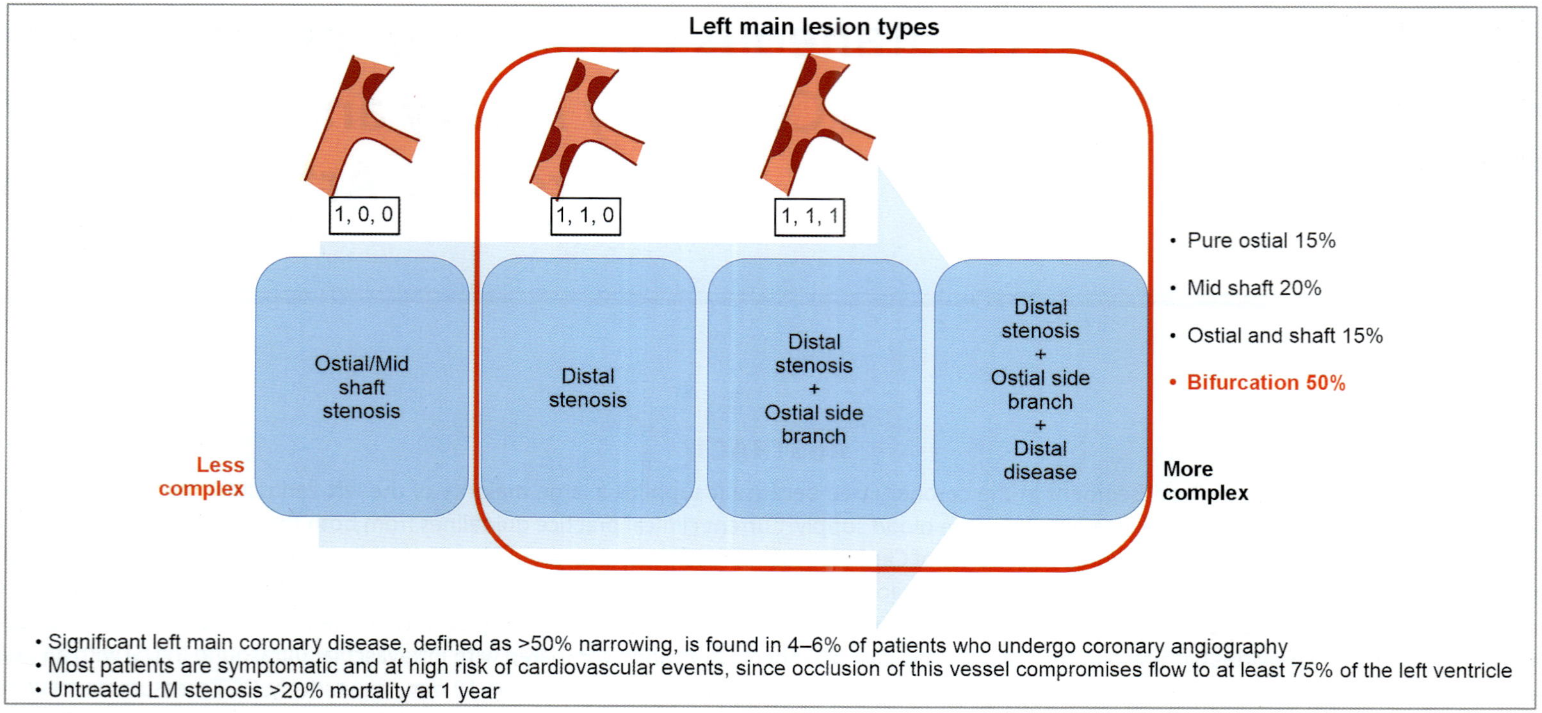

Fig. 1: Spectrum of LMCA disease.

coronary artery disease (CAD) with high surgical risk and a SYNTAX score ≤22, ostium and body of LM, (Class-IIA), and bifurcation (Class-IIB). Current guidelines recommend that intravascular ultrasound (IVUS) be used to assess the severity and optimize the treatment of unprotected LMCA lesions (Class IIa, level of evidence B).[1]

LIMITATIONS OF ANGIOGRAPHY

Assessment of LMCA disease is sometimes very difficult by angiography due to its ambiguity, particularly in complex bifurcation lesions. Noncoaxial alignment, deficient or excessive catheter engagement, contrast jet, and coronary sinus opacification may lead to further confusion in assessing severity by angiography. If LMCA is diffusely diseased due to lack of nondiseased reference segment, there is a possibility of improper assessment of severity of lesion and sometimes difficult to assess due to its branches getting overlapped and impeding angiographic assessment of the severity of distal segment lesions. Severe calcification and eccentric plaque formation results in ambiguous angiographic lesions, thereby leading to misinterpretation of severity of lesion. Reproducibility and accuracy of the angiographic assessment of LM stenosis ≥70% is excellent.[2] Visual estimates of intermediate LM stenosis (30–70%) from coronary angiography have significant interobserver variability which was proved in various clinical and postmortem studies.

Revascularization strategies based solely on the angiographic appearance of LMCAD stenosis of intermediate severity (between 50 and 70%) may be inappropriate and needs to be confirmed with imaging and functional assessment.

Overestimation of ostial minimal lumen area (MLA) due to noncoaxial alignment is shown in **Figures 2 and 3**.

INTRAVASCULAR IMAGING FOR BIFURCATION

As per the histological studies, angiography underestimates one half of the severe LMCA lesions and overestimates one half of the moderate LM lesions. IVUS evaluation reveals higher degree of disease existence compared with angiography and IVUS-derived minimum lumen diameter is the strongest independent predictor of clinical events. Recent evidence suggested a minimal lumen diameter of <2.8 mm of LMCA on IVUS had the highest sensitivity

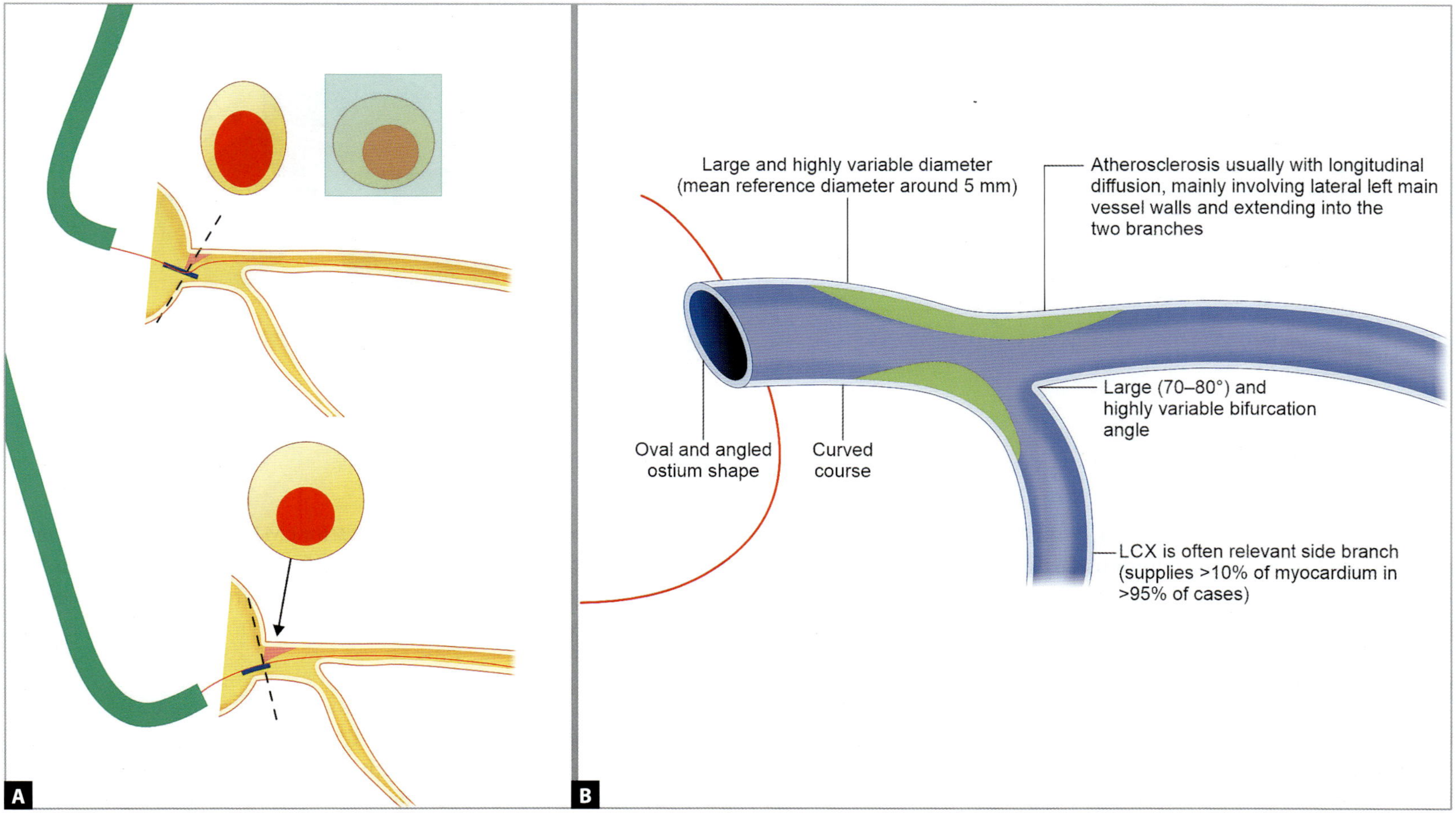

Figs. 2A and B: (A) Overestimation of ostial MLA due to non coaxial alignment; (B) Factors to be considered while doing PCI of LMCA.

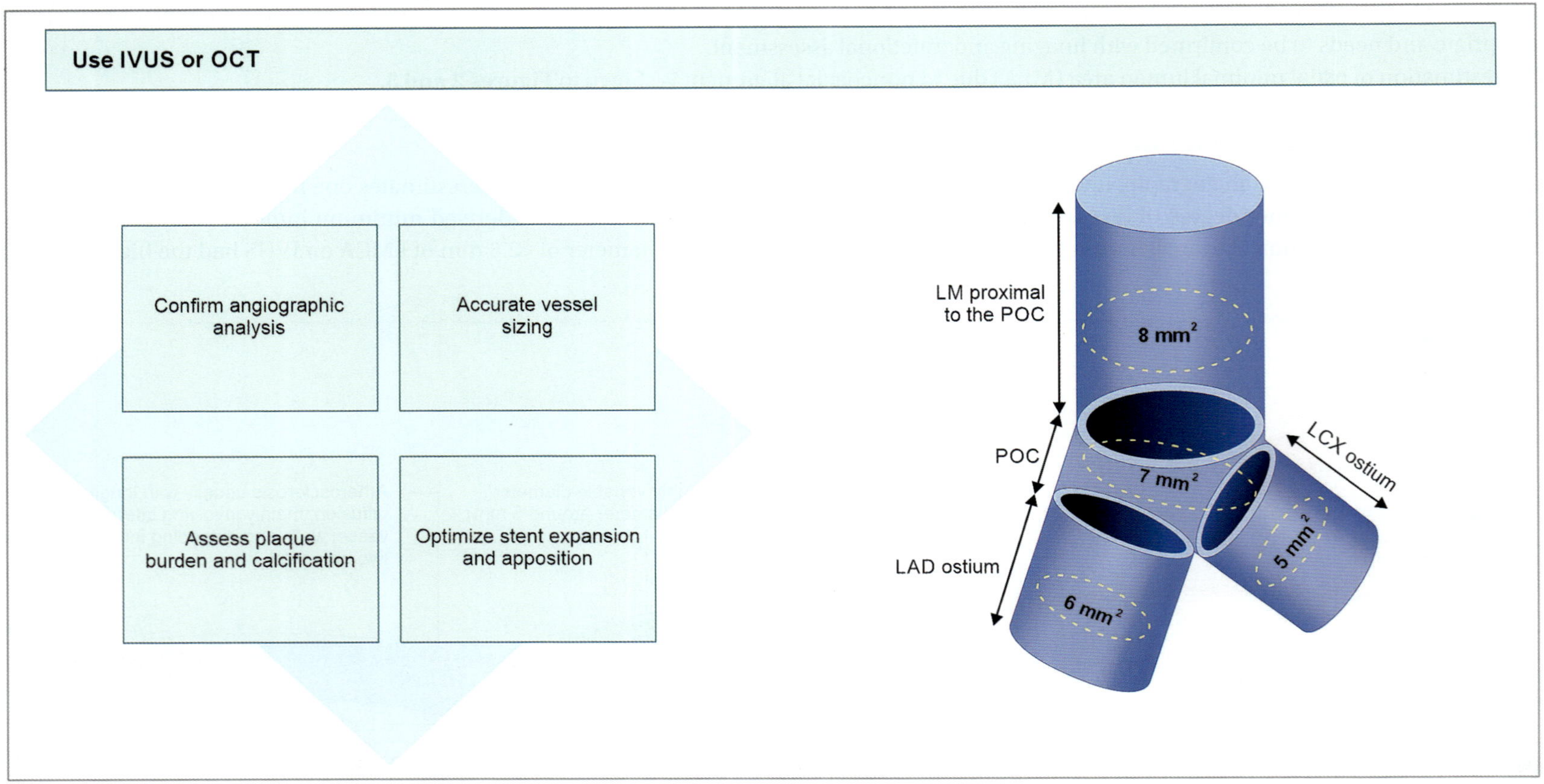

Fig. 3: Usefulness of Intravascular Imaging for PCI of LMCA.

and specificity. In normal LM, MLA is 14.1 mm^2 for women and 16.2 mm^2 for men, requiring an area stenosis of 57–63% for LM lesion to be hemodynamically significant using the prevailing criterion of 6 mm^2 as a cutoff for revascularization[3] **(Fig. 4)**. If MLA of LMCA >6 mm^2 defer PCI of LMCA, if <4.5 mm^2 needs PCI of LMCA and if MLA between 4.5 and 6 mm^2, consider clinical and physiological assessment and PCI recommended if fractional flow reserve (FFR) is <0.8.

REFERENCE VESSEL SIZE ESTIMATION

Basic Principles of Intravascular Imaging for Complex Bifurcation Stenting (Fig. 5)

- *Assessment of plaque (morphology) and full lesion coverage (lesion length and diameter):* 3D-OCT with angio coregistration is very useful in implementing MLD-MAX algorithm by identifying disease extent, landing zones with minimal or no plaque burden, and precise sizing of stents before stent implantation to allow planned full lesion coverage and potentially lower the risk of geographical miss.

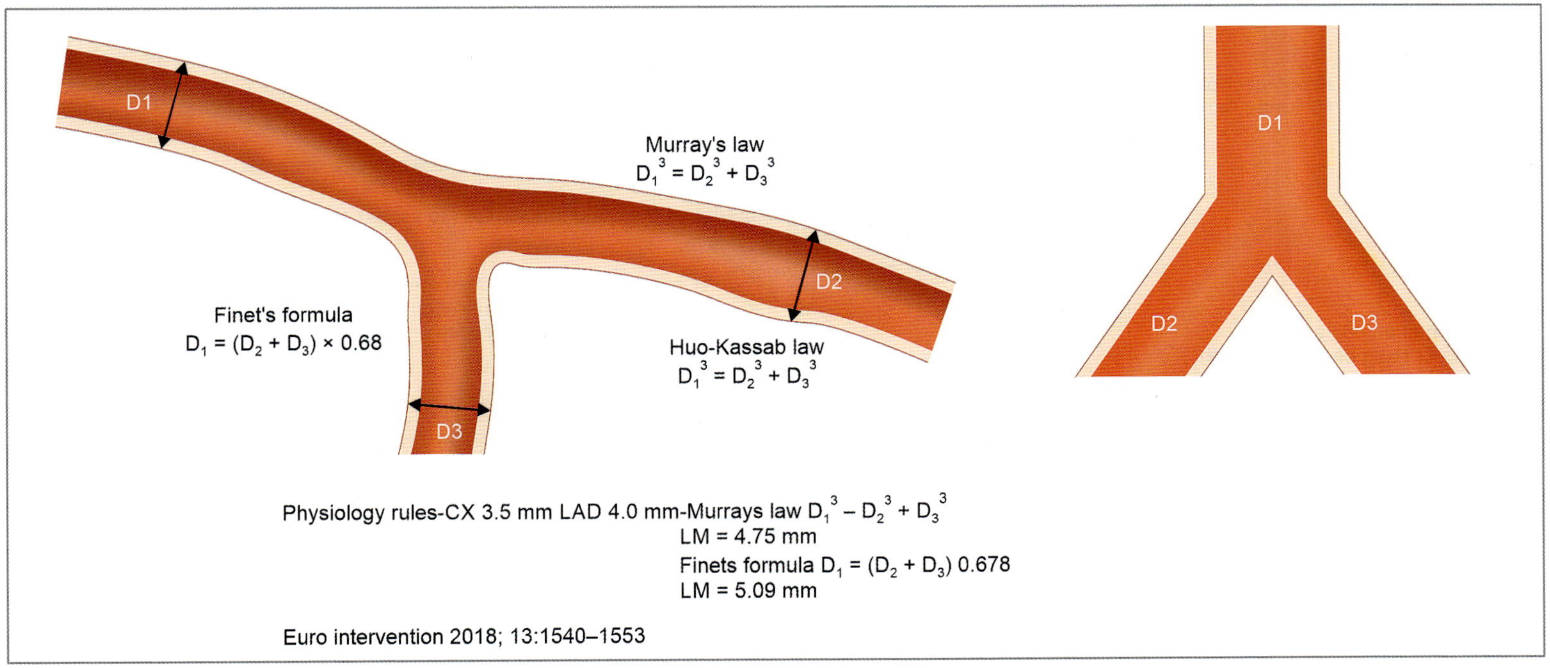

Fig. 4: Bifurcation Law's for angiographic sizing of MV, MB, and SB.
Source: Adapted from Lassen JF, Burzotta F, Banning AP, Lefèvre T, Darremont O, Hildick-Smith D, et al. Percutaneous coronary intervention for the left main stem and other bifurcation lesions: 12th consensus document from the European Bifurcation Club. EuroIntervention. 2018;13:1540-53.

- *Assessment and implementation of MAX of MLD-MAX algorithm:* Look for any significant malapposition, expansion, and medial edge dissection and repeat OCT run to confirm after correcting these predictors of drug-eluting stent (DES) outcome.[4]

ASSESSMENT OF THE LEFT MAIN BIFURCATION PRIOR TO PROVISIONAL STENTING

It defines morphology and distribution of plaque, luminal area of various segments of bifurcation, geometry of carina, and the bifurcation angle to determine procedural plan-provisional versus two-stent technique, any need for plaque modification, and precise sizing of balloons and stents. It may not possible to get the adequate angiographic projections to delineate the ostium of the left circumflex (LCX) due to the limitations of the angiographic equipment movements, which hampers visualization of a short segment or a tight ostium of a LCX stenosis. Sometimes, IVUS pullback of main vessel may not be reliable in assessing ostium of LCX and it may require additional pullback from LCX to assess ostium of LCX. In contrast, OCT is capable of providing accurate assessments of the side branch (SB) ostium from both MV and SB pullbacks. Information about atheroma distribution and type of carina play a crucial role in deciding PCI strategy and minimize the risk of SB occlusion owing to the carina/plaque shift **(Fig. 9A)**. Recent evidence from OCT studies suggested that the plaque accumulates less toward the flow divider region, compared with the opposite wall of bifurcation where low shear area is prevalent. In provisional stenting, SB closure **(Fig. 6)** can be predicted by the type of carina, carina angle (narrow vs. wide) and degree of plaque

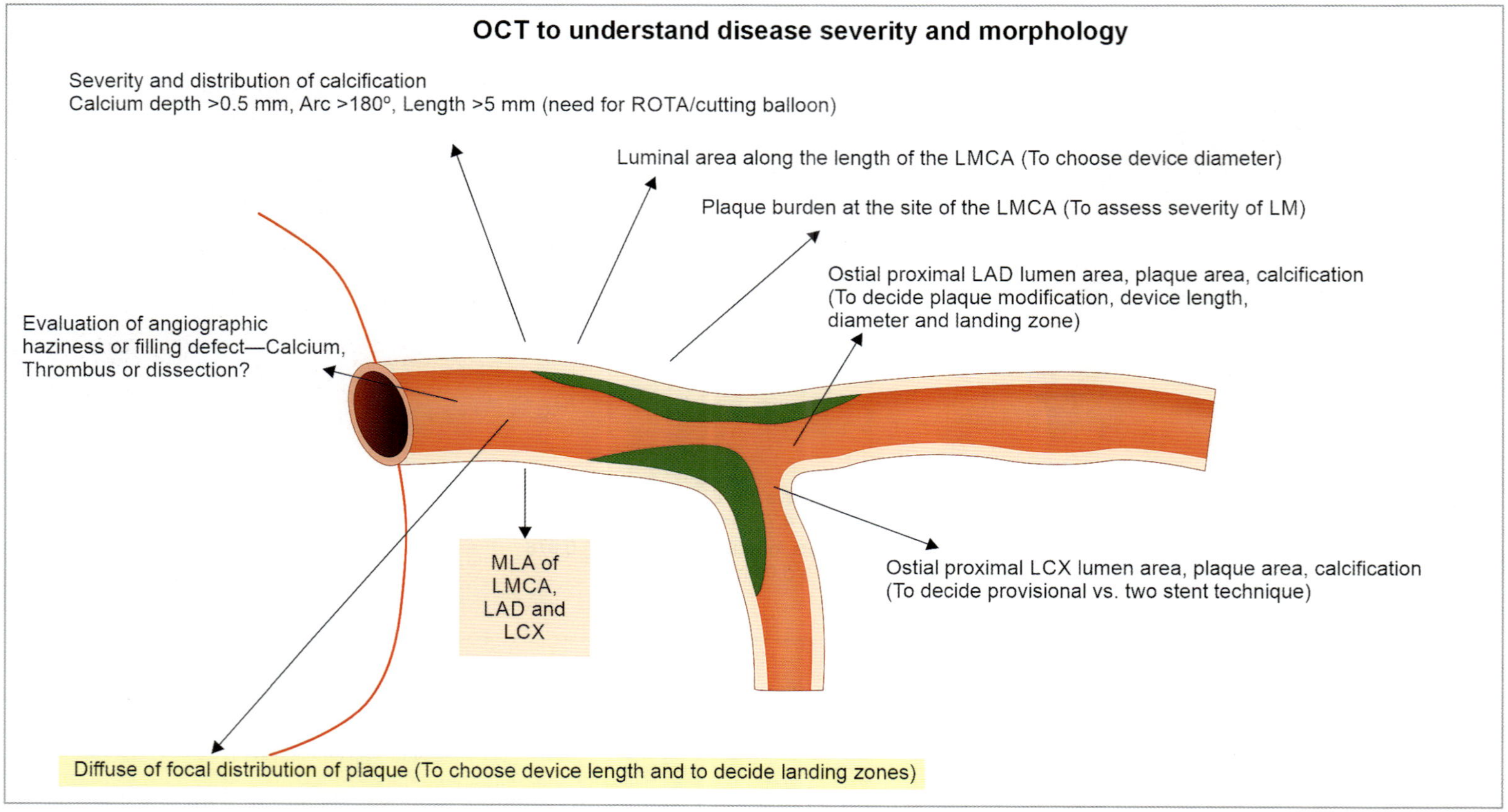

Fig. 5: OCT assessment for PCI of bifurcation lesions.

burden, and elongated carina *("spikey" or "elbow" carina)* on OCT may increase chances of SB closure after the stent implantation in the main vessel which may warrant the placement of guidewire in the SB for protection.[5]

Optical Coherence Tomography Predictors of Side Branch Compromise (Fig. 6)

Optical Coherence Tomography Predictors of Side Branch Complication with Crossover Stenting

Bifurcation evaluation of 49 patients in a recent study showed SB compromise when bifurcation PCI-carina tip angle (CT angle) was 29.5° vs. 65°, BP-CT length-length between proximal branching point to CT 1.2 vs. 2.25 mm. CT-angle and BP-CT length significantly smaller in lesions with SB compromise: 77.3 vs. 16.7%. CT-angle <50° and BP-CT length <1.7 mm, best cutoff values for predicting SB complication after provisional stenting **(Fig. 7)**.

	HR	95% C	p-value
Lumen area at proximal BP	0.96	0.66–1.38	0.81
Theoretical plaque distribution at carina tip	8.53	1.21–59.9	<0.05
CT angle (≤51°)	10.5	1.17–4.4	<0.05
BP-CT length (≤1.75)	19.2	2.27–16.2	<0.01

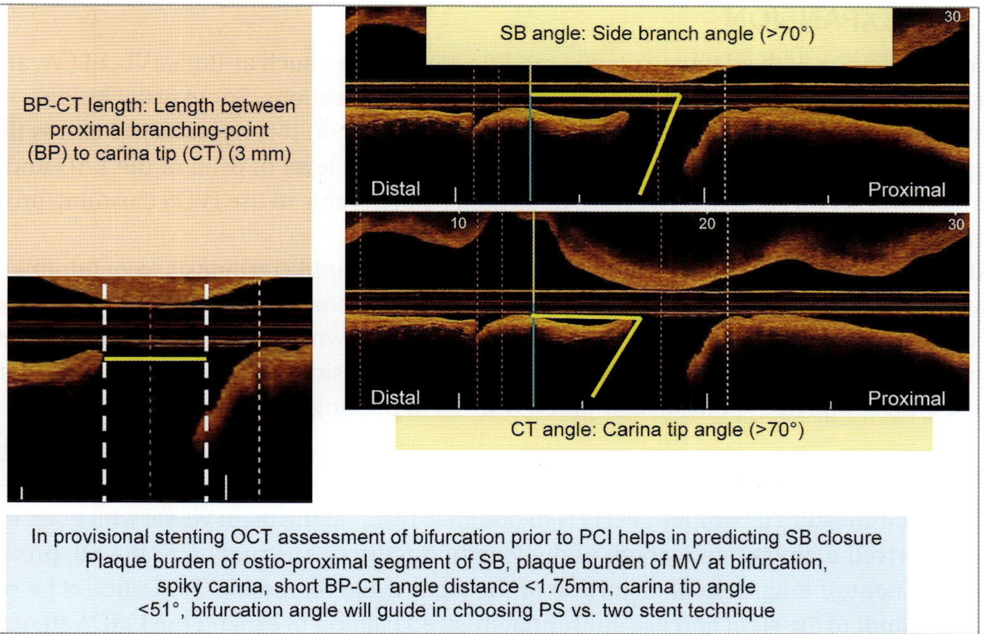

Fig. 6: OCT assessment of bifurcation for predicting SB occlusion.

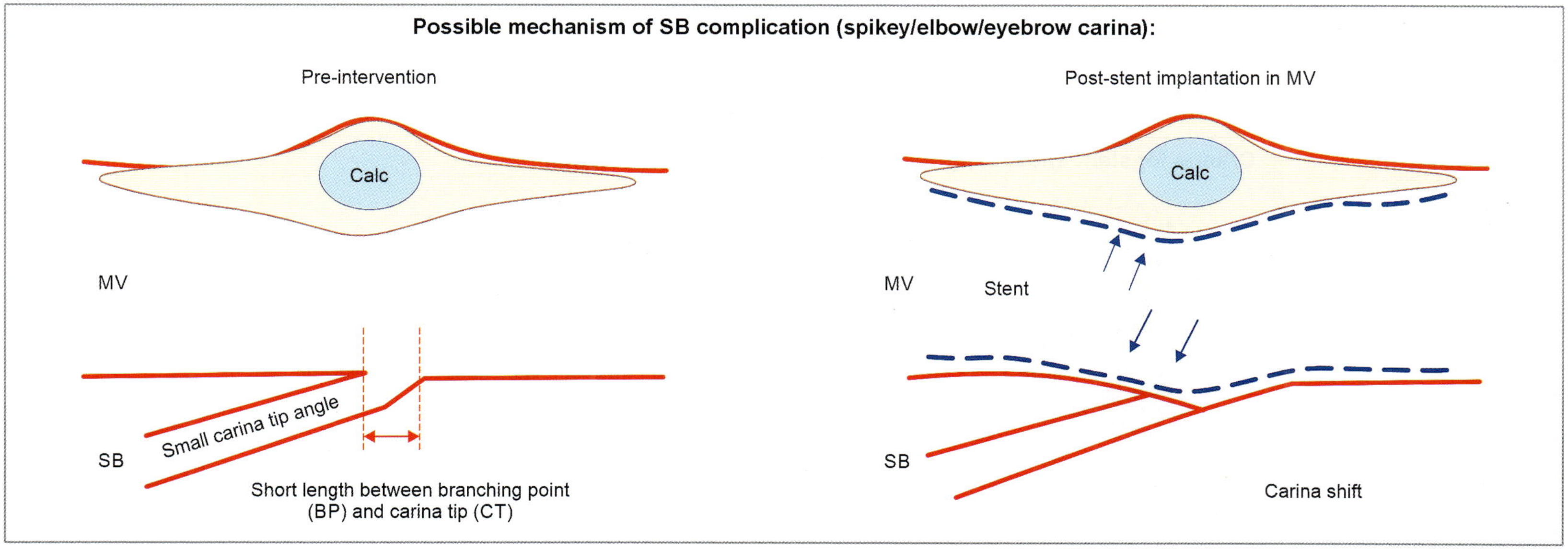

Fig. 7: Possible mechanism of SB complication.

STENT EXPANSION

Lesion preparation with adequate plaque modification devices such as Rota, IVL, ELCA, and OA is very essential prior to stent implantation for adequate expansion and apposition of the stents with low-rate complications. Some ostial lesions, which are often quite very fibrotic, need to be postdilated with cutting or scoring balloons for adequate expansion of the stent. It is necessary to assess the stent expansion at the level of the LMCA, at the level of the *"polygon of confluence"* (merger of the LAD and LCX, at the level of ostia of the LAD and LCX). Assessment of ostium of LMCA will be assessed more accurately with IVUS compared with OCT, it would be preferable to use IVUS if ostium/proximal LMCA is involved. For lesions of mid- and distal-LMCA, either IVUS or OCT can be used for optimization of PCI.[6]

Kang et al. found that the best IVUS predictors of angiographic restenosis were minimal stent areas (MSAs) of <8.2 mm^2 in the proximal LM, <7.2 mm^2 in the polygon of confluence, <6.3 mm^2 in the ostial left anterior descending, and <5.0 mm^2 in the ostial left circumflex **(Fig. 8)**. In the two-stent group the LCX ostium was the most common site of under expansion, when LMCA bifurcation lesions are treated with two-stent strategy. Angiographic restenosis was more frequent in lesions with underexpansion than in lesions without under expansion, even in the two-stent group (restenosis occurred in only 6% of those with complete expansion compared with 6% in the single stent group and 4.5% in nonbifurcation LMCA lesions)[7] **(Fig. 8)**.

Proximal Optimization Technique

Proximal optimization technique (POT) is to optimize result in the main vessel with good expansion and apposition by appropriately sized balloon based on OCT-derived diameter and length of the length. It reduces obstruction to the SB, prevents abluminal placement of guidewire, and reduces chances of development of longitudinal distortion of the stent while recrossing. POT should be performed before SB dilatation, better to know the maximum expansion limit of the stent and use appropriately sized balloon to expand the LMCA stent adequately according to the OCT sizing of LMCA. During POT, placement of the POT balloon across the SB takeoff may push the carina and carinal struts toward the SB ostium and in Y-shaped bifurcation, the area of the SB ostium might be reduced. Thus, final POT performed, the balloon should not cross the SB takeoff **(Fig. 9)**. The OCT-guiding strategy includes OCT sizing of length and diameter of both the stent and the POT balloon **(Figs. 10A and B)**. The stent-landing zone is extended proximally to accommodate the full POT balloon length if possible.

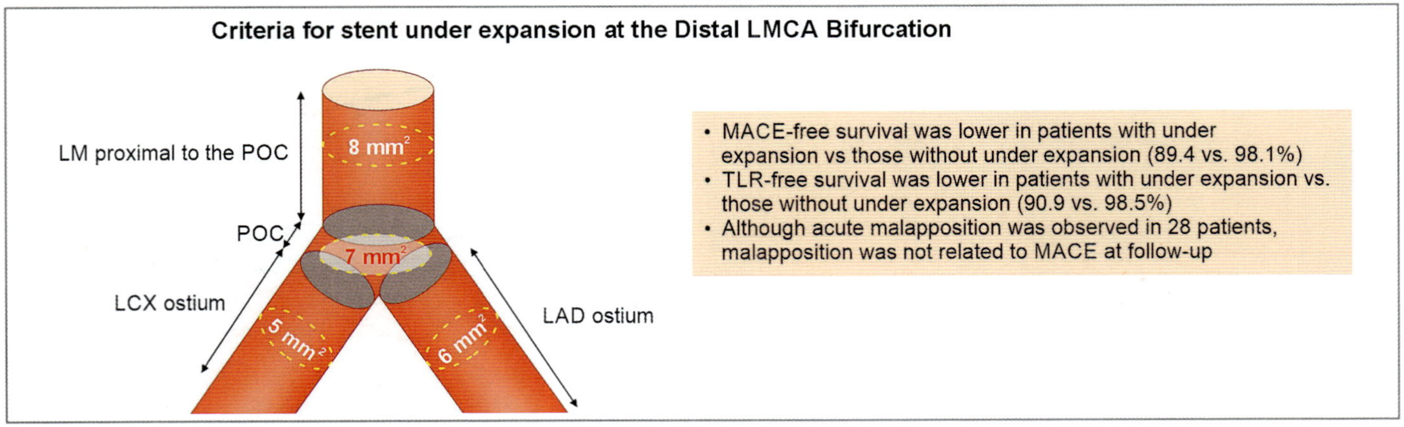

Fig. 8: Criteria for stent under-expansion at the distal LMCA bifurcation.

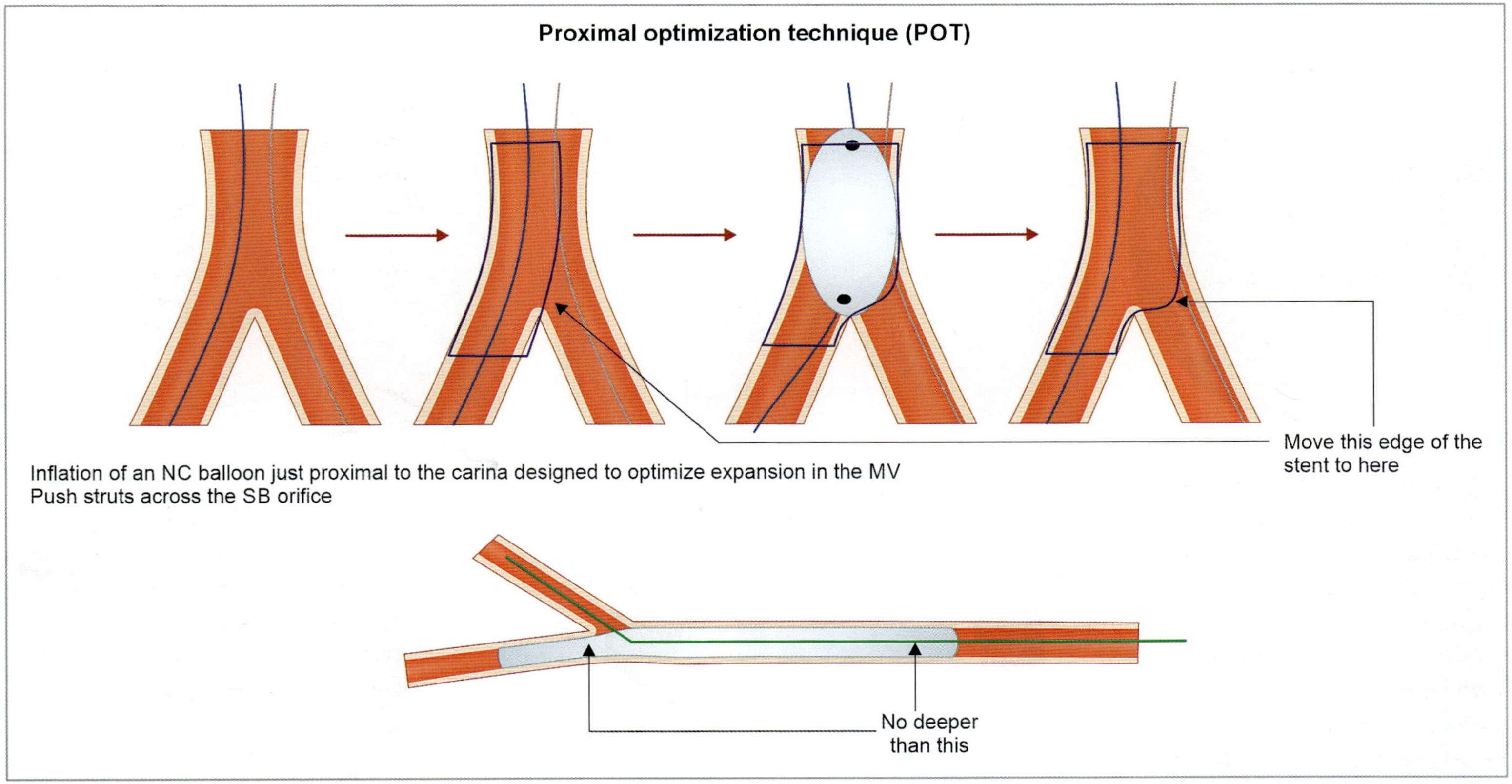

Fig. 9: Proximal optimization technique (POT) - sizing and placement of POT balloon.

Recent NOBLE study **(Figs. 11A and B)** showed evidence of significant reduction of long-term risk in patients who achieved LM MSA of <10.8 mm^2 versus MSA >13.4 mm^2 which emphasized the need for the adequately sized balloon based on either OCT or IVUS for POT to get MSA as much as possible, which is at least 80–90% of the corresponding vessel to produce better acute- and long-term outcomes.

Three-dimensional OCT helps in guiding of distal crossing versus proximal crossing during bifurcation stenting: 3D-OCT with angio coregistration is useful to for the understanding of complex bifurcation anatomy and planning of the procedure during bifurcation PCI. Prior to kissing balloon after stenting, it is important to recross the SB ostium strut cell with a wire in the most distal cell to minimize the risk of pushing struts toward the MV **(Fig. 12)**. Use of OCT is recommended to exclude accidental abluminal rewiring and to assess the position of recrossing wire. The OPTIMUM study demonstrated superiority to angio-guided PCI in terms of incidence of acute ISA (creation of metal carina) in bifurcation segment in 3D-OFDI guided arm, 45% of lesions required second attempt to redirect the wire to the optimal cell.[8]

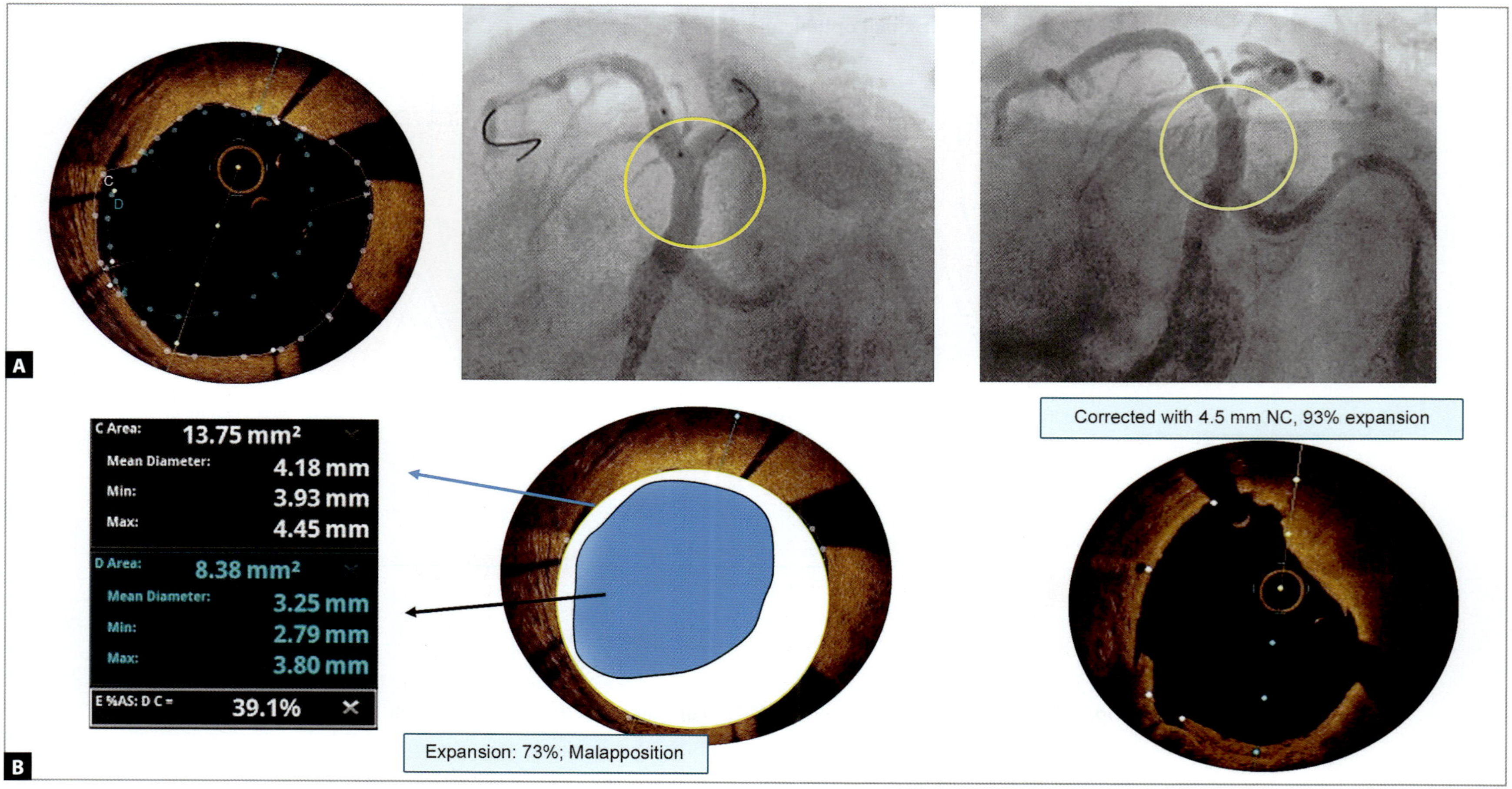

Figs. 10A and B: OCT images before and after mal-apposition.

OPTICAL COHERENCE TOMOGRAPHY ASSESSMENT OF WIRE POSITIONING

Optical coherence tomography guides in recrossing of strut at the ostia of SB, particularly in terms of proximal versus distal, link free versus with link, and any abluminal placement of guidewire **(Figs. 13A and B)**.

Bench studies showed evidence of accidentally crushed stent due to abluminal rewiring and this can be identified by OCT but may not be visible on angiographic images during the procedure.

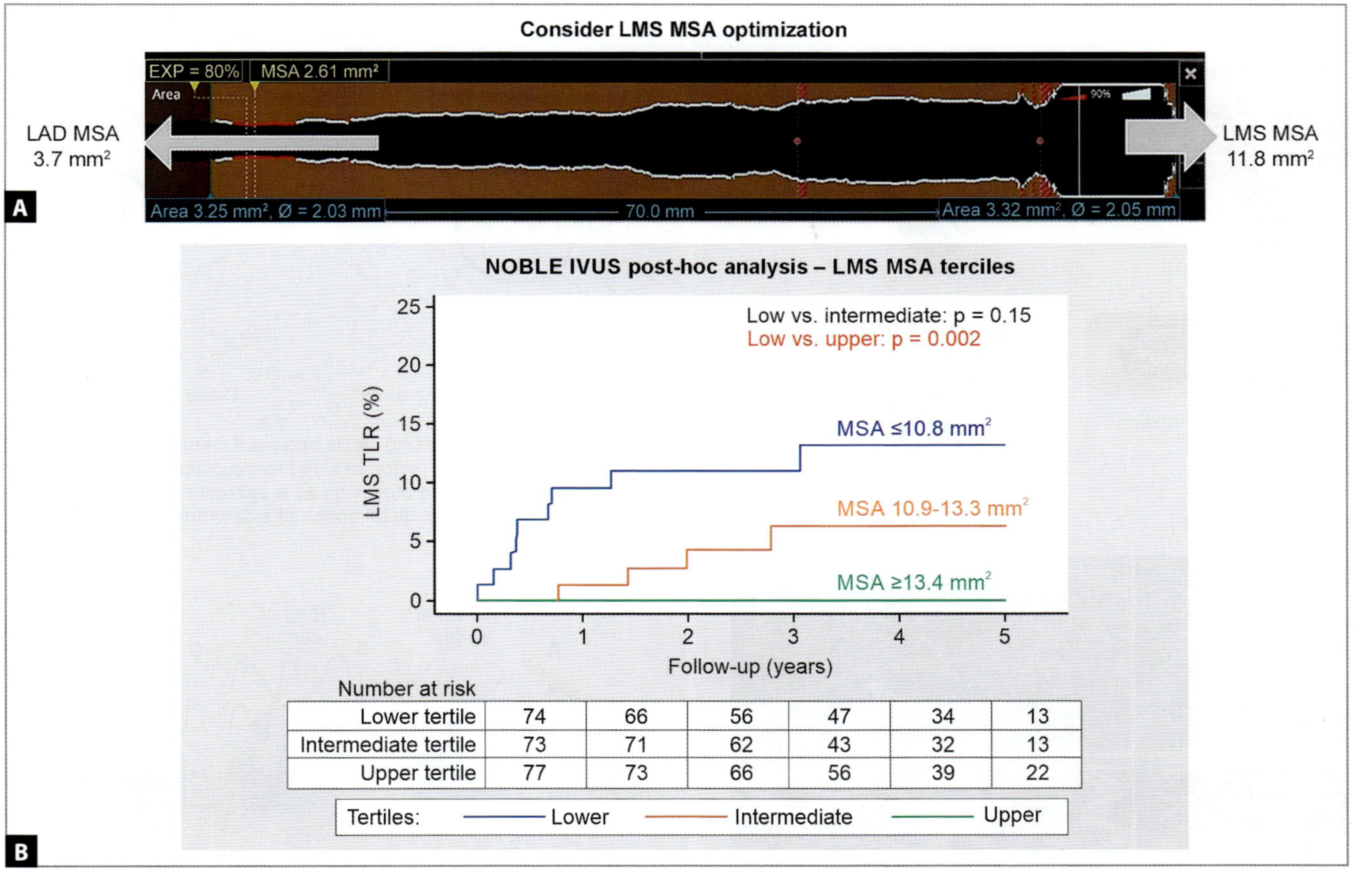

Figs. 11A and B: Recent evidences from NOBLE study about the achievement of Left Main Mean Stent Area.

ACUTE STENT DEFORMATION

Longitudinal stent dislodgment (LSD) is seen as multiple overlapping strut layers within a single stent, often accompanied by stent shortening. IVUS identifies acute stent deformation in about 1.1% of PCI procedure and about half of these are located in the LMCA. Acute LMCA stent deformation was observed in 6.6% of cases of the EXCEL study and ostium of LMCA (81.8%) was the most common site of LSD **(Fig. 14)**.

Figures 15A and B show LSD of ostial LAD stent which was corrected with serial high-pressure NC balloon inflations.

Longitudinal stent deformation should be suspected if there is any difficulty in advancing balloon over the jailed SB and it could be due to narrow cell of the stent across the SB (graded balloon dilatations to open SB strut) or abluminal placement of rewired SB. Preferable to rule out these by OCT or IVUS evaluation before making further attempts of dilatation of SB strut otherwise it may lead worsening of LSD. LSD can be prevented by avoiding guide

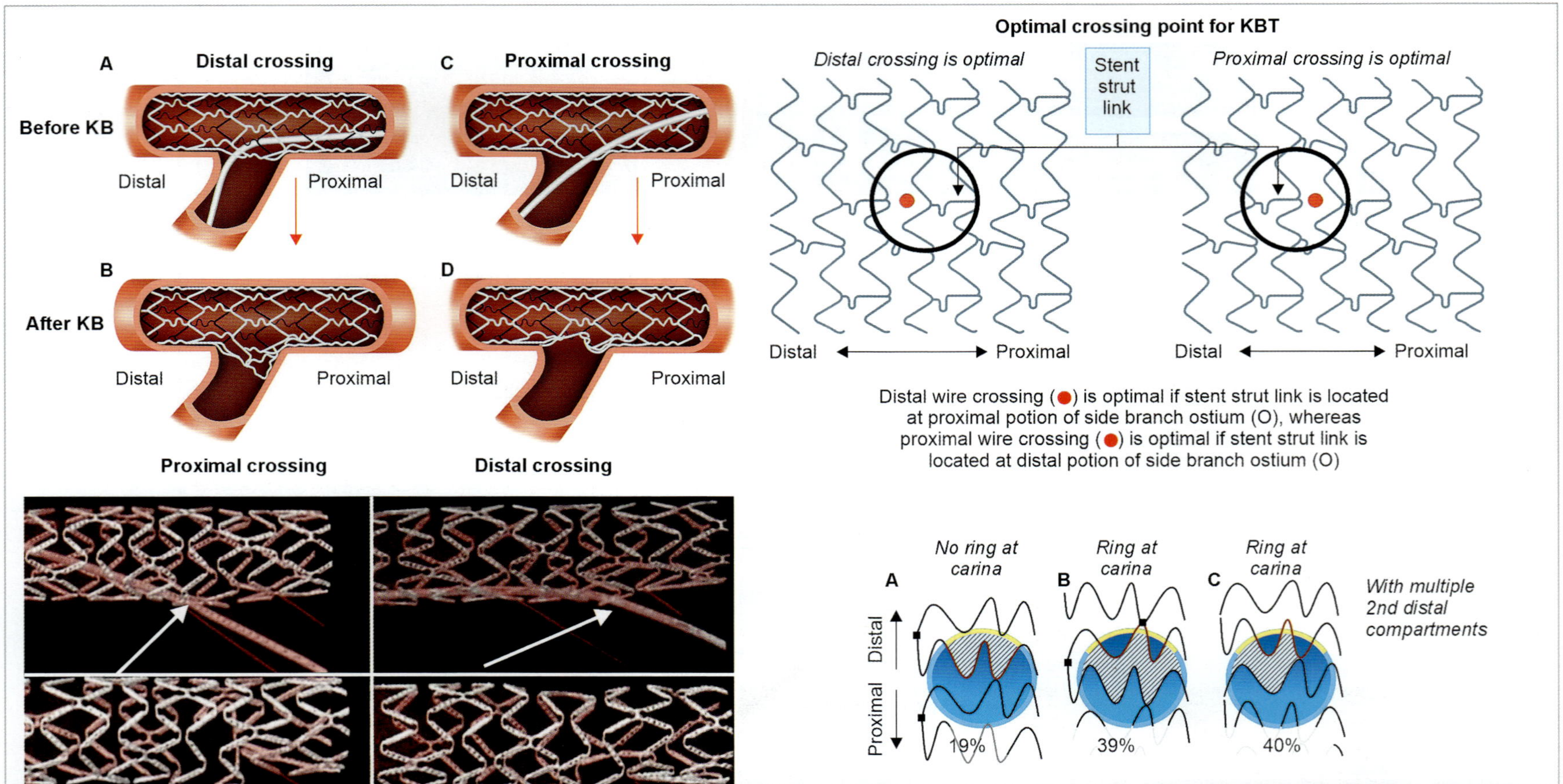

	3D-OFDI, N = 56	Angio, N = 54	p value
Total procedural contrast volume, mL (median)	175.0 (146.3–210.0)	175.0 (125.0–230.0)	0.87

Fig. 12: Usefulness of OCT for wire crossing of proximal vs. distal strut before kissing balloon dilatation.

catheter/guide liner contact with proximal edge of the LM stent, removing jailed wire as early as possible after recrossing SB ostia through stent struts using another guidewire and avoiding sucking of guide catheter while withdrawing balloons, guidewire, and other devices.

LEFT MAIN CORONARY ARTERY STENTING—PROVISIONAL VERSUS TWO-VESSEL STENTING

As per the guidelines, provisional stenting is the most preferred bifurcation technique; however, two-stent technique is preferable when significant disease large SB is present. Preference of provisional versus two-stent technique can be made based on the criteria mentioned in **Box 1** and **Figs. 16A and B**.

Stepwise assessment of OCT in provisional stenting is shown in **Figure 17**.

Provisional Technique

Suitable for most bifurcations, provisional technique requires wiring of both main branch and SB, choose stent sized to distal reference diameter of the branch to be stented and postdilate with balloon matching to distal reference diameter and proximal segment with balloon matching to proximal reference diameter and perform mandatory POT with appropriately sized balloon using OCT or IVUS **(Fig. 18)**. FKB with minimal balloon extension into SB is needed if there is any suboptimal result and stenting of SB can be considered for patients with persistent suboptimal result in spite of FKB inflation.

Side branch treatment after MV stenting is to be considered in provisional stenting if ostial SB stenosis >75% by visual estimate, TIMI flow <III, FFR value ≤0.75–080, and ostial SB stenosis >50% by intravascular imaging.

Different bailout options of provisional bifurcation stenting may be opted as described in **Figure 19**.

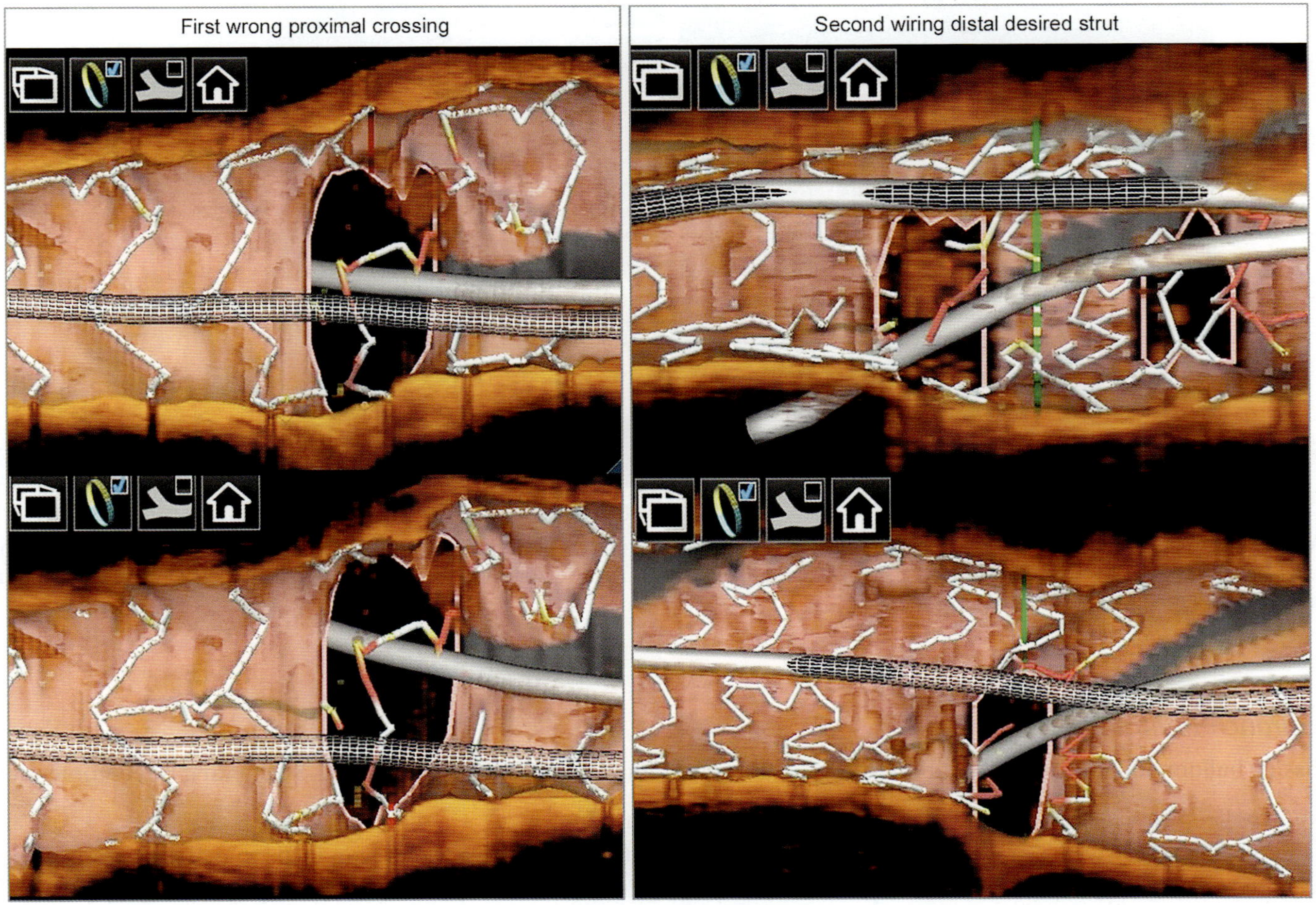

Fig. 13A

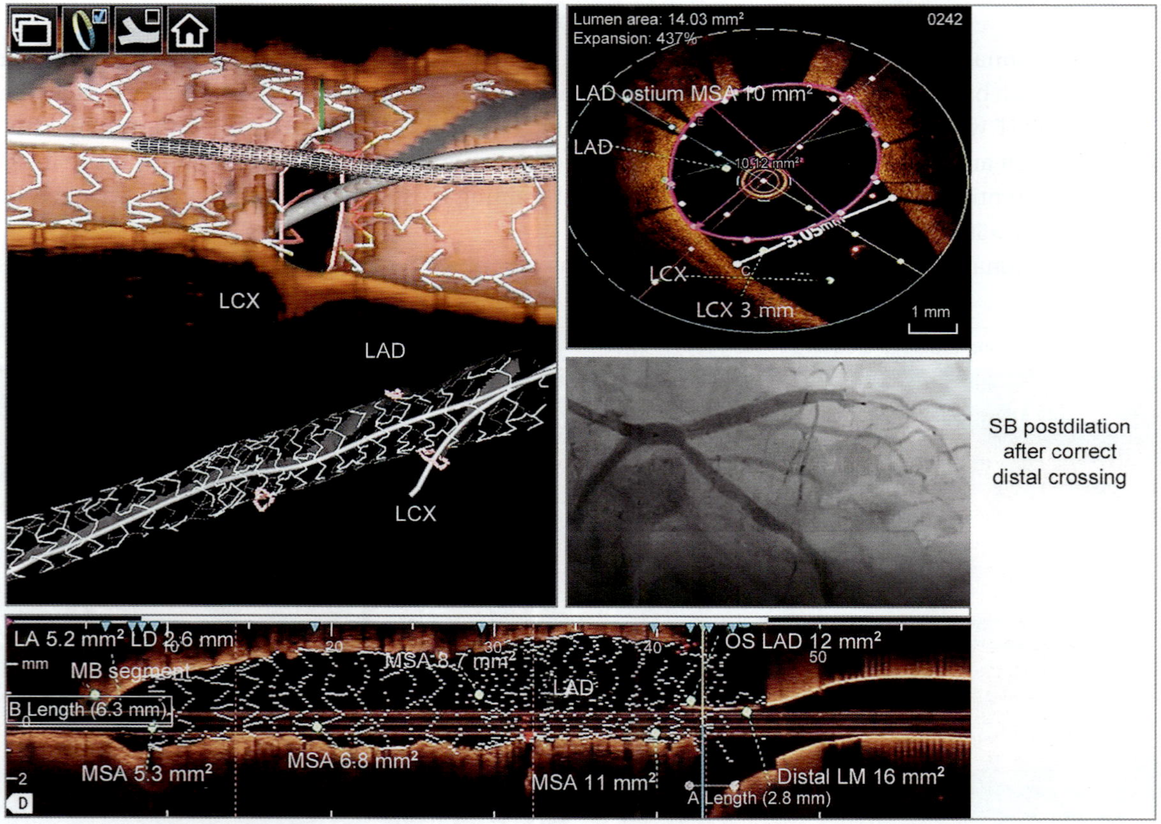

Fig. 13B

Figs. 13A and B: (A) Case examples of SB wire crossing through MB proximal and distal strut; (B) Case example of SB post dilatation after correct crossing through distal strut. *Source:* Adapted from Chen SL, Zhang JJ, Han Y, Kan J, Chen L, Qiu C, et al. Double Kissing Crush Versus Provisional Stenting for Left Main Distal Bifurcation Lesions: DKCRUSH-V Randomized Trial. J Am Coll Cardiol. 2017;70(21):2605-17.

Provisional Side Branch Treatment

Wire exchange, kissing balloon inflation, or SB inflation (re-POT), final POT, and if SB results are still not OK, SB stenting is recommended.

Importance of kissing balloon technique: To create the carina and prevent carina shift.

During FKB, sometimes aggressive kissing carries risk of overexpansion with asymmetrical expansion leads to malapposition of the in the proximal main vessel stent (bottle-neck effect), with increased elliptical shape and elliptical index rather than circular shape and risk of proximal MB underexpansion. This can be rectified by performing re-POT at the end of the procedure.

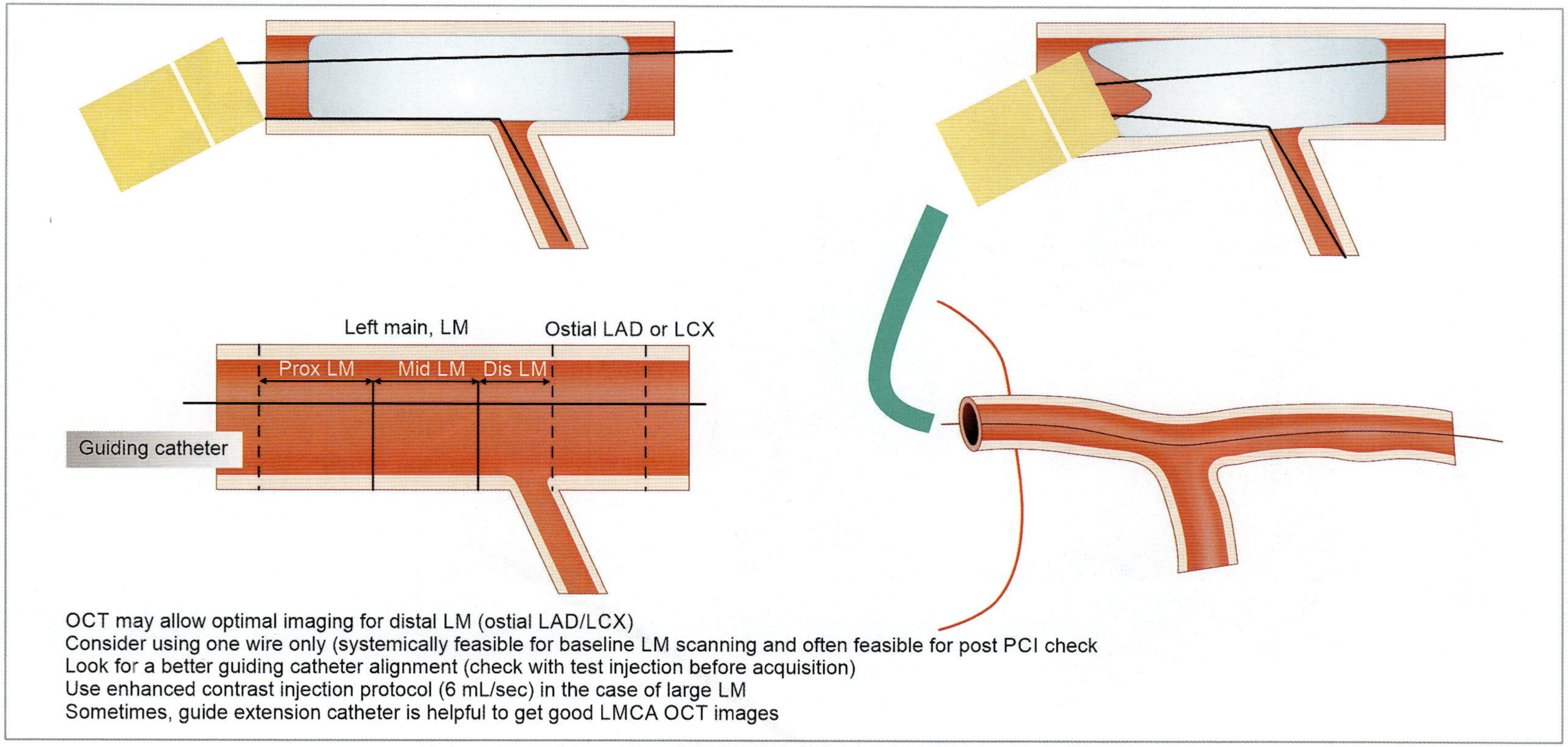

Fig. 14: Tips and Tricks for acquiring good OCT imaging of LMCA.

Steps of OCT during bifurcation percutaneous coronary intervention:

- Perform pre-PCI OCT pullback from main branch and SB—assess plaque extent, volume, and type of plaque. Decide if any plaque modification is required or not.
- Perform OCT before first kissing to assess crossing of wire and SB ostium and sizing of POT balloon and kissing balloons based upon MLA of proximal vessel, main branch and SB.
- Perform OCT before second kissing to assess crossing of SB proximal versus distal strut and any abluminal position of guidewire and SB ostium.
- Final OCT pullback to assess landing zones, any edge dissection, to rule out underexpansion (stent expansion should be >80–90% of corresponding proximal and distal reference lumen areas), malapposition, tissue prolapse, thrombus, geographical miss, and proximal stent deformation.

If MB–SB angle is <90° and inserting the OCT catheter in SB is usually safe, if SB angle >90°, insert only if there is no resistance or difficulty to avoid dissection.

Stepwise assessment of OCT in DK Crush stenting is shown in **Figures 20A and B**.

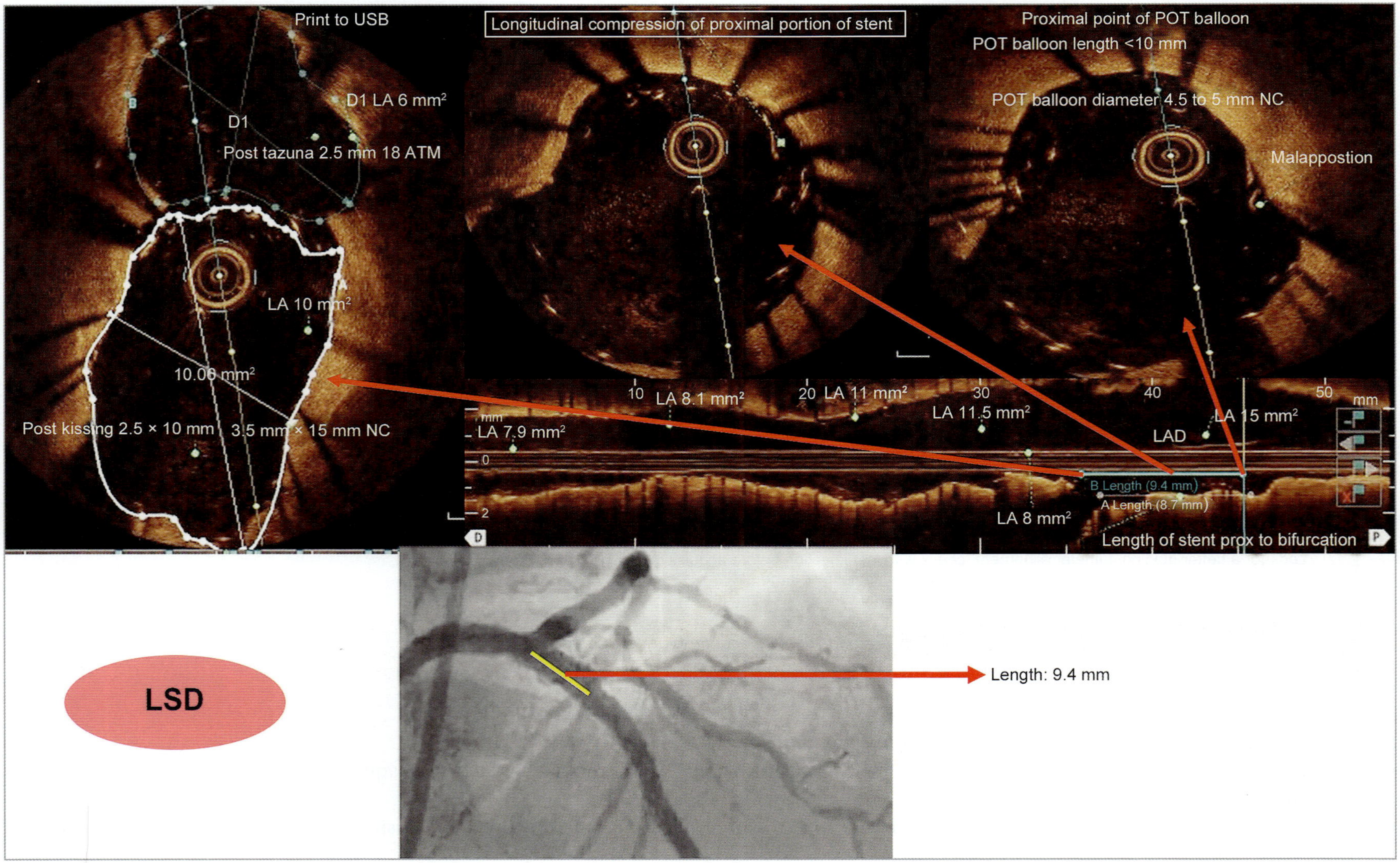

Fig. 15A

LSD at LM produces worst outcomes due to its vast area of supply, and it is usually due to deep seating of guide hitting the proximal edge of the stent.

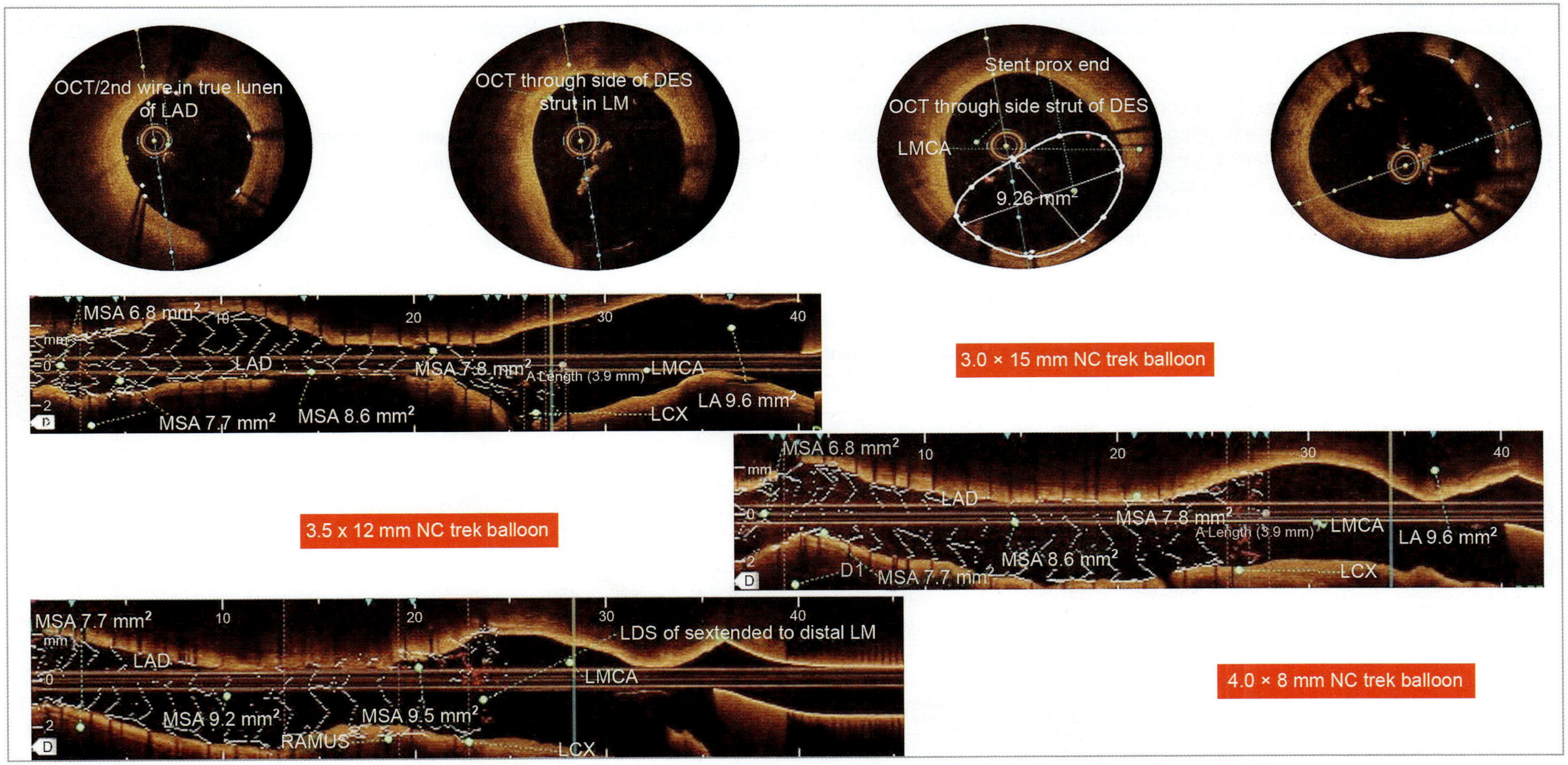

Fig. 15B

Figs. 15A and B: (A) Case example showing LSD of ostial LAD stent which was corrected with serial high pressure NC balloon inflations; (B) LSD of stent due to crossing of the side strut of DES in distal LM entering into true lumen LAD.

Evaluation of crush assessment by OCT is shown in **Figure 20**.

Stepwise assessment of OCT in T-stenting technique (through the stent) is illustrated in **Figures 21 and 24**.

Stepwise assessment of OCT in Culotte-stenting technique is illustrated in **Figures 25A to C**.

Influence of Main Vessel Stent Cell Rewiring on Stent Deformation Following Kissing Balloon Angioplasty

Access to the SB through the strut of a stent is usually possible through two or three different cells. The cell choice affects stent deformation. Bench testing has shown that wire crossing through the strut close to the carina provides better scaffolding of the origin of the SB than proximal crossing that pushes the struts inward toward the main vessel lumen.

BOX 1: LM bifurcation PCI.

- PS is the preferred strategy for treating LM bifurcation as it is faster, requires low contrast, lower radiation exposure due to less procedural complexity, and associated with lower perioperative MI
- Ostial/shaft of left main PCI results are comparable to CABG at 3 and 5 years
- DK crush superior to provisional stenting with LM bifurcations with SB size diameter of 2.5–4.0 mm and SB stenosis >50% with >50% plaque burden
- DK crush technique is the preferred two-stent technique owing to the supportive evidence over the other two-stent techniques
- FKB inflation is mandatory for all two-stent techniques
- Use IVUS or OCT for implementation of MLD-MAX Algorithm.
- Use MCS support for complex bifurcation intervention, especially for patients with depressed EF, single surviving vessel, and unstable hemodynamic status

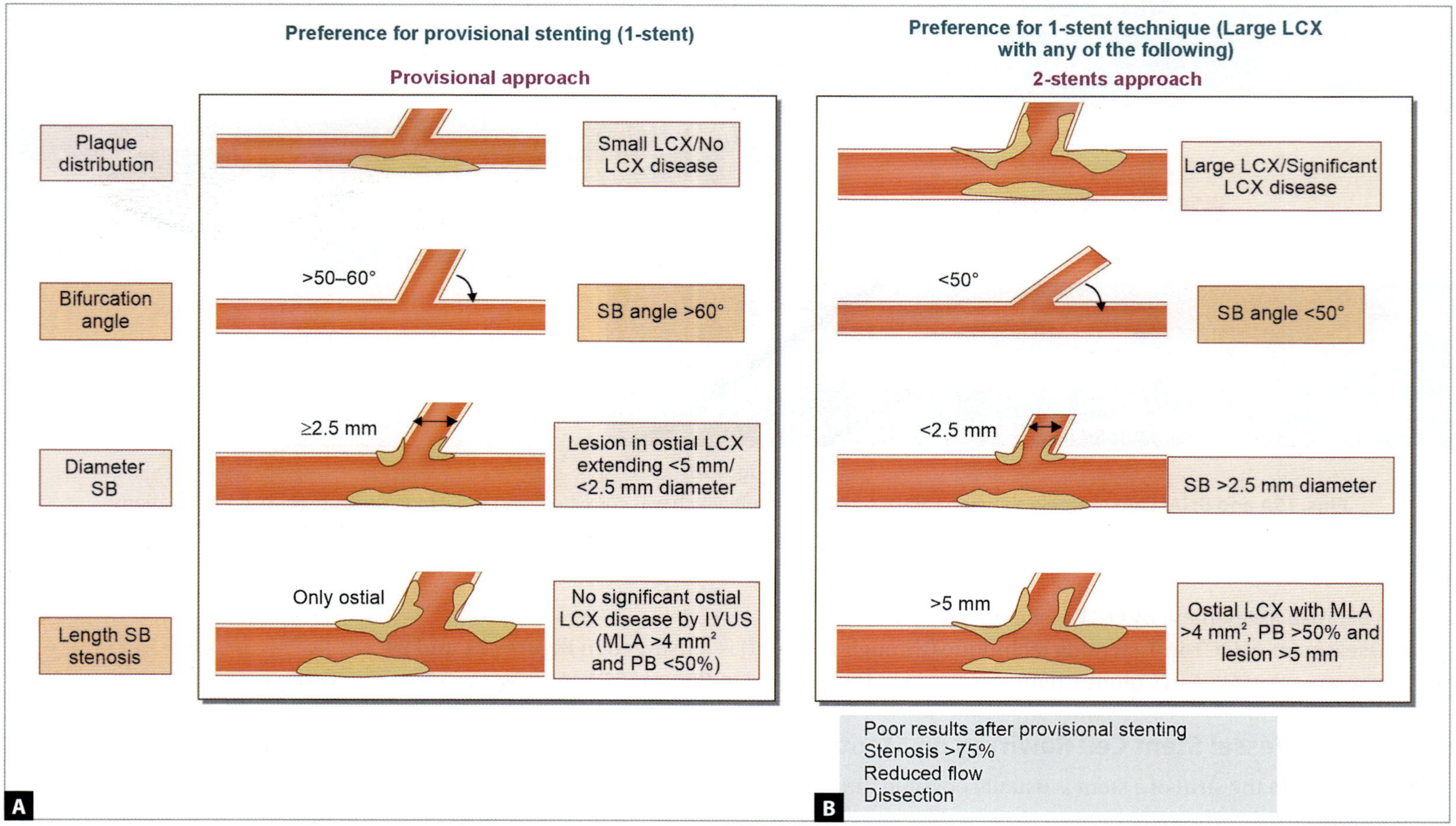

Figs. 16A and B: Recommendations for provisional stenting vs. 2-stent approach to LM PCI.

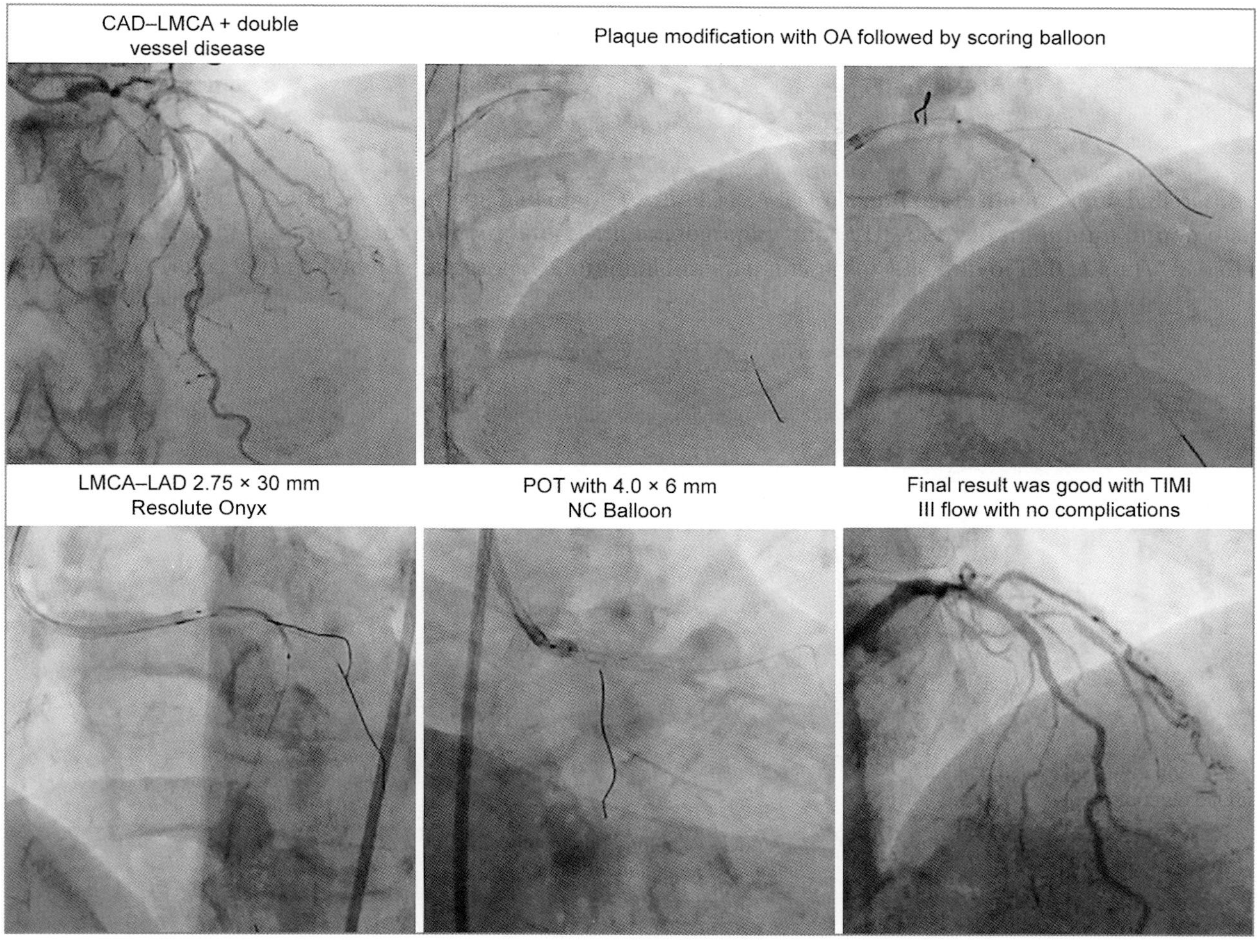

Fig. 17: Case example of provisional stent technique.

Optical coherence tomography assessment for strut crossing—scroll and back to evaluate crossing position: (A) Optimal distal rewiring, (B) Optimal distal rewiring, and (C) Longitudinal view is often useful.

Proximal rewiring appears as a jailed wire proximal to the ostium and follows the proximal vessel wall: (A) Mid-bifurcation, (B) Proximal to SB take off the wire **(Fig. 26)**.

Kissing Balloon Inflation (Fig. 26)

Use NC balloons, sized 1:1 according to the SB and distal MV reference, perform high-pressure sequential kissing inflations before low pressure simultaneous kissing inflation. Simultaneous inflations should be performed with similar pressure in both balloons; exact simultaneous deflation is of

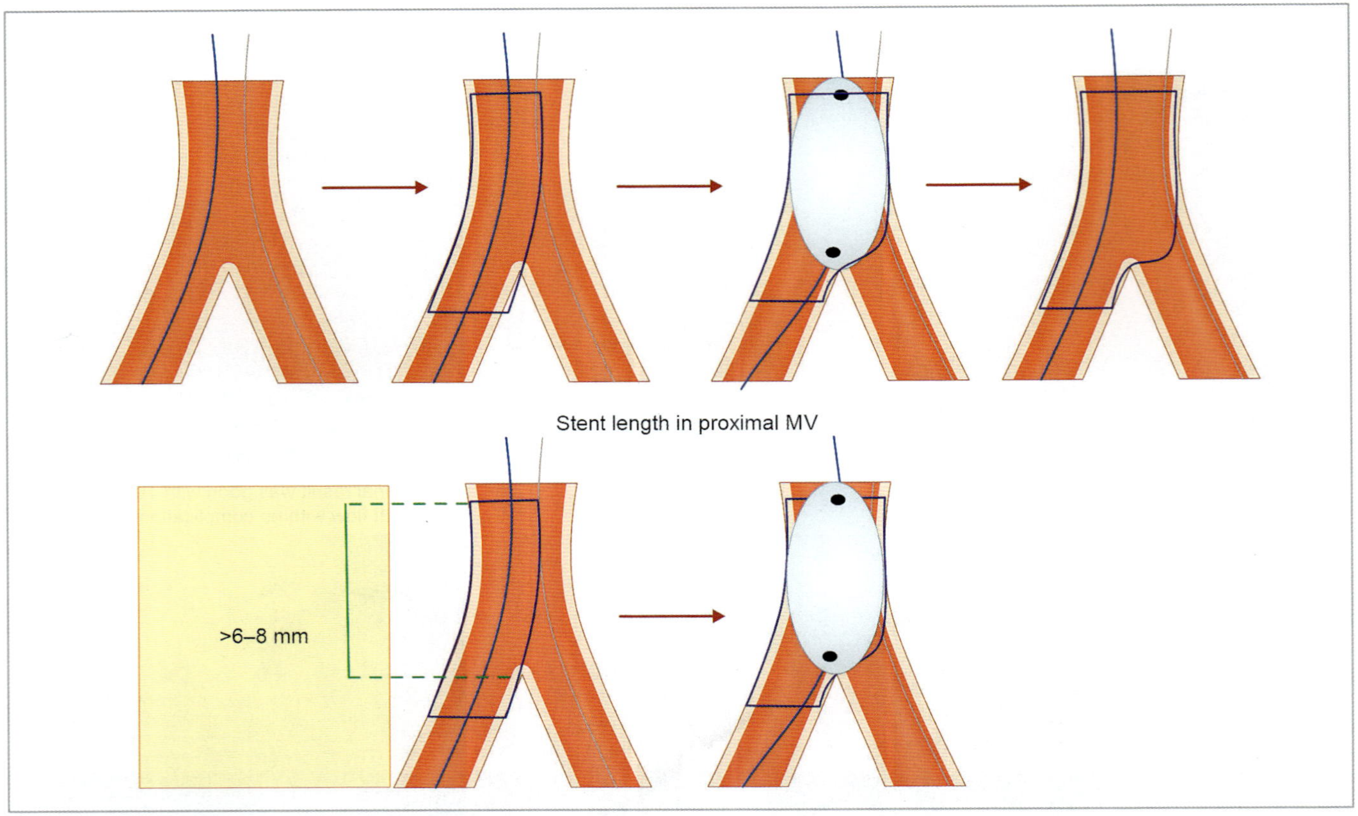

Fig. 18: Step by step approach for provisional stent technique.

utmost importance to ensure the carina is not pushed in the direction of the first deflation balloon. In provisional stenting, avoid extending the SB balloon too distal into the SB. A truly ostial stenosis rarely requires more than a few mm of balloon in the SB.[9]

BIFURCATION AND OSTIAL OPTICAL COHERENCE TOMOGRAPHY MAPPING (BOOM) TECHNIQUE TO TREAT TRUE OSTIAL BIFURCATING DISEASE (FIG. 27)

A novel technique using OCT-guided angiographic coregistration to optimize stent placement in true ostial bifurcation lesion. Precisely identify and map the SB to minimize stent protrusion while ensuring full coverage of the ostium. Using OCT to identify the ostium and coregistration (radio-opaque OCT lens marker) for precise stent deployment with the help of BOOM technique, it is preferred to know the position of stent markers to place it appropriately in ostial location.

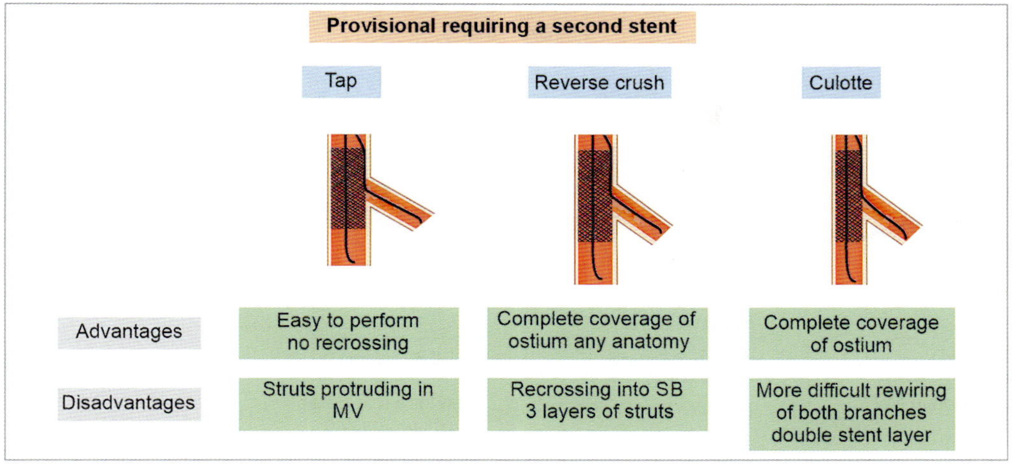

Fig. 19: Bifurcation stenting–bailout options.

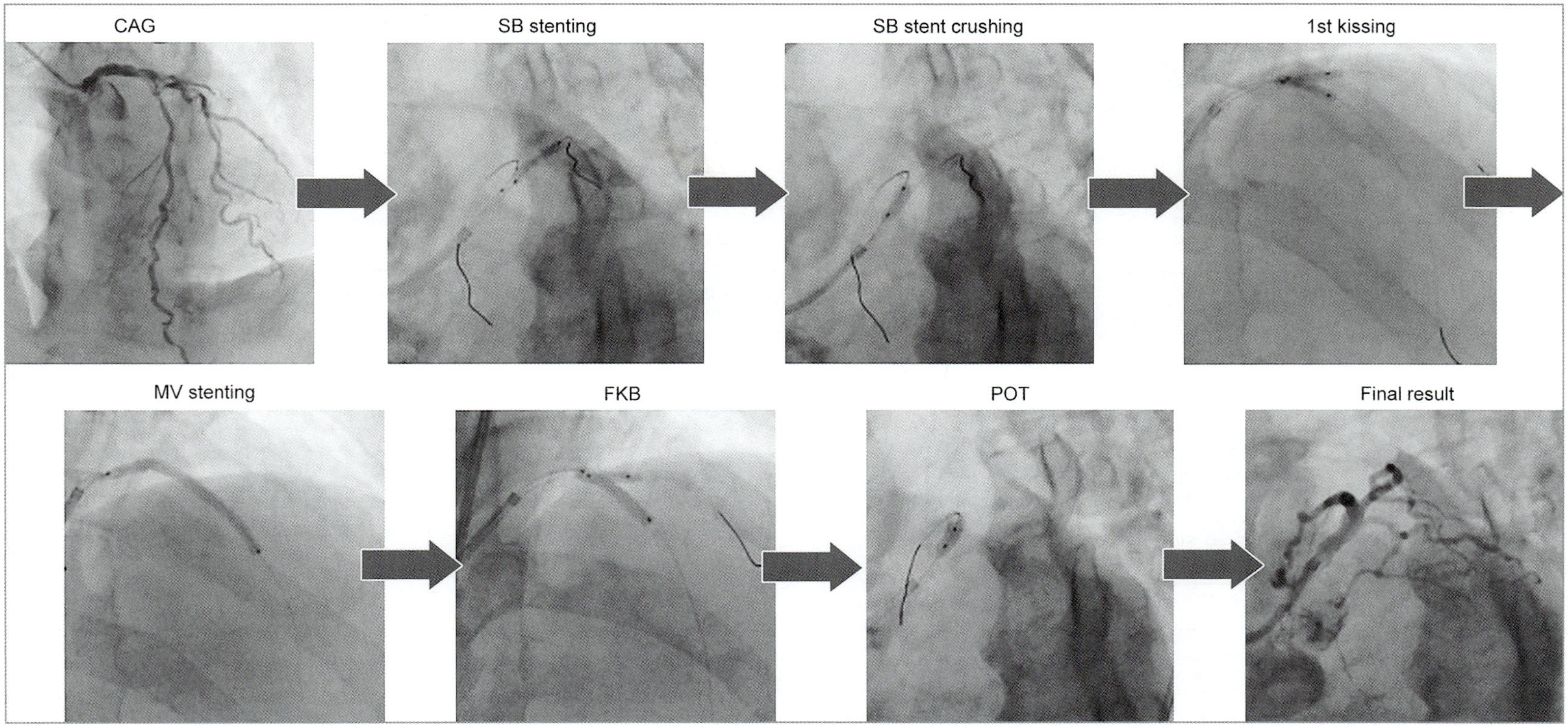

Fig. 20A

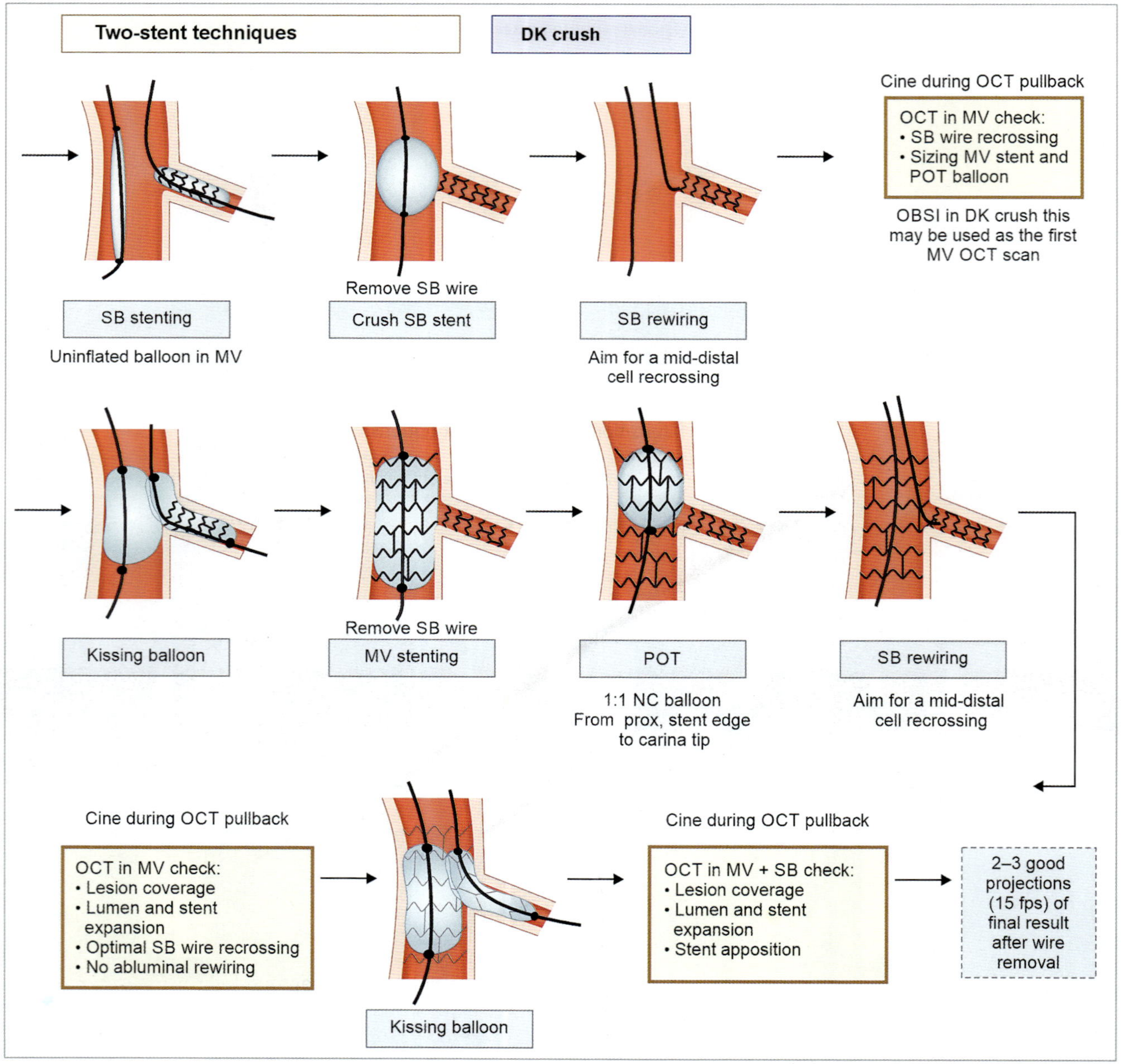

Fig. 20B

Figs. 20A and B: (A) Case example showing DK Crush stent technique; (B) Step by step approach of DK Crush stent technique.

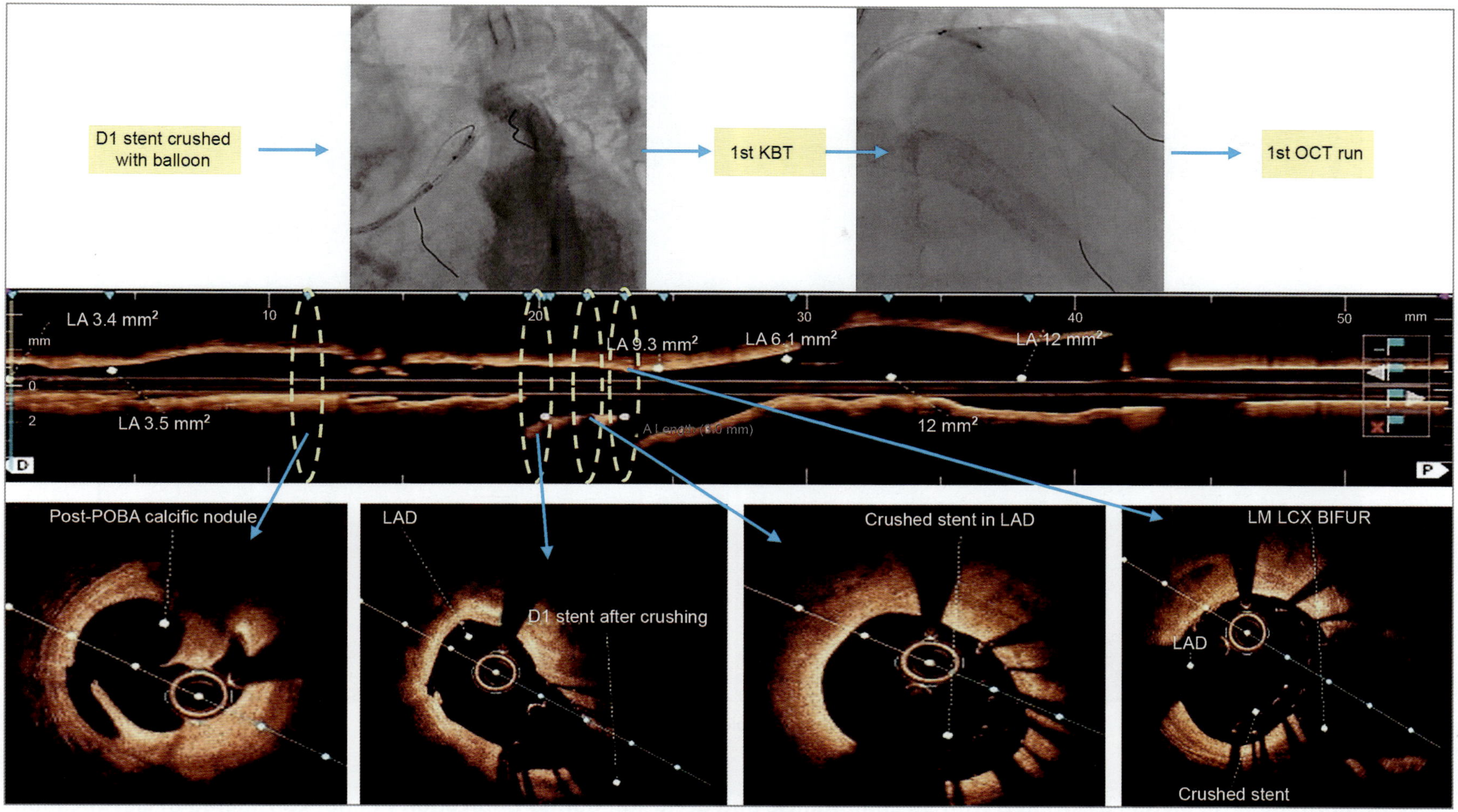

Fig. 21: Evaluation of crush assessment by OCT.

Dragonfly Optical Coherence Tomography Catheter

The BOOM technique will help to optimize results in ostial bifurcation lesions by precise stent placement while minimizing stent protrusion. It is reliable with good reproducibility, the very best of precision PCI **(Fig. 28)**.

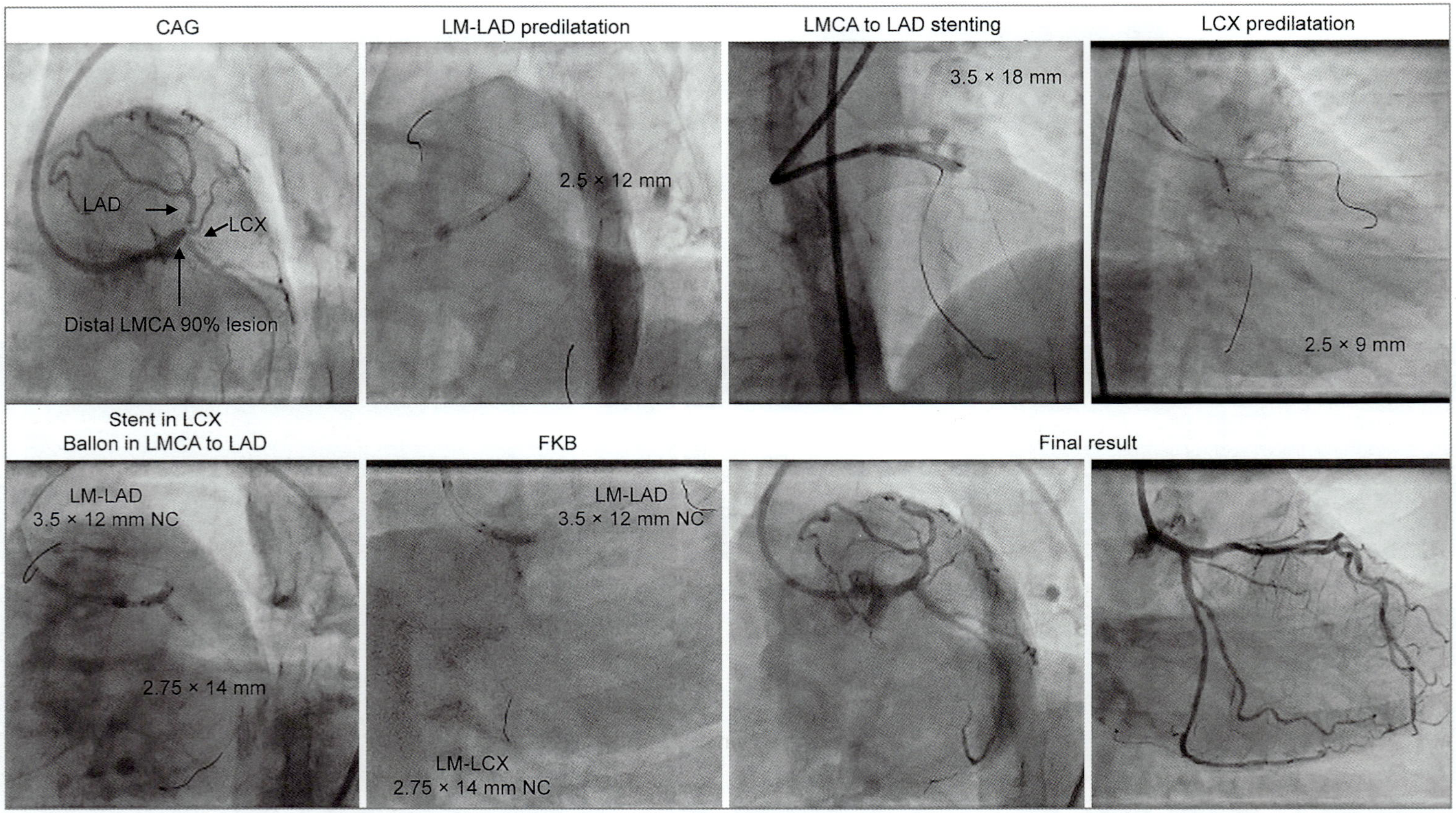

Fig. 22: Case example showing T stenting.

Several morphological factors associated with SB compromise and occlusion during bifurcation PCI not considered in classification systems:

- **Degree of stenosis (worse outcomes with increased severity)**
- **Large plaque burden, eccentric distribution**
- **Diffuse lesion extending from SB ostium**
- **Significant calcification and tortuosity**
- **Shallow angle (Y-shape) between distal branches (<70)**
- **Impaired flow at baseline**
- **Vessel size and corresponding myocardial territory.**

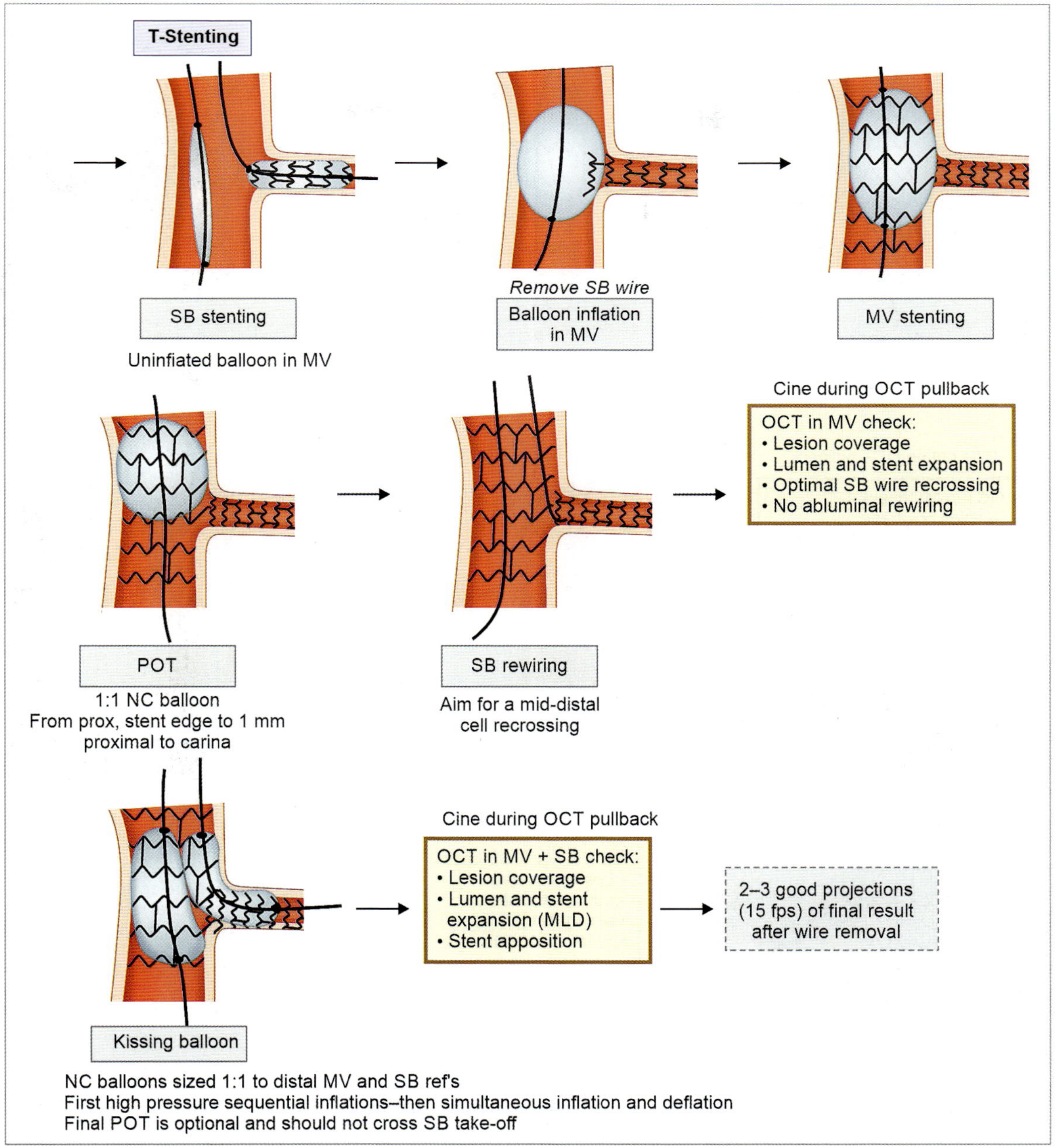

Fig. 23: Stepwise assessment of OCT in T-stent technique.

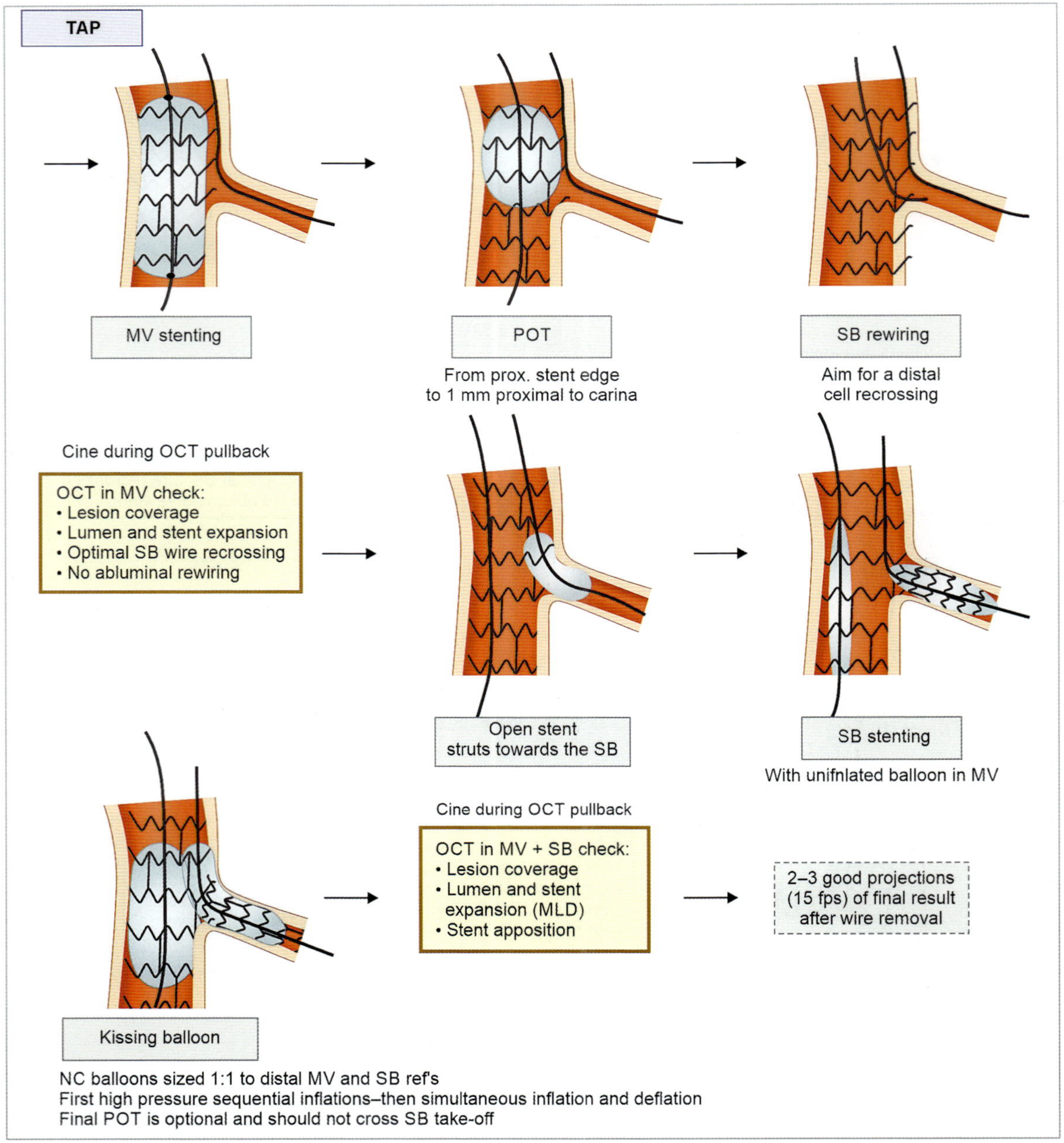

Fig. 24: Stepwise assessment of OCT in T-tap stent technique.

RECENT STUDIES ON OPTICAL COHERENCE TOMOGRAPHY IMAGING IN COMPARISON WITH INTRAVASCULAR ULTRASOUND

Recently published three randomized controlled trials (RCTs), ILUMIEN IV (n = 2,487) and OCTOBER (n = 1,201) studied the clinical impact of OCT guidance compared to angiography alone in complex PCIs, with OCT arms having over 1,200 and 600 patients, respectively. OCTIVUS (n = 2,008) compared OCT to IVUS guidance in the largest head-to-head RCT study evaluating the two imaging modalities, with approximately 1,000 patients in each arm. This recent data cited further highlights the importance of routine use of IV imaging and specifically OCT during PCI procedures.

- *Image-guided PCI improves outcomes versus angiography alone:* IVI-guided PCI with OCT or IVUS reduces TLF by 31%, driven by 46, 20, and 29% reductions in cardiac death, TV-MI, and ID/CD TLR, respectively (all reductions statistically significant), compared with angiography-guided PCI.

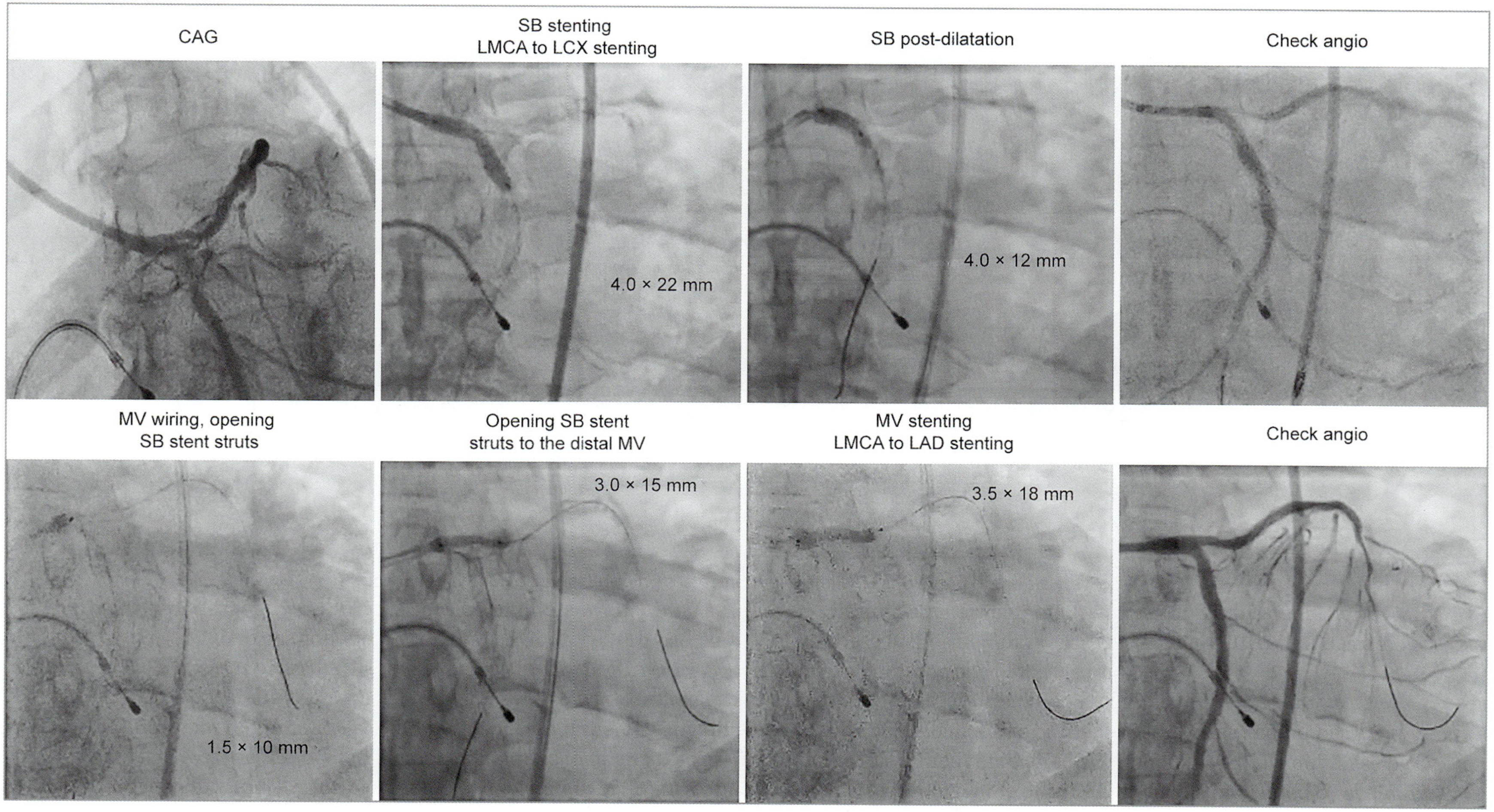

Fig. 25A

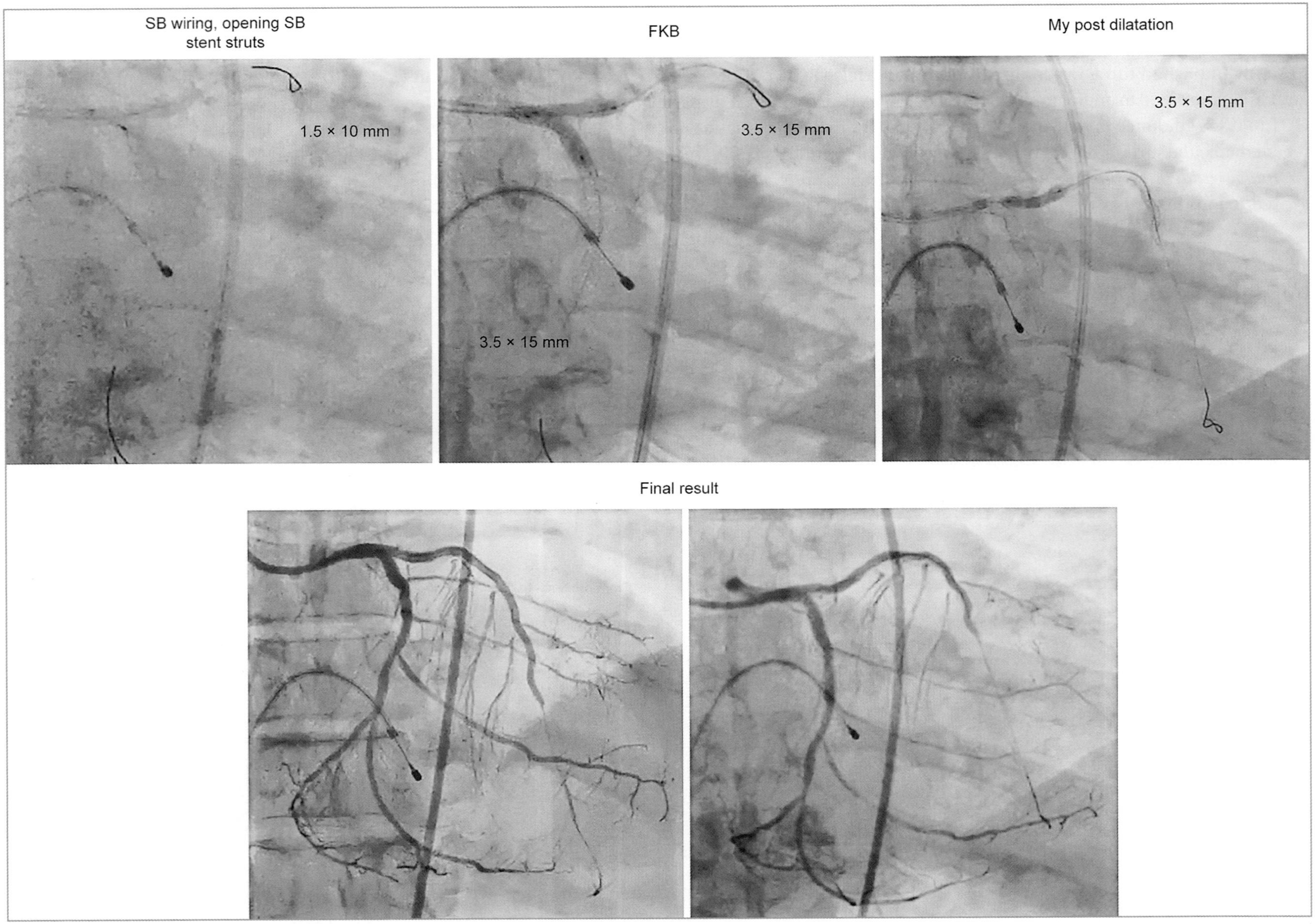
SB wiring, opening SB stent struts
1.5 × 10 mm
FKB
3.5 × 15 mm
3.5 × 15 mm
My post dilatation
3.5 × 15 mm
Final result

Fig. 25B

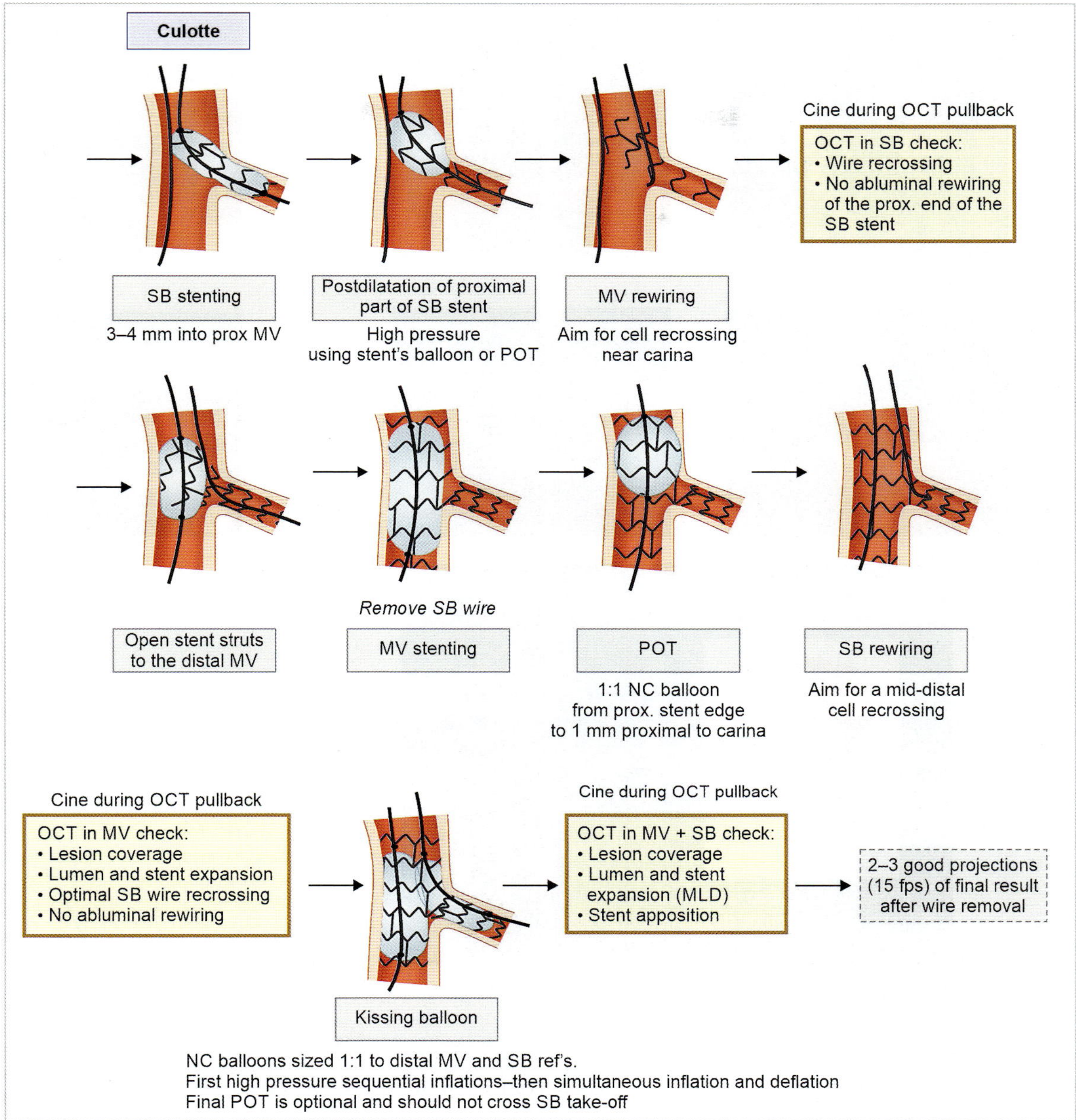

Fig. 25C

Figs. 25A to C: (A) Case example of Culotte stent technique; (B) Case example showing Culotte stent technique; (C) Stepwise assessment of OCT in Culotte stent technique.

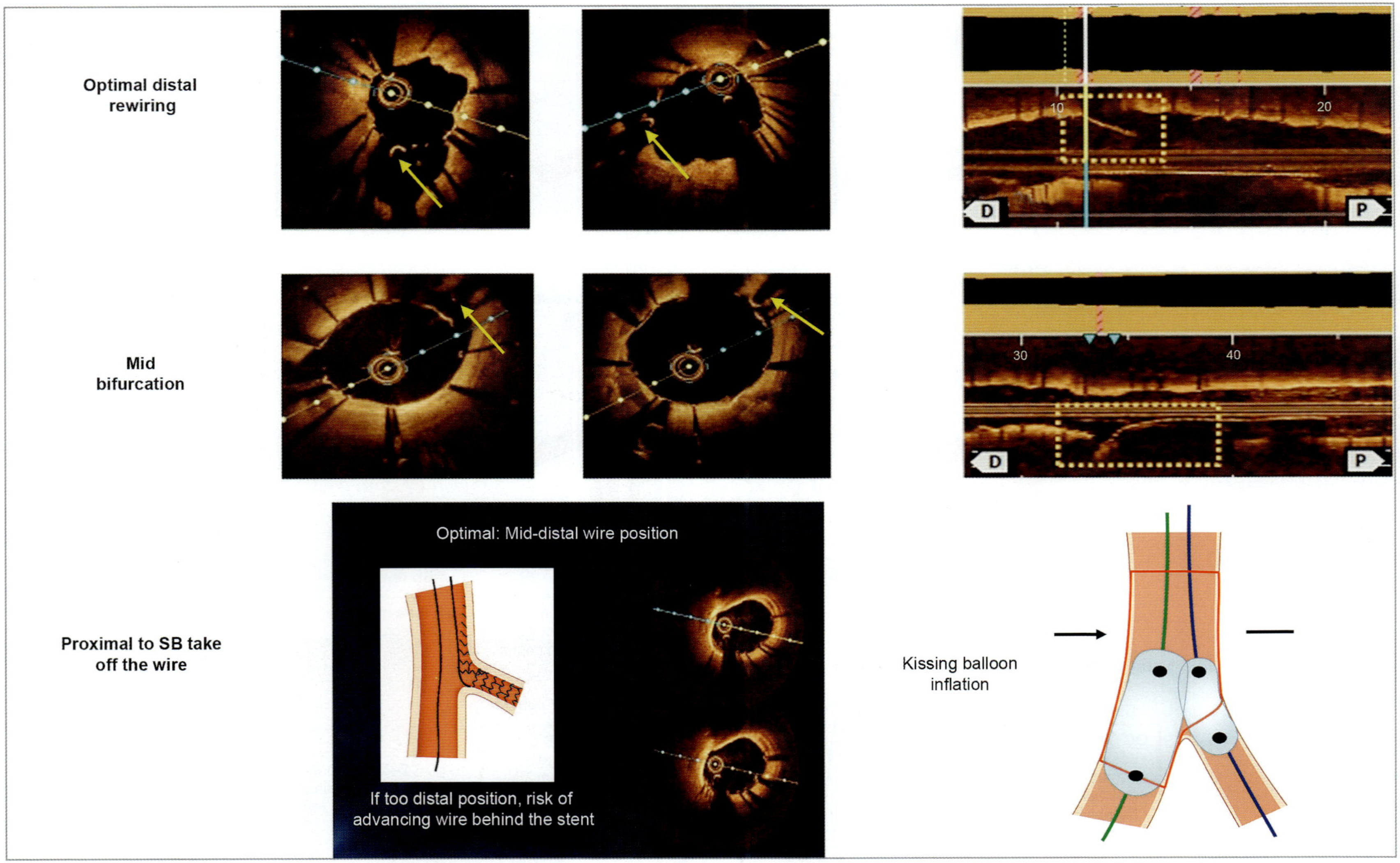

Fig. 26: OCT guidance for crossing SB strut mid vs. distal crossing before kissing balloon.

- *OCT guidance improves procedural outcomes compared to angiography guidance in ILUMIEN IV:* (1) Achieved a larger MSA (met superiority endpoint) and higher stent expansion and (2) reduced complications—fewer occurrences of major dissections, major malappositions, major tissue protrusion, and untreated focal reference segment disease.
- *OCT-guided PCI associated with safety benefits in ILUMIEN IV:* (1) Significantly reduced stent thrombosis by 64% compared to angiography alone (0.5 vs. 1.4%, $p = 0.02$) and (2) numerically lower rates of cardiac death and target vessel myocardial infarction.

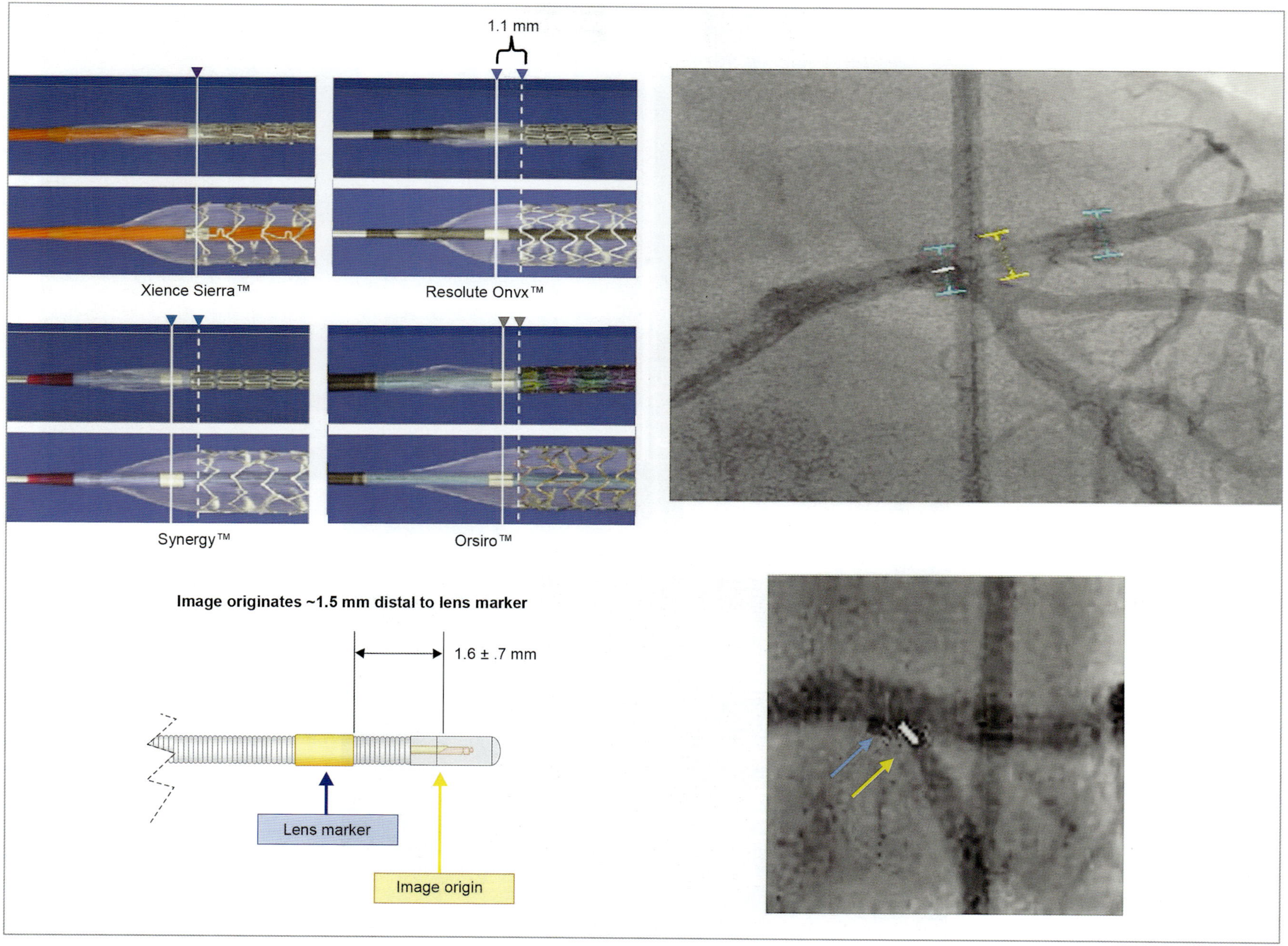

Fig. 27: Bifurcation and ostial optical coherence tomography mapping (BOOM) technique to treat true ostial bifurcating disease.

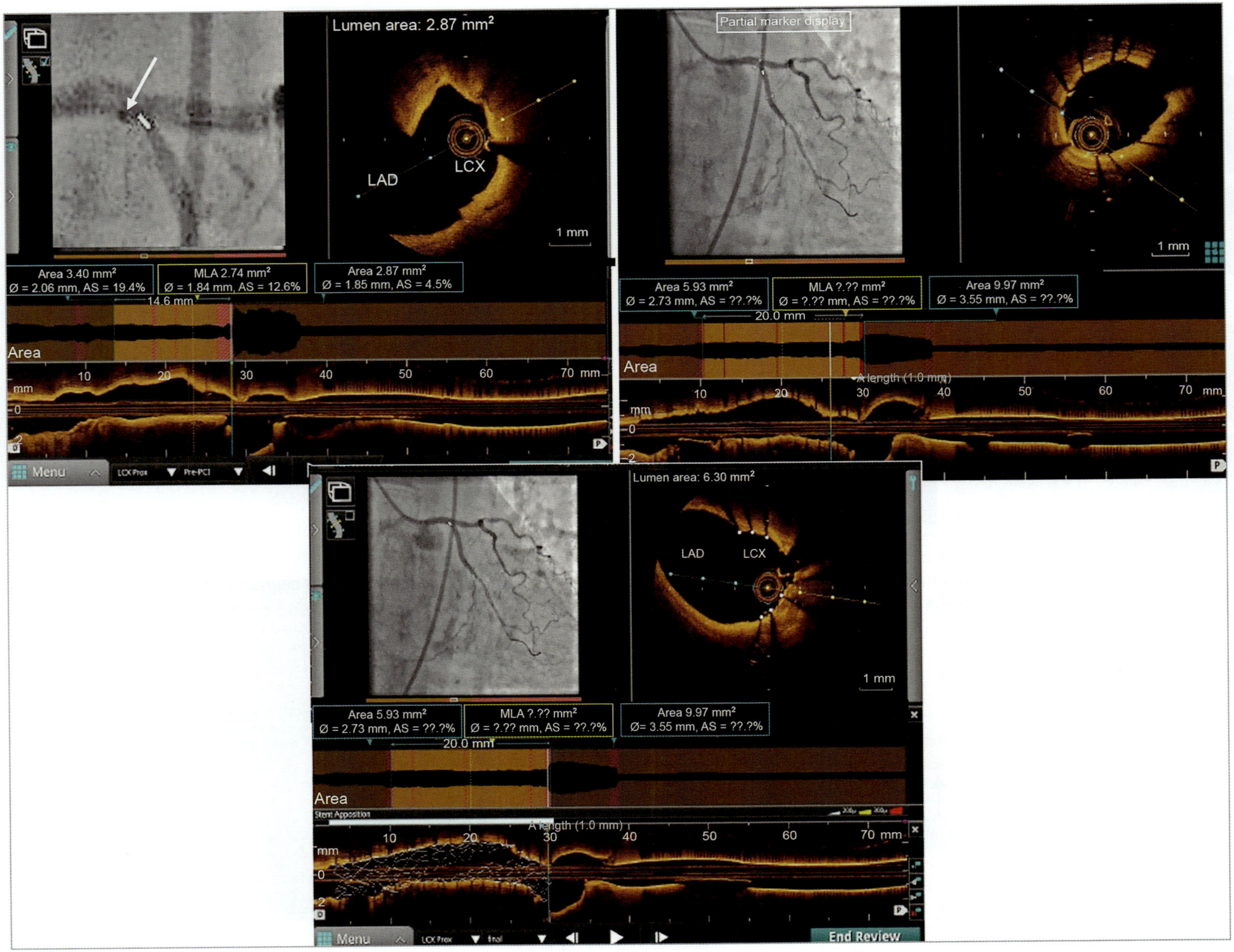

Fig. 28: Dragonfly OCT Catheter.

- *Overall TVF benefit of OCT-guided PCI:* (1) The 2-year rate of TVF in ILUMIEN IV was numerically lower than angiography guidance (7.4 vs. 8.2%, $p = 0.45$), but the difference was not statistically significant largely due to lower than expected and nearly identical rates of TVR between OCT and angiography arms (5.6 vs. 5.6%), a finding possibly impacted by the COVID-19 pandemic. (2) In the OCTOBER trial, OCT guidance demonstrated superiority compared to angiography alone in MACE at 1 year (10.1 vs. 14.1%, $p = 0.035$).
- In *OCTIVUS, OCT guidance demonstrated noninferiority to IVUS in TVF at 1 year* (2.5 vs. 3.1%, $p < 0.001$ for noninferiority), with a numerically lower rate for TVF in the OCT arm.

Rocket study showed that overall, >90% of the quadrants of LM were adequately assessable using OCT. It detected almost 60% more atherosclerotic plaques than angiography and plaques were preponderantly fibrous or fibrocalcific with intimal hyperplasia and is very useful for assessing distal LM lesions and may not be suitable for patients with ostial LM lesions, tortuous, very large, and short LMCA lesions. The latest guidelines of the ESC and European association for cardiothoracic surgery recommended OCT as well as IVUS for procedural optimization as class IIa.[10]

In a patient-level pooled analysis of four registries, IVUS-guided LM PCI is associated with higher freedom from cardiac death, MI, and TLR at 3 years and also showed a significant reduction in stent thrombosis.[8] In recent analysis from the SCAAR study group, IVUS-guided LM PCI was associated with reduction in the composite endpoint of total death rate, need for revascularization and stent thrombosis (HR 0.65, CI 0.50–0.84) and all-cause death.[5]

However, experience and evidence of OCT is limited compared to IVUS which has been widely used for quiet long time in the field of interventional cardiology. CLI-OPCI study of 670 patients showed OCT-guided PCI was superior to angio guided in terms of cardiac death and MI at 1 year (6.6 vs. 13%).[11] The OPINION trial showed noninferiority of OCT-guided PCI in terms of TVF 5.2% in the OCT group versus 4.9% in the IVUS-guided PCI at 12 months follow-up.[12] The ILLUMIEN III study also showed the noninferiority of OCT-guided group versus IVUS group regarding the MSA achieved.[13] The ROCK I study analyzed 267 LM patients and a total of 112 patients had angiographic follow-up at 6 months. A total of 55 patients had OCT guidance and the remaining 57 patients had angio-guided procedures. In the control group, 10 patients (17.5%) underwent LM PCI with IVUS guidance. OCT helped in obtaining optimal stent deployment and improved angiographic outcomes in terms of late lumen loss (LLL), binary restenosis, and percent diameter stenosis after 6 months. In particular, the rate of significant restenosis was only 3.5% in the OCT group, compared to 12.9% in standard care and confirmed the angiographic superiority of OCT guidance during distal LM stenting, when compared to a standard treatment strategy including IVUS in a minority of patients.[14] In the Rocket study, the beneficial impact of OCT guidance on LLL was more relevant in the distal segment of the LM. Dato et al. analyzed 122 patients with intermediate LM lesions, showing the feasibility of OCT in this setting and also showing a good correlation with clinical outcome as regards the initial decision-making process.[15] The LEMON multicenter study of 70 patients showed the efficacy of OCT-guided PCI for mid and distal LM showed that OCT guidance for LM PCI was feasible, safe, and was successful with primary endpoint with procedural success defined as residual stenosis <50% plus TIMI grade 3 flow in all branches plus adequate stent expansion on OCT was achieved in 86% patients. Similarly, OCT showed adequate expansion in 86%, malapposition in 24%, and medial edge dissection in 30%, and it modified operator strategy in 26% of patients with 1-year survival free from major clinical adverse events of 98.6%.[16]

The expert consensus group stated that IVUS and OCT are equivalent and both superior to CAG guidance. OCT guidance is currently proposed by the EBC to support bifurcation lesion PCI and might expand to distal LMS lesion.

CONCLUSION

Vast majority of cases can be managed with provisional stenting strategies and OCT guides in the selection of bifurcation strategy and optimization of bifurcation stent results.

LM bifurcation stenting with OCT is explained in detail in **Flowchart 1**.

Flowchart 1: LM bifurcation stenting with OCT.

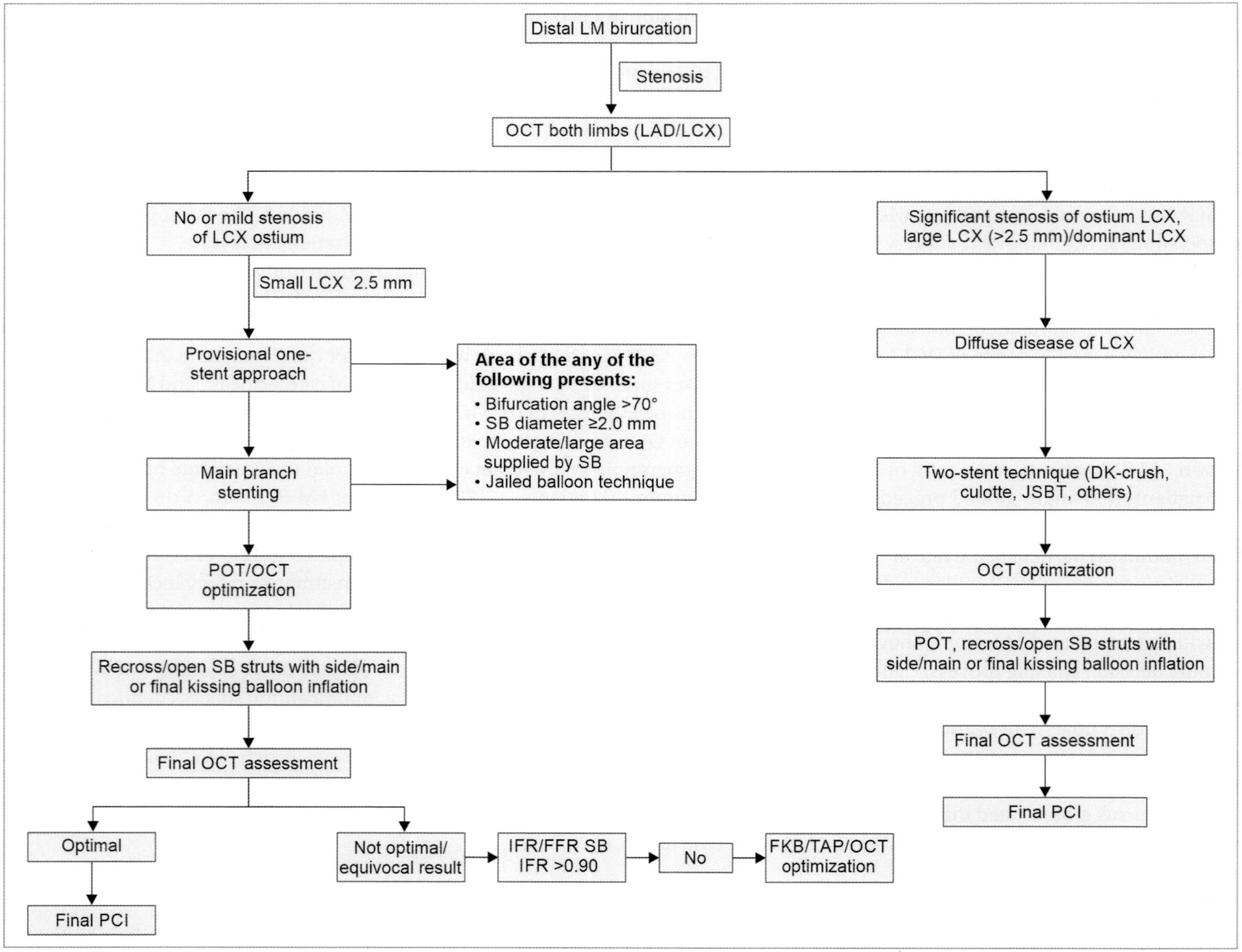

REFERENCES

1. Ye Y, Yang M, Zhang S, Zeng Y. Percutaneous coronary intervention in left main coronary artery disease with or without intravascular ultrasound: a meta-analysis. PLoS One. 2017;12(6):e0179756.
2. Ramadan R, Boden WE, Kinlay S. Management of left main coronary artery disease. J Am Heart Assoc. 2018;7(7):e008151.
3. Chatterjee A, Leesar MA, Hillegass WB. Intravascular ultrasound of normal left main arteries: Insights for stent optimization and standardization. Catheter Cardiovasc Interv. 2019;93(2):239-40.
4. Holm NR, Andreasen LN, Walsh S, Kajander OA, Witt N, Eek C, et al. Rational and design of the European randomized optical coherence tomography optimized bifurcation event reduction trial (OCTOBER). Am Heart J. 2018;205:97-109.
5. Andell P, Karlsson S, Mohammad MA, Götberg M, James S, Jensen J, et al Intravascular ultrasound guidance is associated with better outcome in patients undergoing unprotected left main coronary artery stenting compared with angiography guidance alone Circ Cardiovasc Interv. 2017;10:e004813.
6. Dash D. Stenting of left main coronary artery stenosis: A to Z. Heart Asia. 2013;5(1):18-27.
7. Mehrotra S, Mishra S, Paramasivam G. Imaging during percutaneous coronary intervention for optimizing outcomes. Indian Heart J. 2018;70:S456-65.
8. Gwon HC. Understanding the coronary bifurcation stenting. Korean Circ J. 2018;48(6):481-91.
9. Foin N, Torii R, Mortier P, De Beule M, Viceconte N, Chan PH, et al. Kissing balloon or sequential dilation of the side branch and main vessel for provisional stenting of bifurcations: lessons from micro-computed tomography and computational simulations. JACC Cardiovasc Interv. 2012;5(1):47-56.
10. Price MJ (Ed). Intravascular Imaging: OCT and IVUS, An Issue of Interventional Cardiology Clinics, E-Book. Netherlands: Elsevier Health Sciences; 2015. p. 371.
11. Prati F, Di Vito L, Biondi-Zoccai G, Occhipinti M, La Manna A, Tamburino C, et al Angiography alone versus angiography plus optical coherence tomography to guide decision-making during percutaneous coronary intervention: The Centro per la Lotta contro l'Infarto-Optimisation of Percutaneous Coronary Intervention (CLI-OPCI) study EuroIntervention. 2012;8:823–9
12. Kubo T, Shinke T, Okamura T, Hibi K, Nakazawa G, Morino Y, et al Optical frequency domain imaging vs. intravascular ultrasound in percutaneous coronary intervention (OPINION trial): One-year angiographic and clinical results Eur Heart J. 2017;38:3139–47
13. Ali ZA, Maehara A, Généreux P, Shlofmitz RA, Fabbiocchi F, Nazif TM, et al Optical coherence tomography compared with intravascular ultrasound and with angiography to guide coronary stent implantation (ILUMIEN III: OPTIMIZE PCI): A randomised controlled trial Lancet. 2016;388:2618–28
14. Cortese B, Burzotta F, Alfonso F, Pellegrini D, Trani C, Aurigemma C, et al Role of optical coherence tomography for distal left main stem angioplasty Catheter Cardiovasc Interv. 2020;96:755–61
15. Dato I, Burzotta F, Trani C, Romano A, Paraggio L, Aurigemma C, et al Optical coherence tomography guidance for the management of angiographically intermediate left main bifurcation lesions: Early clinical experience Int J Cardiol. 2017;248:108–13
16. Amabile N, Rangé G, Souteyrand G, Godin M, Boussaada MM, Meneveau N, et al Optical coherence tomography to guide percutaneous coronary intervention of the left main coronary artery: The LEMON study EuroIntervention. 2021;17:e124–31

CASE 1

Nano Crush stenting of LAD-D1

CLINICAL HISTORY

61-year-old male known HTN, presented with compliant of chest pain on exertion on and off for 1 month. ECG suggestive of NSR, 80 bpm, T inversion in V1-V6. Echo was done which revealed normal LV function, CAD - Stable angina

Investigations: Hb-13.3 g/dL, Serum Cr-0.94 mg/dL, eGFR - 88 mL/min.

CAG - SVD with Proximal LAD 95% stenosis. Mid LAD 70–80% stenosis and ostio-proximal D1 90% stenosis.

LMCA engaged with EBU 3.5-6 Fr guiding catheter, LAD lesion crossed with runthrough wire. Diagonal lesion crossed with Sion blue. LAD and D1 lesions pre dilated with 2.0 × 10 mm Ryurei balloon. Prestent OCT in LAD and D1 showing severe calcific plaque and to choose IVL for the plaque modification **(Figs. 29A and B)**.

PROCEDURE

IVL C2 + 3.0 × 12 mm balloon taken and 80 pulses delivered in Proximal LAD and 40 pulses in D1. D1 and LAD lesions dilated with 2.5 × 15 mm wolverine cutting balloon.

Post plaque modification with IVL, OCT assessment taken for selection of the stent in LAD **(Figs. 30A and B)**.

3.0 × 30 mm Resolute Onyx Stent deployed in Mid LAD, 2.75 × 34 mm Resolute Onyx stent deployed in D1 and D1 stent crushed with LAD stent balloon. D1 recrossed with runthrough and struts opened with 2.0 5 10 mm Ryurei balloon. First KBI done with 3.5 × 15 mm Nc Trek balloon in LAD, 3.0 × 15 mm NC Trek balloon in D1, Post dilatation with 3.5 × 15 mm Nc Trek balloon in LAD, 3.0 × 15 mm NC Trek balloon in D1. 3.5 × 26 mm Resolute onyx deployed in Proximal LAD, POT with 4.0 × 08 mm NC Trek. D1 recrossed with run through and struts opened with 2.0 × 10 mm Ryurei balloon. 2nd KBI with 3.5 × 15 mm NC Trek in LAD, 3.0 × 15 mm NC Trek in D1. Re-pot with 4.0 × 08 mm NC Trek **(Figs. 31A and C)**.

Poststenting OCT of LAD and D1 showing well expanded and apposed stent struts with no medial edge dissections. Final result was good with TIMI III flow with no complications

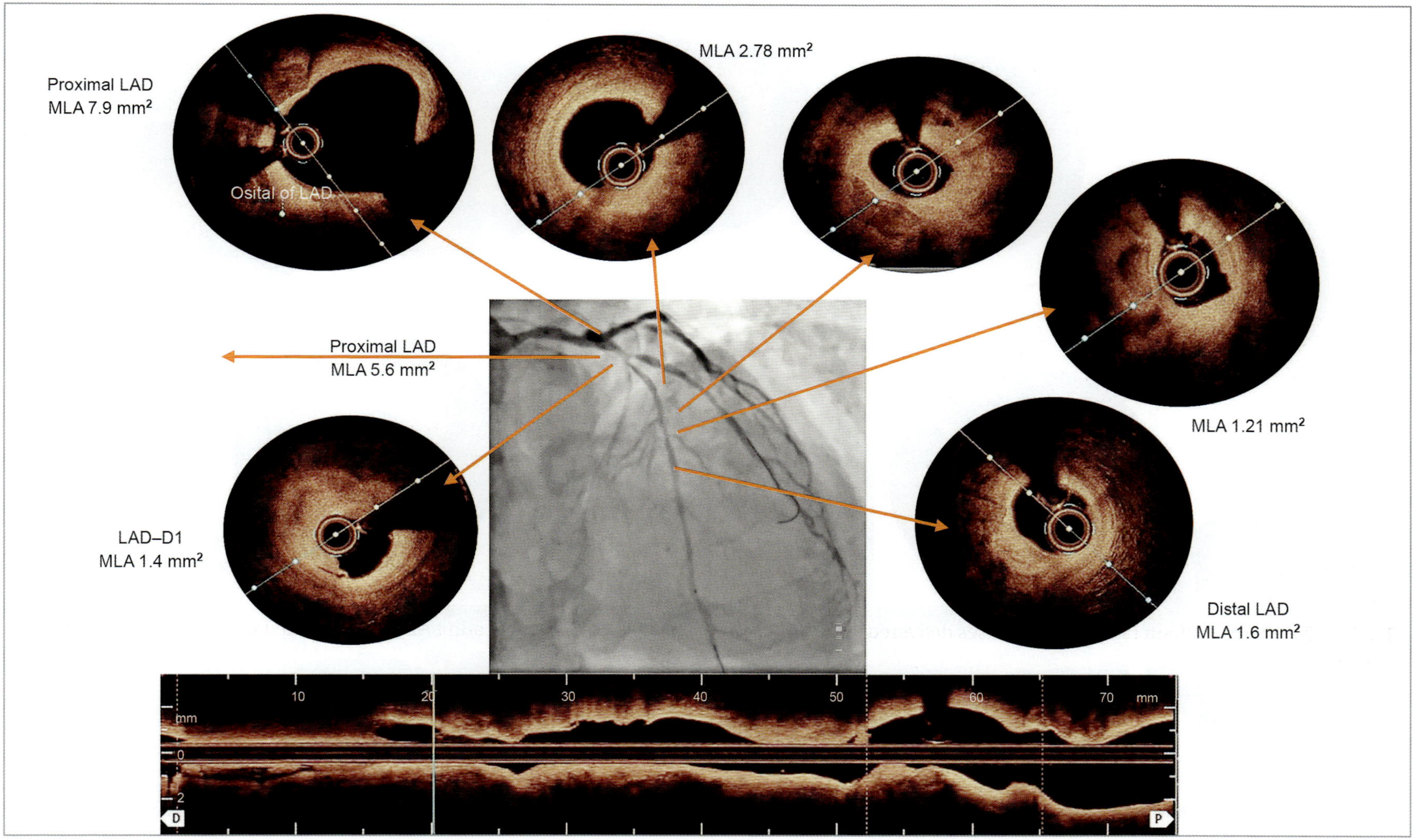
Proximal LAD
MLA 7.9 mm²
Osital of LAD
MLA 2.78 mm²
Proximal LAD
MLA 5.6 mm²
MLA 1.21 mm²
LAD–D1
MLA 1.4 mm²
Distal LAD
MLA 1.6 mm²
10
20
30
40
50
60
70
mm
0
2
D
P

Fig. 29A

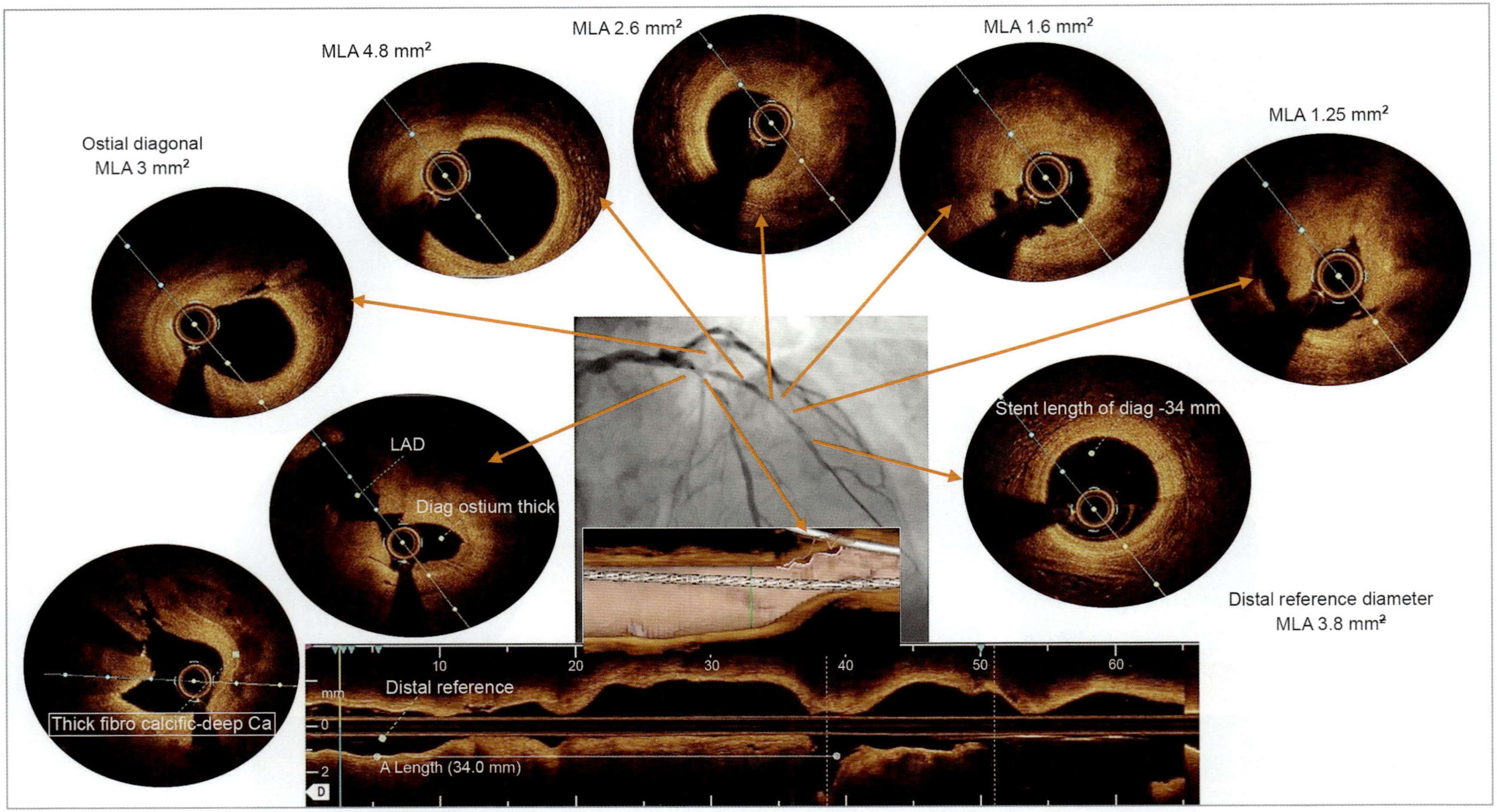

Fig. 29B

Figs. 29A and B: (A) Presenting LAD OCT assessment for plaque modification; (B) Presenting D1 OCT assessment for plaque modification.

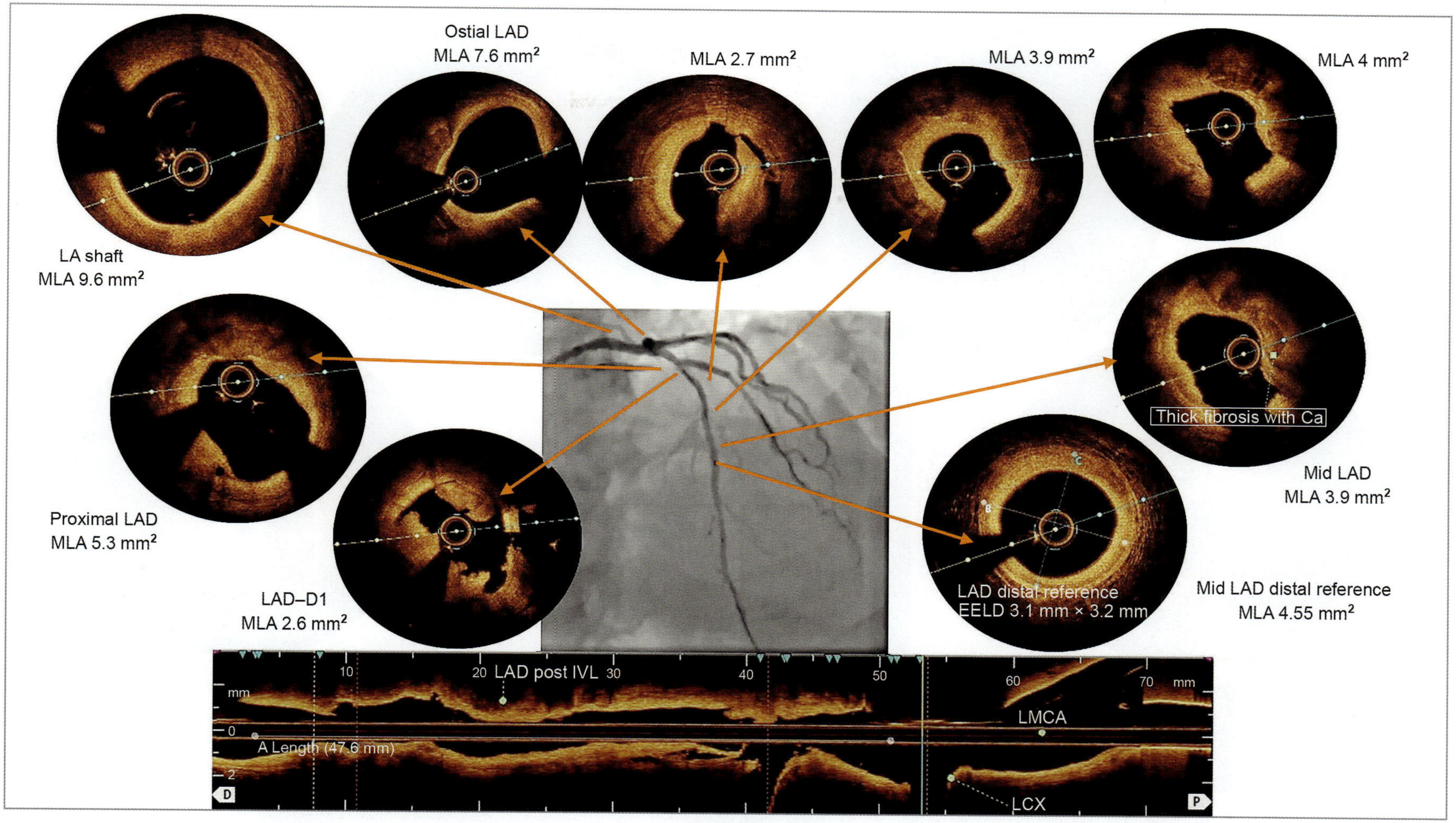

Fig. 30A

Sizing the MB stent based on the proximal MB can result carina shift.

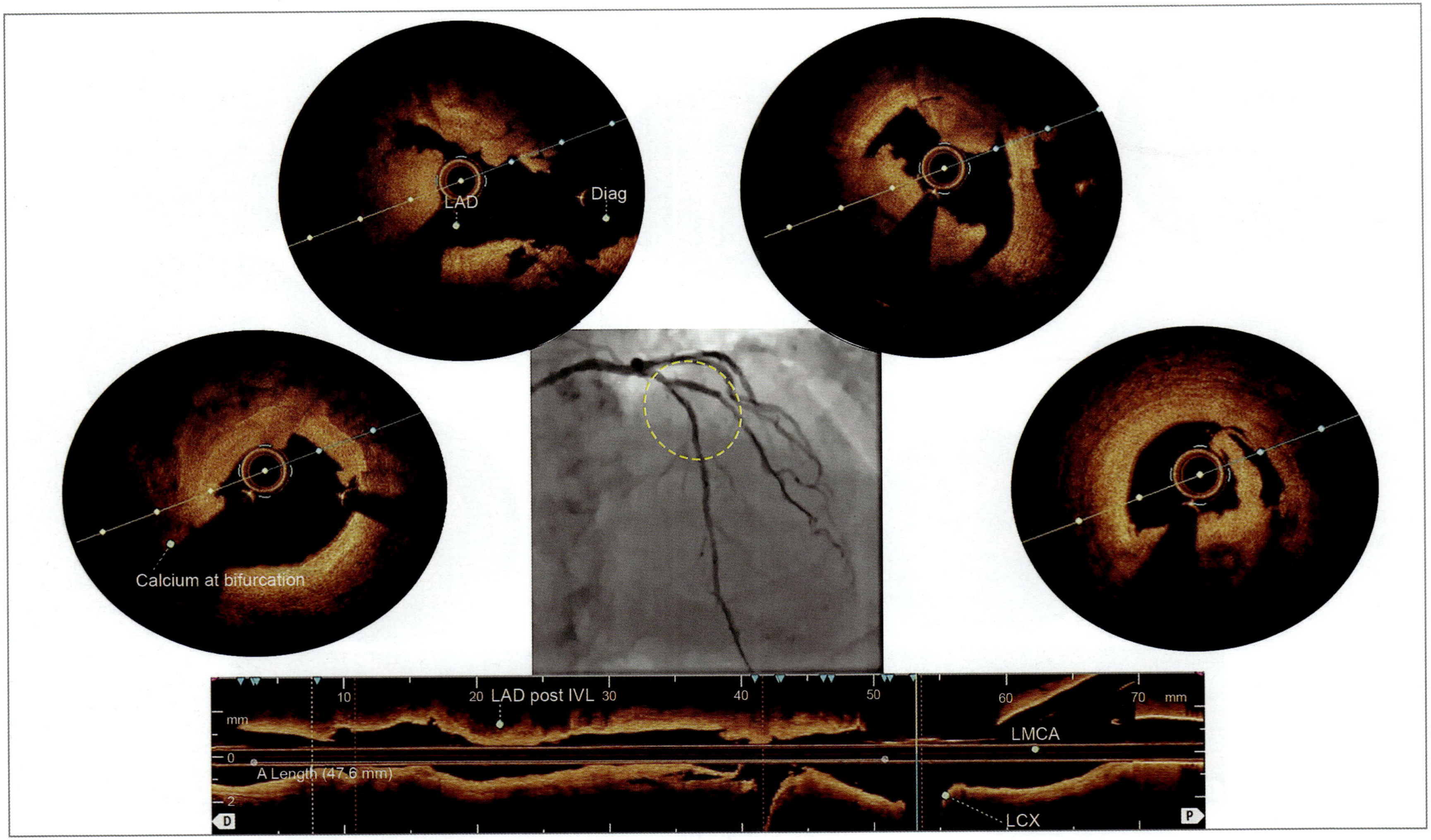

Fig. 30B

Figs. 30A and B: (A) Post plaque modification with IVL, LAD OCT assessment for selection of the stent size; (B) Post plaque modification with IVL calcium fractures.

Sizing on the distal MB respects the bifurcation diameters and prevents carina shifts.

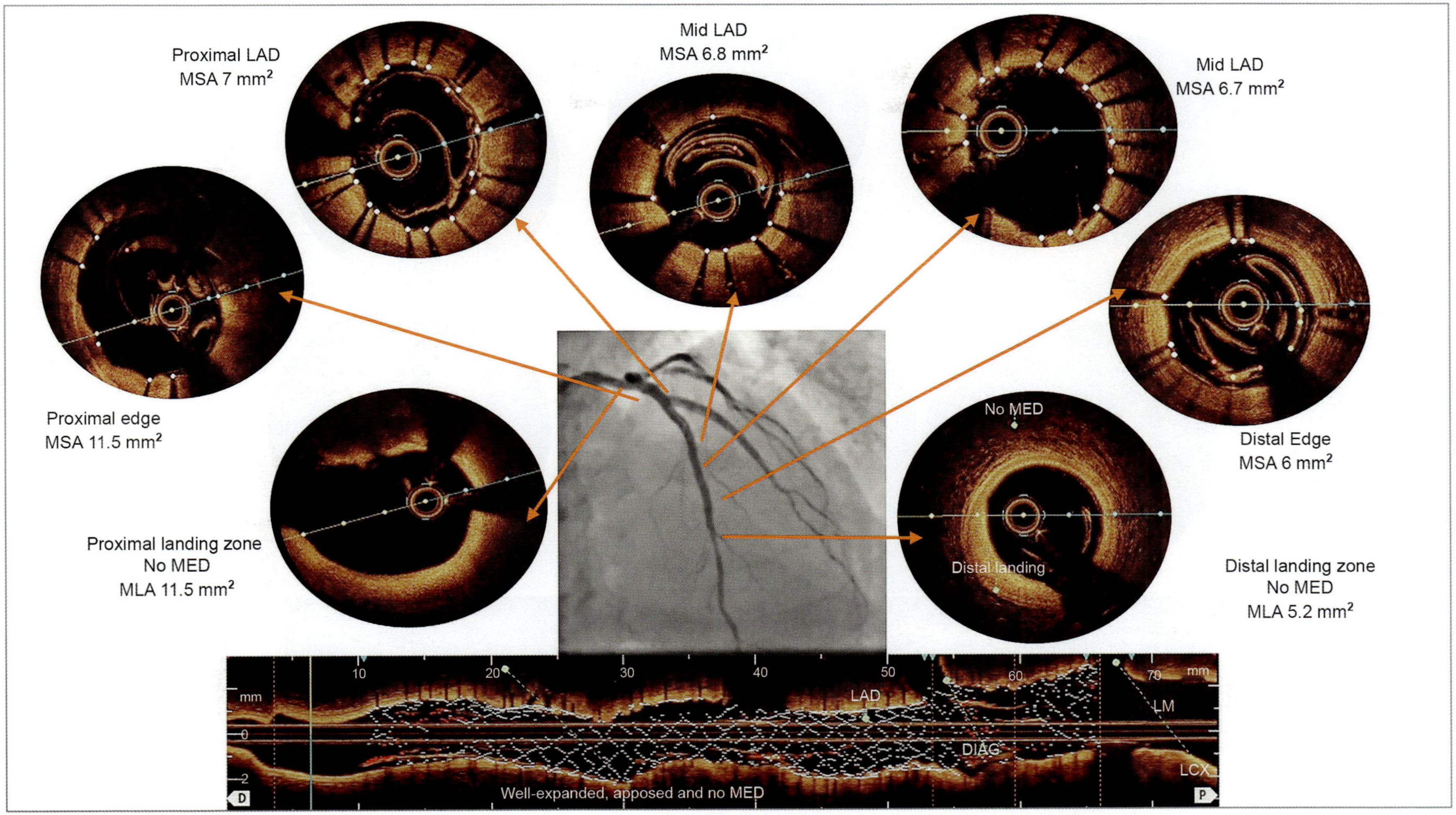

Fig. 31A

DCB angioplasty requires an optimal balloon angioplasty result, which may be assessed using angiography, physiology, or intravascular imaging, followed by DCB application

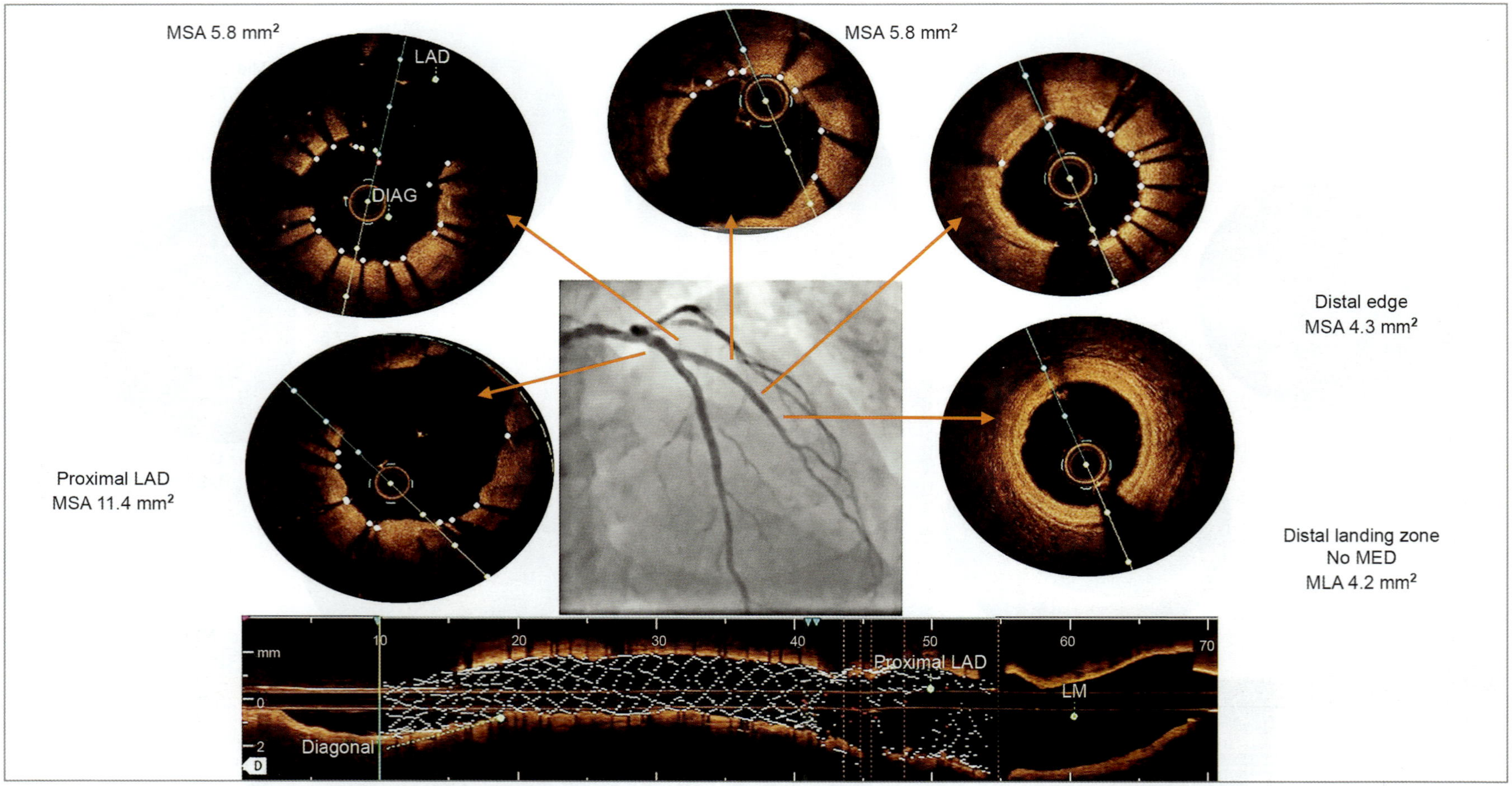

Fig. 31B

IVUS Definition of LSD-Longitudinal stent deformation was defined as multiple layers of stent struts seen in any single cross-section within a single stent.

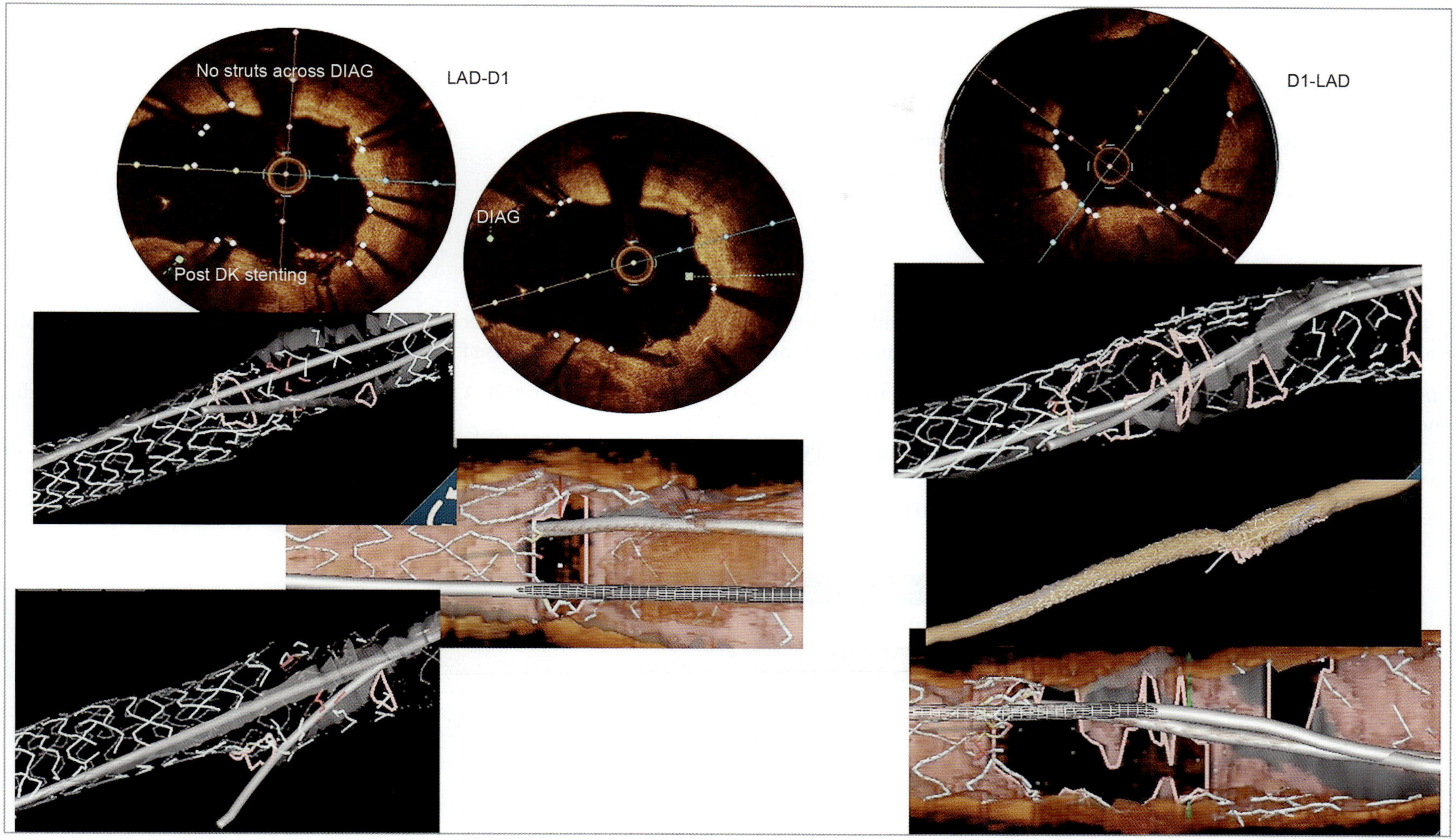

Fig. 31C

Figs. 31A to C: (A) Poststenting OCT assessment showed MAX criteria achieved in LAD; (B) Poststenting OCT assessment showed MAX criteria achieved in D1; (C) Post bifurcation stenting – 3D OCT assessment of stent expansion and SB patency.

CASE 2

OCT-guided precision PCI of LM to LAD provisional stenting and RCA.

CLINICAL HISTORY

A 49-year-old male, a known hypertensive, presented with effort angina for 10 days. ECG—normal, 2D echo—no RWMA, good LV function, EF 60%, TMT was positive for inducible ischemia, came to our hospital with CAG showing LMCA + two vessel disease for further evaluation and management.

Investigations: Hb 14.7 g/dL, RBS 120 mg/dL, Serum Cr 0.9 mg/dL, eGFR 110 mL/min, TCL-88 mg/dL, LDL-53 mg/dL, HDL-31 mg/dL, TGL 240 mg/dL, and VLDL 48 mg/dL.

Planned for PCI of dominant RCA with critical lesion prior to PCI of LM with image guidance to provide adequate backup while performing PCI of LMCA.

Initially planned for provisional stenting of LM to LAD with jailed wiring of LCX and D2 with plaque modification.

BOX 2: Strategy—precision PCI.

- Assessment of plaque **M**orphology
- Any need for plaque modification
- Assessment of vessel sizing for the selection of balloons and stents (**L**-length and **D**-diameter)
- Assessment of **M**edial edge dissection, **A**pposition, and e**X**pansion
- Optimization of DES implantation

PROCEDURE

Right coronary artery was engaged through RRA with JR 3.5–6 Fr guiding catheter, check angio was taken, RCA lesion was crossed with 0.014″ Runthrough wire, and lesion was predilated with 2 × 15 mm Ryurei balloon at 12 atm. Then OCT run pullback was taken which showed severe fibrotic plaque with mild-to-moderate superficial calcium near the site of maximum stenosis **(Figs. 32A and B)**.

Lesion plaque modification with 3 × 15 mm angio sculpt-cutting balloon at 14 atm. Then, RCA stenting was done with 3 × 48 mm Xience Xpedition deployed at 10 atm. Postdilatation was done with 3 × 15 mm NC Trek balloon at 18 atm. Poststenting OCT was done which showed well-expanded and

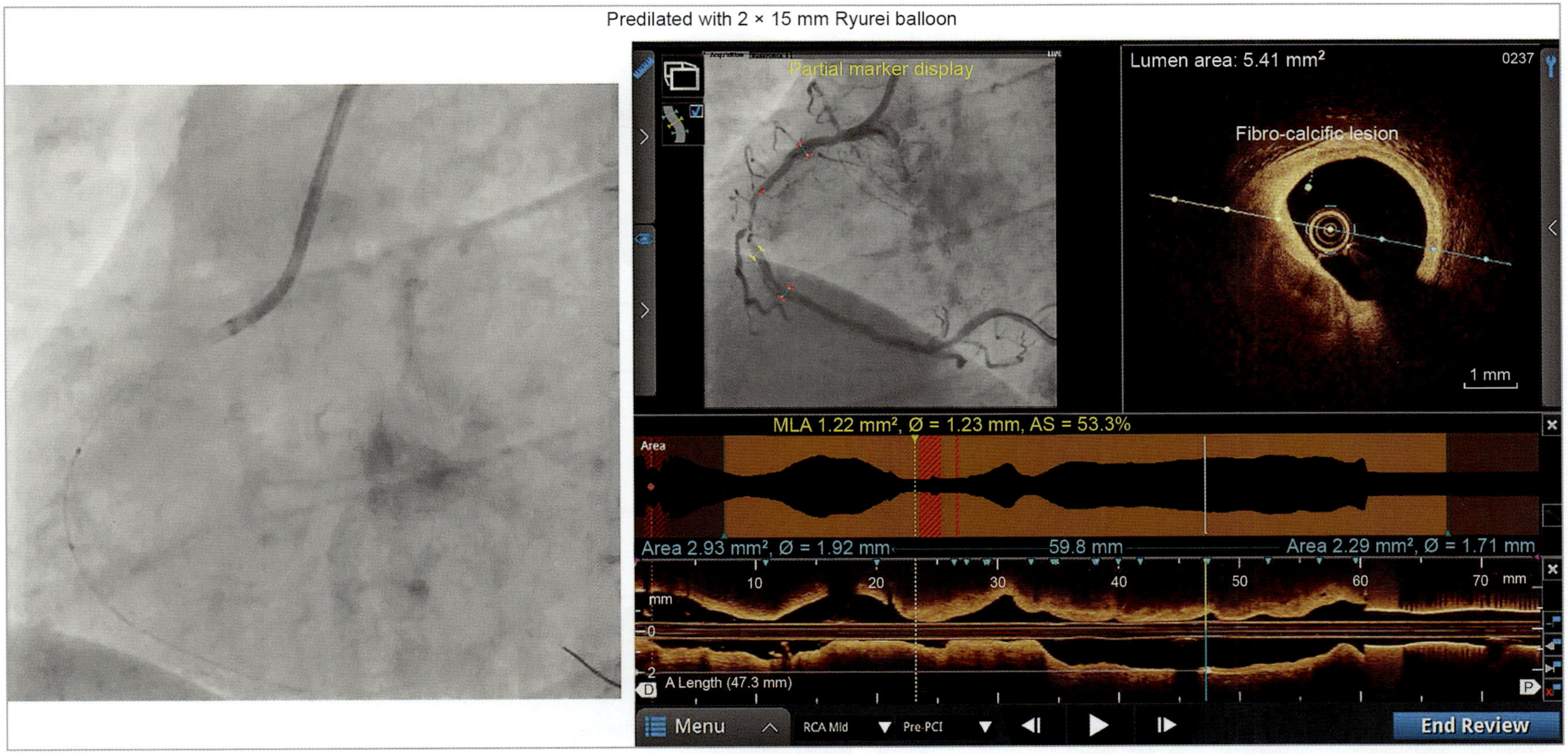

Fig. 32A

The management strategies for total occlusion of the LMCA include thrombolytic therapy, PCI, and emergency CABG. However, patients with left main with Cardiogenic shock (CS) do not benefit from thrombolytic therapy.

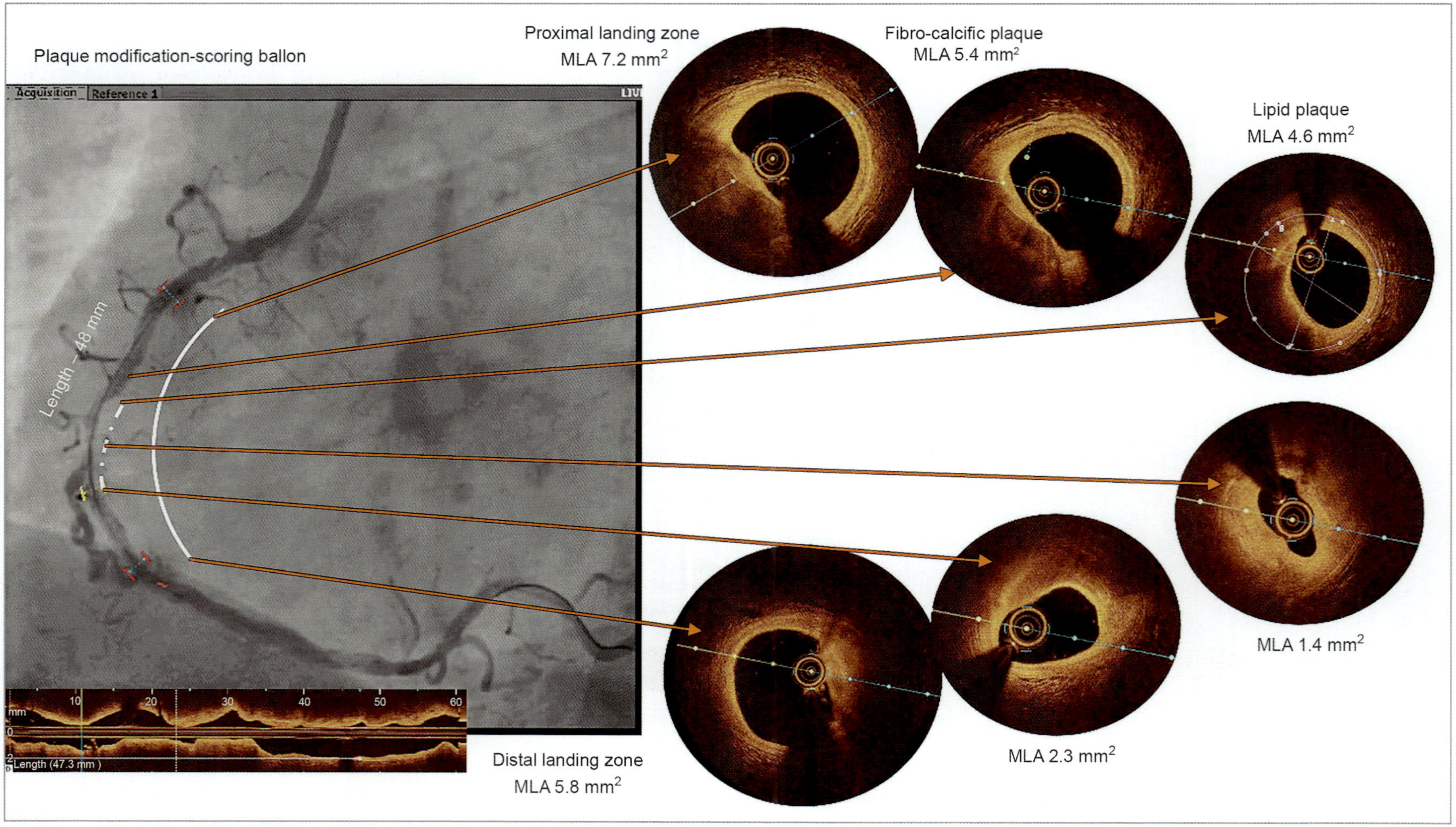

Fig. 32B

Figs. 32A and B: (A) Pre dilatation followed by OCT assessment to RCA; (B) Prestenting OCT - MLD assessment for plaque modification.

apposed stent struts with proximal edge dissection, which was covered by deploying 3.5 × 23 mm Xience Alpine stent overlapping with the previous stent **(Fig. 33A)**.

Postdilatation was done with 3.5 × 15 mm NC Trek balloon at 14 atm. The final result was good with TIMI III flow without complications **(Figs. 33B and C)**.

Left coronary artery was engaged through RRA with EBU 3.5–7 Fr guiding catheter, LAD lesion was crossed with 0.014" Runthrough wire, and LCX lesion was crossed with BMW wire. OCT pullback taken showed fibrotic plaque in mid-LAD and proximal LAD with focal calcified plaque **(Figs. 34A and B)**.

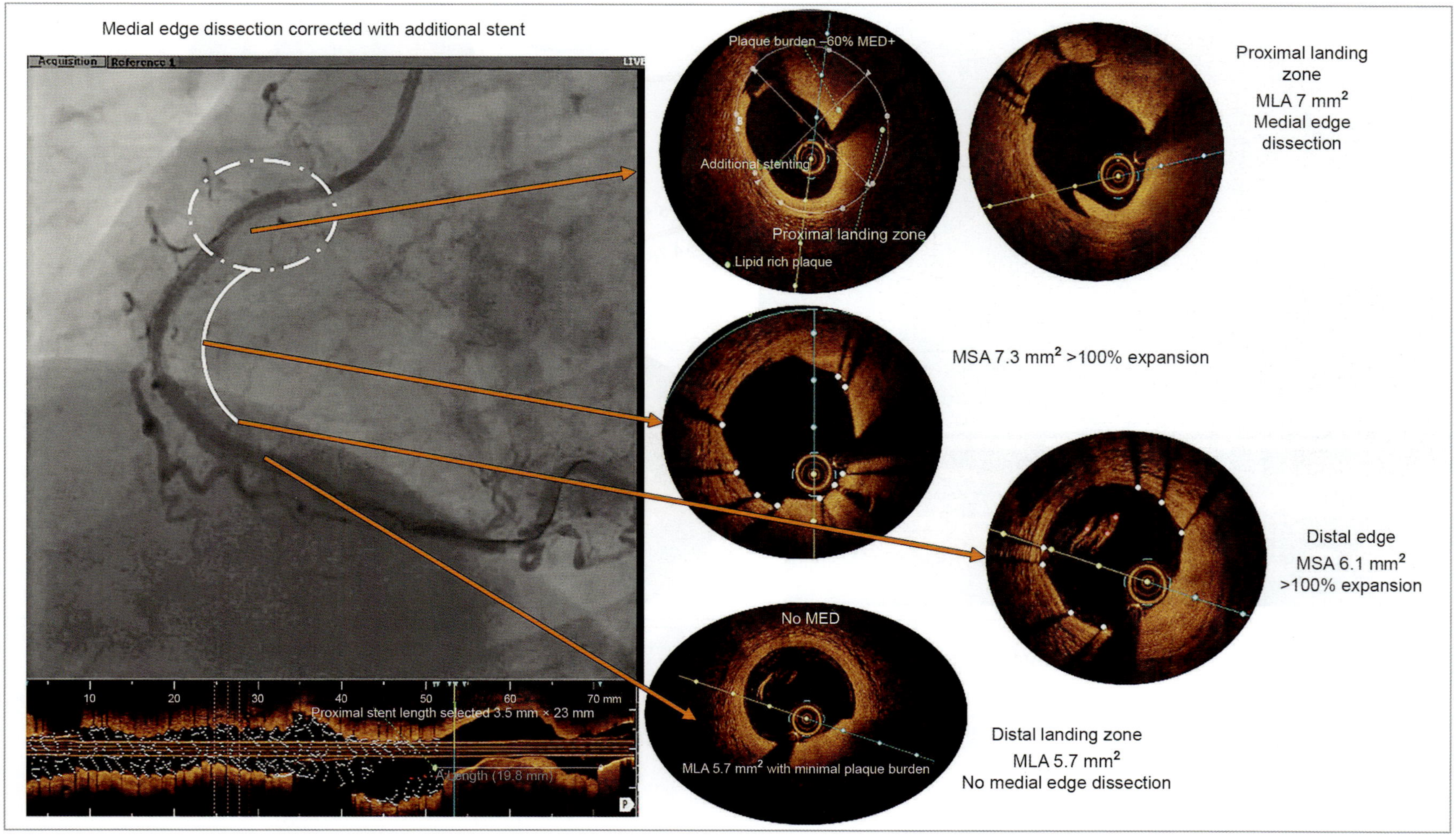

Fig. 33A

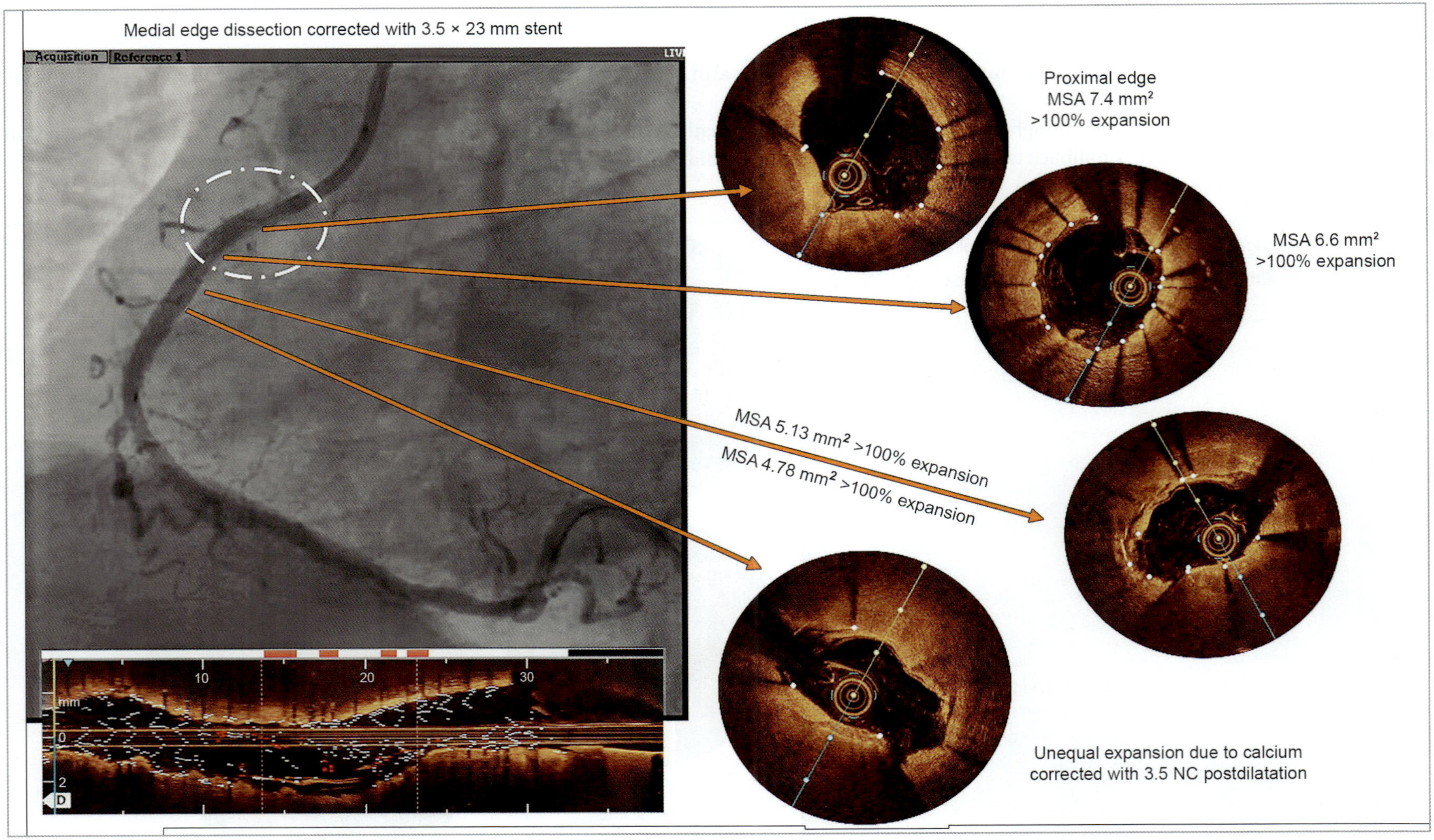
Medial edge dissection corrected with 3.5 × 23 mm stent
Acquisition
Reference 1
10
20
30
mm
0
2
D
Proximal edge
MSA 7.4 mm²
>100% expansion
MSA 6.6 mm²
>100% expansion
MSA 5.13 mm² >100% expansion
MSA 4.78 mm² >100% expansion
Unequal expansion due to calcium
corrected with 3.5 NC postdilatation

Fig. 33B

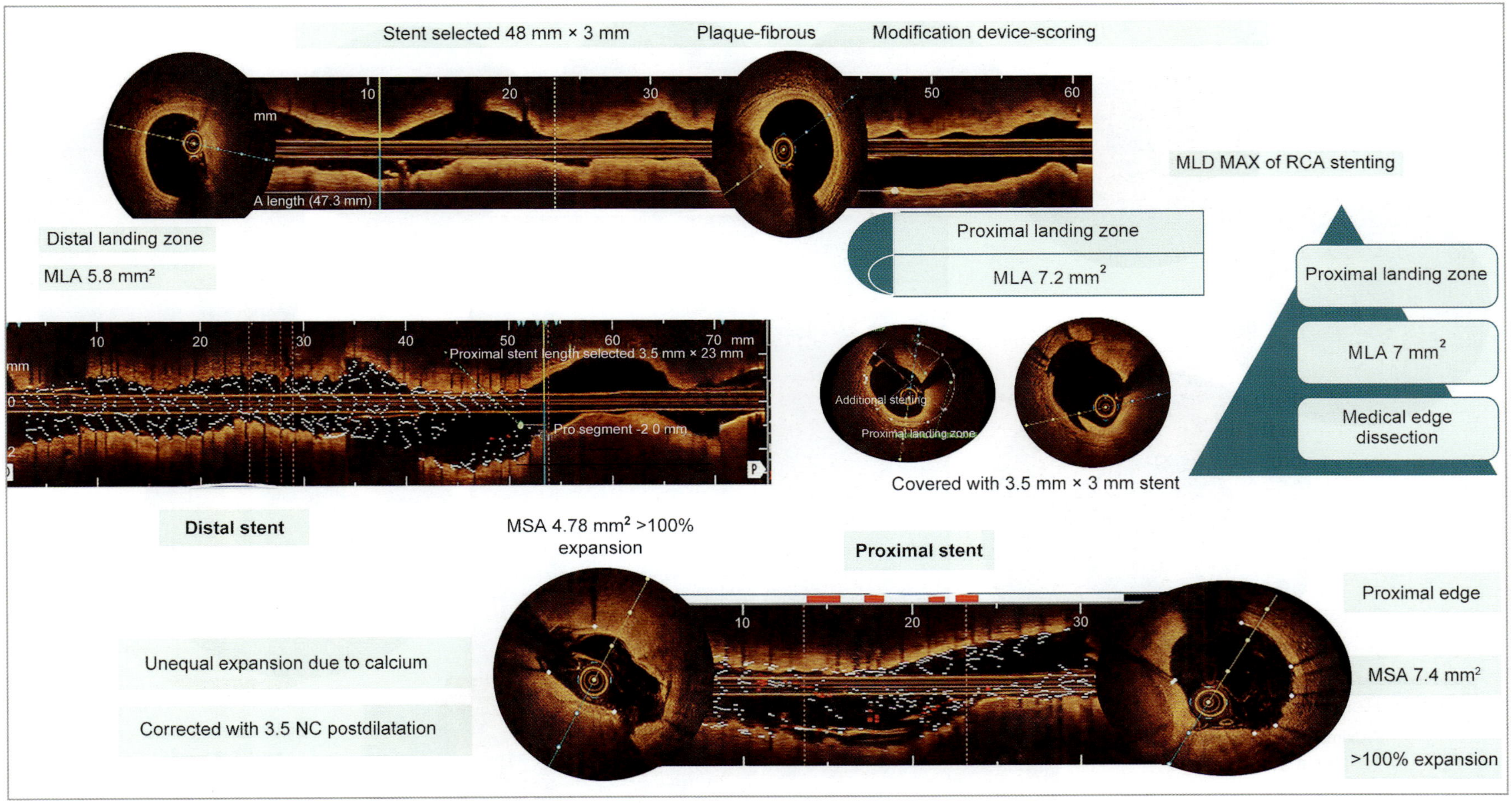

Fig. 33C

Figs. 33A to C: (A) Post proximal RCA stenting showed well apposed and expanded stent struts with proximal medial edge dissection required additional stent placement; (B) Post RCA stenting showed well apposed and expanded stent struts with no medial edge dissection; (C) OCT assessment of RCA for MLD & MAX.

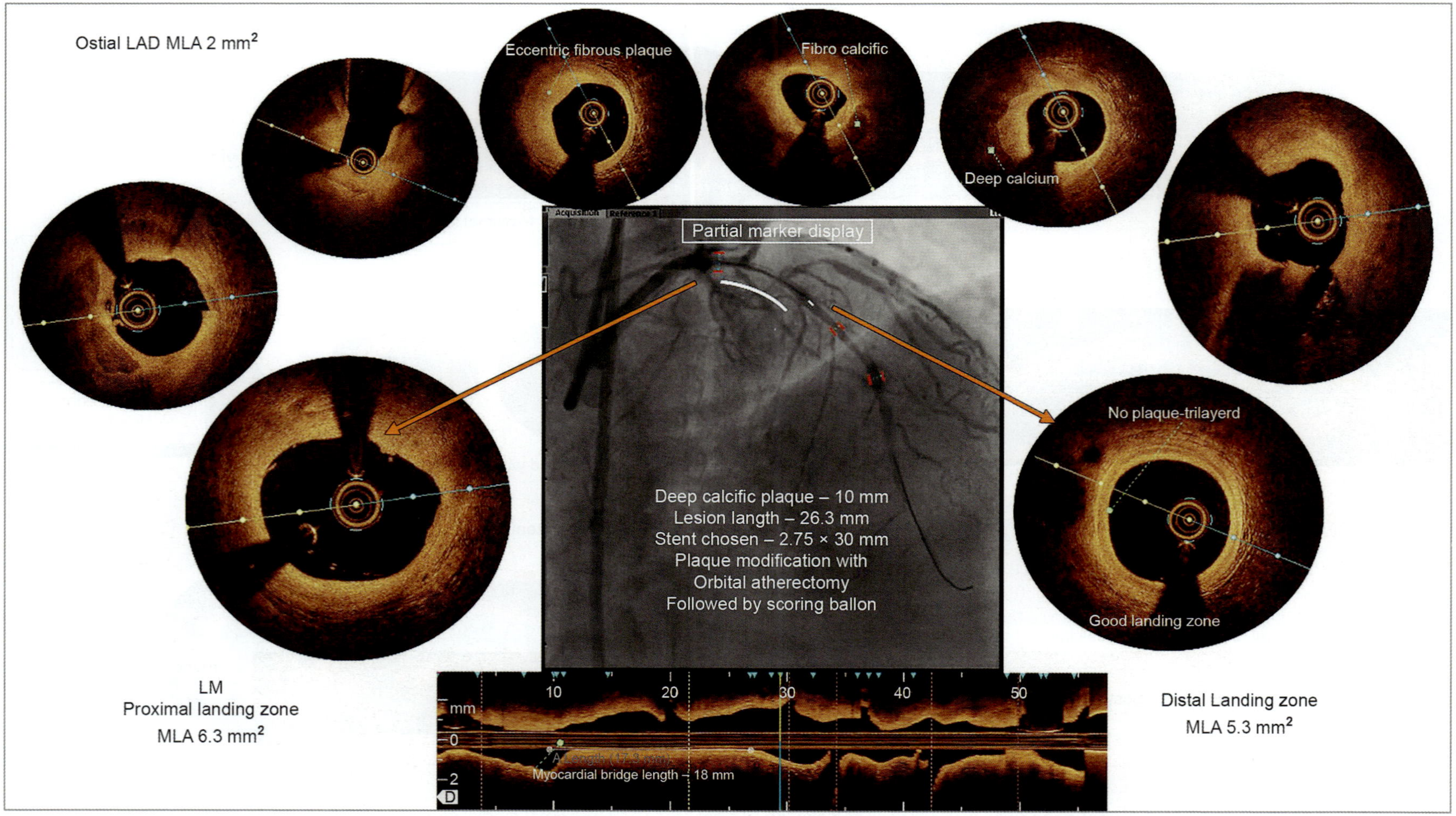

Fig. 34A

Based on results of DEFINE-FLAIR 27 and iFR-SWEDEHEART studies cut off value of iFR for deferring revascularization of lesions is >0.89.

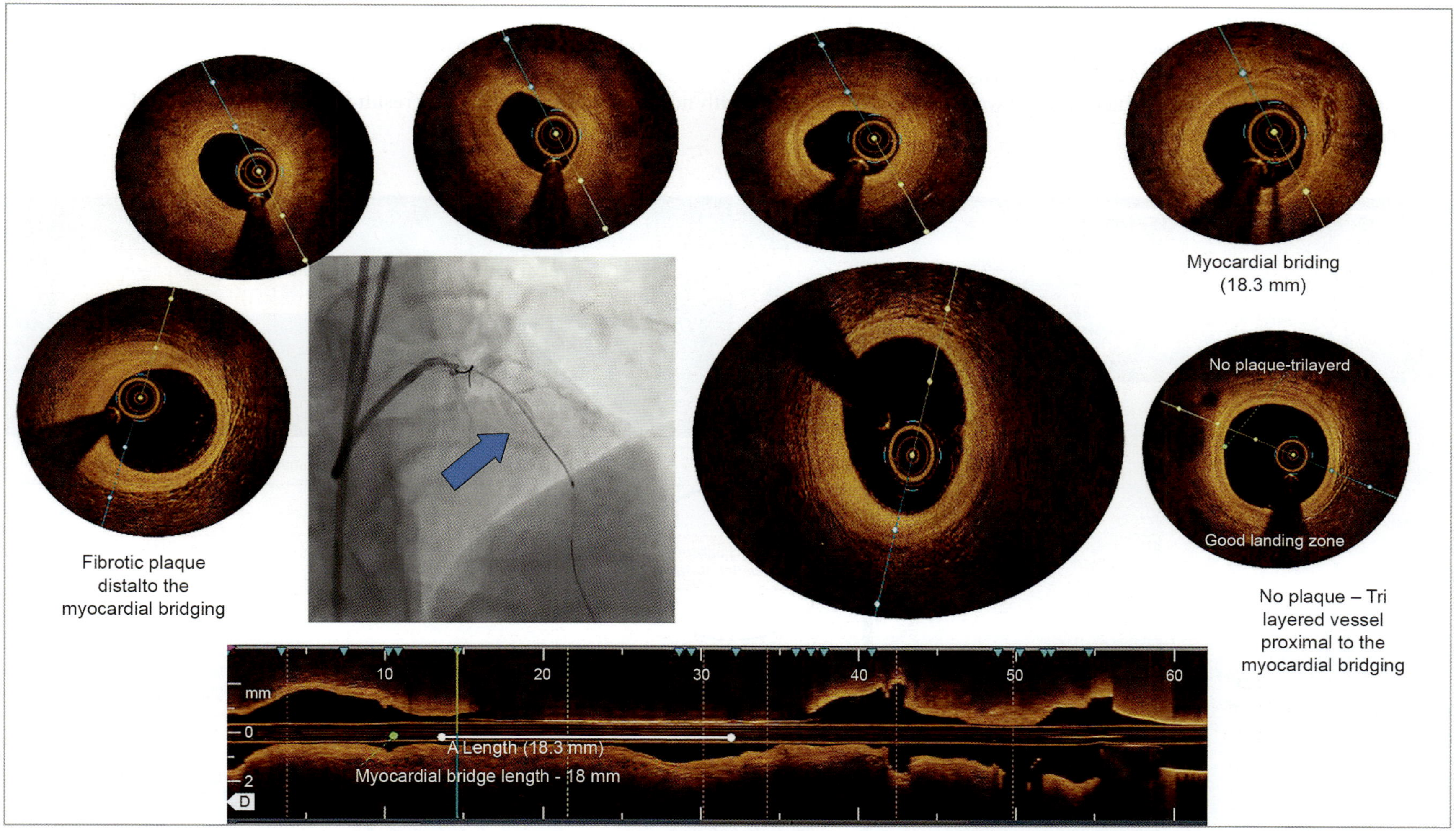

Fig. 34B

Figs. 34A and B: (A) Pre LAD stenting OCT assessment showing severe calcification needs plaque modification with Orbital Atherectomy and selection of stent size; (B) OCT assessment of 18.3mm myocardial bridging in distal LAD.

Plaque modification was carried out with 3 × 15 mm angiosculpt-cutting balloon at 12 atm and second diagonal was crossed with Sion blue wire. Then, LMCA to LAD stenting was done with 2.75 × 30 mm Resolute Onyx stent at 10 atm. Postdilated with 3.0 × 15 mm NC Trek balloon, final POT of LM was done with 4.0 × 06 mm NC balloon at 14 atm **(Fig. 35A)**.

Poststenting OCT was done which showed well-expanded stent struts with no edge dissection. The final result was good with TIMI III flow with no complications **(Figs. 35B to D)**.

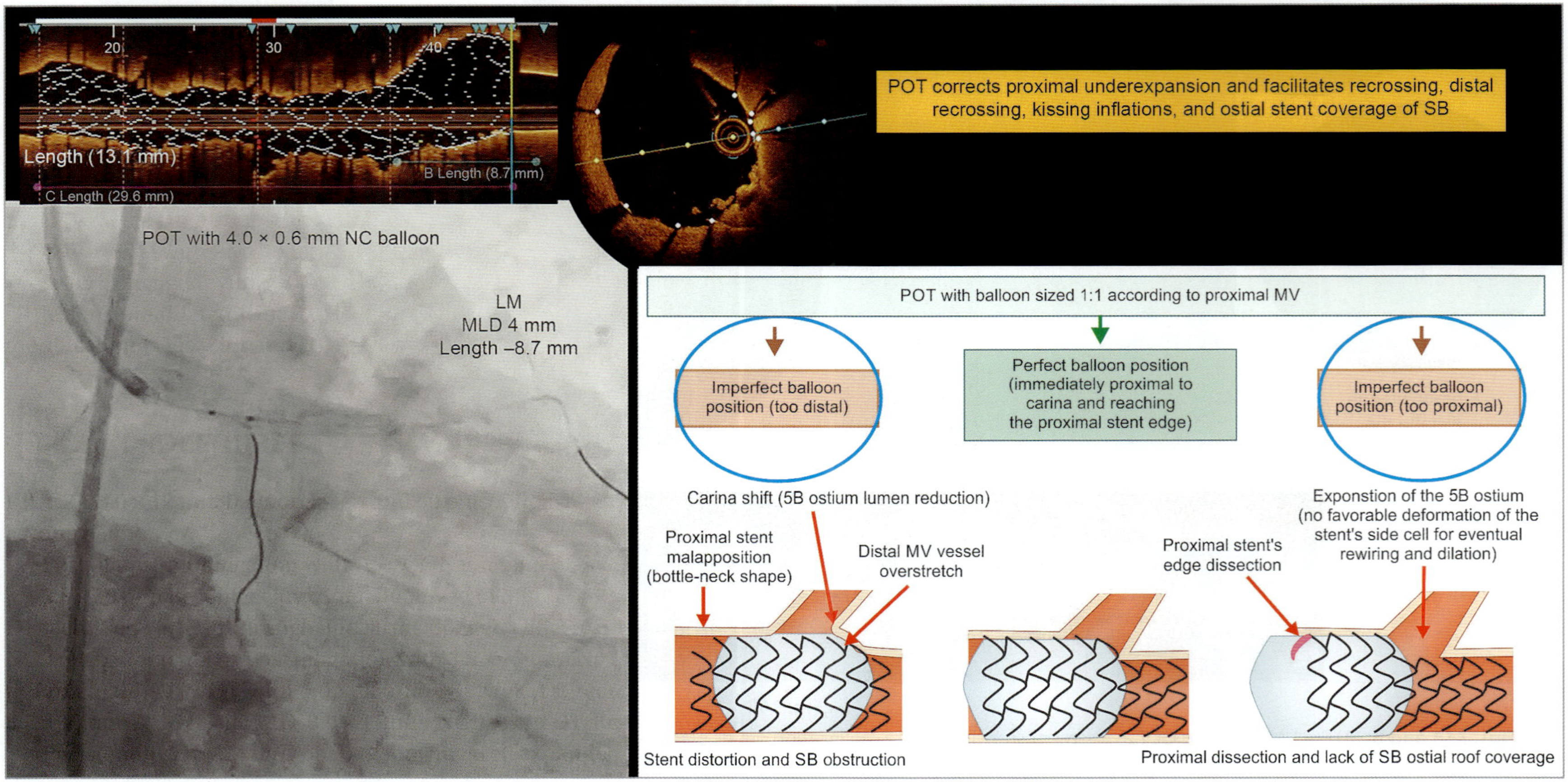

Fig. 35A

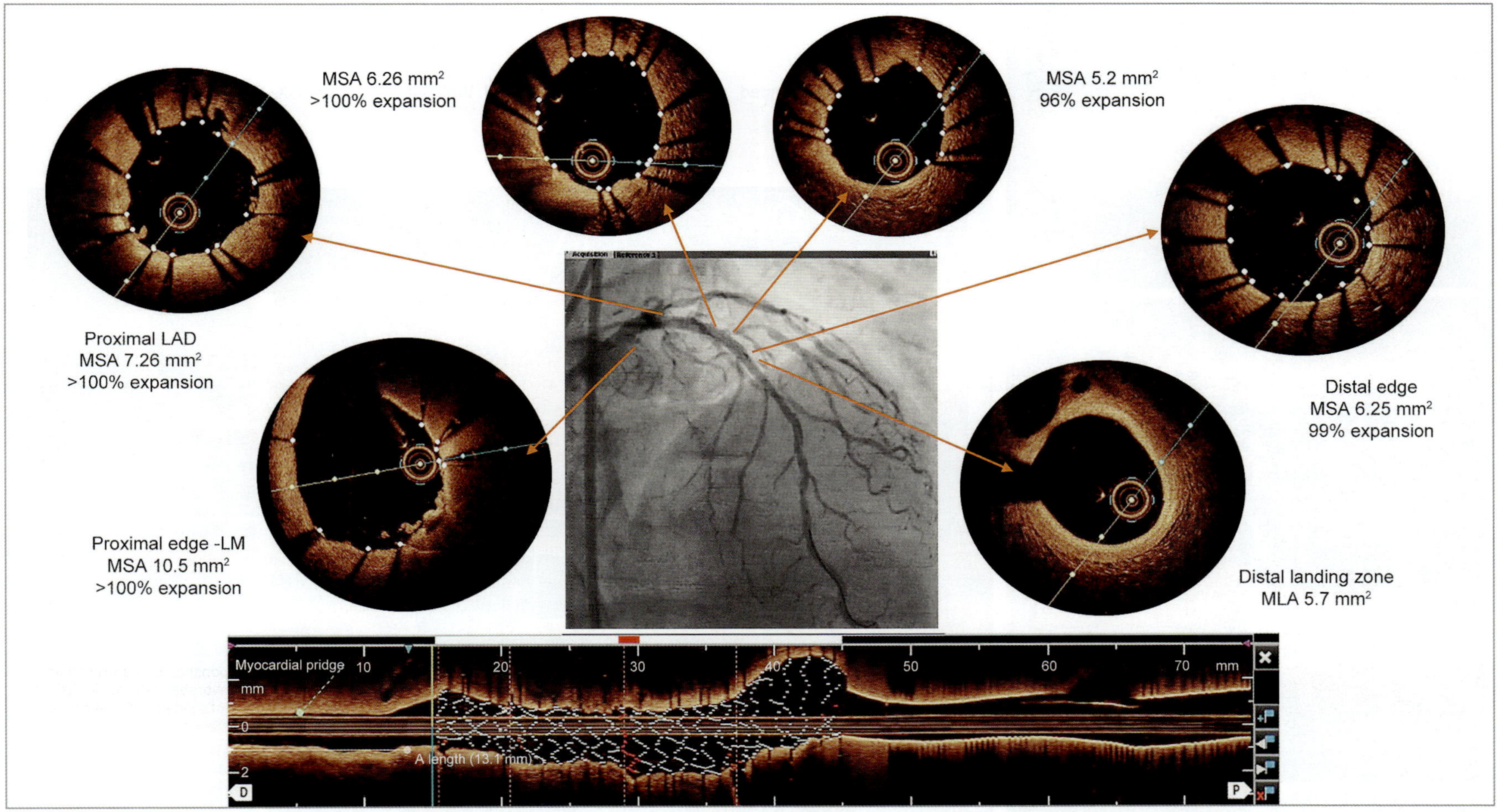

Fig. 35B

Precautions while navigating catheter through Radial access-Respect Natural Curves and Loops of Vessels-Gentle Manipulations, No Force Particularly if There is any resistance, allow catheter to slide gently, use Terumo wire, balloon tracking, external manipulations for loops in RA, deep breathing, turning head and coughing.

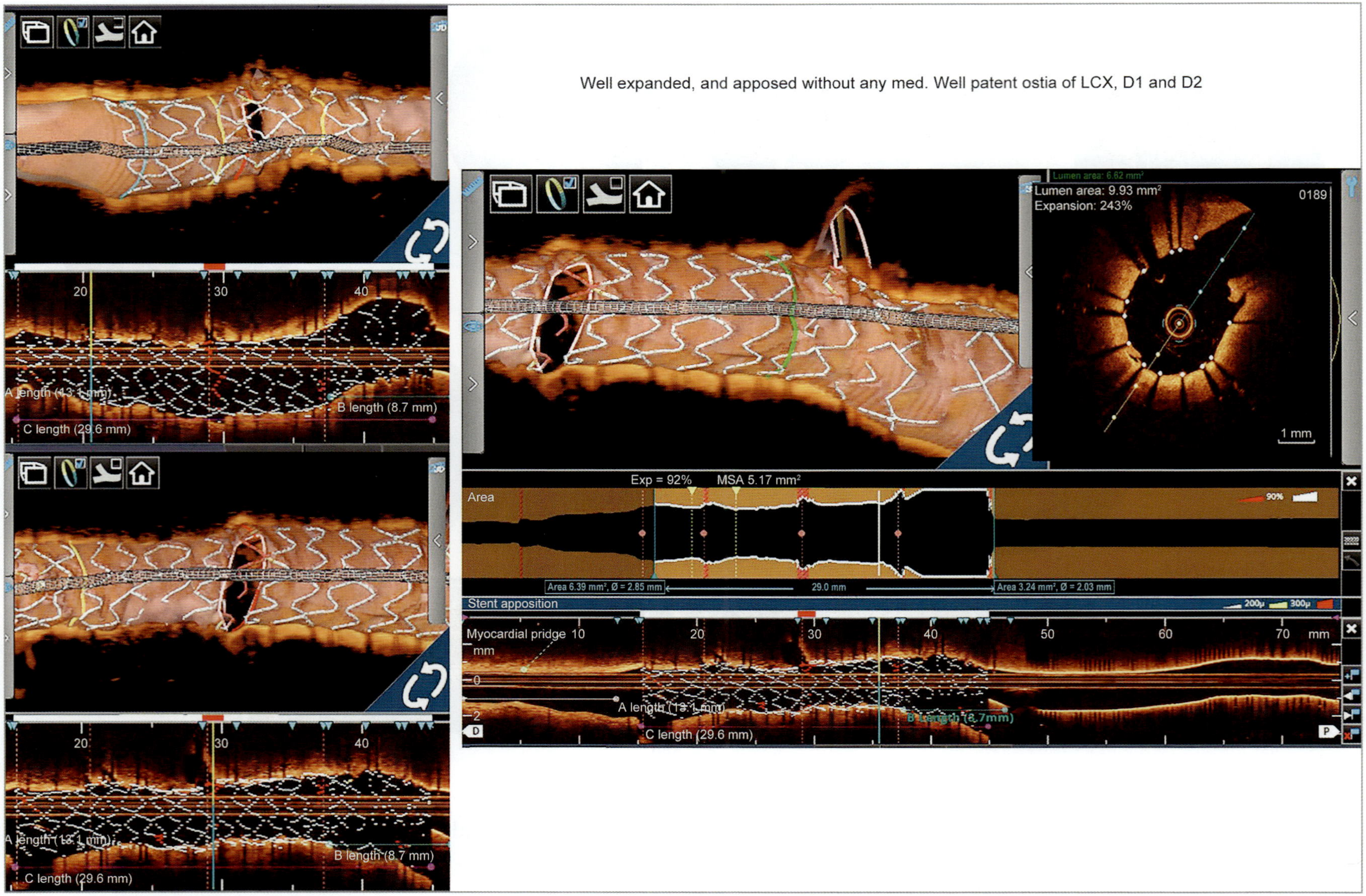
Well expanded, and apposed without any med. Well patent ostia of LCX, D1 and D2
A length (13.1 mm)
B length (8.7 mm)
C length (29.6 mm)
Lumen area: 9.93 mm²
Expansion: 243%
0189
1 mm
Exp = 92%
MSA 5.17 mm²
Area
Area 6.39 mm², Ø = 2.85 mm
29.0 mm
Area 3.24 mm², Ø = 2.03 mm
Stent apposition
Myocardial pridge
mm

Fig. 35C

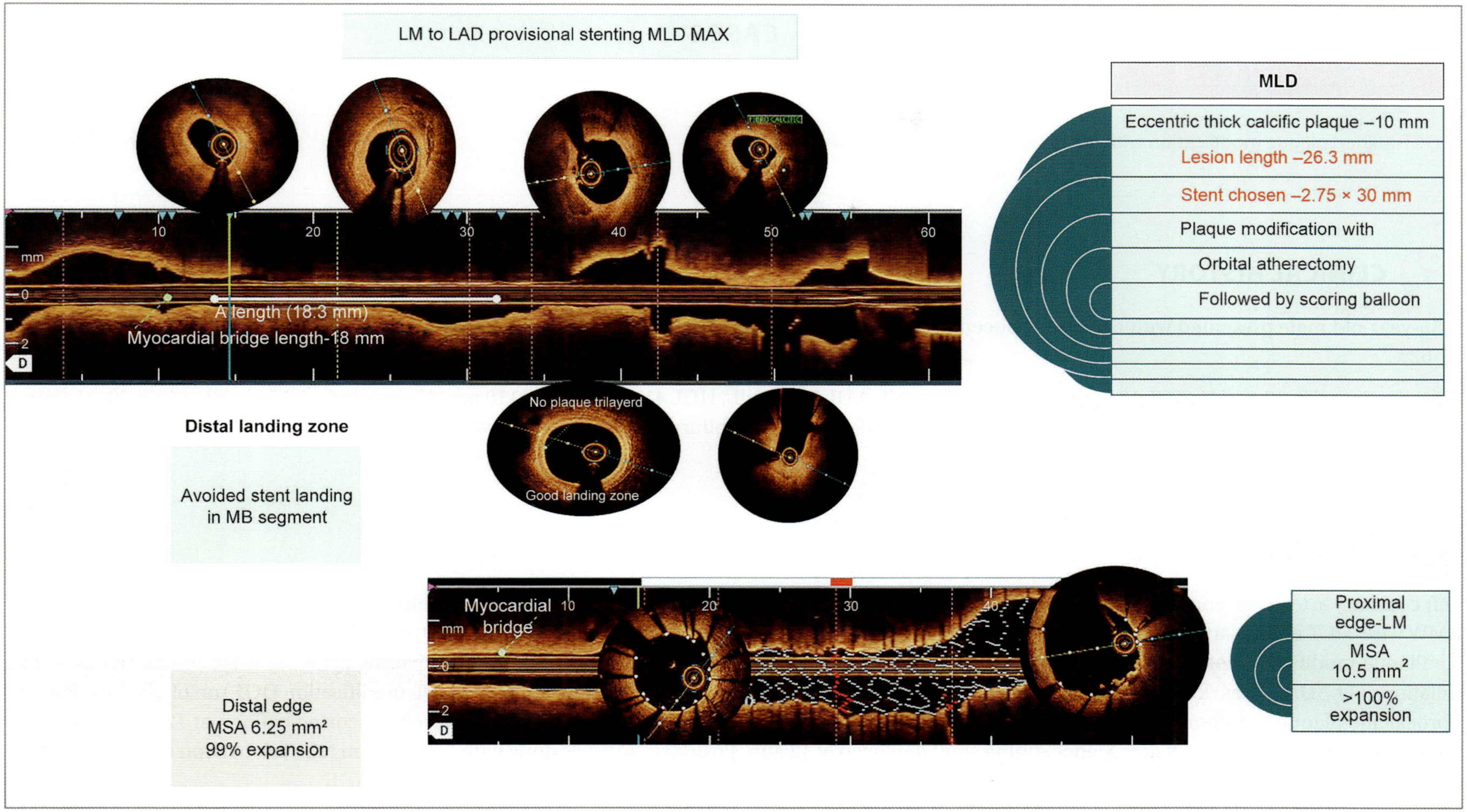

Fig. 35D

Figs. 35A to D: (A) Post OCT assessment for POT balloon sizing; (B) Poststent OCT showing well expanded and apposed stent struts with no medial edge dissections—MAX fulfilled; (C) 3D OCT showing well patent ostia of LCX, D1 and D2; (D) LM to LAD provisional stenting OCT assessment for MLD MAX.

CASE 3

OCT-guided plague modification with IVL of LM and non-LM bifurcations.

CLINICAL HISTORY

A 55-year-old male presented with exercise-induced LBBB, TMT was positive for inducible ischemia. ECG—normal, 2D echo—normal LV function with EF 62%.

Investigations: Hb 13.3 g/dL, TCL 124 mg/dL, TGL 129 mg/dL, LDL 78 mg/dL, HDL 41 mg/dL, RBS 110 mg/dL, Serum Cr 1.17 mg/dL, eGFR 70 mL/min.

Coronary angiography—SVD with proximal LAD 70% calcified stenosis at bifurcation, D1—ostioproximal 70% lesion (1,1,1). FFR study of LAD showed significant LAD disease **(Fig. 36)**.

PROCEDURE

Left coronary artery was engaged with EBU 3.5–7 Fr guiding catheter, LAD lesion was crossed with 0.014″ Runthrough wire. D1 lesion crossed with 0.014″ BMW wire. OCT of LAD and diagonal were done which showed significant fibrocalcific plaque involving LAD and D1 bifurcation site **(Figs. 37A and B)**.

Plaque modification of LAD was done with IVL 3.5 × 12 mm balloon, 80 pulses were delivered, while delivering pulses to LAD, simultaneous kissing inflations of LAD/D1 was done using 3.5 × 12 mm IVL balloon in LAD and 2.5 × 10 mm balloon in D1. Post-IVL modification OCT run of diagonal showed fibrocalcific plaque. Additional plaque modification of LAD lesion was carried out with 3.5 × 15 mm angiosculpt scoring balloon at 12 atm. Then, LAD stenting was done with 3.5 × 28 mm Xience Alpine stent deployed at 12 atm. Postdilatation was done with 3.5 × 12 mm NC Trek balloon at 16-18 atm. POT of LMCA was performed with 4.0 × 15 mm balloon at 12 atm.

Diagonal branch was recrossed again with Runthrough wire. OCT run of diagonal showed significant dissection of the ostioproximal segment of the diagonal branch. Then 2.5 × 15 mm Xience Alpine stent deployed in ostial diagonal using snuggle T-stenting technique **(Figs. 38 and 39)**.

Postdilatation of D1 was done with 2.75 × 12 mm NC Trek balloon. Final kissing balloon dilatation of LAD/D1 was done with 3.5 × 12 mm NC Trek balloon in LAD and 2.25 × 12 mm NC Trek balloon in diagonal. Final OCT run of LAD was taken which showed well-expanded and apposed stent struts with no edge dissection. The final result was good with TIMI III flow without complications **(Figs. 40 and 41)**.

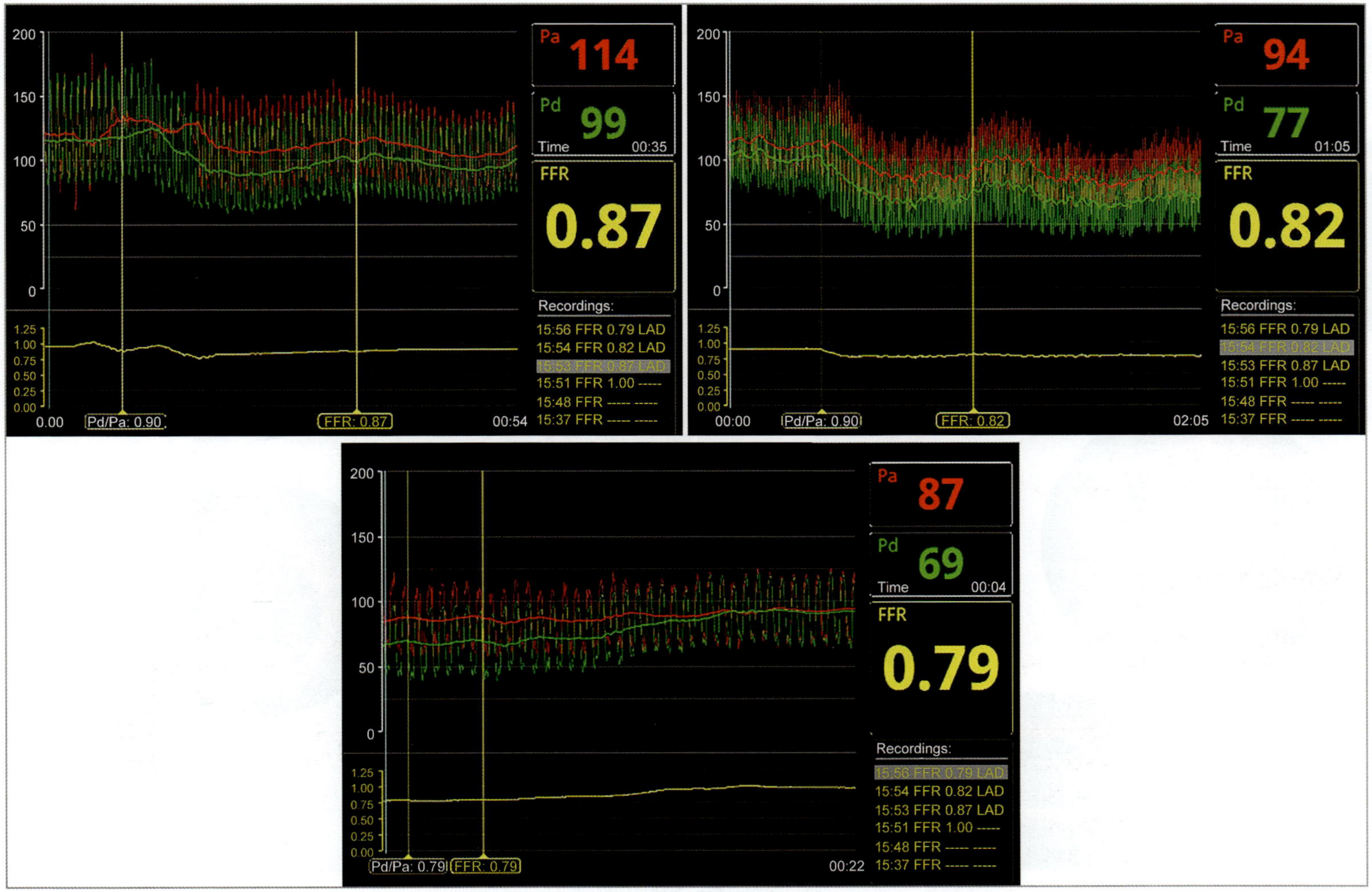

Fig. 36: FFR study of LAD showed significant LAD disease.

The presence of a critical stenosis at one branch can divert flow more to the other branch and influence FFR value (branch steal phenomenon.) As long as the stenosis in the LAD or LCx is not very tight (FFR <0.60), it hardly influences the FFR value of the LM.

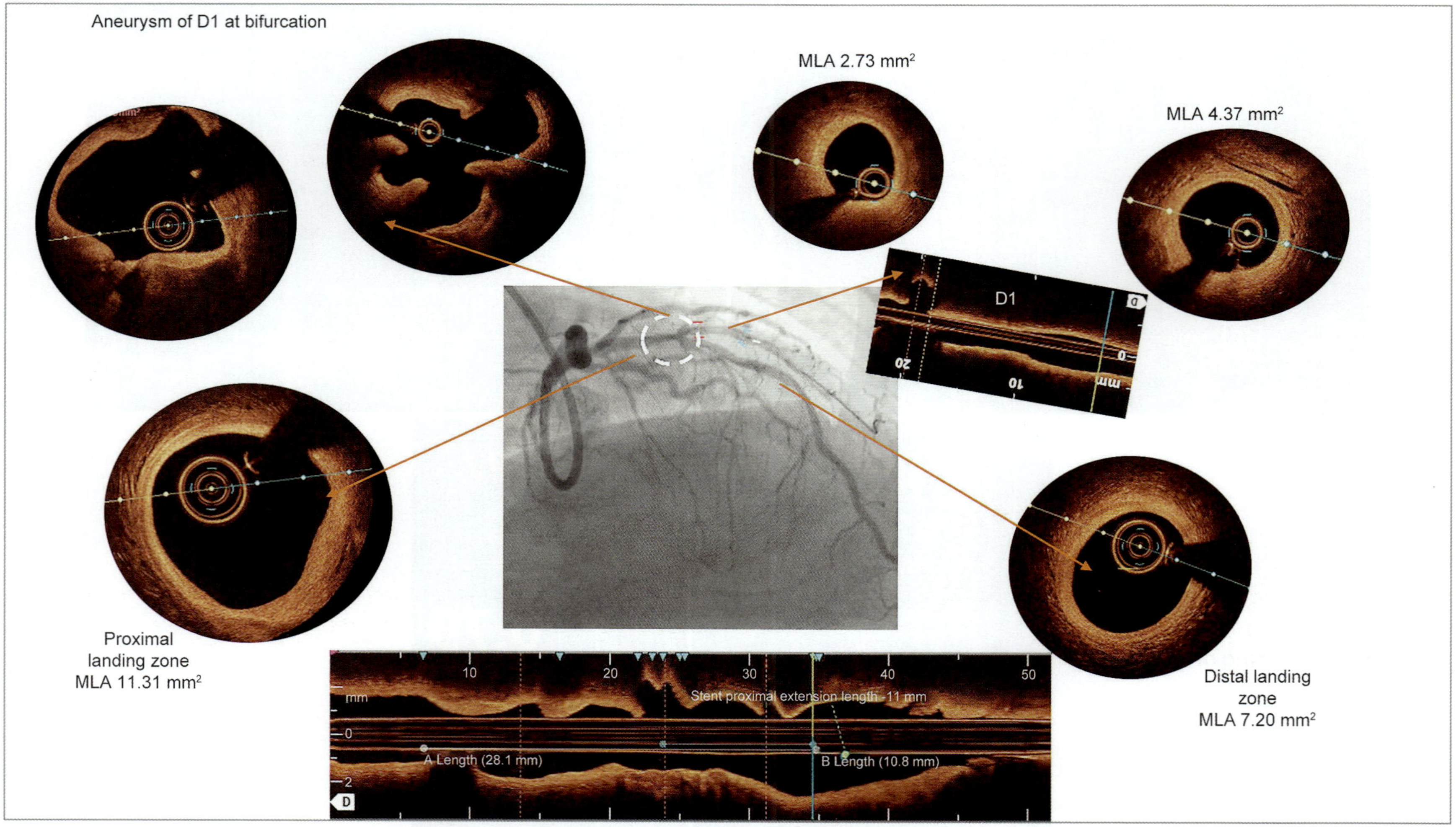

Fig. 37A

During primary PCI, Radial access is preferred over femoral access due to lower all-cause mortality, stroke or non CABG major bleeding at 30 days follow up in MATRIX, and RIVAL studies.

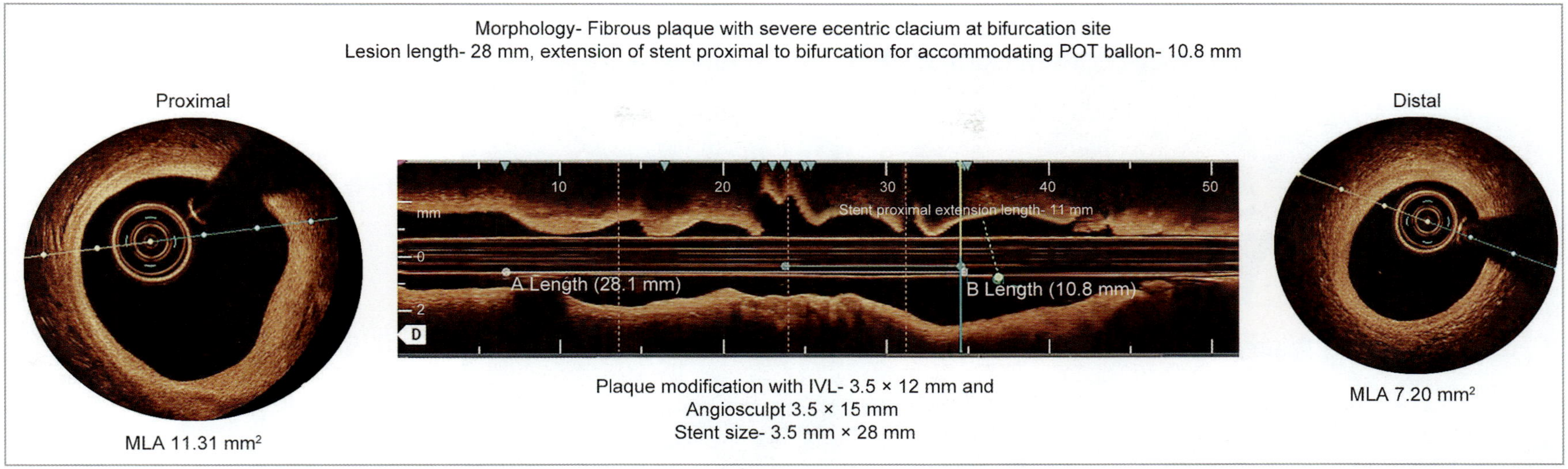

Fig. 37B

Figs. 37A and B: (A) OCT of LAD and diagonal were done which showed significant fibrocalcific plaque involving LAD and aneurysm at D1 bifurcation site; (B) Prestenting OCT for assessment of plaque modification and stent size selection

PCI of LM is emerging as an alternative to CABG especially in patients with low syntax score with suitable coronary anatomy for PCI, and life-saving emergency situations like ACS with hemodynamically unstable, and high risk group patients who are unsuitable coronary anatomy for grafting or due to associated co-morbidities

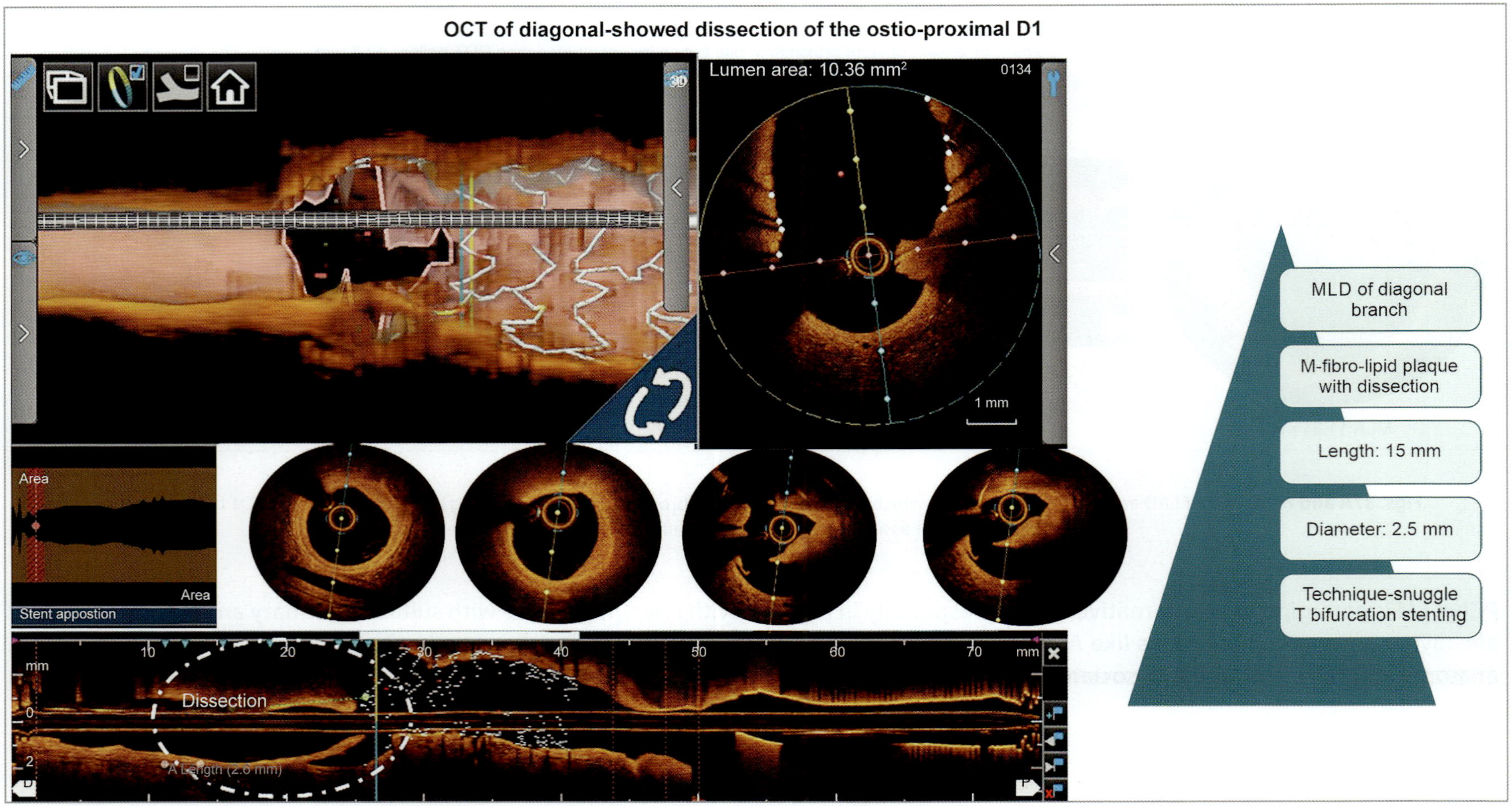

Fig. 38: Ostio-proximal D1 dissection.

POT corrects proximal under-expansion and facilities recrossing, distal recrossing, kissing inflations and ostial stent coverage of SB.

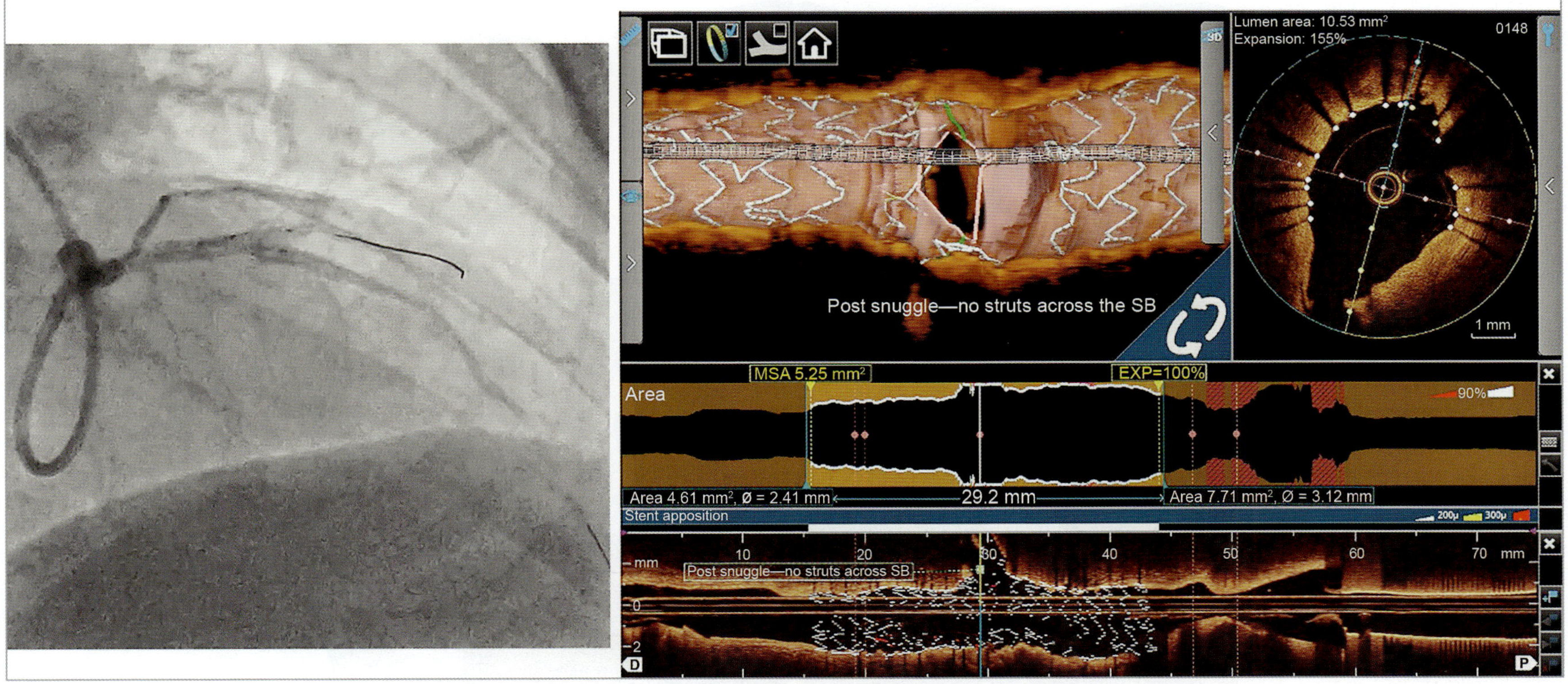

Fig. 39: Post snuggle KB dilatation - well patent D1 ostium free of struts.

Selection of Guide/Long Sheaths/Guide Extension/Radial Access

- Strong back-up guide with good alignment, and if needed Guideliner.
- 7/8 Fr EBU or XB, JL with side hole for ostial left main lesion especially for 2 stent implantation.
- Floating wire/Knuckle wire to keep the GC preferred position avoiding injury and helping good stent position
- Tortuous Ilio-femoral arteries—Long Sheaths.
- Prefer Radial access with Slender sheaths if feasible.

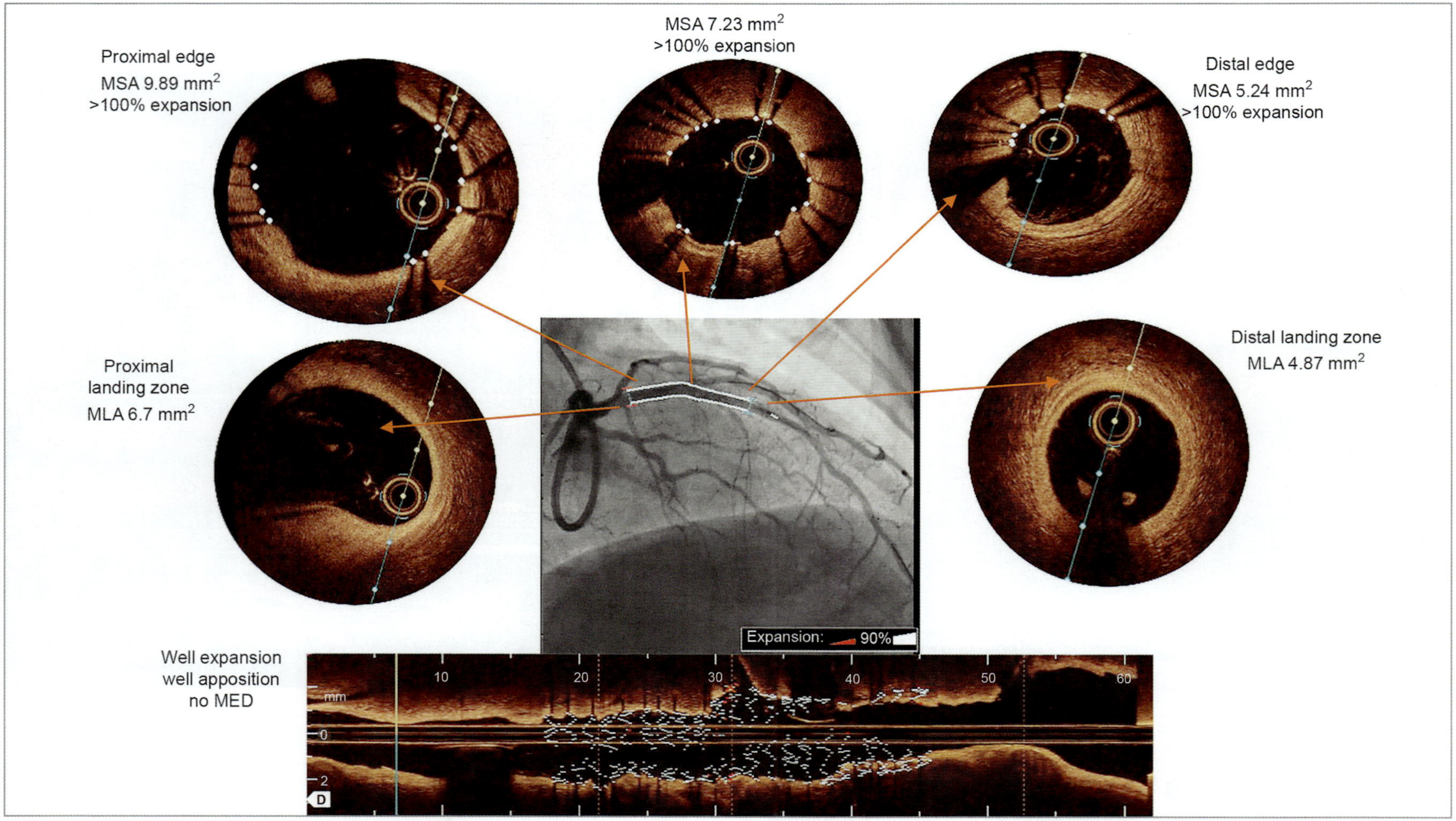

Fig. 40: Poststenting LM-LAD OCT assessment showing well expanded and apposed stent struts with no medial edge dissections.

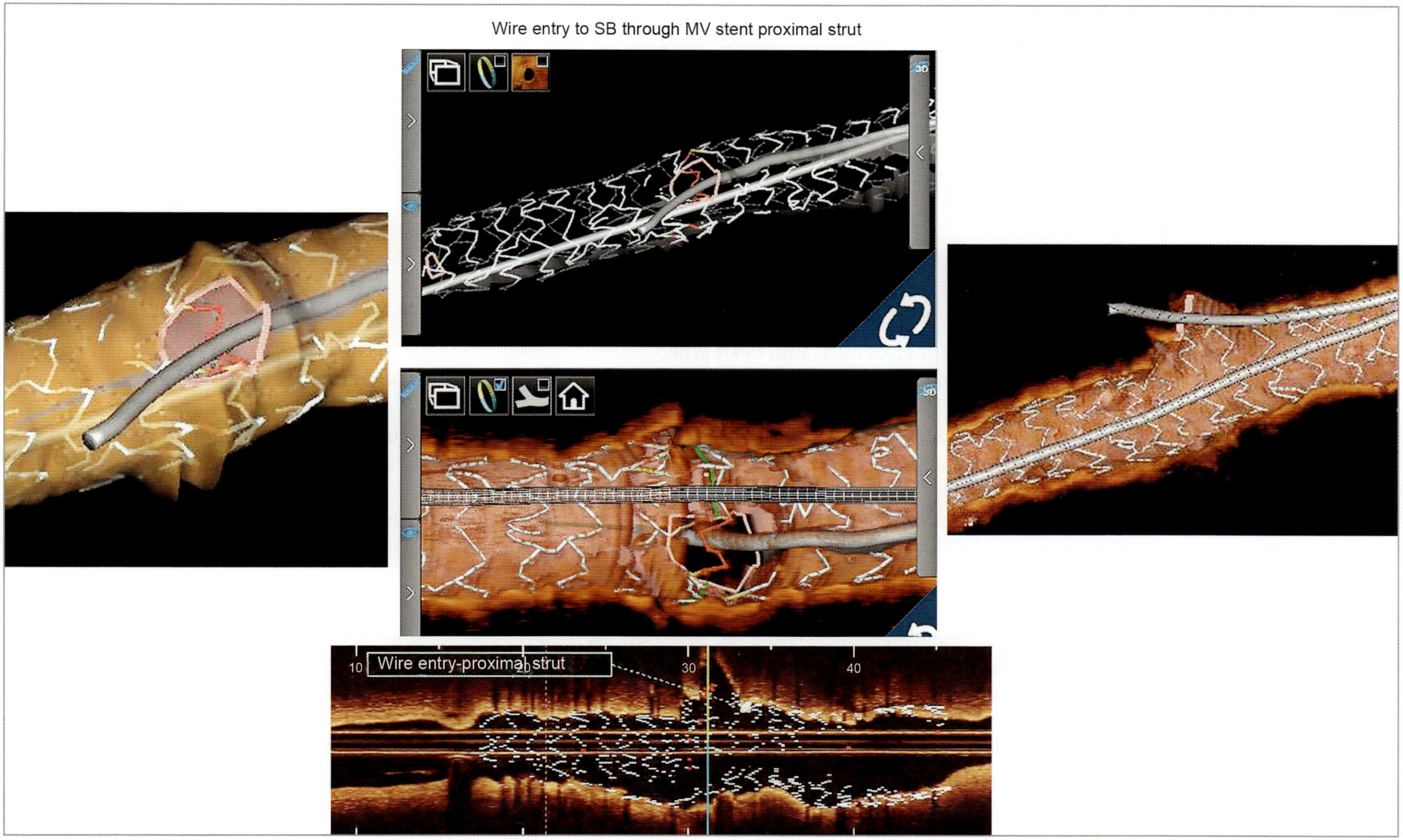

Fig. 41: 3D bifurcation mode - guide wire through proximal strut & well expanded stent.

CASE 4

OCT assessment of LAD and LM.

CLINICAL HISTORY

A 67-year-old male, known HTN presented with c/o on and off chest pain radiating to back. ACS—USA, ECG—NSR, 2D echo—good LV function, 65%.

Investigations: Hb 13.2 g/dL, s Cr 0.85 mg/dL, Trop-I 11.09 ng/L, RBS 199 mg/dL.

CAG-LMCA—distal 50% lesion, LAD—ostial mild plaquing with 30–40% lesion, mid 90% lesion, RAMUS—ostial 90% lesion, LCX—normal, RCA—mid 90% lesion.

Right coronary artery engaged through RRA with JR 3.5-6 Fr guiding catheter, RCA lesion crossed with 0.014″ BMW wire. Predilatation done with 2.0 × 10 mm Ryurei balloon. Then RCA stenting done with 2.75 × 28 mm Xience Xpedition stent deployed at 12 atm. The final result was good with TIMI III flow with no complications.

Left main coronary artery engaged through RRA with EBU 3.5-6 Fr guiding catheter, LAD lesion crossed with 0.014″ BMW wire. Predilatation done with 2.0 × 10 mm Ryurei balloon. OCT showed lipid-rich plaque with white thrombus and lesion length was found to be 23.6 mm **(Fig. 42)**.

PROCEDURE

Dilated with 3.0 × 10 mm angiosculpt cutting balloon. Then mid-LAD stenting done with 4.0 × 23 mm Xience Xpedition stent deployed at 12 atm.

Optical coherence tomography was done which showed proximal stent edge dissection **(Figs. 43 and 44)**. LMCA-LAD stenting done with 4.0 × 18 mm Xience Xpedition stent deployed at 12 atm. Postdilatation done with 5 × 08 mm NC Trek balloon up to 12 atm. Poststenting OCT was done which showed well-expanded stent struts. The final result was good with TIMI III flow with no complications **(Figs. 45 and 46)**.

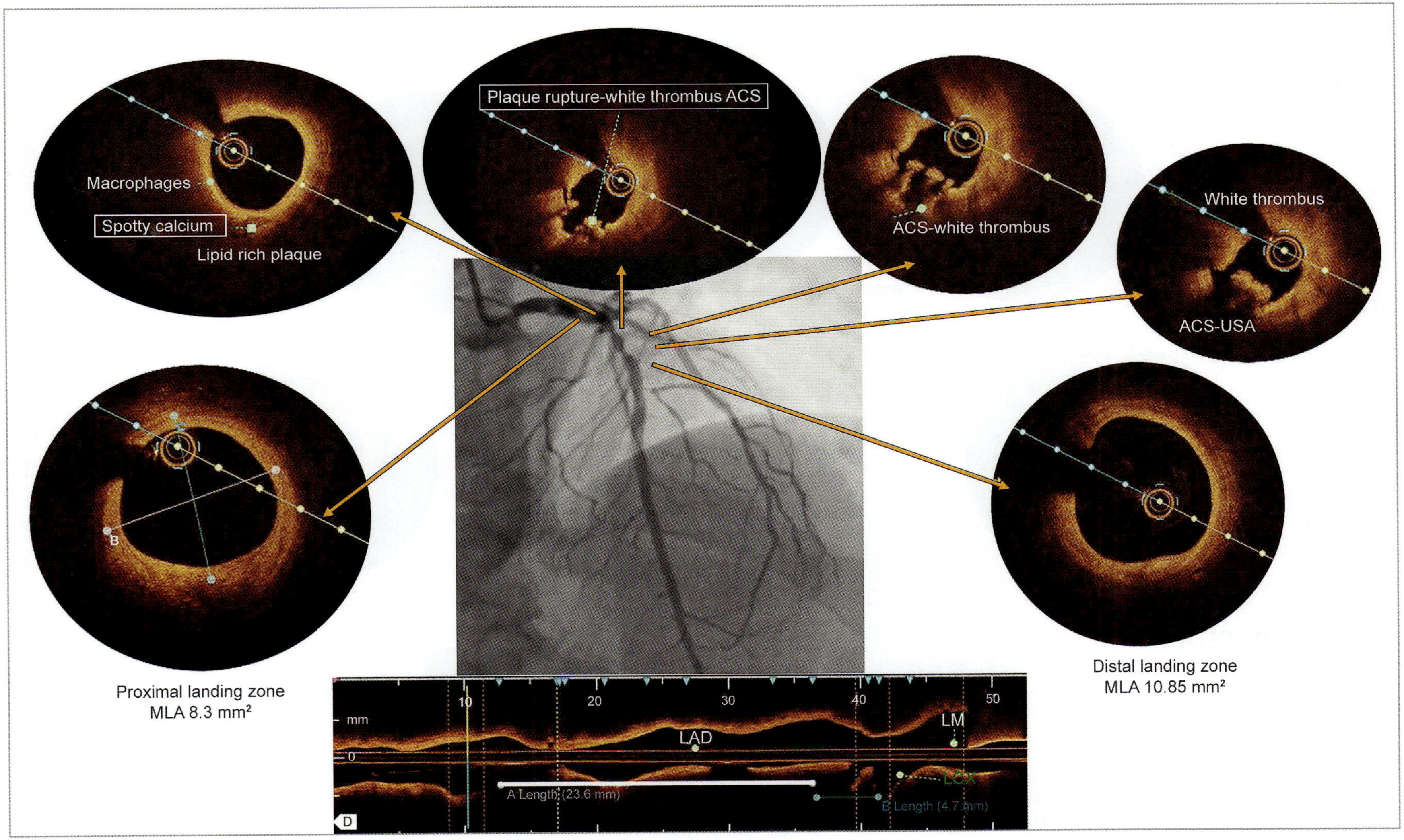

Fig. 42: MLD assessment of LAD - D1 bifurcation.

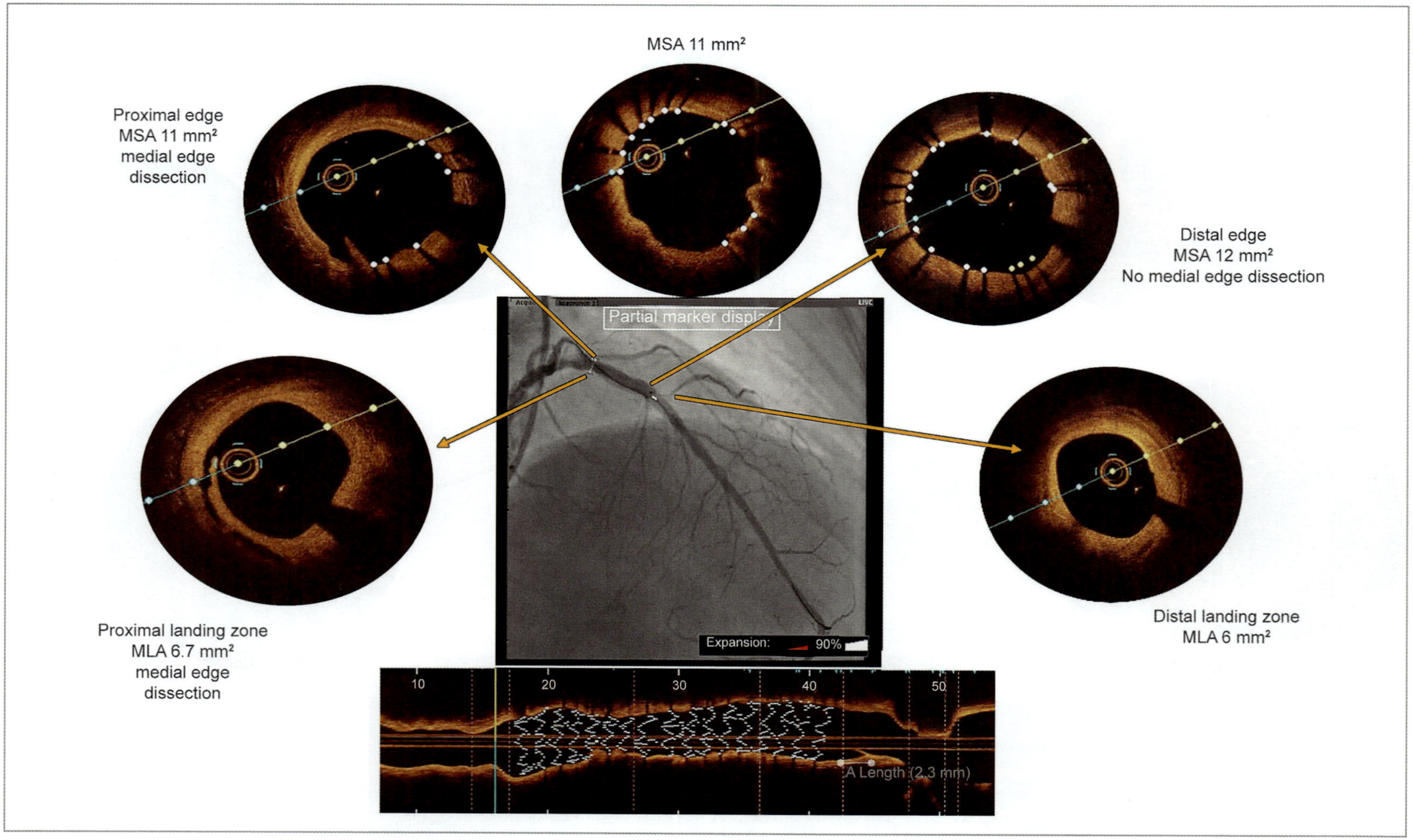

Fig. 43: Poststent OCT for MAX assessment - medial edge dissection at proximal edge.

Careful femoral access site puncture is essential to reduce access related complications:

1. **Meticulous puncture (bony land marks)**
2. **Ultrasound guided**
3. **Fluoroscopy contrast injection guided**
4. **Micro puncture technique.**

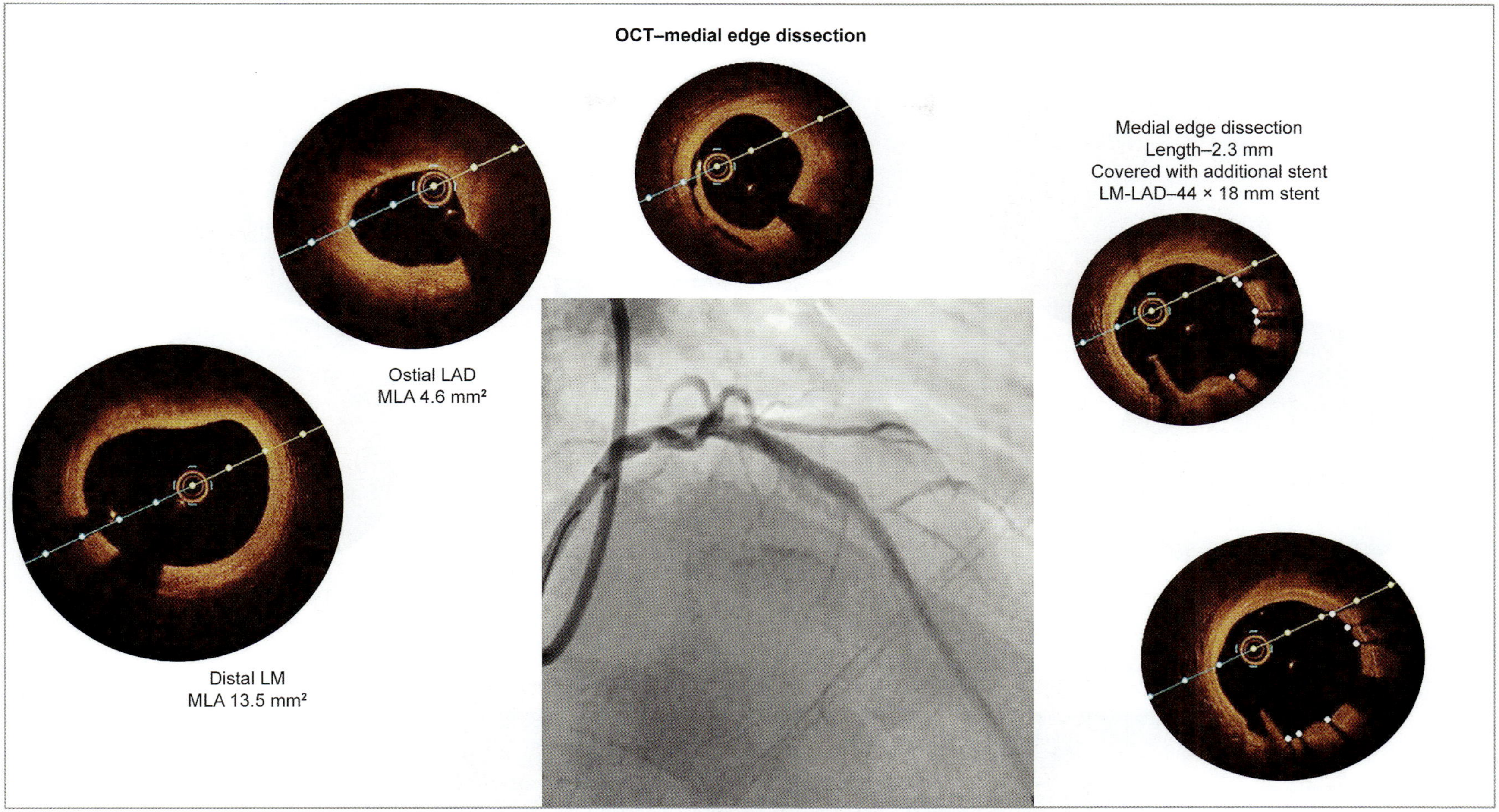

Fig. 44: OCT assessment of medial edge dissection for additional stenting.

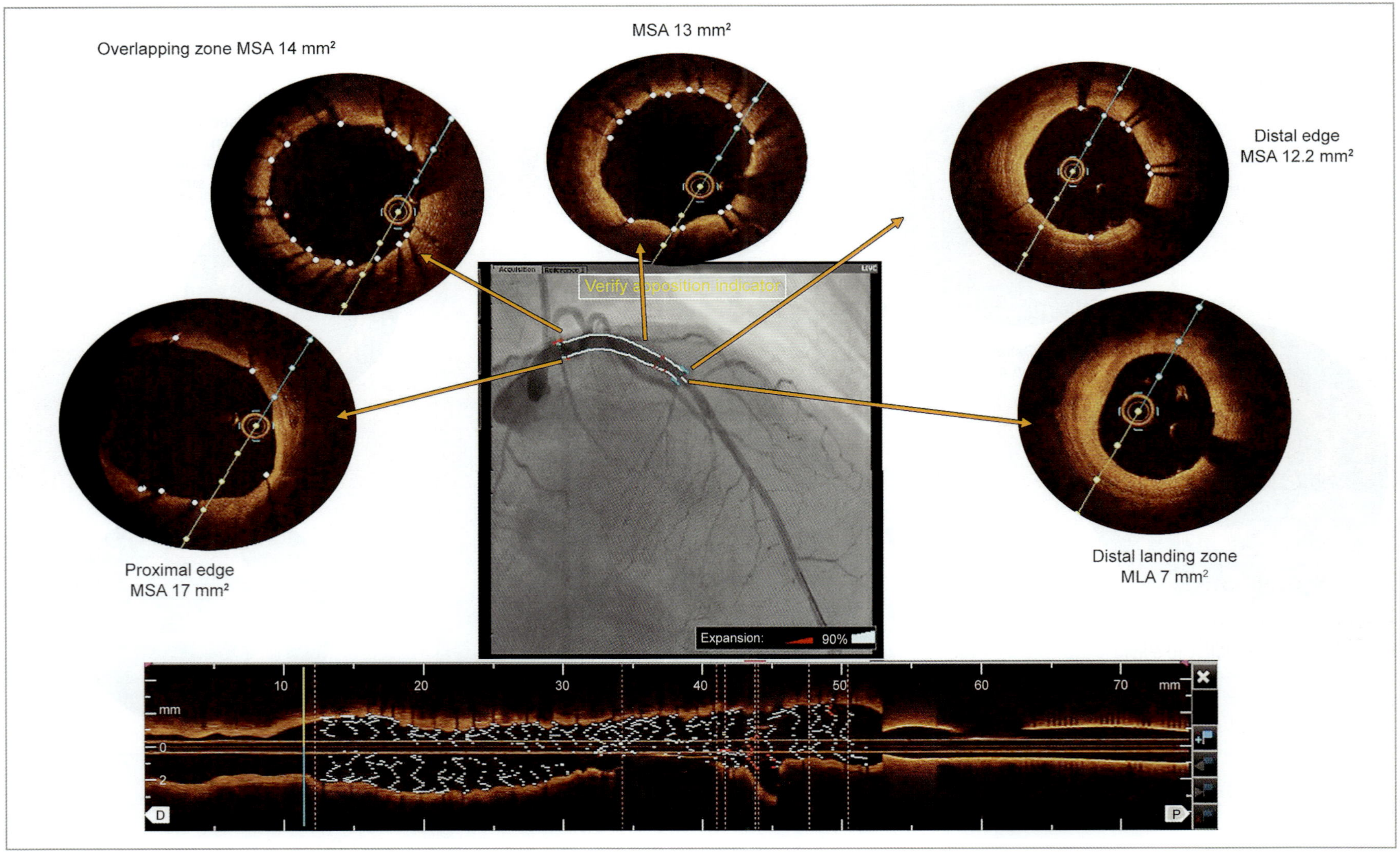

Fig. 45: Final poststenting for MAX assessment.

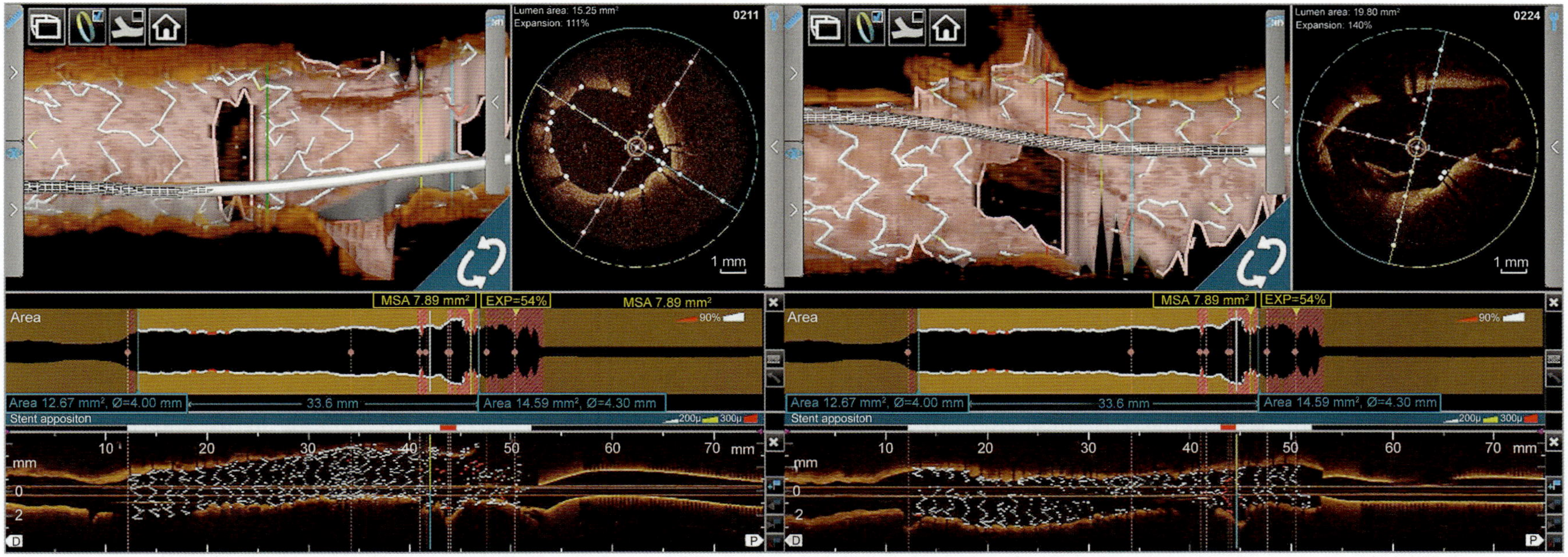

Fig. 46: 3D OCT bifurcation showing patent ostial LCX with free of struts.

Wire Entrapment—Fractured Wire

Within the coronary:

- Pin to the wall with stent
- Pass a 2nd or 3rd wire and entangle the wires and pull it out
- Snare
- Drag out with balloon/guide extender.

CASE 5

OCT assessment of anterior STEMI due to LM thrombosis.

CLINICAL HISTORY

A 49-year-old female, a known diabetic, came with complaints of chest pain, CAD-ACS—evolved AWMI with WP >24 hours, 2D echo—RWMA in LAD territory, mild LV dysfunction with EF 48%.

Investigations: Hb 11.5 g/dL, WBC 10,700 cells/cmm, Trop-I 10.08 ng/mL, NT-pro BNP 1,553 pg/mL, S Cr 0.64 mg/dL, RBS 382 mg/dL, and Hb1Ac 11%.

On day 2, angio revealed ostial LMCA 70–80% thrombotic lesion, mid-LAD 50% lesion, D1 95% lesion with faint flow in view of large thrombus burden with postinfarct angina, immediate stenting was differed, treated with IC thrombolysis with TNK 10 mg and abciximab 10 mL. Plan was to reassess angio before proceeding with LMCA stenting next day **(Figs. 47A to C)**.

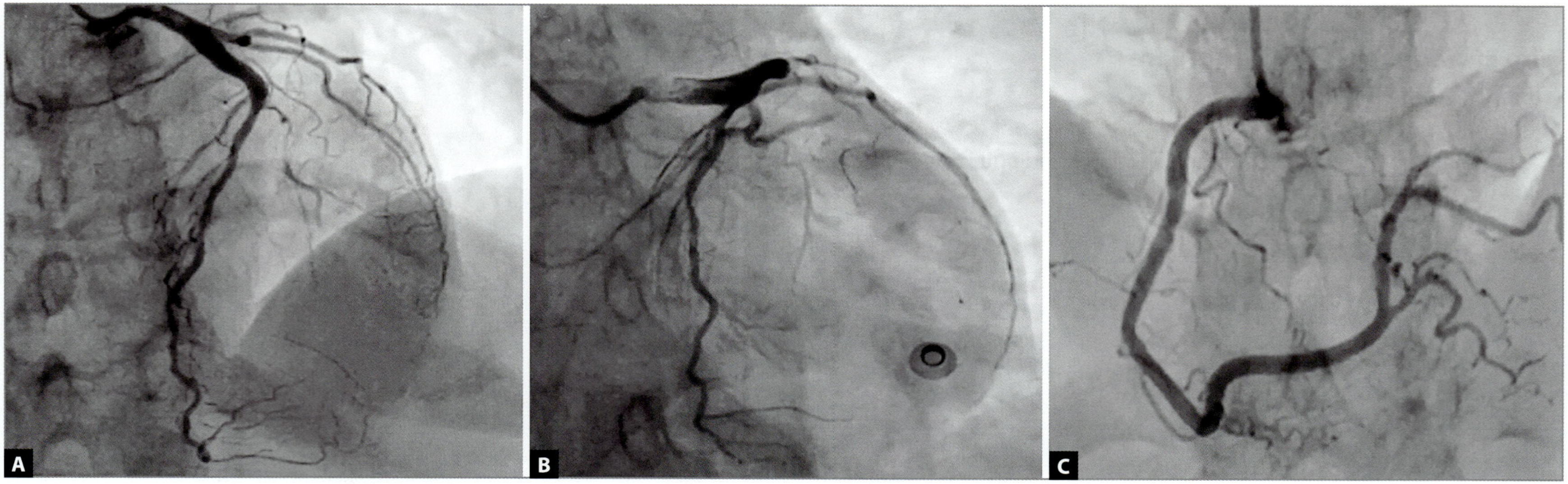

Figs. 47A to C: CAG - thrombus involving ostio-proximal LMCA and total occlusion of diagonal branch.

PROCEDURE

Next day planned for PCI of LMCA with OCT to assess thrombus burden and to evaluate the cause of ACS with STEMI of anterior wall (plaque rupture vs. plaque erosion). LCA engaged with EBU 3.5–7 Fr guiding catheter, angio revealed recanalized thrombus of LMCA with mild narrowing, assessed with OCT **(Figs. 48 to 50)** showed lipid-rich plaque of ostium and proximal LMCA, and totally recanalized LMCA thrombus in D1 ostia at LAD-D1 bifurcation

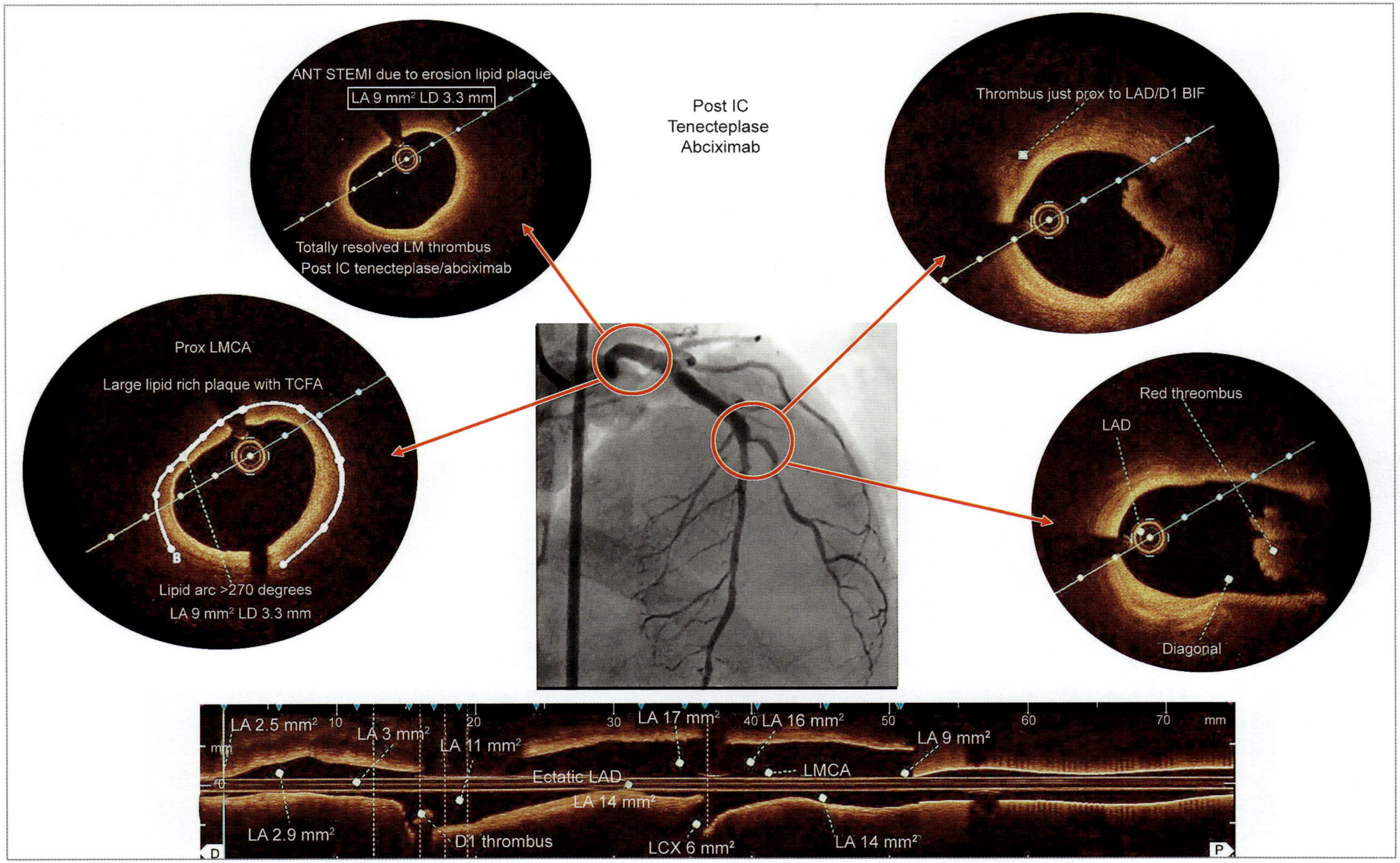

Fig. 48: OCT showing Lipid-rich plaque LMCA with TCFA and Thrombus at LAD-D1 junction.

with markedly improved diagonal flow with radiolucency at the ostium of D1. OCT showed MLA of ostial LMCA was about 9 mm^2, and LAD-D bifurcation showed thrombus in D1 ostium which could be due to embolized thrombus at LMCA site which was treated with additional dose of IC abciximab 10 mL.

On day 3, patient developed abdominal hematoma as Hb dropped to 7.2 g/dL, WBC 15,300. Ultrasound of abdominal hematoma in anterior abdominal wall in right lumbar region and iliac fossa. Two units of PRBC transfused and patient was discharged on 6th day with no complications.

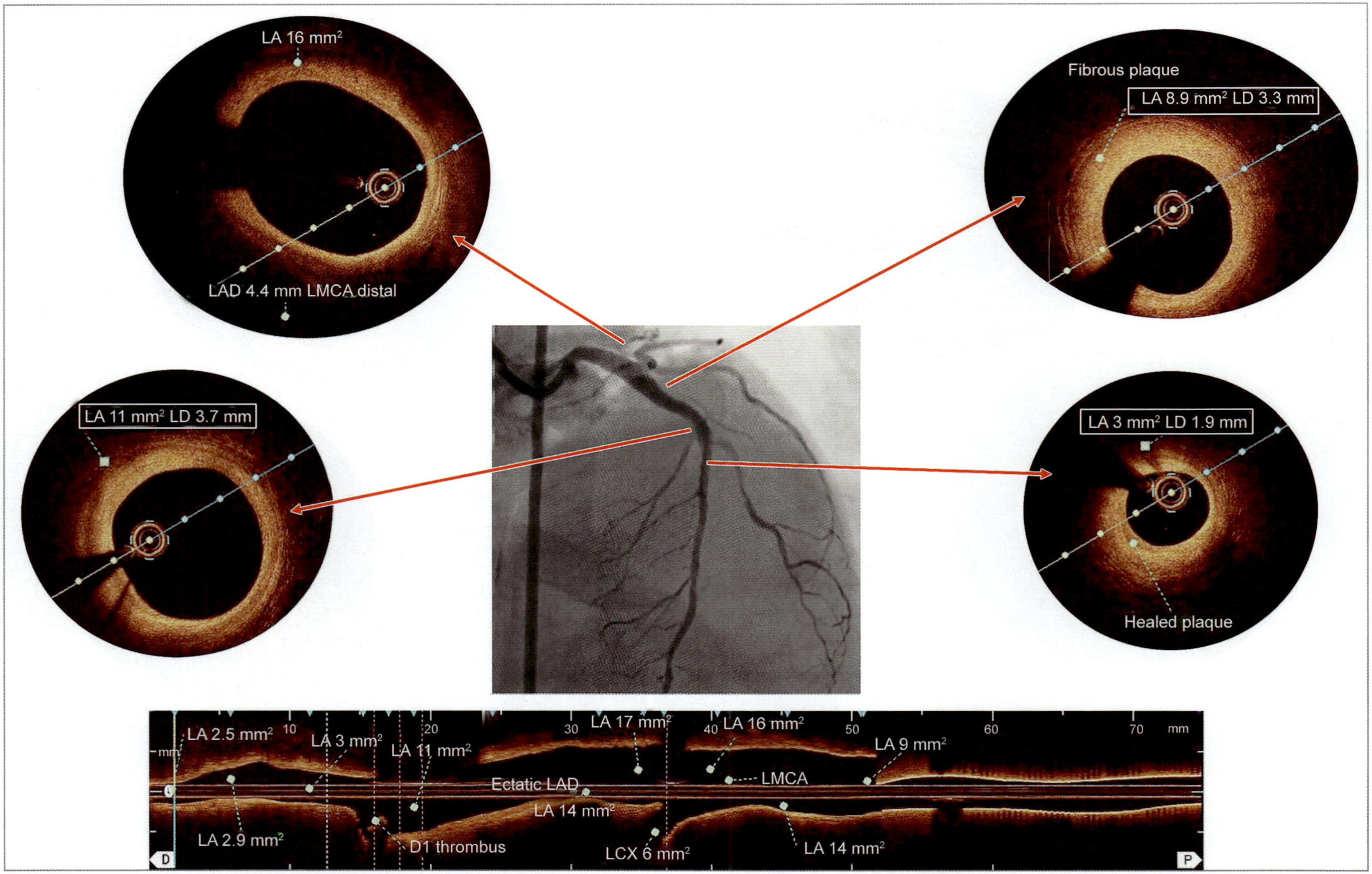

Fig. 49: Well recanalized thrombus of LMCA improved patency of diagonal with TIMI grade III flow of LAD and D1.

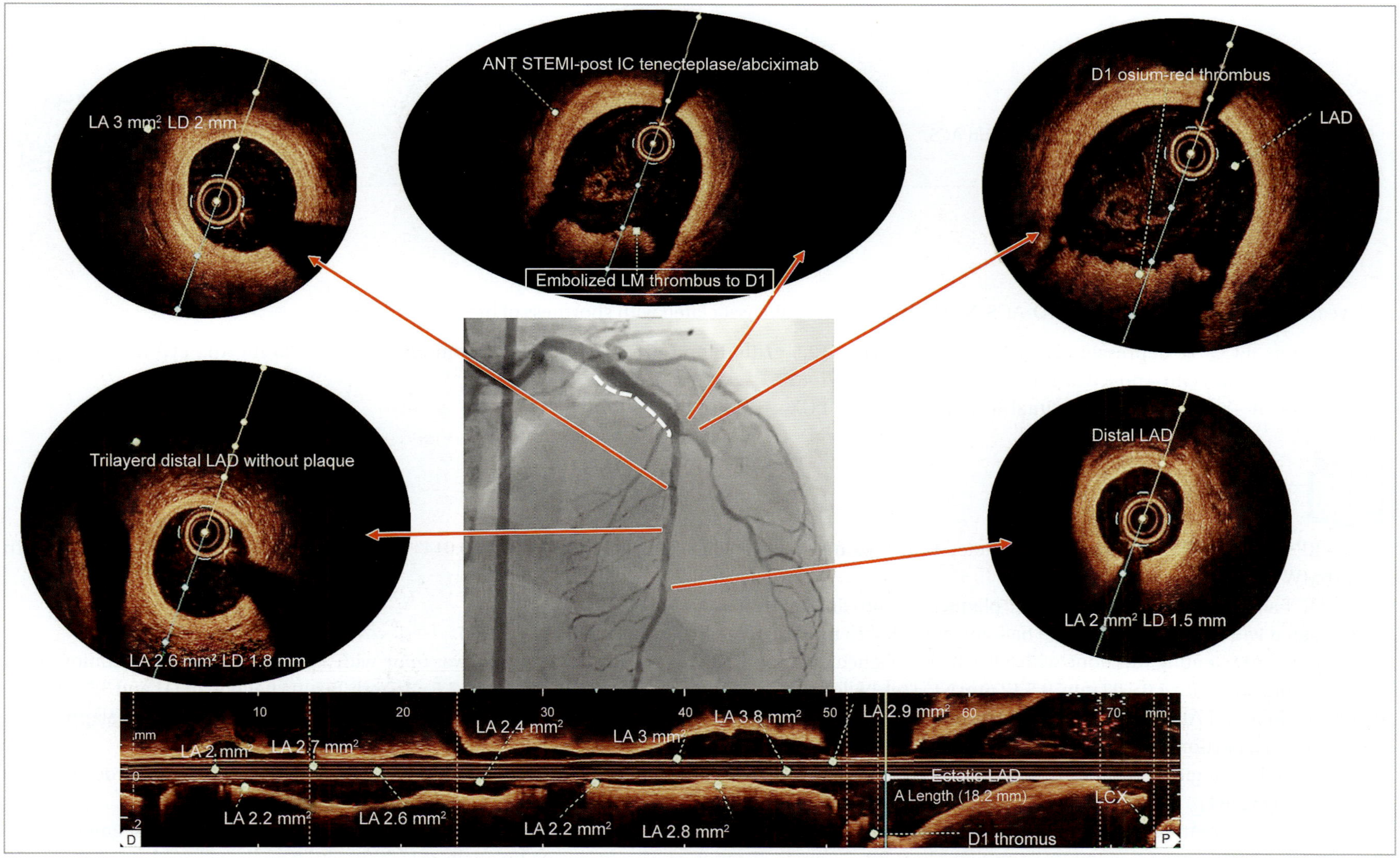

Fig. 50: Visible thrombus with partial recanalization at LMCA and D1 ostium.

CASE 6

Bifurcation PCI-provisional stenting of LAD/D1in ACS.

CLINICAL HISTORY

A 65-year-old male presented with CAD-ACS-NSTEMI and chest pain associated with shortness of breath.

Investigations: ECG-ST depressions in anterior leads, Hb—12.5 g/dL, blood urea—14 mg/dL, serum creatinine—0.83 mg/dL, eGFR—92 mL/min, RBS—86 mg/dL, 2D echo—no RWMA, normal LV function, EF—61%.

CAG-LMCA—normal, LAD—proximal-to-mid 80% lesion, LCX—normal, RCA—normal.

PROCEDURE

Route—RFA, using 7 Fr EBU 3.5 guiding catheter, LAD proximal-to-mid 80% lesion was crossed with 0.014″ × 190 cm Turntrac wire and D1 crossed with 0.014″ BMW wire.

Pre-OCT showed long-segment fibrotic plaque from proximal to mid LAD **(Fig. 51)**.

Predilated with 2.5 × 15 mm Tazuna balloon, and 3.0 × 15 mm AngioSculpt cutting balloon **(Fig. 52)**.

Proximal LAD stenting was done with 3.0 × 48 mm Xience Xpedition stent and distal LAD stenting was done with 3.0 × 12 mm Xience Xpedition stent. Postdilatation done with 4.0 × 08 mm, 3.5 12 mm NC Trek balloons. Kissing balloon dilatation done with 2.5 × 15 mm Tazuna balloon in D1 and 3.5 × 12 mm NC Trek balloon in LAD. Post-OCT showed well-apposed stent struts, no edge dissection, no residual thrombus and 73% expansion with malapposition 39% of proximal portion of the stent which was corrected with 4.5 × 08 mm NC Trek **(Fig. 53)**.

Postprocedure angio view showed well-implanted stents with TIMI-III flow without any dissection. Patient was discharged on 3rd post procedure in a stable status **(Fig. 54)**.

In provisional stenting OCT assessment of bifurcation prior to PCI helps in predicting SB closure. Plaque burden of ostioproximal segment of SB, plaque burden of MV at bifurcation, spiky carina, short BP-CT angle distance <1.75 mm, carina tip angle <51°, bifurcation angle will guide in choosing PS Vs two-stent technique **(Fig. 55)**. Crossing distal strut is very useful before FKB for adequate and optimal scaffolding of stent struts at SB ostium, crossing of proximal strut is associated with malapposition, and improper coverage of SB ostium after FKB **(Fig. 56)**.

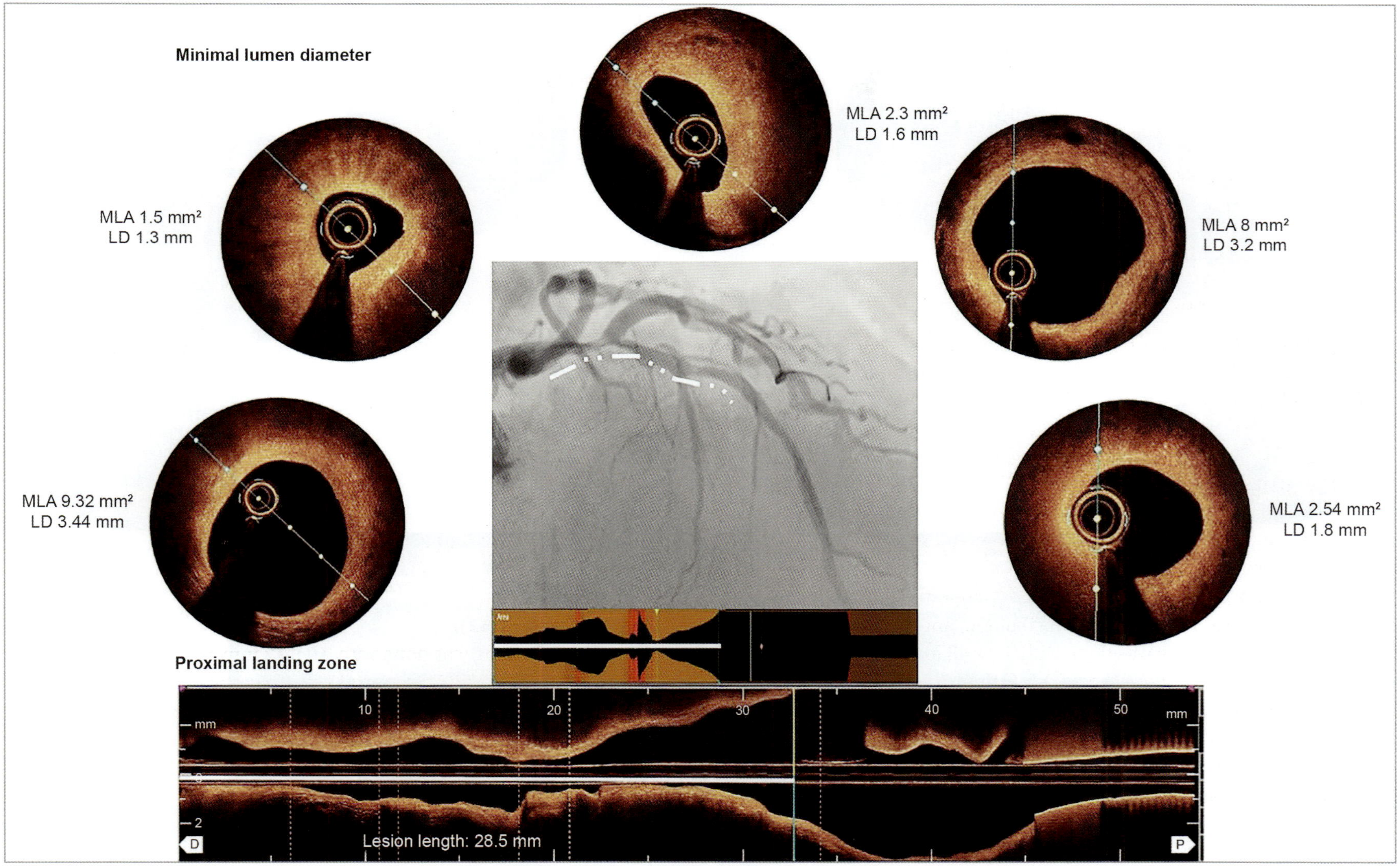

Fig. 51: OCT assessment of MLD of LAD-D1 bifurcation.

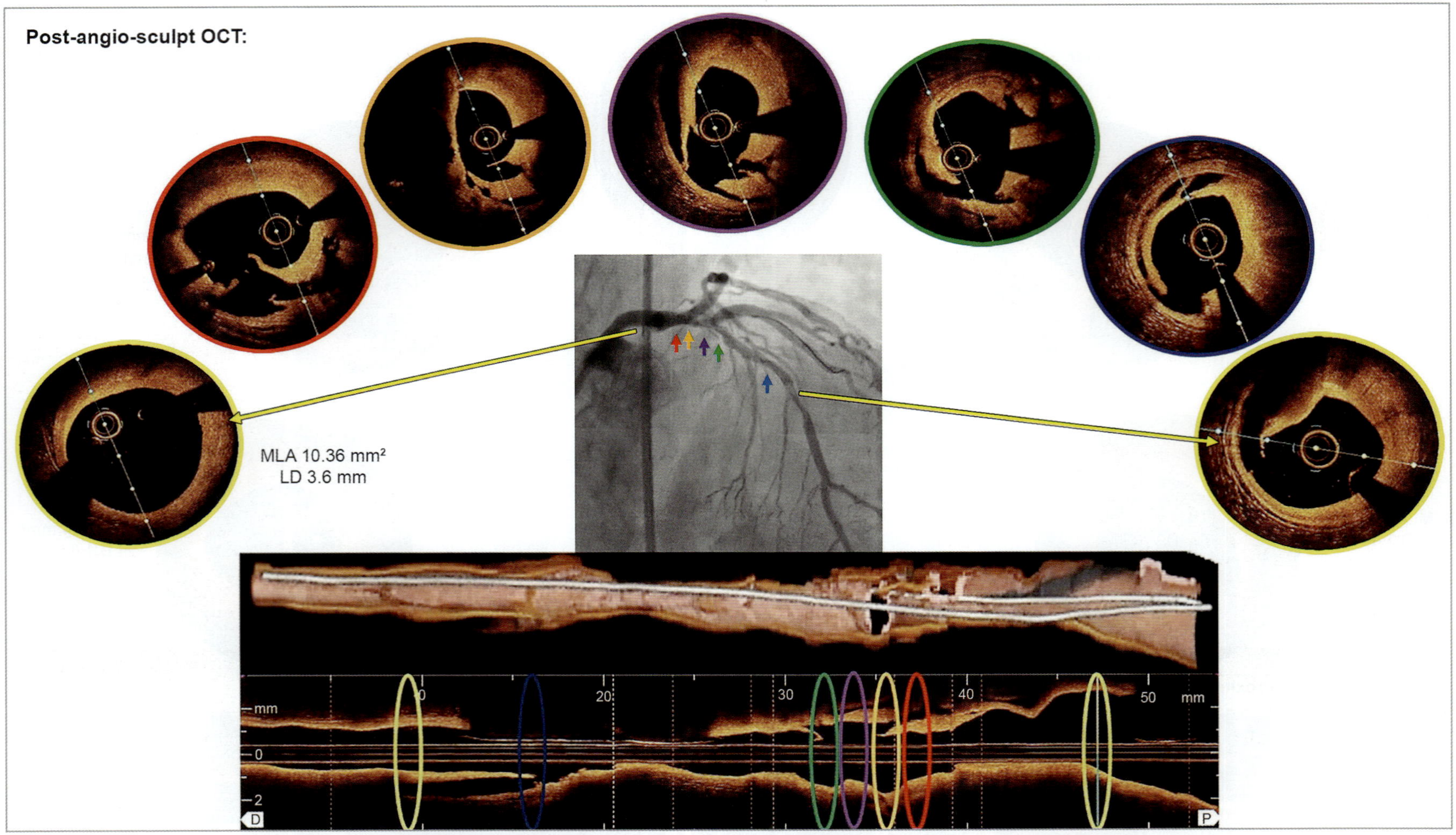

Fig. 52: Post angiosculpt OCT assessment - visible dissections of fibrotic plaque.

CB/SCORING Balloons- Produces Controlled Dissections with less inflammation and better MLA gain, less chances of IMH, and No melon seed effect with thick fibrotic lesions, and very useful for dilating Ostial fibrotic and mild to moderate fibrotic plaques.

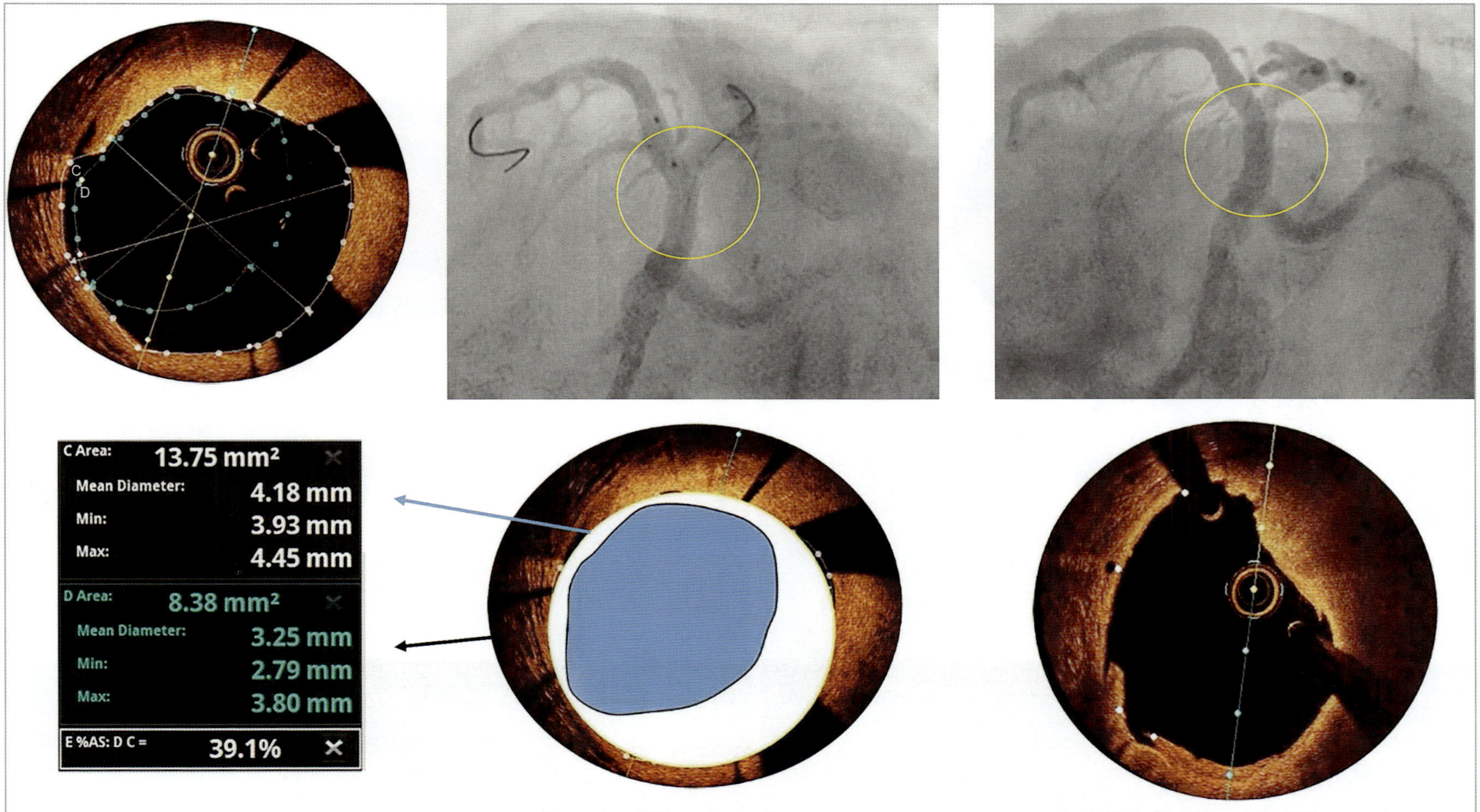

Expansion: 73%; malapposition

Corrected with 4.5 mm NC, 93% expansion

Fig. 53: Poststenting OCT assessment of mal-apposition due to large proximal reference diameter - before and after correction.

Elongation and shortening associated with distorting stent geometry may occur and are known as LSD which is most frequently observed at ostia and bifurcation sites especially in the LMCA.

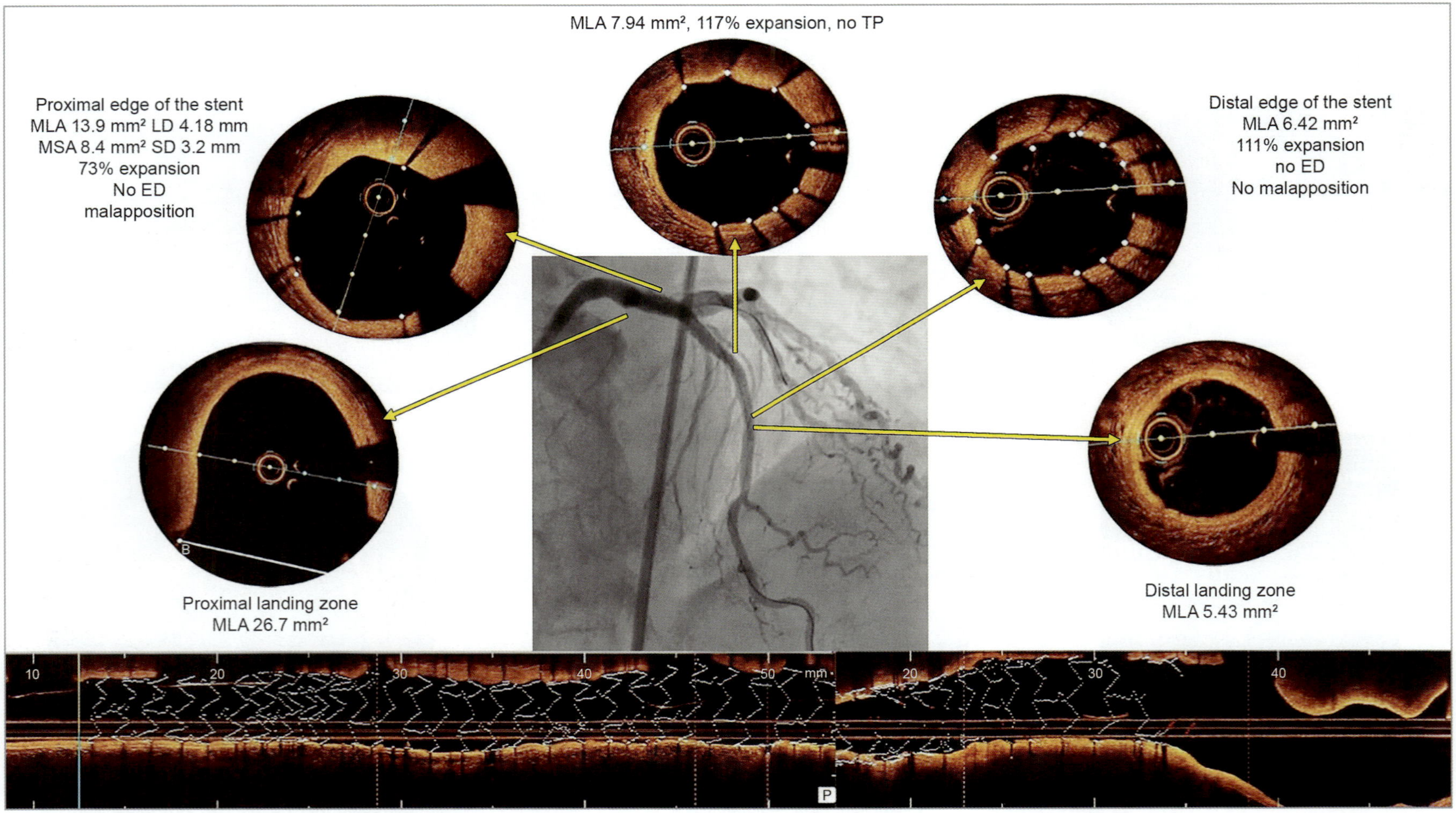

Fig. 54: Poststenting MAX assessment by OCT.

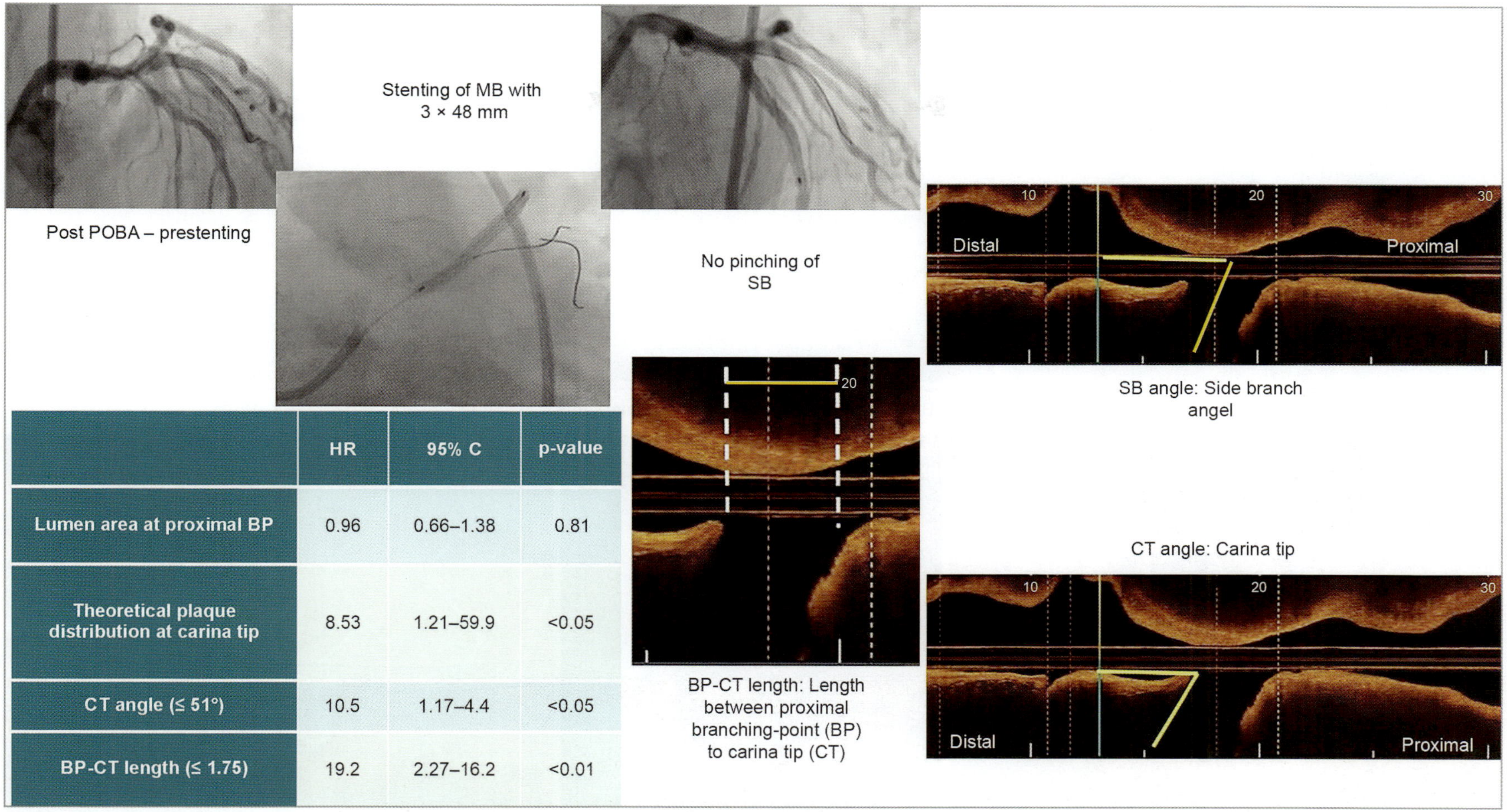

	HR	95% C	p-value
Lumen area at proximal BP	0.96	0.66–1.38	0.81
Theoretical plaque distribution at carina tip	8.53	1.21–59.9	<0.05
CT angle (≤ 51°)	10.5	1.17–4.4	<0.05
BP-CT length (≤ 1.75)	19.2	2.27–16.2	<0.01

Fig. 55: Predictors of SB closure based on OCT imaging.

Recognize a Difficult Bifurcation?

- Angle between MB and sideis not favorable (>90 degrees)
- Complex lesions within the bifurcation like—long lesions, calcification, aneurysm
- Tortuosity or lesion before the bifurcation.

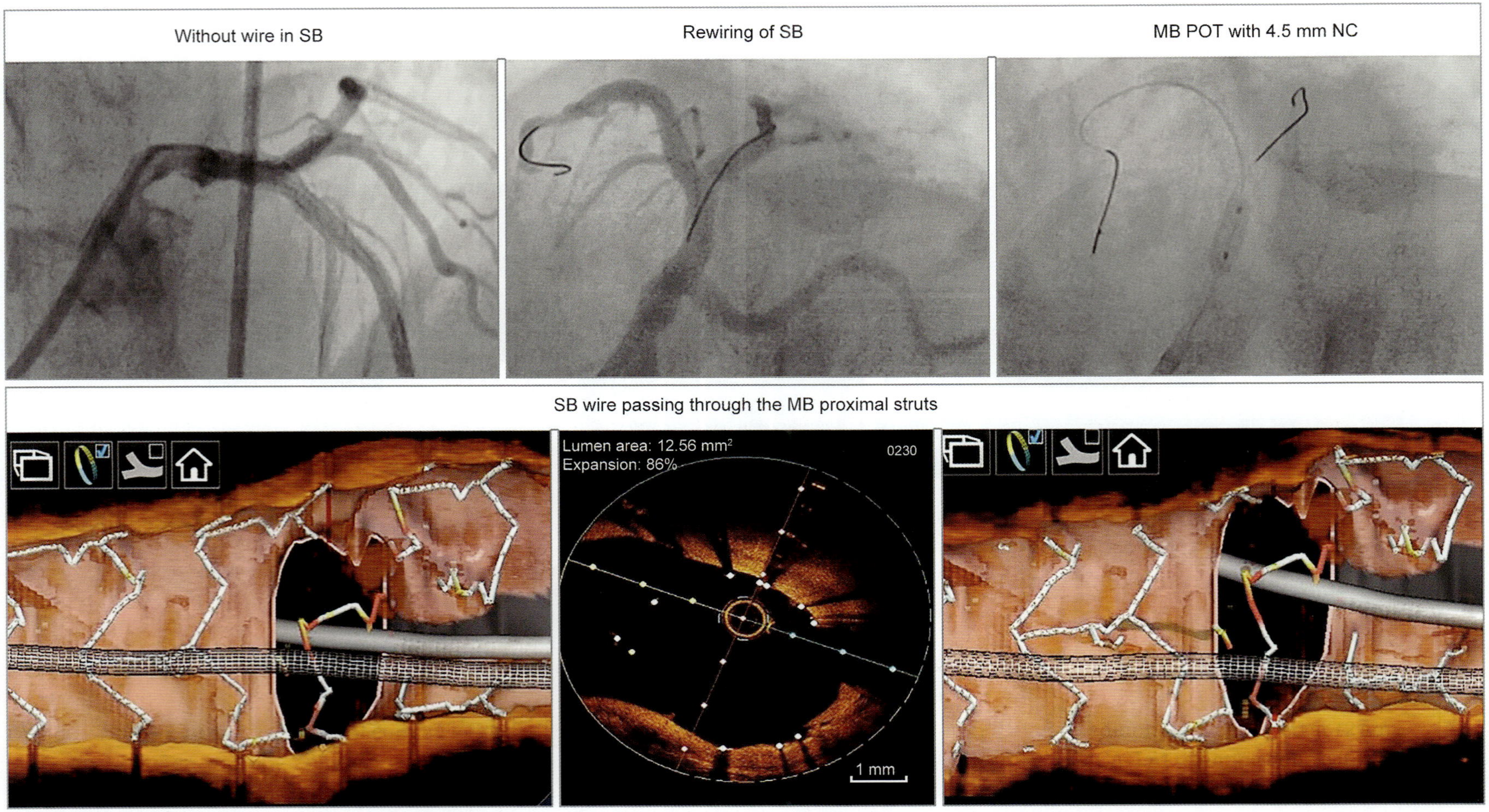

Fig. 56: 3D bifurcation OCT mode showing guidewire crossing through proximal strut.

CASE 7

OCT assessment of LMCA provisional stenting, LAD/D1 DK-crush stenting.

CLINICAL HISTORY

A 61-year-old male known hypertensive, diabetic presented with NSTEMI of inferior wall, chest pain associated with shortness of breath, with past history of PCI of RCA in 2015. ECG—inferior leads ST-depression.

Investigations: RBS—92 mg/dL, blood urea—17 mg/dL, serum creatinine—0.76 mg/dL, eGFR—99. 2D echo—hypokinetic inferior wall, concentric LVH, mild LV systolic dysfunction, EF—51%. CAG-LMCA—mild lesion, LAD—ostial to mid long segment 70-80% lesion, D1—proximal 80% lesion, LCX—normal, RCA—normal.

PROCEDURE

Route—RFA, using 7 Fr EBU 3.5 guiding catheter, LAD was wired with 0.014″ Sion blue wire and 0.014″ Runthrough wire was placed in D1. Preprocedure OCT showed long-segment fibrotic lesion extending from distal LMCA to mid LAD, thick fibrotic long-segment lesion after LAD and D1 bifurcation involving D1 origin, LAD LD—2 × 1.8 mm, D1 LD—1.8 × 1.7 mm, mid LAD tightest portion LD 12 × 1.1 mm fibrolipid plaque **(Fig. 57)**.

LAD and D1 predilated with 2.5 × 12 mm Tazuna balloon, D1 stenting was done with 2.25 × 22 mm Orsiro stent. Stent struts projecting in LAD was crushed with 3.0 × 12 mm NC balloon. D1 was recrossed through distal strut. OCT was done to assess proximal versus distal strut crossing, luminal position of guidewire, and adequately crushed portion of the SB stent in LAD, which confirmed no abluminal position, and crushed portion of the SB stent in LAD (3.0 mm) **(Fig. 58)**.

D1 ostial stent struts opened with 2.0 × 10 mm Tazuna balloon. First kissing balloon dilatation done with 2.5 × 10 mm Tazuan balloon placed in D1 and 3.0 × 12 mm NC Trek balloon placed in LAD. LMCA to LAD stenting was done with 3.0 × 40 mm Orsiro stent. POT of LM was done with 4.0 × 08 mm NC Apollo balloon and LAD post dilated done with 3.0 × 12 mm NC Trek balloon. D1 wire recrossed and struts opened with 2.0 × 10 mm Tazuna balloon. Postprocedure OCT showed well-apposed stent struts and SB wire in luminal position and no edge dissection **(Fig. 58)**. Final kissing balloon dilatation was done with 2.5 10 mm Tazuan balloon in D1 and 3.5 × 20 mm NC Pantera Leo balloon in LAD. Re-POT was done with 4.0 × 08 mm NC Apollo balloon. Postprocedure angio views showed well-implanted stents with TIMI-III flow without any dissection. Patient was discharged on third post procedure in a stable status.

Post-OCT assessment—no edge dissection, no underexpansion, no malapposition, no tissue prolapses, expansion >100% **(Fig. 59)**.

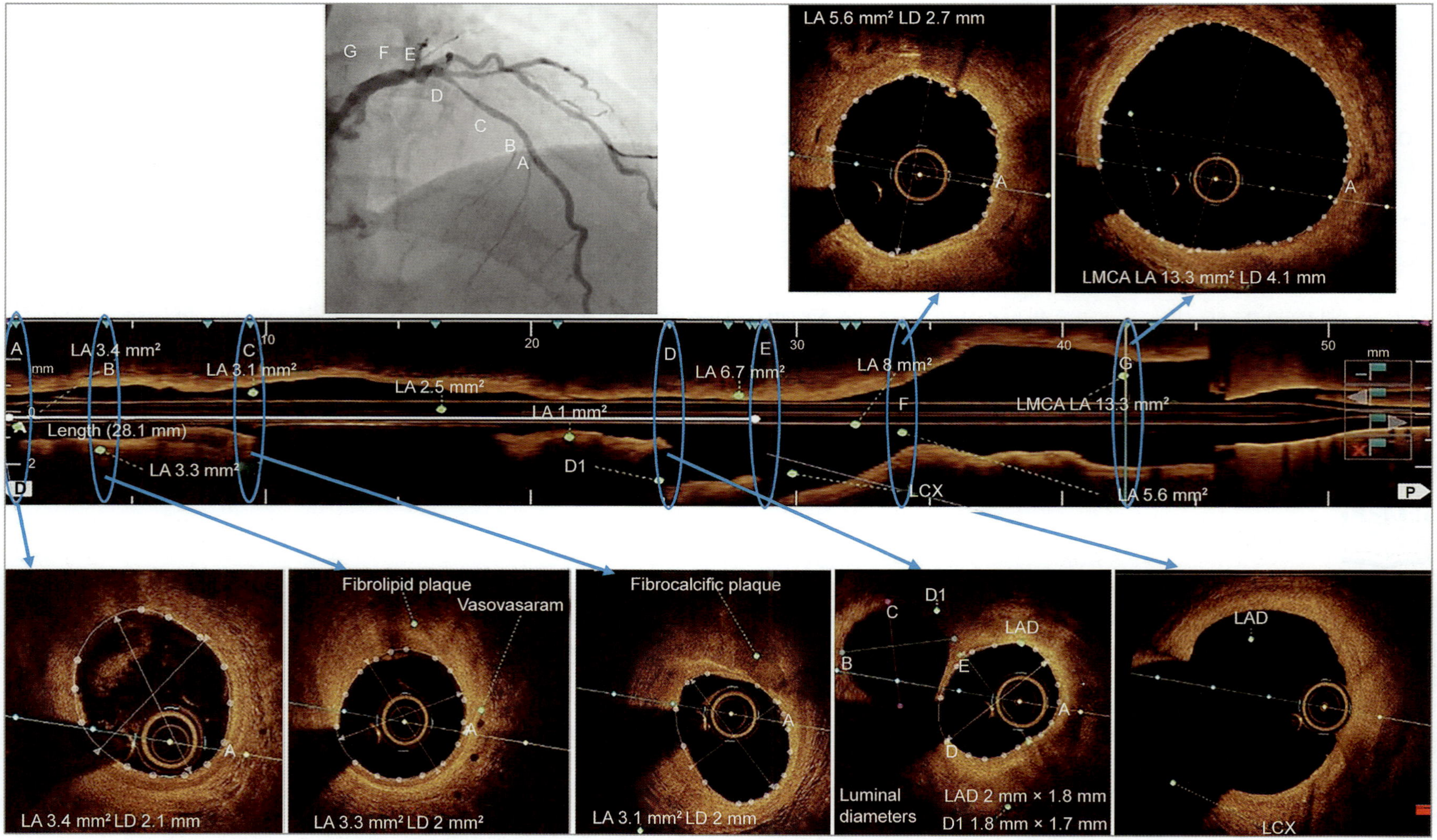

Fig. 57: Prestenting MLD assessment of LM, LAD-D1 bifurcation.

Features of Stent to be Considered During PCI

- Architecture
- Strut thickness
- Polymer
- Expansion.

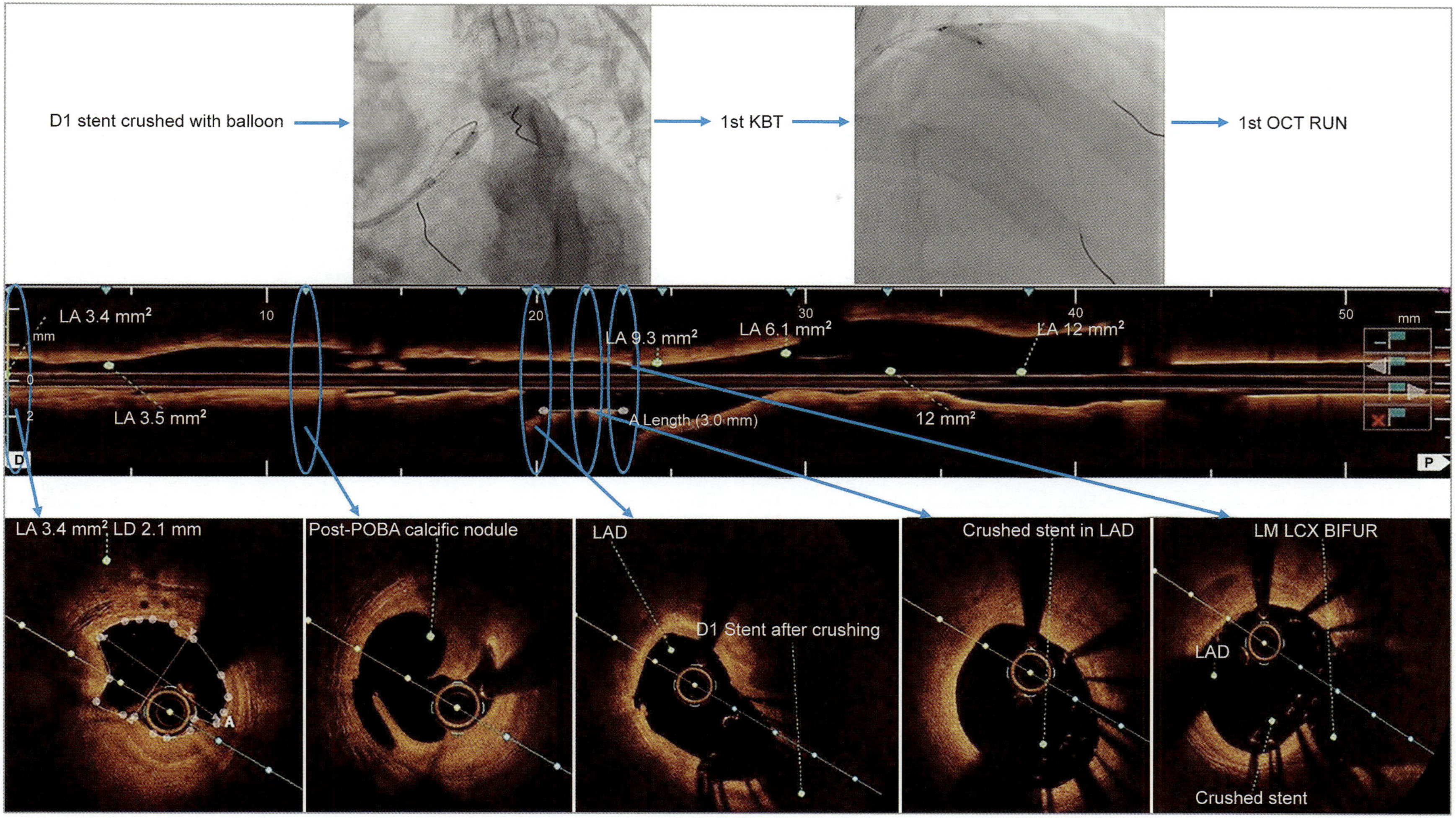

Fig. 58: Post D1 stent crushing - assessment of crushed segment length and adequacy of crushing in LAD.

Repeating POT at the end of the DK crush helps to maintain circular geometry through the bifurcation and reduce SB ostium strut obstruction and strut.

Unlike the first POT, it may be best to keep the distal balloon marker for the re-POT just proximal to the carina to avoid disruption of the bifurcation stent architecture.

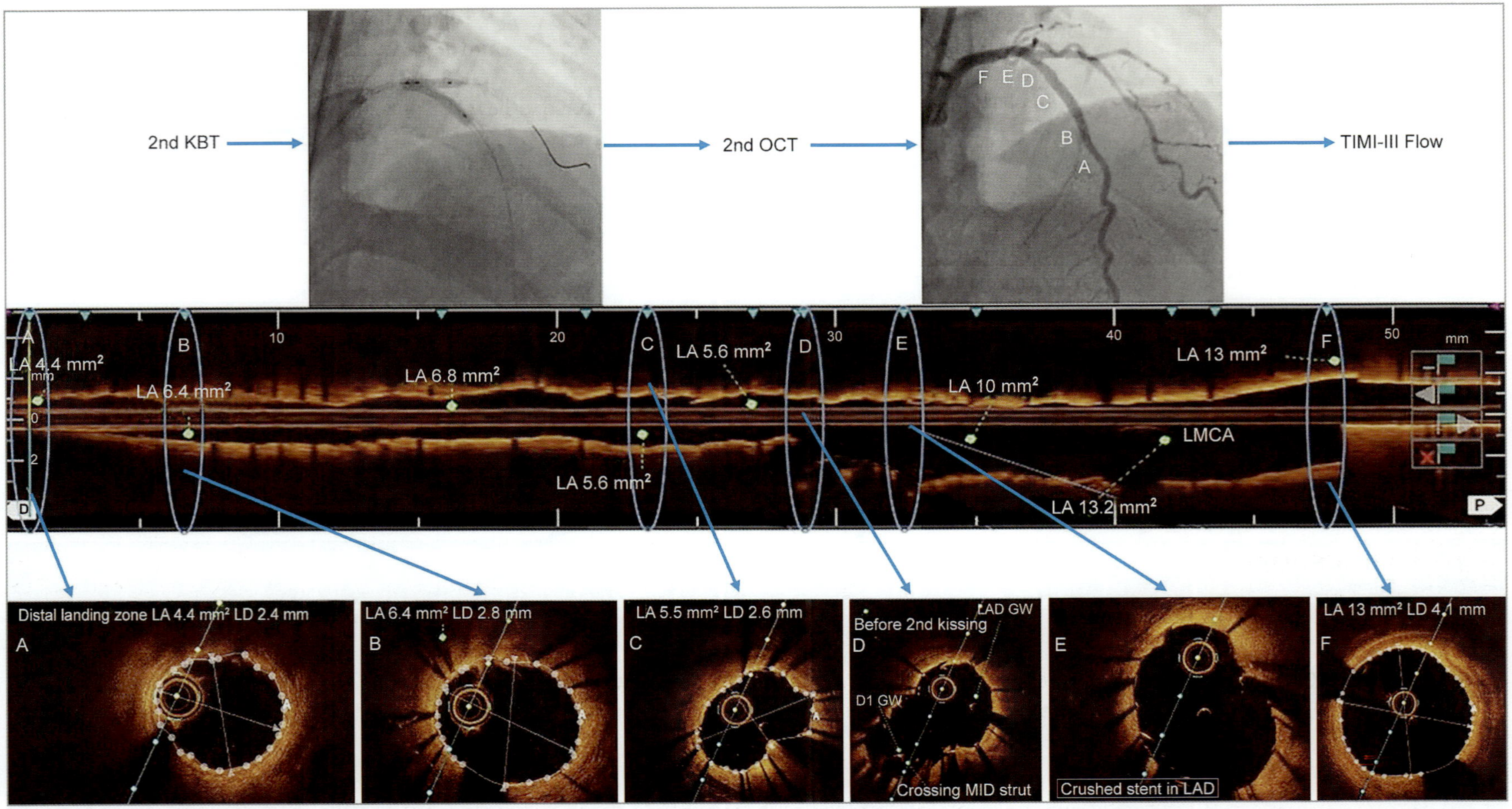

Fig. 59: Poststent MAX assessment by OCT.

SB inflation without POT can distort MB stent.

CASE 8

Provisional stenting of LMCA to LAD.

CLINICAL HISTORY

A 63-year-old male, known hypertensive and diabetic, presented with ACS—USA.

Investigations: ECG—normal, 2D echo—no RWMA, normal LV function, EF—60%. TMT—positive for inducible ischemia. Hb—14.2 g/dL, serum creatinine—1 mg/dL, blood urea—33 mg/dL.

CAG-LMCA—distal 40% lesion, LAD—ostioproximal 70% lesion, LCX—proximal 50% lesion, RCA—mild disease.

Fractional flow reserve—LMCA to LAD positive, LMCA to LCX negative.

PROCEDURE

Right femoral artery—route, 7 Fr EBU 3.5 guiding catheter, LAD lesion was crossed with 0.014″ Sion blue wire, and LCX was crossed with 0.014″ Runthrough wire.

Preprocedure OCT showed tight long-segment lesion from LMCA to proximal LAD **(Figs. 60 and 61)**.

Predilated with 2.5 × 10 mm Tazuna balloon, and LMCA to proximal LAD stenting done with 3.0 × 38 mm Resolute Onyx stent. Postdilatation of LAD with 3.5 × 122 mm NC Apollo and POT of LMCA with 4.5 × 08 mm NC Pantera Leo balloons.

Postprocedure OCT showed fibrotic plaque at edge of stent with area of 3.0 mm **(Fig. 62)**.

Mid LAD stenting done with 3.0 × 12 mm Resolute Onyx stent. Postprocedure angio revealed there was a gap between two stents with dissection which was covered with 3.0 × 08 mm Resolute Onyx stent overlapping proximal and distal stents **(Fig. 63)**.

Postprocedure angio view showed well-implanted stents with TIMI-III flow without any dissection. Patient was discharged on third post procedure in a stable status.

Prior to distal LM bifurcation PCI, FFR evaluation of LAD and LCX were done, FFR study of LCX was negative, and LAD was positive. OCT evaluation of LMCA showed distal LM area was 4.4 mm^2 with significant plaque burden, and luminal area of tightest LAD was 1.8 mm^2. In view of negative LCX FFR study, provisional stenting of LMCA to LAD was performed covering entire diseased segment.

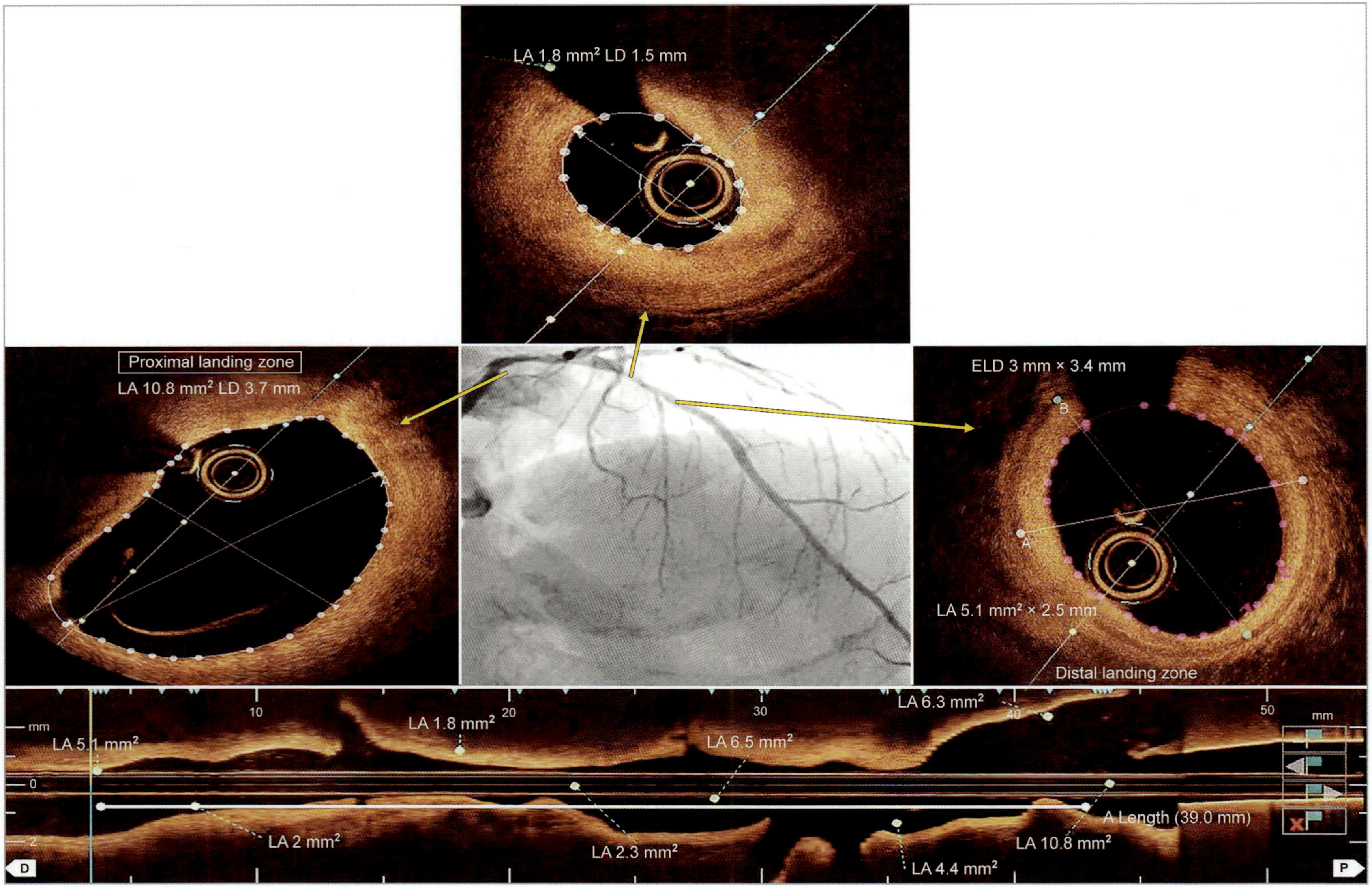

Fig. 60: MLD assessment by OCT of LM-LAD.

LSD is more often missed on angiography images, can be detected with stent boost or IVUS or OCT.

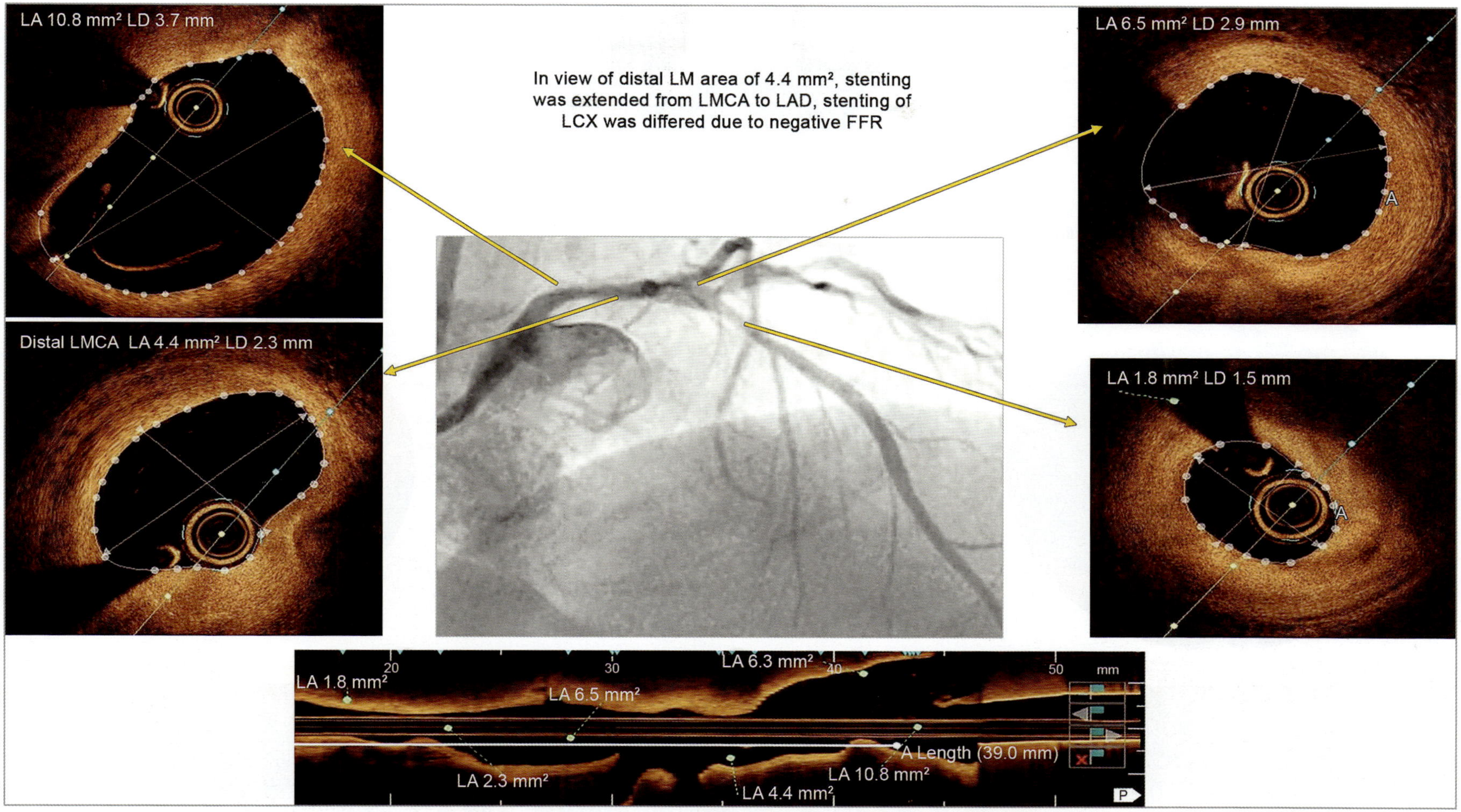

Fig. 61: Provisional stenting of LM-LAD based upon OCT LMCA area.

Bifurcation lesions with a fibrotic plaque at the SB ostium may require adequate plaque modification with cutting balloon (Cutting balloon/Angio sculpt/Score-flex) to achieve adequate expansion of stent.

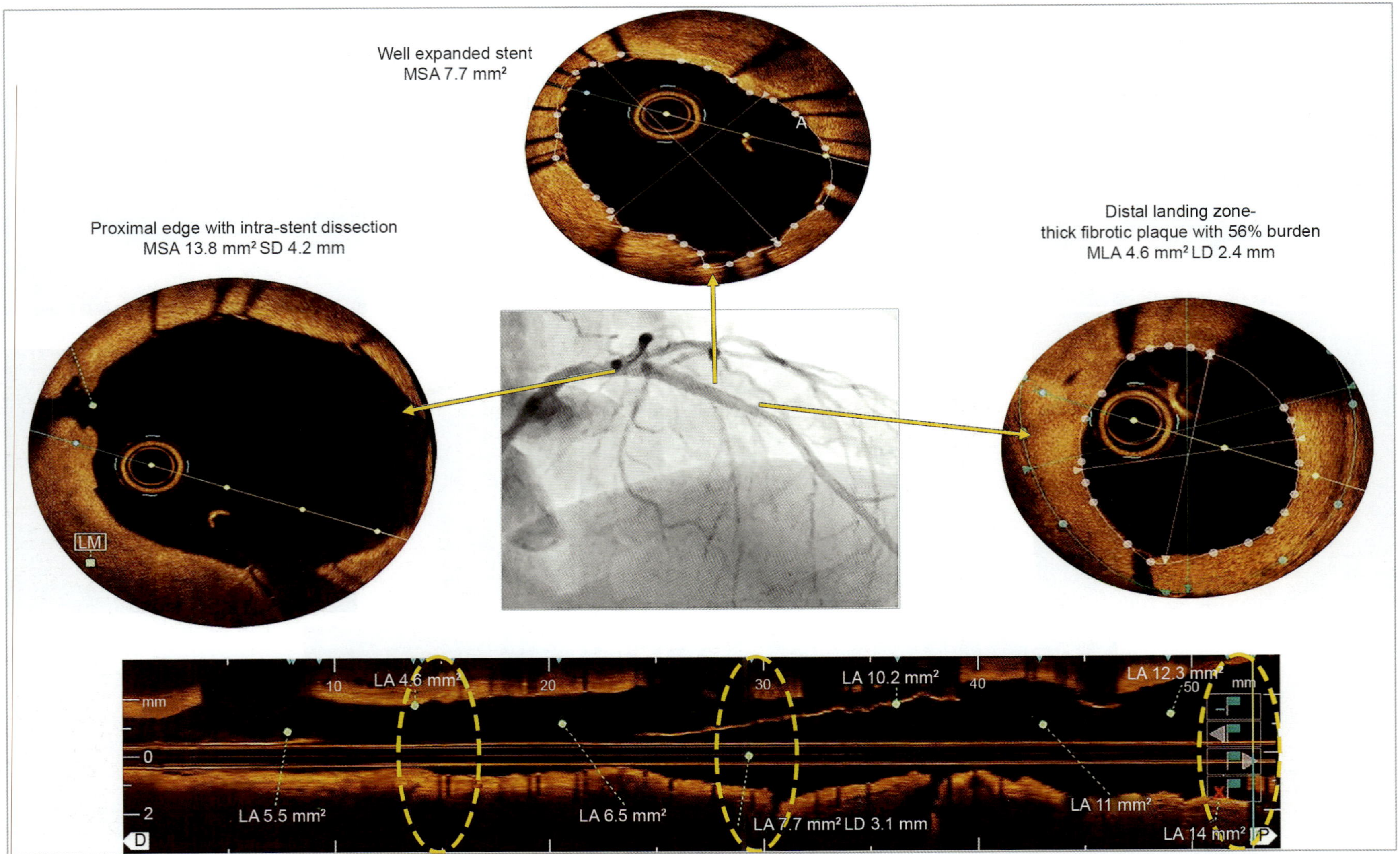

Fig. 62: Poststent MAX assessment of LM-LAD by OCT showing more plaque burden in the distal landing zone requiring additional stenting.

Adequate lesion preparation can be assessed by following criteria prior to DEB delivery: (1) a fully inflated balloon of the correct size for the vessel; (2) less than 30% residual stenosis; (3) TIMI (Thrombolysis in Myocardial Infarction) flow grade 3; and (4) the absence of a flow-limiting dissection.

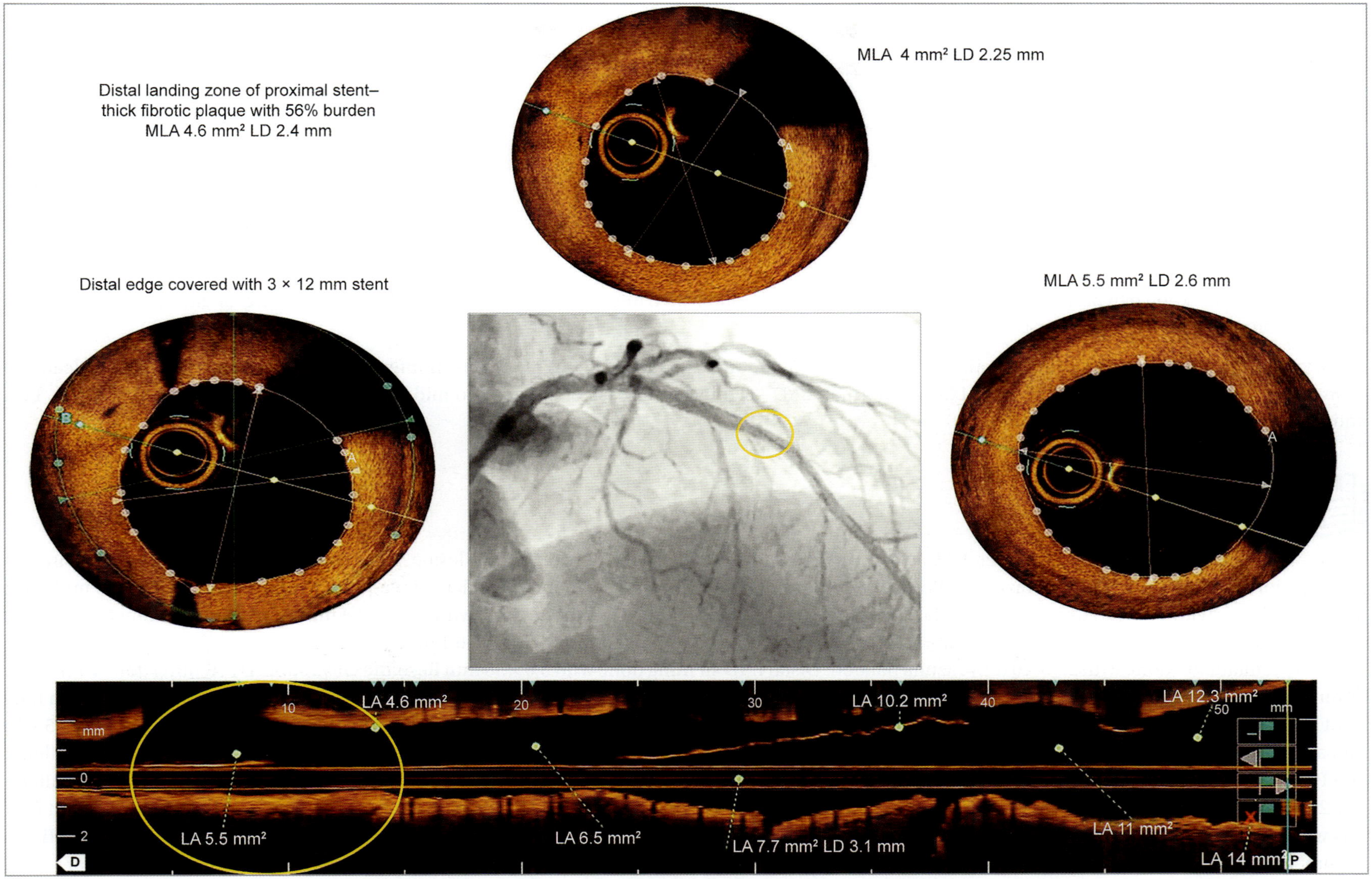

Fig. 63: Detection of plaque burden at distal landing zone.

In diabetics, CAD is more complex, diffuse, and long lesions in smaller calibre vessels with reduced coronary vasodilator reserve, and DCBs may be a favourable alternative to DES.

CASE 9

OCT-guided DK-crush stenting of LAD/D1.

CLINICAL HISTORY

A 55-year-old male, known hypertensive and diabetic, presented with established inferior and posterolateral MI with postinfarct angina. Past history of PCI of LCX (Promus Element 3.5 × 32 mm).

Investigations: Hb—10.8 g/dL, serum creatinine—1.2 mg/dL, blood urea—33 mg/dL. ECG-Q waves in inferior leads with R/S ratio >1 in V1 lead. 2D echo—mild LV dysfunction, EF—52%. CAG-LMCA—normal, LAD—significant disease of proximal to mid LAD with bifurcation lesion of LAD/D1, LCX and RCA—normal.

PROCEDURE

Route—RFA, 7 Fr EBU 3.5 guiding catheter, LAD lesion was crossed with 0.014″ BMW wire and D1 lesion was crossed with 0.014″ Powerturn wire. D1 predilatation done with 1.5 × 10 mm Tazuna balloon. Presenting OCT showed long-segment fibrocalcified plaque extending from proximal to mid LAD, lipid-rich plaque with TCFA >3 quadrants, and cholesterol crystals (high risk of slow flow or no flow) with MLA—3.4 mm^2, and luminal diameter (1.5 mm) of LAD at septal branch origin with deep calcium, LAD proximal to LAD—D1 bifurcation with MLA—6.1 mm^2 **(Fig. 64)**.

LAD predilatation done with 2.0 × 10 mm Tazuna balloon. Distal LAD stenting done with 3.0 × 38 mm Resolute Onyx stent. D1 stenting done with 2.25 × 08 mm Resolute Onyx stent. First kissing balloon dilatation done with stent balloon 2.25 × 18 mm in D1 and 3.0 × 38 mm in LAD. D1 stent crushed with LAD stent balloon. D1 wire removed and recrossed through stent struts and dilated with 1.5 × 10 mm and 2.0 × 10 mm Tazuna balloons. D1 dilated with 1.5 × 10 mm and 2.0 × 10 mm Tazuna balloon. Proximal LAD stenting done with 3.5 × 26 mm Resolute Onyx stent. Postdilated with 3.0 × 12 mm NC Trek balloon, and POT was performed with 4.0 × 08 mm NC Trek balloon. Wire in D1 removed and recrossed, SB stent struts dilated with 1.5 × 10 mm Tazuna balloon and 2.0 × 10 mm Tazuna balloon. Poststenting OCT showed 21% malapposition in proximal LAD 21% with MLA—13.5 mm^2, MSD—10.6 mm. Second POT was with 4.5 × 08 mm NC Trek balloon. FKB of LAD with 3.5 × 15 mm NC trek balloon, and D1 with 2.5 × 10 mm Tazuna balloon, post KBT LAD-MLA—10 mm^2 and D1-MLA—6.0 mm^2, longitudinal compression of proximal portion of stent, length of stent proximal to bifurcation—9.4 mm, POT of LMCA done with 4.5 mm and 5 mm NC balloon. Third POT was done with 5.0 × 08 mm NC Trek balloon. Poststenting OCT was done which showed well-apposed stent struts, no residual stenosis and no thrombosis, proximal edge compression of stent **(Fig. 65)**, Crushed D1 stent length 2.8 mm in LAD **(Fig. 66)**, LSD of proximal edge of the stent post dilated with 5 mm NC **(Fig. 67)**. Postprocedure angio view showed well-implanted stents with TIMI-III flow without any dissection. Patient was discharged on third post procedure in a stable status.

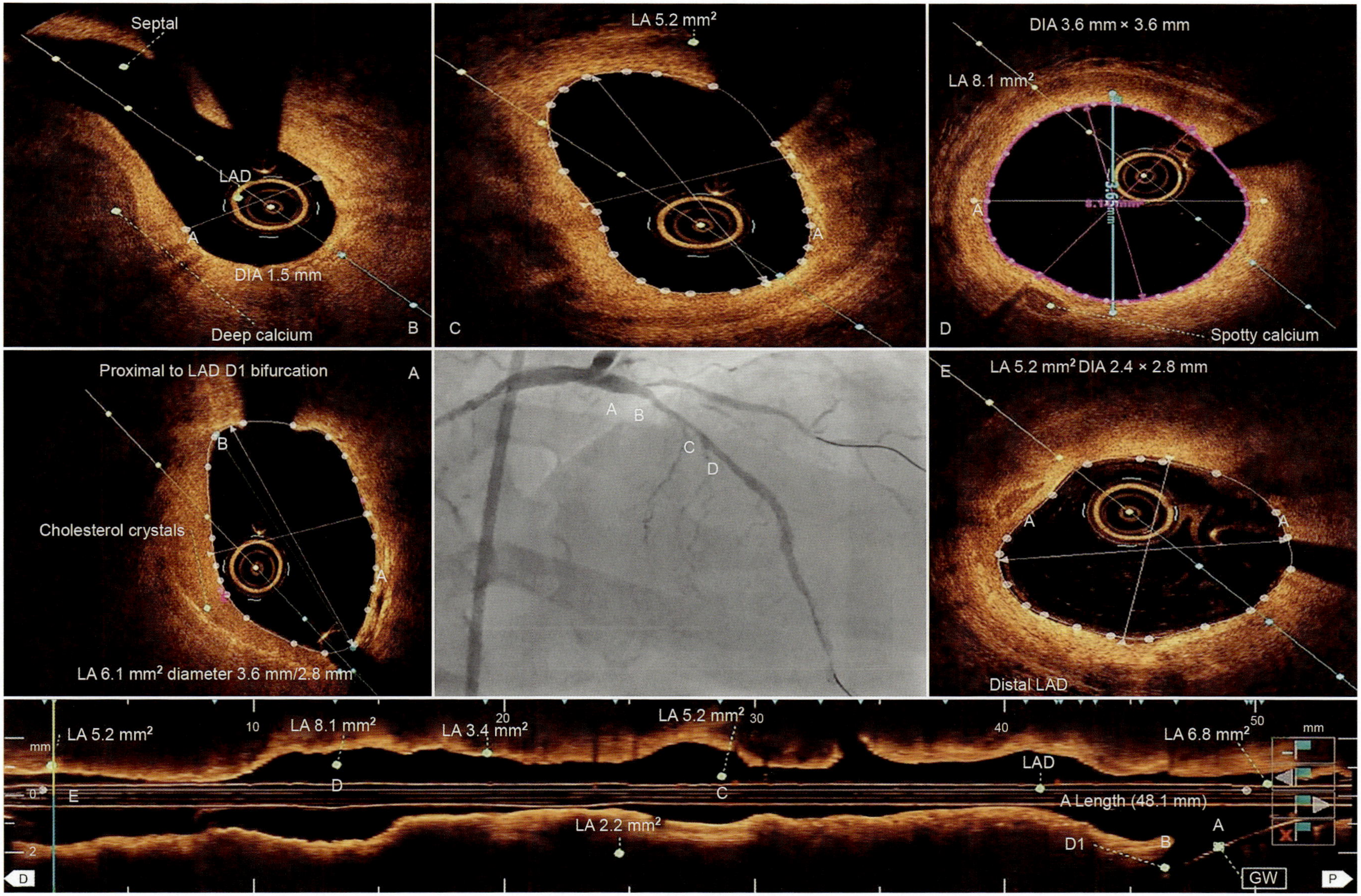

Fig. 64: MLD assessment of LAD-D1 by OCT.

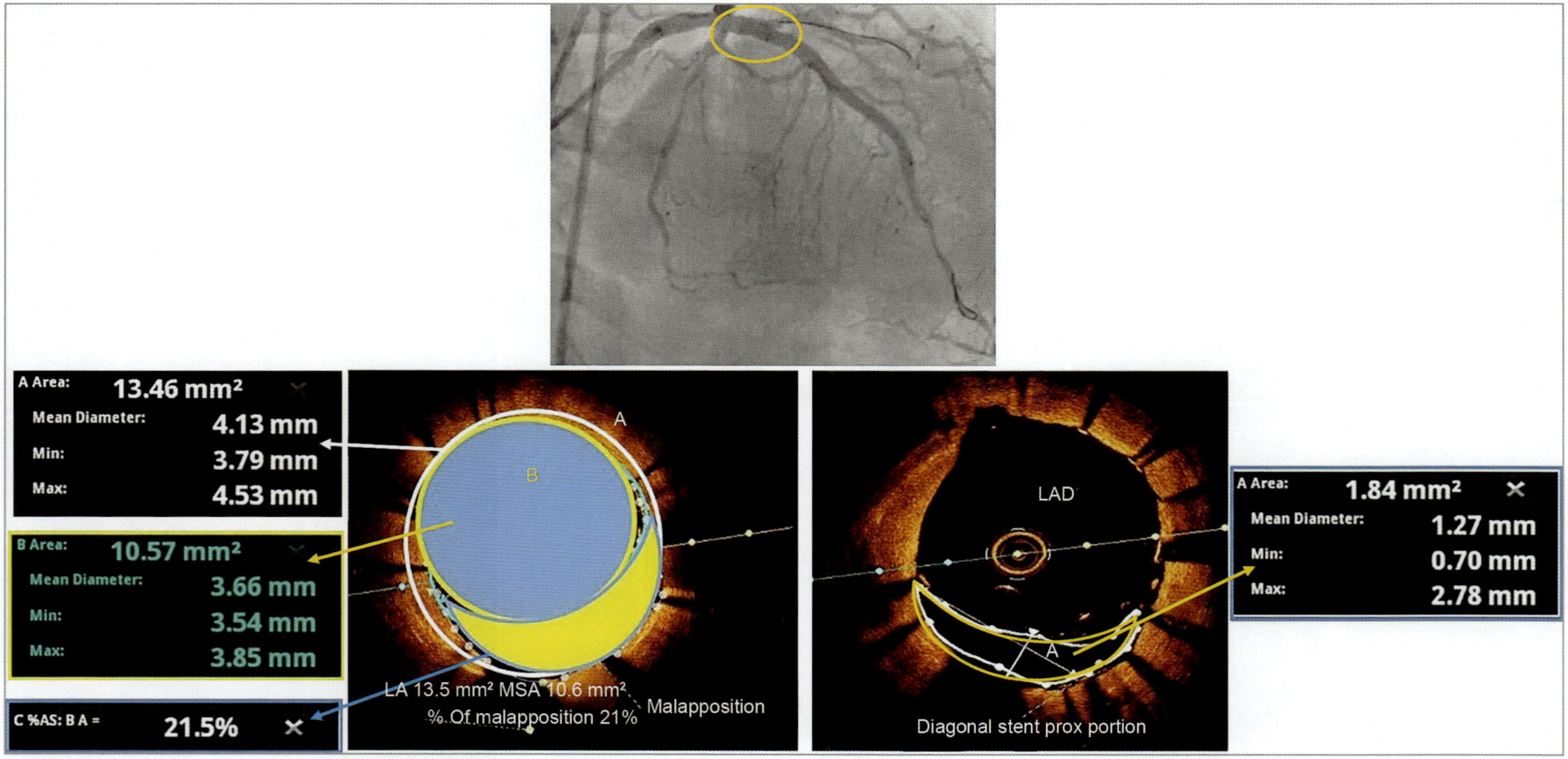

Fig. 65: MAX assessment by OCT - Mal-apposition at proximal edge corrected with upsized balloon.

Acute stent deformation or LSD: IVUS identified acute stent deformation in 1.1%. About half of the stent deformations were located in the LMCA, and 8.3% of 96 LMCA-stented lesions had stent deformation resulting in multiple overlapping strut layers within a single stent, often accompanied by stent shortening. In EXCEL, acute LMCA stent deformation was observed in 33 patients (6.6%) and was most commonly located at the LMCA ostium [27/33 (81.8%)], although struts protruding into the aorta was not a risk factor **(Fig. 68)**.

Any stent can undergo LSD, either lengthening or shortening, LM stent particularly at ostial site more often prone for LSD due to guide catheter manipulations while engaging, deep intubation of guide catheter hitting the proximal edge of the stent while pulling improperly deflated with large NC balloon, jailed wires, imaging catheters. LSD at ostial site of LM is associated with increased MACE rate due to its crucial position, which may result in ISR, stent thrombosis of LM compromising blood supply to major myocardial territory.

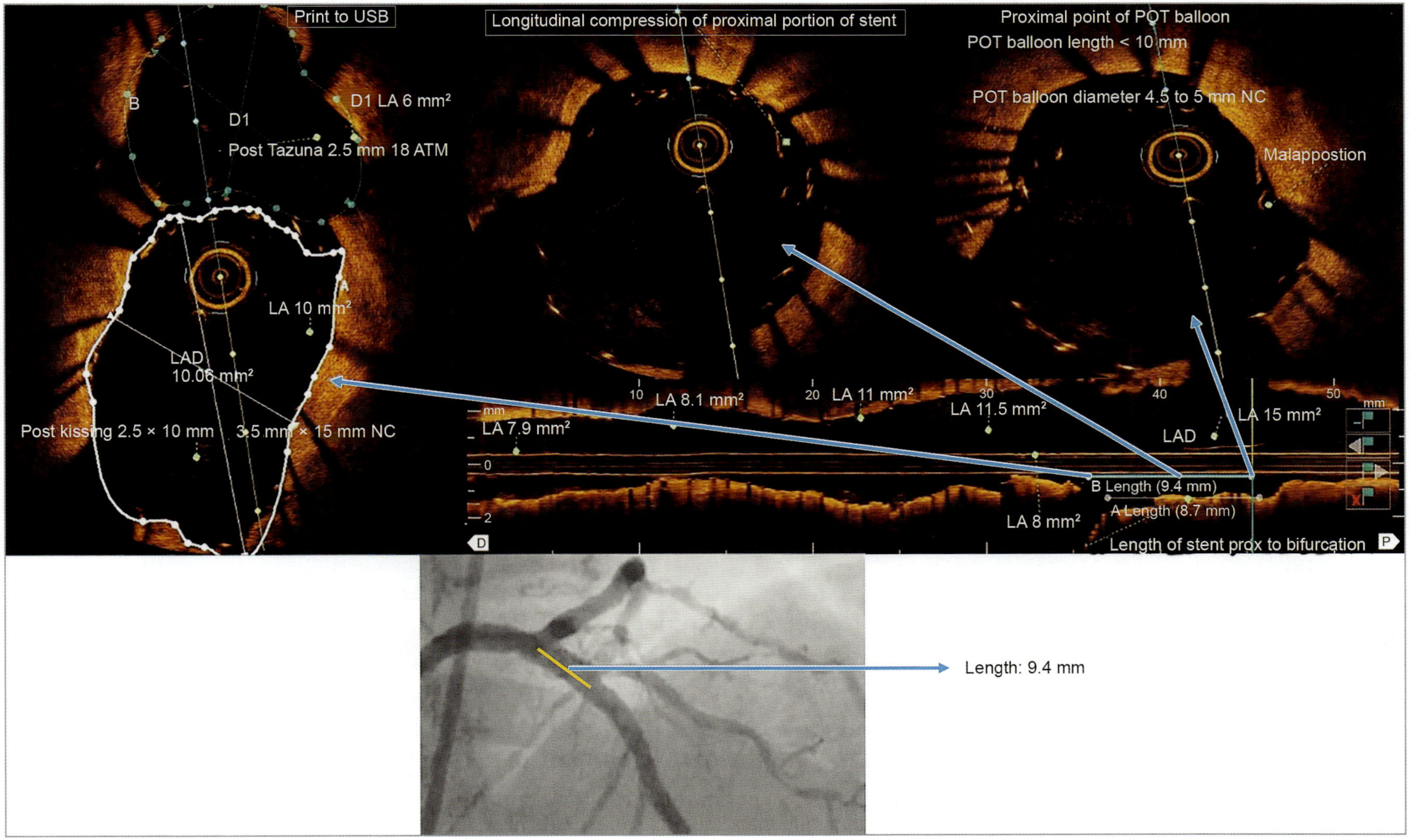

Fig. 66: Proximal edge compression of stent - LSD assessment by OCT.

LSD at LM produces worst outcomes due to its vast area of supply, and it is usually due to deep seating of guide hitting the proximal edge of the stent.

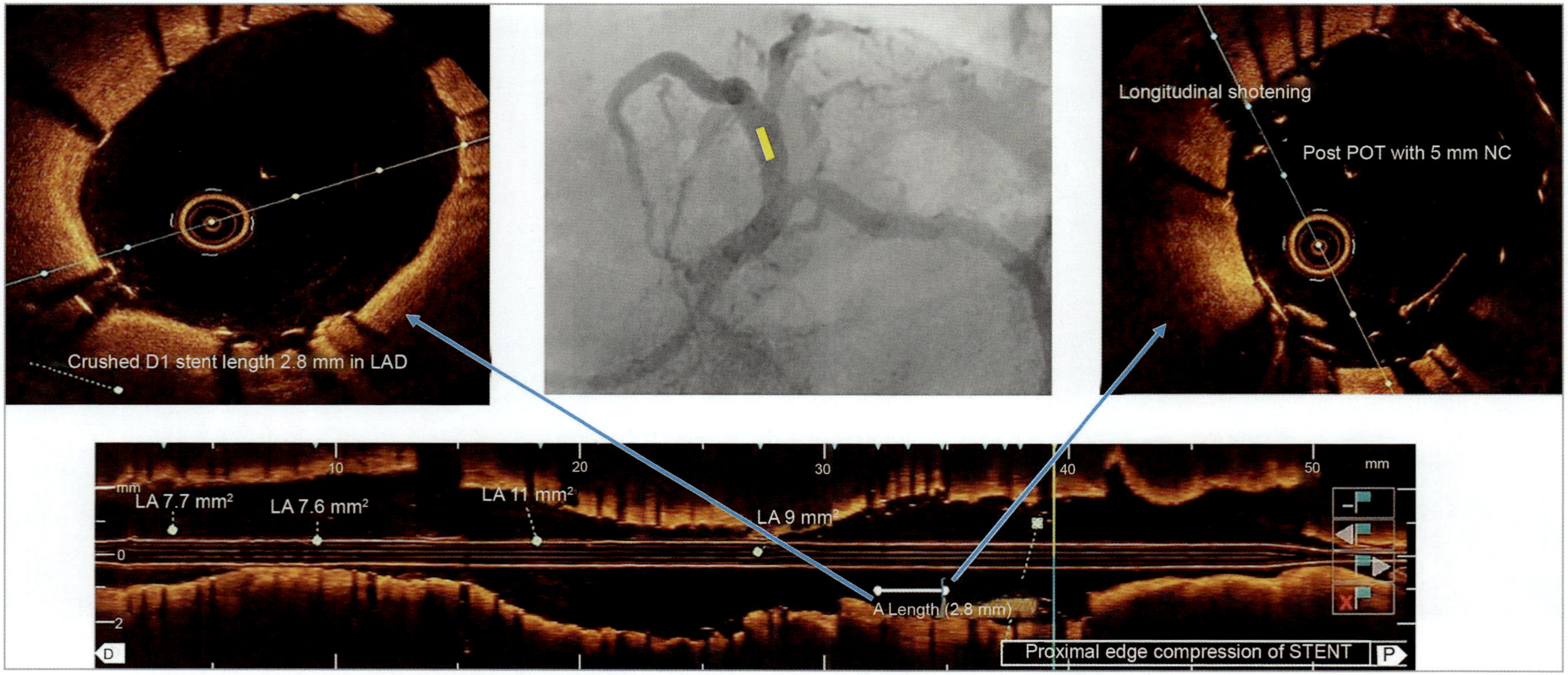

Fig. 67: LSD of proximal edge of the stent postdilated with 5 mm NC.

In EXCEL study acute LMCA stent deformation was observed in 33 pts (6.6%) and was most commonly located at the LMCA ostium (27/33[81%), and it was associated with increased acute and long term MACE rate (28% vs. 13.4%) in terms of increased mortality rate (15.7% vs. 9%), LM related MI (18.9% vs. 4.6%), LM ischemia driven TLR, and stent thrombosis (3.1% vs. 1.1%).

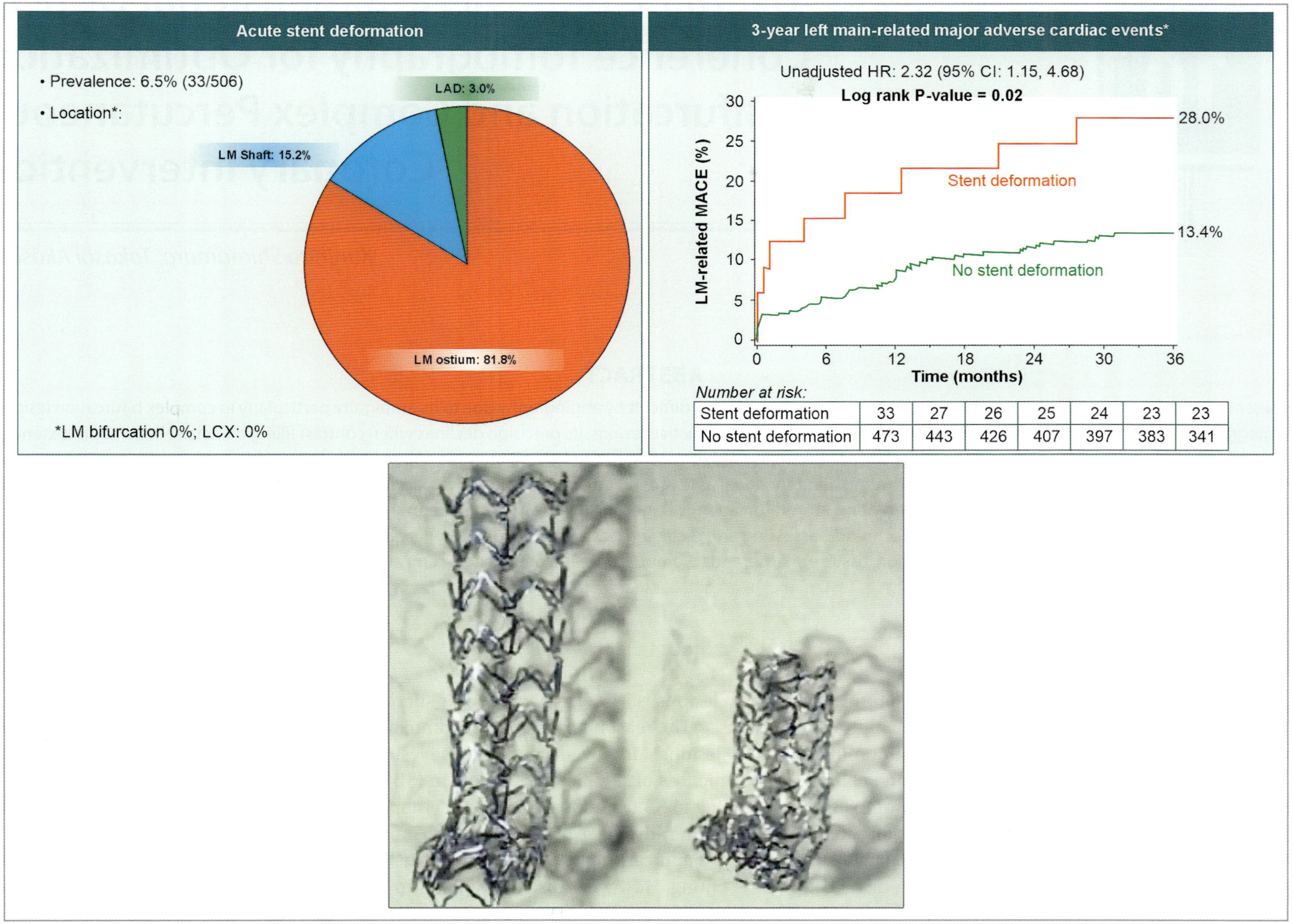

Fig. 68: Acute stent deformation or LSD.

CHAPTER 10

Usefulness of Three-dimensional Optical Coherence Tomography for Optimization of Bifurcation and Complex Percutaneous Coronary Intervention

Kunihiro Shimamura, Takashi Akasaka

ABSTRACT

Assessment of left main coronary artery disease (LMCAD) is sometimes very difficult by angiography due to its ambiguity particularly in complex bifurcation lesions. Angiography is highly accurate when defining critical or very severely obstructive lesions, its precision declines when contrast filling defects or intermediate stenosis are involved. Revascularization strategies based solely on the angiographic appearance of LMCAD stenosis of intermediate severity (between 50 and 70%) may be inappropriate, and needs to be confirmed with imaging and functional assessment. Intravascular imaging particularly intravascular ultrasound (IVUS) and optical coherence tomography (OCT) for distal LMCA and non-LMCA bifurcation is beneficial in assessing plaque morphology, severity assessment, identifying proper landing zones, assessing single versus two stent technique, assessing and rectifying postpercutaneous coronary intervention (PCI) issues such as under-expansion, malapposition, edge dissection, intrastent dissection, tissue prolapse, and thrombus to ensure better short-term and long-term results of current drug-eluting stents (DES) post-PCI results.

INTRODUCTION

Percutaneous coronary intervention (PCI) in coronary bifurcation lesions is associated with lower success rates, higher acute complication rates, and higher event rates in follow-up compared to nonbifurcation lesions.[1-3] The reason for this higher complication and event rate relates to the relationship between anatomy, flow, and atheroma distribution in bifurcation lesions. Moreover, stenting these lesions can be a prolonged procedure and can be technically more demanding. The most common complication is the loss of significant side branch (SB). Main vessel (MV) stenting may enhance the carina displacement and atheroma shift across the SB ostium leading to SB ostium narrowing. Provisional stenting without unnecessary SB stenting is generally recommended in most bifurcation lesions. In this technique, the advantage of kissing balloon inflation (KBI) after MV stenting is controversial.[4-7] KBI should be performed effectively to reduce jailed struts without significant stent deformation in the MV. For optimal KBI, it is important to assess the guidewire recrossing position (generally a distal cell) after stenting. However, it is very difficult to confirm the guidewire recrossing position by conventional angiography, intravascular ultrasound (IVUS), or two-dimensional (2D) optical coherence tomography (OCT). The three-dimensional (3D) reconstruction of OCT is useful for identifying the configuration of an implanted stent, especially at the bifurcation lesion.[8,9] In this chapter, we will introduce the usefulness of 3D-OCT for optimization of bifurcation PCI.

USEFULNESS OF 3D-OCT FOR OPTIMIZATION OF BIFURCATION PCI

A single center experience conducted by Okamura et al. demonstrated that both the strut configuration and rewiring position before SB dilatation affect the incidence of nonapposed struts at the SB orifice after final kissing balloon technique.[10] In this study, classification of configuration of overhanging struts in front of the SB ostium and definition of the most distal cell were shown **(Figs. 1A and B)**. After KBI with the most distal cell rewiring, OCT revealed that the percentage of incomplete stent apposition (ISA) of the free carina type was significantly smaller than that of the connecting to carina type (0.7 ± 0.9% vs. 12.2 ± 6.5%, $p = 0.0074$). Moreover, Okamura et al. investigated the influence of the guidewire recrossing point in the SB assessed by 3D-OCT or 2D-OCT on the incidence of nonapposed struts at the SB orifice, and also clinical and angiographic outcome in the long term in a prospective multicenter registry enrolling 168 bifurcation lesions of 168 patients.[11] In this study, the cases were divided into two groups according to the jailing configuration and rewiring position as follows—link-free and distal guidewire recrossing (LFD) group, cases with both the link-free (LF) type and distal (D) rewiring, and the non-LFD group, which included all other cases **(Fig. 2)**. ISA in the LFD group was significantly smaller than that in the non-LFD group (6.7 ± 5.9% vs. 17.0 ± 10.5%, $p < 0.0001$). The distal recrossing rate was 83%. Proximal recrossing increased ISA compared with distal recrossing, particularly in parallel bifurcations

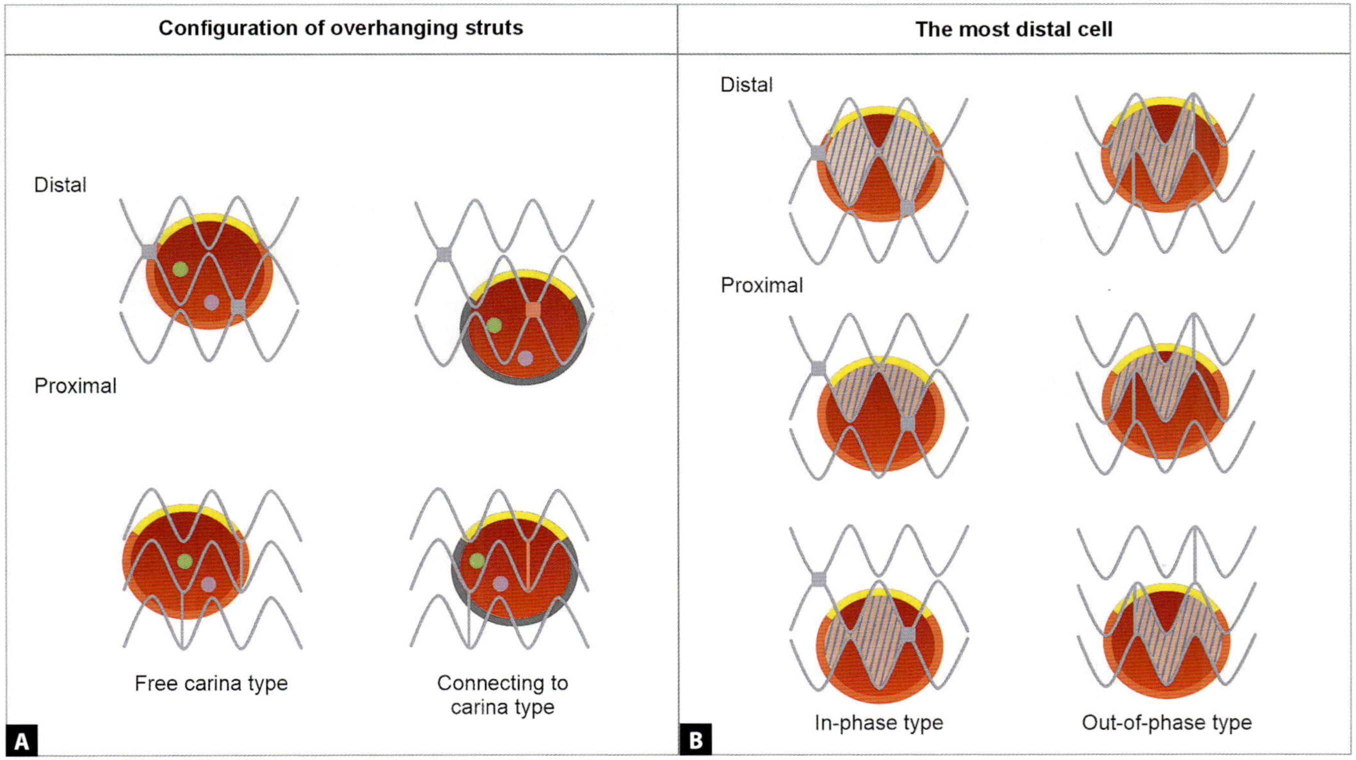

Figs. 1A and B: Classification of configuration of overhanging struts in front of the side branch ostium and definition of the most distal cell. Yellow line indicates the carina, red color indicates the link between hoops connecting to the carina, green and purple dots indicate the distal and proximal recrossing position, and the shaded area indicates the most distal cell.[10]

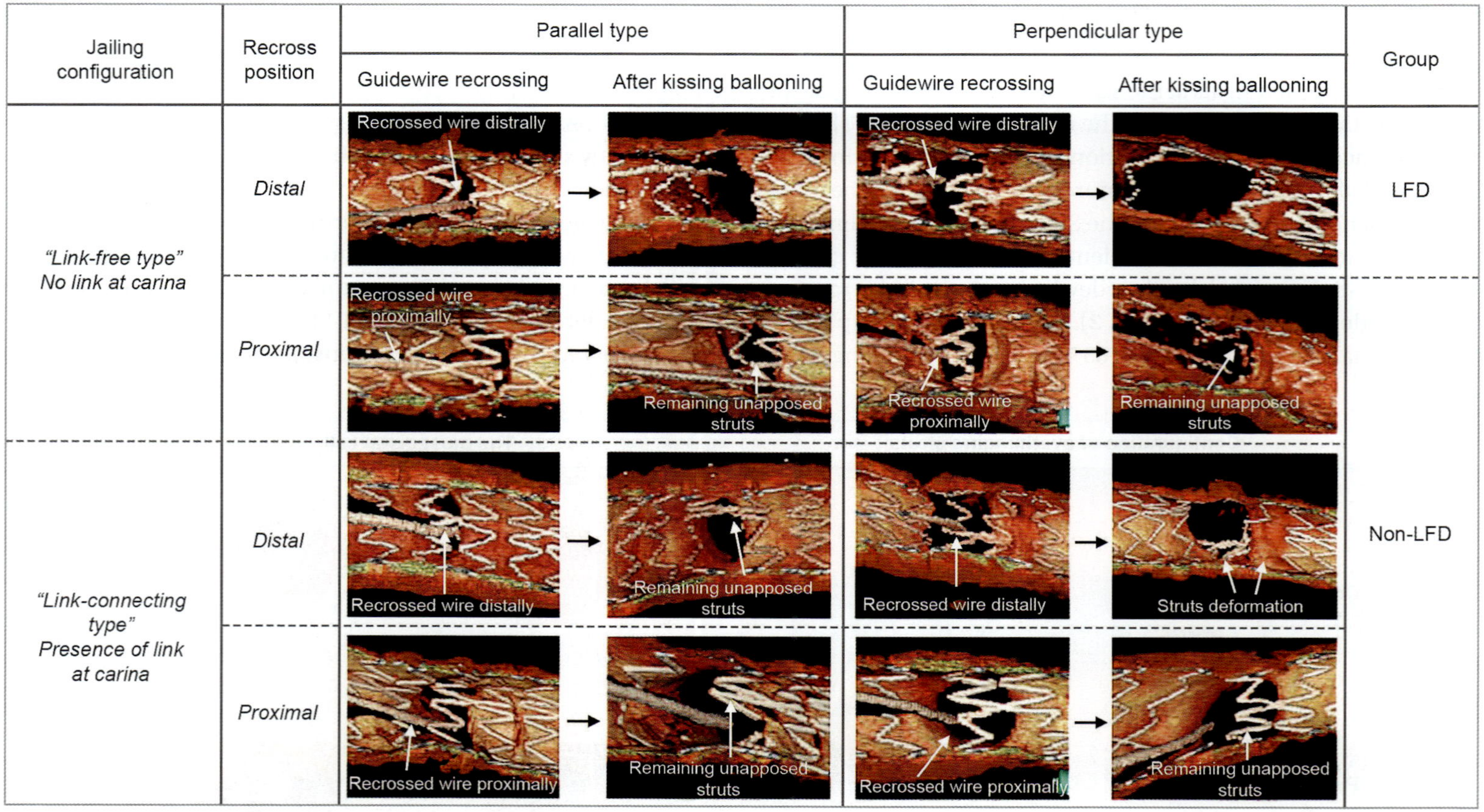

Fig. 2: Pictures according to the jailing configuration, recrossing position and 3D bifurcation type. In the link-free type, if the guidewire was recrossed distally, jailed struts were removed optimally (LFD group). In other cases, unapposed struts at the side branch (SB) ostium and strut deformation were observed (non-LFD group).[11]

(17.1 ± 10.1% vs. 6.3 ± 6.0%, p <0.0001). At follow-up, though event rates did not differ, SB restenosis in the non-LFD group tended to be higher than in the LFD group (20.5% vs. 8.3%, p = 0.1254). Nagoshi et al. evaluated the feasibility and usefulness of 3D-OCT in bifurcation PCI compared with conventional 2D-OCT-guided PCI in 150 bifurcation lesions, retrospectively.[12] Distal guidewire recrossing was achieved at higher rate in 3D-OCT group compared with 2D-OCT group (91.7% vs. 75.6%, p = 0.004). Compared with the 2D group, the incidence of ISA toward the SB in the 3D group tended to be lower in the whole cohort (14.5 ± 13.6% vs. 10.0 ± 9.0%, p = 0.077), and was significantly lower in left main trunk bifurcations (18.7 ± 12.8% vs. 10.3 ± 8.9%, p = 0.014). Independent contributors to ISA were the link-connecting type (β–0.089, p = 0.001) and distal guidewire recrossing (β –0.078, p = 0.001).

Japanese prospective observational study of 3D-OCT-guided bifurcation PCI (Japanese 3D-OCT Bifurcation Registry) which is a prospective multicenter observational study aimed to assess the link between initial results of 3D-OCT-guided bifurcation PCI and subsequent clinical outcomes and to investigate the clinical benefit of 3D-OCT-guided PCI in bifurcation lesions is on-going.[13] This study is going to enroll 600 patients (400 patients SB opening guided by 3D-OCT and 200 patients no SB opening) who have de novo bifurcation lesions and require bifurcation stentings. Primary endpoint is going to be assessed by the incidence of SB restenosis within 1 year after the initial PCIs among those who had optimal SB dilatation, suboptimal SB dilatation, and no SB dilatation. This study will provide the further usefulness of 3D-OCT.

The following is a summary of the suggested 3D-OCT navigation for optimization of provisional stenting in bifurcation lesion:

- Perform 3D-OCT assessment after stent implantation and confirm the configuration of overhanging struts in front of the SB ostium.
- When the configuration is link-free type, perform distal cell rewiring (and confirming this wire is definitely in the distal cell by another 3D-OCT scan) and KBI **(Figs. 3A to G)**.
- When the configuration is link-connecting type, the complete optimization may be difficult even if the rewiring position is carefully selected.

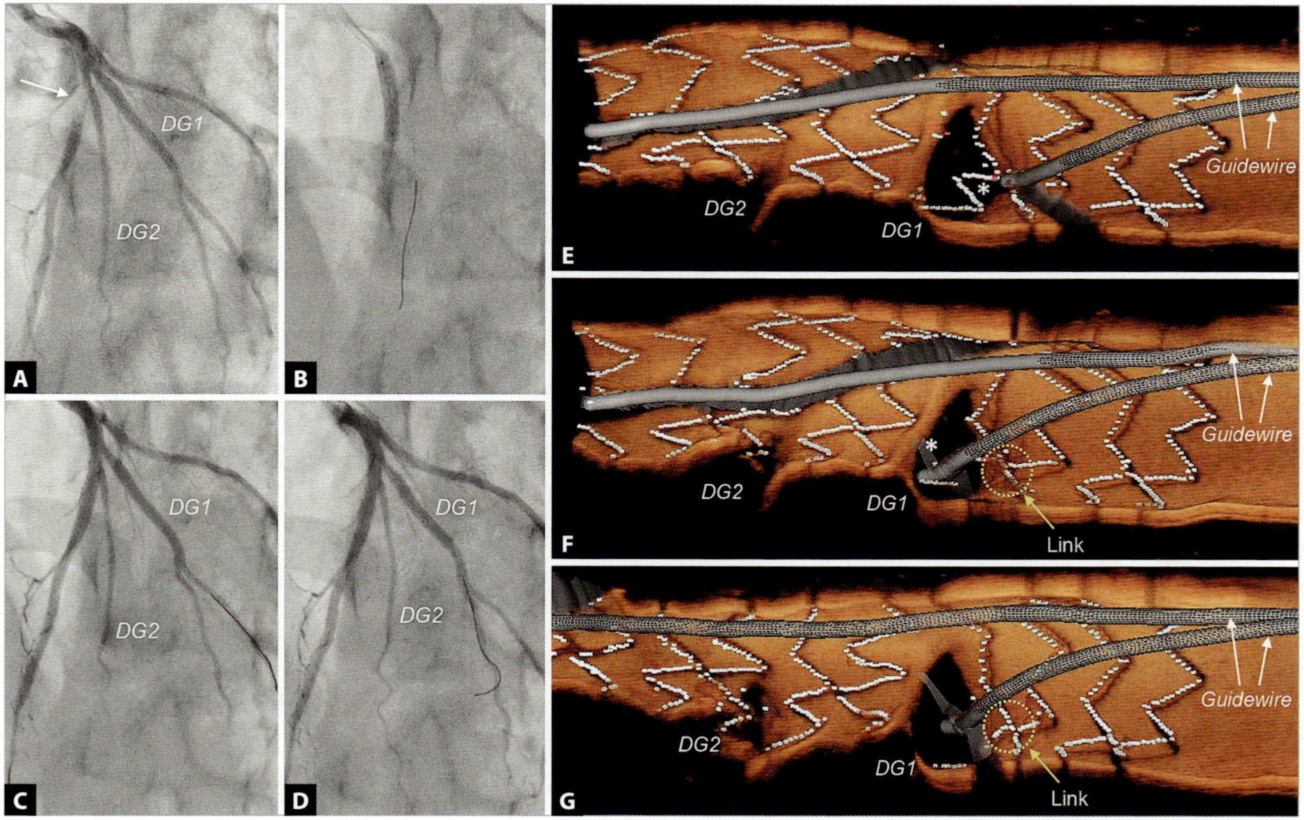

Figs. 3A to G: 3D-OCT guidance for guidewire-recrossing into the appropriate cell and optimization in bifurcation lesion. Coronary angiography (CAG) showed severe bifurcation stenosis of the proximal left anterior descending artery (LAD) and first diagonal (DG1) and second diagonal (DG2) (A, white arrow). A provisional stenting was performed with biodegradable-polymer sirolimus-eluting stent 3.5/18 mm (B). A cell wire recrossing was performed to open the stent struts toward the major side branch (DG1). While CAG was unable to reveal which stent cell was recrossed (C), 3D-OCT image clearly displayed the guidewire crossing into a proximal cell (E, asterisk), with a risk of stent distortion. After guidewire cell recrossing, 3D OCT showed that the guidewire was crossing into a more favorable distal cell (F, asterisk). Kissing balloon inflation was performed. Final CAG showed good stent expansion with appropriate dilation of ostial DG1 (D). Final 3D OCT showed optimal opening of jailed DG1 (G).

SUMMARY

Improvement of clinical outcomes in bifurcation lesion PCI can be expected by the guidance of 3D-OCT, although there are not enough data to support the reduction of the adverse clinical events using 3D-OCT-guided PCI for bifurcation lesions at the moment. The publication of the results of Japanese 3D-OCT Bifurcation Registry is necessary. Moreover, randomized prospective studies with greater number of study population should be planned to demonstrate the improvement of clinical outcome by 3D-OCT-guided PCI for bifurcation lesions in the near future.

REFERENCES

1. Iakovou I, Schmidt T, Bonizzoni E, Ge L, Sangiorgi GM, Stankovic G, et al. Incidence, predictors, and outcome of thrombosis after successful implantation of drug-eluting stents. JAMA. 2005;293:2126-30.
2. Nakazawa G, Yazdani SK, Finn AV, Vorpahl M, Kolodgie FD, Virmani R. Pathological findings at bifurcation lesions: the impact of flow distribution on atherosclerosis and arterial healing after stent implantation. J Am Coll Cardiol. 2010;55:1679-87.
3. Antoniadis AP, Mortier P, Kassab G, Dubini G, Foin N, Murasato Y, et al. Biomechanical Modeling to Improve Coronary Artery Bifurcation Stenting: Expert Review Document on Techniques and Clinical Implementation. JACC Cardiovasc Interv. 2015;8:1281-96.
4. Sgueglia GA, Chevalier B. Kissing balloon inflation in percutaneous coronary interventions. JACC Cardiovasc Interv. 2012;5:803-11.
5. Sgueglia GA, Chevalier B. Randomized comparison of final kissing balloon dilatation versus no final kissing balloon dilatation in patients with coronary bifurcation lesions treated with main vessel stenting: the Nordic-Baltic bifurcation study III. Circulation. 2011;123:79-86.
6. Gwon HC, Hahn JY, Koo BK, Song YB, Choi SH, Choi JH, et al. Final kissing ballooning and long-term clinical outcomes in coronary bifurcation lesions treated with 1-stent technique: results from the COBIS registry. Heart. 2012;98:225-31.
7. Kim YH, Lee JH, Roh JH, Ahn JM, Yoon SH, Park DW, et al. Randomized comparisons between different stenting approaches for bifurcation coronary lesions with or without side branch stenosis. JACC Cardiovasc. Interv. 2015;8:550-60.
8. Farooq V, Serruys PW, Heo JH, Gogas BD, Okamura T, Gomez-Lara J, et al. New insights into the coronary artery bifurcation hypothesis-generating concepts utilizing 3-dimensional optical frequency domain imaging. JACC Cardiovasc Interv. 2011;4:921-31.
9. Farooq V, Okamura T, Onuma Y, Gogas BD, Serruys PW. Unravelling the complexities of the coronary bifurcation: is this raising a few eyebrows? EuroIntervention. 2012;7:1133-41.
10. Okamura T, Onuma Y, Yamada J, Iqbal J, Tateishi H, Nao T, et al. 3D optical coherence tomography: new insights into the process of optimal rewiring of side branches during bifurcational stenting. EuroIntervention. 2014;10:907-15.
11. Okamura T, Nagoshi R, Fujimura T, Murasato Y, Yamawaki M, Ono S, et al. Impact of guidewire recrossing point into stent jailed side branch for optimal kissing balloon dilatation: core lab 3D optical coherence tomography analysis. EuroIntervention. 2018;13:e1785-93.
12. Nagoshi R, Okamura T, Murasato Y, Fujimura T, Yamawaki M, Ono S, et al. Feasibility and usefulness of three-dimensional optical coherence tomography guidance for optimal side branch treatment in coronary bifurcation stenting. Int J Cardiol. 2018;250:270-4.
13. UMIN-CTR Clinical Trial. (2021). Japanese prospective observational study of 3D-OCT guided bifurcation PCI. Available from https://upload.umin.ac.jp/cgi-open-bin/ctr_e/ctr_view.cgi?recptno=R000030721 [Last accessed February, 2024].

CHAPTER 11

Stent Thrombosis

PREVALENCE AND ETIOLOGY OF STENT THROMBOSIS

Acute stent thrombosis (AST) presents with acute myocardial infarction in 75% and cardiogenic shock in 30% of the patients during poststenting follow-up period, and it may necessitate emergency management strategies. Although an approximately 5 million percutaneous coronary interventions (PCIs) are performed worldwide annually, stent thrombosis (ST) is observed in about 0.5–1% of patients during the first year of poststenting period with a 30-day mortality rate as high as 25–30%. Its development is dependent on various risk factors, and proper understanding of these mechanisms by optical coherence tomography (OCT) is very useful in implementing appropriate treatment strategies.

Stent thrombosis can be classified as mentioned in the **Table 1** based on definition of diagnostic criteria for and timing of ST.

TABLE 1: Definition of diagnostic criteria for and timing of stent thrombosis.

Definite ST	Presence of an ACS with angiographic or autopsy evidence of thrombus or occlusion
Probable ST	Unexplained deaths within 30 days after the procedure or acute MI involving the target vessel territory without angiographic confirmation
Possible ST	All unexplained deaths occurring at least 30 days after the procedure
Timing of ST in relaxation to index stent implantation	
Acute ST	Developing between 0 and 24 hours after the index PCI
Subacute ST	Developing between 24 hours and 30 days after the index PCI
Late ST	Developing between 31 and 360 days after the index PCI
Very late ST	Developing later than 360 days after the index PCI

(ACS: acute coronary syndrome; MI: myocardial infarction; PCI: percutaneous coronary intervention; ST: stent thrombosis)

Source: Brancati MF, Burzotta F, Trani C, Leonzi O, Cuccia C, Crea F. Coronary stents and vascular response to implantation: literature review. Pragm Observ Res. 2017;8:137-48.

Definite Stent Thrombosis

Definite ST is defined as the presence of thrombus that develops in the stent or within the 5 mm of landing zones and associated with acute onset of ischemic symptoms at rest, new ischemic changes that suggest acute ischemia or typical increase and decrease in cardiac biomarkers, or the presence of a pathologic confirmation of ST within a 48-hour window.[1]

Probable Stent Thrombosis

Probable ST is defined as the presence of any unexplained death within the first 30 days after stent implantation, in the presence of any MI related to documented acute ischemia in the territory of the implanted stent without angiographic confirmation of ST and in the absence of any other obvious cause, irrespective of the time after the index procedure.

Possible Stent Thrombosis

Possible stent thrombosis is any unexplained death from 30 days after stenting until the end of follow-up.

Almost 75% cases of ST present with very late ST (VLST) while remaining 25% of cases are due to AST, subacute ST (SAST), and late ST (LST) cases. In-hospital mortalities of patients suffering from ST have been reported to be as high as 7.9% for AST and SAST, 3.8% for LST, and 3.6% for VLST. As per the recent evidence, long DAPT therapy compared to short DAPT therapy has been shown to reduce thrombotic events following drug-eluting stent (DES) implantation. However, with slight increase in bleeding risk but does not eliminate total risk of ST. The SCAAR (Swedish Coronary Angiography and Angioplasty Registry) revealed that the cumulative rates of definite ST up to 3 years were 2.0% for bare metal stents (BMS), 2.1% for first-generation DES, and 1.3% for second-generation DES. Although current second-generation DESs have improved stent design with thinner struts, more biocompatible polymers and lower drug load that has decreased ST rates, they have not totally eliminated ST-related mortality and morbidity.

The ST risk factors **(Box 1)** can be classified into four major categories: (1) patient-related, (2) lesion-related, (3) procedure-related, and (4) medication (poststenting)-related clinical problems.[2,3]

Early Stent Thrombosis (≤30 Days) (Figs. 1A to H)

Patients with large thrombotic burden, acute coronary syndromes, impaired coronary flow, and residual disease are at risk of early stent thrombosis (EST), and it has been associated with premature discontinuation of dual antiplatelet therapy (DAPT) during the initial 30 days after stenting.

BOX 1: Risk factors associated with stent/scaffold thrombosis.

Patient-related:	*Lesion-related:*	*Procedure-related:*
• Diabetes	• Thrombotic burden	• Stent malapposition
• Renal failure	• Long lesion	• Under expansion
• Left ventricular dysfunction	• Small vessel	• Stent edge dissection
• Acute coronary syndrome	• Bifurcation	• Neoatherosclerosis
• *CYP2C19* polymorphism	• Calcification	• Two-stent strategy
• Asian ethnicity	• Chronic total occlusion	• First-generation DES
Medication (postprocedure)-related:	• Left anterior descending artery	
Premature discontinuation of DAPT		

(DAPT: dual antiplatelet therapy; DES: drug-eluting stent)

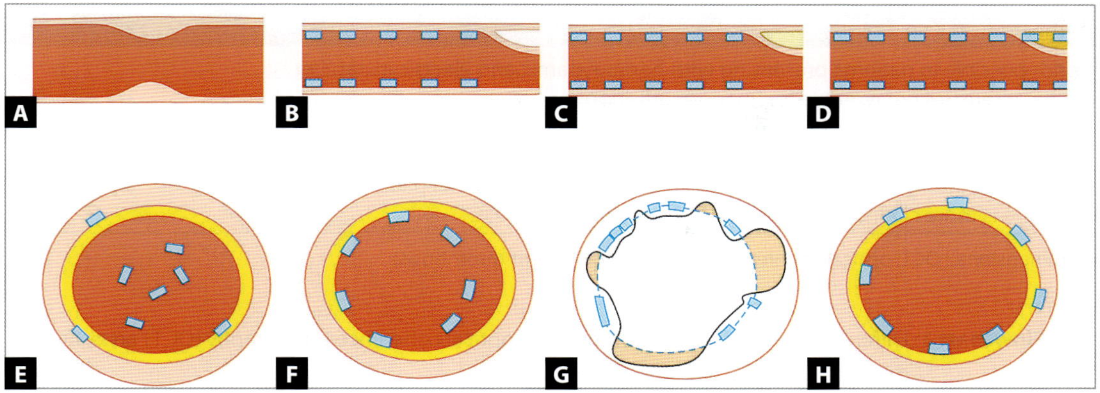

Figs. 1A to H: Mechanisms of early and late stent thrombosis. (A) Under-expansion; (B) Medial edge dissection; (C) Geographical miss; (D) Neoatherosclerosis; (E) Dismantling; (F) Mal-apposition; (G) Evaginations; (H) Uncovered struts

Early stent thrombosis is mainly due to the following procedure-related risk factors:

- *Underexpansion:* Ratio of minimum in stent area/reference vessel area <80%, minimum stet area <5.5 mm^2 by IVUS and <4.5 mm^2 by OCT, residual diameter stenosis >20% **(Fig. 1A)**.
- *Medial edge dissection:* Flow limiting, >200 µm at distal stent edge, angle of the dissection >60°, dissection reaching the media, and longitudinal length >3 mm **(Fig. 1B)**
- *Poor landing zones:* Minimum lumen area <4.5mm^2 and plaque burden >50% **(Fig. 1C)**.

Late stent thrombosis (>30 days)

It is usually attributed to the following risk factors:

- Geographical miss **(Fig. 1C)**
- Neoatherosclerosis **(Fig. 1D)**
- Dismantling **(Fig. 1E)**
- Malposition—strut-vessel wall distance >300 µm, >1 mm in length **(Fig. 1F)**
- Evaginations major when extending ≥3 mm with a depth ≥10% of the stent diameter **(Fig. 1G)**
- Uncovered struts—Number ≥6%, uncovered length >3 mm, and other mechanisms responsible for LST/VLST are hypersensitivity reactions, and impaired re-endothelialization **(Fig. 1H)**.

  Optical coherence tomography evaluation of ST carries certain limitations as described in **Box 2**.

ROLE OF OCT TO IDENTIFY INTRASTENT PATHOLOGY IN STENT THROMBOSIS

- It is useful to understand the possible mechanisms are responsible for the development of ST (e.g., stent under expansion or malapposition, neoatherosclerosis, and uncovered struts) and guiding choosing various treatment strategies **(Flowchart 1)**.
- A tailored and more effective approach for treatment with implementation of MLD MAX Algorithm.

BOX 2: Limitations of OCT in ST.

- OCT is not possible in patients presenting with hemodynamic and electric instability
- Vessel characteristics unfavorable for image acquisition
- Presence of residual thrombus burden in >95% of cases impact the assessment of the Underlying stent and vessel wall findings
- Manual thrombectomy was often required to re-establish target vessel patency before imaging
- Strut fracture is more clearly visible on 3D OCT compared to 2D OCT

(3D: three-dimensional; OCT: optical coherence tomography; ST: stent thrombosis)

Flowchart 1: Different causes of stent thrombosis by optical coherence tomography (OCT) analysis.

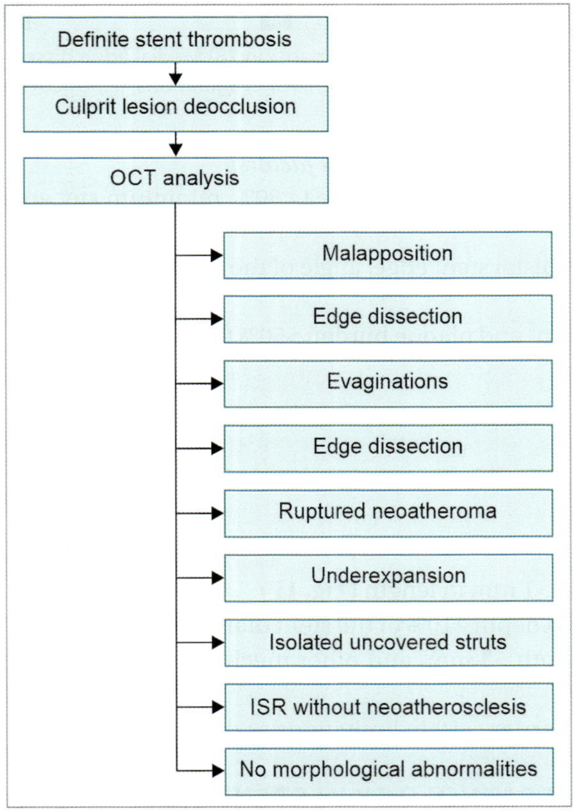

(ISR: in-stent restenosis)

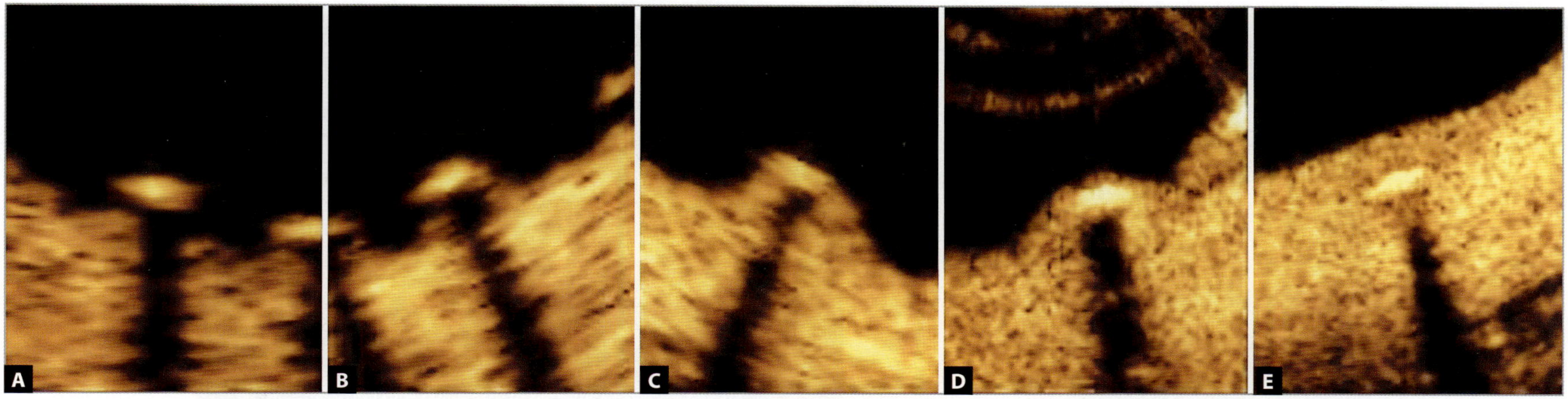

Figs. 2A to E: Classification of strut coverage. (A) Definitely uncovered; (B) Uncovered fibrin; (C) Partially covered; (D) Covered protruding; (E) Covered embedded.

Patients showing genetic abnormality of the *CYP2C19* gene show decreased antiplatelet activity, thereby increasing the tendency to develop ST, and these patients should be treated with other alternative potent P2Y12 inhibitors, such as prasugrel and ticagrelor, which are less influenced by polymorphisms of the *CYP2C19* gene, especially in patients with high-risk multivessel or left main coronary stenting.

Lack of Stent Endothelialization

During follow-up of PCI patients with well-expanded and apposed stent, thrombus may develop on struts without endothelialization. The covered strut is a strut with surrounding tissue beyond the strut surface, whereas the uncovered strut is completely embedded with disruption of lumen contour or partially embedded with extension of strut into lumen.

Although patients with current-generation DES have shown improved **(Figs. 2A to C)** endothelialization **(Figs. 2D and E)** of struts with decreased rate of ST, still some patients may present with ST owing to the partial endothelialization of struts, especially when DAPT therapy is stopped or with prothrombotic state. As per the evidence, an about of 6% of uncovered struts per stent has been associated with an increased risk of ST. Stent strut coverage can be improved by OCT-guided optimal strut apposition, which reduces shear stress at the level of the strut surface.

Stent Thrombosis due to Intrastent Dissection (Fig. 3)

Intrastent dissection is disruption of the luminal vessel surface in the stent segment. It can appear in two forms: (1) Dissection—the vessel surface is disrupted and a dissection flap is visible; (2) cavity—the vessel surface is disrupted, and an empty cavity can be seen. It is most likely due to rupture of new plaque within the stent, with spreading of the dissection plane along the interface between the stent and intima. The magnitude of intrastent necrotic core prolapse and medial tear are also independent predictors of ST.[6]

Malapposition and Undersizing

Malapposed strut produces high shear stress and micro-recirculation that prevent strut coverage by endothelial cells, alter blood viscosity, and stimulate platelet activation and neointimal formation.[7]

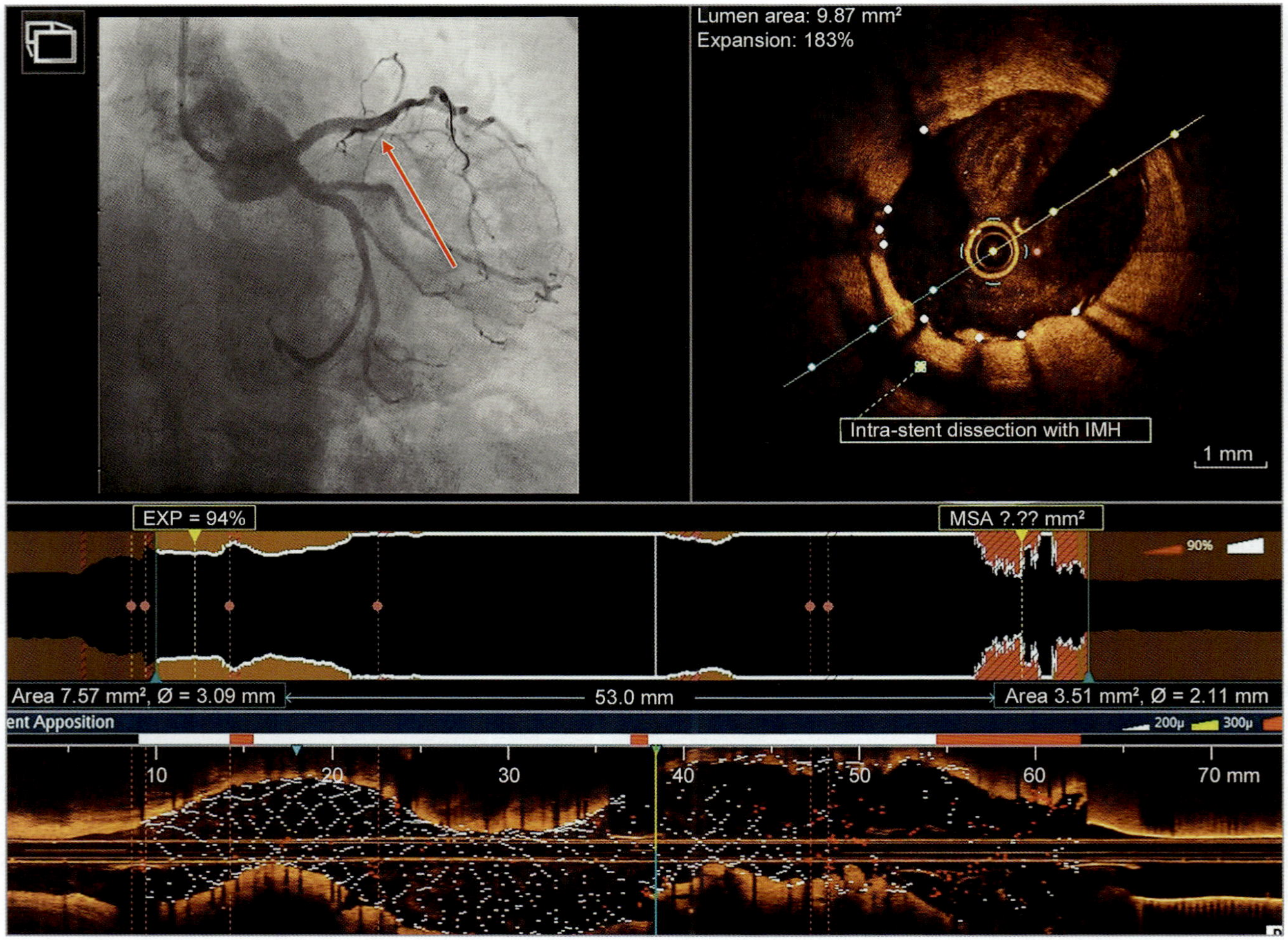

Fig. 3: Intra-stent dissection with IMH.

Late stent malapposition is associated with nearly sevenfold increase in the risk of ST; it is usually due to chronic inflammation and delayed healing as a result of tissue necrosis and erosion adjacent to the strut. The positive remodeling of the arterial wall may cause a stasis of blood flow between the aneurysmatic wall and the stent struts serving as a local nidus for thrombus formation.[4,6]

Coronary Evaginations (Fig. 1G)

Coronary evaginations (CEs) are 10 times more common in first-generation DES compared to second-generation DES, and their presence predict LST. On OCT images, they are visible as finger-like outward bulges of the contour of the vessel lumen between stent struts. The evaginations could be due to

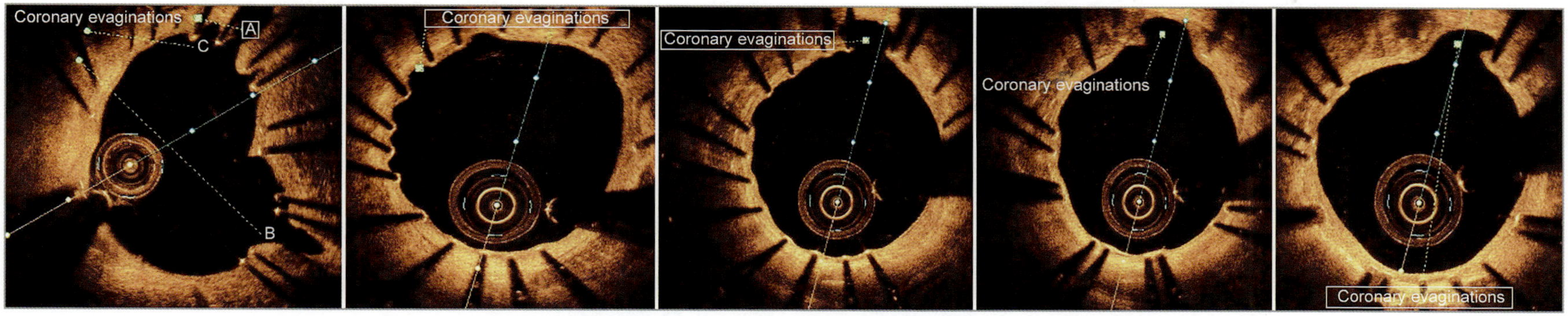

Fig. 4: OCT appearance of coronary evaginations.

inflammatory process in the surrounding area of stent struts **(Fig. 4)**. Prescence of evaginations and malapposition may require prolonged DAPT therapy and sometimes, stenting with covered stent may be useful depending upon the clinical symptoms.[7-9]

Stent Thrombosis—Endothelial Bridges

Formation of endothelial bridges (Ebs) connecting malapposed struts with the vessel lumen as a result of excessive neointimal healing on the abluminal side which produces flow disturbances with high shear stress by the struts leads to stimulation of platelet activation[5] and development of ST.

Stent Thrombosis—Dismantling (Fig. 1E)

Dismantling is a unique phenomenon observed with biovascular scaffolds and which has been reported with both poly-l-lactide-based and magnesium-based biovascular scaffolds. Progressive degradation of the polymer in the post-PCI procedure period may cause the progressive structural disintegration of scaffold that may lead to protrusion of discontinuous struts into the lumen which might cause turbulence and exposure of highly thrombogenic remnants to the blood flow contributing to the ST development. Dismantling has been reported to be 40% of the cases of very late scaffold thrombosis.[10,11]

LOCALIZED HYPERSENSITIVITY REACTIONS OF DRUG-ELUTING STENT

Some cases of LST/VLST in DES could be due to chronic inflammation and hypersensitivity reactions in response to stent components, and the allergenic response varies with the stent metal (e.g., stainless steel vs. chromium). Recent addition of more biocompatible alloys with improvement of specific design also contributed to declining rate of ST with current-generation DES.[12]

Neoatherosclerosis

Neoatherosclerosis is a continuum of the spectrum of neointimal hyperplasia, where in addition to smooth muscle proliferation, lipid deposition, calcification, and intraplaque angiogenesis can occur, similar to a native coronary atherosclerotic plaque. By OCT, neoatherosclerosis typically has heterogeneous signal intensity with diffuse edges and high attenuation suggestive of lipid pools or sharply defined areas of signal attenuation suggestive of calcium deposition. Plaque rupture is sometimes seen as a fissure in the neointimal fibrous cap with communication to the lipid pool; it can occur spontaneously or as a consequence of stent fracture. ST due to neoatherosclerosis tends to occur late following stent implant.[13]

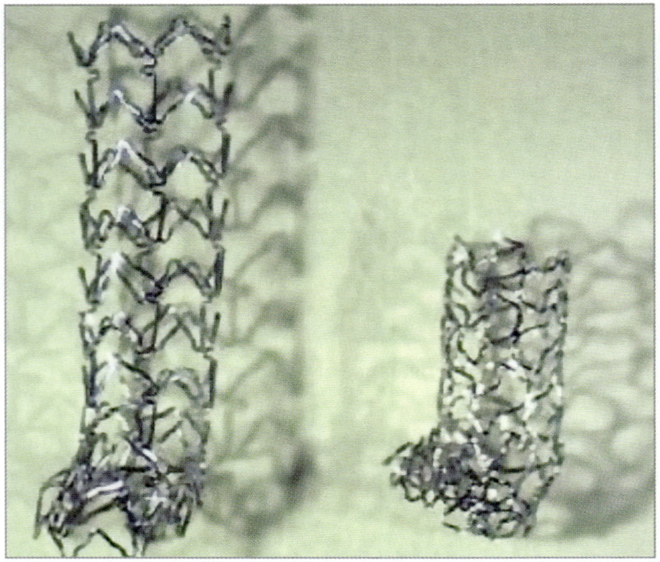

Fig. 5: Longitudinal stent deformation.

Strut Fracture

Strut fracture can be detected on angiography in 2–3% of newer—generation DES. The prevalence of fractures was as high as 22% for DES, and it is associated with stent restenosis, target-lesion revascularization, and ST.

Evaluation of OCT runs can reveal relatively rare contributing mechanisms of in-stent restenosis (ISR), such as stent fracture and longitudinal stent deformation (LSD), which are difficult to diagnose on conventional angiography images.

Longitudinal stent deformation (LSD) is defined as fluoroscopically visible longitudinal shortening of the implanted stent with concertina-like stent strut crowding/deformation **(Fig. 5)**.

The LSD is rare (overall 0.2% of cases), which may be due to guide contact of the stent at the ostium of the coronary during PCI of ostial lesions of left main coronary artery/right coronary artery (LMCA/RCA); it is associated with an increased risk of restenosis and ST. It varies between DES platforms due to variation in radial strength and number of connecting links. OCT imaging is useful in identifying and guides while correcting LSD with additional postballoon dilatations or stenting, thereby improving acute and long-term outcomes of DES.[14,15]

The three registries of ST with OCT evaluation differ to some extent in the patient population studied; the Bern registry focused on cases of VLST in DES, whereas PESTO and PRESTIGE included all cases of ST to study various causes that were responsible for the development of ST **(Table 2)**.

OPTICAL COHERENCE TOMOGRAPHY ASSESSMENT OF THROMBUS IN ACUTE STENT THROMBOSIS

- *Stent thrombus:* As an irregular protruding of signal rich, low backscattering protrusions, or high backscattering protrusions beyond the stent struts into the lumen, with signal-free shadowing and a sharp intensity gap with a dimension of ≥250 μm on the OCT image.
- *Percent thrombus:* Length—calculated as the thrombus length divided by the stent length.
- *Thrombus burden:* Mean thrombus area divided by the mean lumen area.

TABLE 2: Dominant findings identified by OCT imaging at the time of LST/VLST reported in large registries.

Study (year)	*Uncovered struts*	*Malapposition*	*Neoatherosclerosis*	*Severe underexpansion*	*NIH with thrombus*	*Others*
PRESTIGE Registry (2017) LST/VLST% (*n* = 134)	22	14	27	6	13	18
PESTO French Registry (2016) LST/VLST% (*n* = 97)	10	32	28	7	5	18
Taniwaki et al. (2016) VLST% (*n* = 57)	12	35	28	7	2	16

(LST: late stent thrombosis; NIH: neointimal hyperplasia; OCT: optical coherence tomography; VLST: very late ST)

Semiquantitative Assessment of Thrombus by Optical Coherence Tomography

Thrombus was classified as absent (0) or subtending 1, 2, 3, or 4 quadrants in each cross section. Thrombus score was calculated as the sum of each score.

MANAGEMENT OF STENT THROMBOSIS

Optical coherence tomography is helpful in the evaluation and management of ST by assessing the diagnosis, in identifying the underlying mechanism, and in guiding treatment **(Flowchart 2)**.

The ability of OCT to show high-resolution images with clear identification of luminal areas, underexpansion, malapposition, uneven stent struts distribution, or small intrastent thrombotic formations makes it a more useful imaging modality for the optimization of stent implantation to prevent mechanical complications that may result in ST. Mechanical or manual thrombus aspiration may be required prior to acquiring OCT run in patients with totally occlusive ST to get good OCT images for sufficient clearance of blood with contrast injections, and imaging runs should be repeated after thrombus aspiration and before dilatation to determine the mechanism of ST. Primary PCI or thrombolysis should be given as soon as the diagnosis of ST is confirmed to produce effective and early recanalization of culprit vessel to reduce high morbidity and mortality associated with ST. Thrombus aspiration, although almost completely abandoned in the setting of ST-elevation myocardial infarction (STEMI), might be useful in cases of high thrombus burden, and therapy with intracoronary (IC) thrombolytic therapy or glycoprotein IIb/IIIa inhibitors is to be considered depending upon the clinical situation and operators' choice. OCT also quantifies thrombus burden before and after thrombus aspiration and directs further interventional strategy. For example, additional DES implantation is recommended for edge dissections, but this strategy might worsen the problem in cases of underexpansion of the stent and ISR with more than two layers of stents who can be treated favorably with drug-eluting balloon (DEB) application after adequate preparation of the lesion with necessary devices. OCT guides in precise sizing of the stent and balloons for proper deployment of the stents with prolonged inflation at higher pressure to get adequate expansion and apposition that are considered essential to reduce the formation of ST, especially in severely calcific lesions.[16]

Special attention should be paid to assess compliance of drugs; assessment of platelet function is helpful in selecting proper antiplatelet therapy to improve the antiplatelets' efficacy by ruling out resistance to antiplatelets, mainly clopidogrel. Duration of DAPT therapy and/or switching to other potent P2Y12 inhibitors should be considered and weighed against the individual bleeding risk, especially in cases with complex high-risk anatomy or where interventional therapy is not possible, such as patients with persistent aneurysms or evaginations or with persistent underexpansion in spite of multiple attempts to treat it.[17]

Flowchart 2: Management of stent thrombosis.

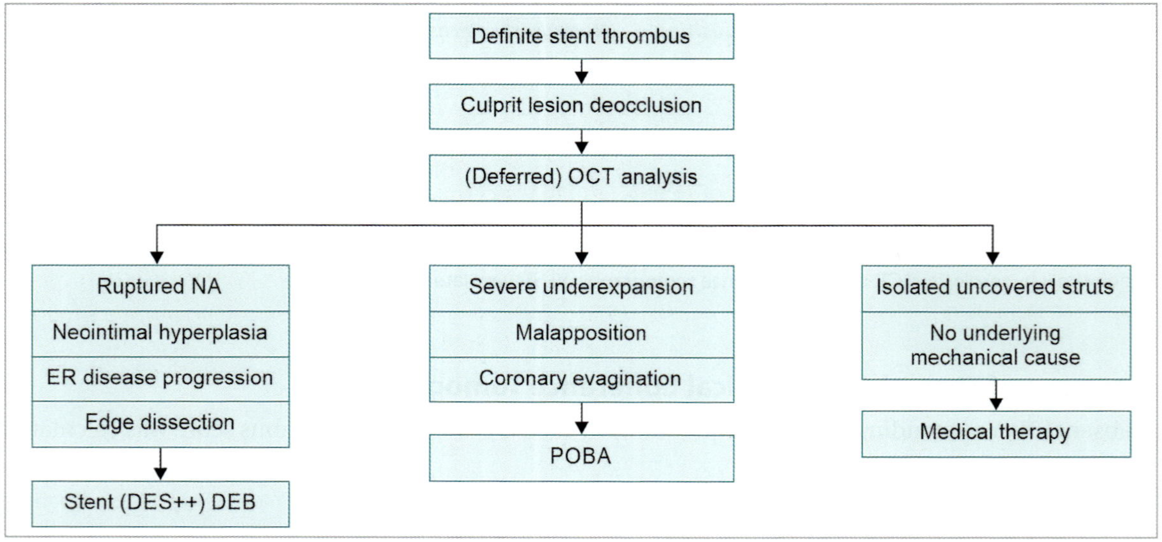

(DEB: drug-eluting balloon; DES: drug-eluting stent; POBA: plain-old balloon angioplasty; OCT: Optical coherence tomography)

PREVENTION AND IMAGING

Recent evidence from various studies has consistently proved that IVUS was associated with a decreased incidence of ST. The CLI–OPCI (Centro per la Lotta contro l'Infarto–Optimization of Percutaneous Coronary Intervention) study and other retrospective studies suggested that OCT findings of suboptimal stent deployment were associated with an increased incidence of ST during 5 years of follow-up, and similar results were reported in the Pan-London registry. The DOCTORS trial that compared OCT-guided with angiography-guided PCI in 240 patients with non-ST-segment elevation ACS with a fractional flow reserve-based analysis demonstrated that postprocedural results were superior in the OCT-guided group. Intravascular image-guided PCI either with IVUS or with OCT is superior to angiography-guided PCI in reducing ST by 50–60%.

REFERENCES

1. Price MJ. Intravascular Imaging: OCT and IVUS, An Issue of Interventional Cardiology Clinics. Philadelphia: Elsevier; 2015. Eur Heart J. 2016;37(15):1217-9.
2. Mori H, Joner M, Finn AV, Virmani R. Malapposition: is it a major cause of stent thrombosis? Eur Heart J. 2016;37(15):1217-9.
3. Wada H, Mattson PC, Iwata H. Stent or scaffold thrombosis: Past, current, and future perspectives. EMJ. 2017;5:55-61.
4. Torrado J, Buckley L, Durán A, Trujillo P, Toldo S, Raleigh JV, et al. Restenosis, stent thrombosis, and bleeding complications: Navigating between Scylla and Charybdis. J Am Coll Cardiol. 2018;71(15):1676-95.
5. Gori T, Polimeni A, Indolfi C, Räber L, Adriaenssens T, Münzel T. Predictors of stent thrombosis and their implications for clinical practice. Nat Rev Cardiol. 2019;16(4):243-56.
6. Algazzar AS, ElSayed AA, Katta AA, Ahmed KS. Early drug eluting stent thrombosis in acute coronary syndromes. Interventional Cardiology. 2018;10(1):17-20.

7. Poon EK, Thondapu V, Hayat U, Barlis P, Yap CY, Kuo PH, et al. Elevated blood viscosity and microrecirculation resulting from coronary stent malapposition. J Biomech Eng. 2018;140(5).
8. Gori T, Jansen T, Weissner M, Foin N, Wenzel P, Schulz E, et al. Coronary evaginations and periscaffold aneurysms following implantation of bioresorbable scaffolds: incidence, outcome, and optical coherence tomography analysis of possible mechanisms. Eur Heart J. 2015;37(26):2040-9.
9. Bezerra HG, Attizzani GF, Costa MA. OCT Made Easy. United States: CRC; 2017.
10. Yamamura S, Fujisue K, Tsujita K, Sakamoto K, Miyazaki Y, Kaikita K, et al. Optical coherence tomography visualization of stent deformation with subsequent thrombus adhesion at very early phase after everolimus-eluting stent implantation: a case report. BMC Cardiovasc Dis. 2016;16(1):116.
11. Okamoto N, Vengrenyuk Y, Baber U, Kini AS. Asymptomatic large thrombus formation in drug-eluting stent 2 days after primary percutaneous coronary intervention in ST-segment elevation myocardial infarction patient. JACC Cardiovasc Interv. 2017;10(23):2461-3.
12. Adriaenssens T, Joner M, Godschalk TC, Malik N, Alfonso F, Xhepa E, et al. Optical coherence tomography findings in patients with coronary stent thrombosis: a report of the PRESTIGE consortium (Prevention of Late Stent Thrombosis by an Interdisciplinary Global European Effort). Circulation. 2017;136(11):1007-21.
13. Sato N, Minami Y, Shimohama T, Kameda R, Tojo T, Ako J. Vascular response and intrastent thrombus in the early phase after drug-eluting versus bare-metal stent implantation in patients with ST-segment elevation myocardial infarction: An observational, single-center study. Health science reports. 2019;2(1):e105.
14. Prati F, Kodama T, Romagnoli E, Gatto L, Di Vito L, Ramazzotti V, et al. Suboptimal stent deployment is associated with subacute stent thrombosis: optical coherence tomography insights from a multicenter matched study. From the CLI Foundation investigators: the CLI-THRO study. Am Heart J. 2015;169(2):249-56.
15. Hamshere S, Byrne A, Guttmann O, Rees P, Bourantas C, Weerakody R, et al. An observational study of clinical outcomes of everolimus-eluting bioresorbable scaffolds comparing the procedural use of optical coherence tomography against angiography alone. Coron Artery Dis. 2018;29(6):482-8.
16. Maehara A, Matsumura M, Ali ZA, Mintz GS, Stone GW. IVUS-guided versus OCT-guided coronary stent implantation: a critical appraisal. JACC Cardiovasc Imaging. 2017;10(12):1487-503.
17. Romagnoli E, Gatto L, La Manna A, Burzotta F, Taglieri N, Saia F, et al. Role of residual acute stent malapposition in percutaneous coronary interventions. Catheter Cardiovasc Interv. 2017;90(4):566-75.

CASE 1

Optical coherence tomography (OCT) evaluation bare metal stents (BMS) stent thrombosis.

CLINICAL HISTORY

A 67-year-old male known hypertensive presented with established inferior wall myocardial infarctions (IWMI) and postinfarct angina associated with giddiness and nausea for 3 days. Acute pulmonary edema was treated with decongestive therapy and CHB treated with TPI. History of PCI of RCA (BMS) in 2002. 2D Echo showed AF during study, RWMA in RCA territory, mild LV function, EF—46%. Coronary angiography (CAG) showed LMCA—normal, separate origin of left anterior descending artery (LAD) and left circumflex artery (LCX), LAD—proximal 50-60% lesion, D1—mild lesion, LCX—proximal segment of obtuse marginal 1 (OM1) 70% lesion with aneurysm, RCA—proximal 99% ISR with acute stent thrombosis, distal 70% lesion, and posterior descending artery (PDA) and PLVB—normal **(Figs. 6A to C)**.

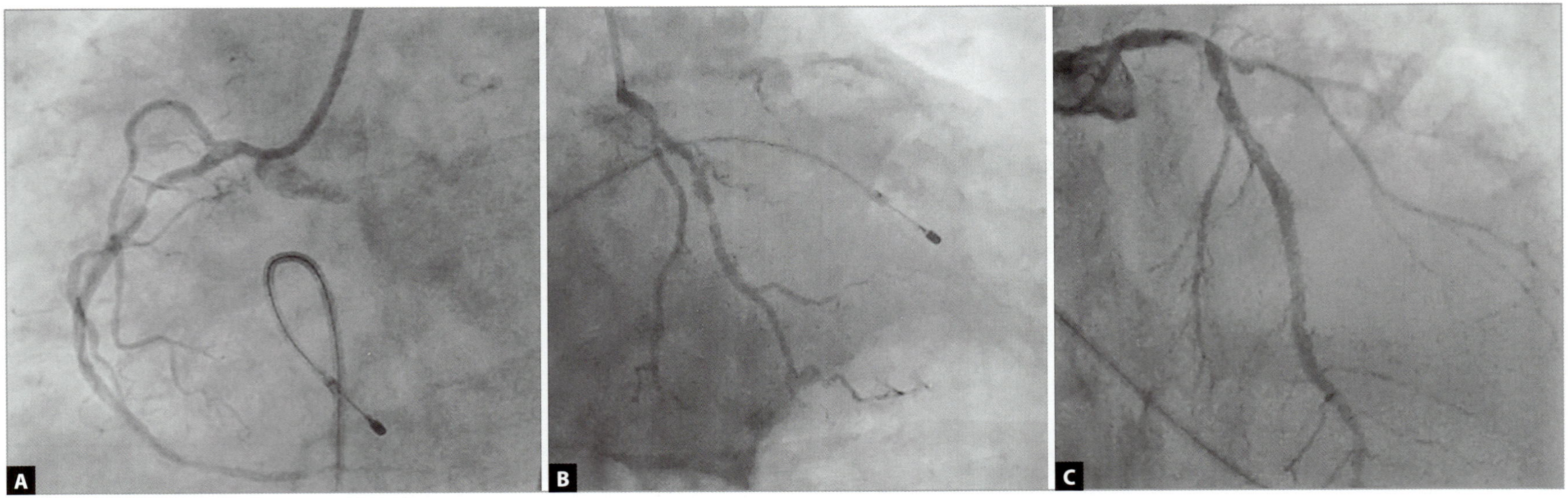

Figs. 6A to C: Coronary angiogram.

PROCEDURE

Percutaneous Coronary Intervention of Right Coronary Artery

Route—RRA, 6 Fr JR 3.5 guiding catheter, RCA ISR lesion was crossed with 0.014″ Sion Blue wire and predilated with 2.0 × 10 mm Tazuna balloon.

Preoptical Coherence Tomography Analysis

Pre-OCT—proximal landing zone: LA—7.9 mm^2, minimal lumen diameter (MLD)—3.1 mm, external luminal diameter (ELD)—4.27 mm/3.4 mm (ELD—3.7 mm), distal landing zone—minimal lumen area (MLA)—5.4 mm^2, MLD—2.6 mm, ELD—3 mm, and lesion length—38.3 mm. Pre-OCT showed red thrombus due to previous uncovered stent struts, neoatherosclerosis with lipid-rich plaque, MLA—6 mm^2, MLD—2.7 mm, area of thrombus—2.5 mm^2, percentage of thrombus area—57%, length of the red thrombus—7.6 mm **(Figs. 7A to C)**.

Proximal RCA stenting was done with 3.0 × 38 mm Resolute Onyx Stent with the help of GuideLiner 6 Fr support, and distal RCA stenting was done with 2.5 × 26 mm Resolute Onyx Stent **(Figs. 8A and B)**. Postprocedure OCT showed 30% malapposition of proximal stent, distal landing zone of proximal stent—thick fibrocalcific plaque—MLA—2.7 mm^2, MLD—1.8 mm. Proximal RCA postdilated with 4.0 × 18 mm balloon.

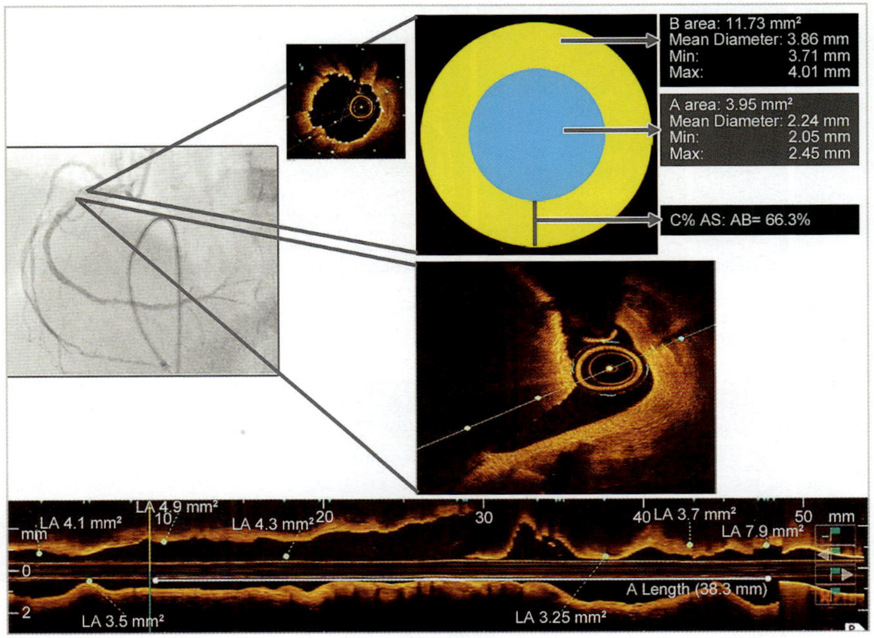

Fig. 7A

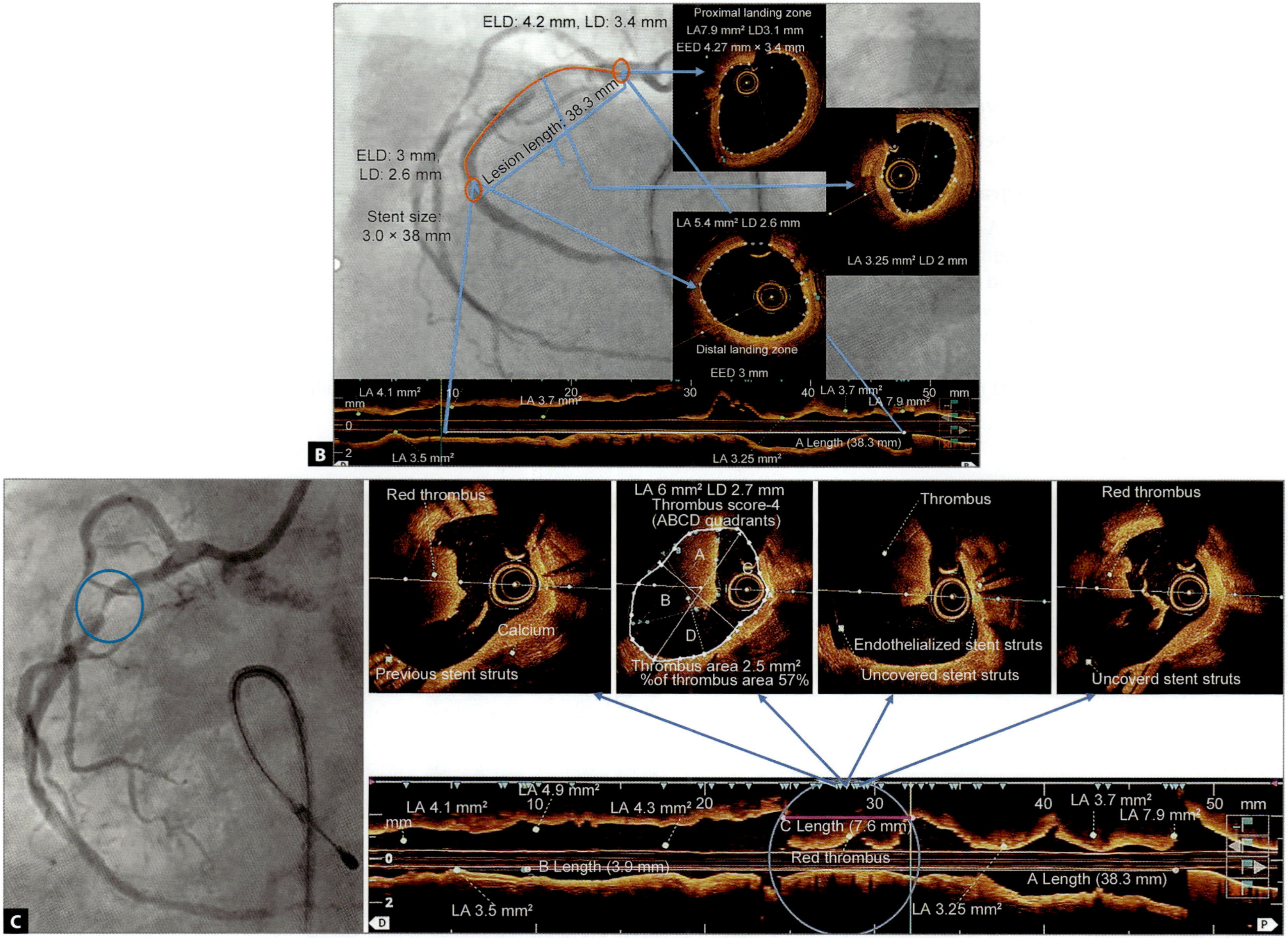

Fig. 7B and C

Figs. 7A to C: (A) Acute inferior STEMI due to stent thrombosis; (B) Plaque burden for plaque morphology; (C) Assessment of red thrombus.

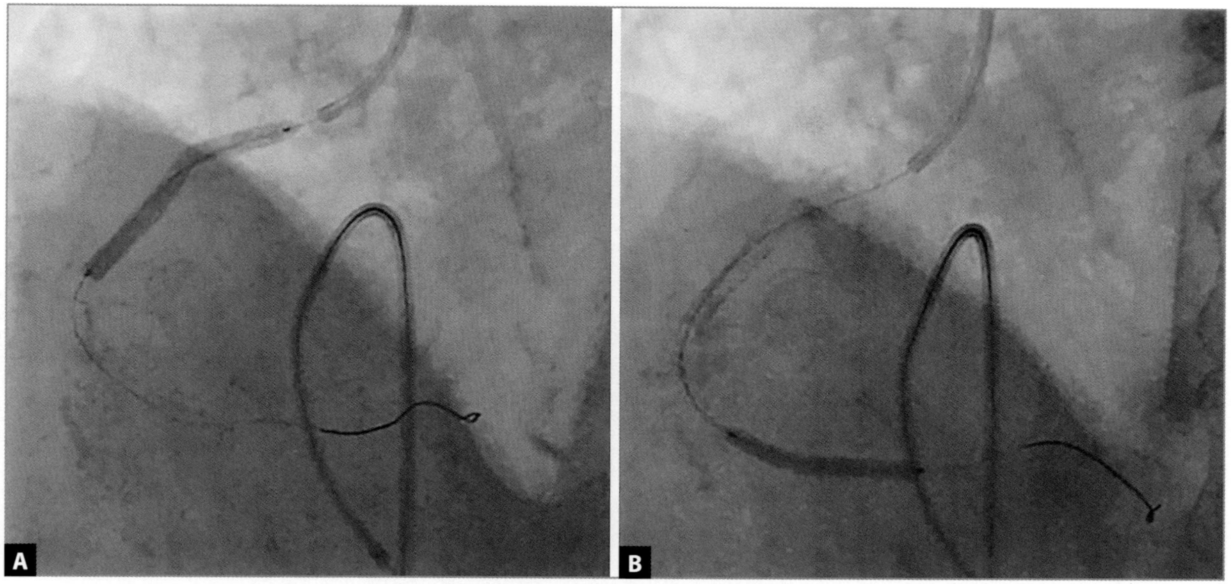

Figs. 8A and B: Stenting of proximal and distal RCA.

Post-OCT assessment proximal portion 30% malapposition—corrected with 4.0 × 18 mm NC **(Fig. 9)**, distal landing zone of proximal stent—thick fibro-calcific plaque—MLA—2.7 mm^2, MLD—1.8 mm which was covered with 2.75 × 30 mm stent (overlapping proximal RCA stent and distal RCA stent) **(Fig. 10)**.

Mid-RCA stenting done with 2.75 × 30 mm Resolute Onyx Stent. The final result was good with TIMI-III flow with no complications **(Figs. 11A and B)**.

Potential Mechanisms of In-Stent Atherosclerosis

- Absent or dysfunctional endothelium due to endothelial denudation poststenting, eluted drug-induced inhibition of reendothelialization, and disturbed flow-induced upregulation of proinflammatory cell migration into intima in a similar but potentially accelerated manner promoting neoatherosclerosis.
- Chronic foreign body inflammatory reaction to metal/polymer of stent with subsequent neovascularization and macrophage recruitment might promote neoatherosclerosis.
- The underlying native atherosclerotic plaque might contribute to in-stent atherosclerotic lesion either directly via expansion through stent struts or indirectly via release of growth factors and chemoattractants (paleoatherosclerosis).

Potential natural history of atherosclerosis and stent failure. Following stenting, the atherosclerotic plaque (neoatherosclerosis or paleoatherosclerosis) might progress gradually or rapidly contributing to ISR. At any time, point, it might rupture or erode leading to stent thrombosis or rapid ISR progression due to recurrent cycles of plaque rupture and healing. These events might occur inside as well as behind the stent. In the latter case, intravascular imaging would merely detect various accompanying findings, such as strut malapposition, stent underexpansion, or coronary evaginations.

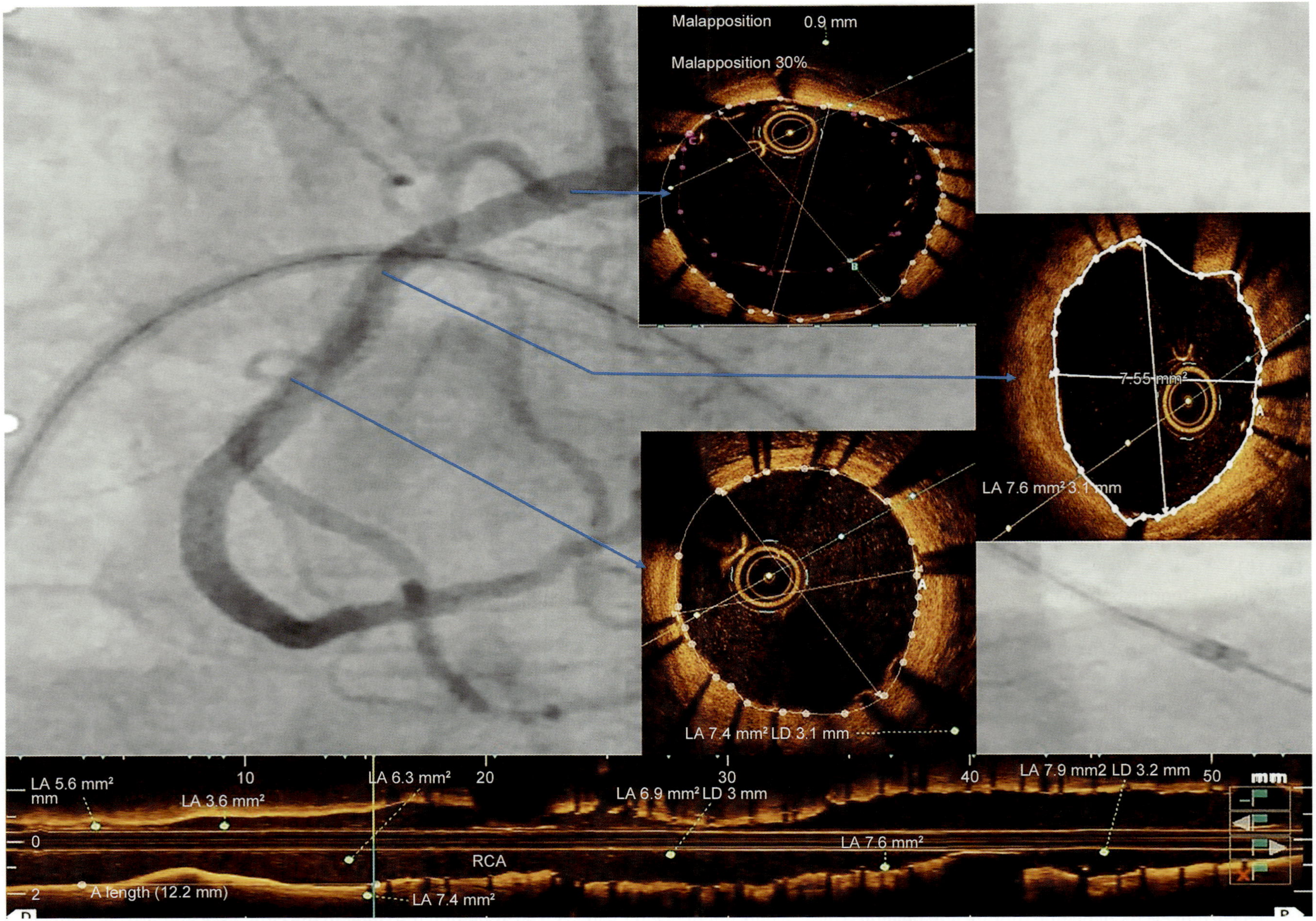

Fig. 9: Poststenting assessment for malapposition, expansion, and edge dissections.

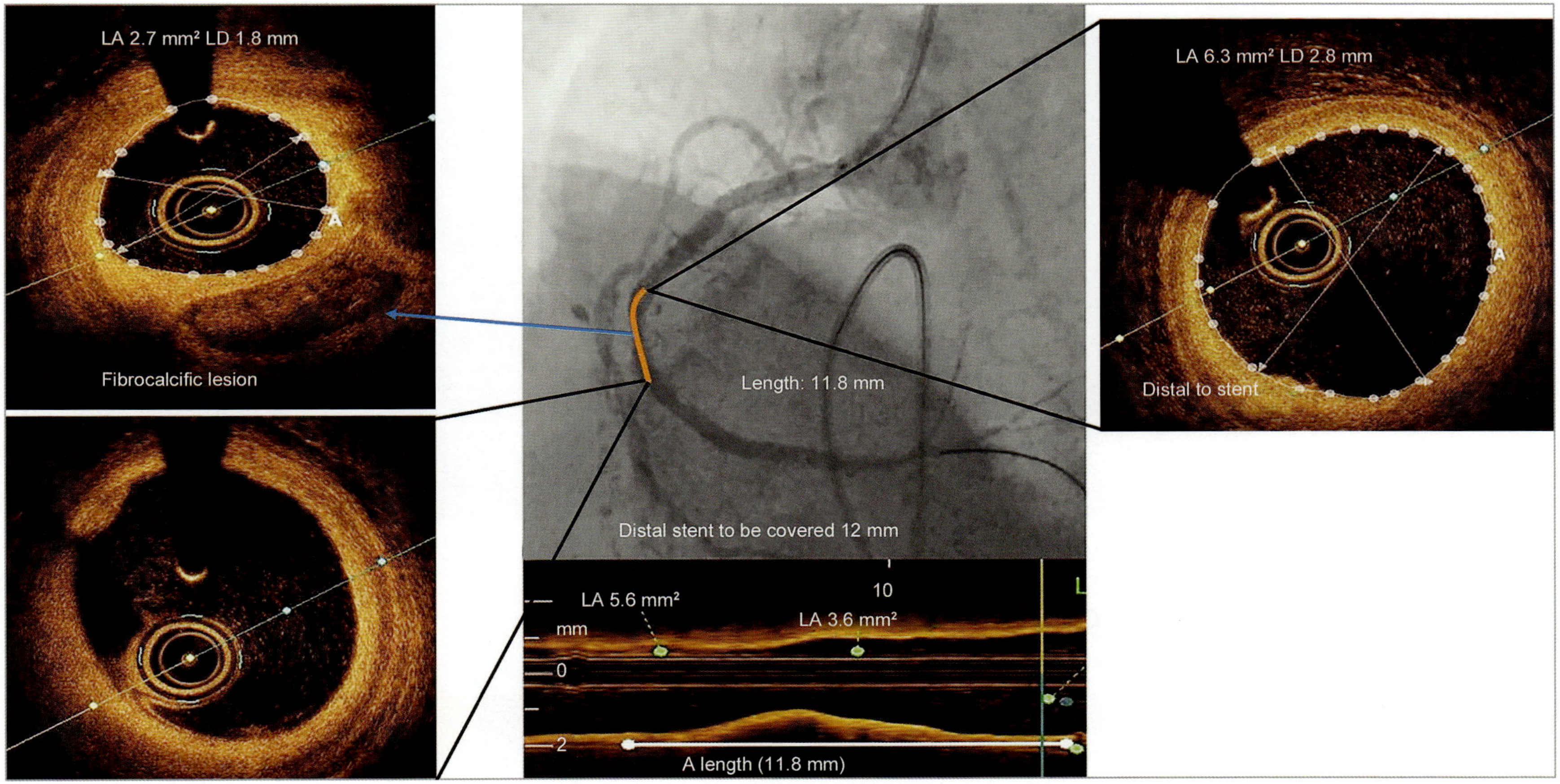

Fig. 10: Plaque between distal edge of proximal stent and proximal edge of distal stent.

Very late events (beyond a year) were similar between BMS and 2nd generation DES-Approximately 1–2%/year, and By Five years, TLF/TVF with Contemporary DES occurs in nearly 1 in 7 patients

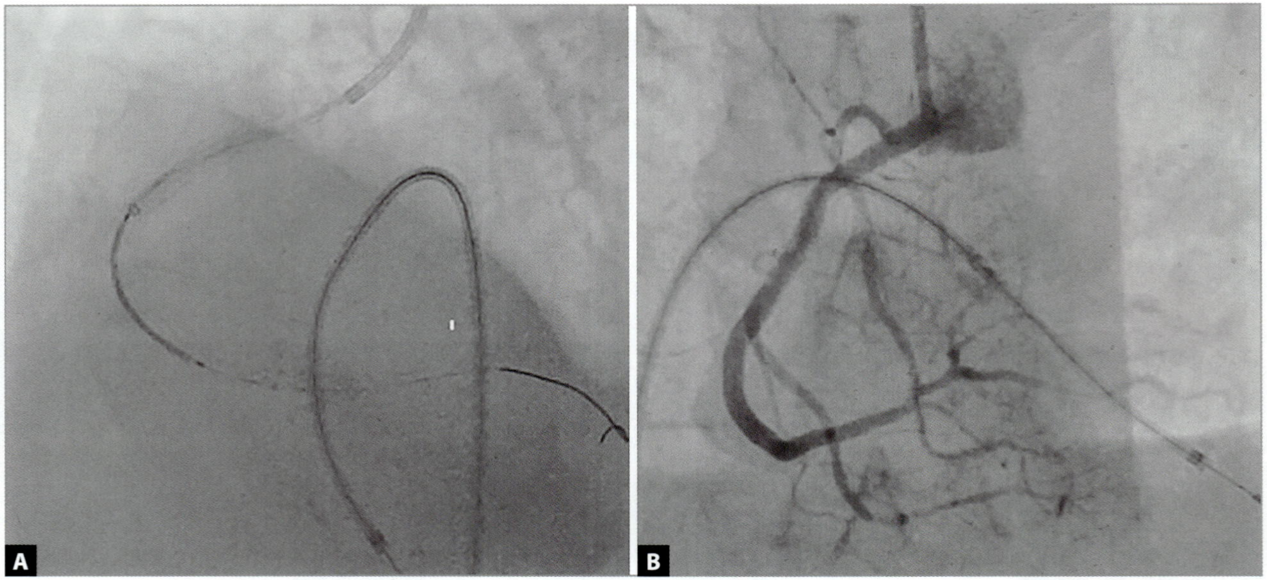

Figs. 11A and B: Mid RCA stenting and final result.

Extend the help of Guide Extension Catheter

- Facilitates placement of devices
- Expedites the procedures
- Limits the extension of IMH
- Useful to trap and retrive the dislodged/broken devices.

CASE 2

Optical coherence tomography (OCT) evaluation of stent thrombosis-inferior ST-elevation myocardial infarction (STEMI).

CLINICAL HISTORY

A 53-year-old male presented with ACS inferior wall STEMI. Past history of PCI of RCA in 2012 (4.5 × 25 mm optima tacrolimus eluting stent to proximal RCA, mid RCA with 3.5 × 20 mm cobalt chromium stent, proximal—mid overlapping stented with 3.5 × 18 mm cobalt chromium stent). ECG-ST elevations and T inversions in inferior leads, 2D echo—good LV function, EF—62%. Hb—13.8 g/dL, S. Cr—0.8 mg/dL, B. urea—20 mg/dL, and estimated glomerular filtration rate (eGFR)—100 mL/min.

Coronary angiography-LMCA—normal, LAD—mid 30-40% lesion, slow flow, LCX—proximal 30-40% lesion with slow flow, RCA—proximal—mid 70-80% ISR, PDA and PLVB—normal **(Figs. 12A to C)**.

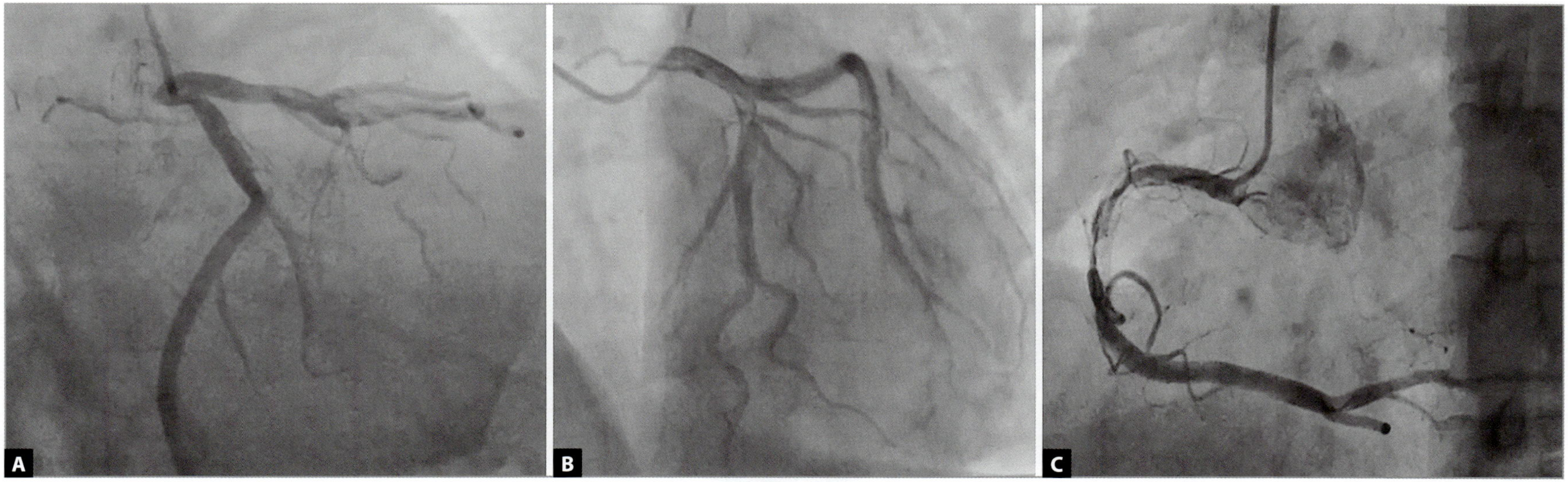

Figs. 12A to C: Coronary angiogram.

PROCEDURE

Route—right radial approach (RRA), 7 Fr JR 3.5 guiding catheter, RCA lesion was crossed with 0.014" Sion Blue wire and predilated with 2.0 × 15 mm Tazuna balloon.

Prestenting OCT showed long segment fibrotic intimal hyperplasia within the stent. Speckled ISR, area of stenosis 80% **(Figs. 13A to C)**.

Predilated with 3.5 × 15 mm NC Trek balloon, proximal stenting was done with 4.0 × 38 mm Resolute Onyx Stent, distal RCA stenting was done with 4.0 × 15 mm Resolute Onyx Stent and postdilated with 4.5 × 12 mm NC Trek balloon.

Predilatation was done with 2.0 × 15mm Tazuna balloon, proximal stenting done with 4.0 × 38 mm Resolute Onyx Stent, distal RCA stenting done with 4.0 × 15 mm Resolute Onyx Stent, postdilatation done with 4.5 × 12 mm NC Trek balloon. Final result is shown in **Figures 14A to E**.

Poststenting OCT crossed with GuideLiner support which showed well-apposed and expanded stent struts with no edge dissection **(Figs. 15A to C)**.

Postprocedure Angio view showed well-implanted stents with TIMI-III flow without any dissection. Patient was discharged on third day post procedure in a stable status.

Comparison of OCT data for BMS and first- and second-generation DES if stent duration <2 years **(Table 3)**.

The major findings were (1) the frequency of neoatherosclerosis was significantly greater in the DES than in the BMS group, (2) longitudinal extension of neoatherosclerosis in the stent segment was significantly less in the DES than in the BMS group, and (3) the minimum fibrous cap thickness was significantly greater in the DES than in the BMS group **(Figs. 16A to B)**.

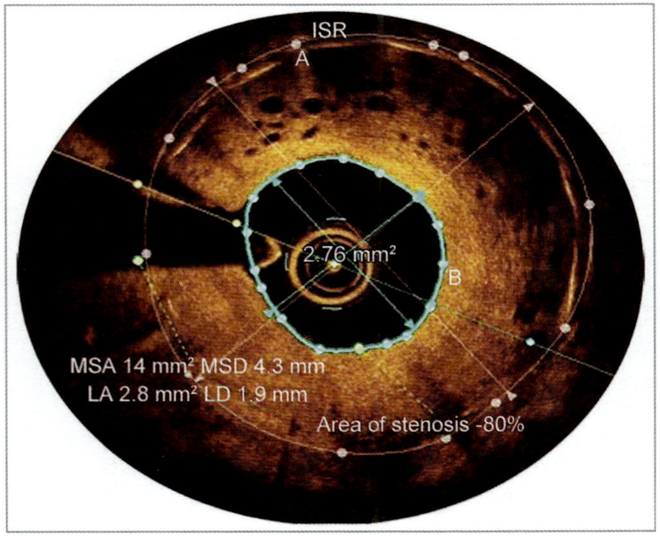

Fig. 13A

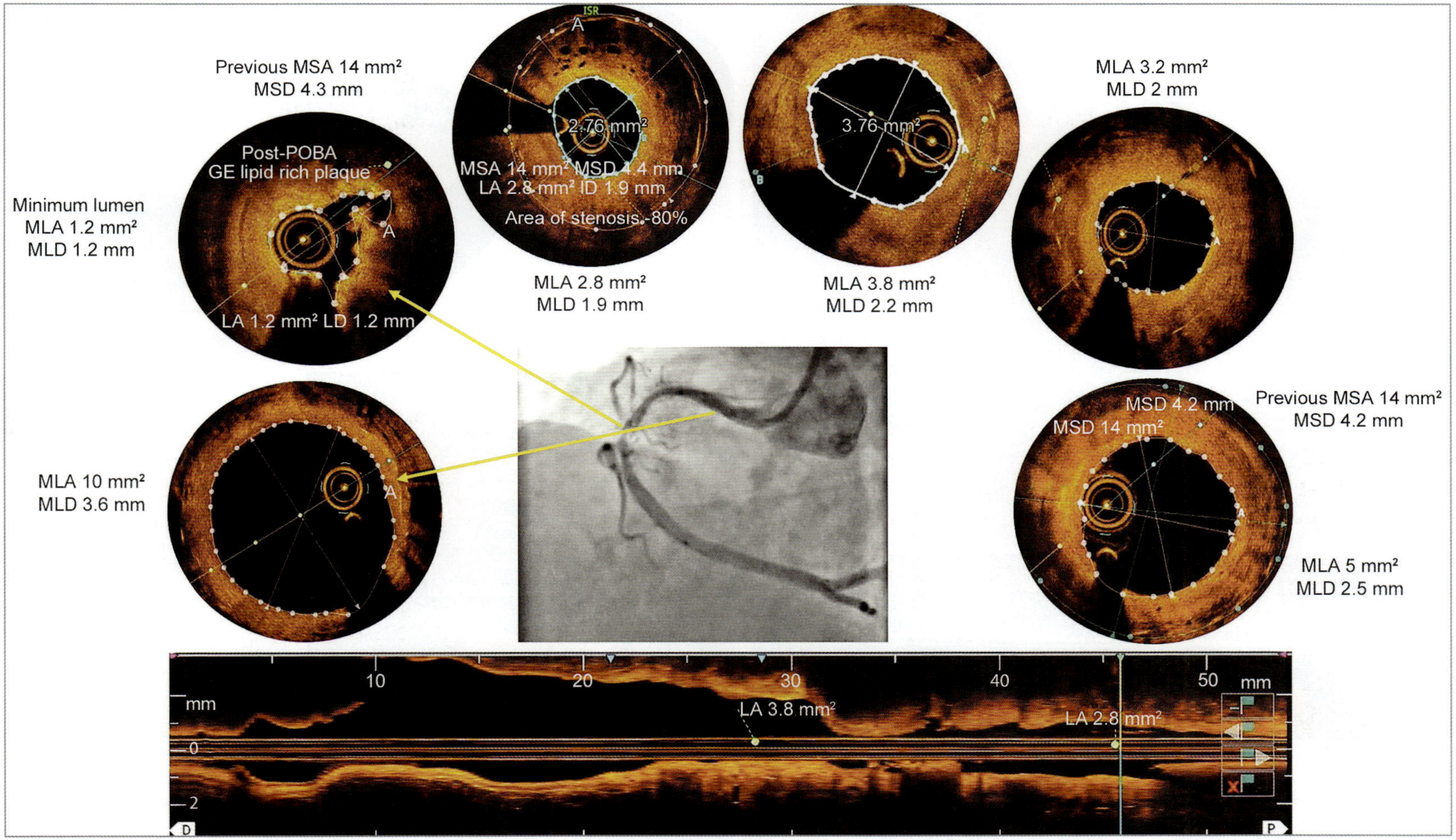
Previous MSA 14 mm²
MSD 4.3 mm
Post-POBA
GE lipid rich plaque
Minimum lumen
MLA 1.2 mm²
MLD 1.2 mm
LA 1.2 mm² LD 1.2 mm
2.76 mm²
MSA 14 mm² MSD 4.4 mm
LA 2.8 mm² ID 1.9 mm
Area of stenosis -80%
MLA 2.8 mm²
MLD 1.9 mm
3.76 mm²
MLA 3.8 mm²
MLD 2.2 mm
MLA 3.2 mm²
MLD 2 mm
MLA 10 mm²
MLD 3.6 mm
MSD 4.2 mm
MSD 14 mm²
Previous MSA 14 mm²
MSD 4.2 mm
MLA 5 mm²
MLD 2.5 mm
LA 3.8 mm²
LA 2.8 mm²

Fig. 13B

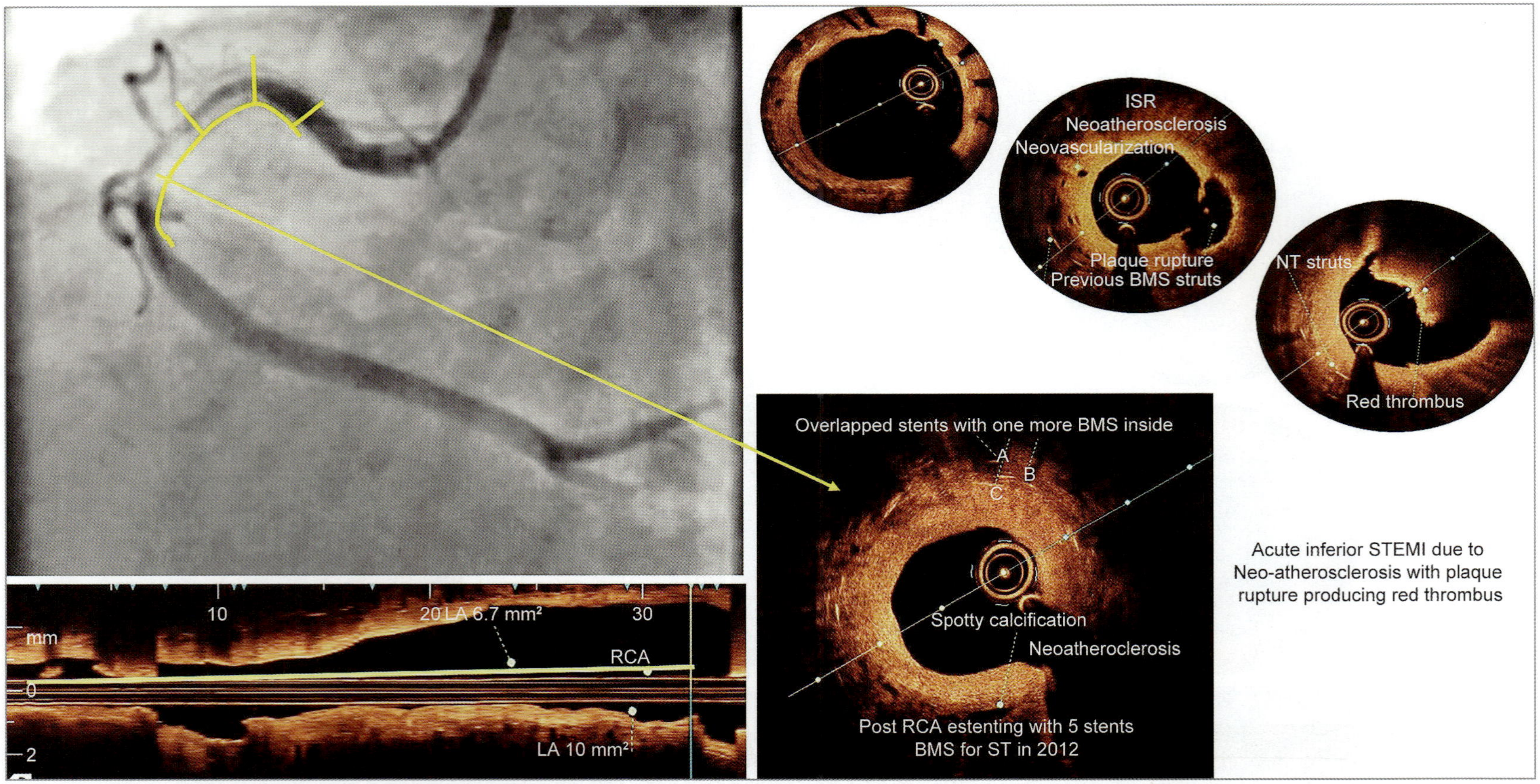

Fig. 13C

Figs. 13A to C: Prestenting OCT assessment: (A) Heterogenous ISR; (B) Speckled ISR; (C) Area of stenosis 80%.

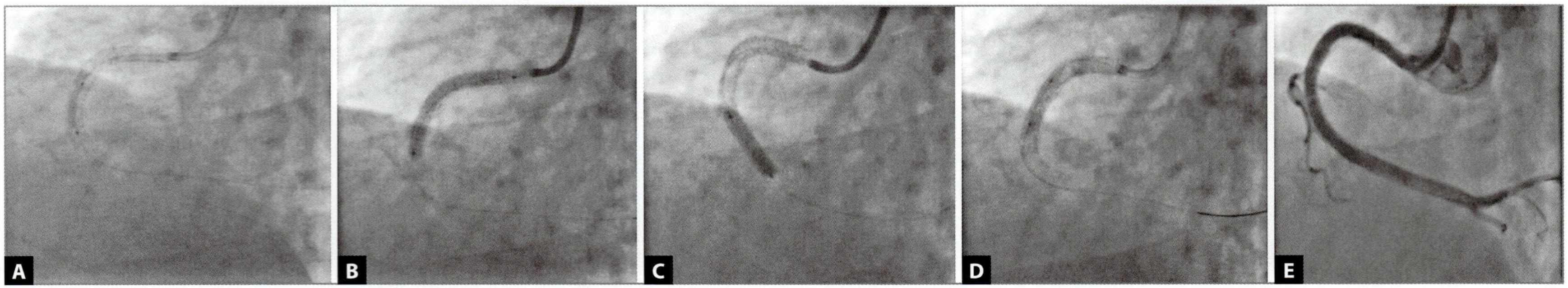

Figs. 14A to E: Predilatation, proximal and distal stenting, postdilatation, and final result.

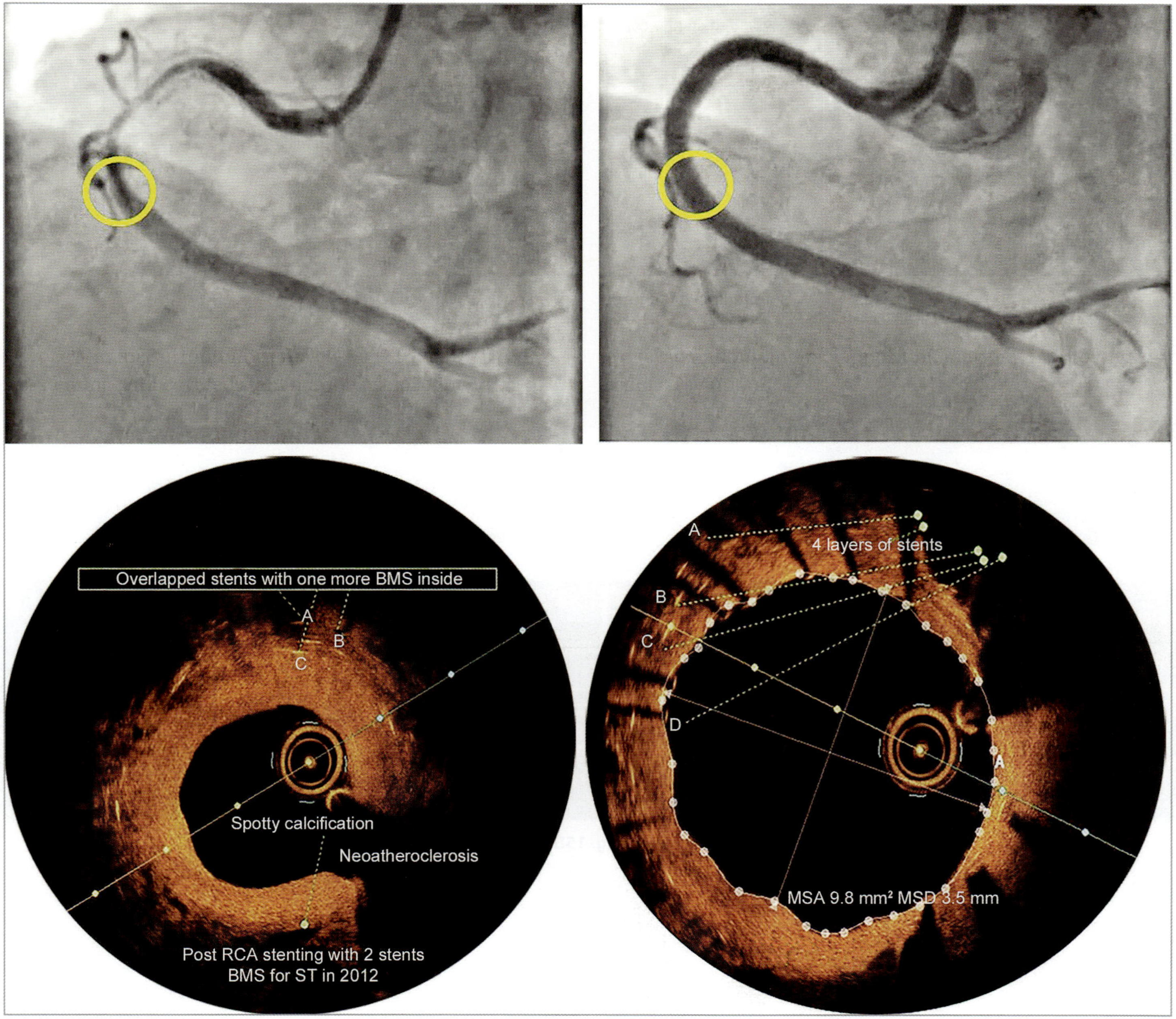

Overlapped stents with one more BMS inside
A
B
C
Spotty calcification
Neoatheroclerosis
Post RCA stenting with 2 stents
BMS for ST in 2012
A
4 layers of stents
B
C
D
A
MSA 9.8 mm² MSD 3.5 mm

Fig. 15A

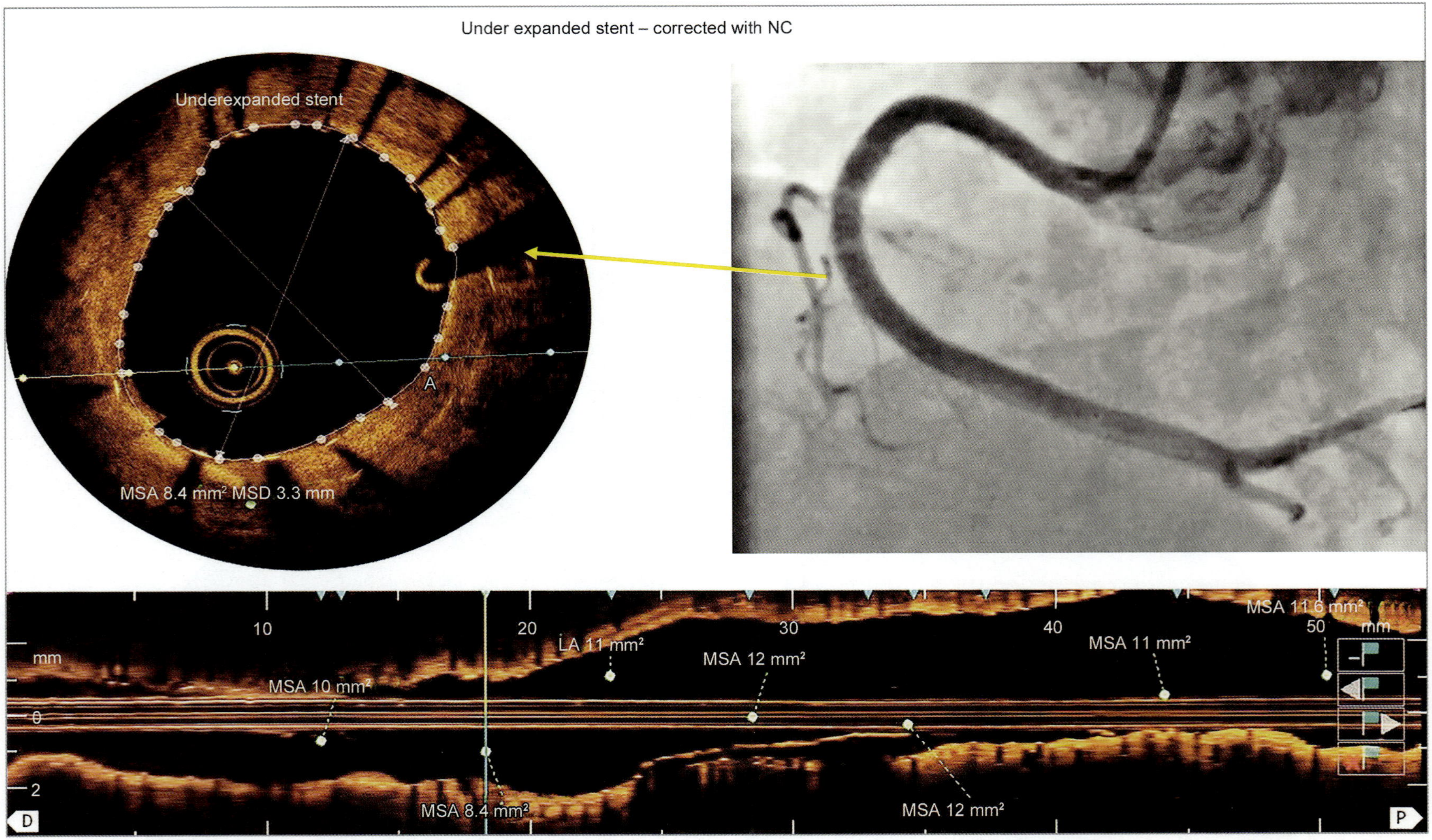
Under expanded stent – corrected with NC
Underexpanded stent
A
MSA 8.4 mm² MSD 3.3 mm
10
20
30
40
50
mm
mm
0
2
LA 11 mm²
MSA 12 mm²
MSA 11 mm²
MSA 11.6 mm²
MSA 10 mm²
MSA 8.4 mm²
MSA 12 mm²
D
P

Fig. 15B

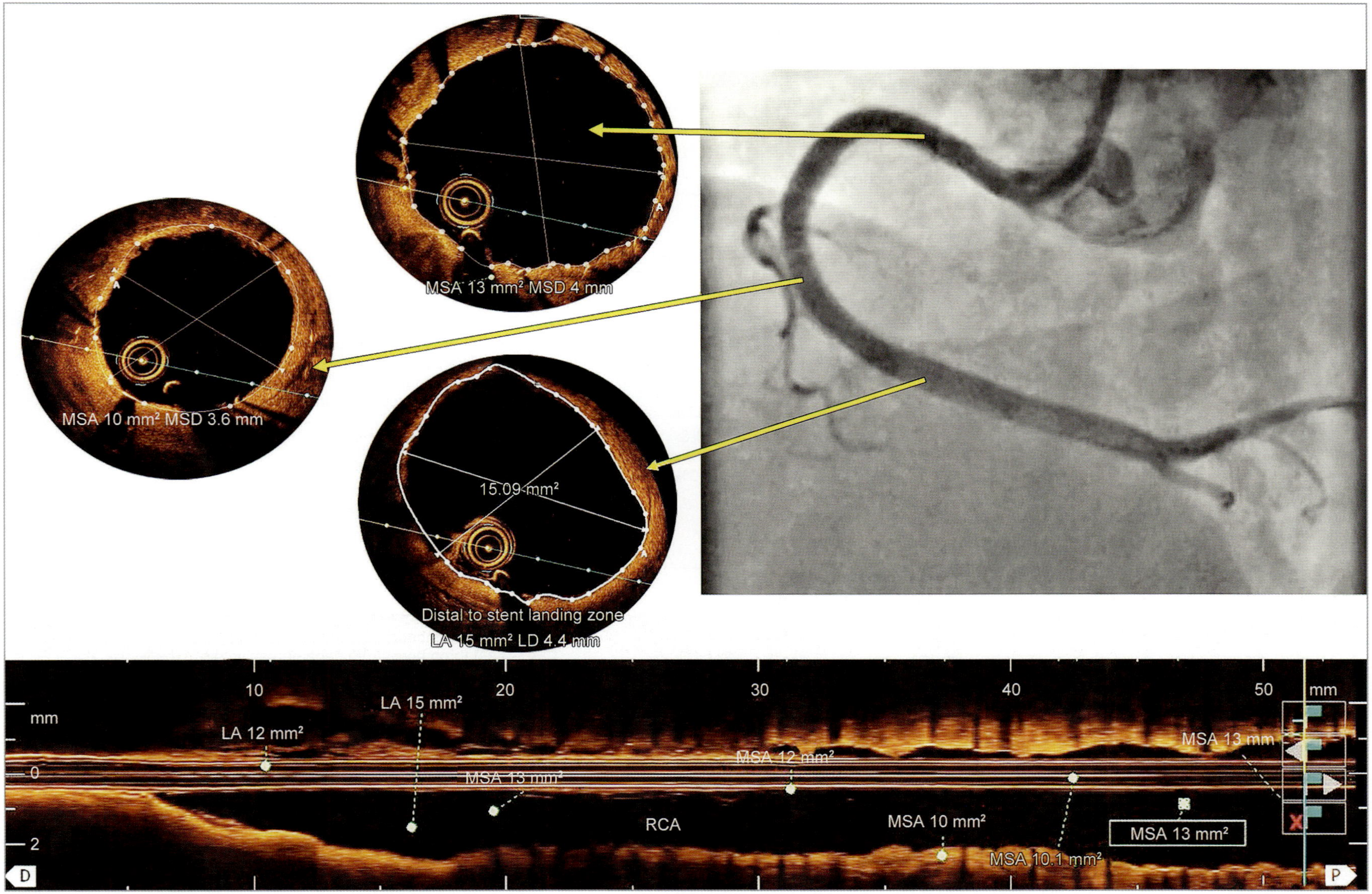

Fig. 15C

Figs. 15A to C: Poststenting OCT assessment: (A) Overlapping zone before stenting (3 layers) and after stenting (4 layers); (B) Underexpanded stent which was corrected with NC; (C) Well-expanded and well-apposed stent without stent edge dissection.

TABLE 3: Comparison of OCT data for BMS and first- and second-generation DES.

	BMS (n = 22)	***First-generation DES (n = 19)***	***Second-generation DES (n = 30)***	***p value***
Neoatherosclerosis	2 (9.2%)	13 (68.4%)	9 (30)	<0.001
Fibrous cap thickness, μm	85 ± 17.1	113 ± 42	131.4 ± 17.3	0.375
Longitudinal extension of neoatherosclerosis, %	30 ± 14.1	19.3 ± 4.7	7.8 ± 12.9	0.041

(BMS: bare metal stent; DES: drug-eluting stent; OCT: optical coherence tomography)

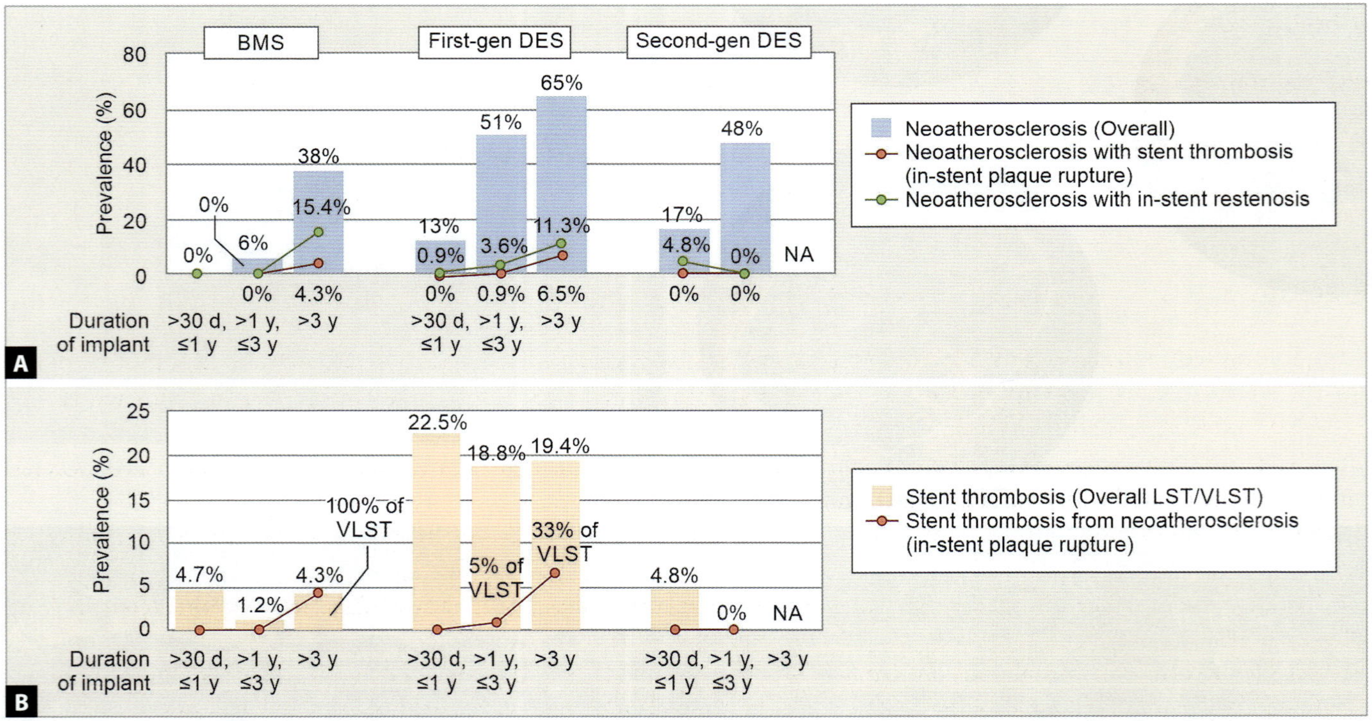

Figs. 16A and B: (A) Prevalence of neoatherosclerosis in BMS, first- and second-generation drug-eluting stents stratified by duration of implant (bar graphs) along with the prevalence of restenosis (green line) and thrombosis (orange line) in the lesions with neoatherosclerosis and late stent failure; (B) Prevalence of overall stent thrombosis, in association with neoatherosclerosis (in-stent plaque rupture).

CASE 3

Stent thrombosis due to Under-expanded severe Calcified LCX.

CLINICAL HISTORY

A 51-year-old male, No comorbidities, Presented with—Acute onset chest pain for 2 hours. ECG—ST ↑ in II/III/aVF with ST↓ V1-V3, 2 D Echo—LV RWMA + EF—45%.

O/I: Hb-15.8 g/dL, Creatinine 0.9 mg/dL, Trop-I-450 ng/mL, CPK-MB-200 IU, LDL—156 mg/dL.

CAG: DVD with Mid LAD 80% calcific plaque, proximal LCX total occlusion.

PROCEDURE

LMCA engaged through RRA with EBU 3.5-6 Fr LCX wired with runthrough and sion blue 0.014 wire in OM branch. LCX lesion pre dilated with Ryurei 2.0 × 10 mm further dilated with 2.5 × 10 mm cutting balloon. Then LCX stenting with 2.5 × 33 mm Xience Alpine, Post dilatation with 2.75 × 12 mm NC trek. Final result was good with TIMI III flow with no complications.

Three hours after PCI patient suddenly developed chest pain with diaphoresis. Check angio showed acute stent thrombosis of LCX lesion crossed with runthrough wire and lesion pre dilated with Ryurei 2.0 × 10 mm.

OCT showed under-expanded stent due to severe circumferential calcification which required adequate plaque modification with IVL **(Figs. 17 and 18)**.

IVL done with 3.0 × 12 mm balloon 80 pulses delivered with guide plus backup. Post IVL OCT showed gain in the luminal area and fractures of calcium due to IVL **(Fig. 19)**.

Further dilated with 3.0 × 15 mm NC trek balloon. OM crossed with run through wire and pre dilated with 1.5 × 10 mm Ryurei balloon. Kissing balloon dilatation with 2.0 × 10 mm balloon in OM and 3.0 × 15 mm balloon in LCX. Final OCT run showed well expanded and apposed stent struts with no medial edge dissections. Final result was good with TIMI III flow **(Fig. 20)**.

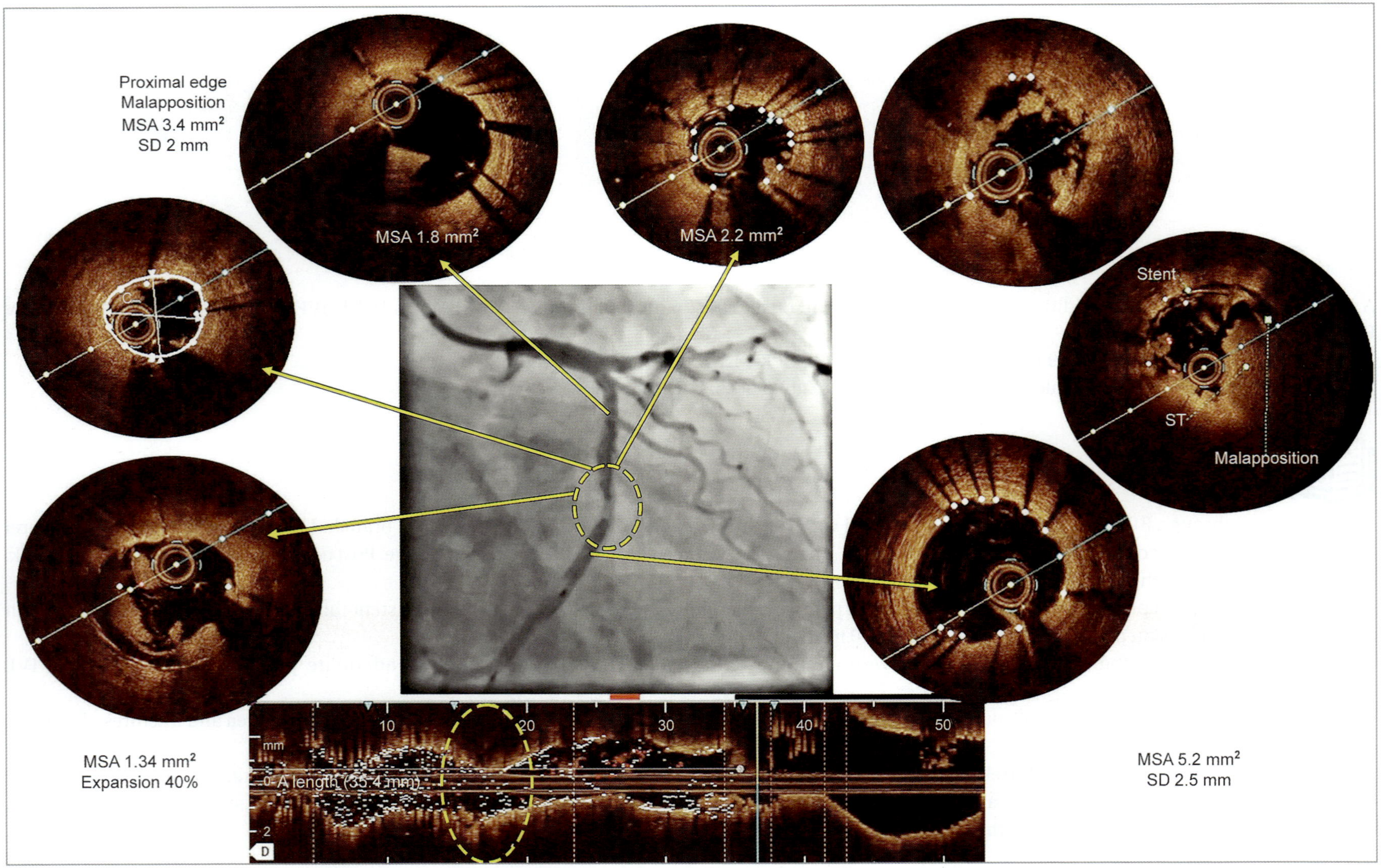

Fig. 17: OCT showing Acute stent thrombosis due to under-expansion and malapposition.

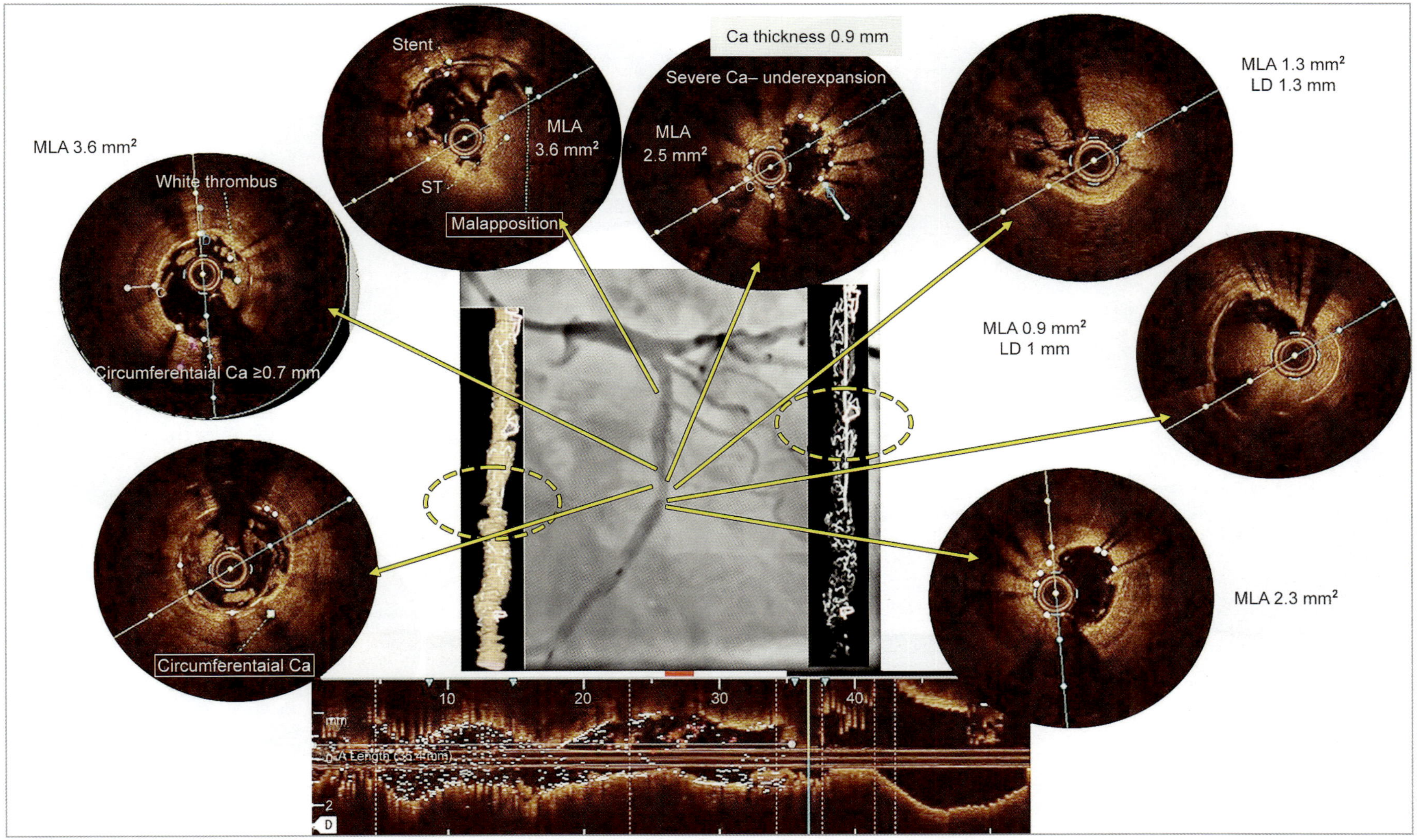

Fig. 18: OCT showing underexnanion and malapposition due to severe calcium.

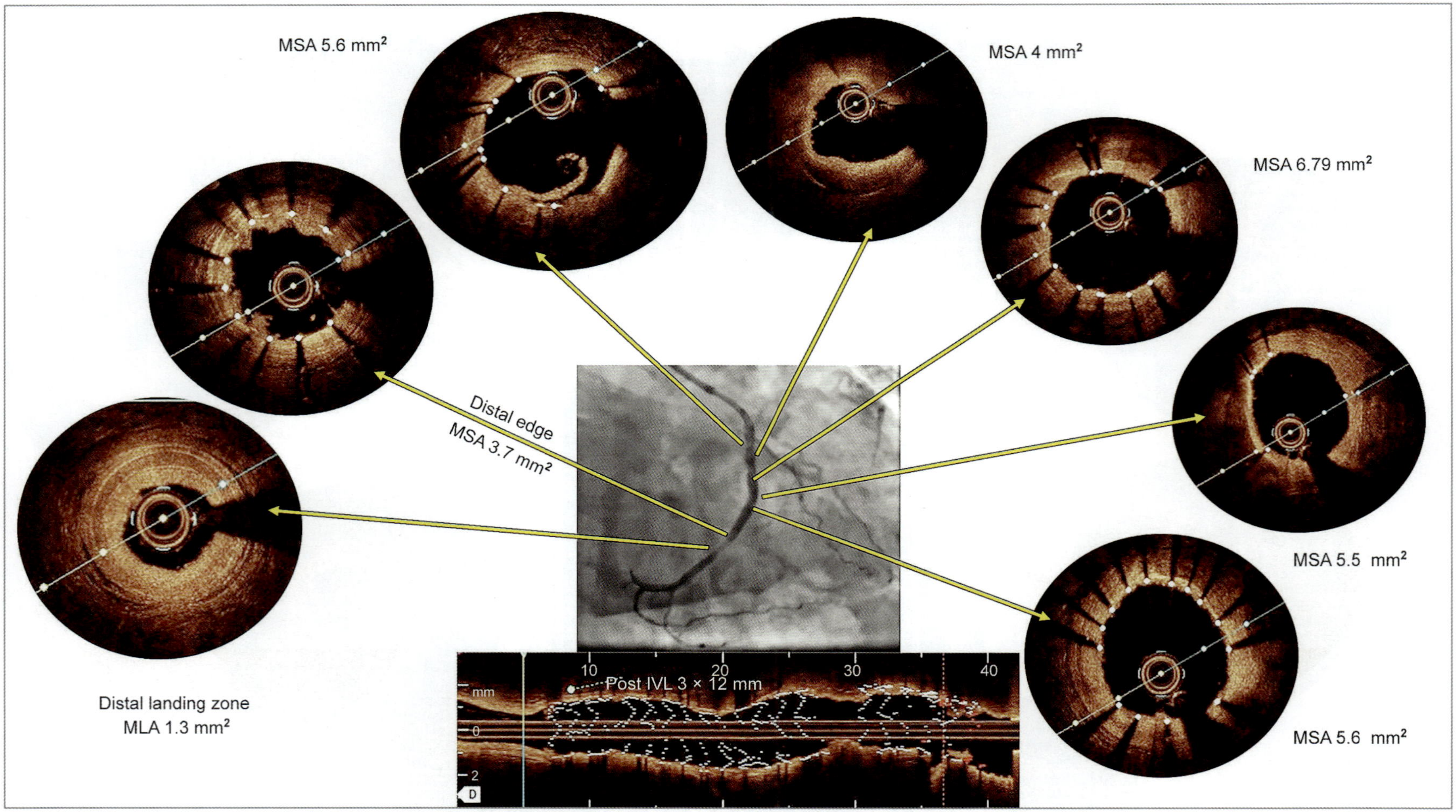

Fig. 19: Post IVL OCT showing adequate luminal gain and fractures.

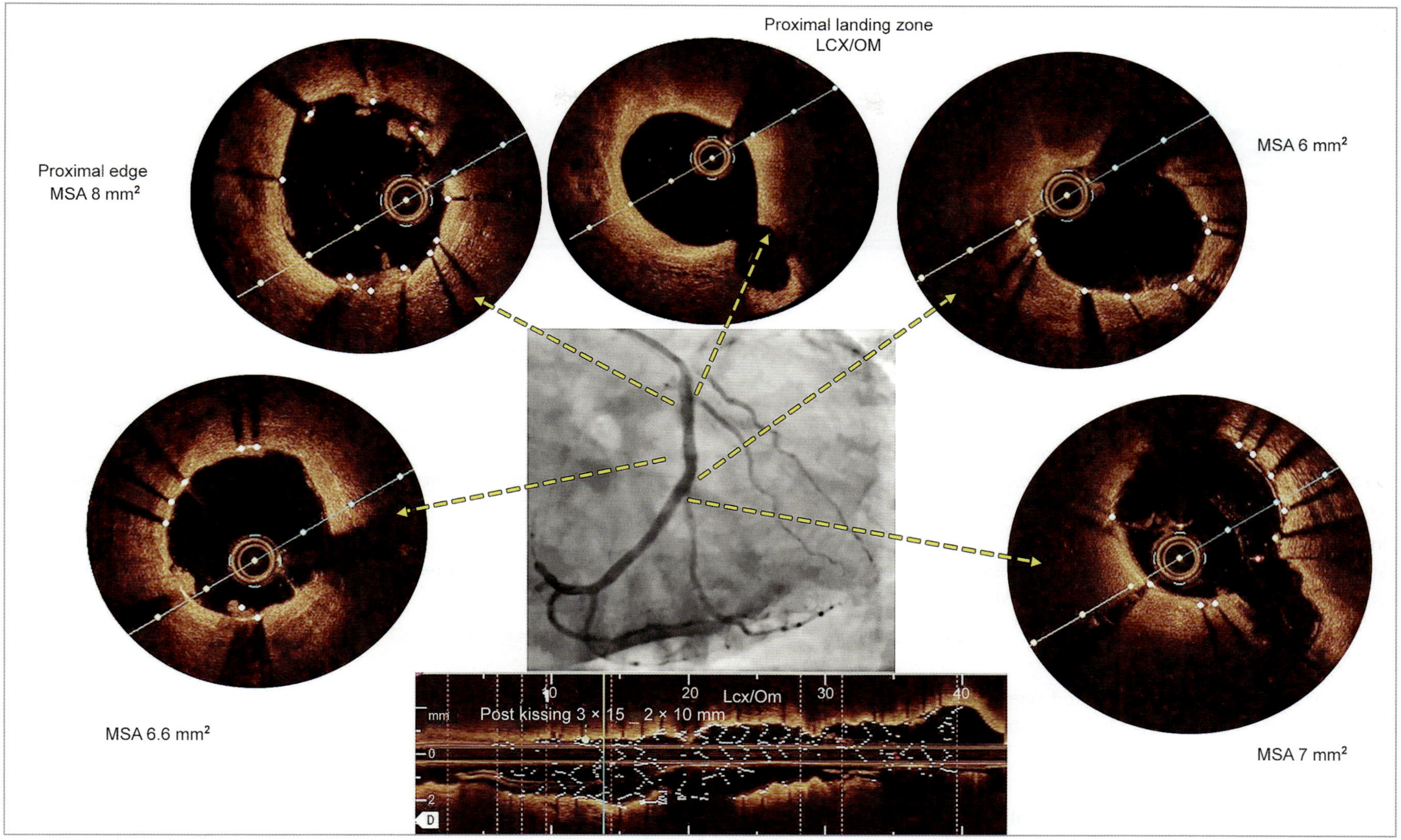

Fig. 20: Final OCT showing well expanded and apposed stent struts with no edge dissections.

CHAPTER 12

In-Stent Restenosis

ABSTRACT

Stent restenosis is observed in about 10% and 5–7% of all patients who underwent percutaneous coronary intervention (PCI) with drug-eluting stent (DES) in the USA and Europe respectively. In-stent restenosis (ISR) may present with various clinical presentations like asymptomatic status to symptomatic acute coronary syndrome (ACS) including myocardial infarction (MI) and sudden events. Neointimal proliferation is responsible for majority of cases during the first 2 years of poststenting period whereas neoatherosclerosis for maximum number after 2 years of DES stenting. Optical coherence tomography (OCT) plays a pivotal role in the evaluation and management of ISR because of its high-resolution images.

In-stent Restenosis

Stent restenosis is usually due to the progressive re-narrowing of a stented coronary artery lesion due to arterial damage with subsequent neointimal tissue proliferation leading to ischemic symptoms when it reaches to significant narrowing.

ANGIOGRAPHIC ISR

Coronary stenosis within the stented segment or landing zones consisting of 5-mm segments adjacent to the stent of >50% of the vessel diameter as determined by coronary angiography **(Table 1)**.

CLINICAL ISR

Significant ISR presenting with any one of these findings: (1) Evidence of ischemia on ECG, (2) evidence of positive result on physiological assessment, (3) significant luminal narrowing on intravascular imaging, and (4) restenosis producing ≥70% luminal narrowing.

Although most of the patients may present with stable ischemic heart disease, still some may present with symptoms and signs of ACS due to gradual narrowing of the lumen or neoatherosclerotic plaque rupture with thrombus formation.

Neointimal proliferation is responsible for the majority of cases of stent restenosis during the initial 2 years of poststenting follow-up period. After 2 years of stenting, it is most often due to progression of neoatherosclerosis with lipid intima and less frequently calcification inside the stented segment.[1]

Initial studies of PCI showed restenosis rate of 20–30% with BMS, and 5–15% with first-generation DES at 12 months follow-up. On the contrary,[2] PCI studies involving second-generation DES revealed ISR of <5% at 12 months. As per the evidence available, DES produces early development of

TABLE 1: Mehran's angiographic classification of ISR.

Type of ISR	*Characteristics*	*Occurrence*
I-Focal	Length <10 mm	42%
IA	The articulation or gap between stents	
IB	The proximal or distal margin	
IC	The body of the stent	
ID	Multifocal	
II-Diffuse	Length >10 mm, not exceeding the edges of the stent	21%
III-Proliferative	Exceeding the edges of the stents	30%
IV-Occlusive	Total occlusion with TIMI-0	7%

TABLE 2: Clinical classification of ISR.

Patient factors	*Lesion factors*	*Periprocedural risk factors*
Diabetes mellitus	Complex B2/C lesions	Suboptimal apposition
Renal insufficiency	Long lesions >20 mm	Underexpansion of the stent
ACS	Artery diameter <3 mm	Post-PCI MLD <3 mm
	CTO	Implantation of multiple stents
	Ostial lesions	Stent fractures
	Bifurcation lesions	Type of stent BMS/DES
	Lesions in venous bypass recurrent restenosis	

neoatherosclerosis and more often focal in nature, especially seen at the stent edges, overlapped, underexpanded, and stent fractures segments **(Table 2)**.

Angiographic patterns of restenosis have been described previously as focal, diffuse, stent edge, and occlusive without highlighting ISR mechanisms. In contrast, OCT illustrates various mechanisms responsible for the ISR and even shows the details of its distribution and composition of neointima in relation to stent.

ISR RISK FACTORS

Refer **Table 2**.

OCT IMAGE ANALYSIS

Neointimal hyperplasia area can be estimated after acquiring stent area and luminal area at various sites of restenosis segment and the percent NIH area is calculated as:

(NIH area/stent area) ×100 (NIH = stent area – lumen area)

Various factors related to patient, procedure, and stent might play a key role in the development of ISR **(Fig. 1A)**. However, procedure-related factors, like (1) small MSA—underexpansion, (2) malapposition, (3) inflow/outflow tract disease, (4) overlapped stent segments, (5) residual PB, (6) edge dissection, (7) intramural hematoma, and (8) stent fracture, are responsible for the majority of the correctable causes of ISR. OCT imaging during PCI enables operator to identify and helps in rectifying these factors thereby improves acute and long-term outcomes of PCI with DES implantation.

Optical coherence tomography can identify various morphological features of restenosis: Bare stent restenosis is seen as high-volume homogeneous signal tissue. On the contrary, DES restenosis is visible as layered pattern or homogeneous tissue types **(Flowchart 1, Table 3, and Fig. 1B)**.

MORPHOLOGICAL TYPES OF RESTENOSIS

- *Homogeneous type:* Seen as a uniform optical properties and high-backscattering and low-attenuation characteristics due to the high content of smooth muscle cells and collagen fibers which is associated with major adverse cardiovascular events (MACE) rate of 2.9%
- *Heterogenous type:* Appears as a speckled pattern of neointima speckled with areas of high and low backscattering distributed throughout the tissue, fibrin accumulation, organized thrombus, and inflammation and it is associated with MACE rate of 13.7%
- *Layered type* ***(Fig. 2E)****:* Visible as a concentric layer with different optical properties, an adluminal high scattering layer and an abluminal low scattering layer and this pattern is associated with a MACE rate of 7.3%
- *Peri-strut low intensity area (PLIA):* Appears as an area surrounding the stent struts with homogeneous lower intensity than the surrounding tissue

Restenosis tissue backscatter may be seen as high type in which the majority of tissue shows high backscatter and appears bright or low type, where the majority of tissue is seen as low backscatter and appears dark or black.

Uniform neointimal proliferation with microvessels, layered pattern with multiple microvessels in the dark layer overlying the stent struts, multilayered pattern are shown in **Figures 3A to C**.

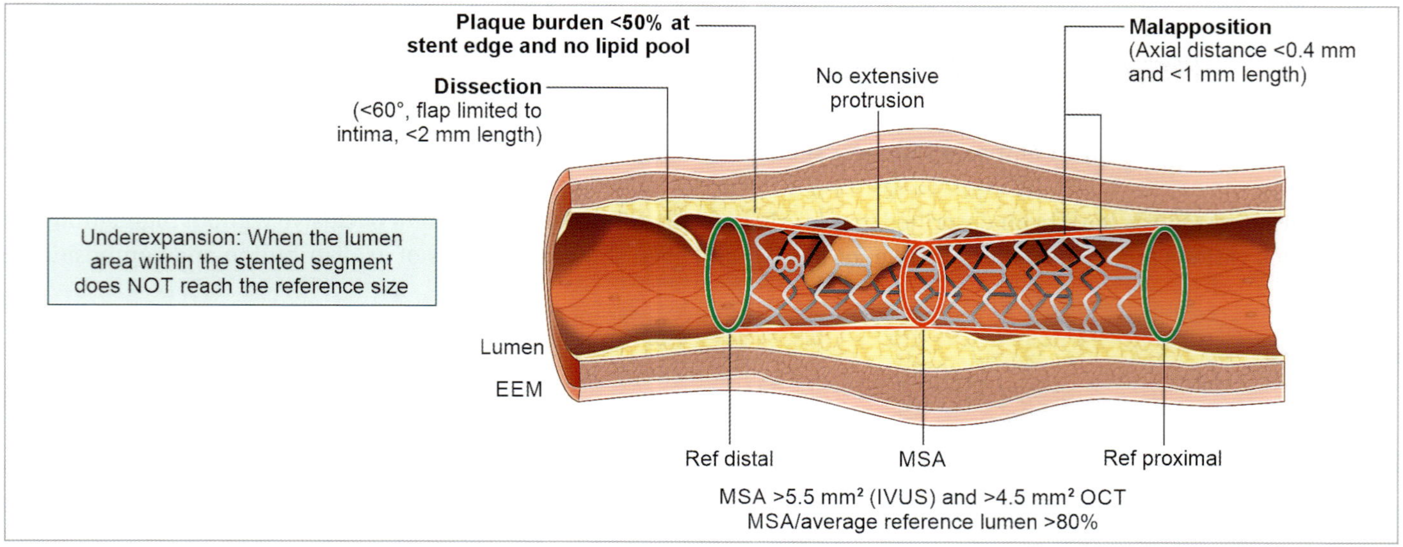

Fig. 1A

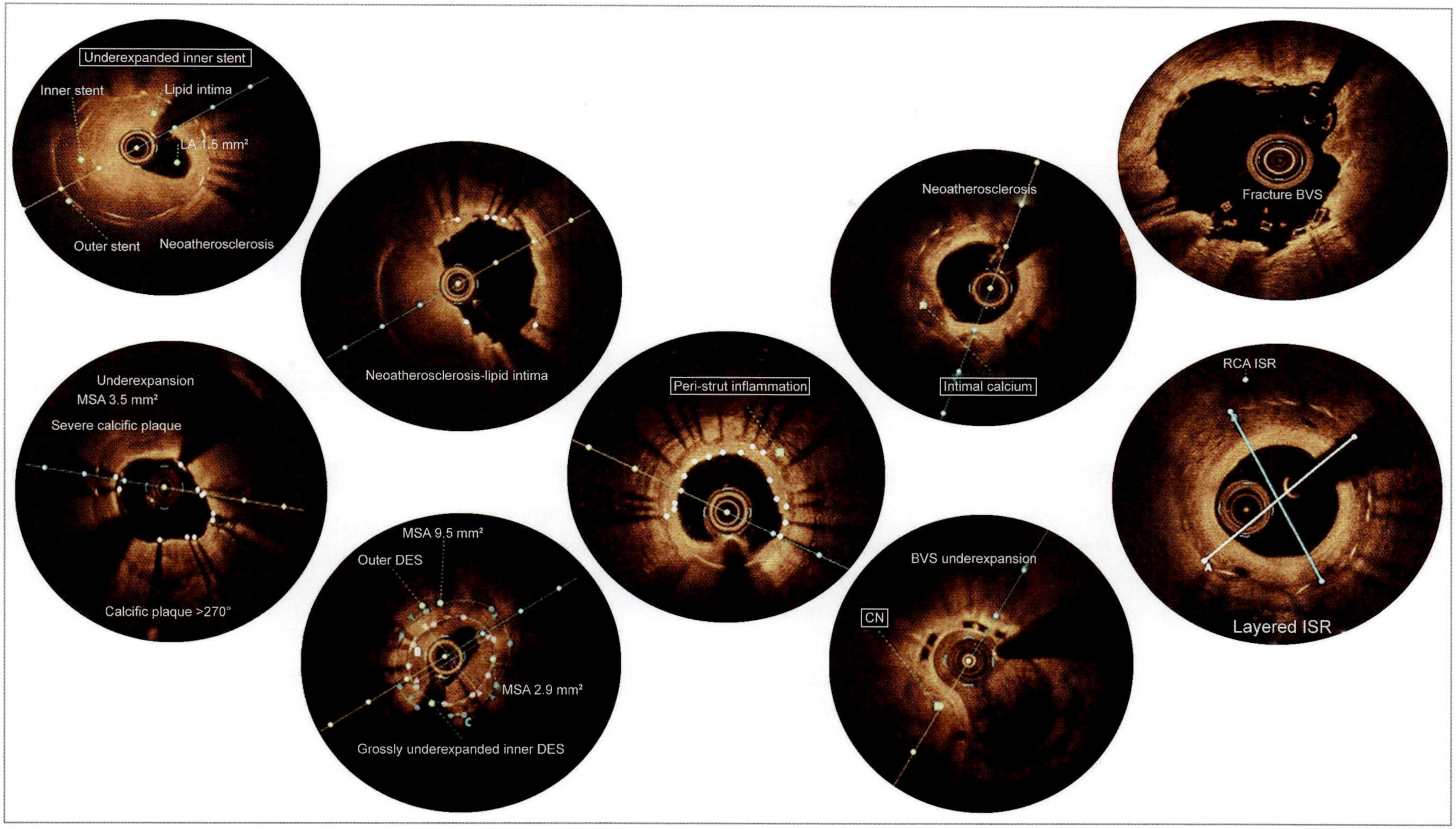

Fig. 1B

Figs. 1A and B: Predictors of DES outcomes by ESC.

Source: Shlofmitz E, Iantorno M, Waksman R. Restenosis of Drug-Eluting Stents: A New Classification System Based on Disease Mechanism to Guide Treatment and State-of-the-Art Review. Circ Cardiovascular Interv. 2019;12:e007023.

Flowchart 1: OCT classification of restenosis.

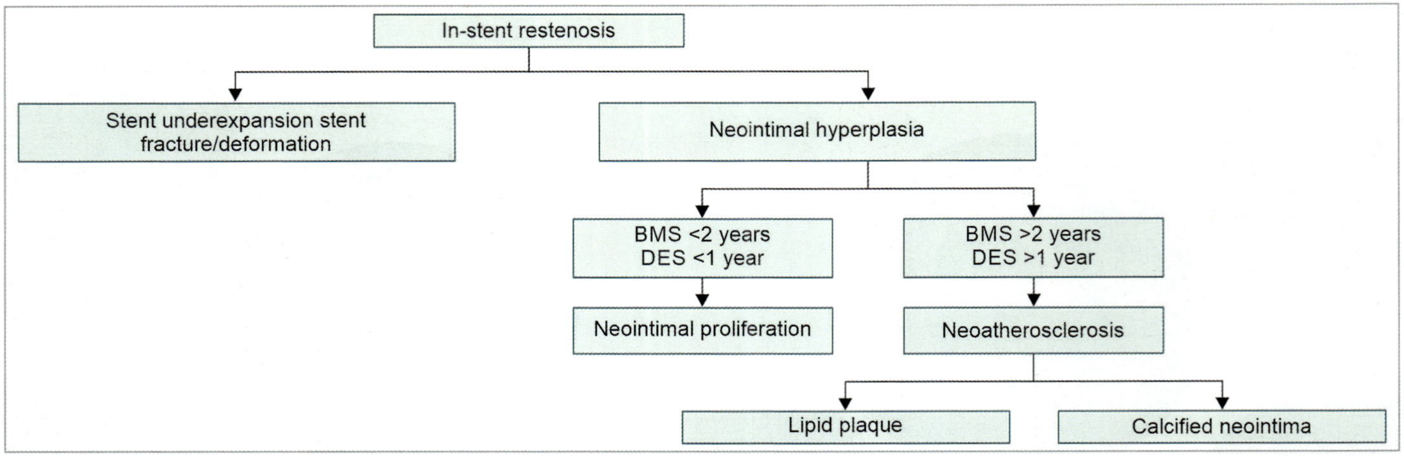

TABLE 3: ISR classification.[4]

Type	*Definition*		*Treatment options*
I	Mechanical	Underexpansion (type IA)	High pressure balloon
		Stent fracture (type IB)	DES
II	Biologic	Intimal hyperplasia (type IIA)	Balloons, DCB, DES, VBT
		Neoatherosclerosis, noncalcified (type II B)	DCB and DES
		Neoatherosclerosis, calcified (type II C)	Scoring balloon, ELCA, RA
III	Mixed pattern, combined mechanical, and biologic etiology		High pressure balloon with DCB, DES, or VBT
IV	CTO		DCB or DES, VBT for multiple layers, CABG
V	>2 layers of stent		Balloon, DCB, VBT, CABG

Optical coherence tomography runs helps in identifying various types of restenotic tissue morphologies and other details like microvessels, macrophage infiltration, lipid accumulation, in-stent calcification, or neointimal rupture with thrombus. ISR of first-generation DES is most often due to neointimal hyperplasia and stent under expansion. Patients with first-generation DES, manifests with neoatherosclerosis early and in some patients, it might be due to durable polymer. Even ISR cases of second-generation DES are mainly due to neointimal hyperplasia and stent under expansion[3] in spite of improved stent designs with biodegradable polymer and polymers with more biocompatible features.

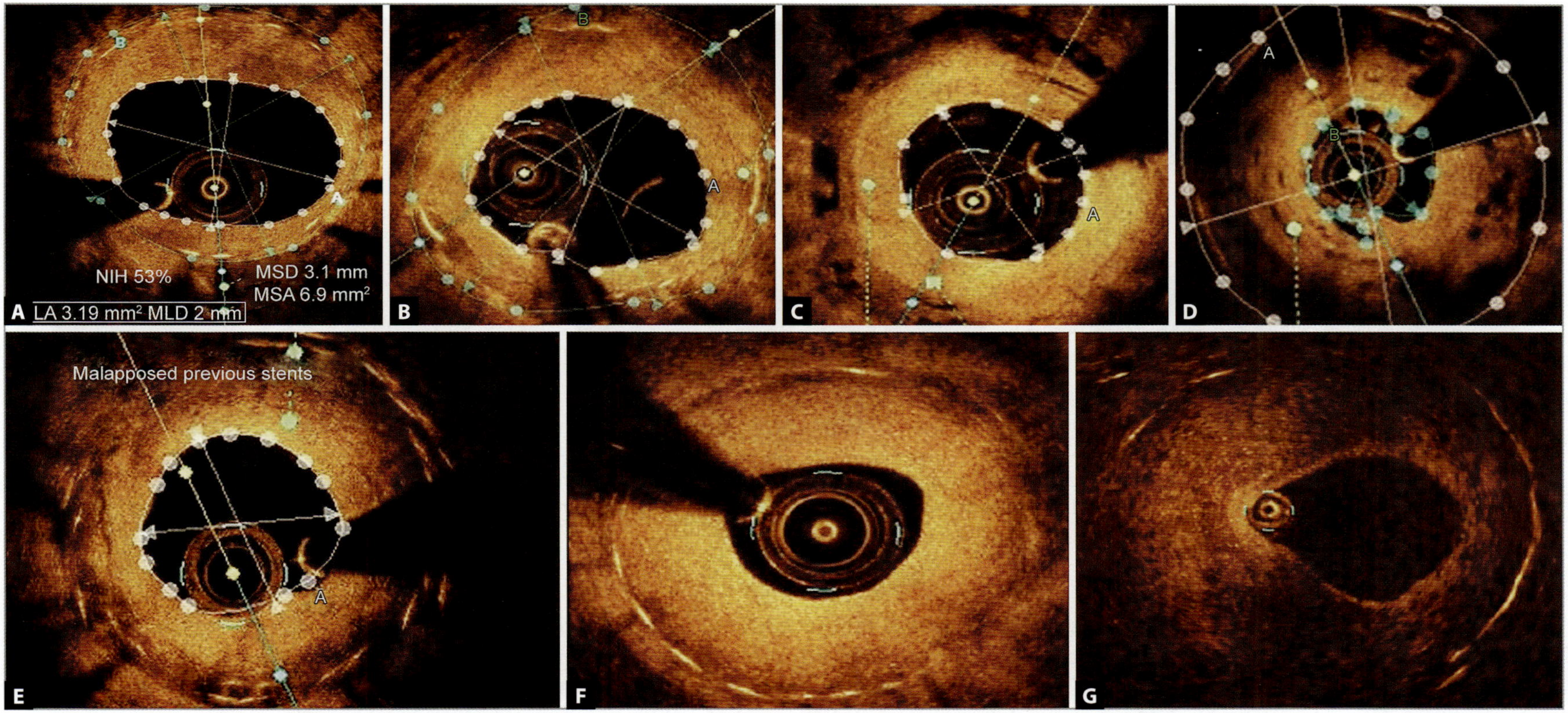

Figs. 2A to G: *Types of restenotic tissue structure:* (A to C) homogenous type; (D) heterogeneous type; (E) layered type; (F) restenotic tissue backscatter high type; (G) restenotic tissue backscatter low type.

Homogeneous neointima is largely seen within the entire stent in patients of both the early ISR and late ISR groups, whereas neoatherosclerosis associated with TCFA is the dominant morphology at the MLA site in the late ISR patients. The external elastic lamina is well seen at the ISR site which is well-delineated behind the stent struts which is useful for precise sizing of the vessel and devices, and to assess adequate expansion of the stent.

NEOATHEROSCLEROSIS

Optical coherence tomography: It is very useful in detecting neoatherosclerosis, differentiates lipid intima from calcific intima for decision-making and useful in decision-making about plaque modification strategies. Lipid neointima is observed in 67% of restenotic patients, seen as a signal-poor area with vague borders and overlying signal-rich bands, whereas calcific neointima is seen as well-delineated, signal-poor regions with sharp borders **(Figs. 4A and B)**.

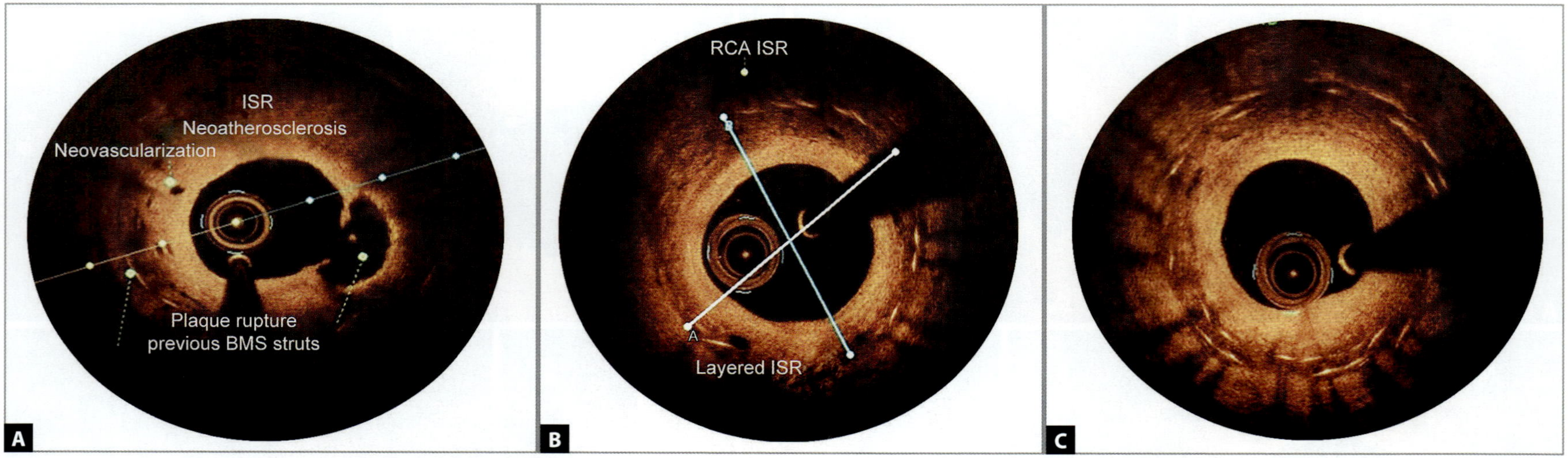

Figs. 3A to C: Early neointima to neoatherosclerosis. (A) Uniform neointimal proliferation with microvessels; (B) Layered pattern with multiple microvessels; (C) Multilayered pattern.

NEOATHEROSCLEROSIS IN DES

Lipid-rich intima of neoatherosclerosis may show macrophage infiltrations and neovascularization similar to lipid-rich plaques of native vessel atherosclerosis, and microvessels are often associated with plaque hemorrhage and its density is more in patients with advanced lesions of ISR.[5]

Thrombus was defined as a mass protruding into the lumen with a shadow effect due to poor transmission of infrared rays by red thrombus.[6]

In stent neoatherosclerosis with calcification was defined as a well-delineated, signal-poor region with sharp borders with neoatherosclerosis.

Patients with neoatherosclerosis are prone to develop higher number of MACE; e.g., composite of death, myocardial infarction, and target lesion revascularization (TLR) compared to those without NA.

STENT EDGE RESTENOSIS

Stent edge restenosis—Restenosis in landing zones adjacent to the proximal and distal border of the stent. Edge restenosis may be due to negative vessel remodeling, progression of plaque at the stent edges, and neointimal hyperplasia.

Stent edge restenosis mostly due to poor landing zones specially with lipid-rich plaques or plaque burden >50% and uncovered significant medial edge dissection due to high inflations of oversized balloon or stent at the time of index procedure **(Figs. 5A and B)**.[7] It can be prevented by landing in normal zones or zones with minimal plaque burden and by covering significant edge dissections with adequate length of additional stent.

Lipid arc in stent edge segments at post-PCI, and larger the lipid plaque the greater the risk of ISR.

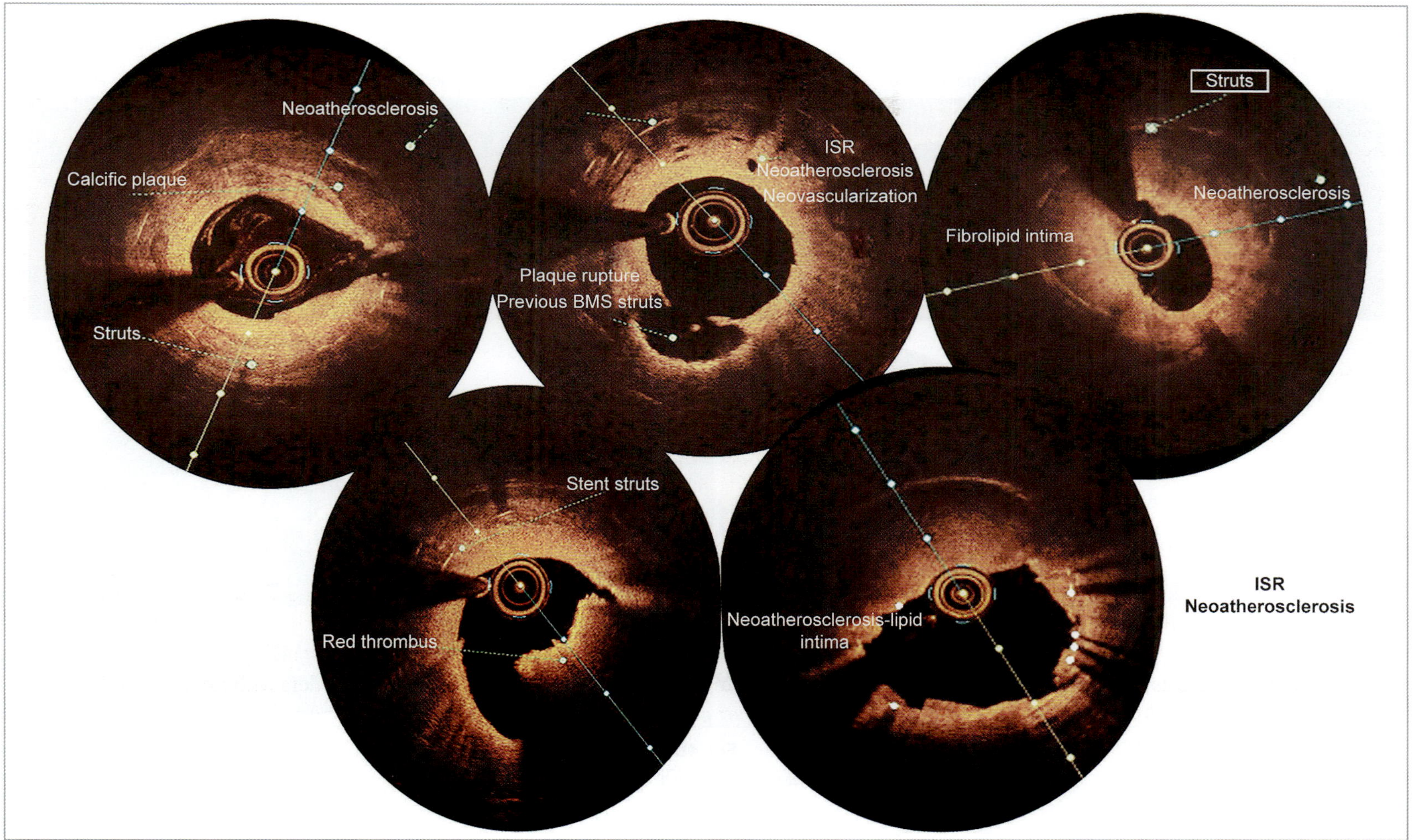
Neoatherosclerosis
Calcific plaque
Struts
ISR
Neoatherosclerosis
Neovascularization
Plaque rupture
Previous BMS struts
Struts
Neoatherosclerosis
Fibrolipid intima
Stent struts
Red thrombus
Neoatherosclerosis-lipid
intima
ISR
Neoatherosclerosis

Fig. 4A

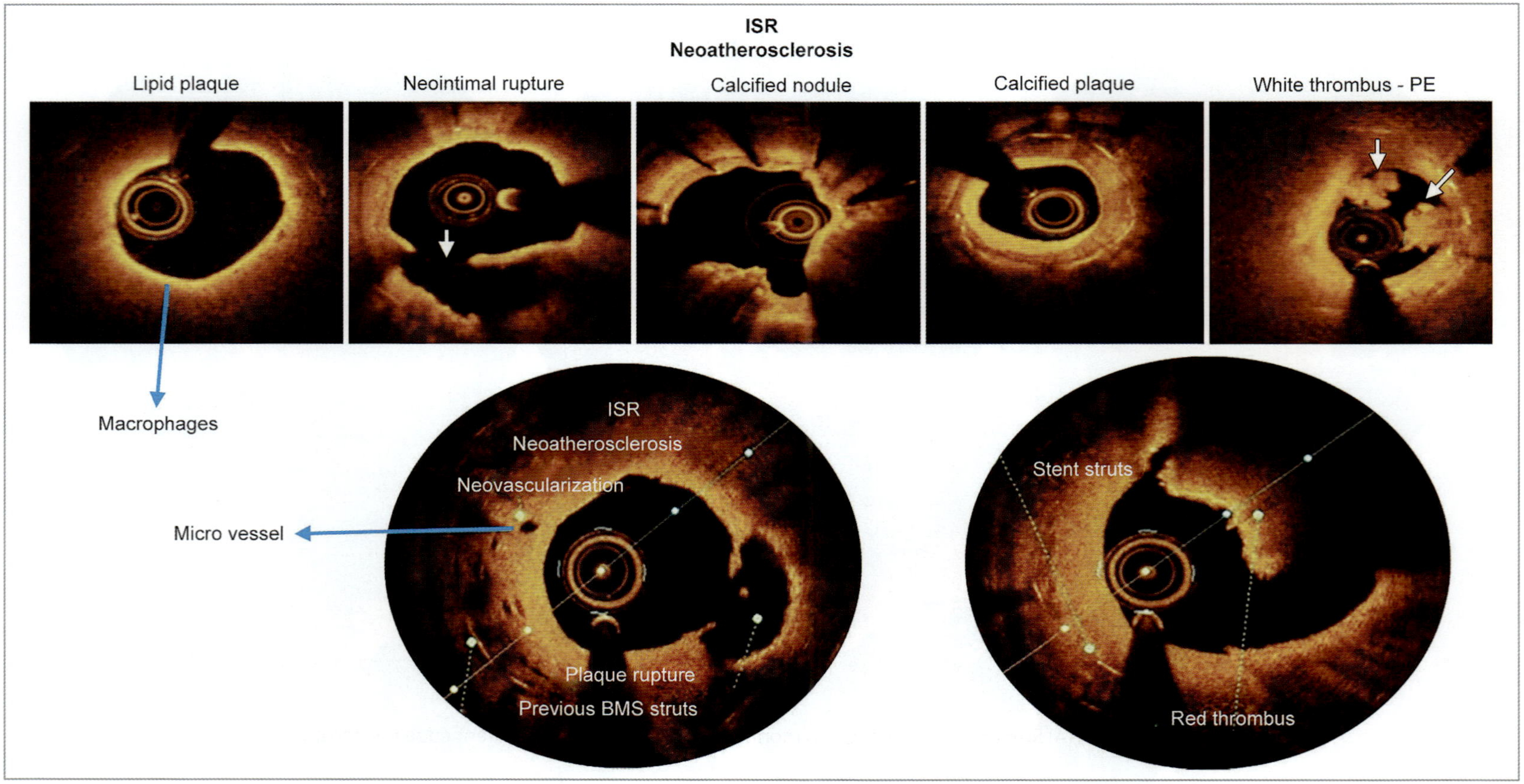

Fig. 4B

Figs. 4A and B: Different morphological types of neoatherosclerosis.

OCT-GUIDED MANAGEMENT OF ISR

The ISR may be due to underlying stent failure, such as uncovered struts, underexpansion, stent malapposition, edge dissection, and neoatherosclerosis. OCT gives insight into various mechanisms of ISR and helps in selecting various treatment strategies to manage ISR and ST patients.

TREATMENT OF ISR

Medical Treatment

Asymptomatic patients of ISR with negative FFR value should be managed medically with regular follow up for any recurrence of symptoms. Guideline-directed optimal control of lipids in cases of neoatherosclerosis with nonobstructive lipid intima reduced MACE rates at 12 months' follow-up (TLR 4.2% vs. 29.9%).[8]

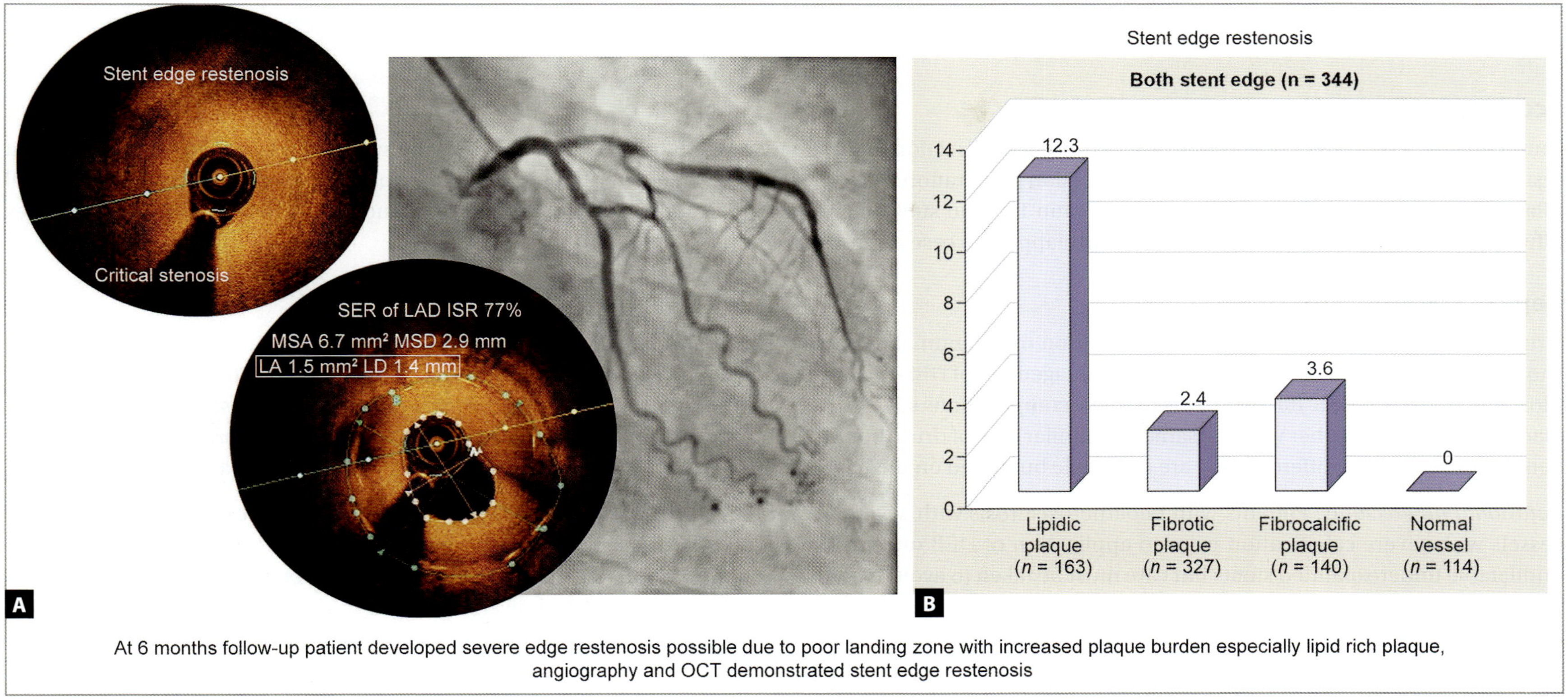

Figs. 5A and B: (A) Stent edge restenosis at 6 months follow-up; (B) Causes of stent edge restenosis.

Balloon Angioplasty

High-pressure plain balloon angioplasty using noncompliant (NC) or OPN NC balloons may be useful for restenotic focal lesions, underexpansion, and if short dual antiplatelet therapy (DAPT) duration is required due to high bleeding risk or other compelling reasons. Balloon slippage outside the stent can lead to edge dissections and suboptimal outcomes and this can be avoided by the use of a scoring/cutting balloon (CB).[9]

DCBs—As per the European Society of Cardiology (ESC)/European Association for Cardio-Thoracic Surgery (EACTS) guidelines, DCBs are considered as a class I indication for the treatment of ISR. As per the recent evidence, DEB results are better with prolonged balloon inflation times >60 seconds, a balloon: artery ratio >0.9, and additional usage of CB/scoring balloon to prepare the lesion. DCBs results are superior to repeat DES for patients with recurrent ISR due to multilayered DES and not inferior to DES stenting for other cases of ISR. Optimal lesion preparation is necessary before applying DEB to produce better acute and long-term results and it should not be used for the lesion preparation. During PCI, optimal result is to be confirmed with angiography and if necessary, with FFR or OCT/IVUS and if the result is suboptimal, stenting of ISR is recommended instead of DEB.

Optical coherence tomography is useful in assessing appropriate balloon diameter and size, and for the selection of the site to be treated to avoid reinjury of well-healed portions of the neointima. OCT evidence that may favor DEB over re-DES stenting includes the presence of a major side branch, multiple layers of prior stent implants, and small stent diameter. However, evidence of extensive intrastent with well-expanded and deeply embedded in the vessel wall, nonuniform stent strut distribution due to placement of the stent in a highly angulated segment, and the inability to achieve a stent-like result with balloon dilatation favor additional DES implantation.

Scoring/Cutting Balloons

Cutting balloon scores the plaque with well-controlled dissection planes therefore reduces elastic recoil, facilitate stent delivery and expansion. In-stent restenosis of ostial bifurcation lesions requires lesion preparation with CB or scoring balloon to allow adequate expansion and luminal gain before optimal dilatation with an NC balloon (balloon–artery ratio 1:1) and subsequent DEB application avoids the risk of more metallic struts resulting from complex bifurcation stenting or avoids repeated stent overlapping in cases of in-stent restenosis.[10,11]

Repeat Stenting with DES

Drug-eluting stent produces a profound inhibition of neointimal proliferation, thereby reduces neointimal hyperplasia associated with BMS-ISR and it should be considered as a treatment option. Management of DES-ISR is more challenging, and carry worse prognosis compared with patients of BMS-ISR. Most of the cases of DES-ISR due to mechanical complications such as stent under-sizing, edge dissection or stent fracture and these can be managed by placing another DES either with the same or a similar type of drug (homo-DES approach) or a different type of drug (hetero-DES approach). As of now, the benefits of choosing a different drug are debatable but based on the hypothesis that it may eliminate drug resistance or polymer-related problems.

Rotational atherectomy: Patients with neoatherosclerosis with severe neointimal calcification require adequate plaque modification similar to native vessels with severe calcification prior to application of DEB or redo DES stenting. Case series have also demonstrated the successful use of RA for undilatable underexpanded stents but care must be taken to avoid burr-related complications such as burr entrapment and burr stall **(Table 4)**.

In-Stent Restenosis (ROSTER) trail of ISR of BMS compared rotational atherectomy to POBA showed reduction in the amount of restenosis tissue and the rate of TLR at follow-up. Contrarily, In-Stent Restenosis trial (ARTIST) showed lower restenosis rates, an improved clinical outcome with POBA compared to RA group.

Intravascular lithotripsy: It is very useful in ISR due to underexpanded stents with deep calcium where it can address deep-seated calcium beneath the stent struts by emitting microbubbles generated due to sonic pressure waves and very useful to modify severe superficial intimal calcifications of neoatherosclerosis that are balloon crossable but balloon undilatable.

Excimer Laser Coronary Angioplasty

It (photoablation) uses light to breakdown, vaporize, and remove matter, and very helpful in patients with resistant stent underexpansion and ISR with uncrossable lesions.

Intracoronary Brachytherapy

Intracoronary radiation inhibits cell proliferation in the vessel wall and favors late remodeling by preventing adventitial fibrosis at the injury site. Brachytherapy has been shown to be inferior to DES but may be an option for patients with recurrent ISR. However, its results are not favorable compared to DEB.

Coronary artery bypass graft (CABG) should be considered to patients with recurrent ISR involving major coronary arteries supplying large area of myocardium with good distal vessel segments suitable for bypass grafting particularly those with a diffuse ISR lesions, especially without any comorbidities. ISR lesions of saphenous vein grafts can be managed with a therapeutic option of a DES or DEB or brachytherapy, but preferable option is to treat native vessel disease with PCI if it is suitable **(Box 1)**.

TABLE 4: Management of ISR—randomized clinical trials of DCB on treatment of ISR.

Author/trial	*Previous stent*	*Treatment*	*Number*	*Angiographic follow-up*	*Clinical follow-up*
Scheller et al.	BMS	DCB versus POBA	52	LLL: 0.03 ± 0.48 mm (DCB) versus 0.74 ± 0.86 mm (POBA), $p = 0.002$ at 6 months	MACE: 4% (DCB) versus 31% (POBA), $p = 0.01$ at 12 months
Unverdorben et al.	BMS	DCB versus DES-P	131	• LLL: 0.17 ± 0.42 mm (DCB) versus 0.38 ± 0.61 mm (DES), $p = 0.03$ • Binary restenosis rate: 7% (DCB) versus 20% (DES), $p = 0.06$ at 6 months	MACE: 9% (DCB) versus 22% (DES), $p = 0.08$ at 12 months
RIBSV	BMS	DCB versus DES-E	189	MLD: 2.01 ± 0.60 mm (DCB) versus 2.36 ± 0.60 mm (DES), $p < 0.001$ at 9 months	MACE: 8% (DCB) versus 6% (DES), HR: 0.76, $p = 0.60$ at 12 months
Habara et al.	DES	DCB versus POBA	50	• LLL: 0.18 ± 0.45 mm (DCB) versus 0.72 ± 0.55 mm (POBA), $p = 0.001$ • Binary restenosis rate: 8.7% (DCB) versus 62.5% (POBA), $p < 0.001$ at 6 months	MACE: 4% (DCB) versus 40% (POBA), $p = 0.005$ at 12 months
PEPCAD-DES	DES	DCB versus POBA	110	• LLL: 0.43 ± 0.61 mm (DCB) versus 1.03 ± 0.77 mm (DES), $p < 0.001$ • Binary restenosis rate: 17.2% (DCB) versus 58.1% (POBA), $p < 0.001$ at 6 months	MACE: 17% (DCB) versus 50% (POBA), $p < 0.001$ at 12 months
PEPCAD China ISR	DES	DCB versus DES-P	220	LLL: 0.46 ± 0.51 mm (DCB) versus 0.55 ± 0.61 mm (DES), p for noninferiority <0.001 at 9 months	TLF: 17% (DCB) versus 16% (DES), $p = 0.52$ at 12 months
ISAR-DESIRE 3	DES	DCB versus DES-P versus POBA	402	DS: 38.0 ± 21.5% (DCB) versus 37.4 ± 21.7% (DES) versus 54.1 ± 25.0% (POBA), p for noninferiority = 0.007 (DCB vs. DES), p for superiority <0.001 (other vs. POBA) at 6–8 months	MACE: 24% (DCB) versus 19% (DES) versus 46% (POBA)
RIBS IV	DES	DCB versus DES-E	309	MLD: 1.80 ± 0.60 mm (DCB) versus 2.03 ± 0.70 mm (DES), $p < 0.01$ at 6–9 months	MACE: 18% (DCB) versus 10% (DES), HR: 0.58, $p = 0.04$ at 12 months

(BMS: bare-metal stents; DCB: drug-coated balloons; DES: drug-eluting stents; DES-E: everolimus drug-eluting stents; DES-P: paclitaxel drug-eluting stents; DS: diameter stenosis; HR: hazard ratio; ISR: in-stent restenosis; LLL: late lumen loss; MACE: major adverse cardiac events; MLD: minimal lumen diameter; POBA: plain old balloon angioplasty; TLF = target lesion failure)

BOX 1: OCT tips and tricks for ISR evaluation.

- Useful to assess mechanism of ISR and plaque morphology
- Precise sizing of stent with IVI is very important in preventing ISR
- Highlights the underlying mechanisms responsible for ISR—malapposition, underexpansion, edge problems, neoatheroma
- Helps in identifying the calcification inside or outside the stent—confirms the stent expansion prior to finishing the procedure
- Aim for achieving stent expansion of >80–90% of the corresponding reference diameter without malapposition and medial edge dissection
- Look for stent fractures/overlapped segments/gap between stents and manage appropriately

REFERENCES

1. Alraies MC, Darmoch F, Tummala R, Waksman R. Diagnosis and management challenges of in-stent restenosis in coronary arteries. World J Cardiol. 2017;9(8):640.
2. Byrne RA, Joner M, Kastrati A. Stent thrombosis and restenosis: what have we learned and where are we going? The Andreas Grüntzig Lecture ESC 2014. Eur Heart J. 2015;36(47):3320-31.
3. Hong SJ, Lee SY, Hong MK. Clinical Implication of Optical Coherence Tomography-Based Neoatherosclerosis. J Korean Med Sci. 2017;32(7):1056-61.
4. Alfonso F, Byrne RA, Rivero F, Kastrati A. Current treatment of in-stent restenosis. J Am Coll Cardiol. 2014;63(24):2659-73.
5. Jinnouchi H, Kuramitsu S, Shinozaki T, Tomoi Y, Hiromasa T, Kobayashi Y, et al. Difference of Tissue Characteristics Between Early and Late Restenosis After Second-Generation Drug-Eluting Stents Implantation—An Optical Coherence Tomography Study. Circ J. 2017;81(4):450-7.
6. Otsuka F, Byrne RA, Yahagi K, Mori H, Ladich E, Fowler DR, et al. Neoatherosclerosis: overview of histopathologic findings and implications for intravascular imaging assessment. Eur Heart J. 2015;36(32):2147-59.
7. Ino Y, Kubo T, Matsuo Y, Yamaguchi T, Shiono Y, Shimamura K, et al. Optical coherence tomography predictors for edge restenosis after everolimus-eluting stent implantation. Circulation: Cardiovascular Interventions. 2016;9(10):e004231.
8. Her AY, Shin ES. Current management of in-stent restenosis. Korean Circ J. 2018;48(5):337-49.
9. Atkinson T, Bagai J, Faisal Latif MD. (2019). Tips and Tricks for Management of in-stent restenosis. Available from https://scai.org/tips-and-tricks-management-stent-restenosis [Last accessed February, 2024].
10. Bezerra H, Costa M, Attizzani G. OCT Made Easy. United States: CRC Press; 2017.
11. Alfonso F, Pérez-Vizcayno MJ, Hernández R, Bethencourt A, Martí V, López-Mínguez JR, et al. Long-term clinical benefit of sirolimus-eluting stents in patients with in-stent restenosis: results of the RIBS-II (Restenosis Intra-stent: Balloon angioplasty vs. elective sirolimus-eluting Stenting) study. J Am Coll Cardiol. 2008;52(20):1621-7.

CASE 1

OCT-guided PCI of ISR of LM bifurcation.

CLINICAL HISTORY

A 72-year-old female, known diabetic, hypertensive with Parkinson's disease staying alone without any domestic help presented with NSTEMI of anterior wall with complaints of chest pain, breathlessness, and hypotension. ECG-ST depressions and T inversions in V2-V4 leads, 2D Echo-RWMA in LAD territory, mild LV dysfunction with 48%.

Investigations: Hb—11.8 g/dL, serum creatinine—1.31 mg/dL, eGFR—41 mL/min, RBS—131 mg/dL.

Coronary angiogram (CAG): Distal LM 40%, proximal LAD 60% and mid 95% stenosis. LCX—normal, RCA—ostioproximal 80% and mid 95% lesion **(Fig. 6)**.

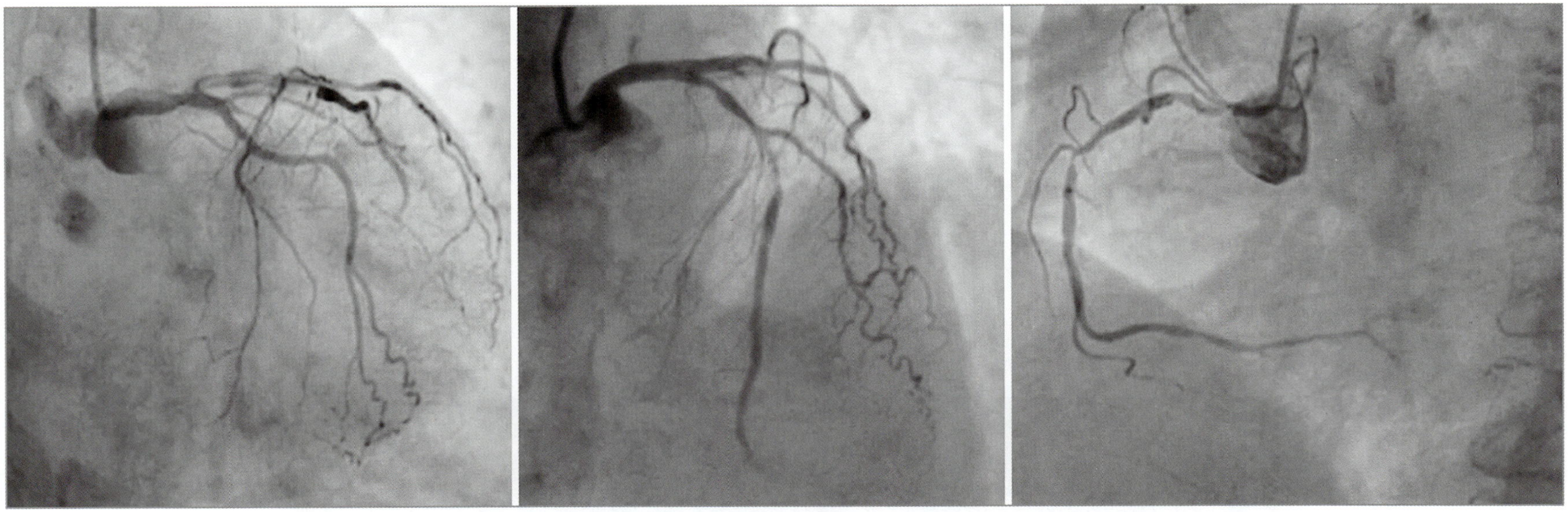

Fig. 6: Coronary angiogram showing LCX, LAD & RCA.

PROCEDURE

Left coronary artery was engaged with XB 3.5–7 Fr, LAD was crossed with BMW wire, LCX was crossed with Runthrough wire, and lesion was predilated with 2.0 × 10 mm Tazuna balloon. Subsequently, LMCA to LAD stenting was done with 2.75 × 48 mm Xience Xpedition, POT of LMCA was performed with 4.0 × 08 mm NC Trek balloon. LCX wire removed and recrossed through the stent struts, postdilatation of LAD stent was done with 3.5 × 08 mm NC Trek balloon.

Poststent OCT run showed malapposition at the proximal edge of the stent in LM. Re-POT of LM stent was done with 4.0 × 08 mm NC Trek. Final result was good with TIMI-III flow and without any complications **(Figs. 7 and 8)**.

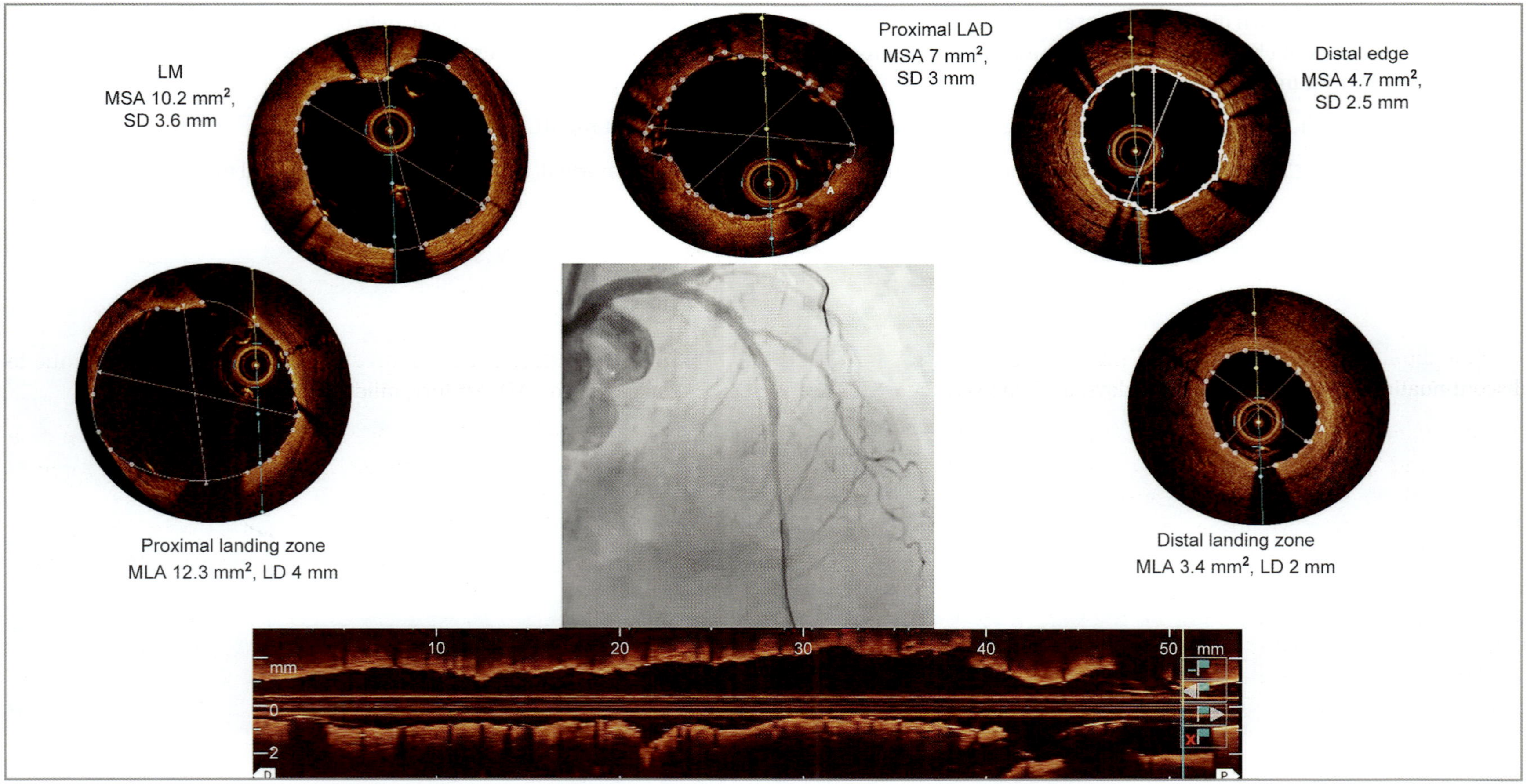

Fig. 7: Poststenting OCT showing well opposed stent struts.

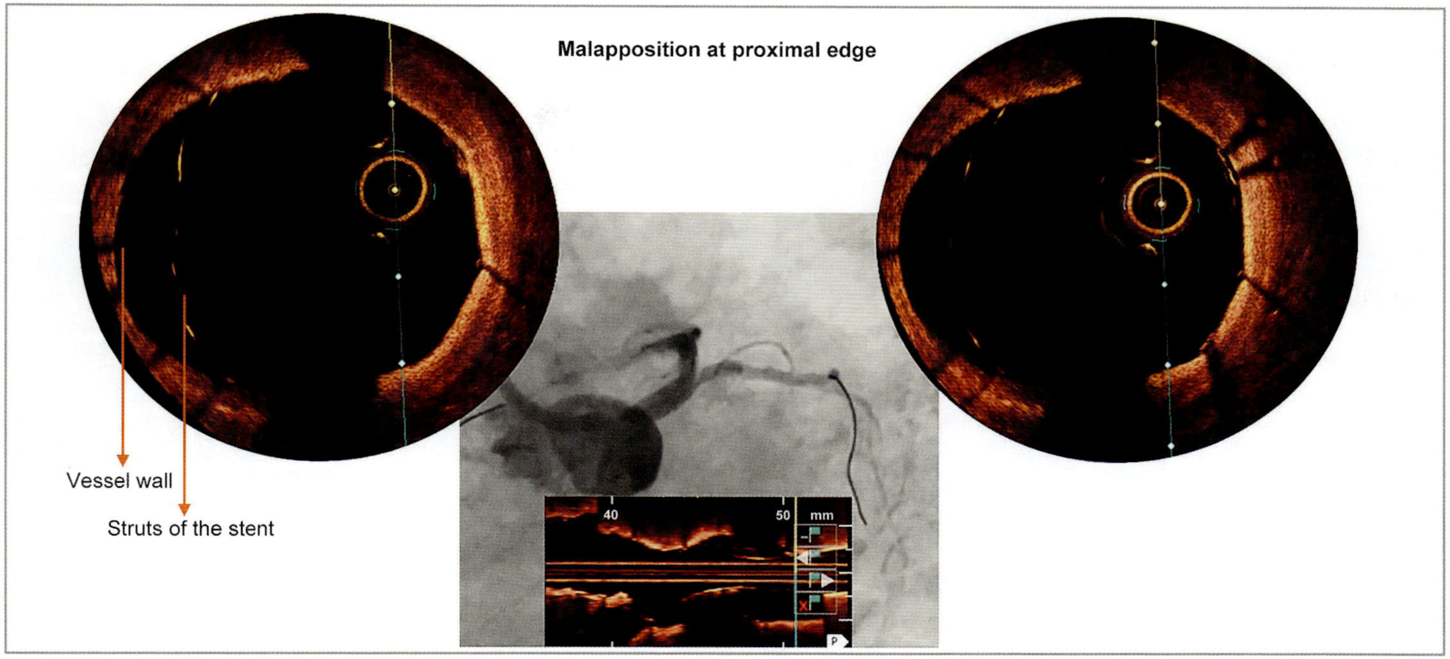

Fig. 8: Poststenting OCT showing malapposition at the proximal edge which was corrected with POT 4 mm NC.

Nine months later, she presented with ACS, NSTEMI, acute severe chest pain associated with shortness of breath (SOB), and hypotension due to discontinuation of DAPT therapy for 15 days, ECG showed acute ST-T changes, 2D Echo-RWMA in LAD territory, mild LV dysfunction, EF—48%.

Investigations: Hb—11.3 g/dL, Trop I-186 ng/L, serum creatinine—1.26 mg/dL, RBS—152 mg/dL, HbA1C—7.5%. CAG-LAD showed acute total occlusion, 99% narrowing of ostioproximal LCX and RCA—80% stenosis of ostioproximal to midsegment stenosis. In view of acute occlusion of LM bifurcation with hypotension, IABP-supported PCI was planned for better hemodynamic support during PCI **(Figs. 9 and 10)**.

Left coronary artery was engaged with EBU 3.5 7 Fr, Runthrough was placed in LAD, and Sion blue in LCX. Predilatation was done with 2.75 × 15 mm. Kissing balloon dilatation of LM bifurcation was done with 3 mm Apollo balloon in LAD, and 2.5 mm Ryurei balloon in LCX. Plaque modification prior to stenting was carried out with 3 × 10 mm AngioSculpt balloon **(Figs. 11 and 12)**.

Mid LAD ISR was treated with DEB angioplasty using 3 × 33 mm ALEX balloon and LCX stenting done with 2.75 × 12 mm Resolute Onyx stent, FKB of LM bifurcation was with 3.5 × 12 NC balloon in LCX and 3.5 × 38 mm ALEX DEB, and repeat FKB was done with 3.5 mm NC in LAD, 3 mm NC in LCX. Final POT of LM was performed with 4.5 × 8 mm NC Trek and check angio showed significant plaque in distal LAD which was stented with 2.5 × 15 mm R. Onyx stent. Final result was good with TIMI-III flow without any complications **(Figs. 13 to 15)**.

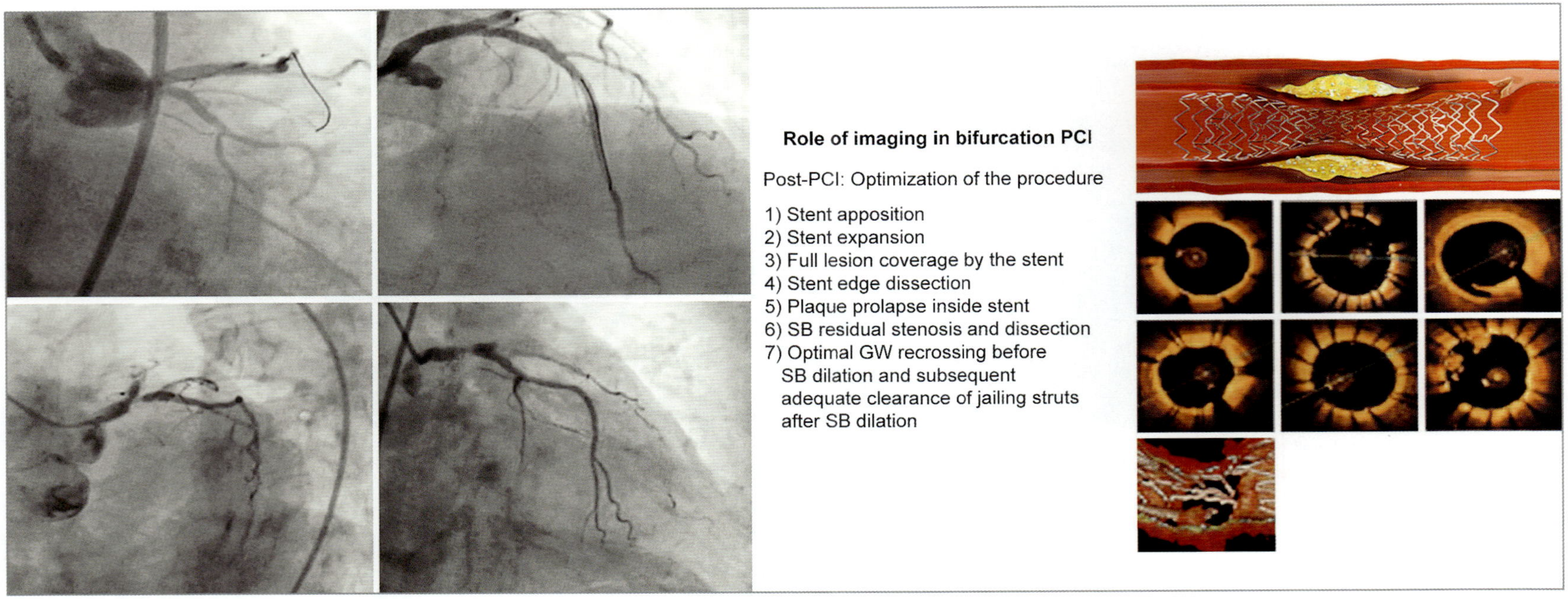

Fig. 9: Coronary angiography at 9 months follow-up and role of imaging in bifurcation PCI.

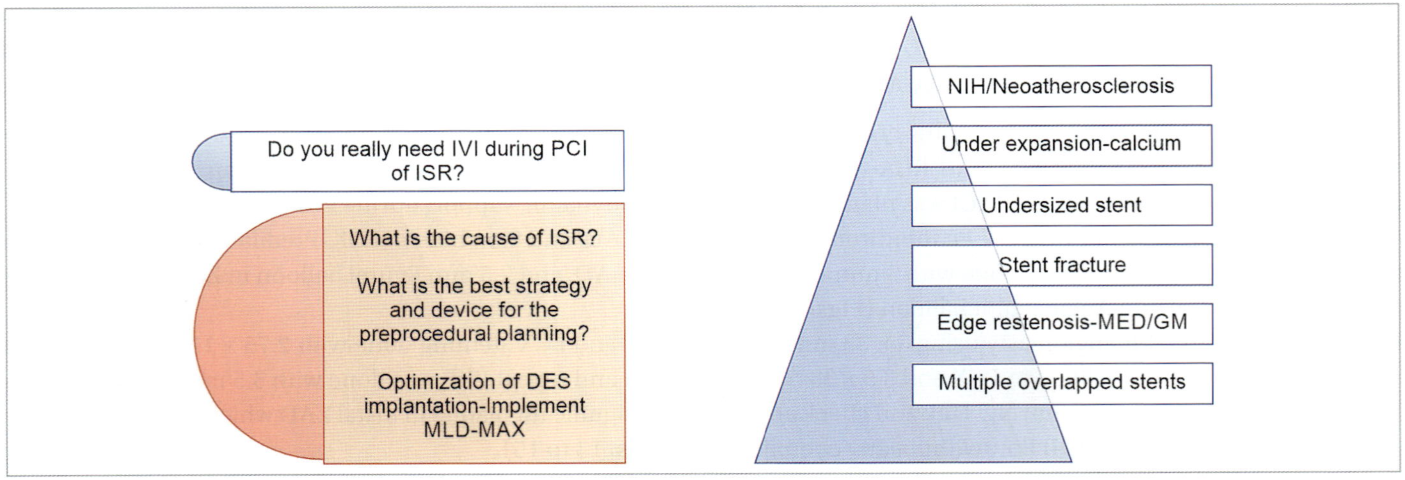

Fig. 10: OCT-guided management of ISR. (DES: drug eluting stent; GM: geographical miss; IVI: intra vascular imaging; ISR: in-stent restenosis; MED: medial edge dissection; MLD: morphology, length, diameter; MAX: medial edge dissection, apposition, expansion; PCI: percutaneous coronary intervention)

Source: Waksman R, Iantorno M. Refractory in-stent restenosis: Improving outcomes by standardizing our approach. Curr Cardiol Rep. 2018;20(12):140.

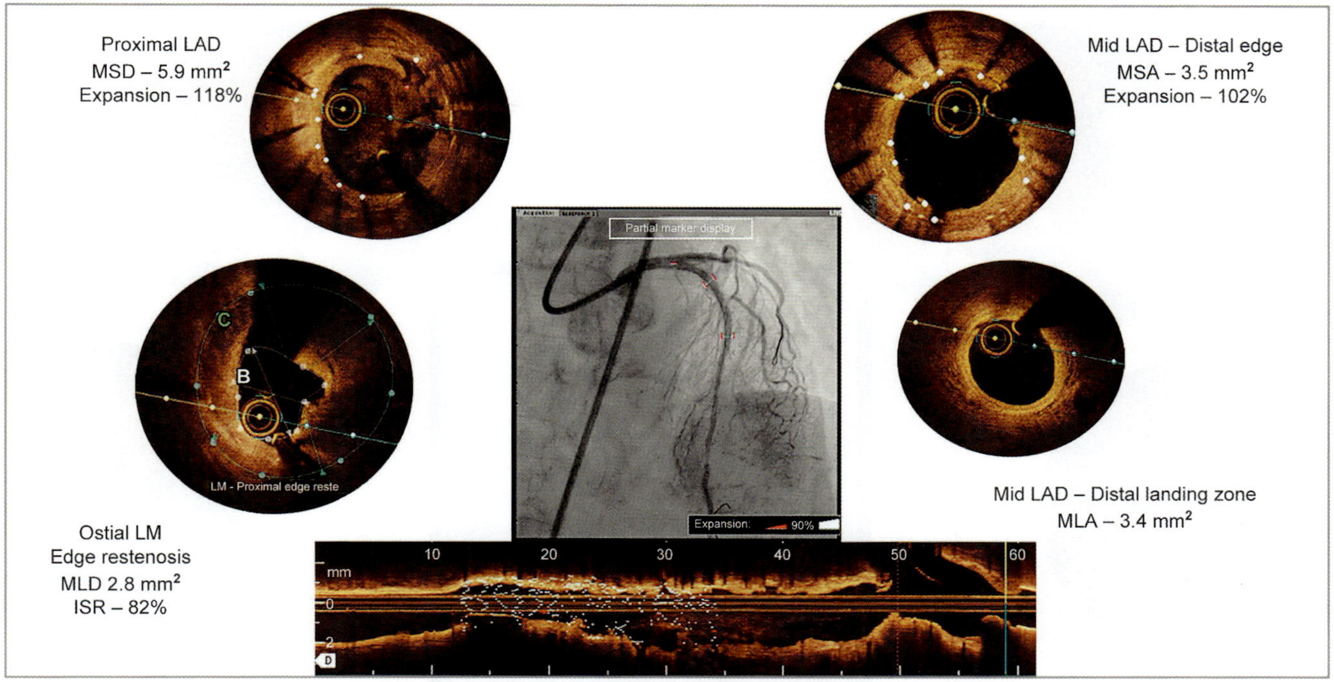

Fig. 11: Presenting OCT showing stent edge restenosis at LM bifurcation.

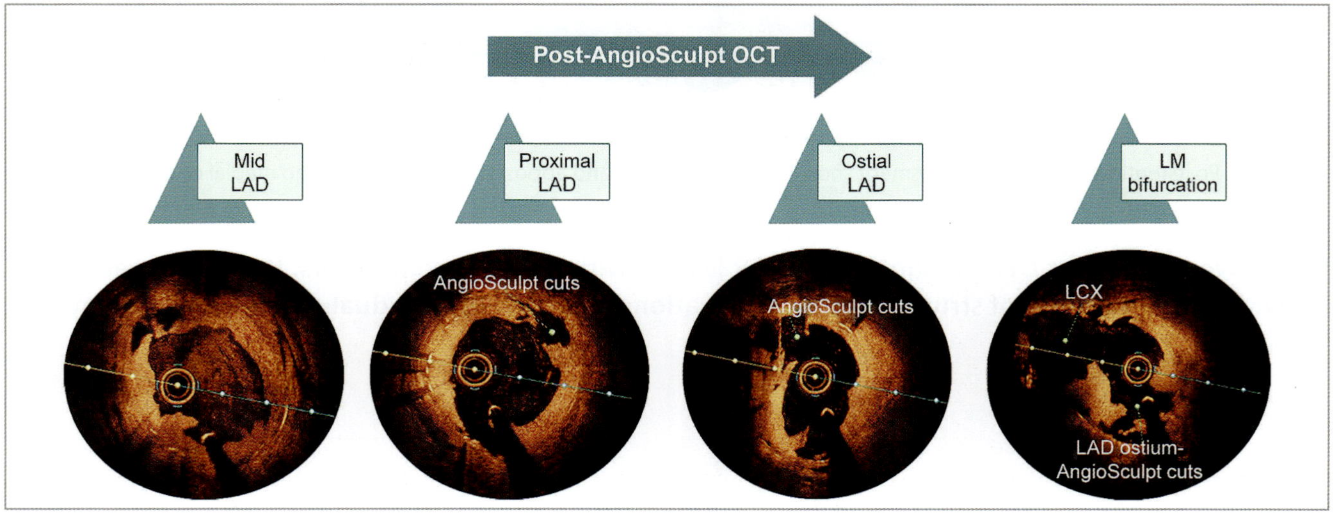

Fig. 12: Post angiosculpt cuts seen by OCT.

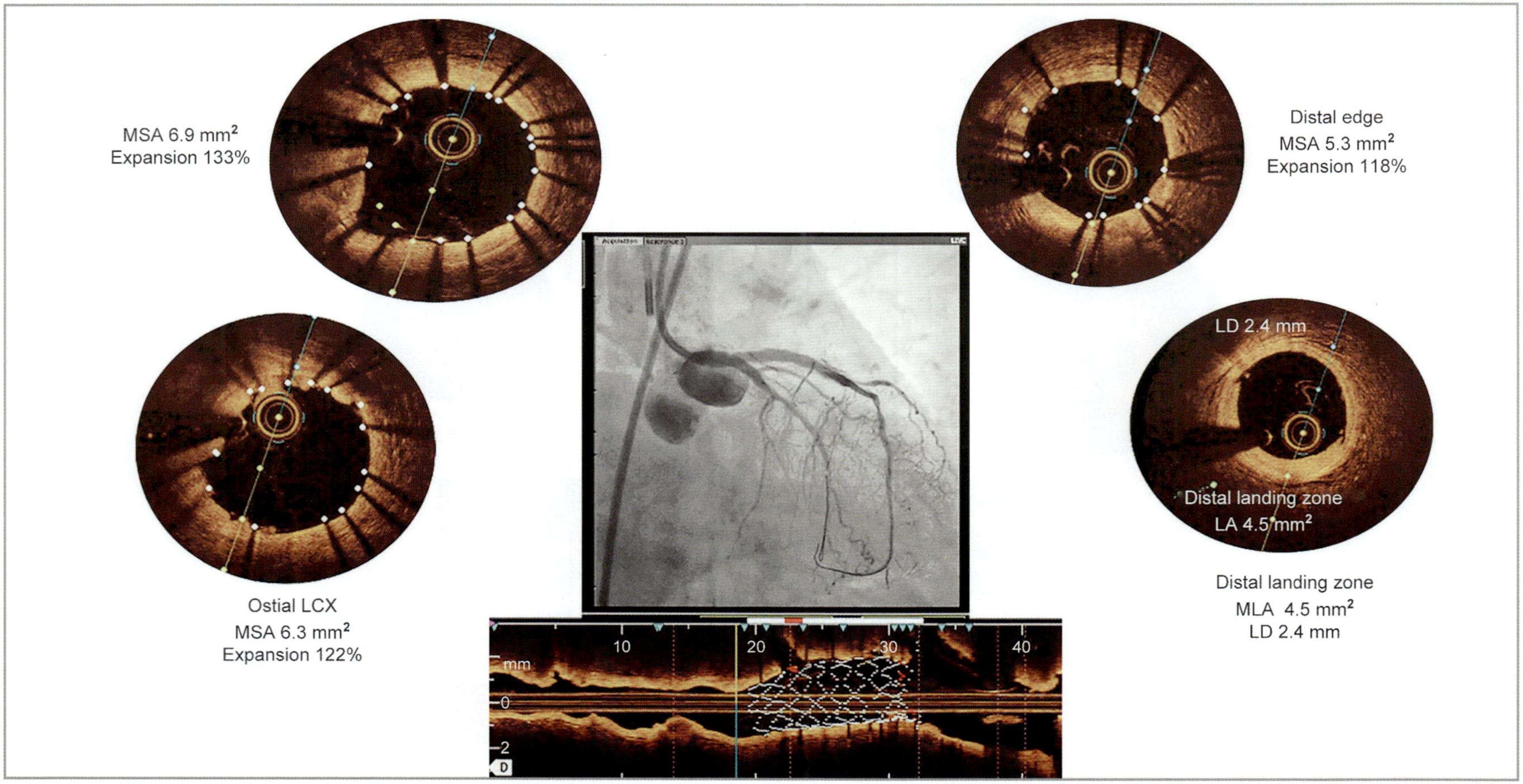

Fig. 13: Poststenting of LCX OCT assessment showing well expanded and apposed stent struts with no medial edge dissections.

The DCB is preferred over the repeat DES implantation in ISR lesions with multiple stent layers, those with relevant side branches to avoid jailing of SB with additional layer of struts, and clinical situations requiring shorter dual-antiplatelet therapy.

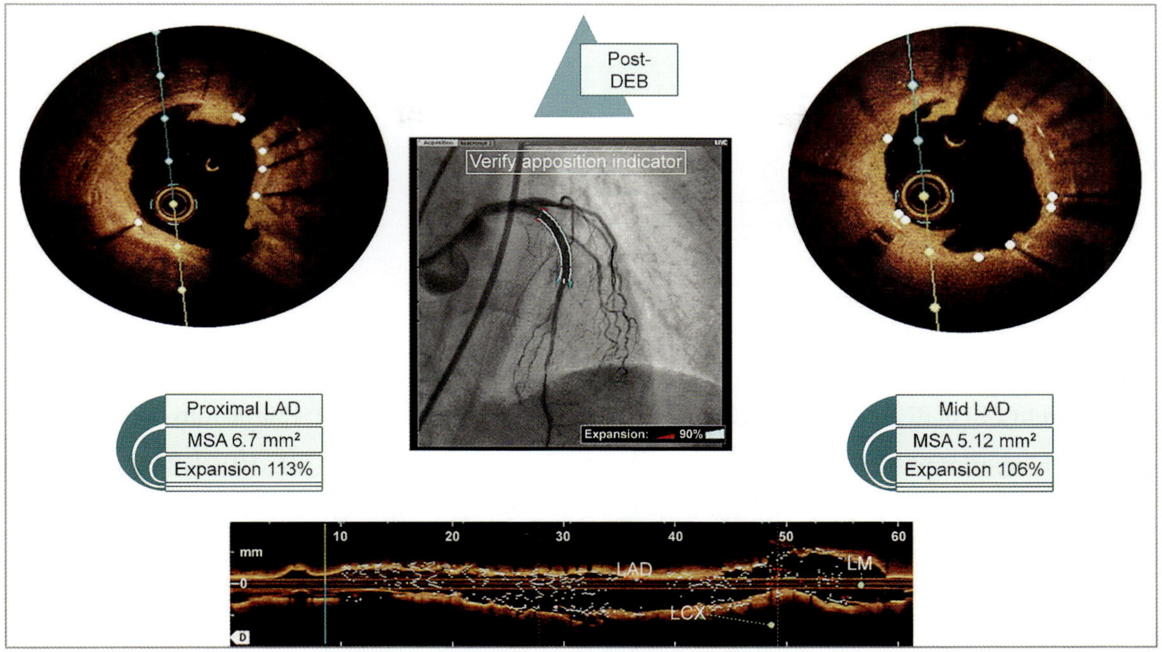

Fig. 14: Post LAD DEB OCT assessment of proximal and mid LAD. (DEB: drug eluting balloon)

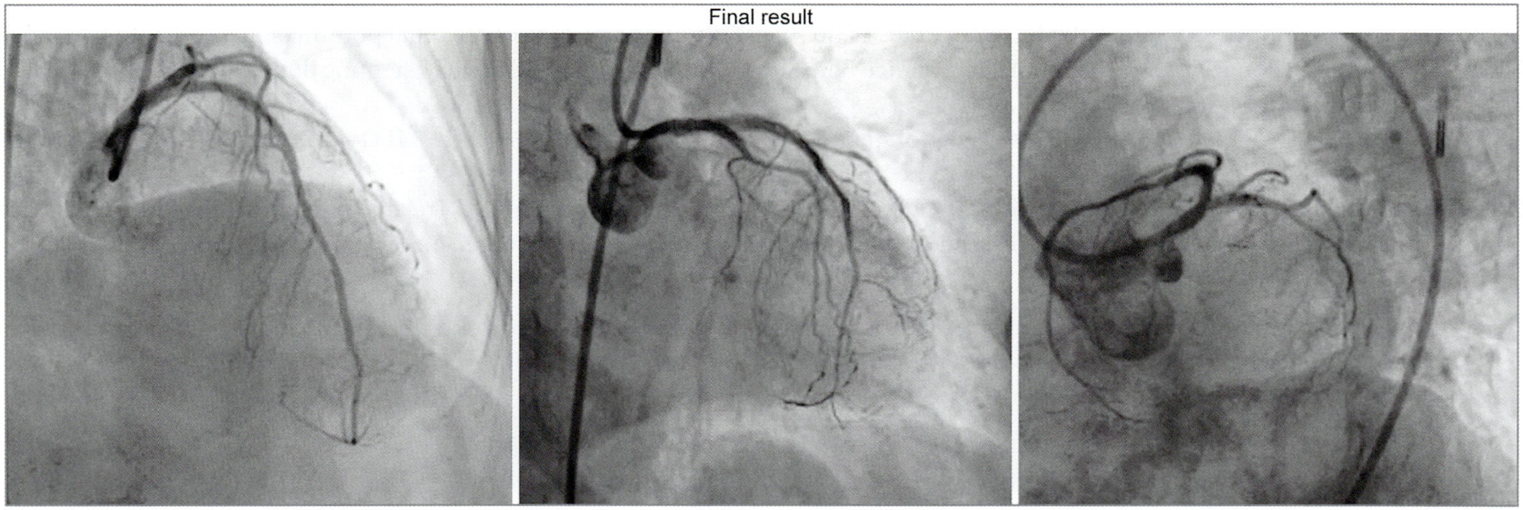

Fig. 15: Final result.

CASE 2

OCT assessment of diffuse ISR of RCA.

CLINICAL HISTORY

A 62-year-old female, known hypertensive, euglycemic, presented with USA, recent onset of chest pain and SOB. Past history of (H/o) old inferolateral wall myocardial infarction, underwent PCI of RCA with DES in 2014. On examination PR-84/min, BP: 130/90 mm Hg, Heart-S^1+, S^2+, $S3^0$, $S4^0$, lungs—clear.

Investigations: Hb—11.2 g%, serum creatinine—0.5 mg/dL, blood urea—23 mg/dL, RBS—148 mg/dL, HIV, HBSAG, HCV—negative. ECG—old IWMI, 2D Echo-dilated LV, global hypokinesia of LV, moderate MR, severe LV dysfunction, EF—35%. CAG—LMCA, LAD, and LCX—Normal, RCA—diffuse long-segment severe ISR **(Figs. 16A and B)**.

PROCEDURE

Right femoral artery (RFA)—route, 7 Fr-3.5 JR guiding catheter, RCA lesion could not be crossed with 0.014 Sion blue, fielder XT, Gaia I wires, finally crossed with Gaia II wire and exchanged with Sion blue. Predilated with 1.25 × 10 mm, 2.0 × 10 mm and 2.5 × 10 mm Tazuna balloons **(Fig. 16C)**.

Optical coherence tomography study showed diffuse ISR of RCA and severe fibrotic narrowing of proximal portion of PLV **(Figs. 17A to D)**.

Distal RCA to PLV stenting done with 2.5 × 32 mm Yukon Choice Elite Stent (DES). Proximal to mid RCA stenting done with 3.5 × 40 mm Yukon Choice Elite Stent (DES) **(Figs. 16D and E)**.

Post-OCT showed distal RCA—malapposition of distal edge of stent—0.39 mm, 38% with MLA—5.9 mm^2, MLD—2.7 mm, MSA—5.9 mm^2, MSD—2.1 mm **(Figs. 18A and B)**.

Distal RCA to proximal RCA postdilatation done with 2.5 × 12 mm, 3.0 × 12 mm, and 3.5 × 12 mm NC Trek balloons. Postprocedure angio view showed well-implanted stents with TIMI-III flow without any dissection **(Figs. 16F to H)**. Patient was discharged on third postprocedure day in a stable status.

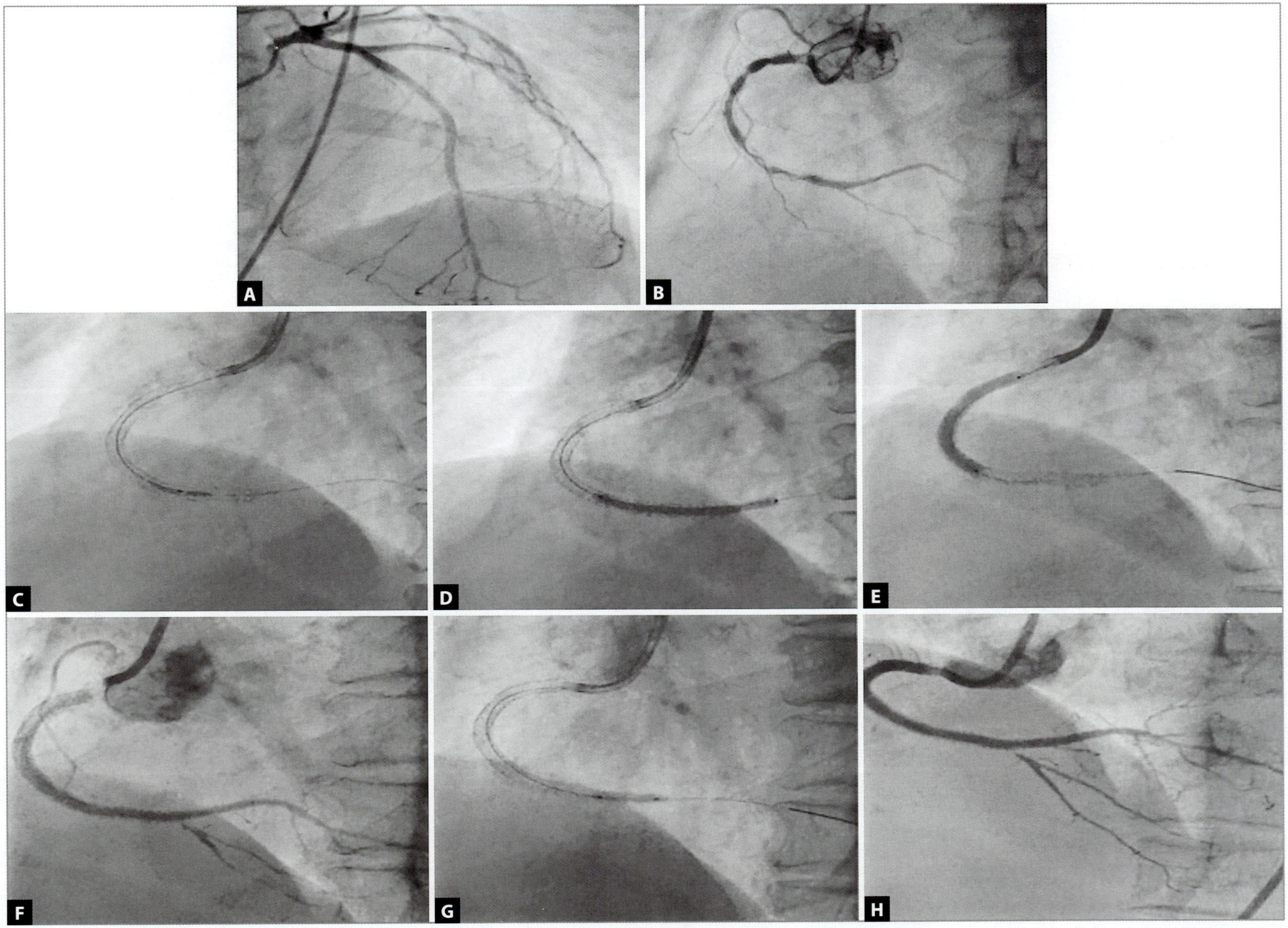

Figs. 16A to H: Coronary angiogram and angioplasty of RCA. (A): CAG—LMCA, LAD, and LCX— Normal, (B): RCA—diffuse long segment severe ISR, (C) Predilatation done with 1.25 × 10 mm, 2.0 × 10 mm and 2.5 × 10 mm Tazuna balloon; (D) Distal RCA stenting done with 2.5 × 32 mm Yukon choice elite stent; (E) Proximal to mid RCA stenting done with 3.5 × 40 mm Yukon choice elite stent; (F) Distal and mid RCA stent mild residual; (G) Distal RCA to proximal RCA post dilatation done with 2.5 × 12 mm, 3.0 × 12 mm and 3.5 × 12 mm NC trek balloons; (H) Final result.

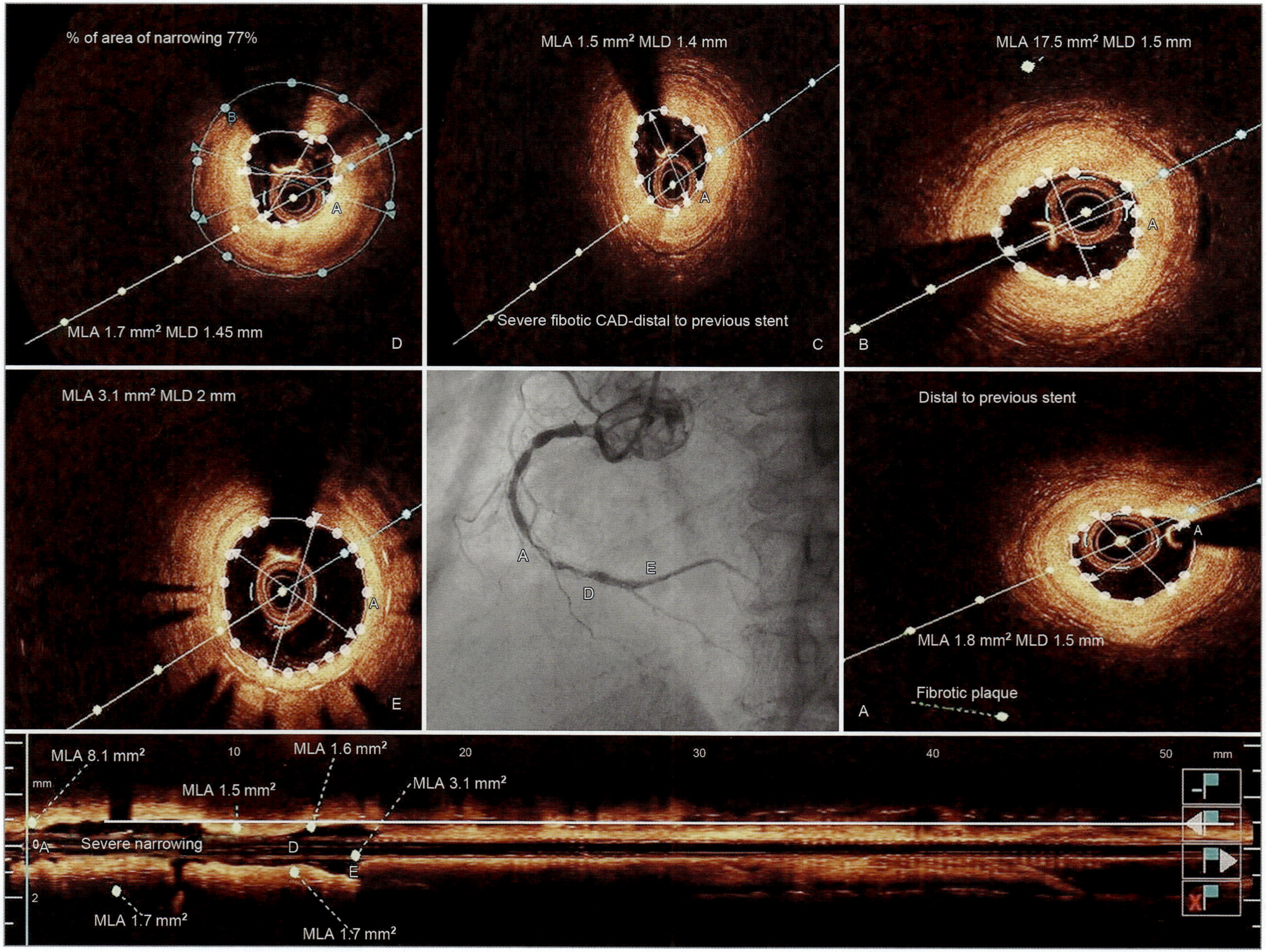
% of area of narrowing 77%
MLA 1.7 mm² MLD 1.45 mm
D
MLA 1.5 mm² MLD 1.4 mm
Severe fibotic CAD-distal to previous stent
C
MLA 17.5 mm² MLD 1.5 mm
B
MLA 3.1 mm² MLD 2 mm
E
Distal to previous stent
MLA 1.8 mm² MLD 1.5 mm
Fibrotic plaque
A
MLA 8.1 mm²
MLA 1.6 mm²
MLA 1.5 mm²
MLA 3.1 mm²
Severe narrowing
MLA 1.7 mm²
MLA 1.7 mm²

Fig. 17A

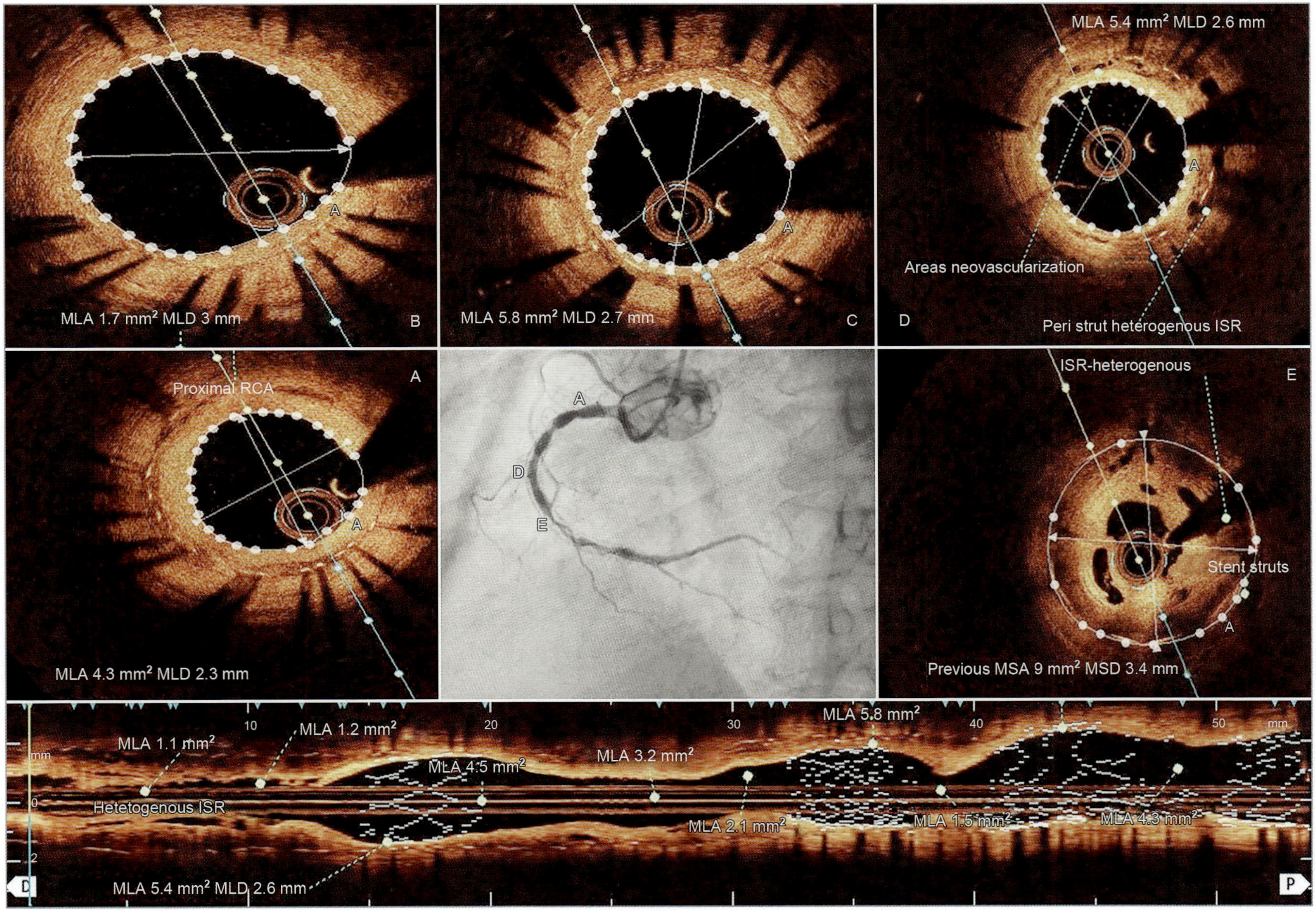
MLA 1.7 mm² MLD 3 mm
B
MLA 5.8 mm² MLD 2.7 mm
C
MLA 5.4 mm² MLD 2.6 mm
Areas neovascularization
Peri strut heterogenous ISR
D
Proximal RCA
A
MLA 4.3 mm² MLD 2.3 mm
A
D
E
ISR-heterogenous
E
Stent struts
Previous MSA 9 mm² MSD 3.4 mm
MLA 1.1 mm²
MLA 1.2 mm²
MLA 4.5 mm²
MLA 3.2 mm²
MLA 5.8 mm²
Hetetogenous ISR
MLA 2.1 mm²
MLA 1.5 mm²
MLA 4.3 mm²
MLA 5.4 mm² MLD 2.6 mm
D
P

Fig. 17B

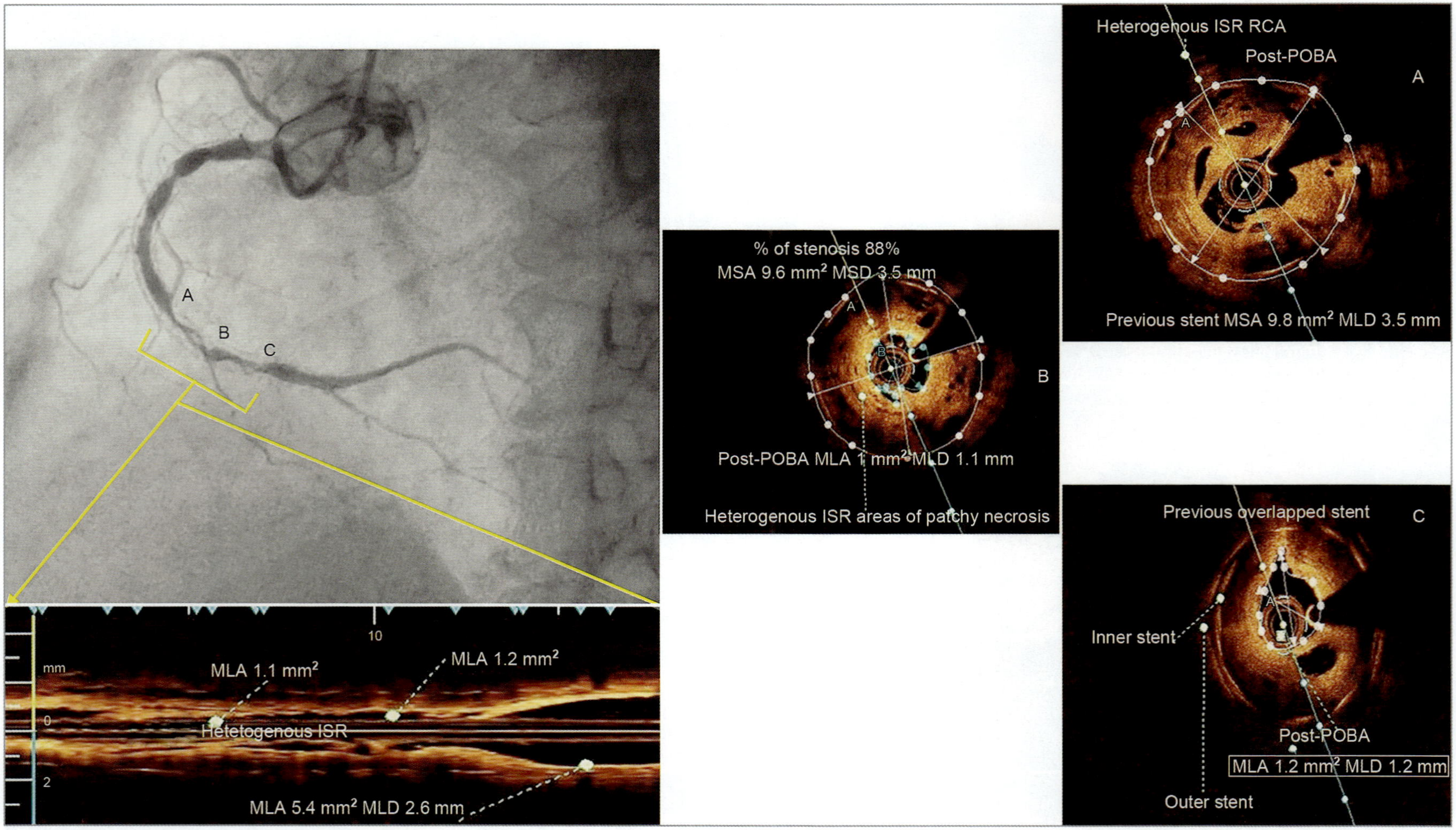

Fig. 17C

2021 ACC/AHS/SCAI Coronary Vascularization Guidelines

>2a, C-LD, In patients with stent failure, IVUS or OCT is reasonable to determine the mechanism of stent failure.

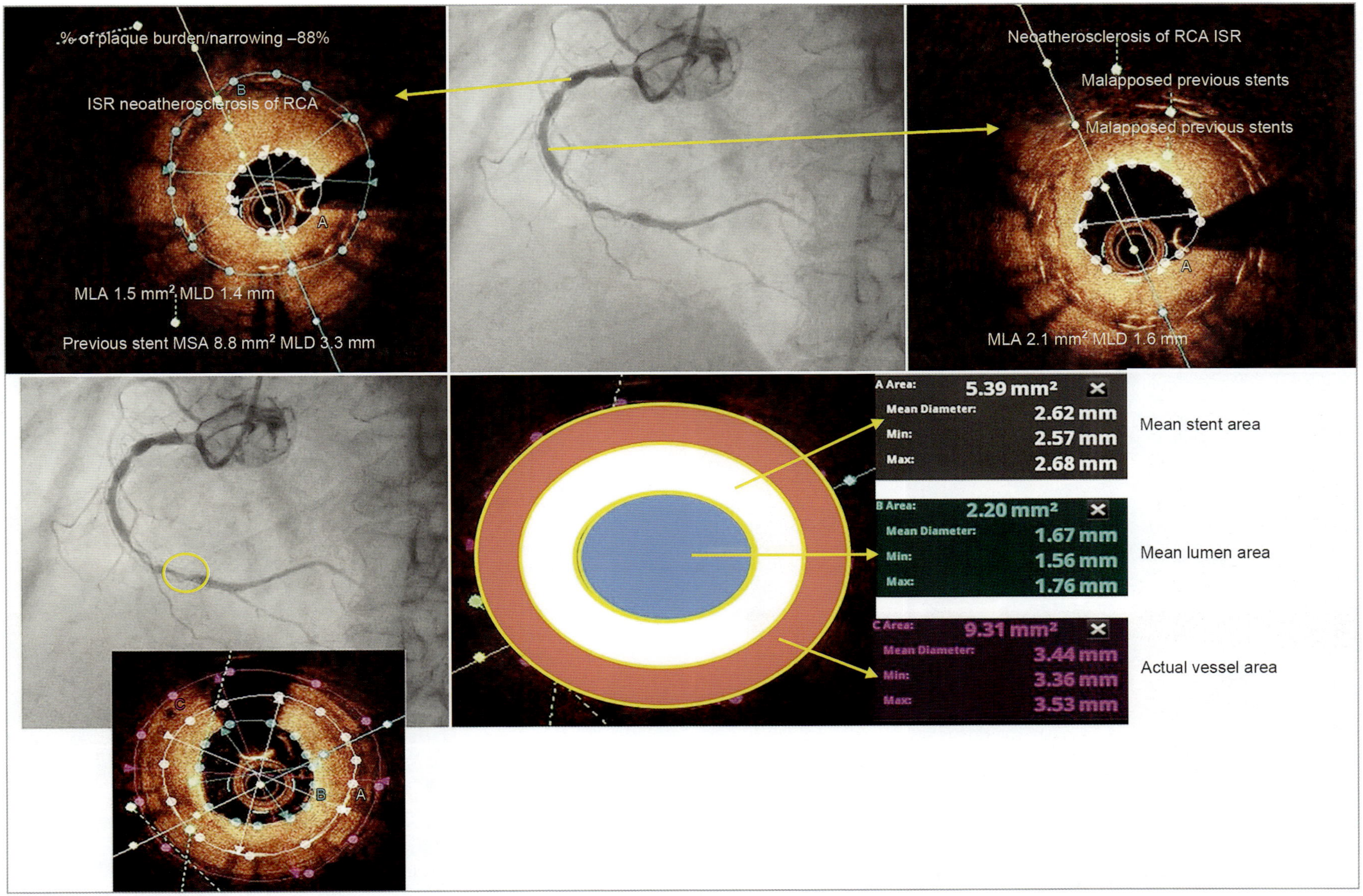

Fig. 17D

Figs. 17A to D: (A) Prestenting OCT assessment of distal RCA; (B) Prestenting OCT assessment of proximal RCA; (C) OCT assessment of Mid RCA ISR segment; (D) OCT assessment of various segments of RCA for ISR.

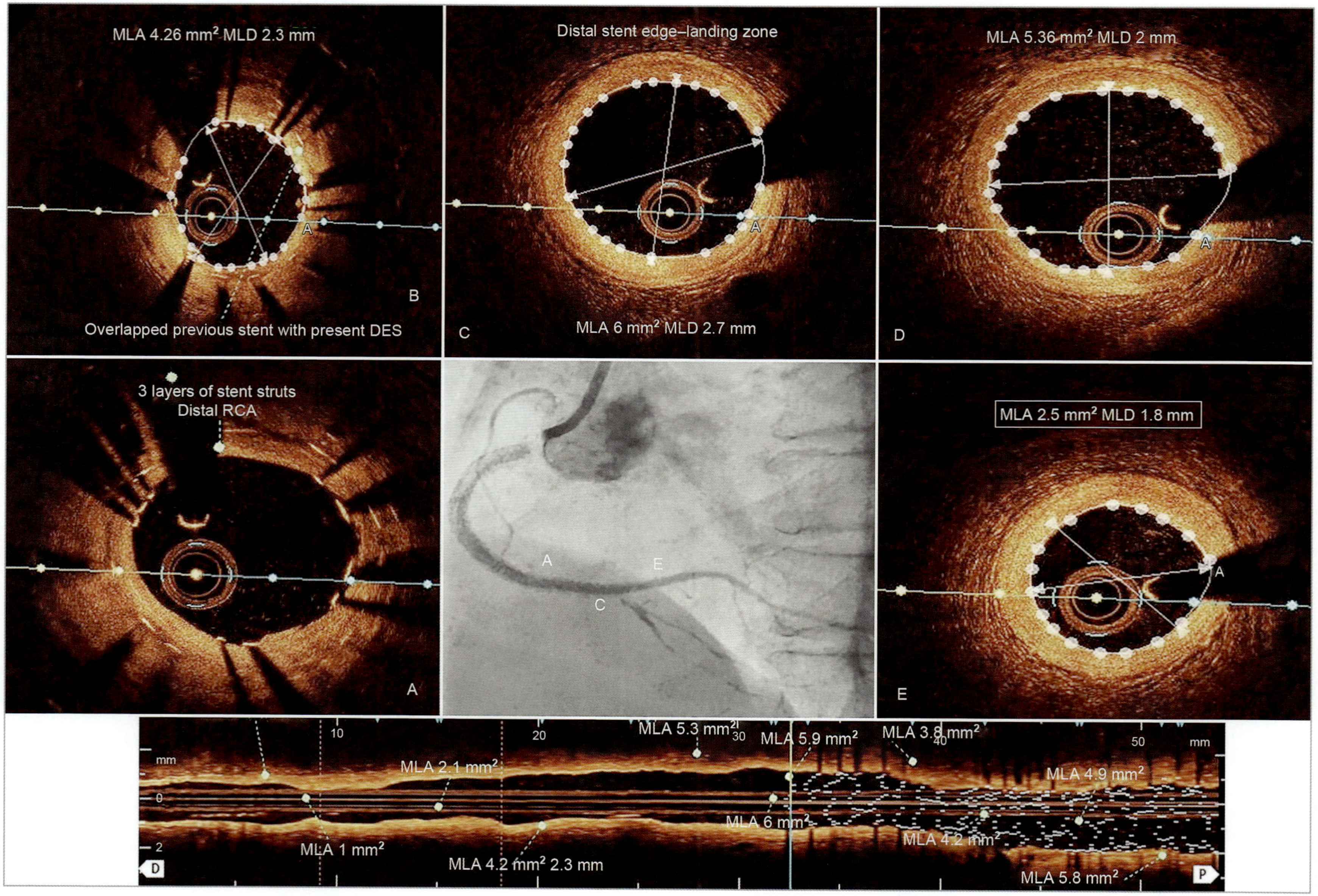
MLA 4.26 mm² MLD 2.3 mm
B
Overlapped previous stent with present DES
Distal stent edge–landing zone
C
MLA 6 mm² MLD 2.7 mm
MLA 5.36 mm² MLD 2 mm
D
3 layers of stent struts
Distal RCA
A
MLA 2.5 mm² MLD 1.8 mm
E
MLA 2.1 mm²
MLA 1 mm²
MLA 4.2 mm² 2.3 mm
MLA 5.3 mm²
MLA 5.9 mm²
MLA 3.8 mm²
MLA 6 mm²
MLA 4.9 mm²
MLA 4.2 mm²
MLA 5.8 mm²
D
P

Fig. 18A

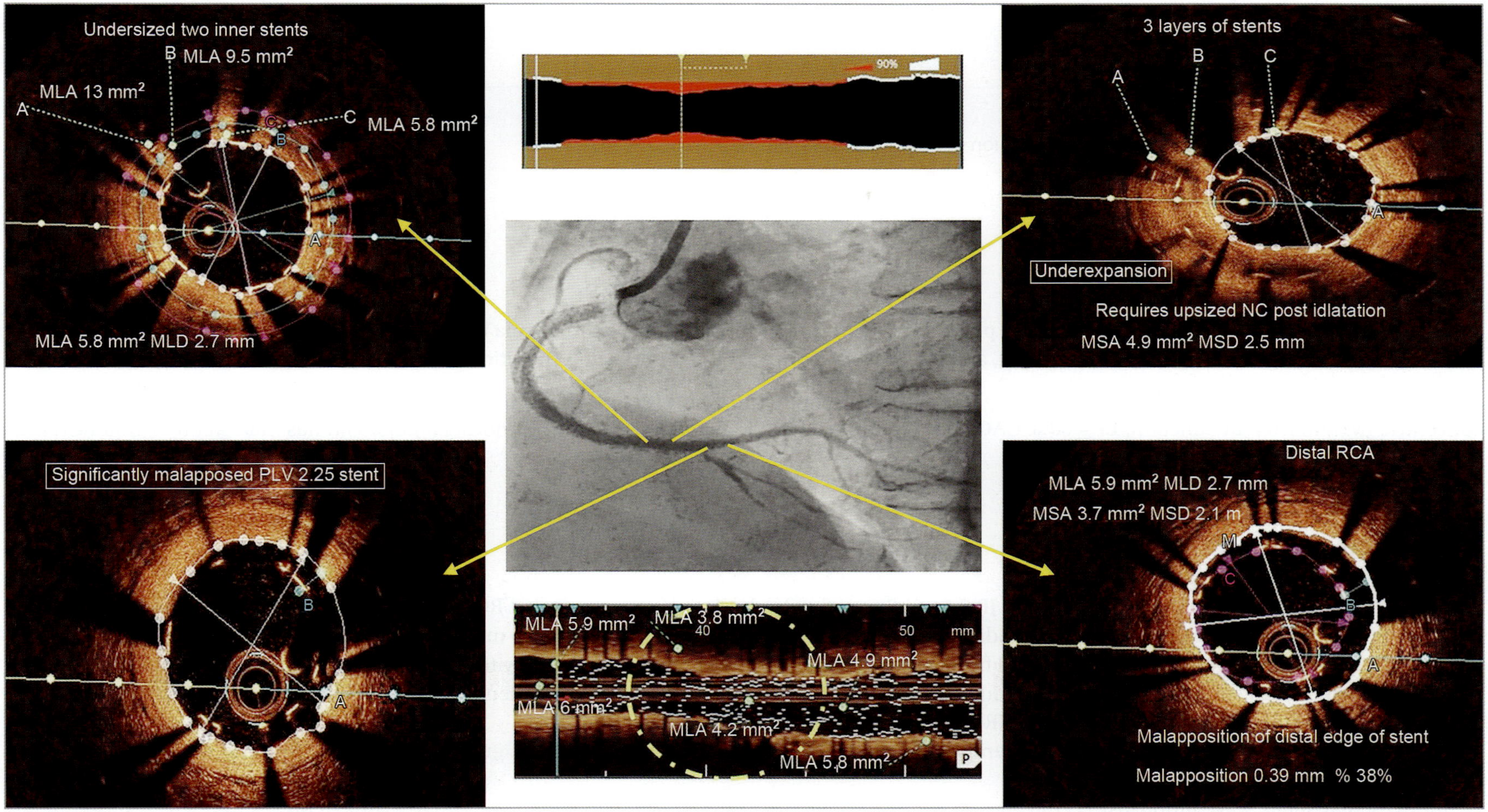

Fig. 18B

Figs. 18A and B: (A) Post distal RCA stenting; (B) Post RCA OCT showed under-expansion and malapposition.

CASE 3

Plaque modification with IVL and PCI of total occlusion of RCA due to DES-ISR.

CLINICAL HISTORY

A 62-year-old male, known hypertensive, diabetic, presented with recent onset of rest and effort angina for 15 days. Underwent IVUS-guided Rota stenting of distal RCA with **(Figs. 19A to E)** 3 × 12 mm stent, and proximal RCA with 3.5 × 48 mm Xience Xpedition stent 7 months back for CAD—unstable angina.

Investigations: Hb—10.6 g/dL, blood urea—10 mg/dL, serum creatinine—0.63 mg/dL, eGFR—106 mL/min, RBS—109 mg/dL, 2D Echo—no RWMA, concentric LVH, normal LV function, EF—60%. CAG-LMCA—normal, mid LAD mild disease, LCX—normal, major OM has mild stenosis, mid RCA total occlusion due to ISR **(Figs. 19F to H)**.

PROCEDURE

Route—RRA (Slender Terumo sheath), using 7 Fr JR 3.5 guiding catheter, check angiogram revealed RCA mid 100% ISR lesion, crossed with 0.014" Sion blue wire with Corsair microcatheter support. Predilatation done with 2.0 × 10 mm Tazuna, 2.5 × 15 mm NC Trek balloons. Pre-OCT showed ISR due to neoatherosclerosis with areas of lipid plaque, and fibrocalcific plaque **(Fig. 20A)**, underexpansion with MSA of 3.1 mm^2 against distal MSA of 5.73 mm^2 (56% eXpansion) due to severe deep calcium behind stent struts. Large atherosclerotic plaque burden behind stent struts may also contribute to future progression of atherosclerotic plaque leading to ISR—paleo atherosclerosis **(Figs. 20B and C)**.

In-stent neoatherosclerosis was more frequently observed in the L-ISR group than in E-ISR group, and the E-ISR group more frequently had homogeneous neointima than the I-ISR group.

Intravascular shock wave lithotripsy (IVL) **(Figs. 21A and B)** done with 3.5 × 12 mm balloon inflated up to 4 atm 10 pulses were given subsequently balloon inflated up to 6 atm. Eight cycles of IVL (80 pulses) were given to the area of tight narrowing **(Figs. 22A and B)**. Guidezilla support was used to place IVL catheter due to difficulty in placing IVL catheter. Post-OCT study showed cuts in the fibrocalcific plaque of neoatherosclerosis with shock waves **(Fig. 23)**.

Stenting done with 3.5 × 38 mm Resolute Onyx with Guideliner support. Postdilatation done with 3.5 × 15 mm OPN NC balloon up to 40 atm **(Figs. 22C and D)**. Final OCT showed well-apposed stent struts, no edge dissection, and no residual thrombus **(Figs. 24A and B)**. Postprocedure angio view showed well-implanted stents with TIMI-III flow without any dissection **(Fig. 22E)**. Patient was discharged on third postprocedure in a stable status.

Intravascular lithotripsy consists of a balloon catheter that uses sonic pulses to fracture calcified tissues with virtually no debris production, avoids the trauma produced by blades and burrs and their related risk, still offering an effective disruptive action on calcium.

- IVL device—12 mm long balloon catheter with three emitters inside the balloon between two radiopaque markers.
- It has a profile smaller than other modifying balloons, quite comparable to a NC balloon and is available in seven sizes ranging from 2.5 to 4.0 mm (for severely calcified balloon uncrossable lesions, atherectomy seems to be a better choice).

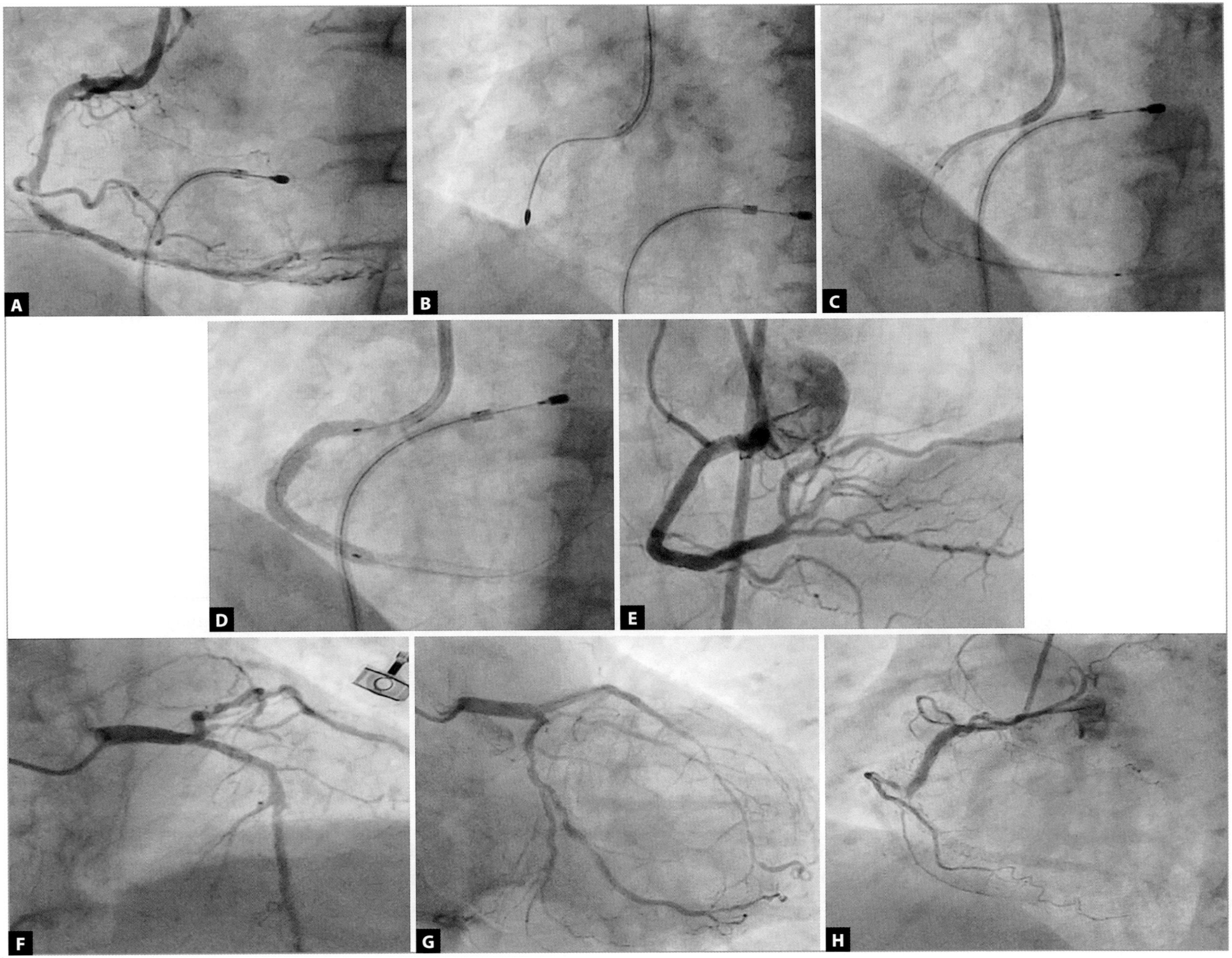

Figs. 19A to H: (A to E) ROTA and image guided coronary angioplasty 7 months before; (F to H) current admission coronary angioplasty.

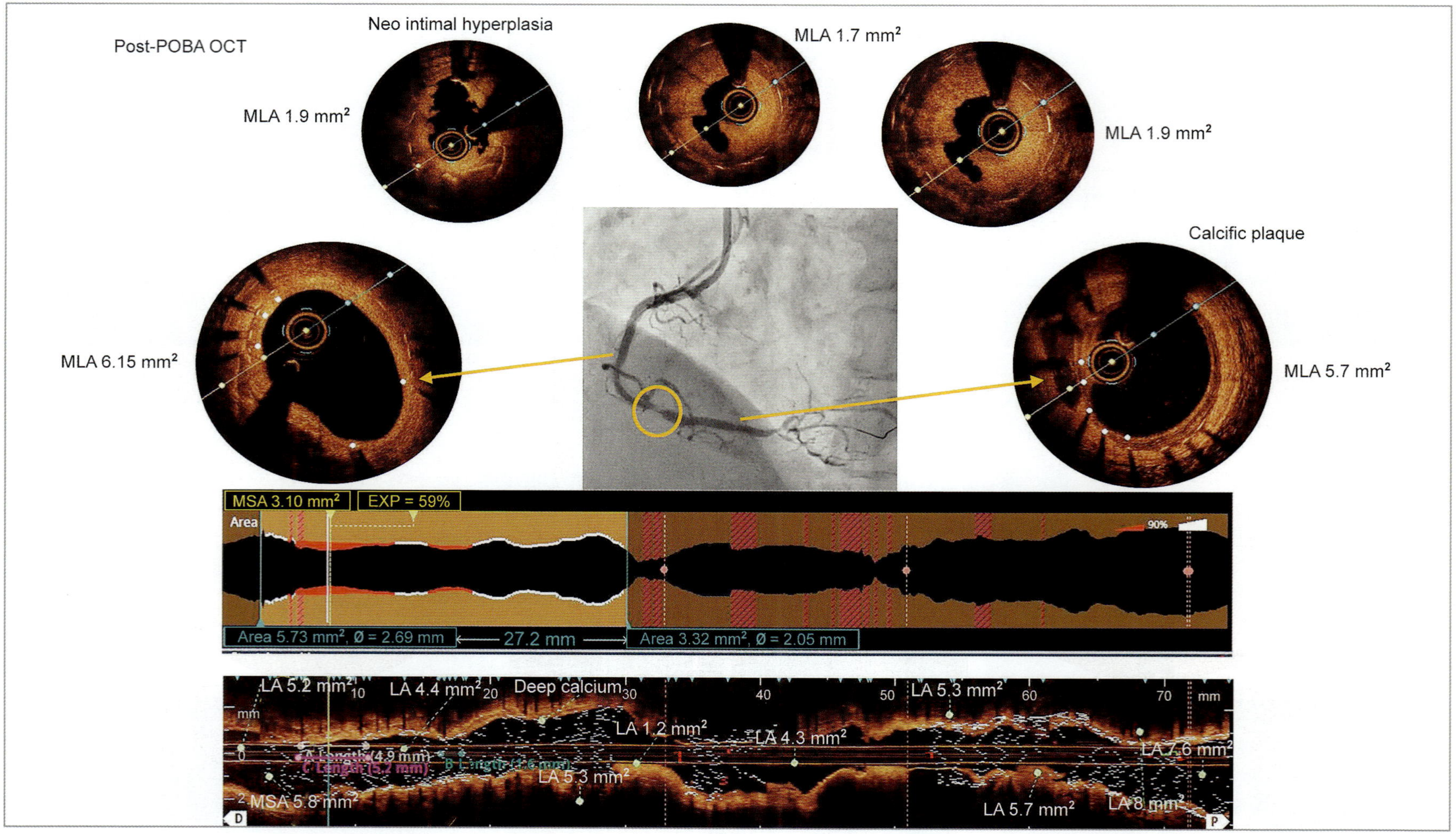

Fig. 20A

Agent DIE trial: **Prospective, randamized, multicenter, superiority trial across 40 US centres (*N* = 600)**

- ***Key inclusion criteria:*** **BMS or DES ISR; lesion length—<26 mm, RVD—>2.0 to <4.0 mm**
- ***Key exclusion criteria:*** **Recent STEMI, bifurcation, LM, SVG, or oriental graft, thrombus in target vessel.**

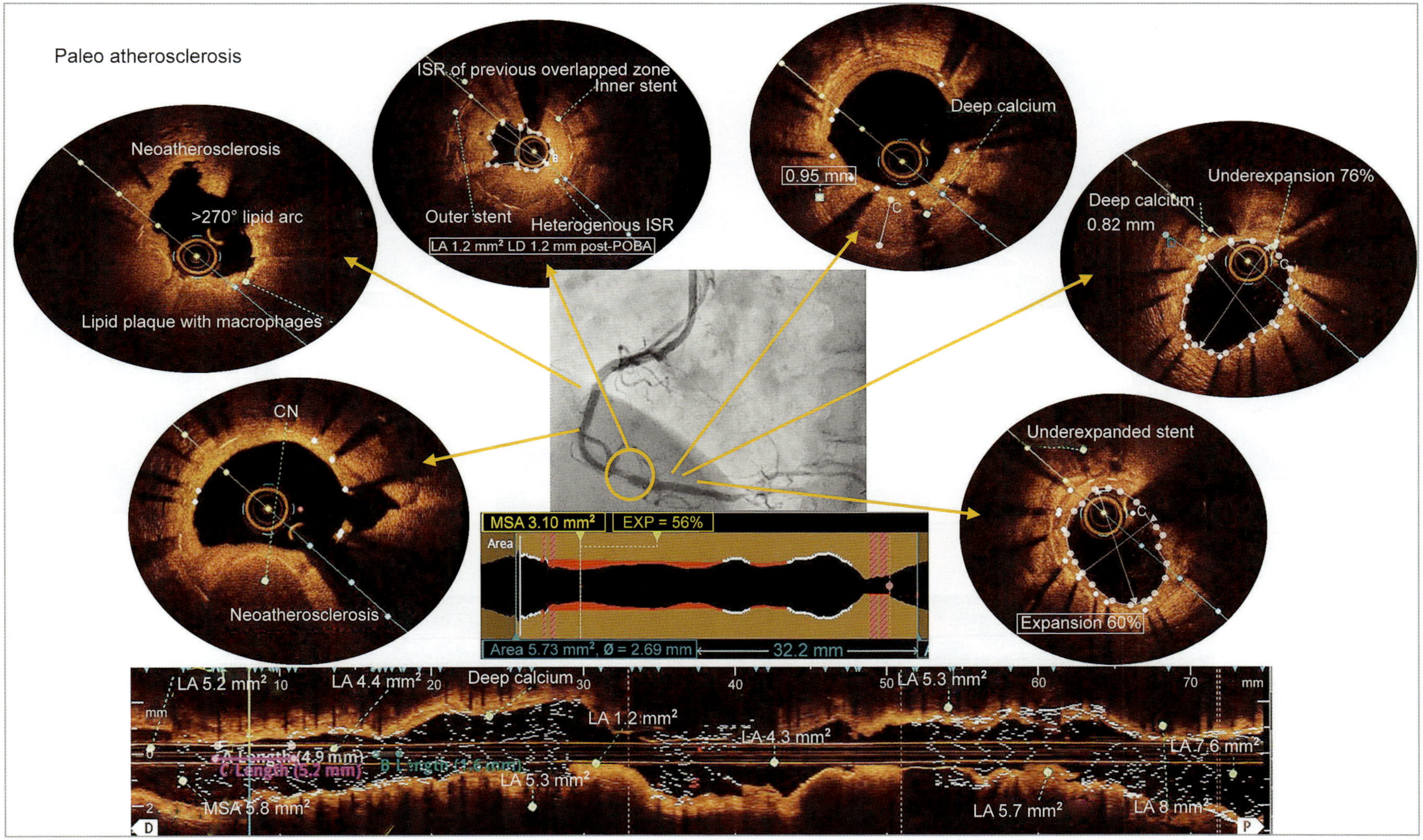

Fig. 20B

Agent DIE trial: **Prospective, randamized, multicenter, superiority trial across 40 US centres (*N* = 600)**

- **2:1 randomization after successful pre-dilatation of target lesion**
- **Agent DCB—*n* = 406, balloon angioplasty—*n* = 194.**

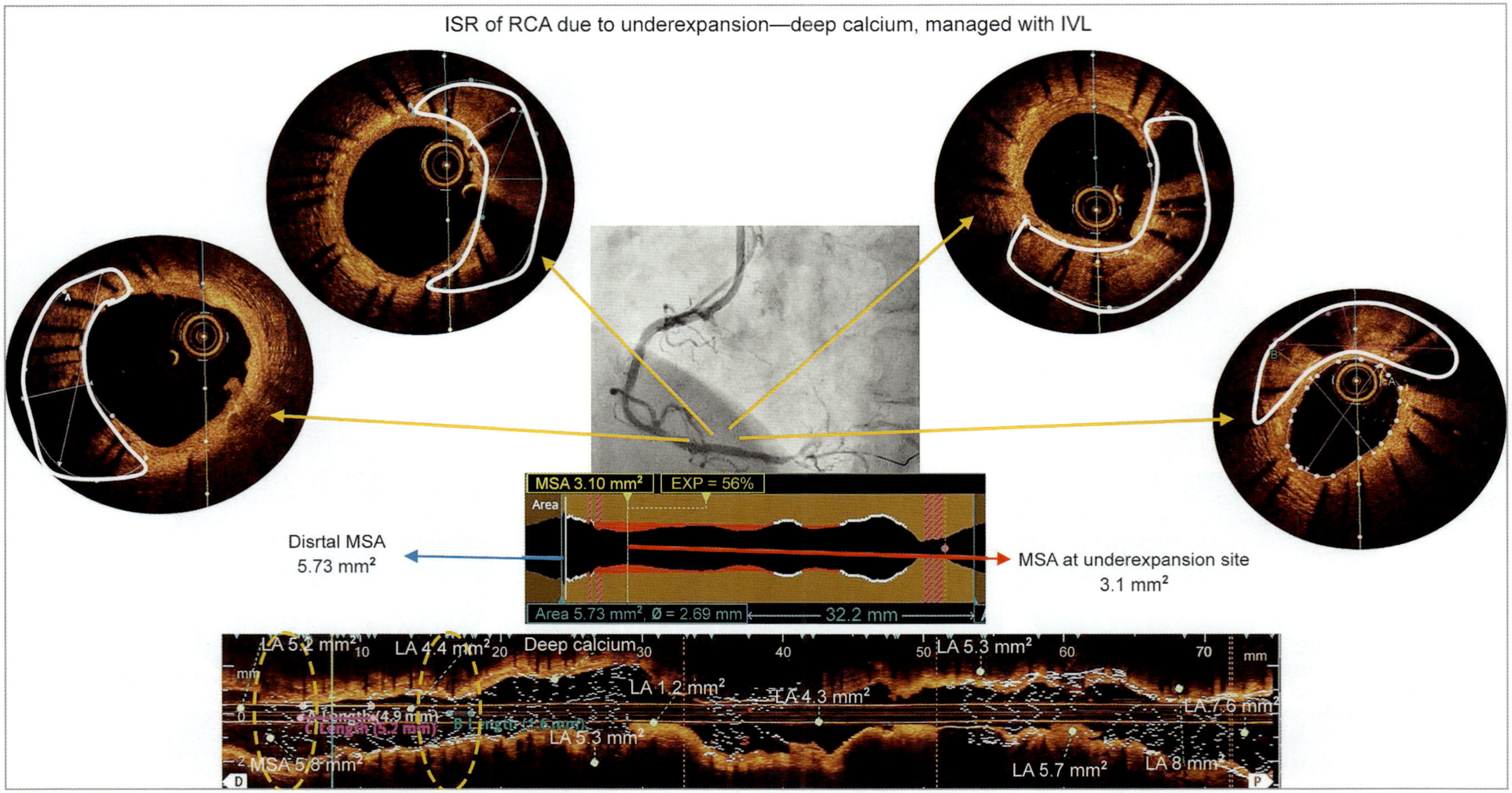

Fig. 20C

Figs. 20A to C: Pre-OCT. (A) ISR due to neoatherosclerosis with areas of lipid plaque, and fibrocalcific plaque; (B) paleo atherosclerosis; (C) underexpansion with MSA of 3.1 mm^2 against distal MSA of 5.73 mm^2 (56% eXpansion) due to severe deep calcium behind stent struts.

Agent DIE trial: **Prospective, randamized, multicenter, superiority trial across 40 US centres (*N* = 600).**
Targe lesion failure at 12 months follow-up showed 17.9% in agent DCB group and 28.6% in balloon angioplasty group.

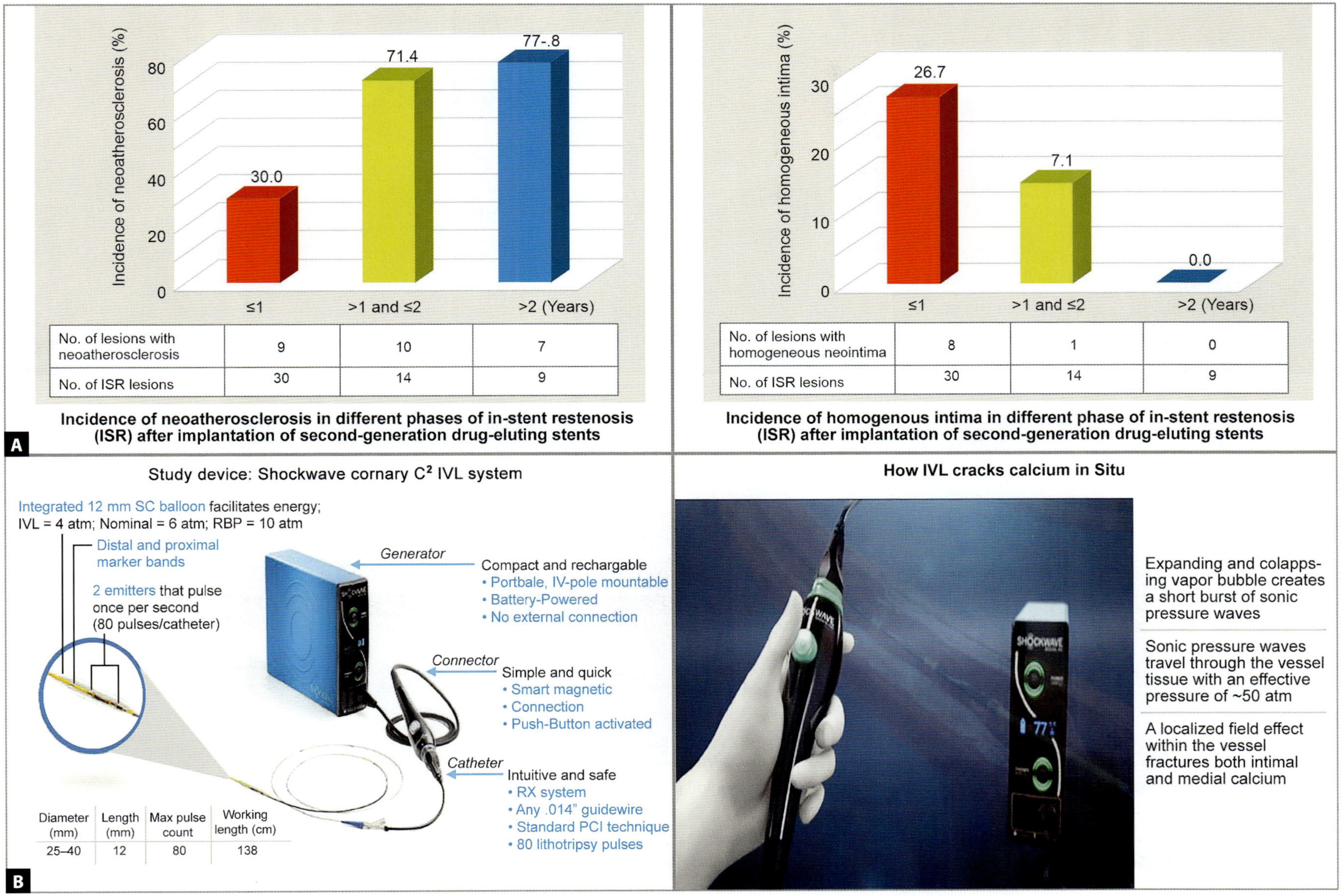

Figs. 21A and B: Intravascular shock wave lithotripsy. (IV: intravenous; PCI: percutaneous coronary intervention; RBP: rated burst pressure; SC: semicompliant)

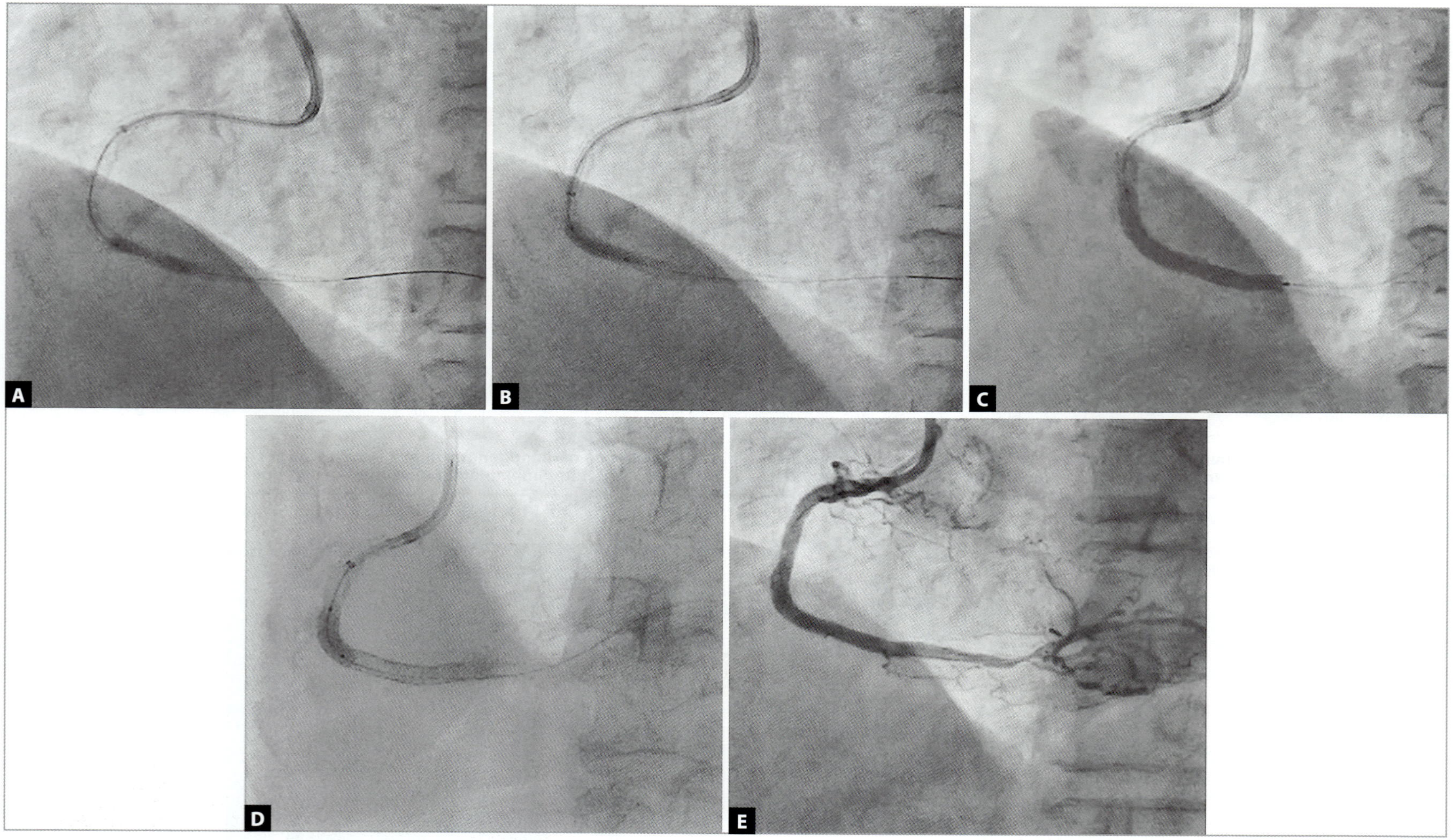

Figs. 22A to E: Coronary angioplasty. (A and B) IVL balloon dilatation; (C) stenting; (D) OPN NC balloon dilatation; (E) final result.

Calcified neoatherosclerosis: **IVI → plaque modification with CB/SB/IVL/RA → DES or DEB → Final IVI.**

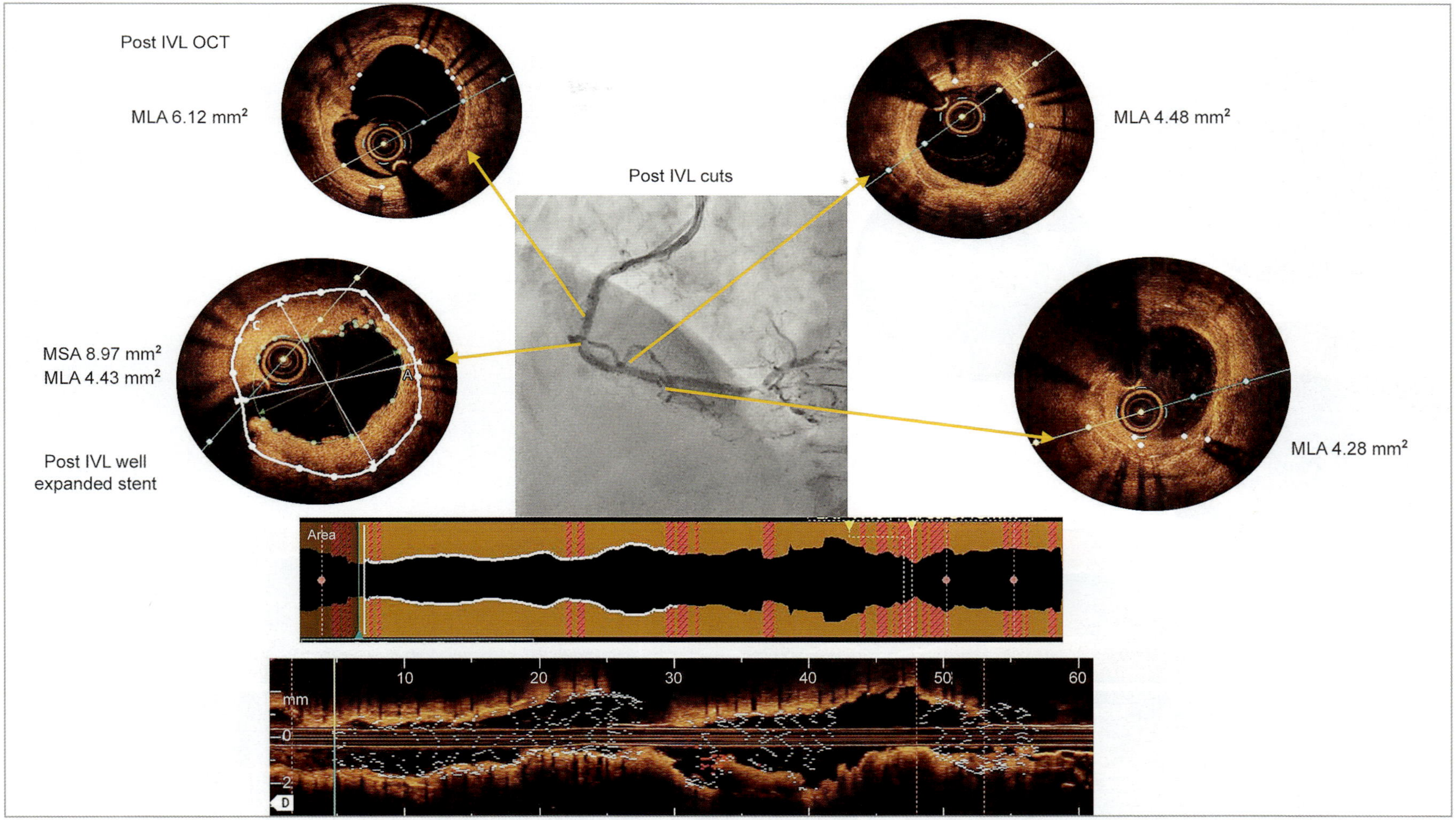

Fig. 23: Post-IVL OCT study showed cuts in the fibrocalcific plaque of neoatherosclerosis with shock waves.

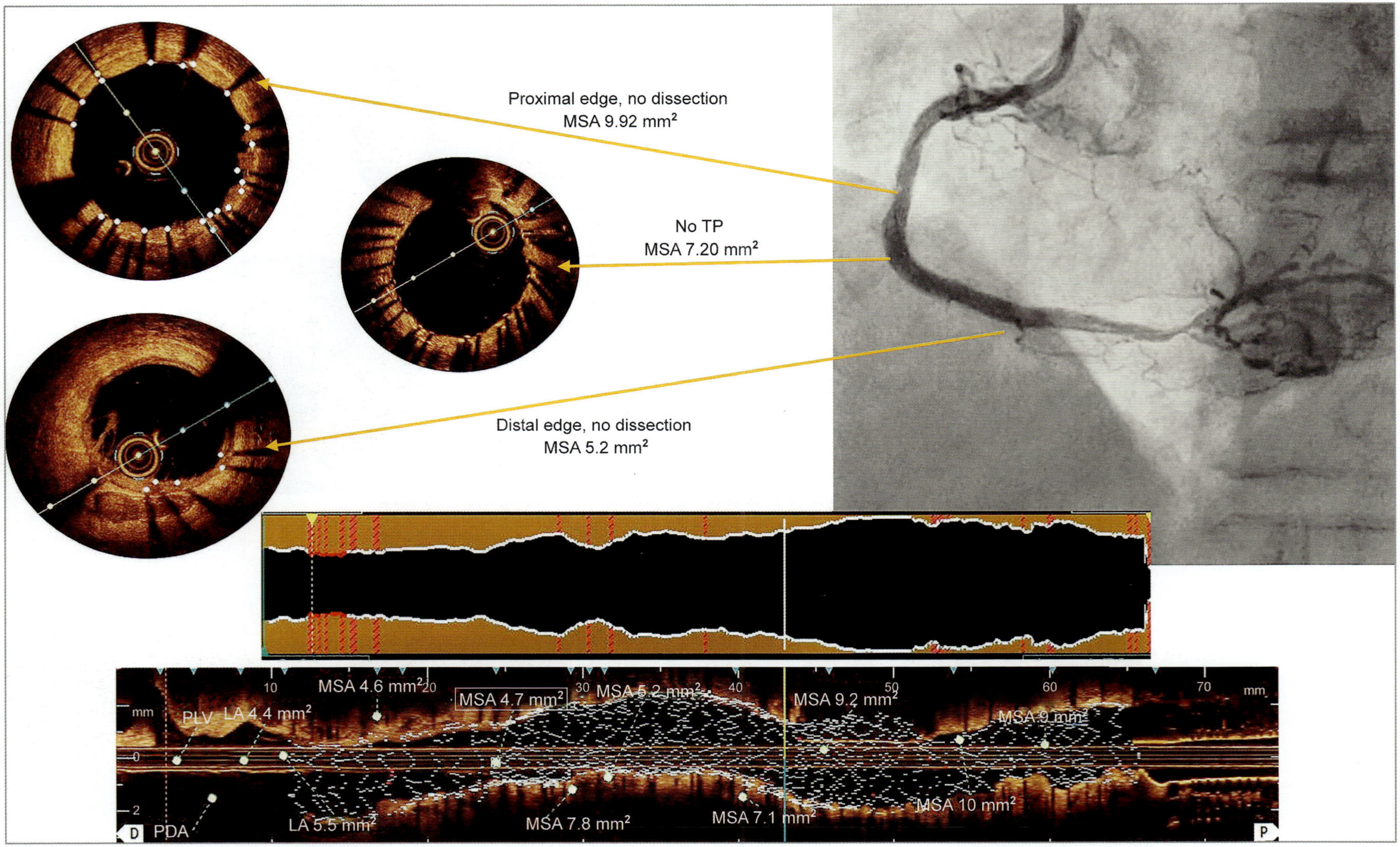
Proximal edge, no dissection
MSA 9.92 mm²
No TP
MSA 7.20 mm²
Distal edge, no dissection
MSA 5.2 mm²
MSA 4.6 mm²
MSA 4.7 mm²
MSA 5.2 mm²
MSA 9.2 mm²
MSA 9 mm²
PLV
LA 4.4 mm²
PDA
LA 5.5 mm²
MSA 7.8 mm²
MSA 7.1 mm²
MSA 10 mm²
D
P

Fig. 24A

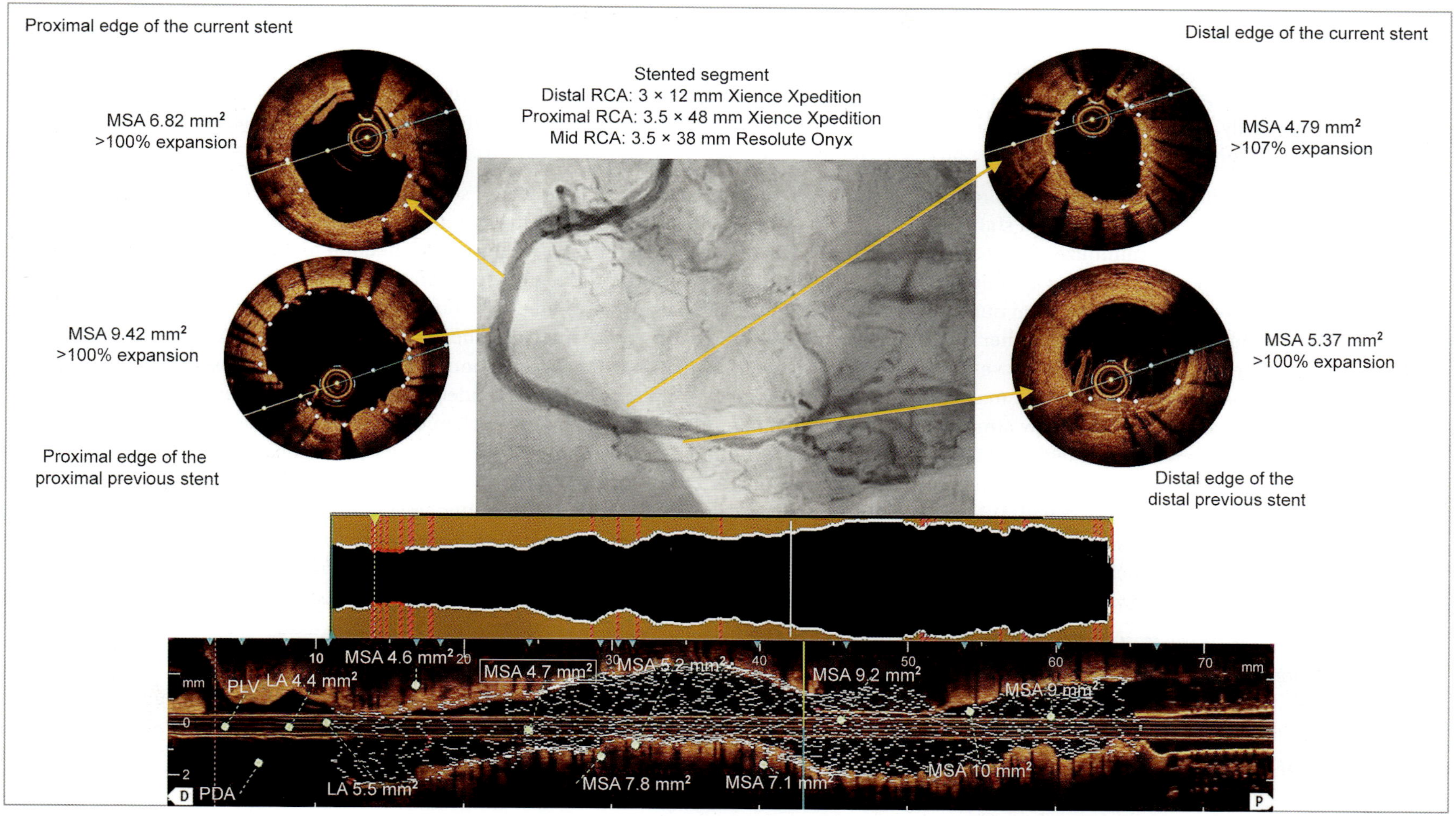

Fig. 24B

Figs. 24A and B: Final OCT showed well-apposed stent struts, no edge dissection, and no residual thrombus.

- IVL delivers an electrical discharge at the emitters vaporizes the fluid generating a series of circumferential ultrashort pulses of high-intensity acoustic energy, which, by virtue of its compressive and decompressive components, results in effective circumferential modification of calcific atheroma, selectively interact with calcified plaques even in their inner adventitial layer.
- Unlike RA/OAS, IVL can be used with more than a guidewire to protect side branches; its effect might theoretically extend to calcified side branches ostia and, reportedly, it can be used with the kissing balloon technique because of the presumed ability of IVL to propagate across a second balloon.
- IVL is associated with a very low complication rate (no perforation, nor slow/no flow phenomenon).

Technique of IVL: Does not require any special training as the IVL balloon-based device is delivered similar to standard catheter-based PCI. The IVL catheter was passed across the lesion over a standard 0.014″ guidewire. IVL balloon, sized 1:1 to the reference artery, was inflated to 4 atm, to allow contact with the vessel wall but minimize static barotrauma, and 10 pulses were delivered followed by further dilation to the nominal pressure of 6 atm. The IVL treatment was repeated providing a minimum of 10 pulses in the target lesion with interval deflation to allow for distal perfusion and overlap of calcified segments as needed. If the maximum number of pulses (80 per catheter) were delivered but lesion preparation was incomplete (i.e., incomplete expansion of the balloon by angiography), further IVL catheters with the same or different diameter balloon could be used. In addition, different diameter IVL balloons could be used when significant vessel tapering was present throughout the target lesion. If any difficulty in crossing the IVL catheter across the lesion, advised to use buddy wire, small balloon (1.5 mm), or guide catheter extension (Guideliner/Guidezilla/mother and child technique). IVL has no guidewire bias, performed at low atmospheric pressure balloon inflation, minimizing mechanical vascular trauma. Side branch protection using a guidewire may be easily performed using IVL, without risk of wire entrapment or severing as may occur with rotational or orbital atherectomy.

Calcified plaques with deep concentric calcium depositions remain resistant to these traditionally available plaque modification devices, in this particular scenario, IVL might be very useful. IVL has ability to fracture a calcified plaque outside an underexpanded stent, allowing appropriate stent expansion at subsequent high-pressure dilatation particularly ISR due to underexpansion associated with severe calcification.

The OCT studies showed calcium fracture as the predominant mechanism of action of IVL, the number of fractures was proportional to the magnitude of calcification. Calcium fracture was identified in 78.7% of CAC plaques, with multiple fractures in more than half of the lesions.

Treatment algorithm for a calcified lesion employing intracoronary imaging: Rotational atherectomy is considered when an imaging catheter cannot pass the calcified lesion. Lesion modification by atherectomy devices are considered when intracoronary imaging findings indicate criteria with risk of stent under expansion, such as calcium arc (>180°), thickness (>500 µm) or insufficient lesion expansion (remaining indication) by balloons including NC balloon, OPN balloon and scoring devices. Once the lesion is pretreated with balloon or atherectomy devices, imaging should be performed to confirm the success of lesion preparation by detecting the presence of fracture and dissection and assessing the stent size **(Fig. 25)**.

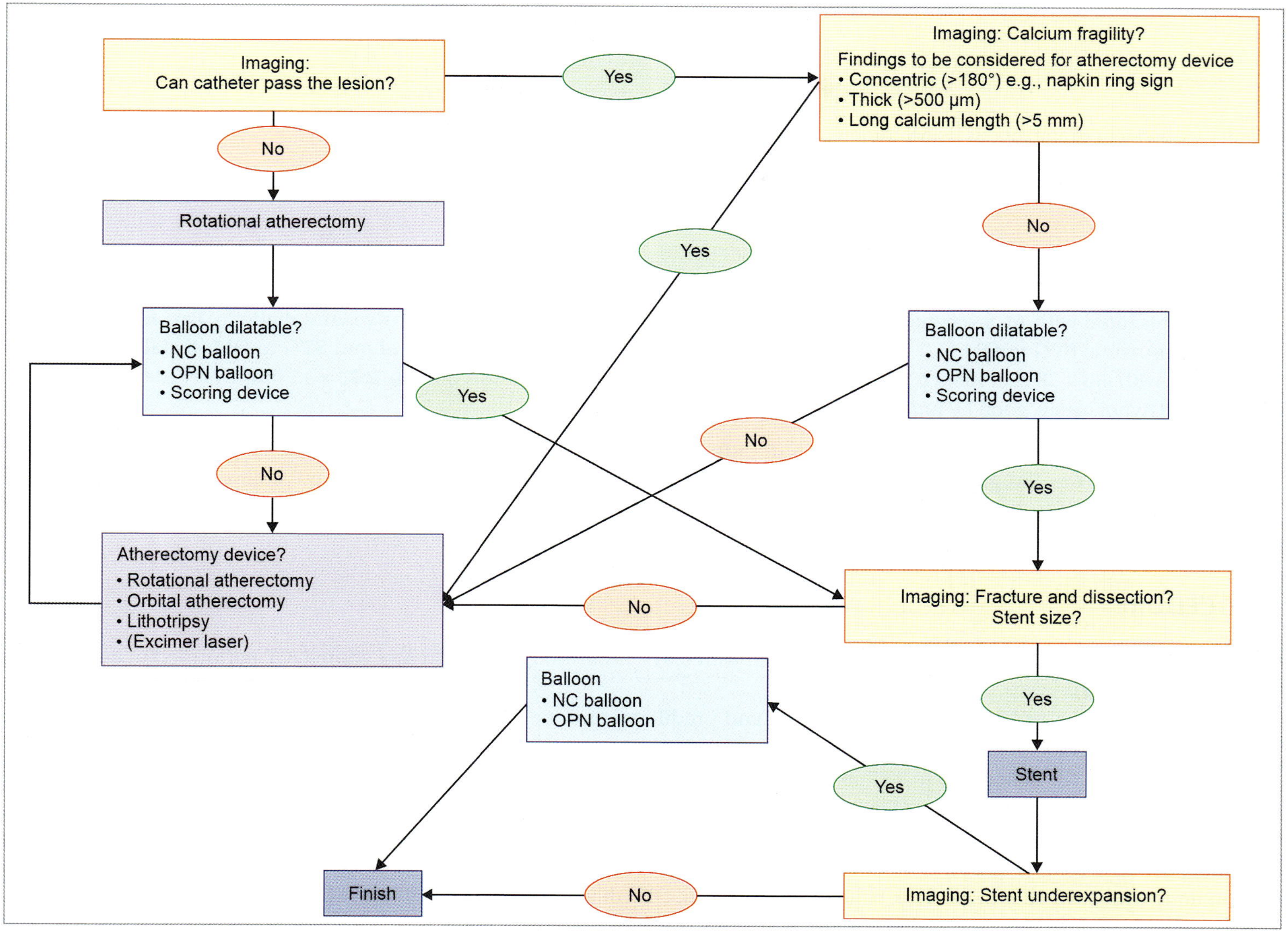

Fig. 25: Treatment algorithm for a calcified lesion employing intracoronary imaging.

CASE 4

ISR of SVG graft—assessment of ambiguous lesion, thrombus versus calcified lesion with stent fracture.

CLINICAL HISTORY

A 63-year-old male presented with ACS-recent onset angina of 1-month duration, known hypertensive, and diabetic. Past history of CABG in 1998, PCI with stenting of proximal SVG to OM (4.0 × 28 mm Synergy stent) in 2016. PCI with stenting of mid SVG to OM (distal to the patent stent has tight stenosis covered with 4.0 × 38 mm Xience Prime stent) in 2017. PCI of native RCA (2.5 × 30 mm, 2.25 × 15 mm Orsiro stents) with ROTA in 2017. 2D Echo—inferior wall hypokinesia, good LV function, EF—62%.

Investigations: Hb—13.7 mg/dL, serum creatinine—0.74 mg/dL, RBS—212 mg/dL. CAG-LAD diffuse disease, LCX—proximal total occlusion and RCA proximal to mid mild ISR, SVG to OM graft showing 80% ISR on angio suggestive of ambiguous lesion with possibility of thrombus or calcified lesion, SVG-D1—mid 80–90% lesion, LIMA-LAD patent graft, RA graft to PDA—occluded **(Fig. 26)**.

PROCEDURE

Route—RFA, 7 Fr JR 3.5 guiding catheter, SVG ISR lesion crossed with 0.014″ Runthrough wire. Preprocedure OCT performed to assess ambiguous ISR lesion of SVG **(Figs. 27A and B)**.

As balloon could not cross, Guideliner support was used and predilatation done with 2.0 × 15 mm Tazuna balloon up to 16 atm, scoring with 3.0 × 10 mm AngioSculpt balloon up to 12 atm for plaque modification of CN with Guideliner support, could not be dilated adequately with CB, then lesion dilated with 3.0 × 10 mm OPN NC balloon up to 45 atm with Guideliner support. After multiple high pressure OPN NC dilatations **(Figs. 28A to C)** OCT showed adequately expanded diseased segment **(Fig. 29)**.

Restenting with 3.5 × 18 mm Resolute Onyx stent deployed at ISR site with previous stent fracture up to 18 atm **(Fig. 28D)**. Poststenting OCT showed mild malappostion of stent **(Fig. 30)**.

Postdilatation done with 4.0 × 12 mm NC Trek balloon up to 12 atm. DEB dilatation with 3.5 × 30 mm Magic Touch balloon at 12 atm (dilated twice for 1 minute each). Postprocedure angio views showed well-implanted stents with TIMI-III flow without any dissection **(Figs. 28E to G)**.

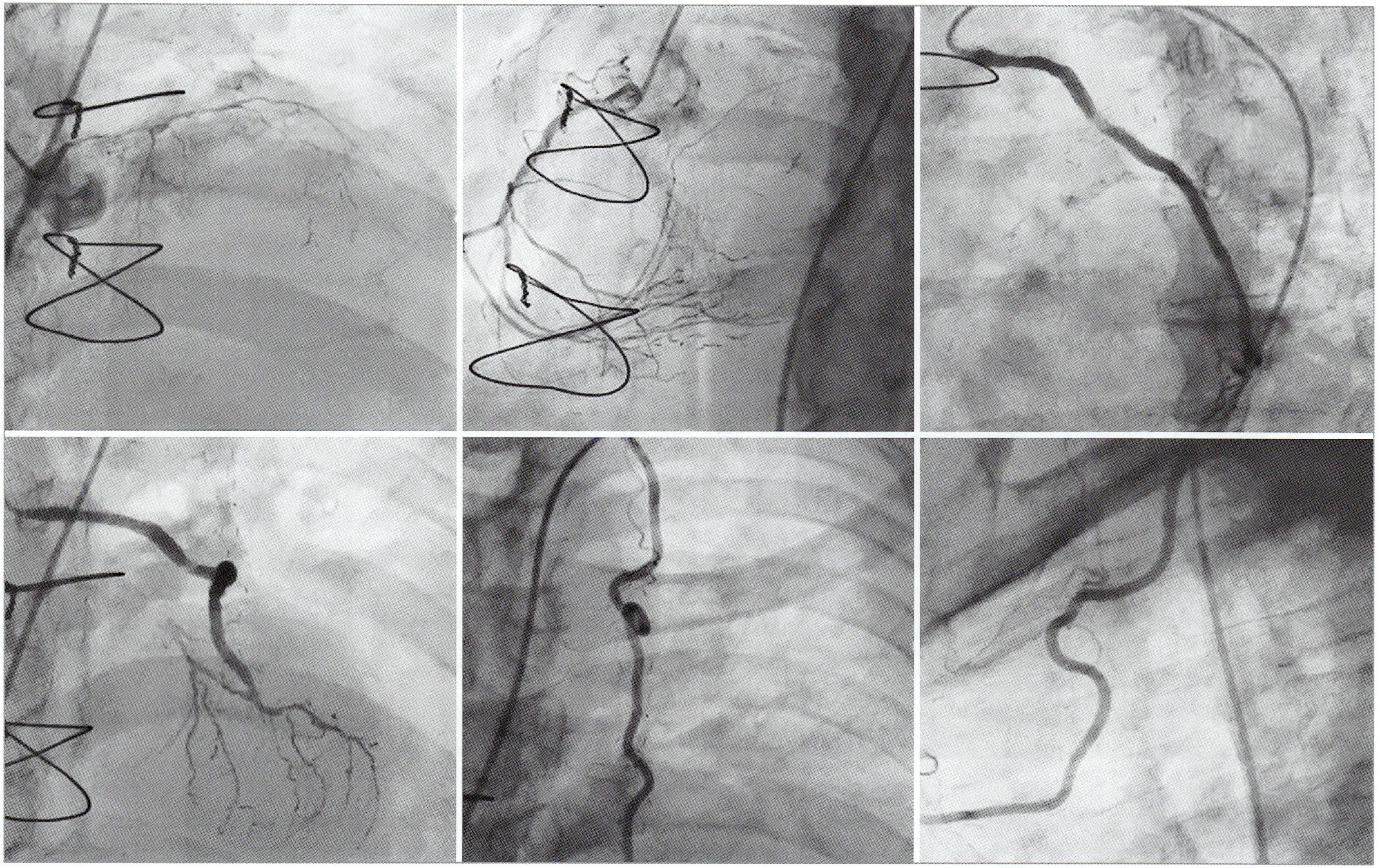

Fig. 26: Coronary and graft angio.

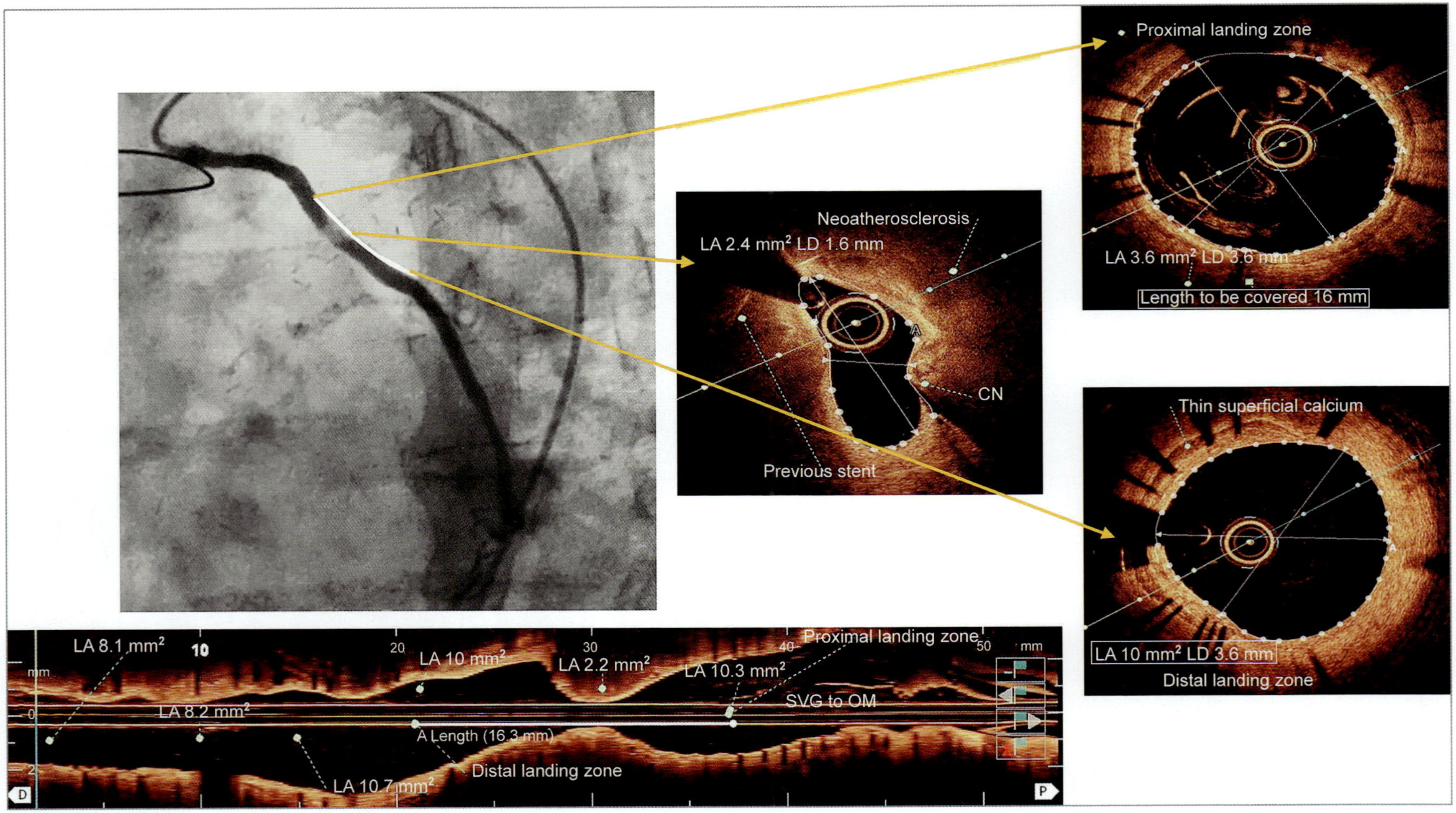

Fig. 27A

Patterns of ISR

- I: FOCAL
- IA: Articulation or Gap, IB: Margin, IC: Focal Body, ID: Multifocal.

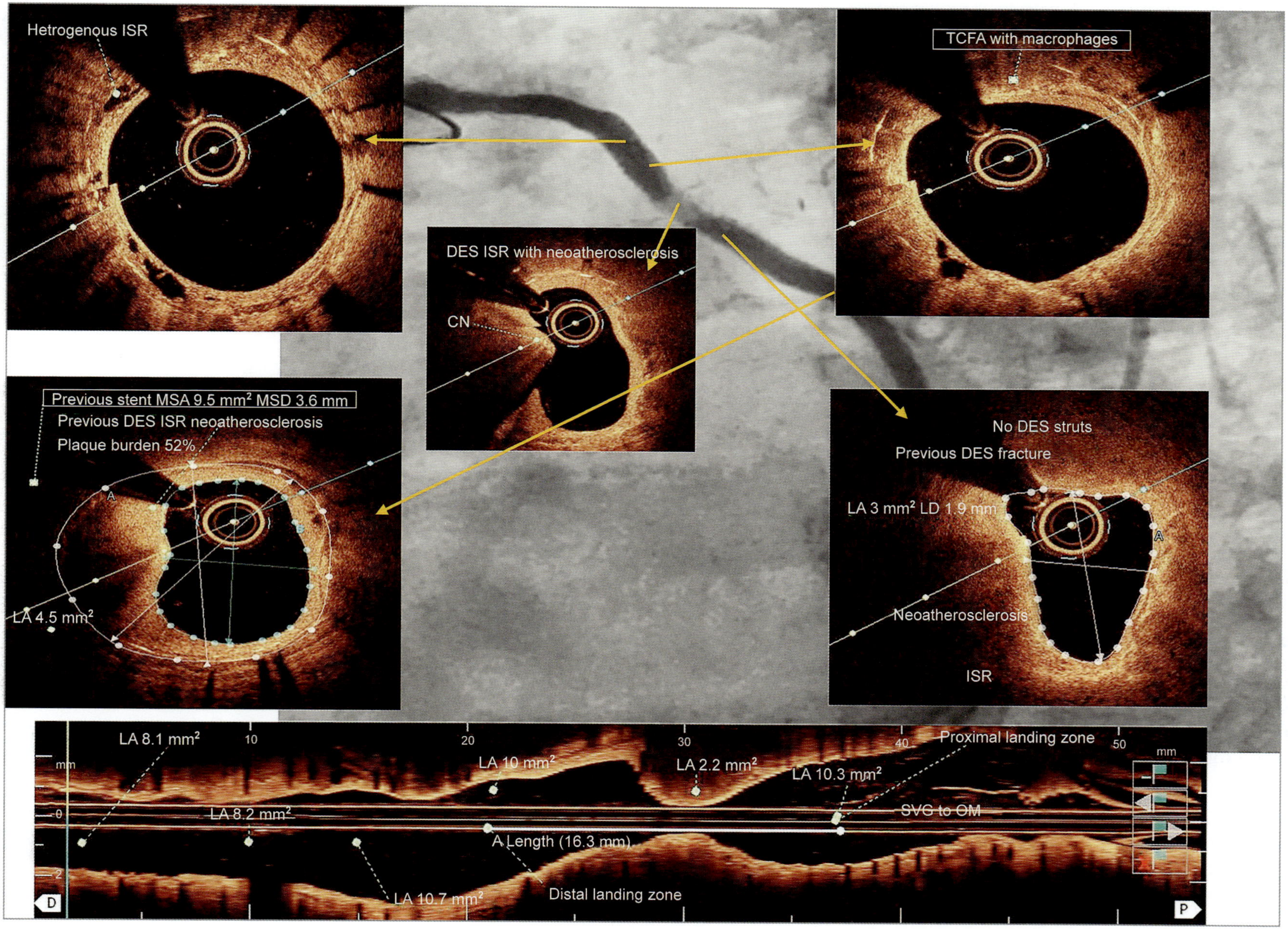

Fig. 27B

Figs. 27A and B: Prestent OCT. (A) Assessment for devise selection; (B) Assessment for plaque morphology.

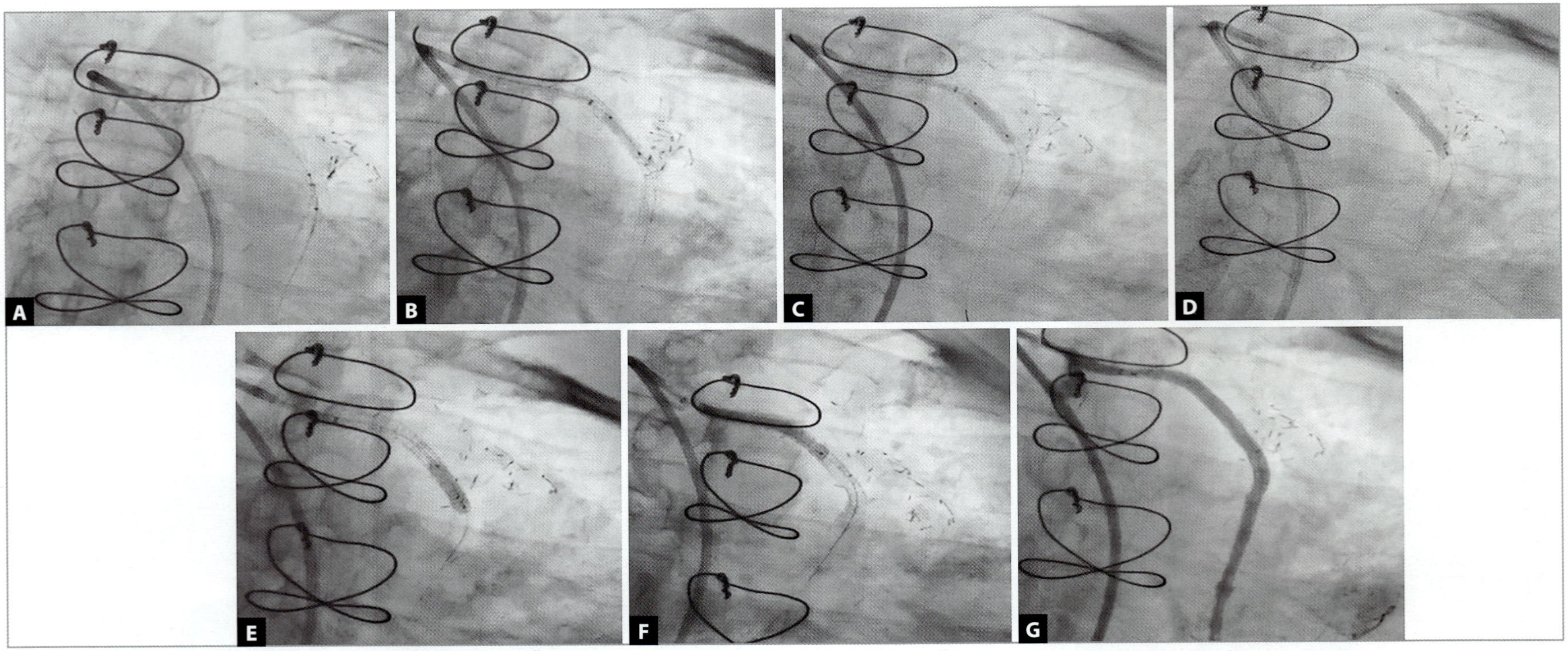

Figs. 28A to G: Coronary angioplasty. (A) Guideliner crossing; (B) Angio-sculpt balloon dilatation; (C) OPN NC high pressure balloon dilatation; (D) Stenting; (E) Postdilatation; (F) DEB dilatation; (G) Final result.

Patterns of ISR

- II, III, IV: Diffuse
- II: Intra-stent
- III: Prolifirative
- IV: Total Occlusion.

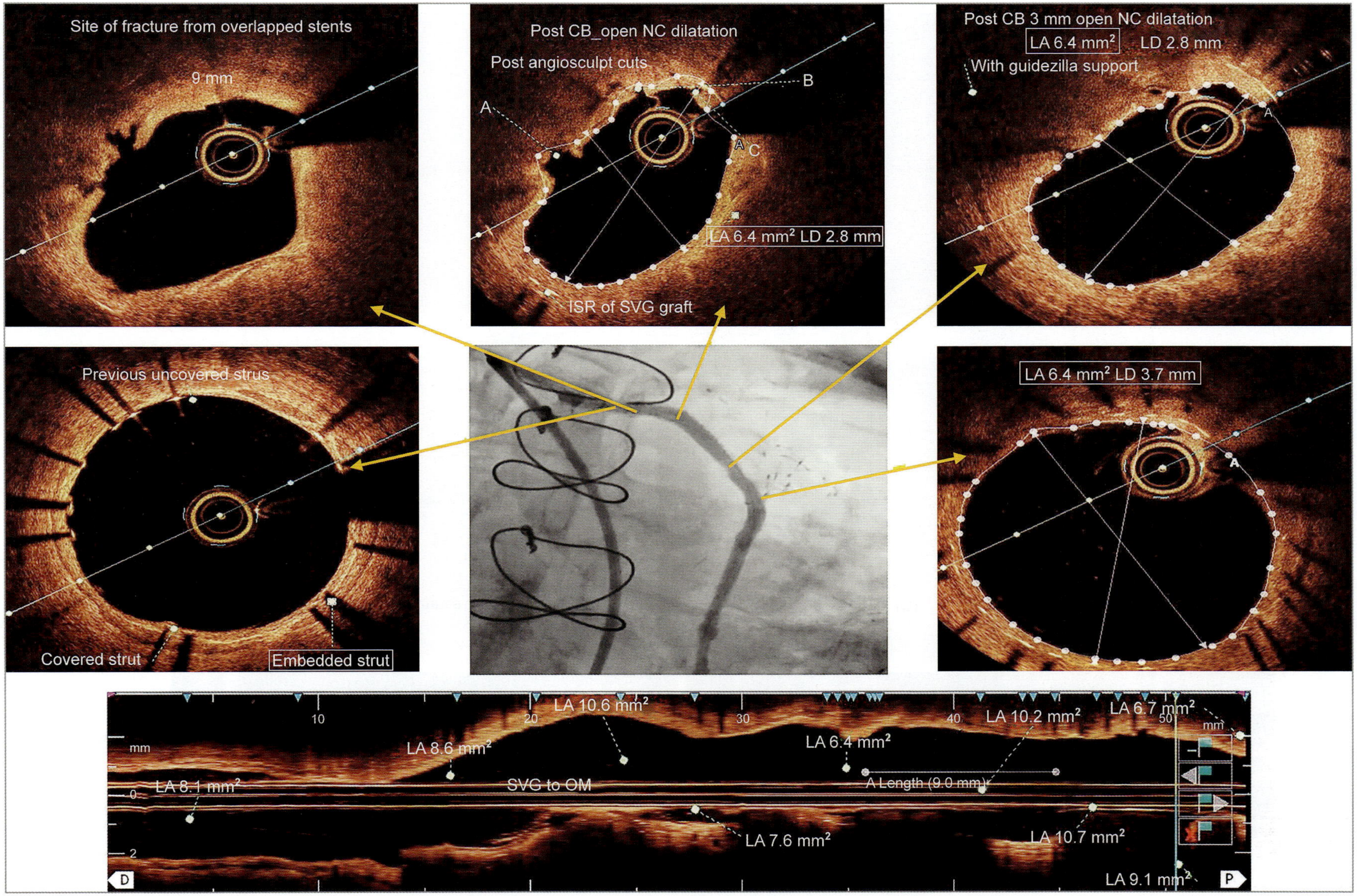

Fig. 29: Post OCT showed adequately expanded diseased segment.

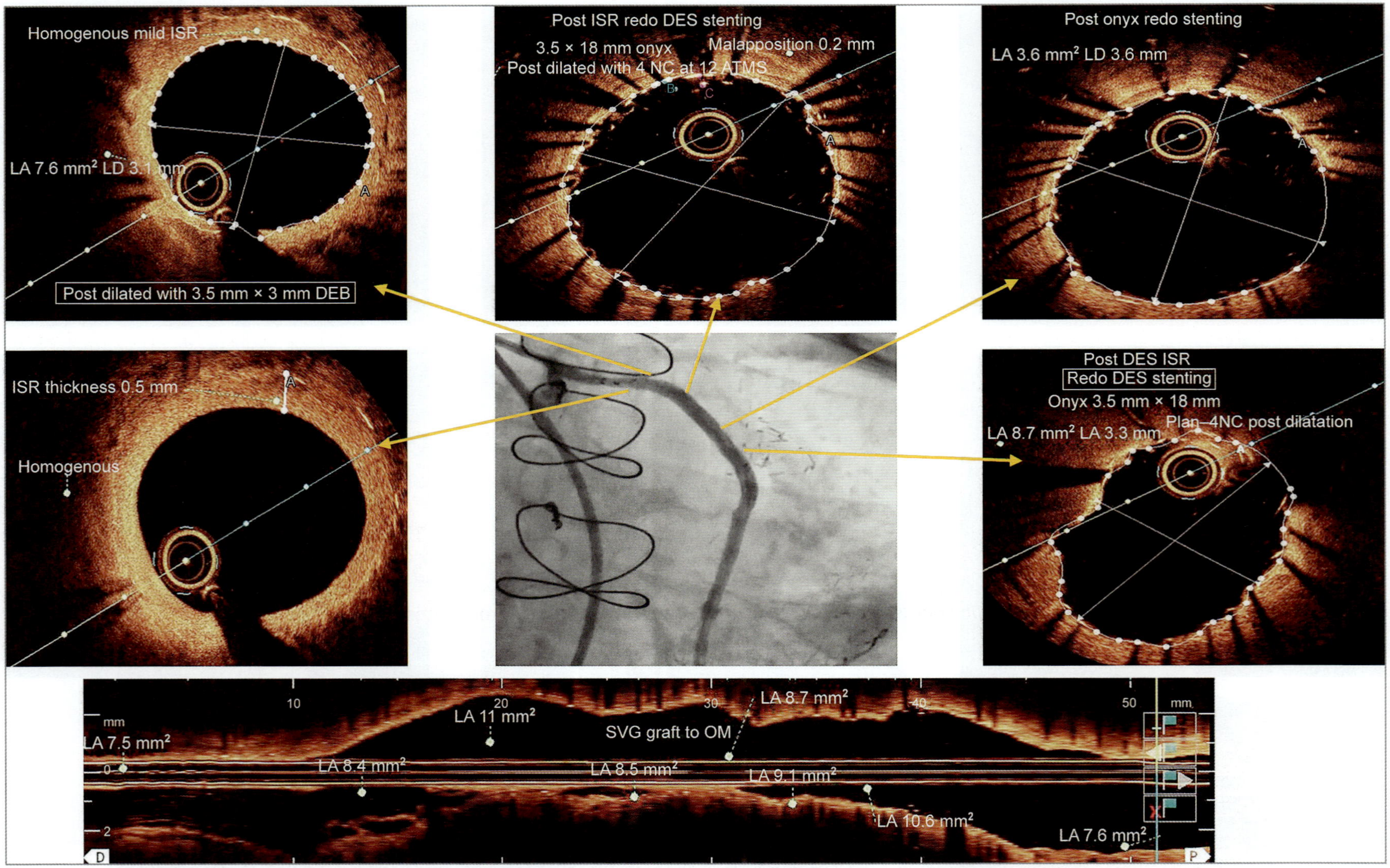

Fig. 30: Post stenting OCT showed mild malapposition of stent.

CASE 5

PCI with DES stenting of BVS-ISR.

CLINICAL HISTORY

A 75-year-old male presented with ACS—unstable angina, chest pain radiating to left arm for 2 weeks. Patient underwent PCI with BVS stenting of LAD 2 years before (2013). ECG-T-inversions in anterolateral leads. 2D Echo—No RWMA with normal LV function, EF—64%. Coronary angiogram revealed BVS ISR of proximal LAD **(Fig. 31A)**.

PROCEDURE

Right radial approach, using 6 Fr EBU 3.5 guiding catheter, pre-OCT showed ISR of BVS **(Fig. 32)**.

Predilated with 3 × 15 mm Trek balloon. Mid LAD stenting done with 3 × 34 mm resolute integrity and proximal lesion overlapping stenting done with 3.5 × 12 mm resolute integrity **(Figs. 31B and C)**. Postdilated with 3.5 × 15 mm, 4 × 15 mm, and 4.5 × 12 mm NC Trek balloons.

Post-OCT showed well-apposed and well-expanded stent struts with no edge dissections **(Fig. 33)**. Postprocedure angio showed well-implanted stents with TIMI-III flow without any dissection **(Fig. 31D)**. Patient was discharged on fourth postprocedure in a stable status.

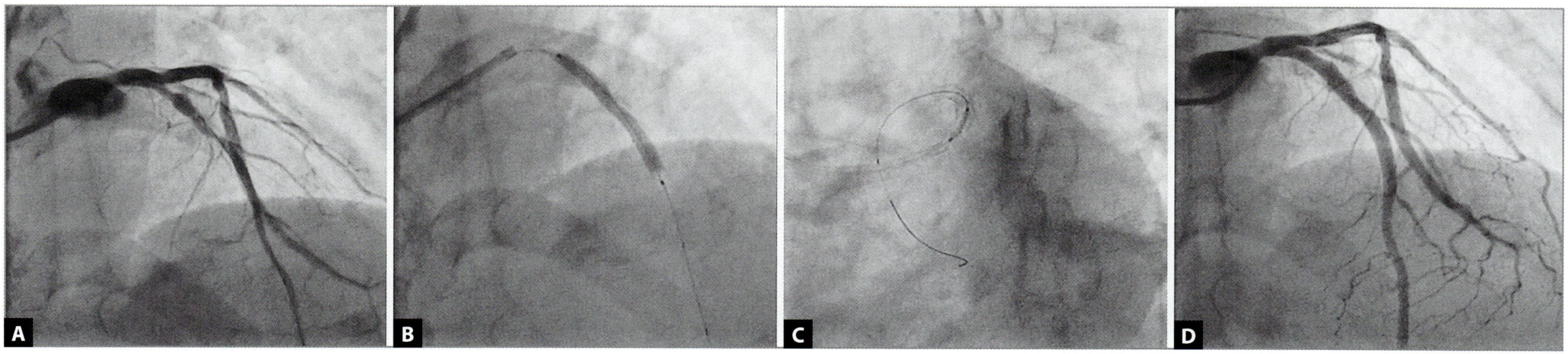

Figs. 31: (A) Coronary angiogram revealed ISR; (B) Mid LAD stenting; (C) Proximal stenting; (D) Final result.

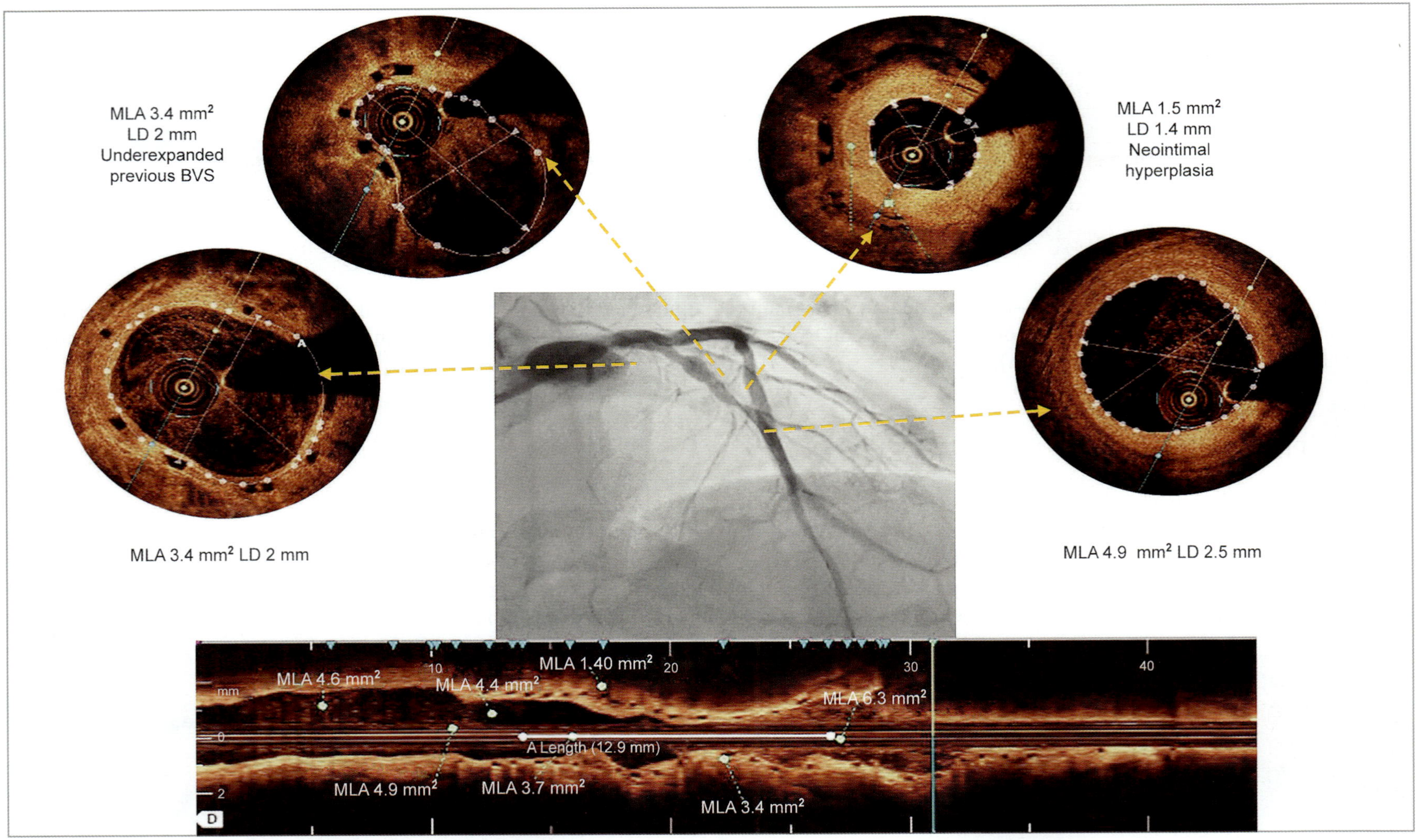

Fig. 32: Presenting OCT assessment for device selection and plaque morphology.

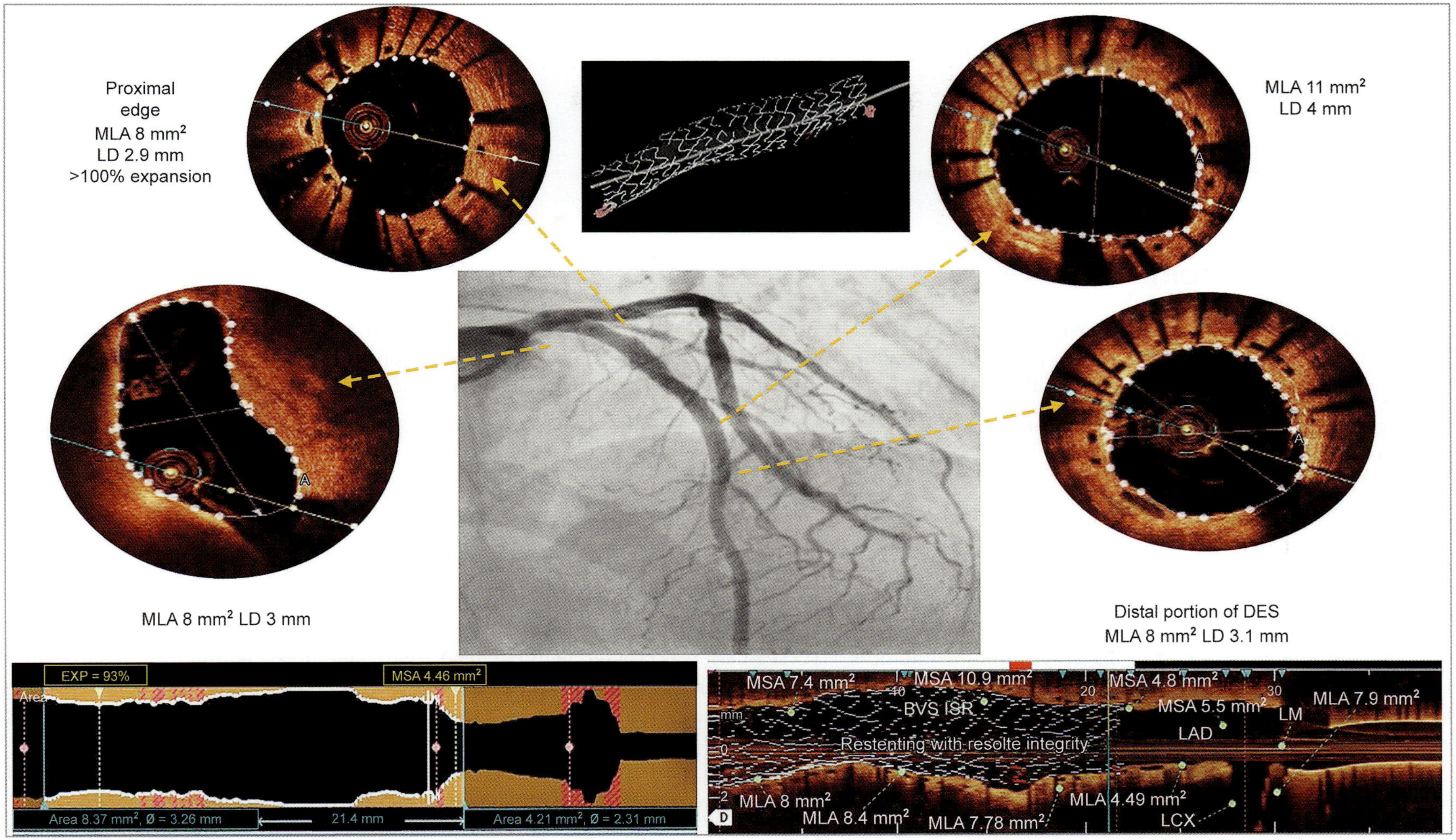

Fig. 33: Poststenting OCT assessment showed no medial edge dissection with well expanded and apposed stent struts.

CASE 6

ISR of RCA-scoring + DEB.

CLINICAL HISTORY

A 64-year-old male, known diabetic with old anterior wall MI, presented with exertional angina and SOB of 1-month duration. H/o PCI of LAD 8 years before with DES but details of the procedure were not available. He underwent angiographic evaluation 2 months earlier to present admission which revealed single-vessel disease, ISR with CTO of mid LAD. He was admitted for PCI of mid LAD under OCT guidance.

Investigations: ECG-QS complexes in anterior leads—Hb—13 g/dL, serum creatinine—0.9 mg/dL, GFR—85, HbA1c—8.6, 2D Echo—RWMA+ with moderate LV dysfunction, EF—38%.

PROCEDURE

Percutaneous coronary intervention of total occlusion of mid LAD stent was performed through right radial approach using 7 Fr, EBU guide catheter. Initially, Runthrough guidewire used to cross the lesion with Finecross microcatheter but could not cross. Then, Fielder XT wire was to cross the CTO segment with microchannel tracking. After multiple attempts, CTO segment was crossed with Fielder XT wire and advanced microcatheter beyond CTO segment in distal LAD. Placement of microcatheter in the true lumen of distal LAD was confirmed with contrast injection before placing Runthrough wire and removed microcatheter. LAD lesion was serially dilated with 1.5 × 2 × 10 mm Ryurei balloons to get adequate OCT images with adequate contrast clearance. Pre-PCI, OCT run was acquired to assess any need for plaque modification prior to stenting.

Optical coherence tomography analysis revealed critical fibrolipid plaque of proximal LAD and neoatherosclerosis with calcific intima in the proximal stent segment, lipid intima in the distal segment of ISR, and severe fibrotic plaque distal to ISR segment **(Figs. 34A to C)**.

There was atherosclerotic involvement of ostium and LM with bifurcation and carina tip angles >90° and bifurcation to carina tip distance is 2.2 mm **(Fig. 34D)**.

Total lesion length was 52 mm starting from ostium of LAD, proximal reference luminal diameter—3.5 mm, and distal reference diameter—3.0 mm **(Fig. 34E)**.

Plaque modification of the proximal segment was performed with 3.5 × 12 mm AngioSculpt and distal segment of the lesion was done with 3 × 12 mm AngioSculpt scoring balloons. Post scoring angio views showed well-prepared lesion, OCT run was taken to see adequacy of plaque modification which revealed scoring-induced well-controlled dissections with increased luminal area **(Fig. 35)**.

Subsequently, distal segment of the lesion was stented with 3 × 28 mm Xience Alphine and proximal segment was covered with 3.5 × 26 mm Xience Alphine stent with overlap of 2–3 mm. Stented segment was postdilated with high-pressure balloon inflations using 3.5 mm balloon at 16–18 atm inflations. Post stent angio views showed well-dilated and implanted stents. Final OCT run revealed well-expanded and apposed stents without any medial edge dissections. Poststent angio views showed TIMI-III antegrade flow without any residual stenosis or dissection **(Fig. 36)**.

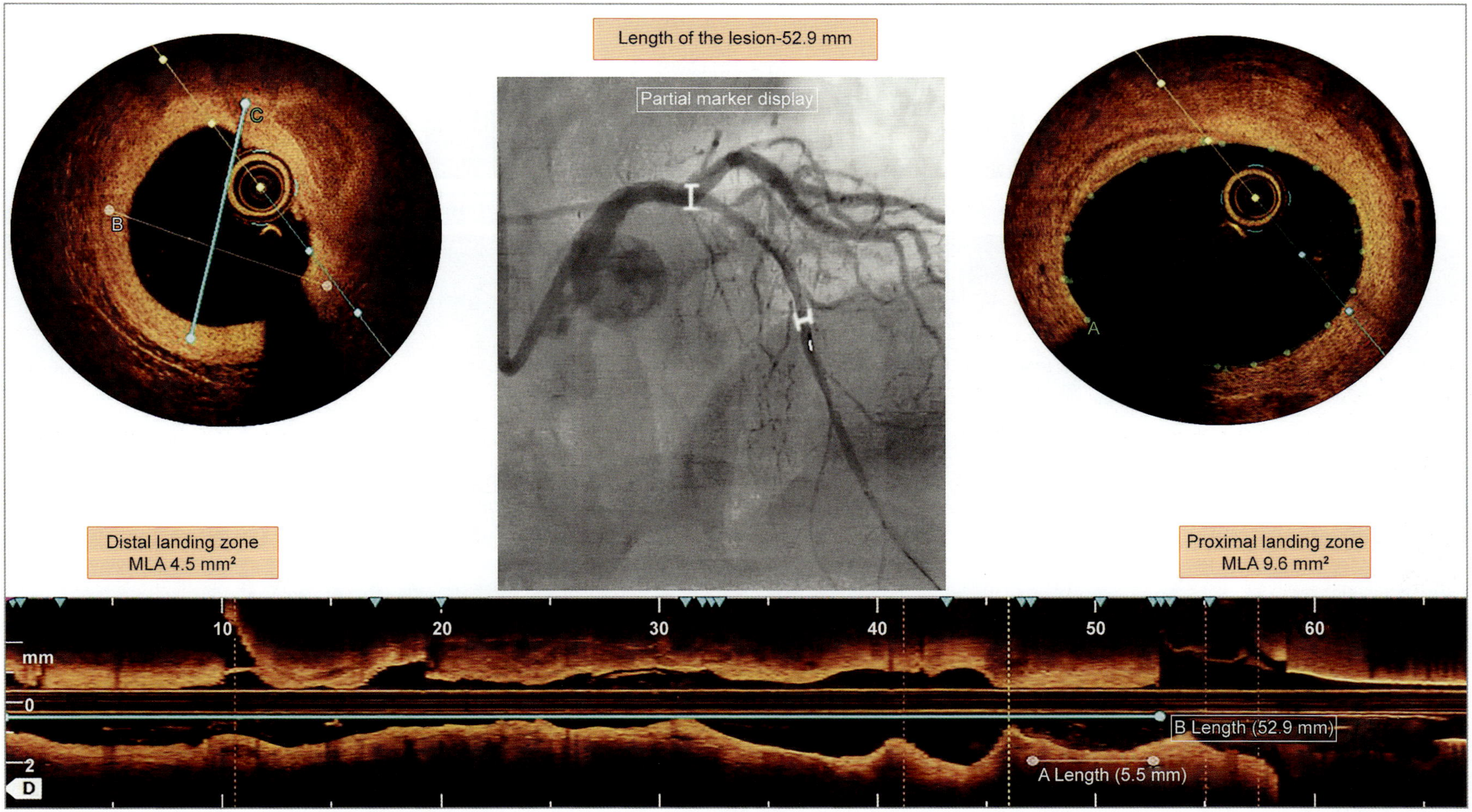

Fig. 34A

PCI of LM is emerging as an alternative to CABG especially in patients with low syntax score with suitable coronary anatomy for PCI, and life-saving emergency situations like ACS with hemodynamically unstable, and high risk group patients who are unsuitable coronary anatomy for grafting or due to associated co-morbidities.

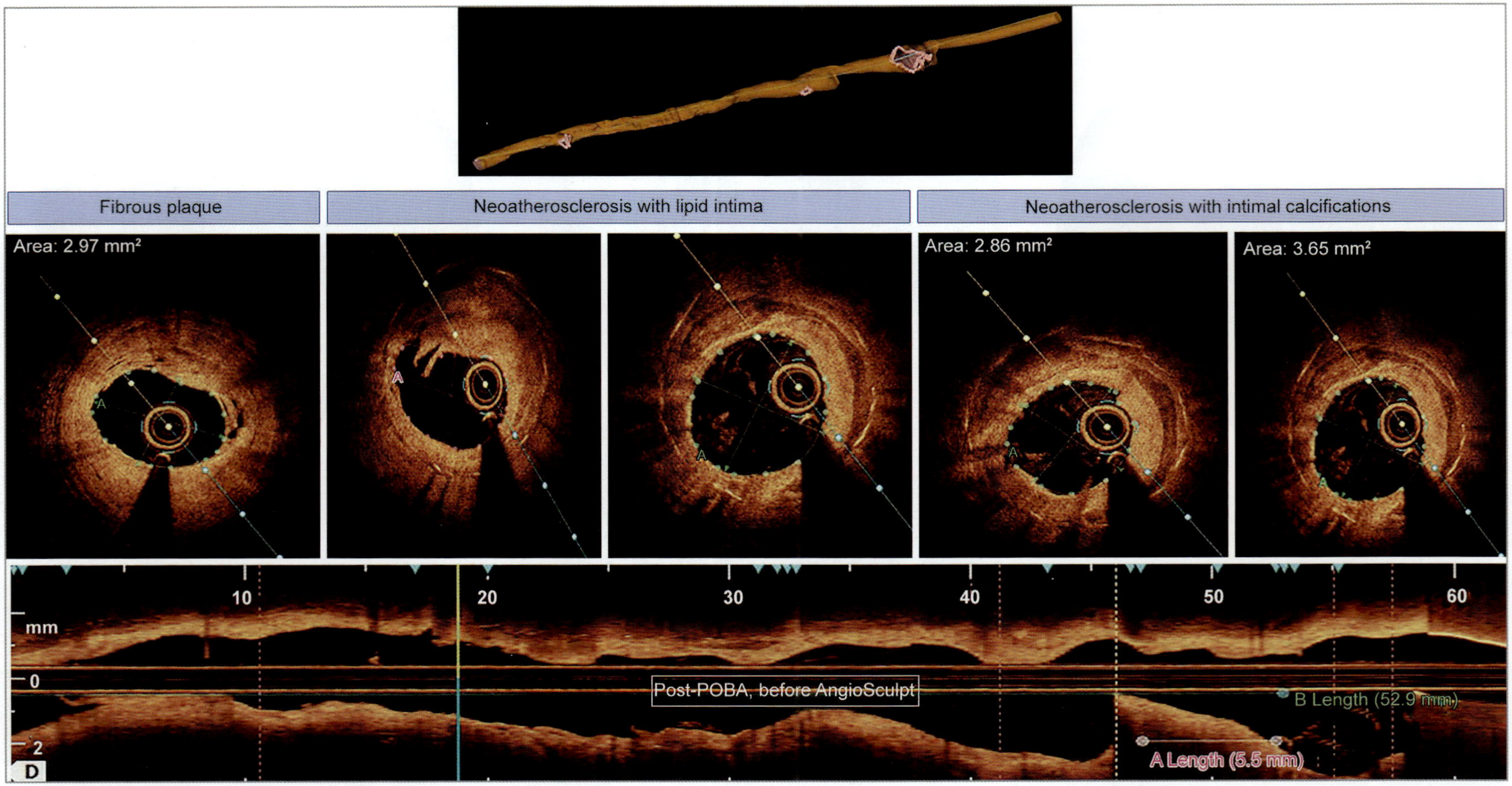

Fig. 34B

If the FFR is between 0.81 and 0.85, then the hemodynamic significance of the LM lesion cannot be accurately determined if the combined FFR of the LM and the downstream disease is ≤0.45. In such situations, IVUS or OCT imaging assessment of mean luminal areas will be helpful to decide whether revascularization is required or not?

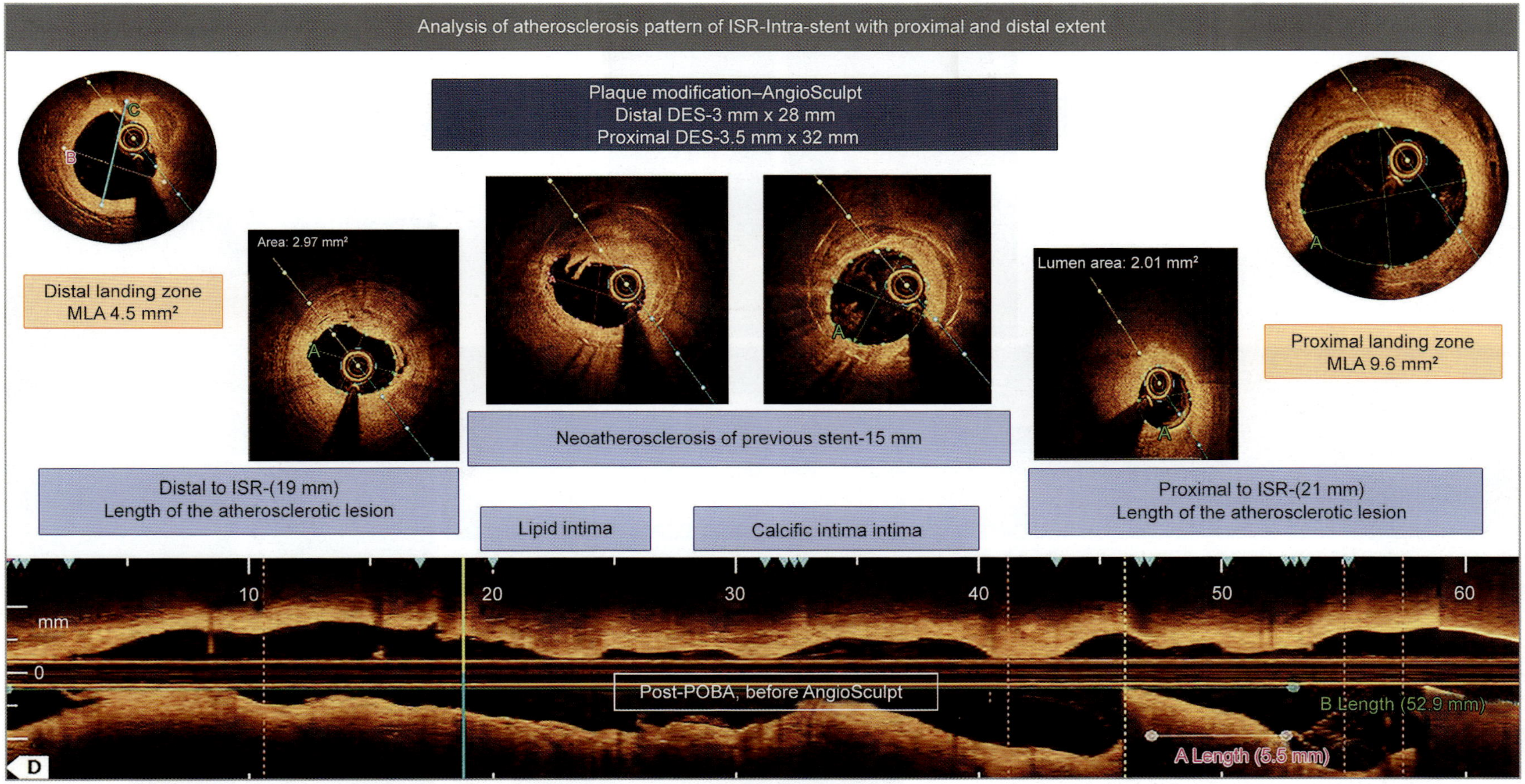

Fig. 34C

For all practical purposes, CABG is the main mode of revascularization procedure for significant LMCA disease unless contraindicated or unsuitable for surgery due to better long term results particularly in diabetics, and in patients with complex coronary anatomy.

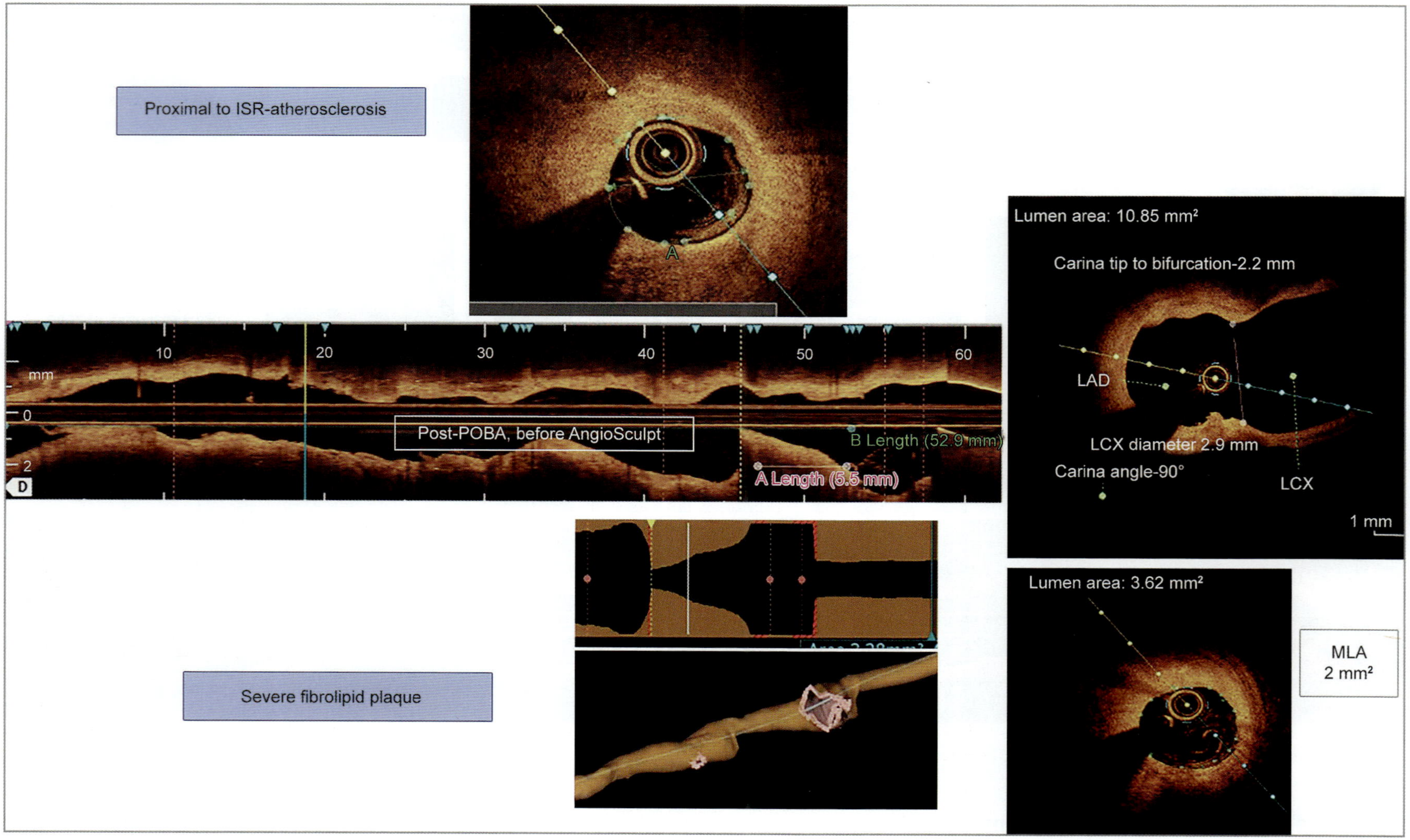
Proximal to ISR-atherosclerosis
A
10
20
30
40
50
60
mm
0
2
D
Post-POBA, before AngioSculpt
B Length (52.9 mm)
A Length (5.5 mm)
Lumen area: 10.85 mm²
Carina tip to bifurcation-2.2 mm
LAD
LCX diameter 2.9 mm
Carina angle-90°
LCX
1 mm
Severe fibrolipid plaque
Lumen area: 3.62 mm²
MLA
2 mm²

Fig. 34D

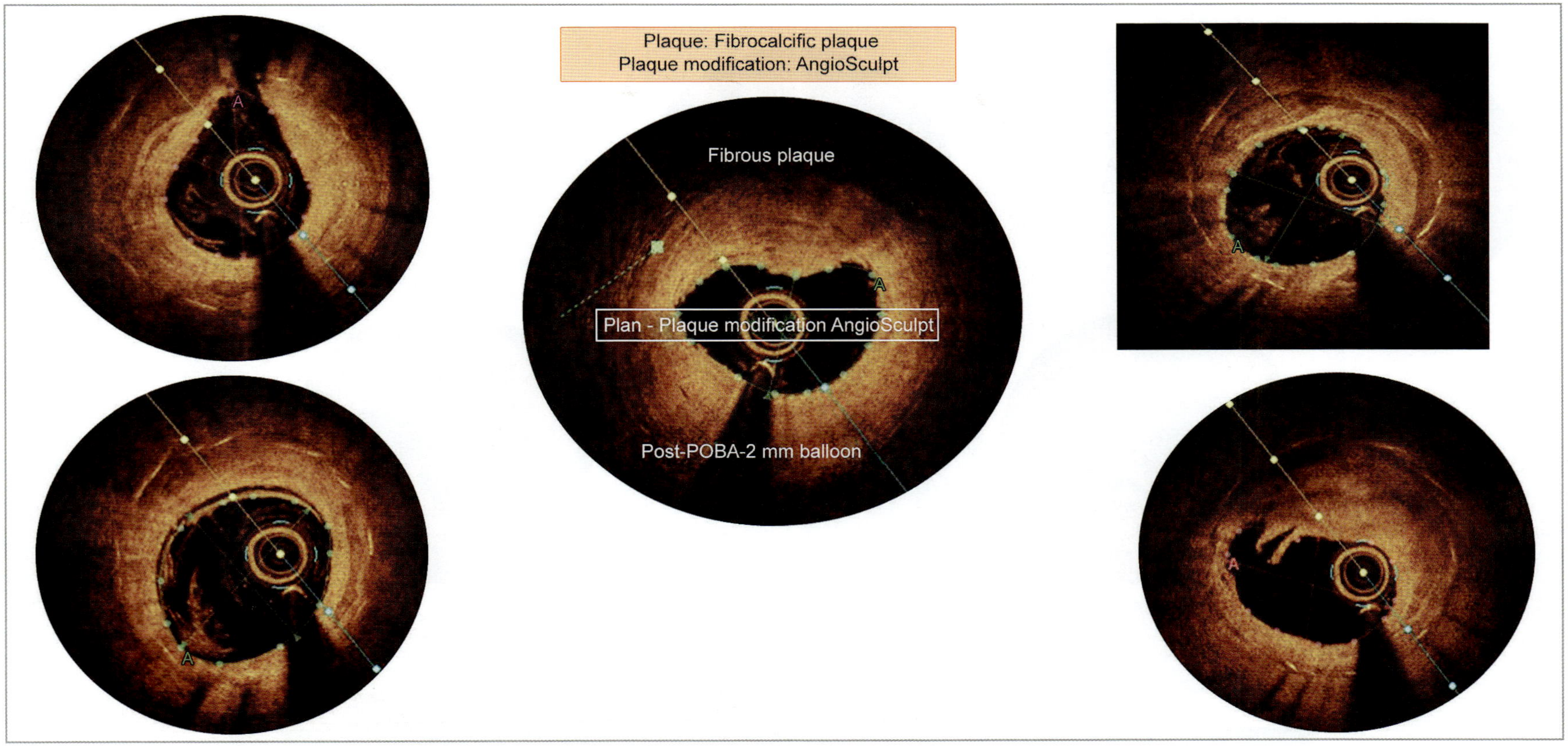

Fig. 34E

Figs. 34A to E: (A) Post-POBA OCT assessment for lesion length and diameter; (B) Post-POBA OCT assessment for plaque morphology; (C) Analysis of atherosclerosis pattern of ISR with proximal and distal extent; (D) Post-POBA OCT assessment at LAD-LCX bifurcation; (E) Post-POBA OCT assessment for plaque morphology to choose plaque modification device.

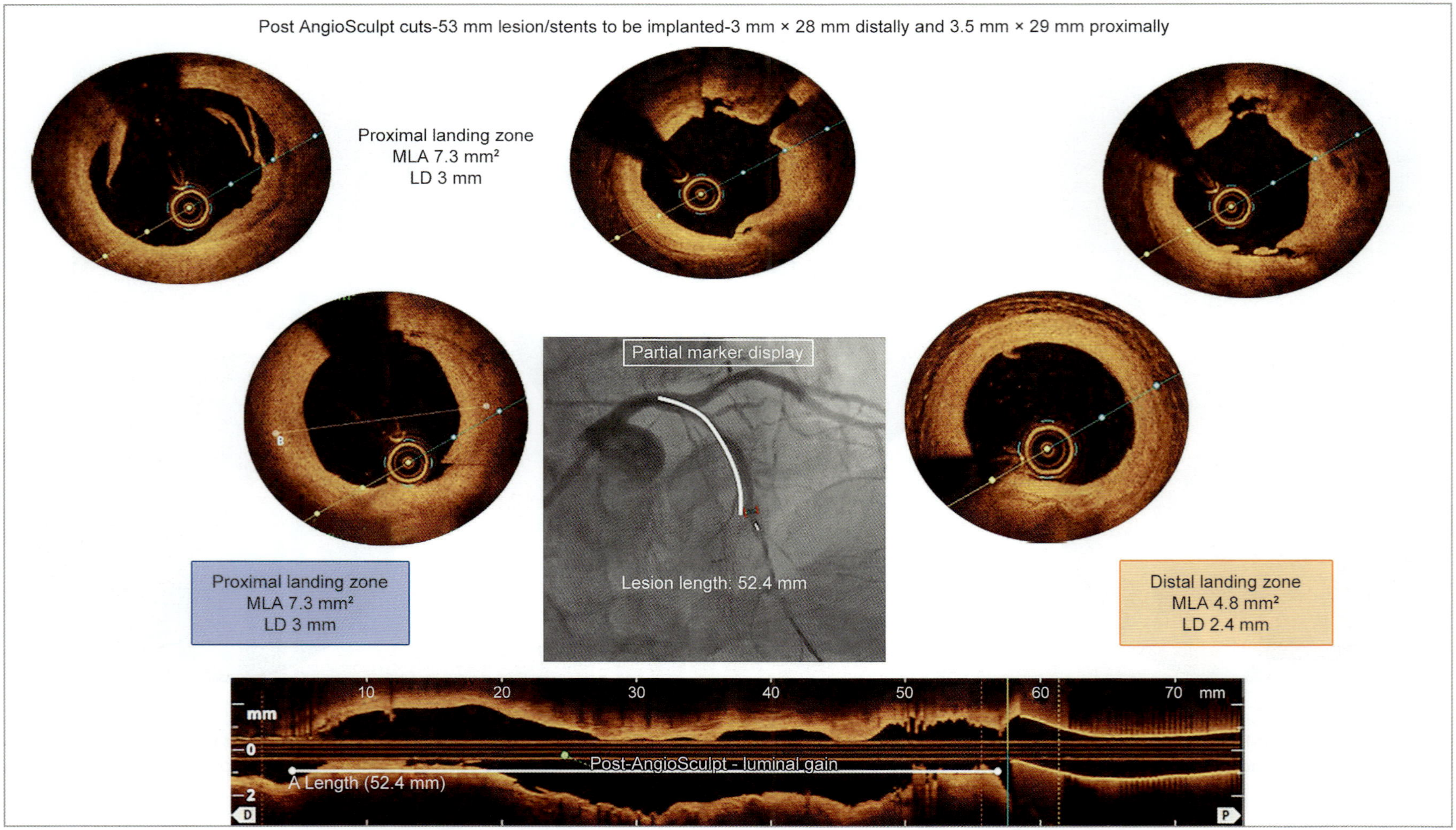

Fig. 35: Post angiosculpt OCT for proximal and distal landing zone to select the device.

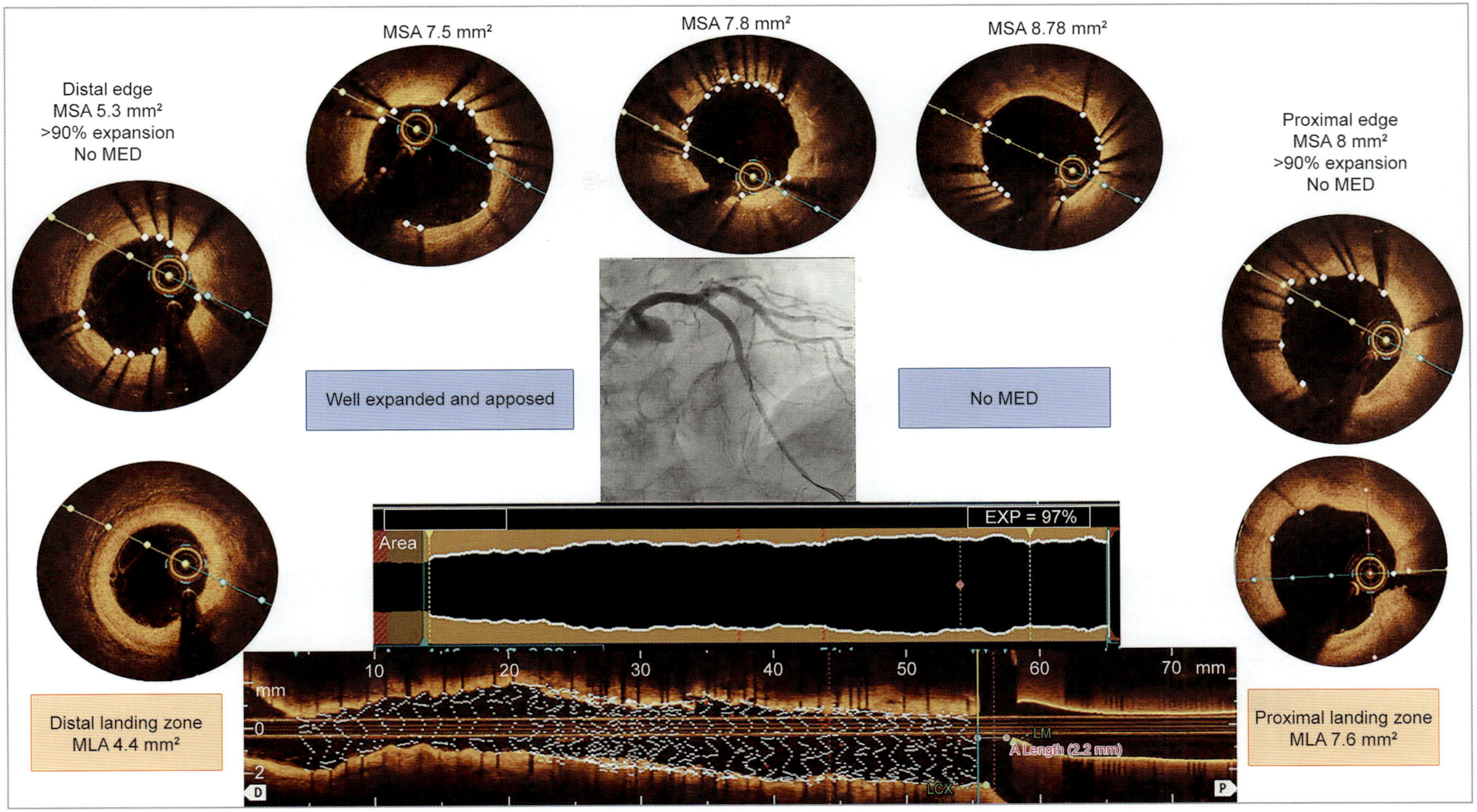
MSA 7.5 mm²
MSA 7.8 mm²
MSA 8.78 mm²
Distal edge
MSA 5.3 mm²
>90% expansion
No MED
Proximal edge
MSA 8 mm²
>90% expansion
No MED
Well expanded and apposed
No MED
EXP = 97%
Area
10 20 30 40 50 60 70 mm
mm
0
2
LM
LCX
Distal landing zone
MLA 4.4 mm²
Proximal landing zone
MLA 7.6 mm²

Fig. 36A

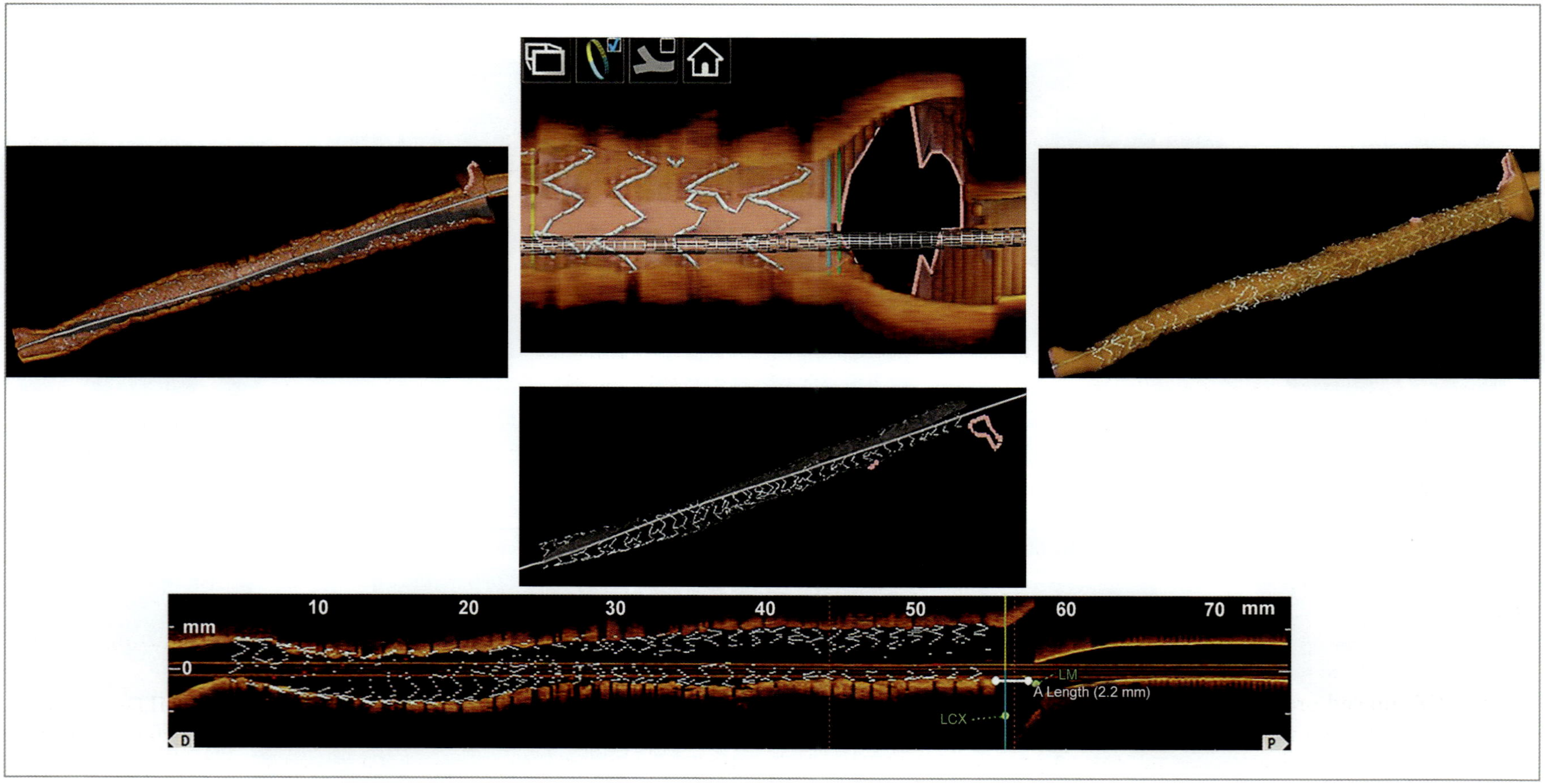

Fig. 36B

Figs. 36A and B: (A) Poststenting OCT assessment showing well expanded and well apposed stent struts with no medial edge dissection; (B) 3D OCT analysis of MAX - no MED, no malapposition and good expansion.

CASE 7

OCT assessment of ISR of ostial LMCA and ISR of RCA.

CLINICAL HISTORY

A 72-year-old male, known hypertensive, presented with ACS-NSTEMI, chest pain associated with SOB. ECG-ST depression in anterior leads, 2D Echo—no RWMA, normal LV function, EF—60%. Previous TMT positive for inducible ischemia.

Investigations: RBS—168 mg/dL, blood urea—62 mg/dL, serum creatinine—1.31 mg/dL, eGFR—54. CAG—90% ISR of LMCA, CTO of LAD ostium, mid and distal LAD filling retrogradely from RCA, LCX—patent stents of proximal and mid LCX, RCA-ISR of proximal segment 70%–80%, PDA, and PLVB—normal **(Fig. 37)**.

PROCEDURE

PCI of LMCA: RFA—route, 7 Fr JL 3.5 guiding catheter, 0.014″ Sion blue wire placed in LCX. Predilatation done with 2.5 × 10 mm Tazuna balloon. Preprocedure IVUS showed severe ISR. Pre-OCT of LCX to LMCA.

Pre-OCT showed proximal LMCA three layers of stents, inside one covered stent for earlier perforation with MLA—8.4 mm^2, MLD—3.26 mm, distal LMCA dissection with MLA—3.96 mm^2, MLD—3.75 mm, ISR of LMCA after POBA with 2.5 and 3.5 mm balloon previous stent area—15.1 mm^2, MLD—4.39 mm, percentage of stenosis—59%, LMCA near ostium earlier uncovered segment with MLA—8.3 mm^2, MLD—3.2 mm **(Figs. 38A and B)**.

Predilatation done with 3.5 × 10 mm AngioSculpt balloon followed by DEB dilation with 3.5 × 30 mm Magic Touch (DEB). LMCA stenting done with 4.0 × 15 mm Orsiro stent **(Fig. 39)**.

Post-OCT showed stent at LMCA ostium, previous stent MLA—14.8 mm^2, MLD—4.3 mm, LMCA underexpanded stent struts with previous stent MLA—7.6 mm^2, MLD—3.12 mm, proximal LCX MLA—7.2 mm^2, MLD—3.0 mm **(Fig. 40)**.

Postdilatation done with 4.5 × 12 mm NC Trek balloon. Postprocedure angio views showed well-implanted stents with TIMI-III flow without any dissection **(Fig. 39)**.

PCI of RCA: RFA—route, 6 Fr JR 3.5 guiding catheter, lesion was crossed with 0.014″ Sion blue wire. Predilatation done with 2.5 10 mm Tazuna balloon, and CB with 3.5 × 10 mm. Preprocedure OCT showed severe ISR, ostium MLA—6.4 mm^2, MLD—2.8 mm, dissection more than 60° and proximal RCA MLA—7.1 mm^2, MLD—3 mm **(Fig. 41)**. Drug eluting balloon dilatation done with 3.5 × 25 mm Magic Touch balloon. Proximal RCA stenting done with 3.5 × 15 mm Orsiro stent **(Fig. 42)**. RCA post-OCT showed near ostium MLA—7.6 mm^2, MLD—3.12 mm, post-CB and DEB dissection MLA—6.18 mm^2, MLD—2.65 mm, proximal RCA MLA—8.1 mm^2, MLD—3.2 mm **(Fig. 43)**. Postprocedure angio views showed well-implanted stents with TIMI-III flow

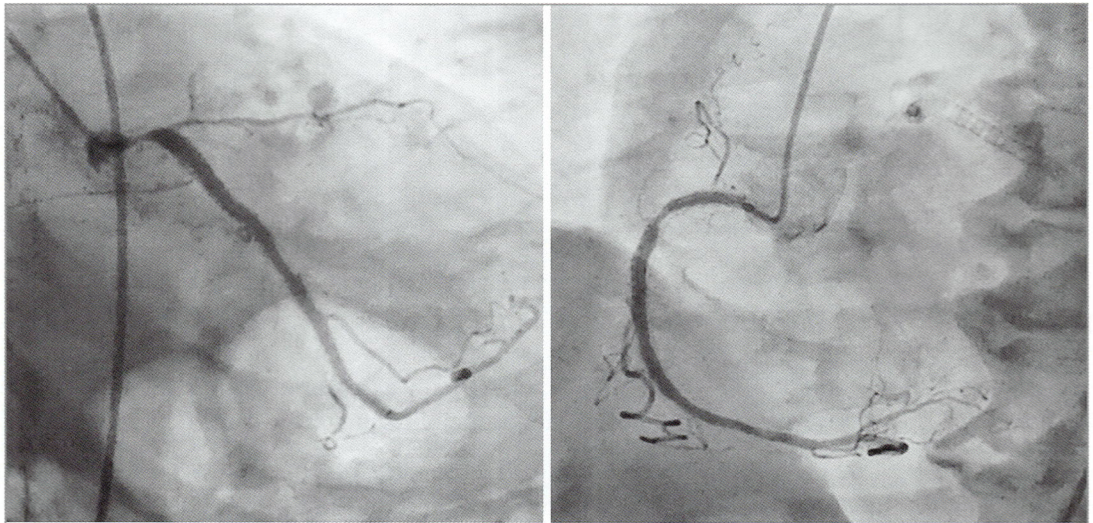

Fig. 37: Coronary angiogram.

without any dissection. Left femoral artery sheath injection was taken, suggestive of grade III perforation. Then through left radial artery exchange length Terumo wire was placed in left femoral artery. Balloon tamponade of left CIA and EIA done with 6 × 50 mm Mozac PTA balloon proximal to SFA perforation **(Fig. 44)**. Under local anesthesia femoral artery and femoral vein repair was done. Check shoot, no extravasation at the site of perforation. Patient was discharged on 5th postprocedure in a stable status.

Many times it would be difficult to obtain optimal images of LM ostium due to guide position, inadequate clearance of contrast, and deep seating of guide in short LMCA. Good LMCA ostial images can obtained by high-flow contrast injections (i.e., 6 mL/s), keeping proximal marker of OCT catheter keeping in proximal LAD, with good alignment of guide catheter with LMCA. This patient underwent PCI of LMCA 4 years earlier with recent onset of angina evaluated with repeat coronary angiogram which showed tight ostioproximal LMCA ISR. OCT revealed underexpansion of the stent, and uncovered ostial segment of LMCA with previous stent resulting in severe ISR. PCI of LMCA was done with DES covering ostial portion of LMCA with adequate expansion of previously under expanded stent. Patient has been undergoing medical management without any CV symptoms for the past 2 years.

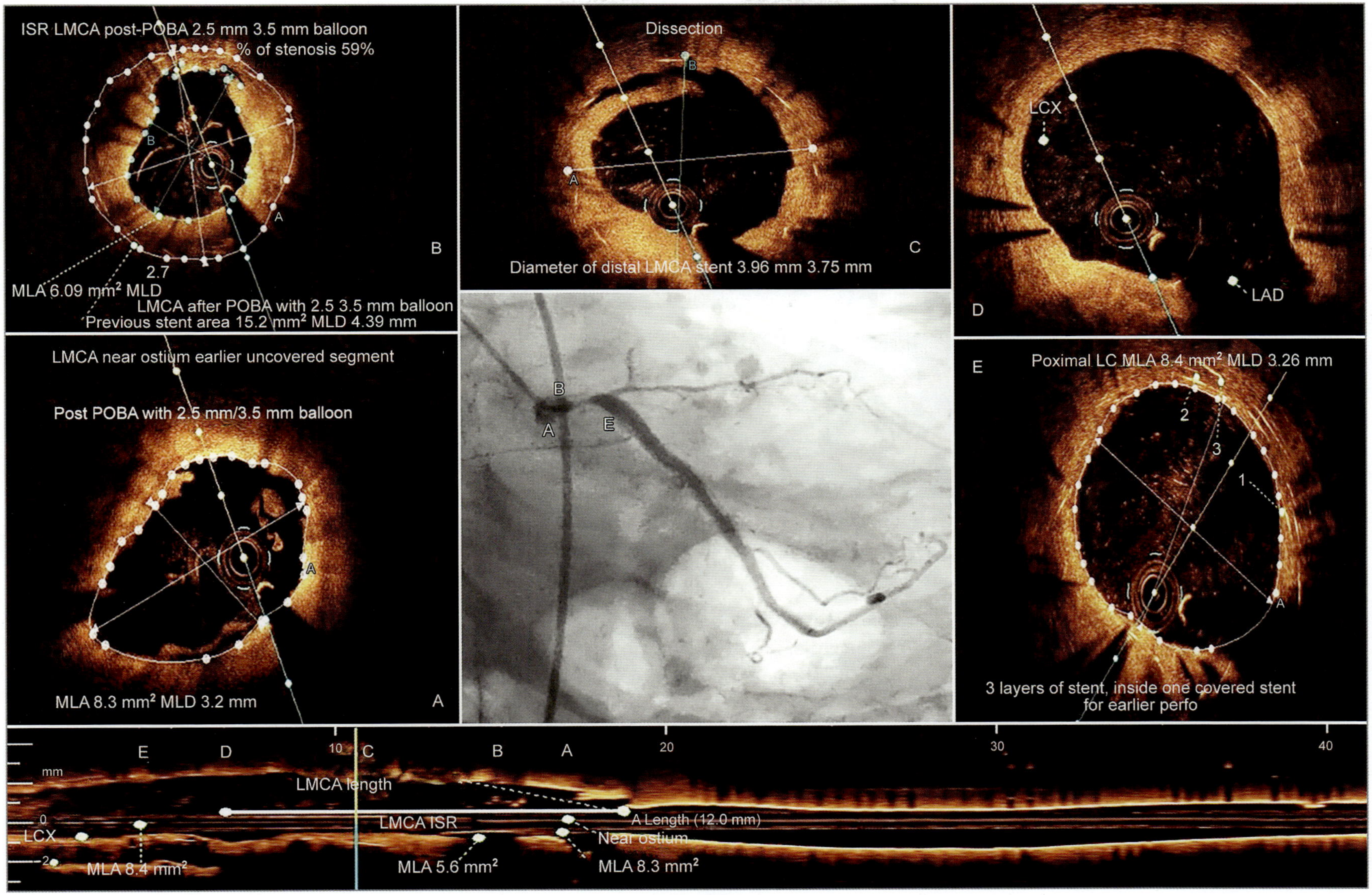
ISR LMCA post-POBA 2.5 mm 3.5 mm balloon
% of stenosis 59%
B
2.7
MLA 6.09 mm² MLD
LMCA after POBA with 2.5 3.5 mm balloon
Previous stent area 15.2 mm² MLD 4.39 mm
Dissection
C
Diameter of distal LMCA stent 3.96 mm 3.75 mm
LCX
LAD
D
LMCA near ostium earlier uncovered segment
Post POBA with 2.5 mm/3.5 mm balloon
MLA 8.3 mm² MLD 3.2 mm
A
B
A
E
E
Poximal LC MLA 8.4 mm² MLD 3.26 mm
3 layers of stent, inside one covered stent
for earlier perfo
E D 10 C B A 20 30 40
mm
LMCA length
A Length (12.0 mm)
LMCA ISR
Near ostium
LCX
MLA 8.4 mm²
MLA 5.6 mm²
MLA 8.3 mm²

Fig. 38A

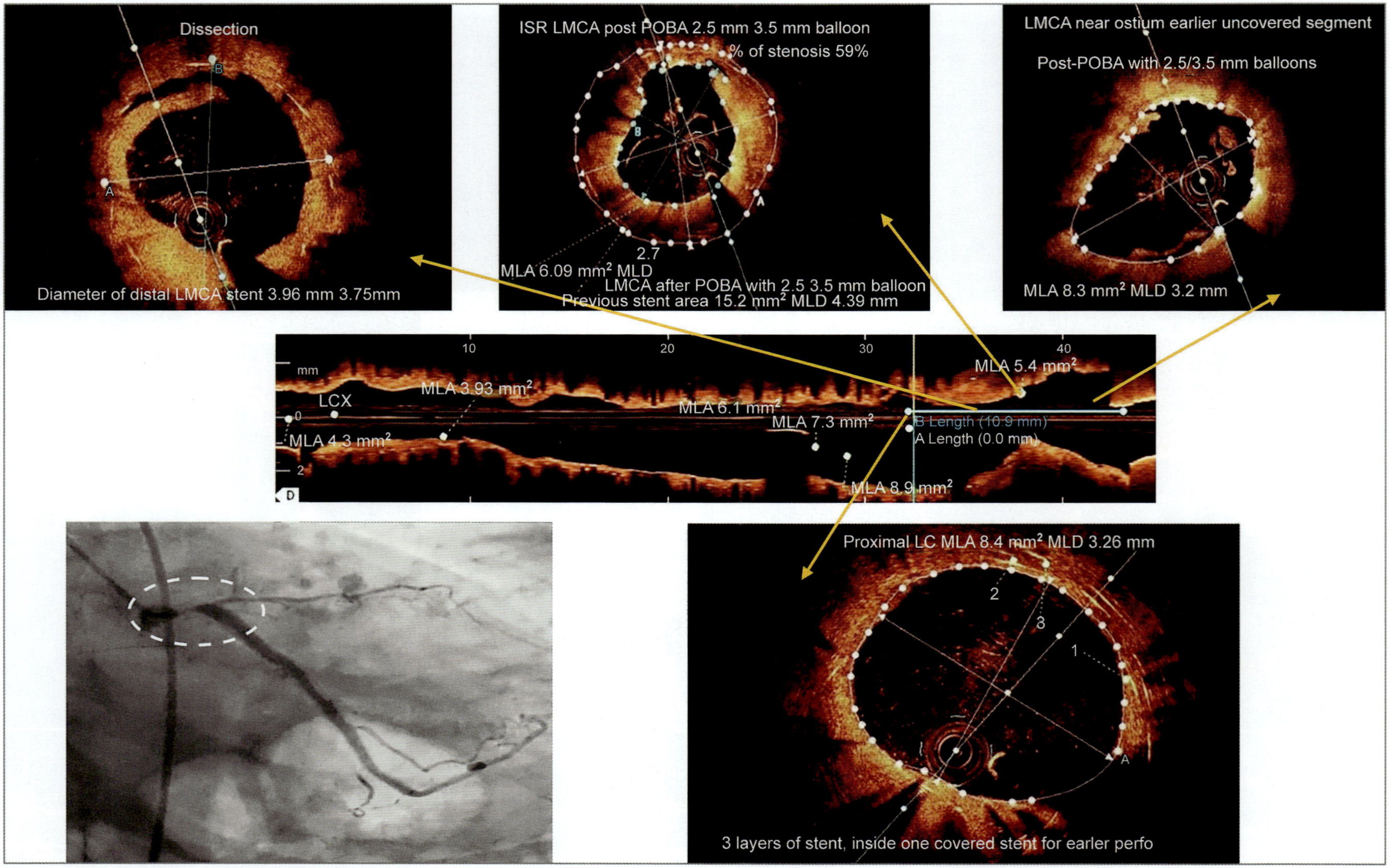

Fig. 38B

Figs. 38A and B: A presenting OCT assessment of LM-LCX. (A) For devise selection; (B) Analysis of ISR segment.

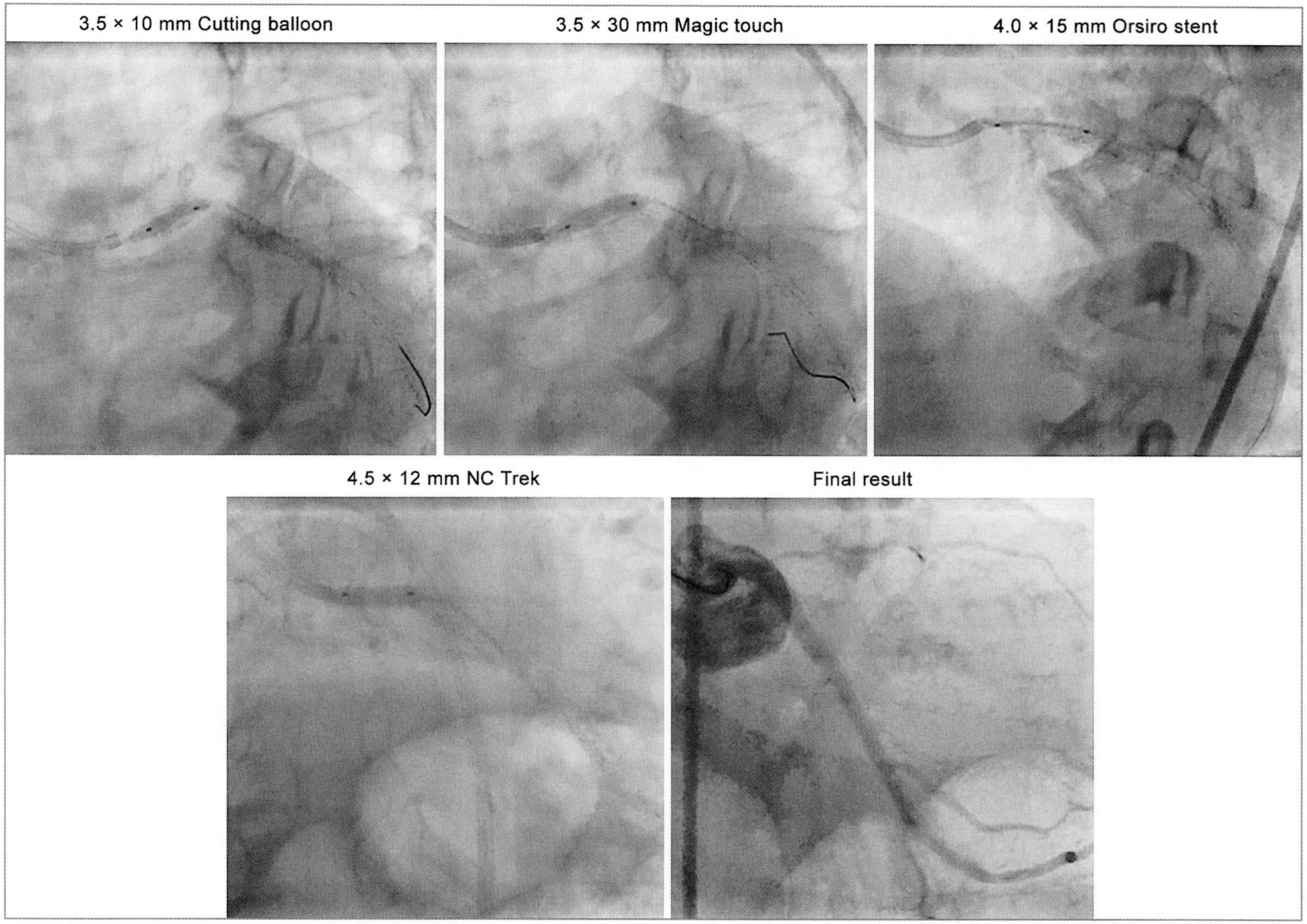

Fig. 39: Coronary angioplasty of LMCA-LCX segment with cutting balloon, DEB, stent and post dilatation.

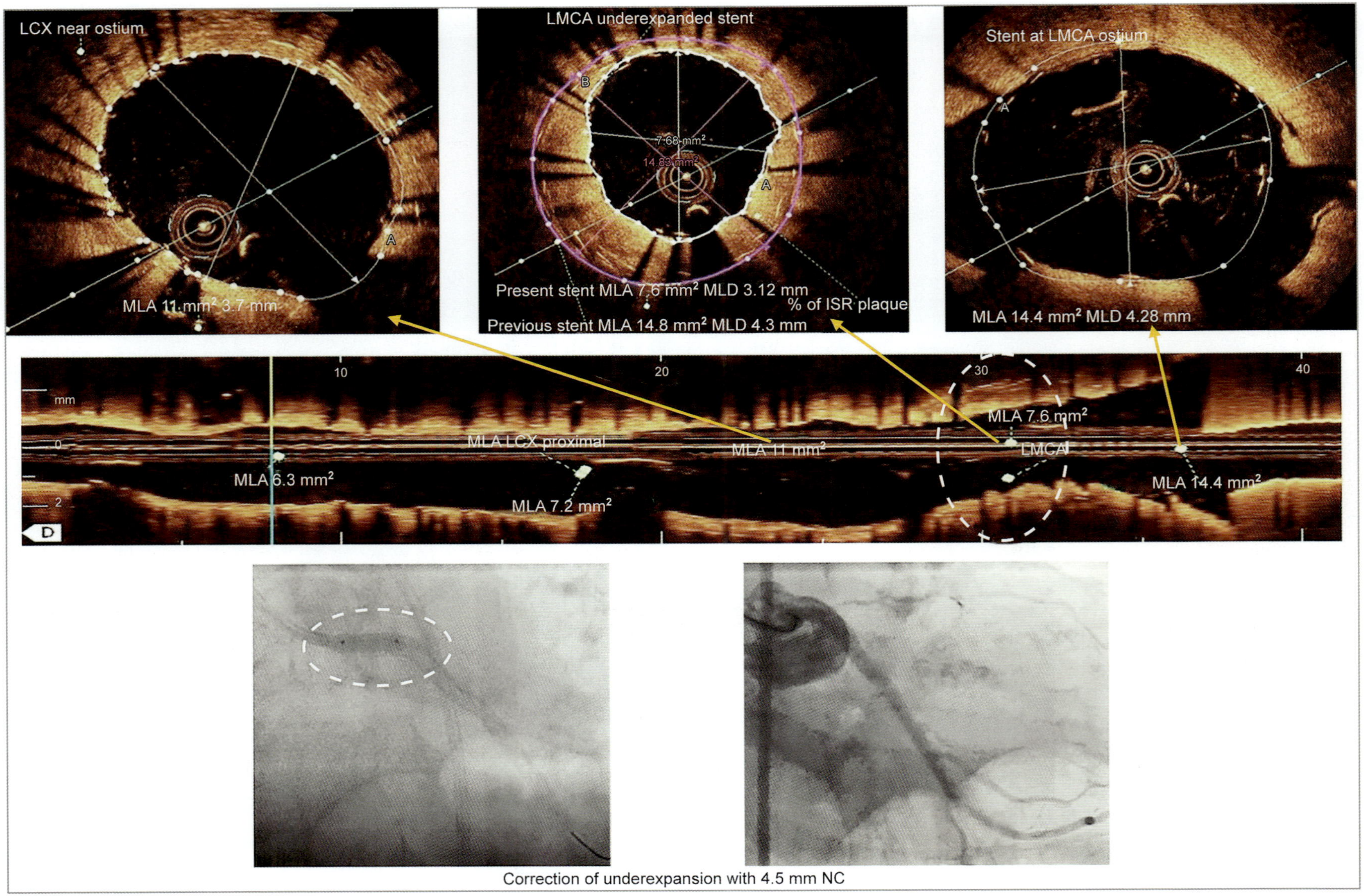

Fig. 40: Poststent OCT assessment showed malapposition in LM segment which was corrected with higher balloon.

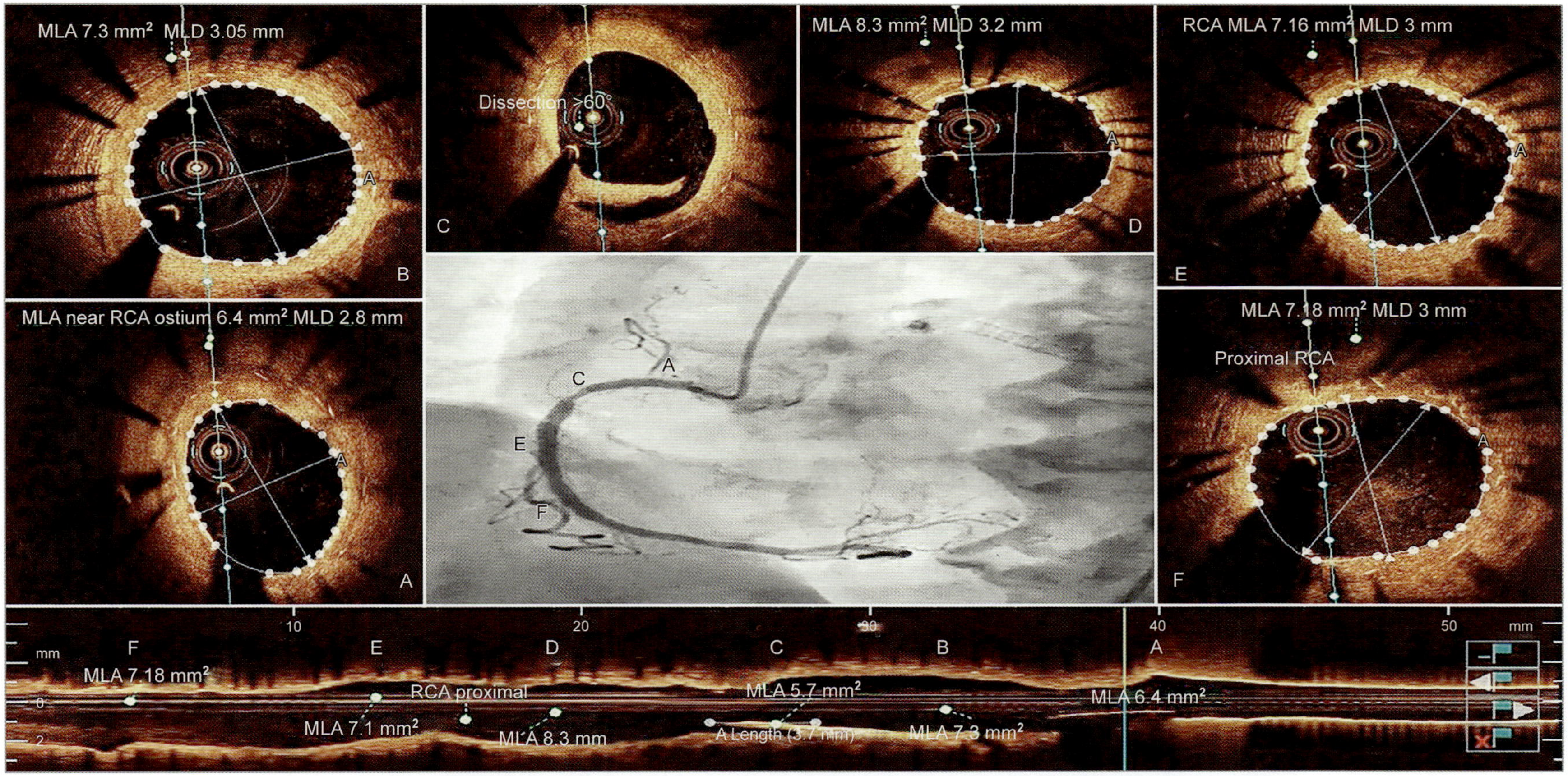

Fig. 41: Prestenting OCT assessment of RCA for plaque morphology and device selection.

New generation DESs are recommended for STEMI patients based on the evidence of lower TLR and ST in the exmination and the comfortable AMI studies.

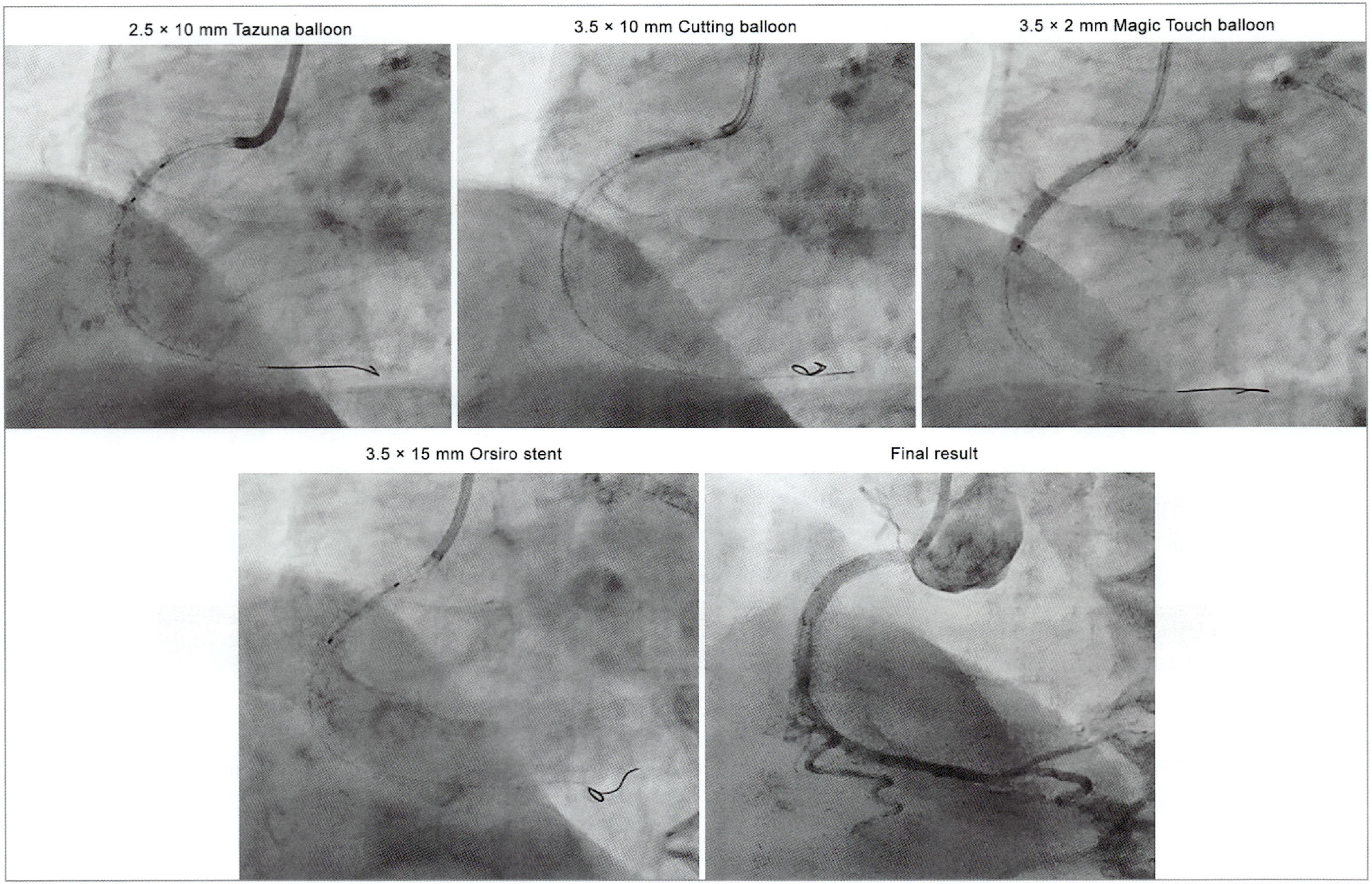

Fig. 42: Coronary angioplasty of RCA ISR segment with cutting balloon, DEB, stent.

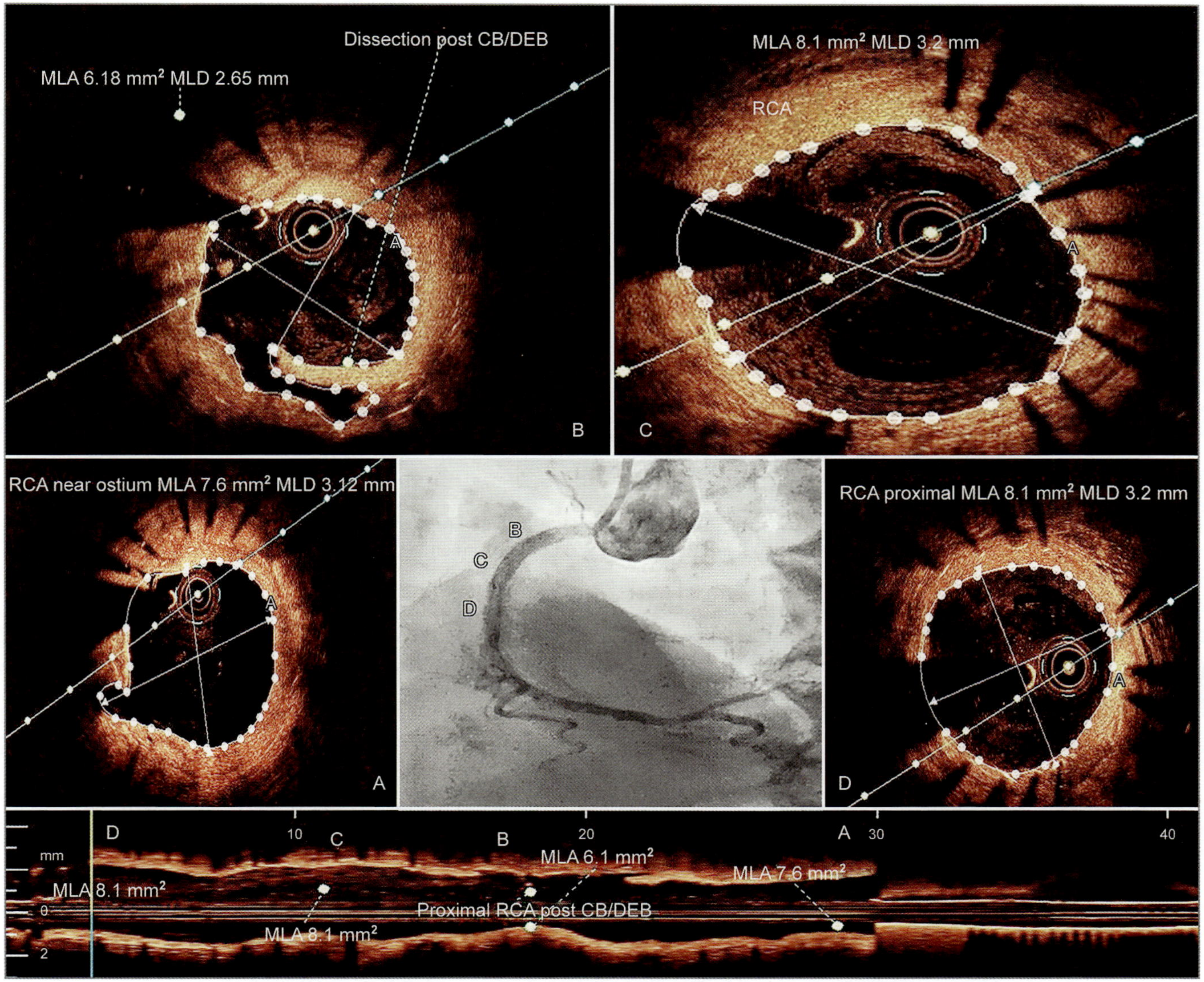

Fig. 43: Poststent OCT assessment showed well apposed and expanded stent struts.

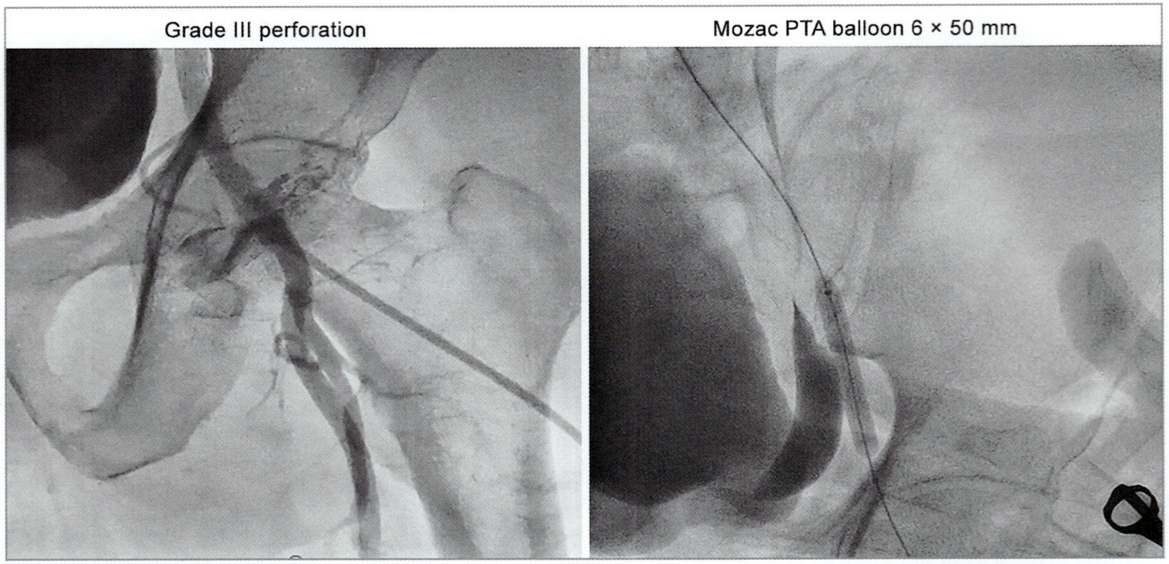

Fig. 44: Post procedure Left femoral artery sheath injection was taken, suggestive of grade III perforation and balloon tamponade of left CIA and EIA done with 6 × 50 mm Mozaic PTA balloon proximal to SFA perforation.

Majority of Acute Total Occlusion of Left Main coronary Artery (ATOLMA) patients with STEMI, who reach hospital will be with right dominance, and they carry a better prognosis than left dominance due to less myocardial necrosis and presence of well-developed collaterals from RCA.

CASE 8

ISR of LAD.

CLINICAL HISTORY

A 70-year-old, male, known diabetic, hypertensive with diabetic peripheral neuropathy, past H/o CABG and PCI of LMCA-OM and LCX:DK crush, right LL superficial thrombophlebitis presented with slurring speech, and giddiness; diagnosis: UTI (C/S pseudomonas PDR) and sepsis (blood C.S—*E. coli*).

Investigations: Hb—11.21 g/dL, RBS—146 mg/dL, serum creatinine—1.33 mg/dL, eGFR—54 mL/min, CRP—132.3 mg/L, Trop-I 518 → 4,300 ng/L, D-dimer 731 ng/mL.

CAG-native TVD with 80% ISR in LCX, LIMA—LAD: Patent graft, RA-PDA: 90% stenosis.

PROCEDURE

Left main coronary artery engaged with EBU 3.5-6 Fr guiding catheter, check angio taken, lesion crossed with 0.014" Runthrough wire. 0.014" BMW wire placed in OM. OCT run was taken which showed ISR (NIH) of stent with MSA 2.5 cm^2 **(Figs. 45A and B)**.

Lesion predilated with 2.0 × 15 mm Ryurei balloon, 2.5 × 15 mm AngioSculpt at 12 atm and 3.5 × 15 mm NC balloon.

Kissing balloon dilatation done with 2.75 × 15 mm NC Trek balloon in LCX and 2.75 × 20 mm NC balloon in OM at 14 atm. Then DEB done with 2.75 × 40 mm Magic Touch balloon in LCX deployed at 06 atm for 1 minute, 2.5 × 40 mm Magic Touch balloon in OM at 06 atm for 1 minute. Kissing inflation of DEB done at 06 atm for 2 inflation × 30 minutes. Post-OCT was done which showed well-expanded stent with MSA 4.0 cm^2. The final result was good with TIMI-III flow with no complications **(Figs. 46A and B)**.

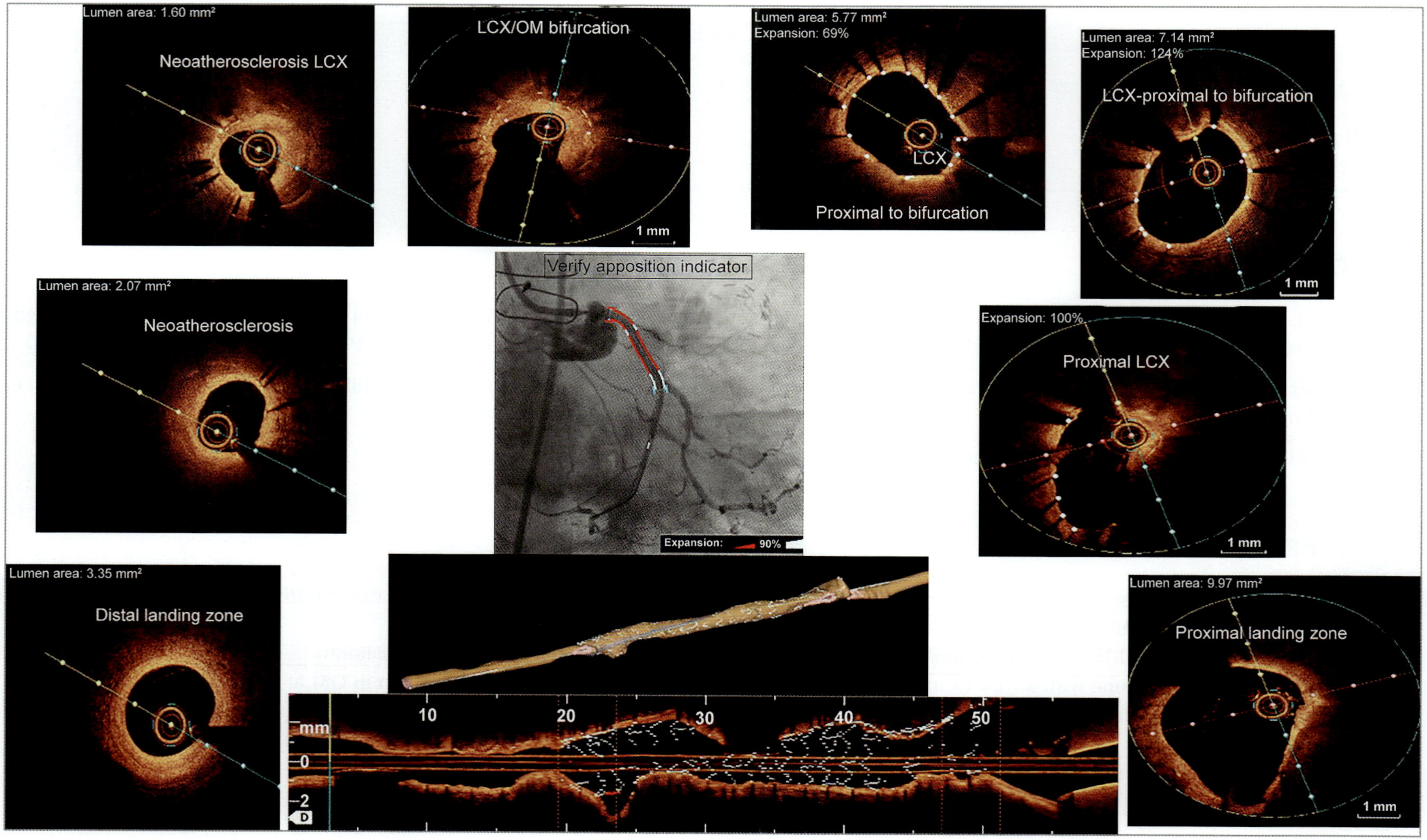
Lumen area: 1.60 mm²
Neoatherosclerosis LCX
LCX/OM bifurcation
1 mm
Lumen area: 5.77 mm²
Expansion: 69%
LCX
Proximal to bifurcation
Lumen area: 7.14 mm²
Expansion: 124%
LCX-proximal to bifurcation
1 mm
Lumen area: 2.07 mm²
Neoatherosclerosis
Verify apposition indicator
Expansion: 90%
Expansion: 100%
Proximal LCX
1 mm
Lumen area: 3.35 mm²
Distal landing zone
Lumen area: 9.97 mm²
Proximal landing zone
1 mm
mm
0
-2
D
10
20
30
40
50

Fig. 45A

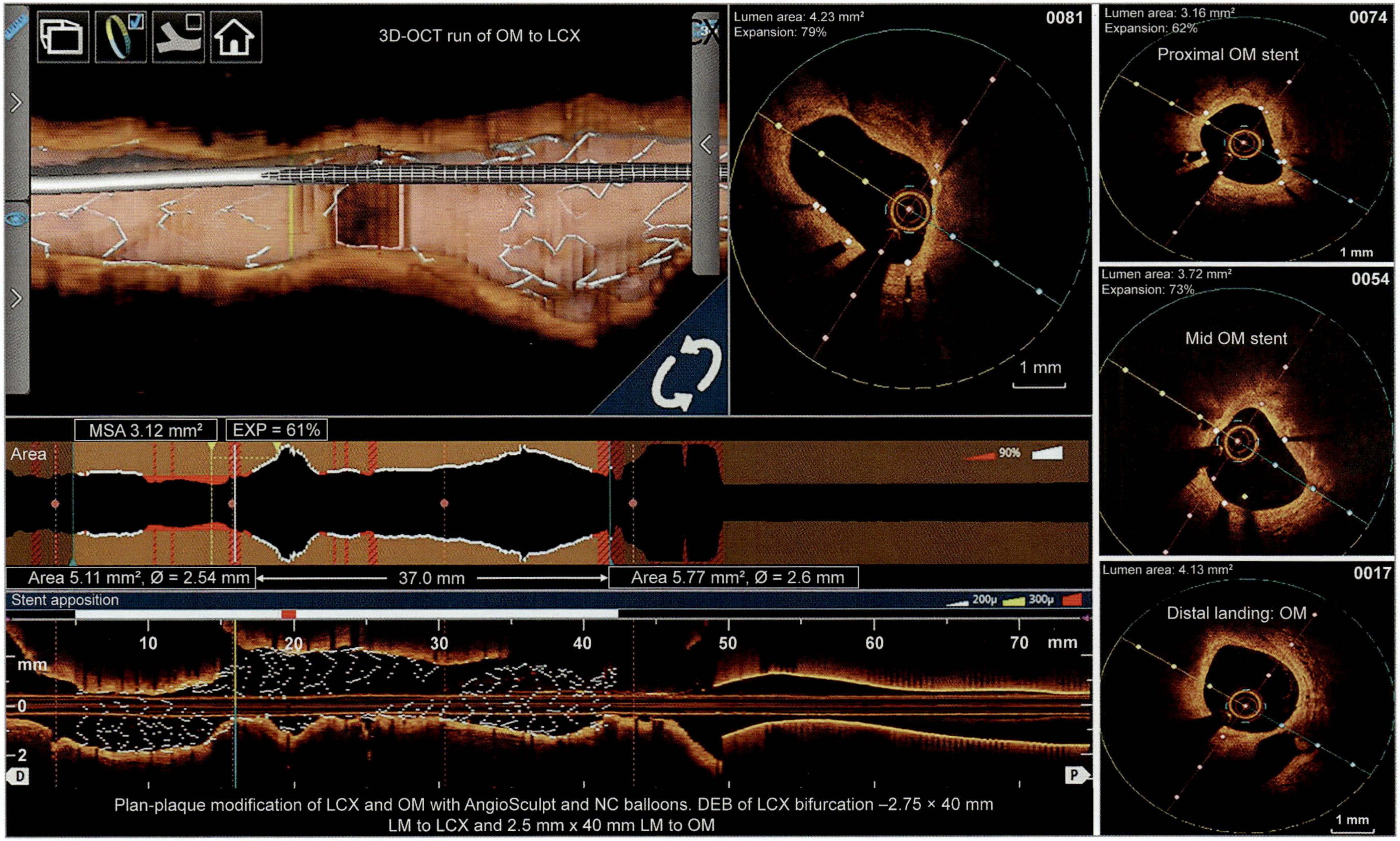

Fig. 45B

Figs. 45A and B: (A) Presenting OCT analysis showing neo atherosclerosis; (B) Presenting OCT analysis for plaque modification followed by Drug eluting balloon (DEB) dilatations.

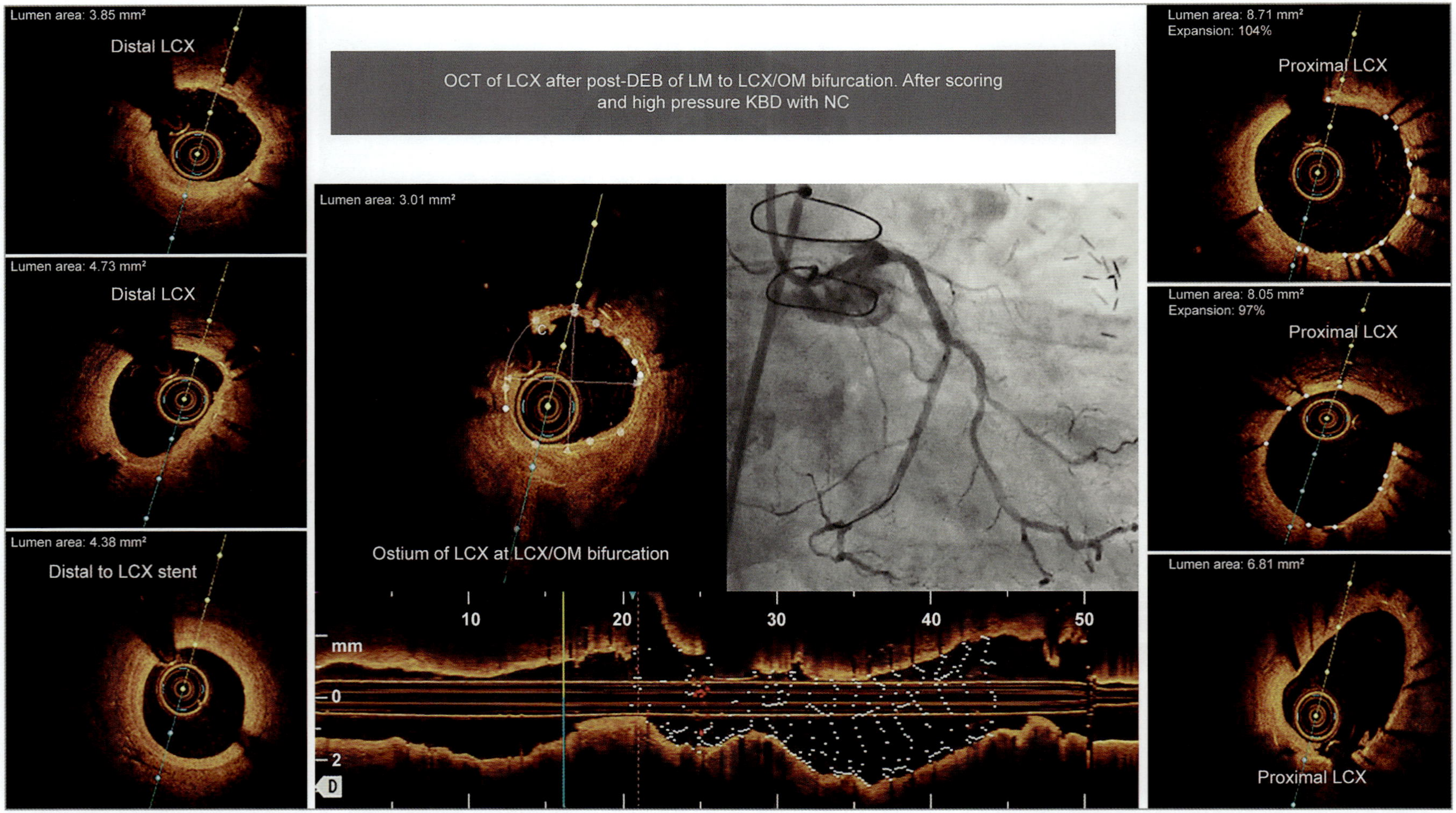
Lumen area: 3.85 mm²
Distal LCX
Lumen area: 4.73 mm²
Distal LCX
Lumen area: 4.38 mm²
Distal to LCX stent
OCT of LCX after post-DEB of LM to LCX/OM bifurcation. After scoring and high pressure KBD with NC
Lumen area: 3.01 mm²
Ostium of LCX at LCX/OM bifurcation
10
20
30
40
50
mm
0
2
D
Lumen area: 8.71 mm²
Expansion: 104%
Proximal LCX
Lumen area: 8.05 mm²
Expansion: 97%
Proximal LCX
Lumen area: 6.81 mm²
Proximal LCX

Fig. 46A

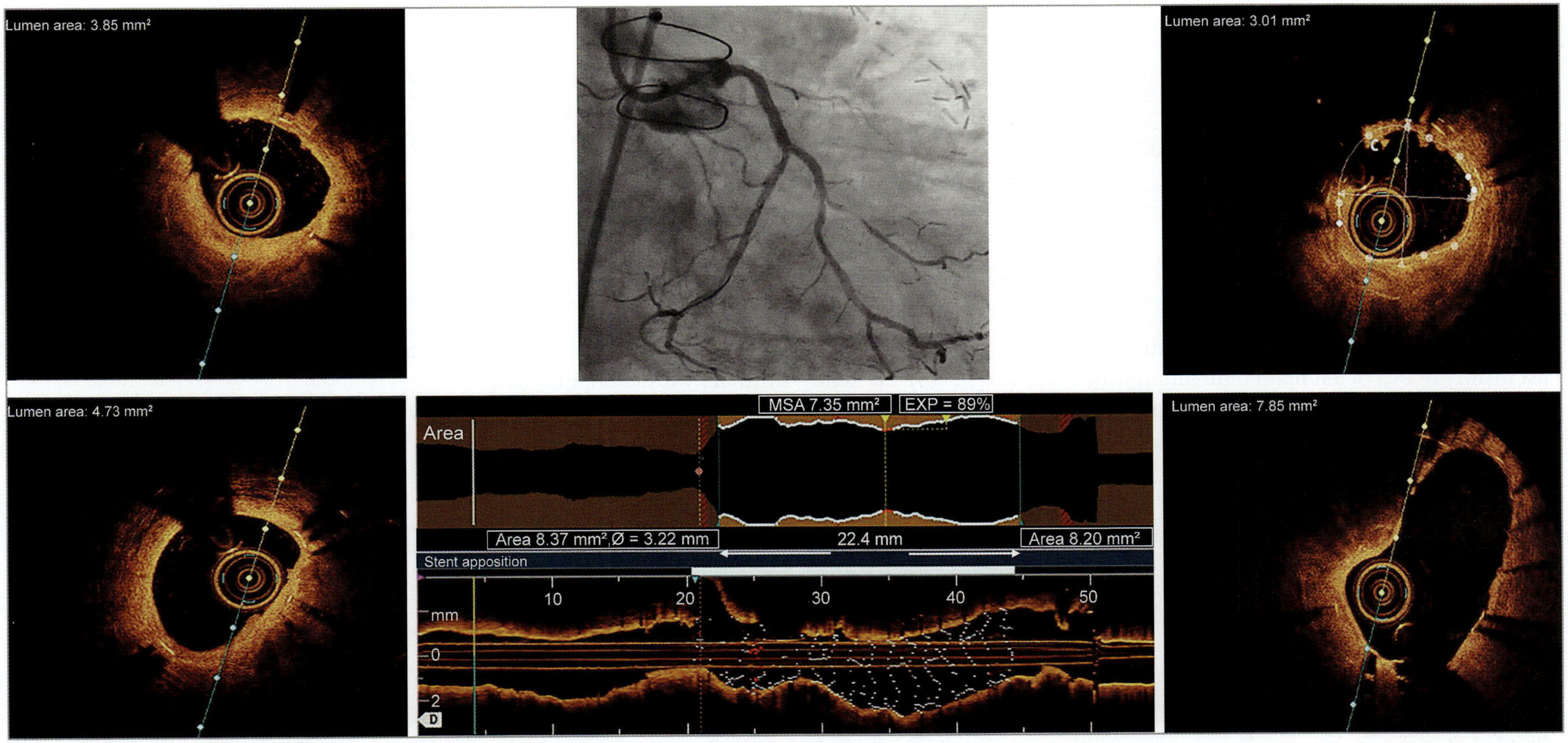

Fig. 46B

Figs. 46A and B: (A) Post DEB OCT analysis of LCX; (B) Post DEB OCT analysis of LCX showing well expanded & apposed stent struts.

DES with thinner struts have:

- Increased flexibility
- Easier delivery
- Comformability
- Quicker endothelialization
- Less side-branch coverage.

CASE 9

OCT guided PCI of ISR of LCX following LMCA bifurcation.

CLINICAL HISTORY

A 64-year-old female, known hypertensive, diabetic with strong family history of CAD, presented with unstable angina, chest pain associated with SOB. Past history of PCI of left main bifurcation with T-stenting (2015). 2D Echo—normal LV function, EF—60%.

Coronary angiogram-LMCA—Proximal 20–30% lesion, LAD—mild lesion with patent stent, ISR of LCX with total occlusion, distal vessel filling retrogradely, RCA mild lesion **(Fig. 47)**.

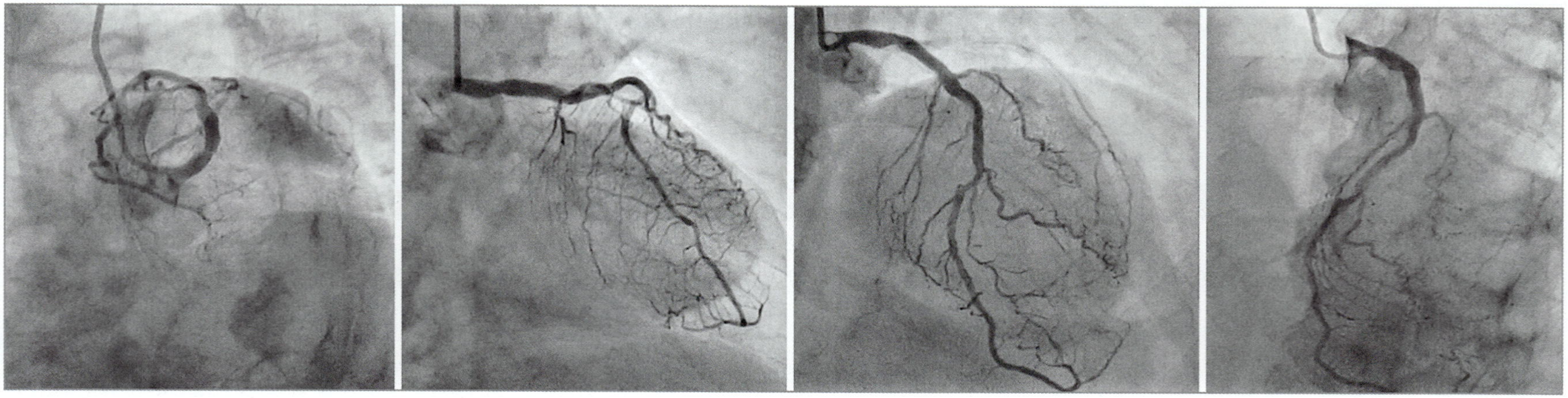

Fig. 47: Coronary angiogram.

PROCEDURE

RFA—Route, 7 Fr-3.5 EBU guiding catheter, LCX lesion was crossed with 0.014 Fielder XT wire using microcatheter, LAD lesion was crossed with 0.014 Fielder FC. Predilatation of LCX done with 1.25 × 10 mm and 2.25 × 10 mm Tazuna balloons. Distal LCX portion of previous DES dilated with 2.5 × 15 mm DEB Magic Touch. Mid LCX which was not covered with stent earlier stented with 2.75 × 18 mm Yukon Choice Elite Stent overlapping distal portion of proximal LCX stent and proximal portion of distal stent. Kissing balloon dilatation of LM bifurcation done with 3.0 × 20 mm Magic Touch balloon placed in LAD and 2.5 × 15 mm Magic Touch balloon placed in LCX **(Fig. 48)**.

Post-KB with DEB OCT study—very tight residual stenosis of LCX ostium **(Fig. 49)**.

Plan—to perform plaque modification of LCX ostium—scoring with AngioSculpt.

Postdilatation done with 3.5 × 10 mm NC Trek balloon and 2.5 × 12 mm AngioSculpt **(Fig. 50)**. Post scoring LCX ostium very well-expanded with MLA of 5.6 mm^2, MLD—2.7 mm. Final kissing balloon dilatation done with 3.5 × 10 mm NC Trek balloon LAD and 3.0 × 10 mm NC Trek balloon LCX.

Postcutting OCT analysis: Post-OCT was done which showed well-apposed stent struts, no residual stenosis, and no thrombosis **(Figs. 51A to E)**.

Postprocedure angio view showed well-implanted stents with TIMI-III flow without any dissection. Patient was discharged on third post procedure in a stable status **(Fig. 52)**.

Optical coherence tomography helped us in achieving adequate expansion of LCX ostium, underexpansion is the most common cause of ISR, and stent thrombosis in complex LM bifurcation lesions, and LCX is the most common site of underexpansion which occurs in 33% of patients. It would be preferable to achieve post bifurcation PCI MSA of LM >8 mm^2, LM confluence >7 mm^2, LAD ostium >6 mm^2, and LCX ostium >5 mm^2 or aim to achieve mean reference diameter of stented area at least >80% compared to proximal and distal reference areas. Underexpansion in two stent technique (46%) is assessed with increased incidence of ISR compared to single stent technique (6%) **(Fig. 53)**.

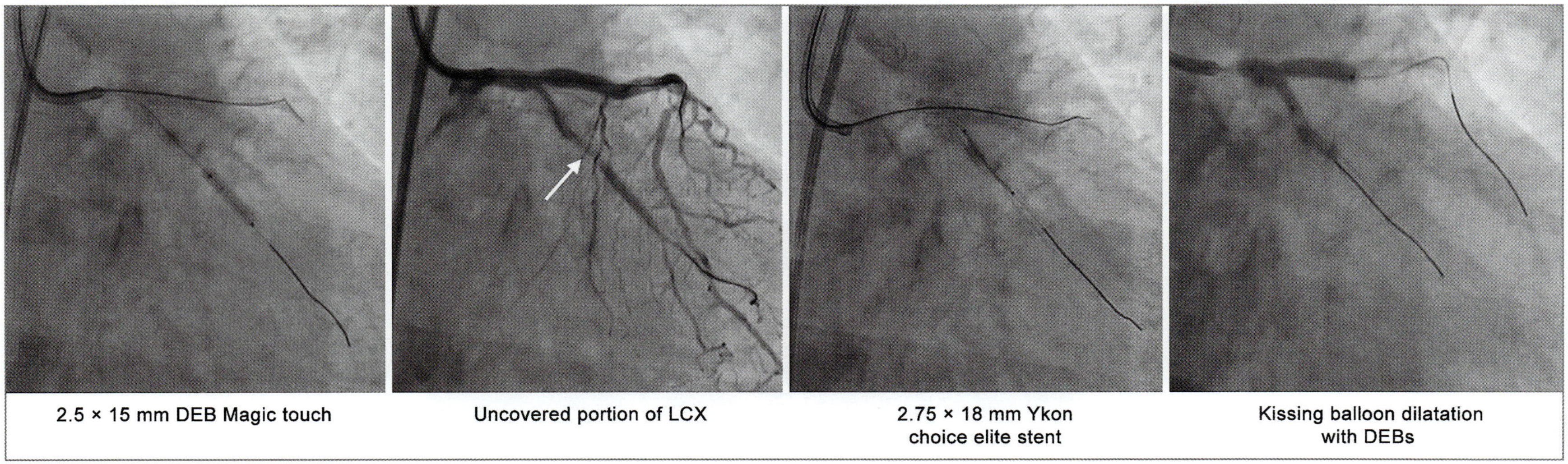

Fig. 48: Angioplasty of LCX ISR segment with DEB and DES and kissing balloon dilatation with DEBs in LAD and LCX.

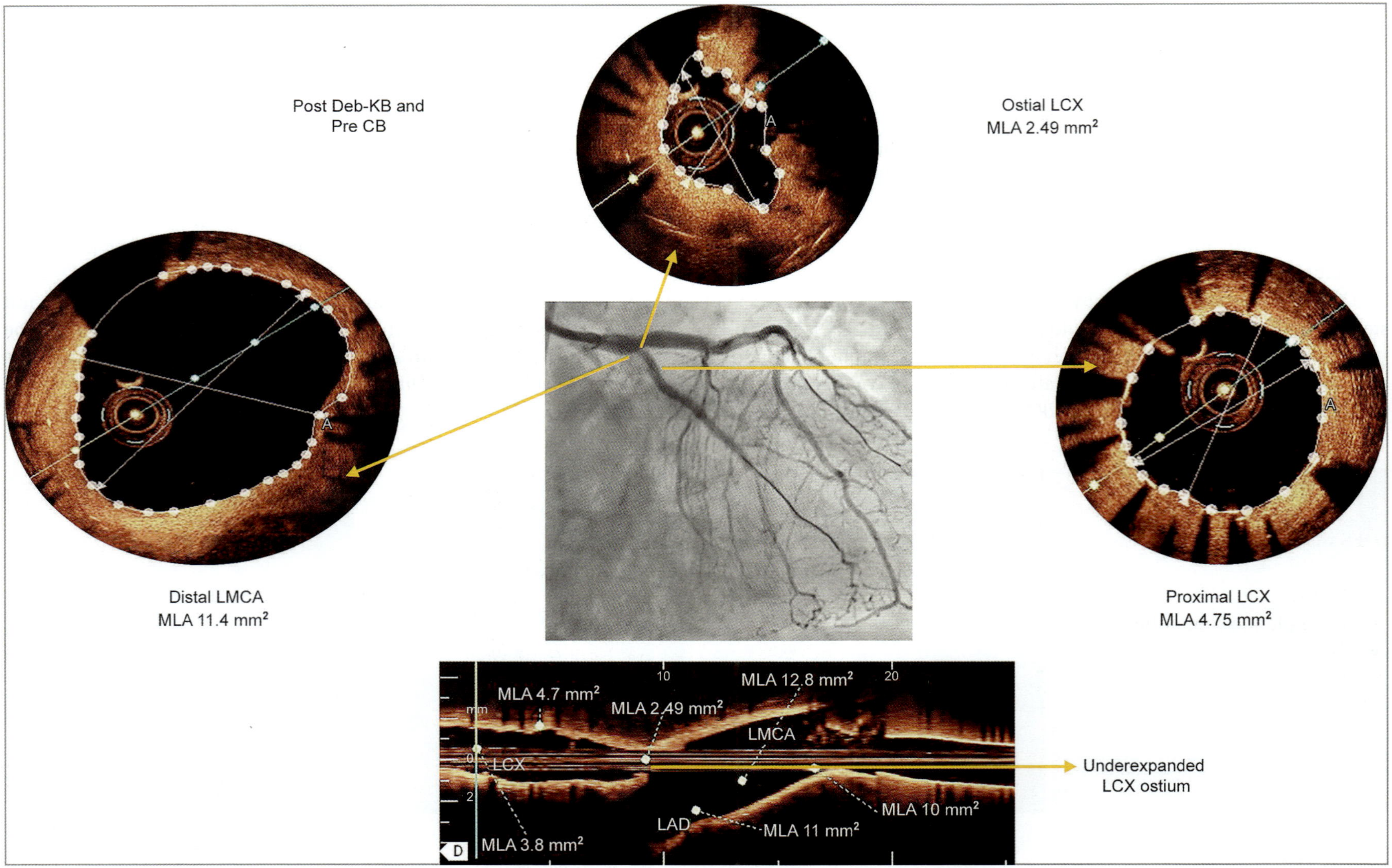

Fig. 49: Post KB with DEB OCT study-very tight residual stenosis of LCX ostium.

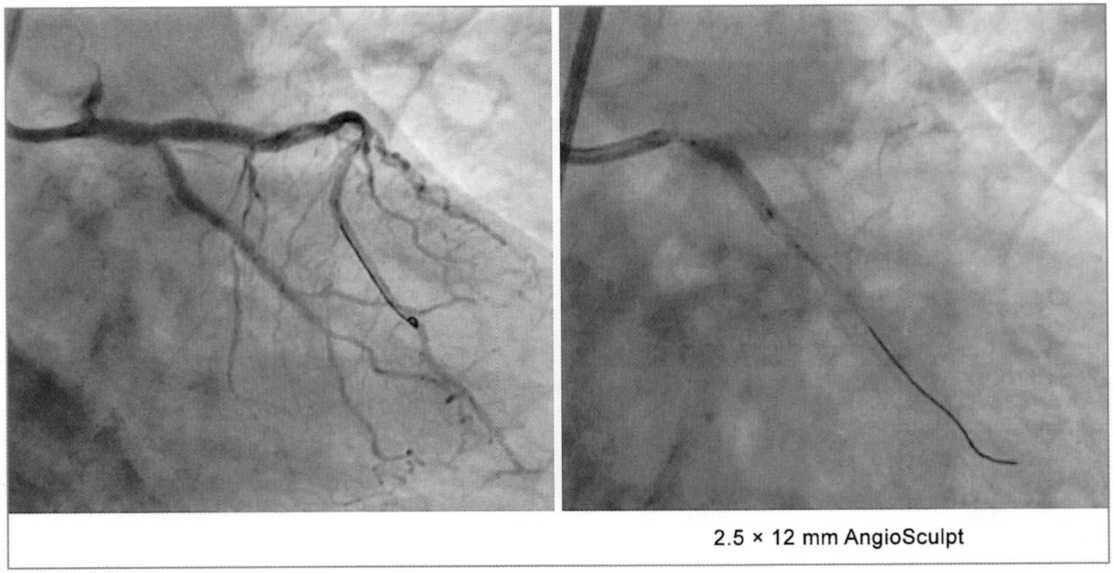

Fig. 50: Plaque modification of LCX ostium-scoring with AngioSculpt.

DES with thicker struts:

- Higher radial force
- Larger strut coverage
- More plaque containment
- Less recoil
- More symmetrical expansion.

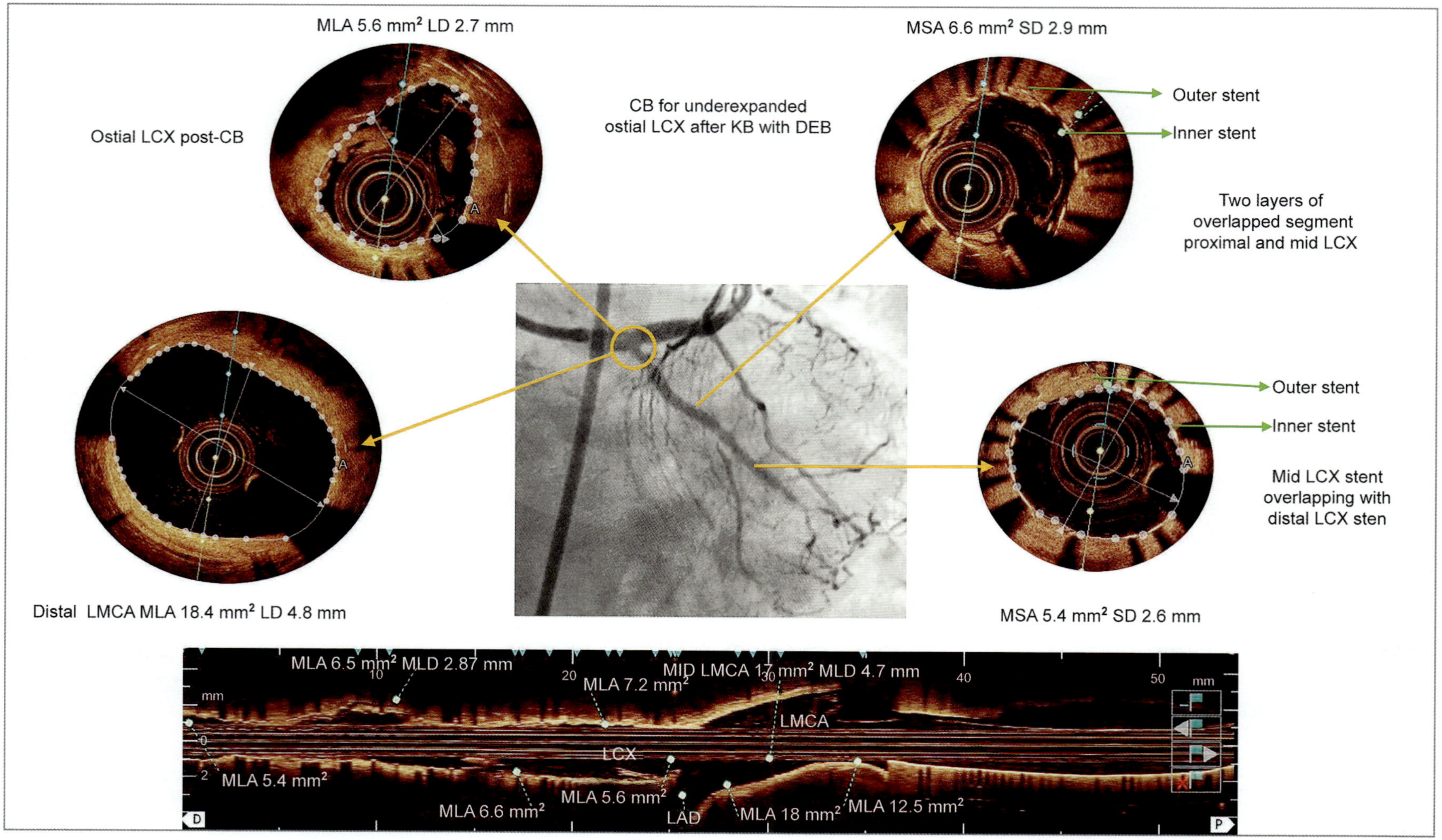

MLA 5.6 mm² LD 2.7 mm
Ostial LCX post-CB
A
CB for underexpanded ostial LCX after KB with DEB
MSA 6.6 mm² SD 2.9 mm
Outer stent
Inner stent
Two layers of overlapped segment proximal and mid LCX
A
Distal LMCA MLA 18.4 mm² LD 4.8 mm
Outer stent
Inner stent
A
Mid LCX stent overlapping with distal LCX sten
MSA 5.4 mm² SD 2.6 mm
MLA 6.5 mm² MLD 2.87 mm
10
20
MLA 7.2 mm²
MID LMCA 17 mm² MLD 4.7 mm
30
40
50
mm
mm
LMCA
LCX
0
2
MLA 5.4 mm²
MLA 6.6 mm²
MLA 5.6 mm²
LAD
MLA 18 mm²
MLA 12.5 mm²
D
P

Fig. 51A

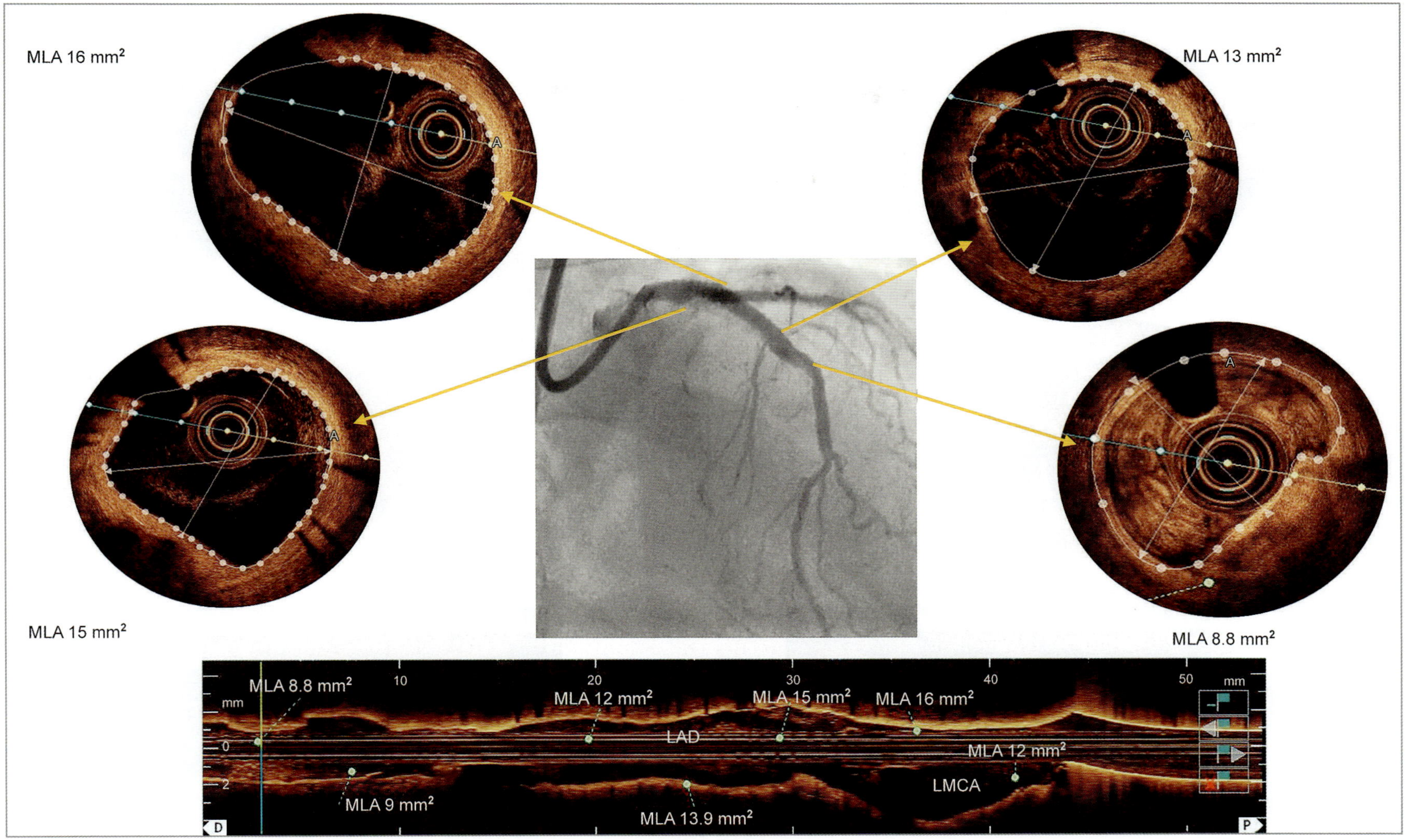
MLA 16 mm²
MLA 13 mm²
MLA 15 mm²
MLA 8.8 mm²
MLA 8.8 mm²
MLA 12 mm²
MLA 15 mm²
MLA 16 mm²
MLA 12 mm²
LAD
LMCA
MLA 9 mm²
MLA 13.9 mm²
mm
10
20
30
40
50
D
P

Fig. 51B

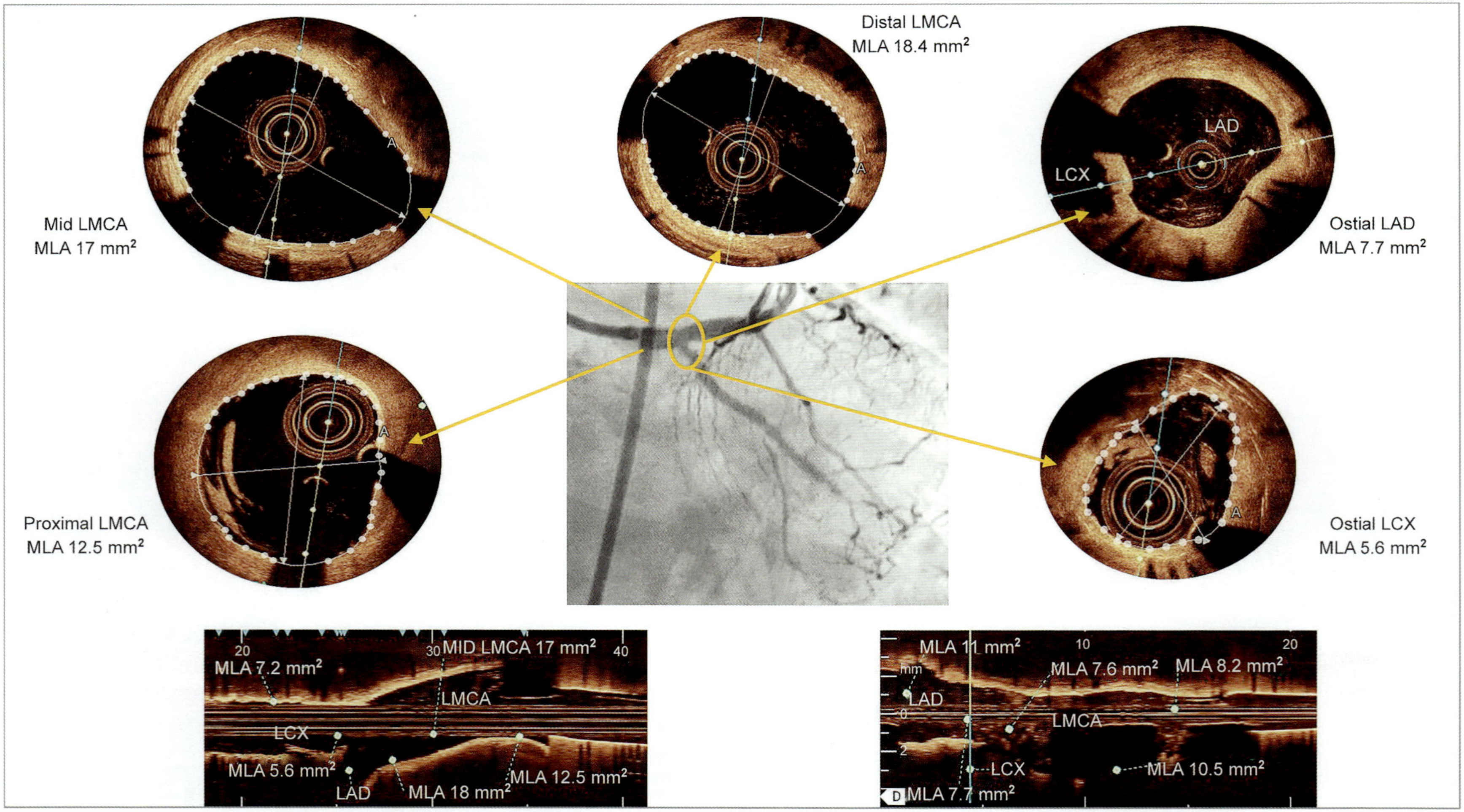

Distal LMCA
MLA 18.4 mm²
Mid LMCA
MLA 17 mm²
LAD
LCX
Ostial LAD
MLA 7.7 mm²
Proximal LMCA
MLA 12.5 mm²
Ostial LCX
MLA 5.6 mm²
MID LMCA 17 mm²
MLA 7.2 mm²
LMCA
LCX
MLA 5.6 mm²
LAD
MLA 18 mm²
MLA 12.5 mm²
MLA 11 mm²
MLA 7.6 mm²
MLA 8.2 mm²
LAD
LMCA
LCX
MLA 10.5 mm²
MLA 7.7 mm²

Fig. 51C

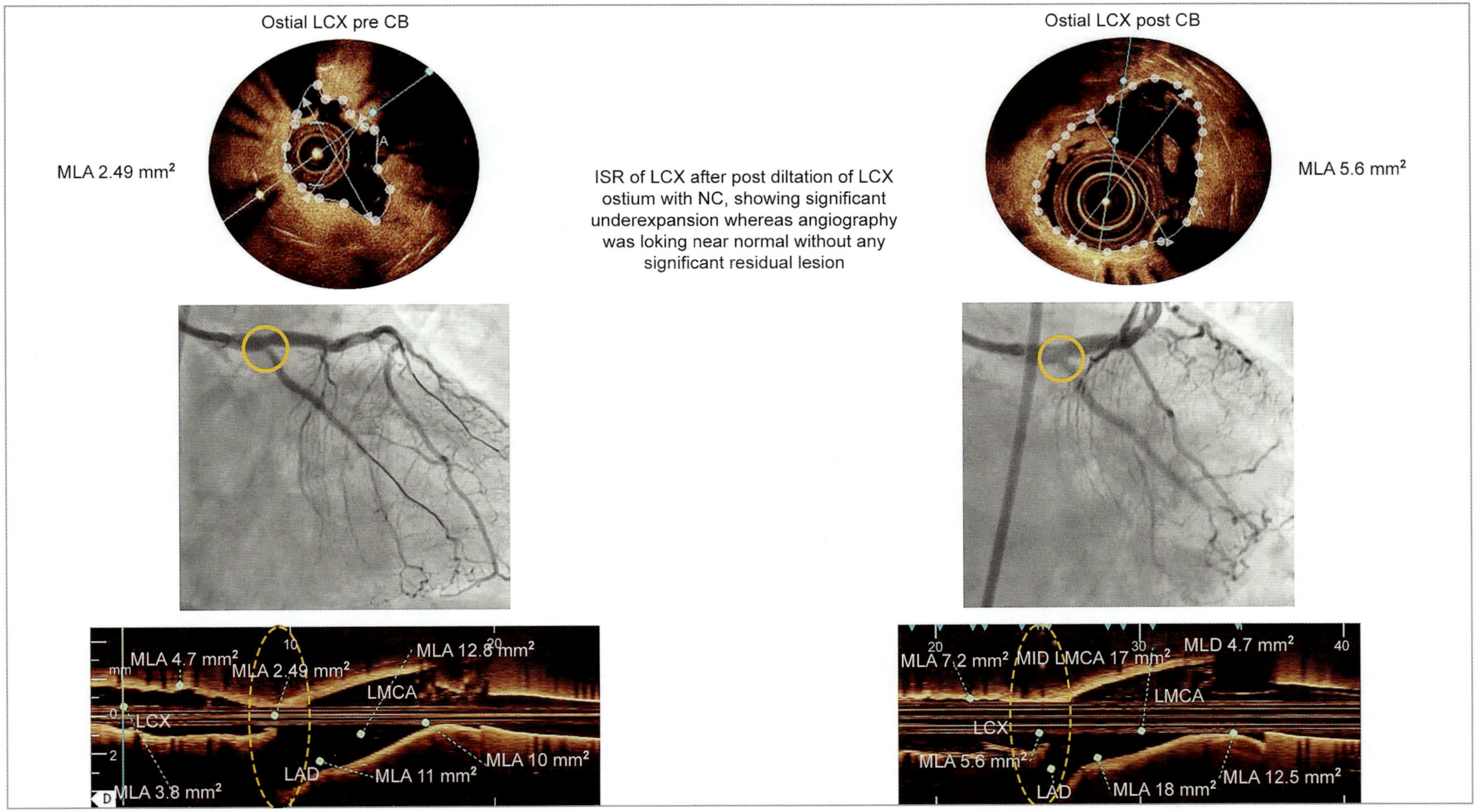
Ostial LCX pre CB
MLA 2.49 mm²
Ostial LCX post CB
MLA 5.6 mm²
ISR of LCX after post diltation of LCX ostium with NC, showing significant underexpansion whereas angiography was loking near normal without any significant residual lesion
MLA 4.7 mm²
MLA 2.49 mm²
MLA 12.8 mm²
LMCA
LCX
MLA 3.8 mm²
LAD
MLA 11 mm²
MLA 10 mm²
MLA 7.2 mm²
MID LMCA 17 mm²
MLD 4.7 mm²
LMCA
LCX
MLA 5.6 mm²
LAD
MLA 18 mm²
MLA 12.5 mm²

Fig. 51D

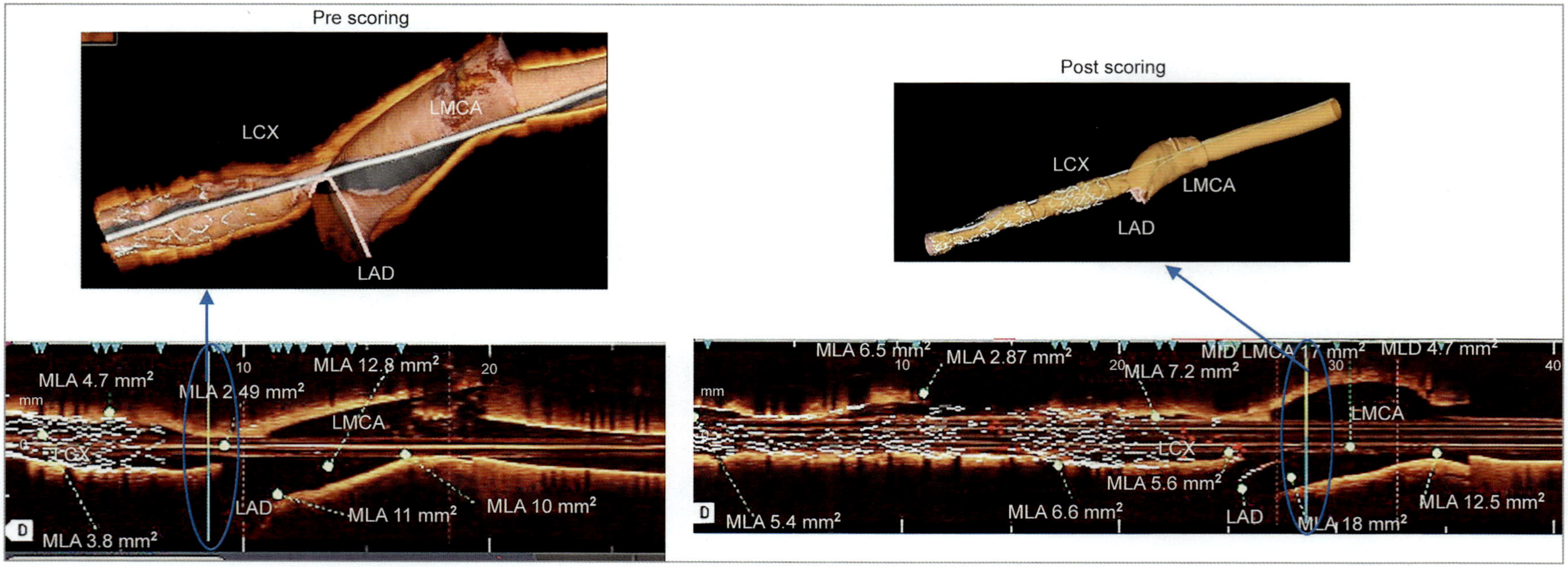

Fig. 51E

Figs. 51A to E: Poststent and scoring OCT assessment showed. (A) Well expanded and well apposed LM-LCX segment; (B) Patent stent segment in LM-LAD; (C) OCT assessment of LM and LM bifurcation segment involving ostium of LAD and LCX; (D and E) Assessment of ostial LCX segment pre and post cutting balloon.

In vessels with lipid rich soft plaques , lesion preparation using a semi- or noncompliant balloon with a balloon-to-artery ratio of 1:1 is recommended, and the lesion is not adequately dilated with semi-compliant balloon, use NC balloons or cutting and scoring balloons to prepare the lesion well especially in the presence of moderate to severe fibro-calcific lesions.

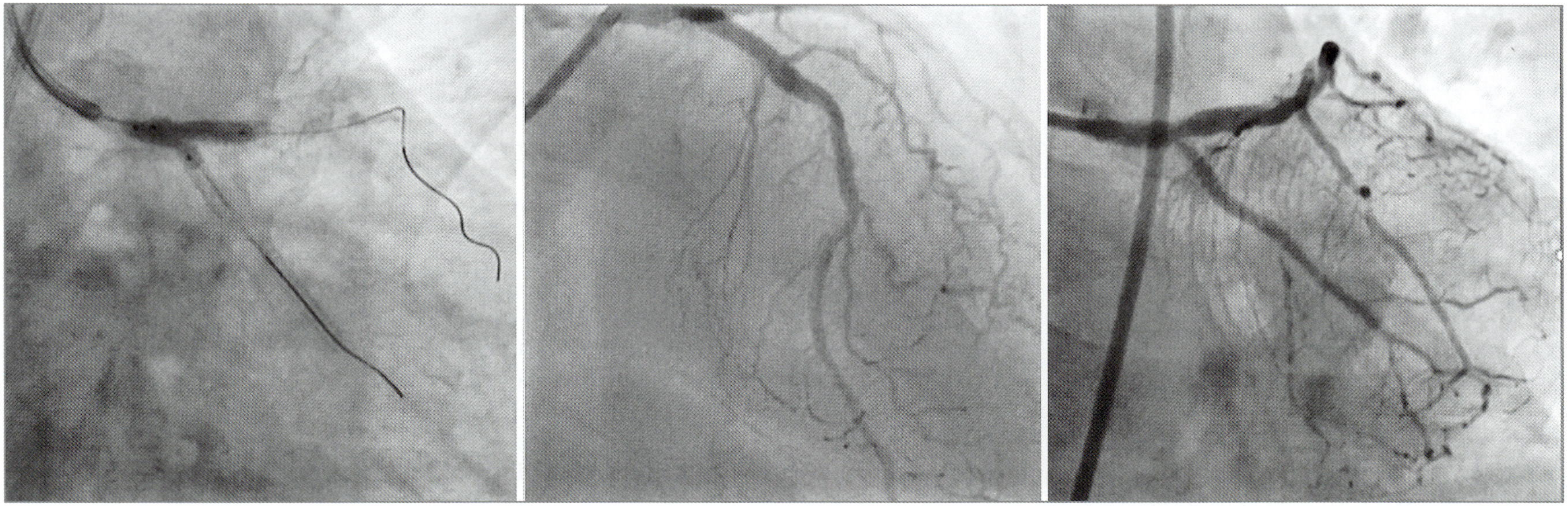

Fig. 52: Final kissing balloon and final result.

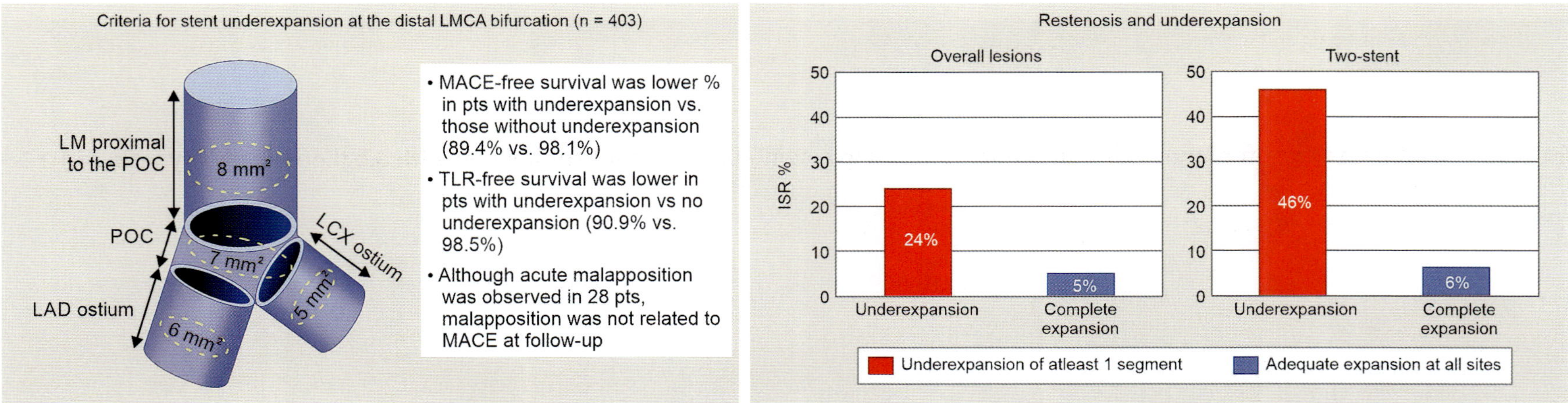

Fig. 53: Criteria for stent under-expansion at distal LM and in two-stent technique.

CASE 10

OCT-guided PCI of provisional stenting of LMCA to LCX for recurrent ISR of LCX (post-BVS ISR for BVS stenting of post-DES ISR).

CLINICAL HISTORY

A 55-year-old male, known hypertensive, diabetic presented with chest pain associated with SOB, chronic kidney disease (CKD), and hypothyroidism. Past history of PCI of RCA and LCX in 2012 and PCI of CTO of LCX (ISR) in 2015 (3.0 × 28 mm BVS in distal LCX and 3.5 × 28 mm BVS in proximal LCX). CAD—Unstable angina, Hb—12.6 g/dL, blood urea—27 mg/dL, serum creatinine—1.24 mg/dL, eGFR—65 mL/min. 2D Echo—no RWMA, good LV function, EF—62%.

Coronary angiogram-LMCA—normal, LAD—normal, LCX—ostioproximal 60–70% ISR, mid and distal OM mild lesion, RCA—proximal to mid stent mid luminal loss, PDA and PLVB—Normal **(Fig. 54)**.

Fractional flow reserve to LCX showed significant disease with baseline value—0.94, after adenosine—0.73 **(Fig. 55)**.

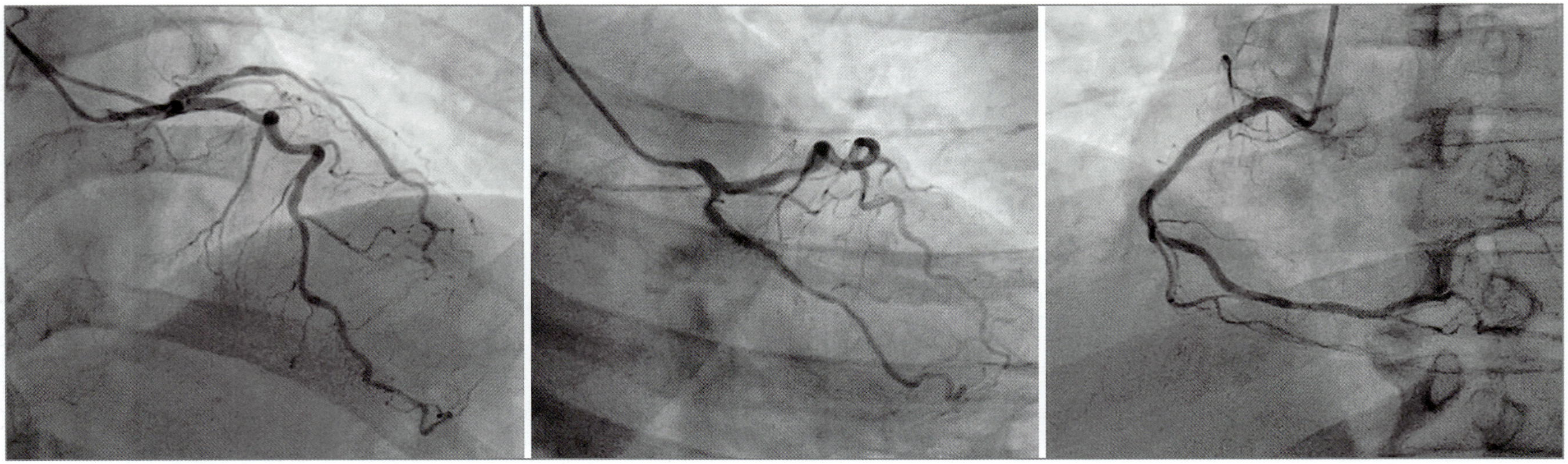

Fig. 54: Coronary angiogram.

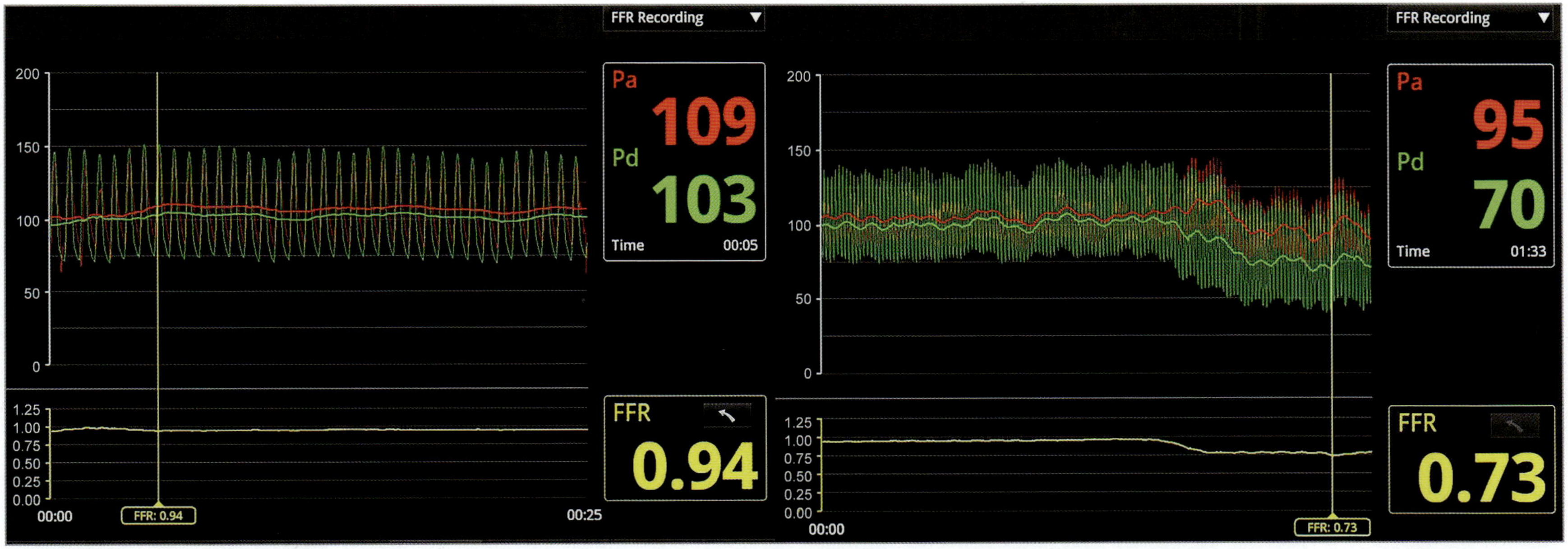

Fig. 55: FFR study of LCX segment showed positive result.

PROCEDURE

Route—RFA, using 7 Fr EBU 3.5 guiding catheter, angiogram revealed proximal LCX 60–70% ISR, tried to cross the lesion with 0.014″ BMW, Fielder FC, but finally crossed with Runthrough wire. Pre-OCT showed severe ISR of LCX with disappeared BVS struts, previous stent MSA—10 mm^2, MSD—3.6 mm, MLA—1.5 mm^2, MLD—1.4 mm and fibrotic plaque in ostial LCX **(Figs. 56A and B)**.

Distal LCX stenting done with 3.0 × 38 mm Resolute Onyx stent. LMCA to LCX stenting done with 3.5 × 26 mm Resolute Onyx stent. Postdilatation done with 3.0 × 15 mm, 2.5 × 15 mm NC Trek balloons. POT of LMCA was done with 4.0 × 08 mm NC Trek balloon. Check angio showed residual LCX lesion; it was dilated with 3.0 × 10 mm OPN NC balloon **(Fig. 57)**. Post OCT study showed distal portion of the distal LCX stent MLA-4.7 mm^2, MLD-2.4 mm, proximal edge of distal stent MLA—5.5 mm^2, MLD—2.6 mm, distal edge of proximal stent with MLA—6.2 mm^2, MLD—2.8 mm, ostium of LCX with MLA—9.3 mm^2, MLD—3.4 mm, LMCA MLA—12 mm^2, MLD—3.8 mm **(Figs. 58A to C)**. Uncovered mid LCX segment (6.1 mm) between two stents stented with 3.5 × 12 mm Resolute Onyx stent. Guidewire recrossed into LAD through stent struts and kissing balloon inflation done with 3.0 × 15 mm NC Trek balloon in LCX and 3.0 × 12 mm NC Trek balloon in LAD. LMCA postdilatation done with 4.0 × 08 mm NC Trek balloon. Postprocedure angio view showed well-implanted stents with TIMI-III flow without any dissection. Patient was discharged on third postprocedure in a stable status **(Fig. 57)**.

NA is defined as atherosclerotic changes in neointimal tissue. It is characterized by the presence of clusters of lipid-laden foamy macrophages with or without necrotic core formation and/or calcification within the neointimal tissue of stented segments. Characteristics of NA include macrophage infiltration, lipid accumulation, in-stent calcification, or neointimal rupture.

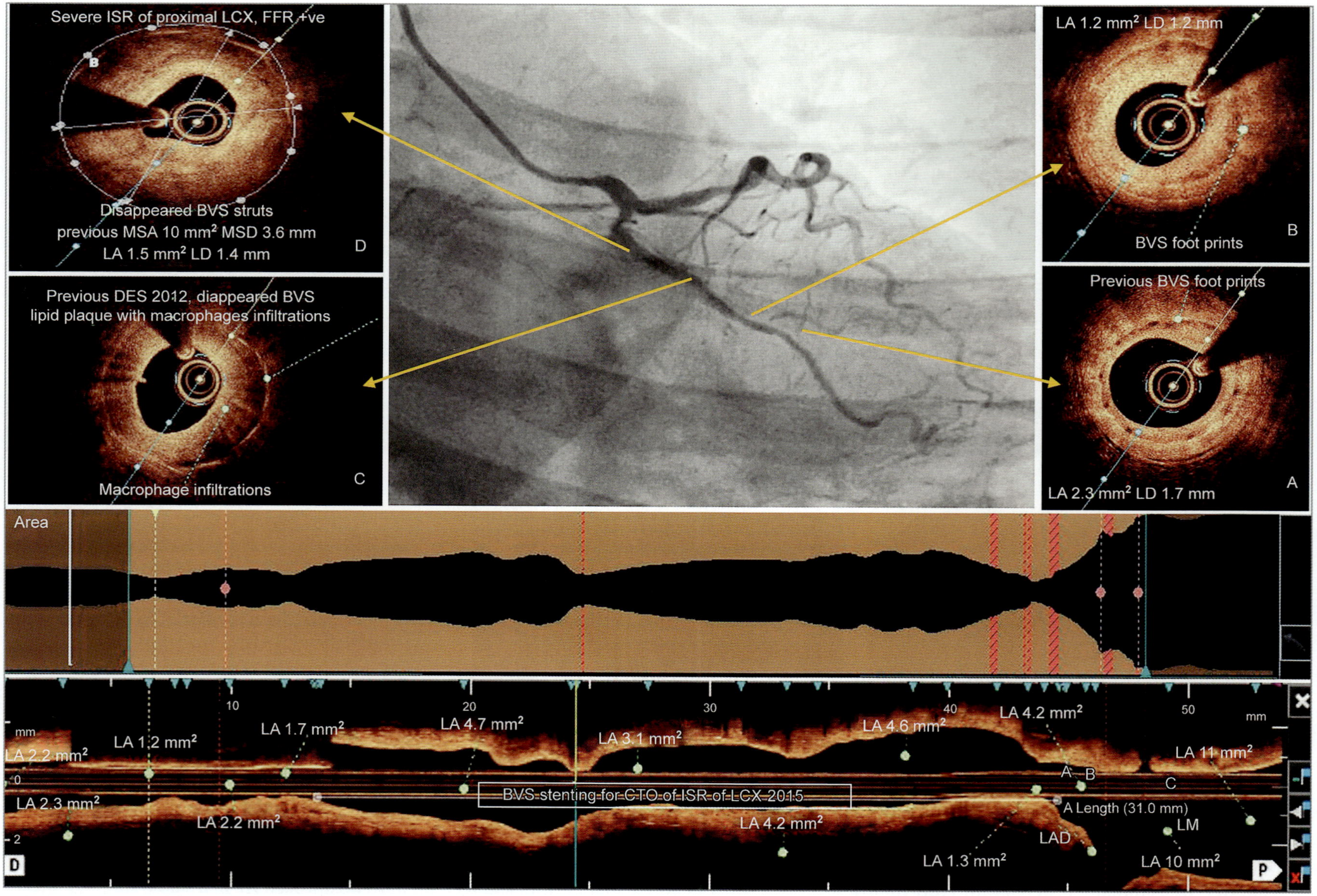

Severe ISR of proximal LCX, FFR +ve
Disappeared BVS struts
previous MSA 10 mm² MSD 3.6 mm
LA 1.5 mm² LD 1.4 mm
D
Previous DES 2012, diappeared BVS
lipid plaque with macrophages infiltrations
Macrophage infiltrations
C
LA 1.2 mm² LD 1.2 mm
BVS foot prints
B
Previous BVS foot prints
LA 2.3 mm² LD 1.7 mm
A
Area
LA 2.2 mm²
LA 1.2 mm²
LA 1.7 mm²
LA 4.7 mm²
LA 3.1 mm²
LA 4.6 mm²
LA 4.2 mm²
LA 11 mm²
BVS stenting for CTO of ISR of LCX 2015
LA 2.3 mm²
LA 2.2 mm²
LA 4.2 mm²
A Length (31.0 mm)
LAD
LM
LA 1.3 mm²
LA 10 mm²

Fig. 56A

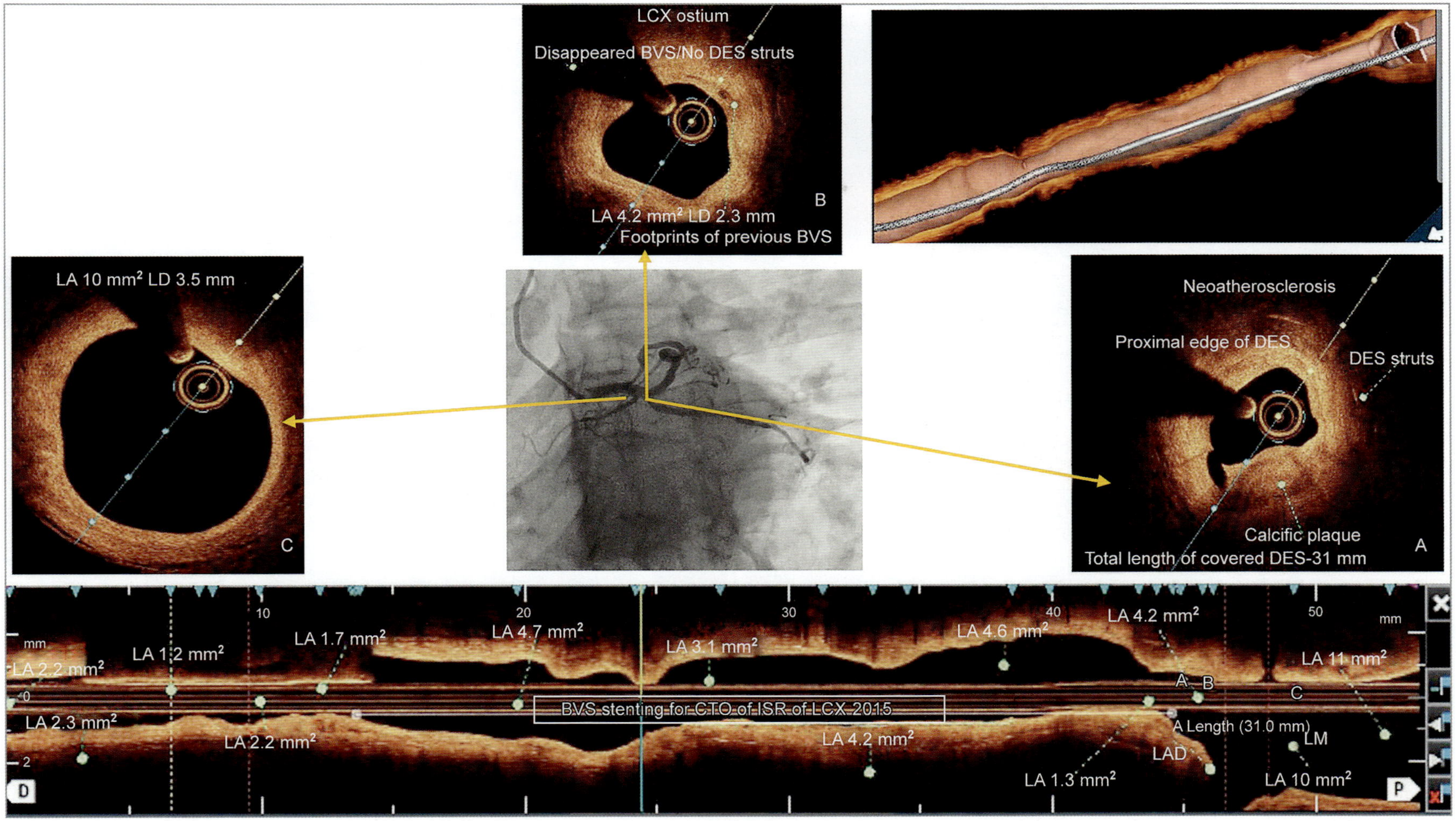

Fig. 56B

Figs. 56A and B: Prestenting OCT assessment. (A) Proximal to distal OCT segment; (B) Distal LM to proximal LCX.

Optical coherence tomography-defined NA is mainly confined to lipidic or calcific neointima. Lipidic neointima is shown as diffusely bordered, signal-poor regions with overlying signal-rich bands. Calcific neointima shows well-delineated, signal-poor regions with sharp borders.

Risk factors of NA include (1) longer time interval to follow-up, when we used OCT to evaluate the incidence of NA that developed after short post-DES implantation durations, early NA was also observed in 6.4% of 482 DES-treated lesions within 12 months after stent implantation (at a median post-implantation follow-up of 9.1 months); (2) current smoking; (3) CKD; (4) absence of angiotensin-converting enzyme inhibitors or angiotensin II receptor blockade usage.

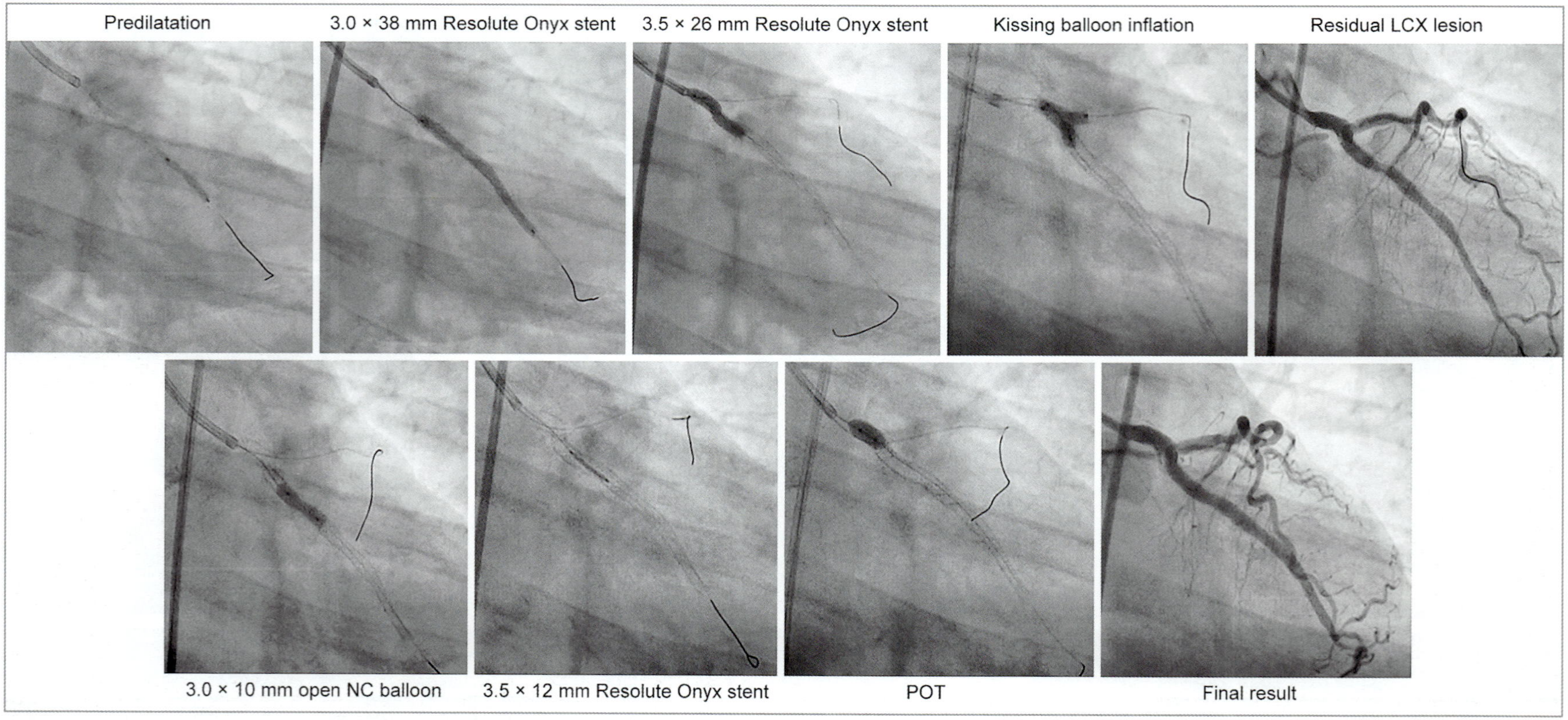

Fig. 57: Coronary angioplasty.

Patients with NA versus without NA had a higher rate of TLR (92.6% vs. 77.6%) and stent thrombosis (14.8% vs. 0%). In addition, based on data from the Kobe University Hospital OCT registry, the incidence of MACE; (e.g., composite of death, myocardial infarction, and TLR) was significantly higher in patients with NA versus those without NA (36.9% vs. 9.3%). This was mainly driven by an increase in the rate of cardiac death (6.5% vs. 0%) and TLR (30.4% vs. 7.7%).

Compared to patients with stable angina, patients with unstable angina show higher incidences of unstable OCT findings, including TCFA-containing neointima, neointima rupture, and thrombus. OCT-defined rupture of lipidic neointima was observed in patients with VLST.

Diffuse ISR of LCX was assessed with FFR study with IV adenosine infusion (140 µg/kg/min), resting FFR 0.95 and post IV adenosine 0.73. OCT revealed disappeared BVS struts at ostial LCX and other segments of LCX with evidence of footprints of disappeared previous BVS struts. LCX ostium was uncovered with previous DES which is grossly underexpanded during previous PCI which resulted in severe ISR. In view of severe ostial ISR with multiple areas of under expansion, provisional stenting of LMCA-LCX was done with restenting of LCX and high-pressure inflation using 3 mm OPN NC balloon at 45 atm with adequate expansion of stent.

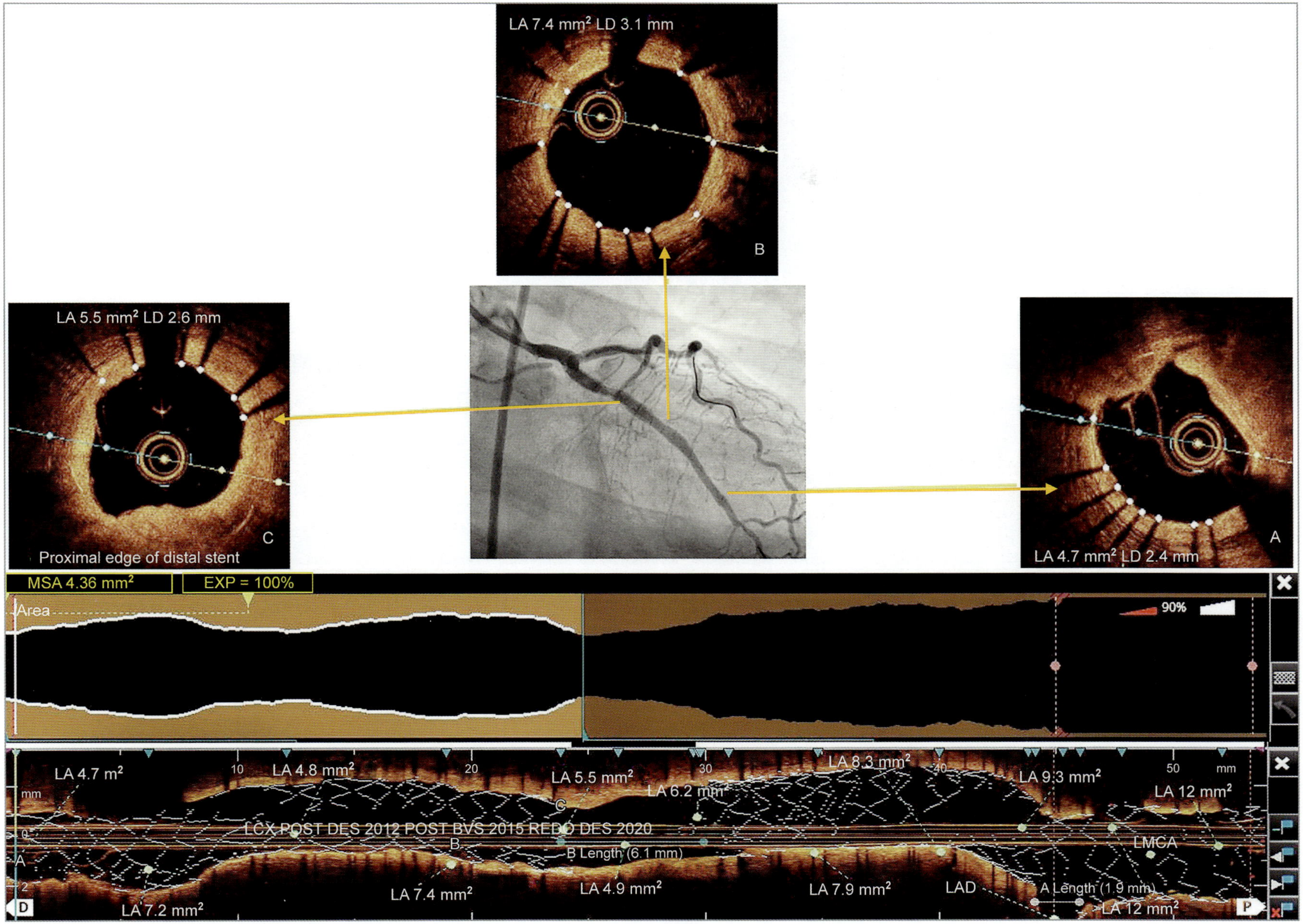
LA 7.4 mm² LD 3.1 mm
B
LA 5.5 mm² LD 2.6 mm
C
Proximal edge of distal stent
A
LA 4.7 mm² LD 2.4 mm
MSA 4.36 mm²
EXP = 100%
Area
90%
LA 4.7 m²
LA 4.8 mm²
LA 5.5 mm²
LA 6.2 mm²
LA 8.3 mm²
LA 9.3 mm²
LA 12 mm²
LCX POST DES 2012 POST BVS 2015 REDO DES 2020
B Length (6.1 mm)
LMCA
LA 7.2 mm²
LA 7.4 mm²
LA 4.9 mm²
LA 7.9 mm²
LAD
A Length (1.9 mm)
LA 12 mm²

Fig. 58A

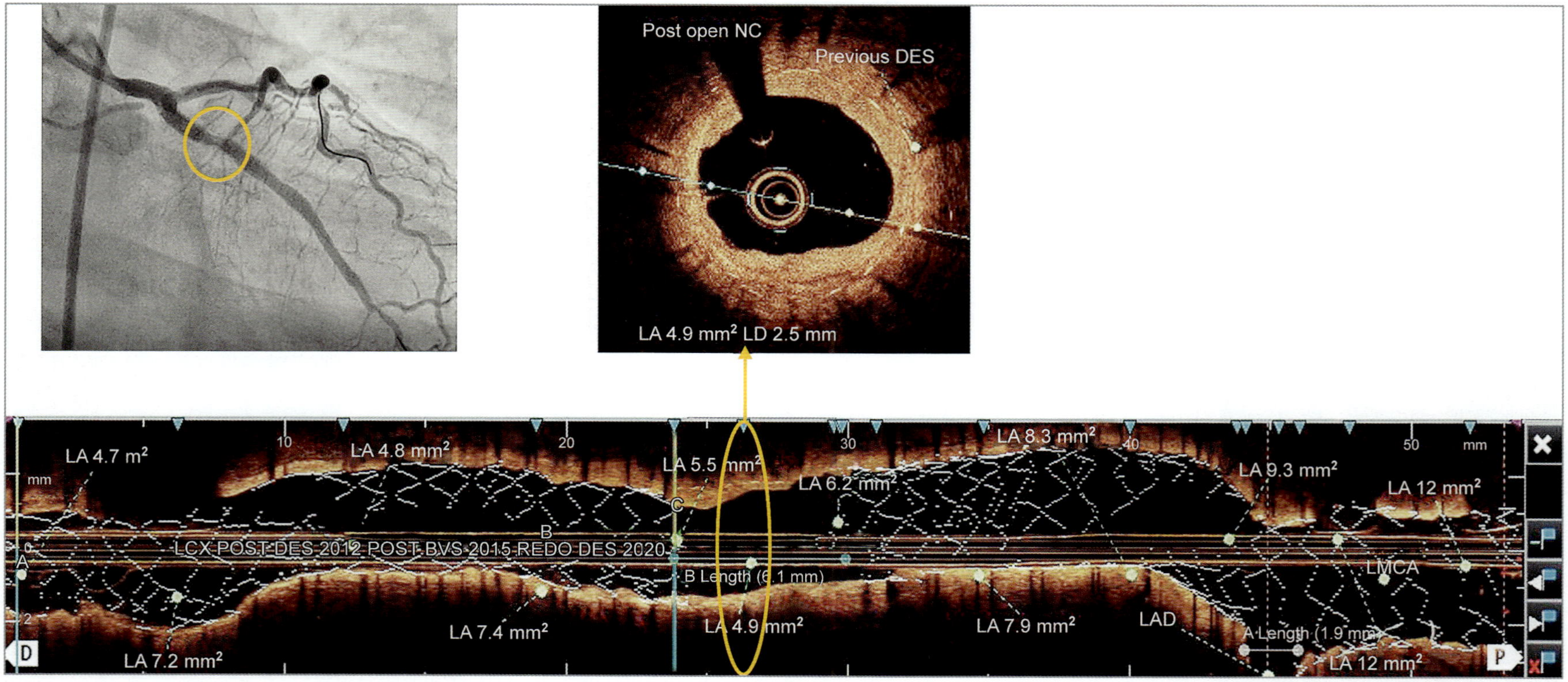

Fig. 58B

DCB angioplasty requires an optimal balloon angioplasty result, which may be assessed using angiography, physiology, or intravascular imaging, followed by DCB application.

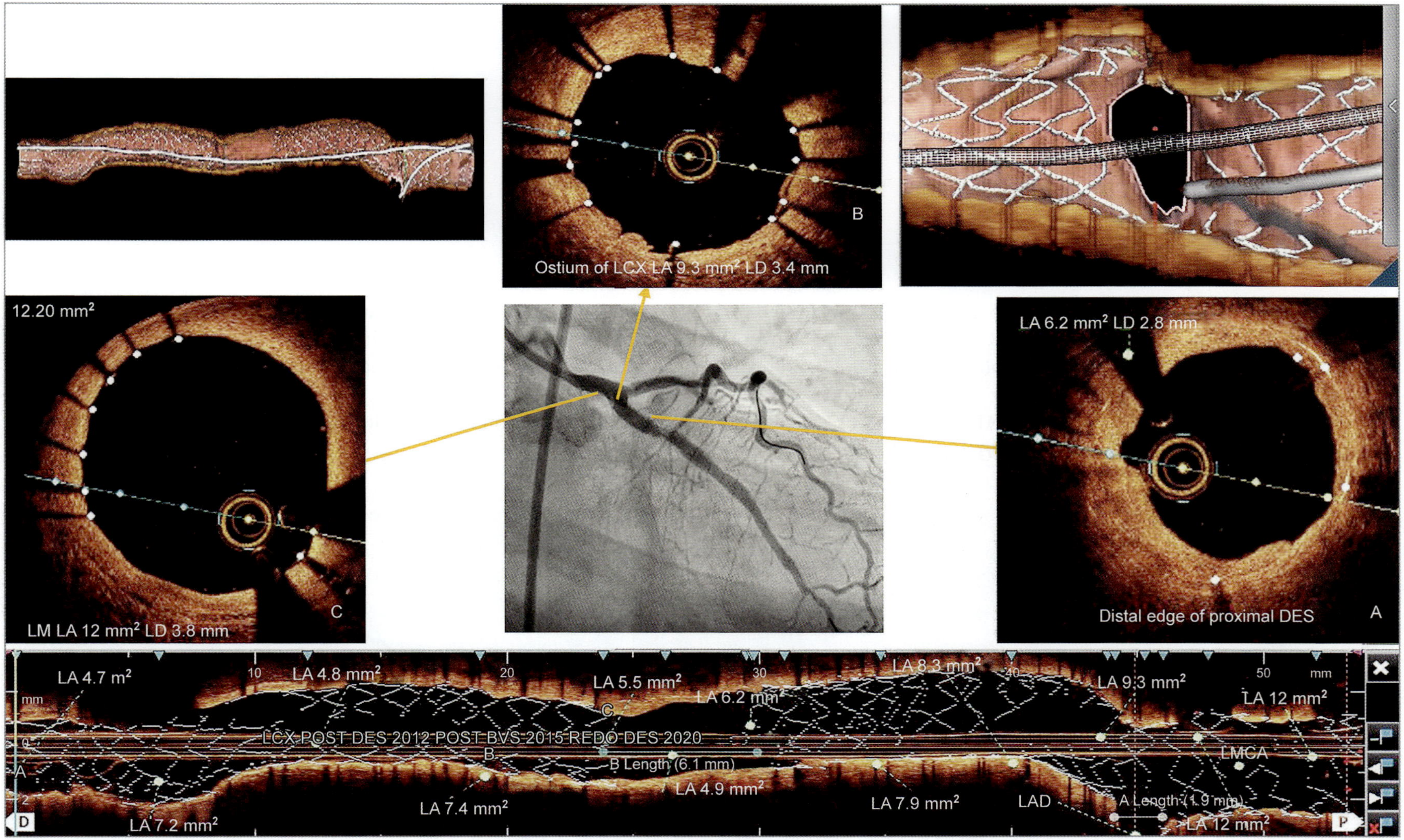

Fig. 58C

Figs. 58A to C: Poststent OCT. (A) Assessment of distal LCX stent segment; (B) Uncovered mid LCX segment between two stent segments; (C) Assessment of distal LM-LCX stent segment.

CASE 11

PCI of diffusely calcified LAD-underexpansion corrected with OPN NC.

CLINICAL HISTORY

A 55-year-old male presented with chest pain associated with SOB for 1 week. Past history of PCI of LAD with BMS in 2013 and PCI of LAD and LCX with DES in 2014. ECG showed poor R wave progression, T inversion V5, V6, L-I and AVL. 2D Echo—thin and hypokinetic distal IVS, apex, and anterior wall, dilated LV, moderate LV systolic dysfunction, EF—38%. Investigation: Hb—14.4 g/dL, serum creatine—0.5 mg/dL, eGFR—116 mL/min, blood urea—23 mg/dL, RBS—97 mg/dL.

Coronary angiogram-LMCA—normal, LAD—proximal 40% lesion, mid long segment 80% lesion before stent, moderate ISR of LAD stent, distal mild disease, LCX and RCA—mild disease **(Fig. 59)**.

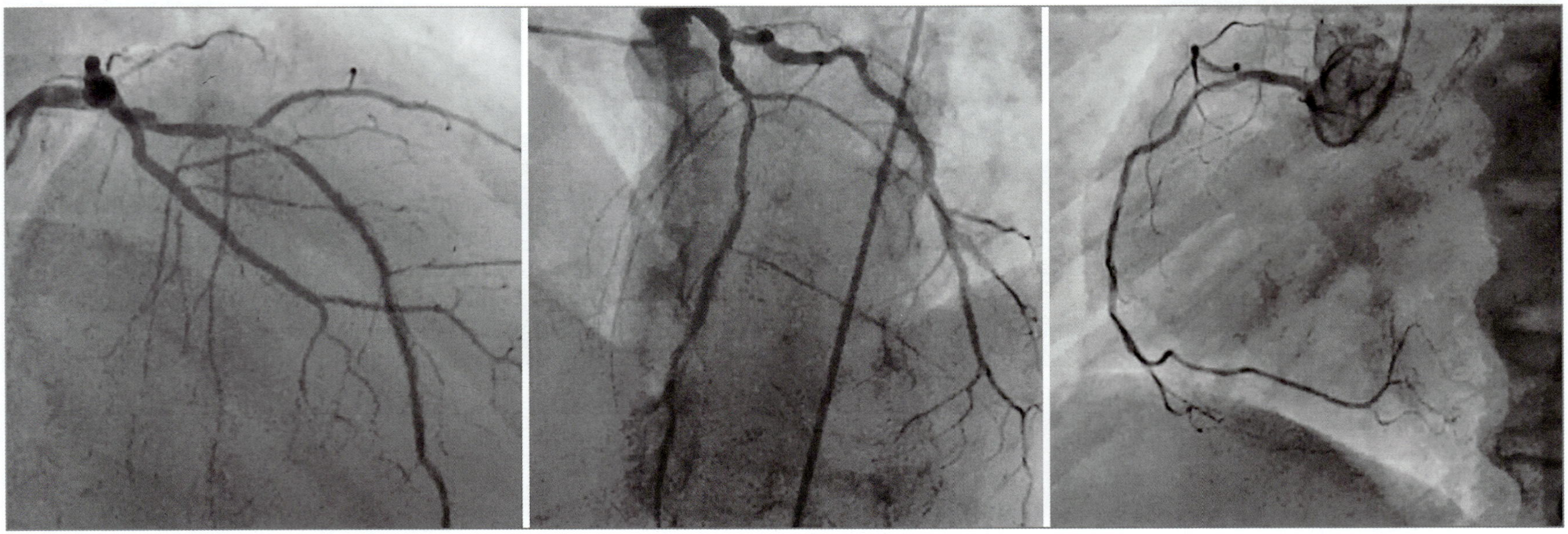

Fig. 59: Coronary angiogram.

PROCEDURE

RRA—route, 6 Fr EBU 3.5 guiding catheter, LAD lesion was crossed with 0.014″ Runthrough wire. Predilatation done with 2.0 × 15 mm and 2.5 × 10 mm Tazuna balloons **(Fig. 60)**.

Pre-OCT showed proximal to mid LAD long segment fibrocalcific lesion, and ISR of mid LAD **(Figs. 61A to C)**.

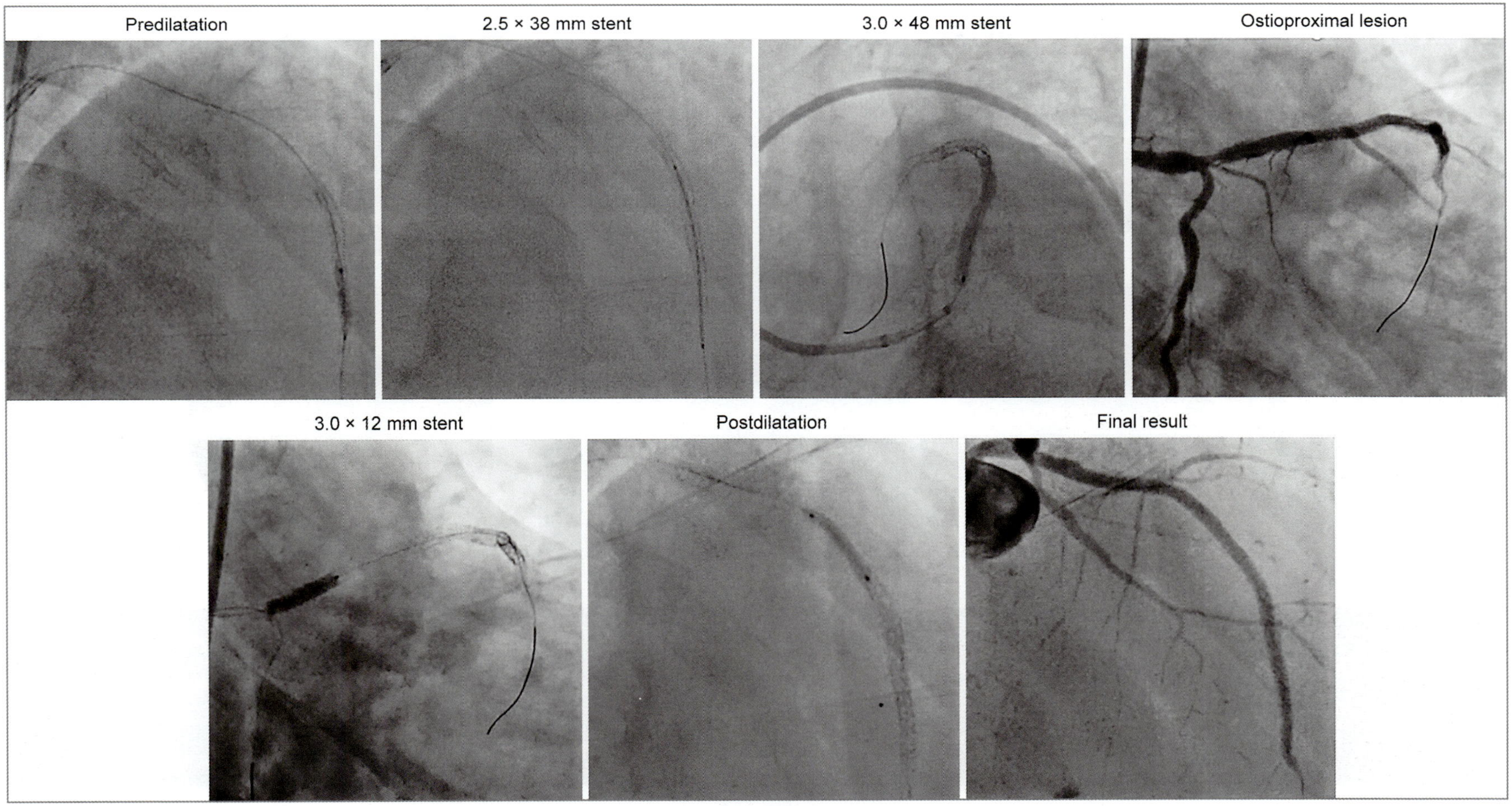

Fig. 60: Coronary angioplasty.

Distal stenting done with 2.5 × 38 mm Resolute Onyx stent. Proximal stenting done with 3.0 × 48 mm Resolute Onyx stent. Poststenting check angio showed ostioproximal residual lesion then stenting done with 3.0 × 12 mm Yukon Choice Flex stent with Guideliner support. Postdilatation done with 3.0 × 10 mm NC Trek balloon **(Fig. 60)**.

Post-OCT showed underexpansion of mid LAD stent **(Figs. 62A to C)**.

Postdilated with 2.5 × 15 mm OPN NC balloon. Postprocedure angio view showed well-implanted stents with TIMI-III flow without any dissection **(Fig. 60)**. Patient was discharged on third postprocedure day in a stable status.

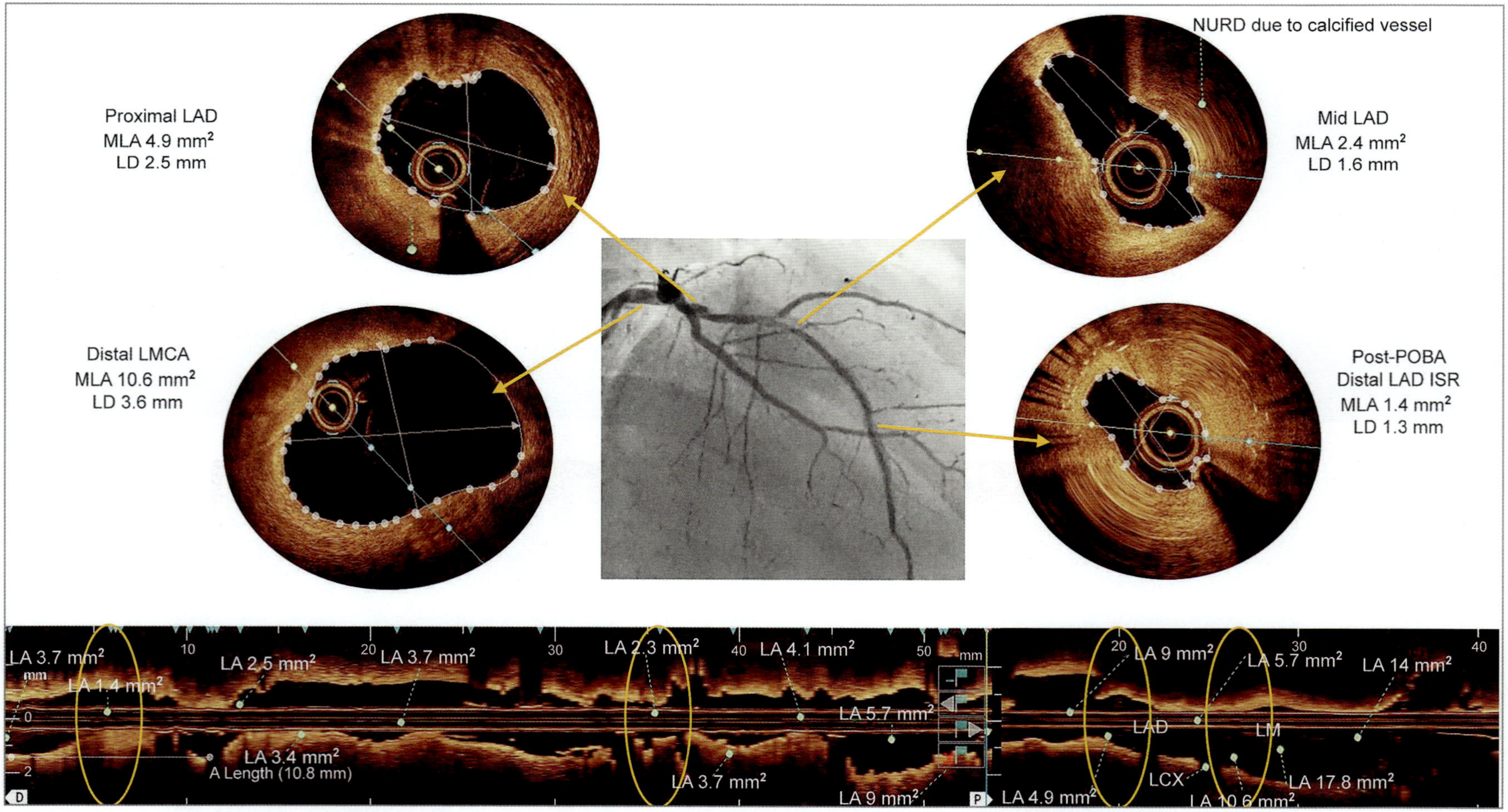

Fig. 61A

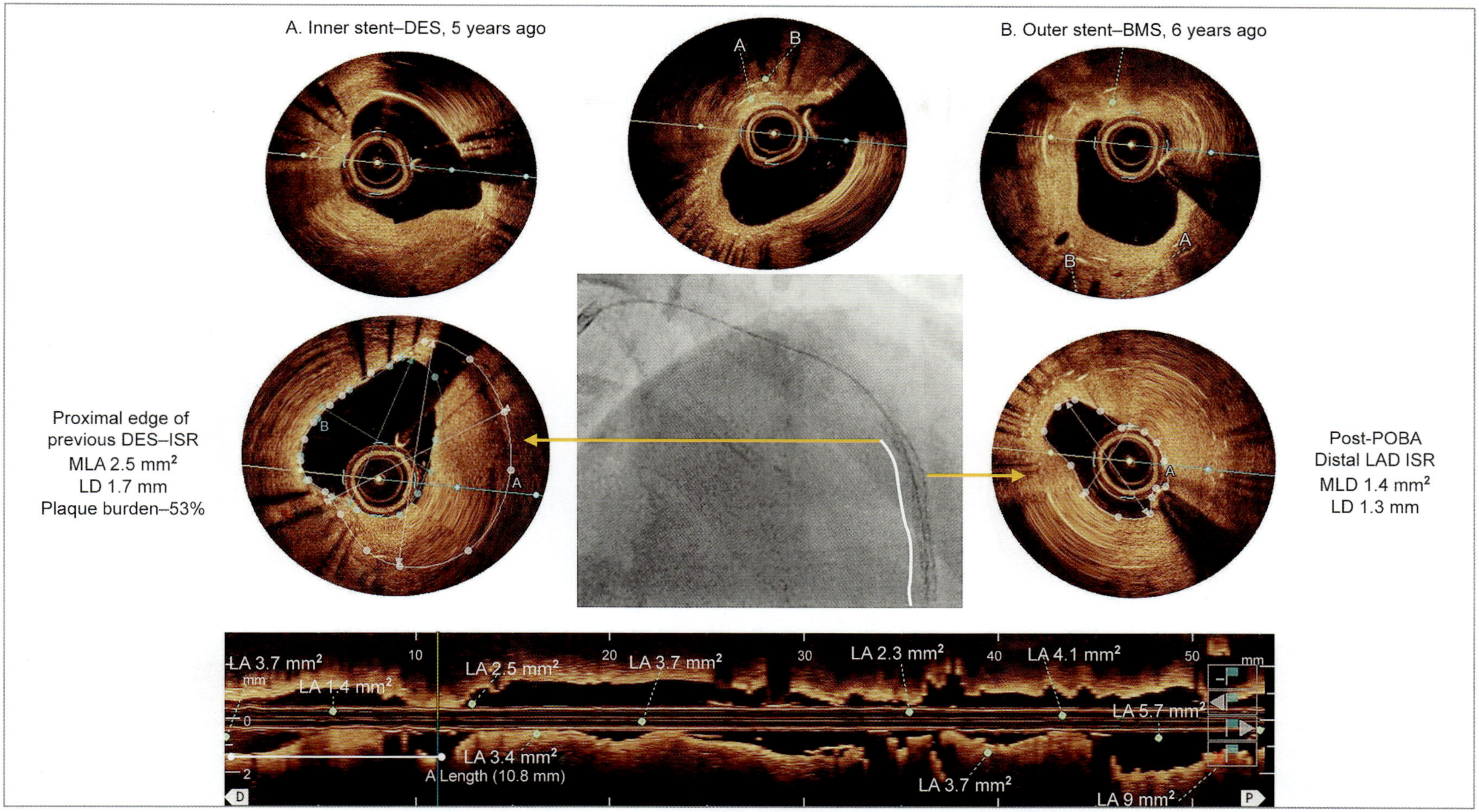

Fig. 61B

Different DCB strategies are also recommended for the management of bifurcation lesions:

- DCB in SB and DES in main branch (MB); and
- DCBs in both MB and SB.

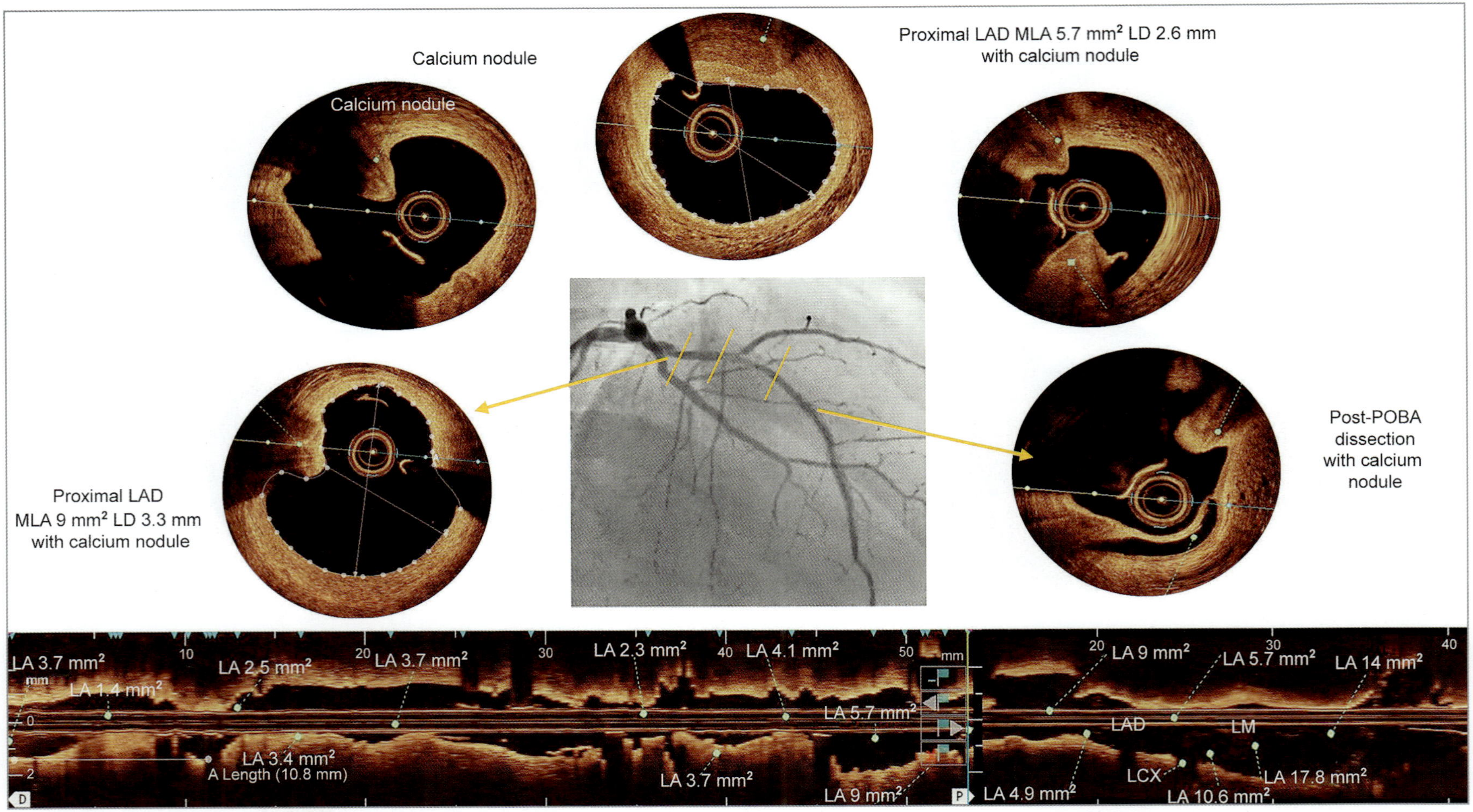

Fig. 61C

Figs. 61A to C: Prestent OCT assessment. (A) Of proximal to mid segment; (B) Distal segment assessment; (C) Plaque morphology.

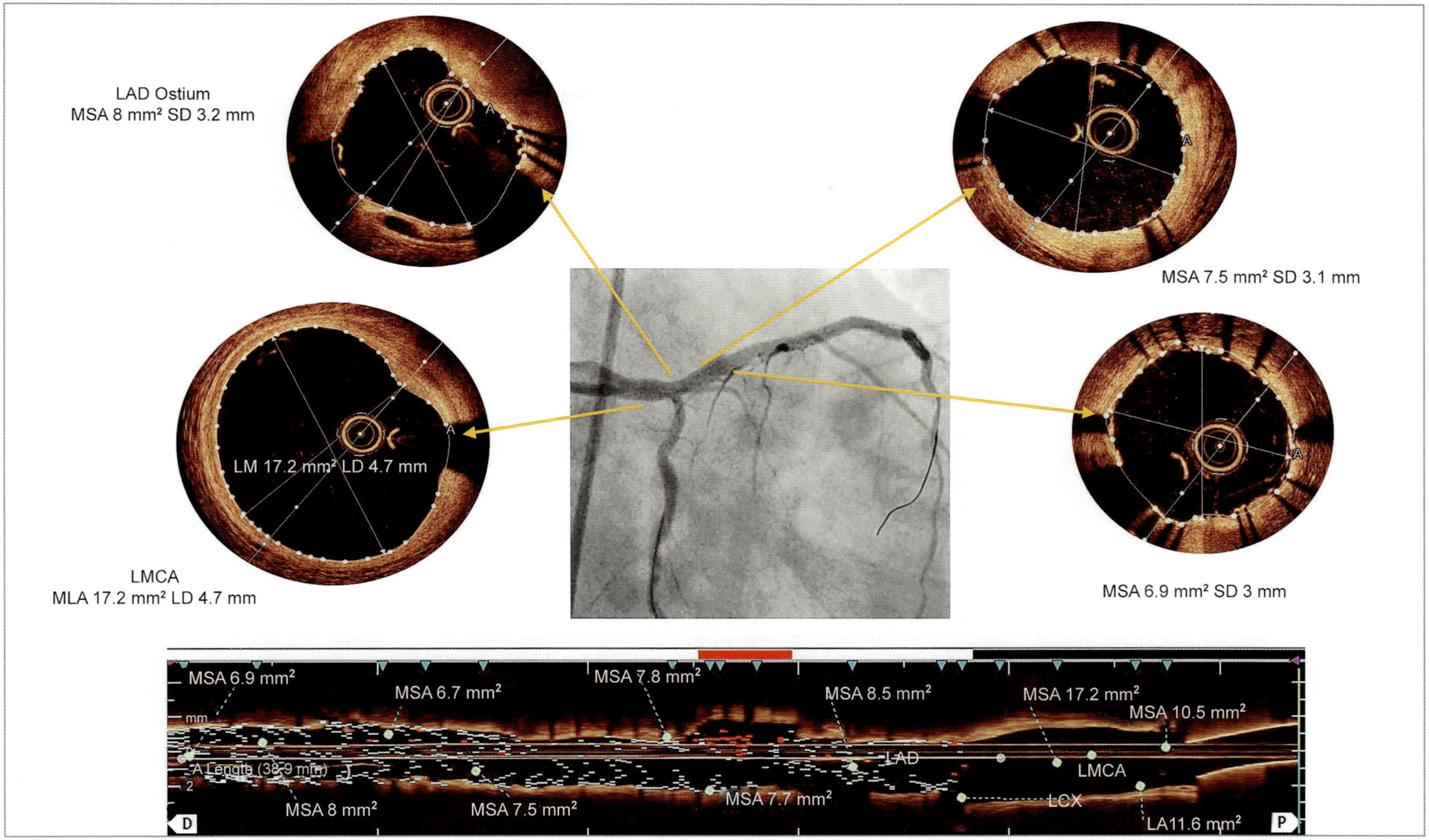
LAD Ostium
MSA 8 mm² SD 3.2 mm
MSA 7.5 mm² SD 3.1 mm
LM 17.2 mm² LD 4.7 mm
LMCA
MLA 17.2 mm² LD 4.7 mm
MSA 6.9 mm² SD 3 mm
MSA 6.9 mm²
MSA 6.7 mm²
MSA 7.8 mm²
MSA 8.5 mm²
MSA 17.2 mm²
MSA 10.5 mm²
LAD
LMCA
LCX
MSA 8 mm²
MSA 7.5 mm²
MSA 7.7 mm²
LA11.6 mm²
D
P

Fig. 62A

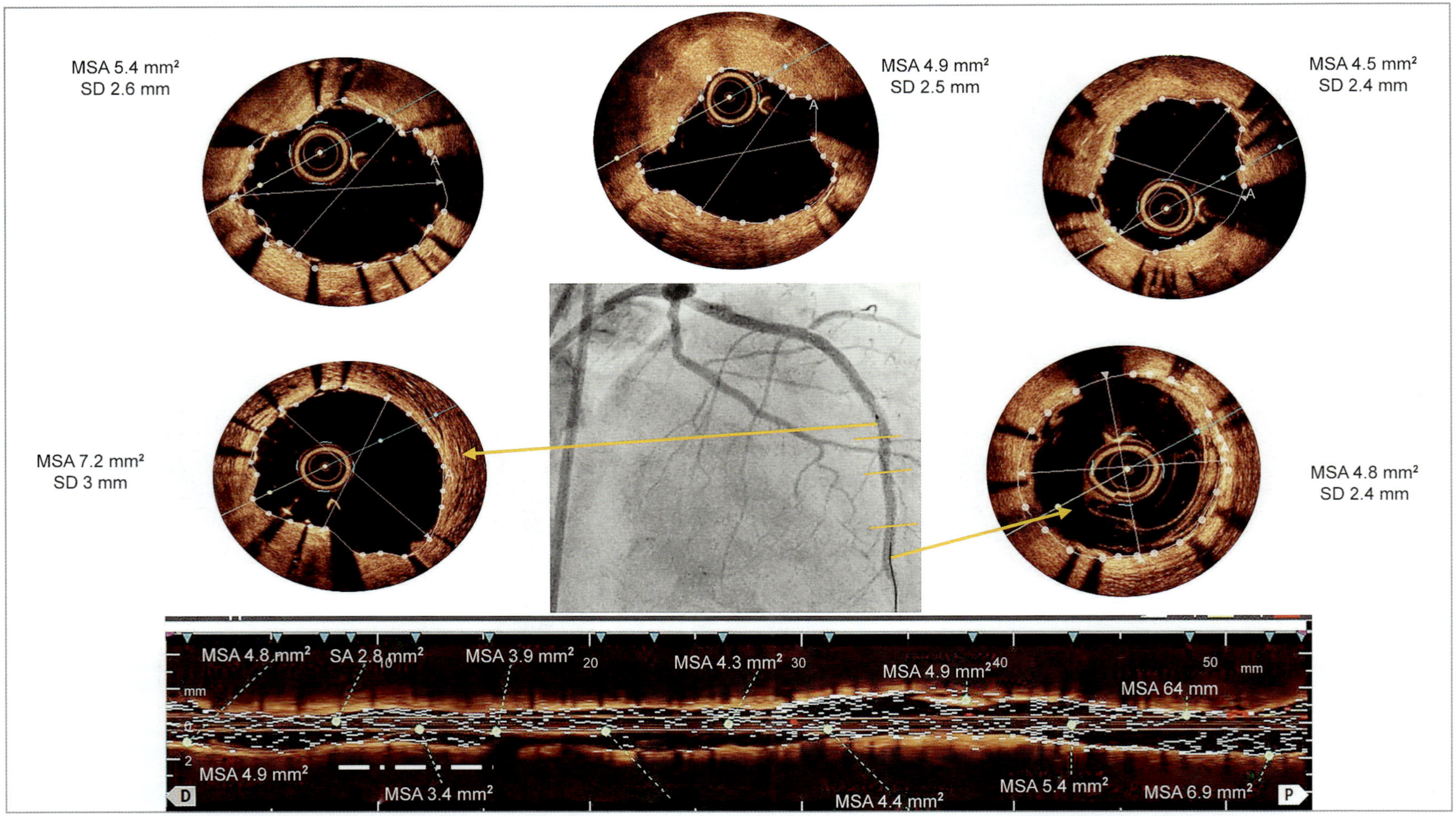

MSA 5.4 mm²
SD 2.6 mm
MSA 4.9 mm²
SD 2.5 mm
MSA 4.5 mm²
SD 2.4 mm
MSA 7.2 mm²
SD 3 mm
MSA 4.8 mm²
SD 2.4 mm
MSA 4.8 mm²
SA 2.8 mm²
MSA 3.9 mm²
MSA 4.3 mm²
MSA 4.9 mm²
MSA 64 mm
MSA 4.9 mm²
MSA 3.4 mm²
MSA 4.4 mm²
MSA 5.4 mm²
MSA 6.9 mm²
D
P

Fig. 62B

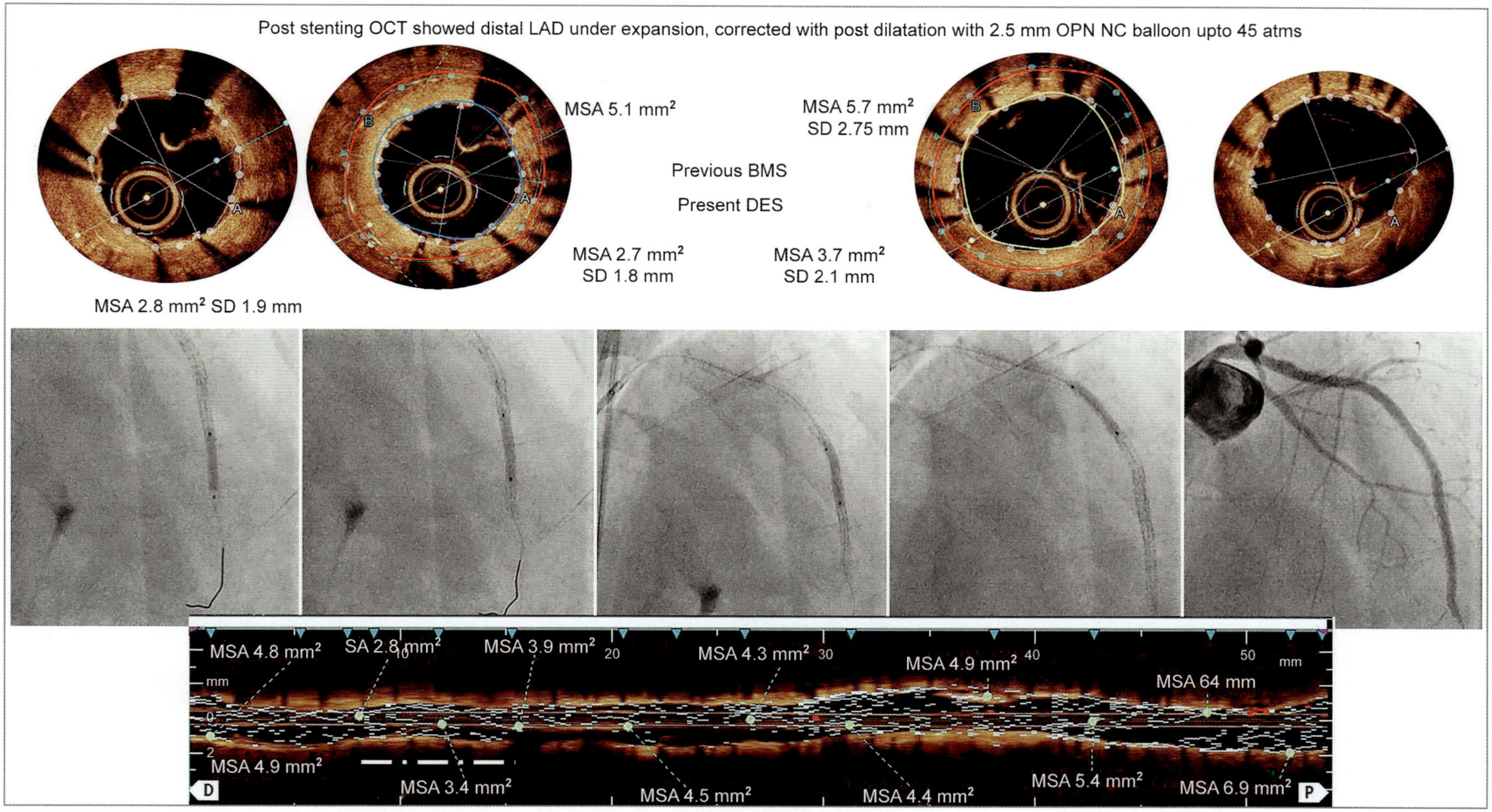

Fig. 62C

Figs. 62A to C: Poststent OCT assessment. (A) Distal LM-proximal LAD segment; (B) Distal LAD segment; (C) Distal LAD stent under-expansion was corrected with high-pressure NC balloon.

CASE 12

OCT-guided PCI of RCA ISR.

CLINICAL HISTORY

A 64-year-old male, known diabetic and hypertensive presented with ACS—unstable angina, ECG—normal, 2D Echo—no RWMA, normal LV function, EF—65%.

Investigations: Hb—13.3 g/dL, serum creatinine—0.59 mg/dL with eGFR—107 mL/min. CAG—two-vessel disease, mid LAD—long segment mild disease, mid RCA ISR 90% lesion **(Fig. 63)**.

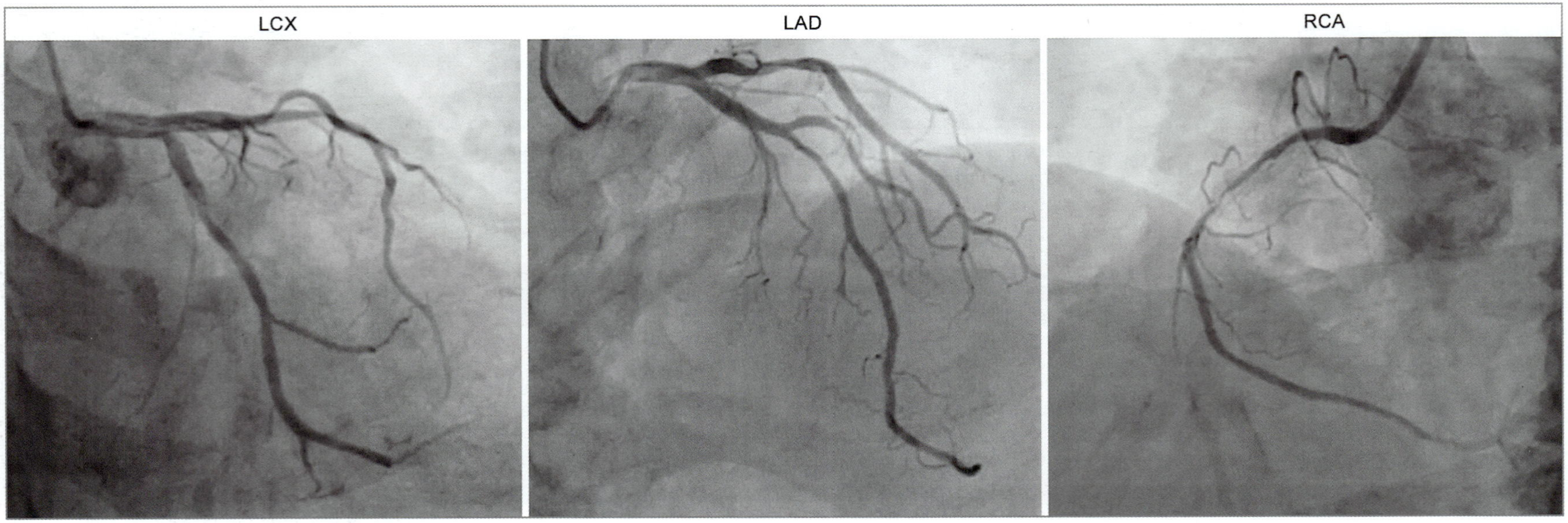

Fig. 63: Coronary angiogram.

PROCEDURE

Right radial approach using Slender sheath (Terumo), RCA engaged with JR 3.5–7 Fr guiding catheter, lesion crossed with BMW wire and predilated with 1.5 × 10 mm, 2.25 × 15 mm Tazuna and 3.0 × 12 mm NC Trek balloon **(Fig. 64)**. Prestenting OCT revealed ISR of RCA due to

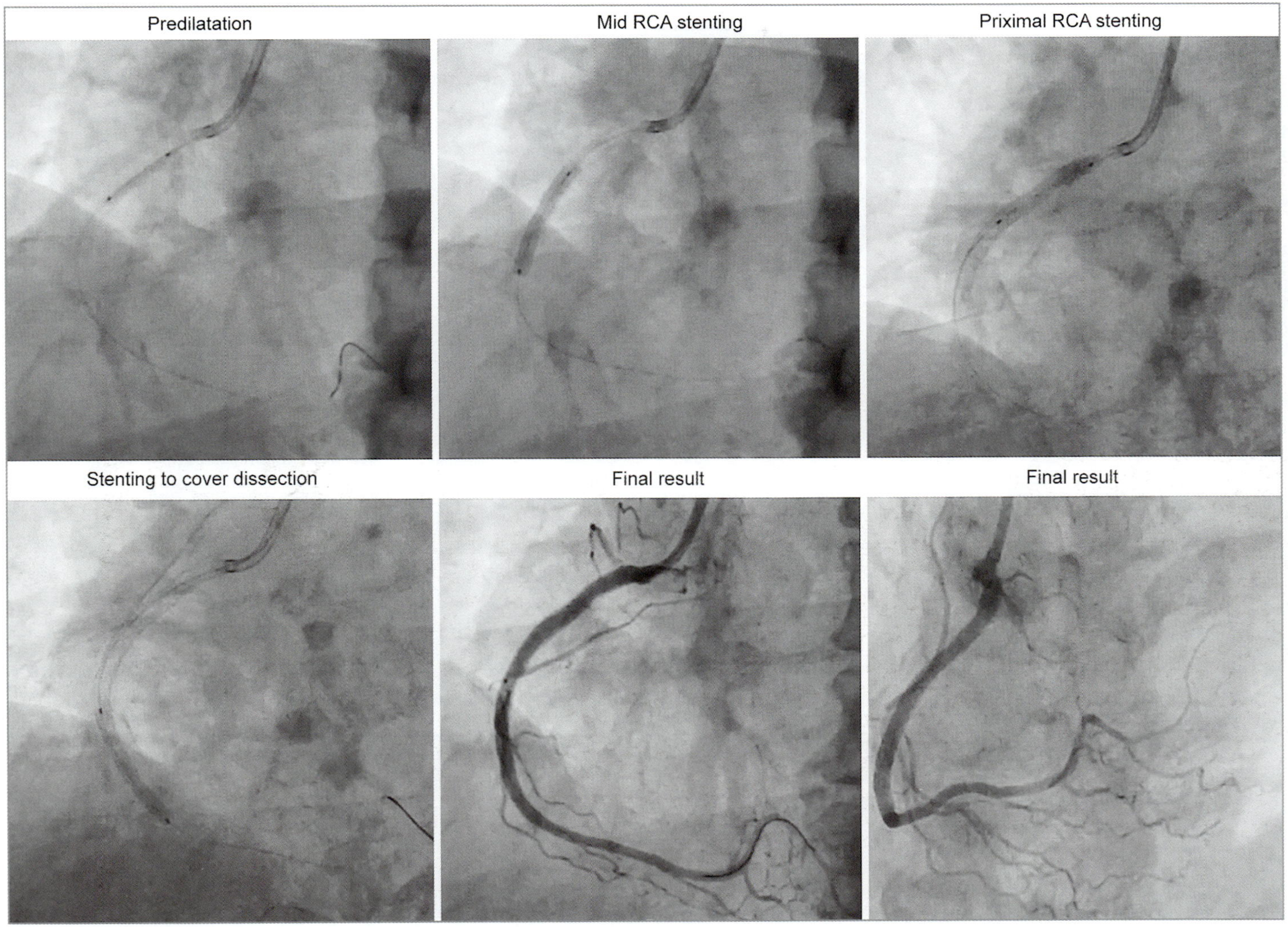

Fig. 64: Coronary angioplasty with DES.

neoatherosclerosis with neointimal calcific plaque **(Figs. 65A to C)**. Then mid RCA stenting done with 3.5 × 22 mm Resolute Onyx stent and postdilated with 3.5 × 22 mm NC balloon. Proximal RCA stenting done with 4.0 × 22 mm Resolute Onyx stent was due to thick fibrotic plaque at proximal landing zone **(Fig. 64)**. Poststenting OCT showed significant medial edge dissection distal to stent in mid RCA due to fibrotic plaque of distal landing zone **(Figs. 66A and B)**. Hence, dissection covered with 3.0 × 22 mm Resolute Onyx stent. The final result was good with TIMI-III flow with no complications **(Fig. 64)**.

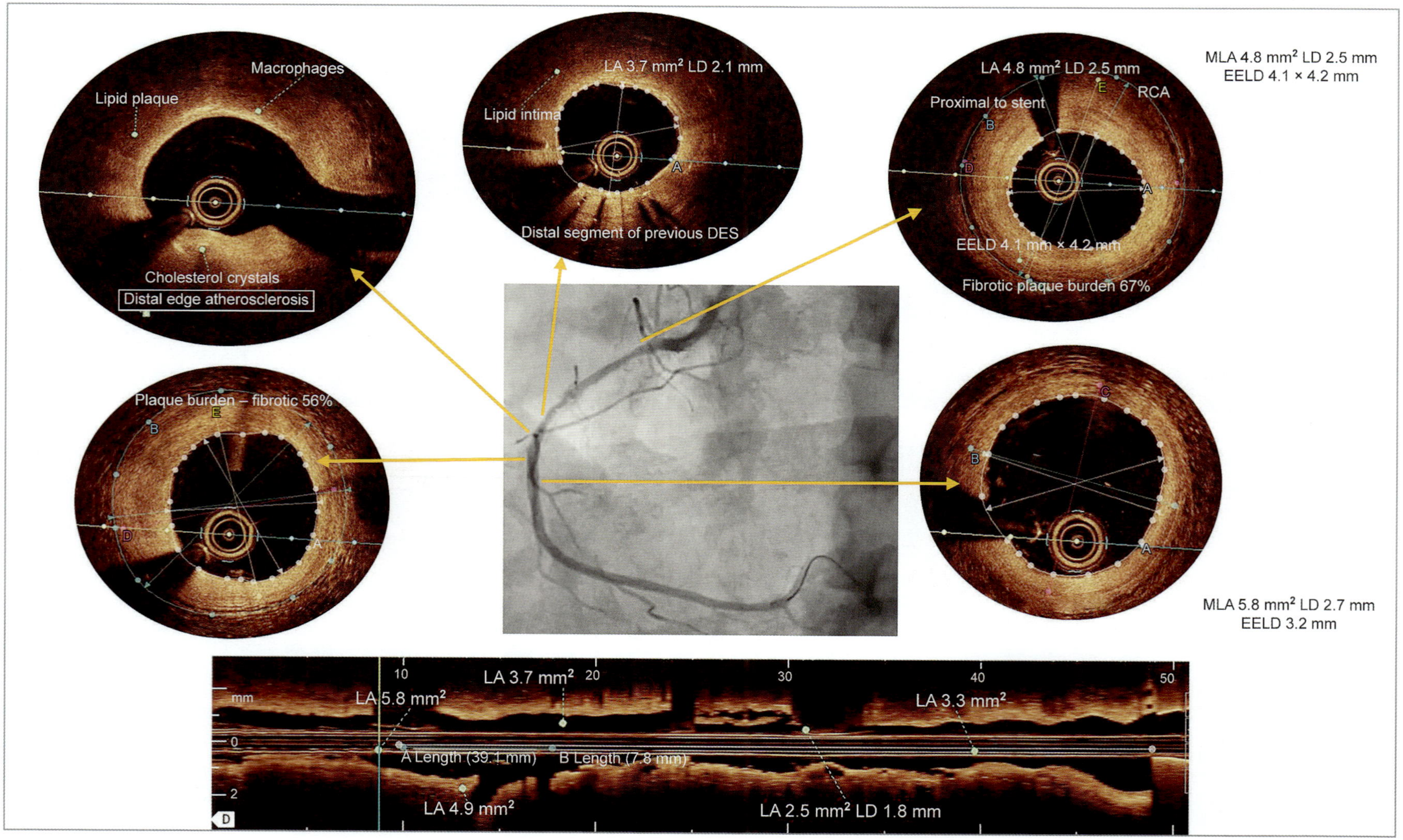

Fig. 65A

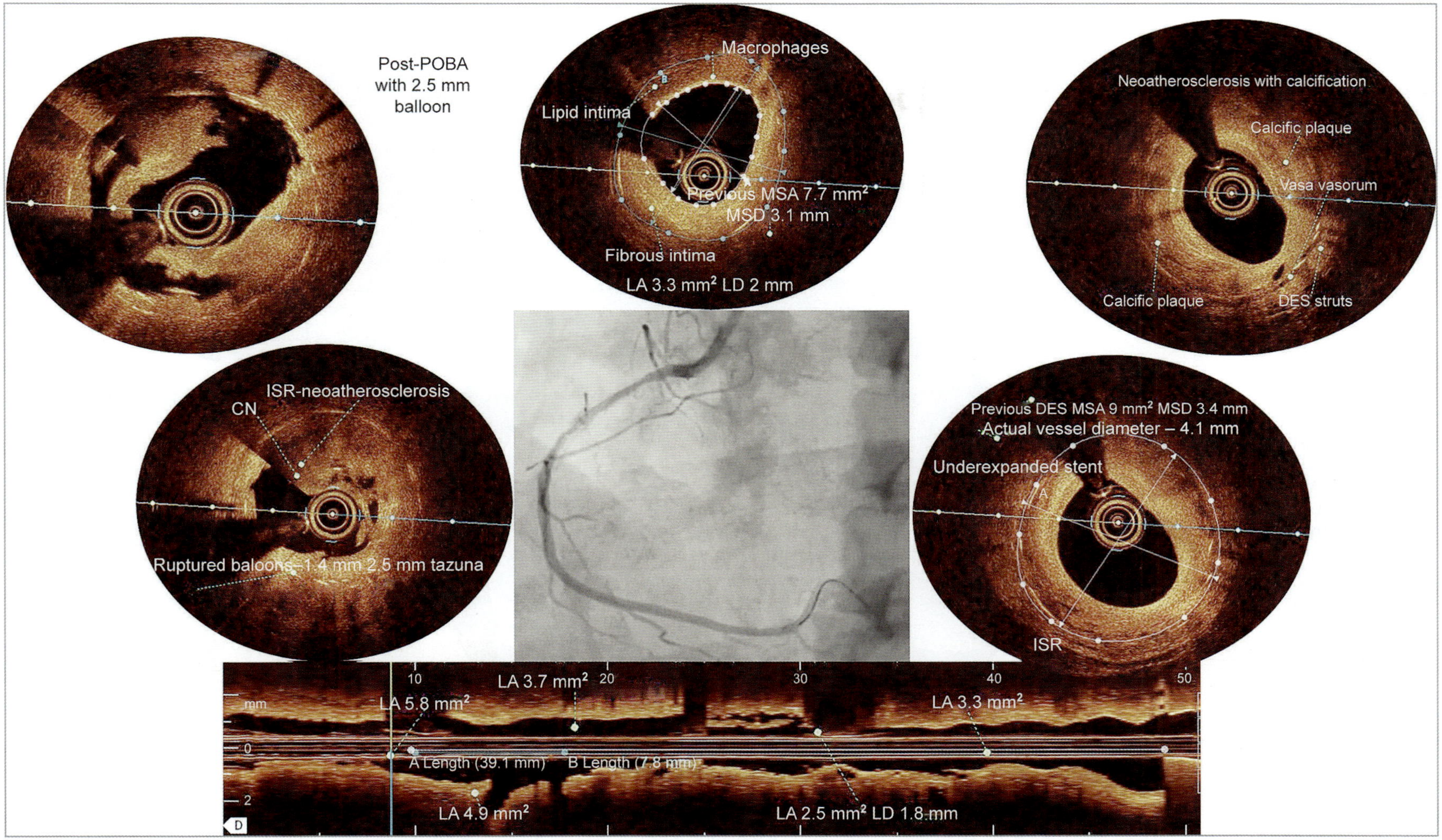
Post-POBA
with 2.5 mm
balloon
Macrophages
Lipid intima
Previous MSA 7.7 mm²
MSD 3.1 mm
Fibrous intima
LA 3.3 mm² LD 2 mm
Neoatherosclerosis with calcification
Calcific plaque
Vasa vasorum
Calcific plaque
DES struts
ISR-neoatherosclerosis
CN
Ruptured baloons-1.4 mm 2.5 mm tazuna
Previous DES MSA 9 mm² MSD 3.4 mm
Actual vessel diameter – 4.1 mm
Underexpanded stent
ISR
LA 3.7 mm²
LA 5.8 mm²
LA 3.3 mm²
A Length (39.1 mm)
B Length (7.8 mm)
LA 4.9 mm²
LA 2.5 mm² LD 1.8 mm

Fig. 65B

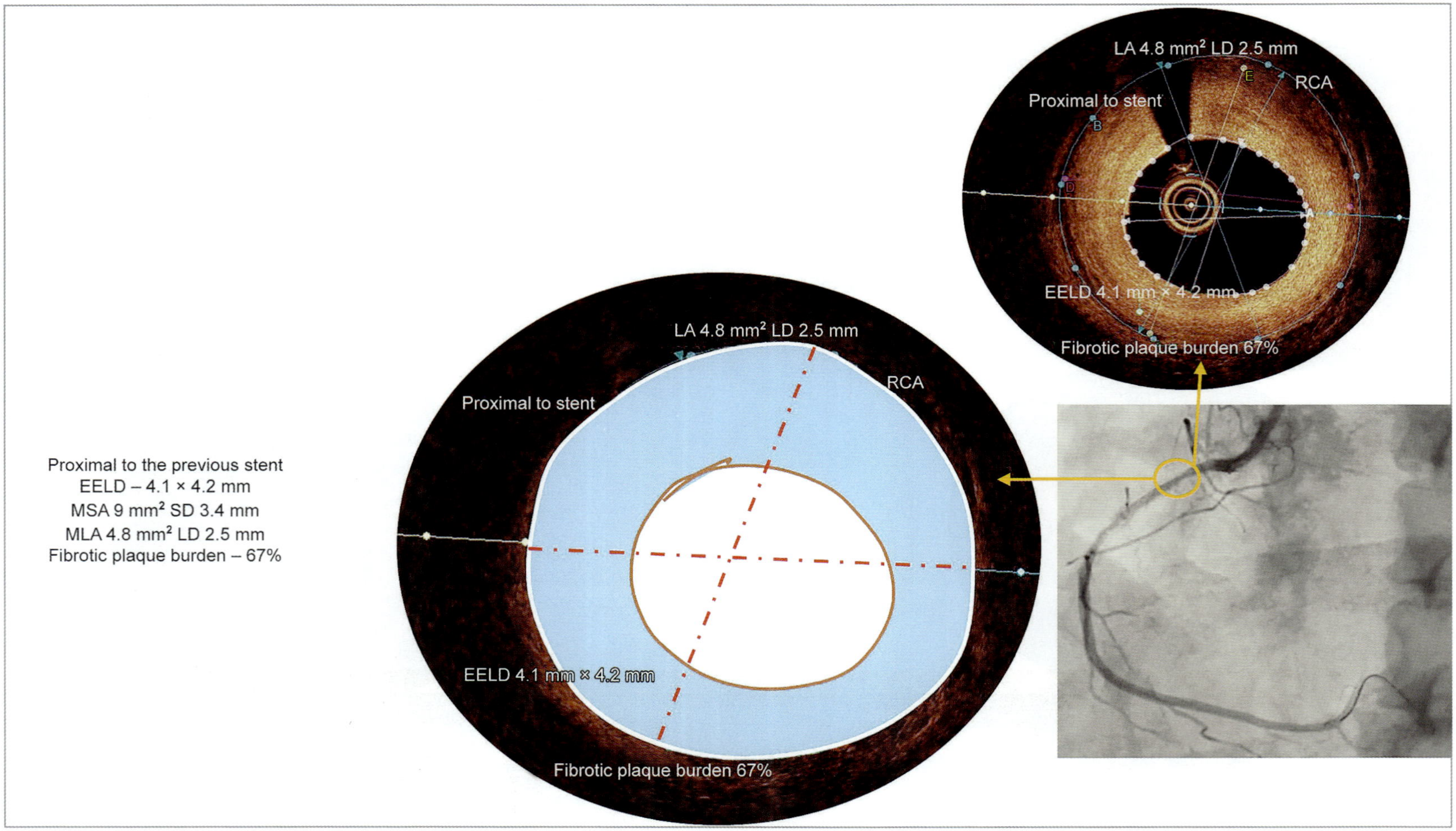

Fig. 65C

Figs. 65A to C: Prestent OCT assessment. (A) For device selection; (B) For plaque morphology; (C) Assessment of ISR segment proximal to previous stent.

Optical coherence tomography study revealed ISR of RCA due to severe neoatherosclerosis with calcification, >180° calcific plaque, and eccentric calcific nodule with thick fibrotic plaque burden. Prestent lesion preparation was done with high-pressure NC balloon inflations prior to stent implantation which resulted in adequate expansion of stent; further prolonged poststent balloon inflations were carried out with high pressure NC balloons to avoid recoiling with adequate expansion. OCT imaging showed thick fibrotic plaque burden in the proximal to the stent landing zone; hence it was covered with proximal overlapping stent using 4.0 × 22 mm stent. Poststenting imaging showed distal significant medial edge dissection due to thick fibrotic plaque at distal landing zone. Imaging helped us assessing plaque morphology, choosing device length and diameter, covering entire diseased segment, identifying significant medial edge dissections and rectifying it with additional stenting.

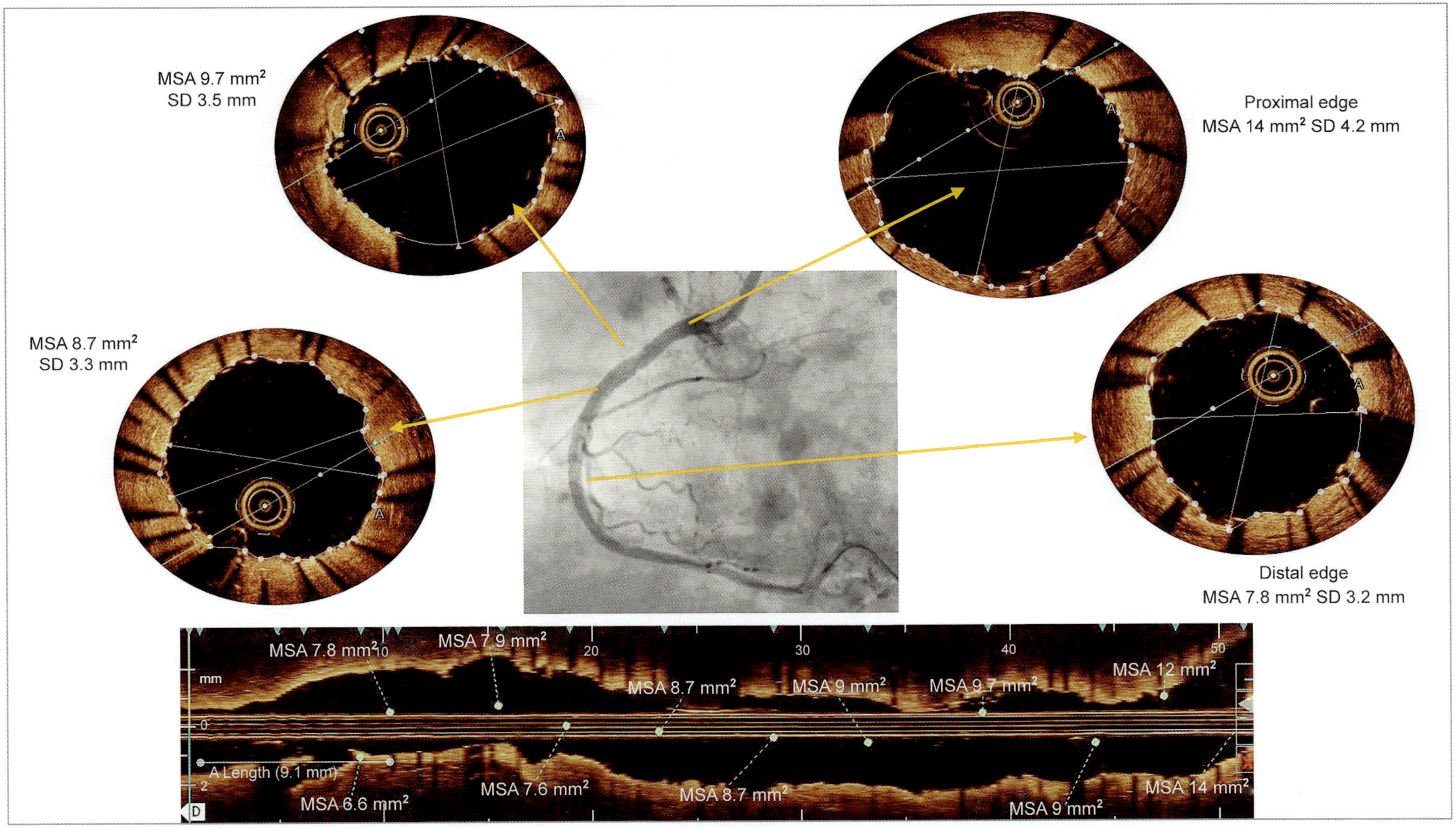

Fig. 66A

Post PCI assessment of FFR suggests:

- Residual Ischemia despite angiographically successful result
- Indicate prognosis of Post PCI patients during follow-up – higher the FFR value(>0.87), better the prognosis
- Pull back study can identify site responsible for ischemia like under expanded stent or uncovered diseased segments beyond stent edges.

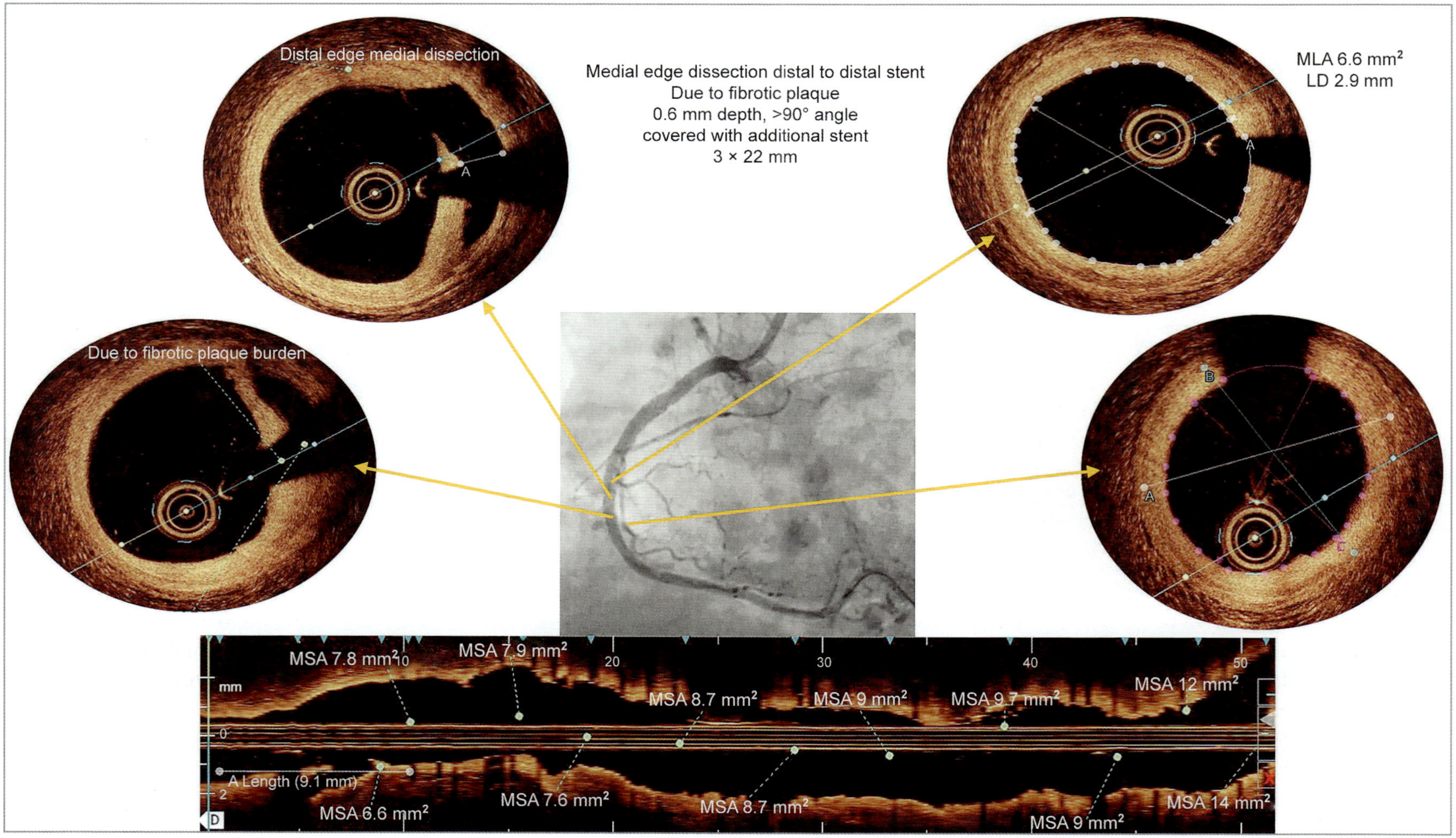

Fig. 66B

Figs. 66A and B: (A) Poststent OCT assessment showed well expanded and well apposed entire stent length with no medial edge dissection at proximal end; (B) Distal stent edge dissection was noted which was covered with additional stent.

CHAPTER 13

Recanalized Thrombus

INTRODUCTION

Recanalized thrombus, usually seen as an ambiguous lesion on angiographic images, is seen less often in regular clinical practice. It is often confused with other clinical conditions such as fresh thrombosis by plaque rupture/erosion, spontaneous coronary artery dissection, coronary aneurysm, or severe calcific lesion. Intravascular imaging is very useful in making differential diagnosis and guides in appropriate device-based therapy.[1]

Optical coherence tomography (OCT) is preferable to intravascular ultrasound (IVUS) because spatial resolution is 10-fold greater (10 μm). It can thus confirm a diagnosis of spontaneous recanalized coronary thrombus (SRCT) when angiography is ambiguous.

Three major findings of radiotherapy (RT):

1. Common angiographic findings such as multiple irregular filling defects and intraluminal haziness were not specific for recanalization.
2. On OCT, the recanalization of organized thrombi was characterized by multiple small channels divided by thin septa communicating with each other; OCT imaging in such cases reveals "spider web", "Swiss cheese", "lotus root", or "honeycomb" a pattern due to the presence of multiple intraluminal channels within the thrombus. The pathognomonic feature is the morphology of circular channels separated by thin septa, unlike in dissection, which is characterized by true and false channels that are intraluminal and in communication, Nonpenetration of these channels in subintimal space with intact intimal layer differentiates them from spontaneous coronary dissection, as the latter has subintimal channels.[2]
3. Despite the neovascularization process, most of these lesions were functionally significant.

LIMITATIONS OF ANGIOGRAPHY IN SYNCHROTRON RADIATION CORONARY ANGIOGRAPHY

Previously reported study stated that most of the present patients (67%) were symptomatic (angina pectoris and/or dyspnea). 9 of the 10 asymptomatic patients were assessed on functional tests, which all proved positive, whereas angiography identified only 9 patients (30%) with >50% (30%) and 3 (10%) with >70% stenosis. Moreover, estimated lumen reduction varied from 28% to 100% in the 15 patients with functional test, which indicated ischemia in all cases. There was thus discordance between the ischemia and the stenosis induced by the lesion on angiography. In these patients, quantitative coronary angiography (QCA) assessment of stenosis was poorly predictive of the ischemia induced by SRCT.[2]

OCT optical coherence tomography indicated lumen reduction between 20% and 93%, but there was no clear association with stenosis severity or coronary flow. The present discordance between lumen reduction and symptomatic impact may be due to the tortuosity of the channels. Downstream hemodynamic impact cannot be assessed from cross-sectional imaging and is probably underestimated on angiography, as seen from the symptomatic impact in the previous series. Despite atypical morphology, this treatment option is technically feasible and associated with a low rate of failure.[3,4]

RECANALIZATION OF ORGANIZED THROMBI DEMONSTRATED BY CORONARY CT ANGIOGRAPHY COMPARED WITH OCT

The flap-like lesion showing signal-poor, darker tissue in the deeper portion corresponds to what has been described by pathology as proteoglycan-collagen-rich areas that separate the multiple blood-filled channels. The "Swiss cheese" pattern of the lumen suggests the recanalization of organized thrombi.[5]

REFERENCES

1. Kang SJ, Nakano M, Virmani R, Song HG, Ahn JM, Kim WJ, et al. OCT findings in patients with recanalization of organized thrombi in coronary arteries. JACC Cardiovasc Imaging. 2012;5(7):725-32.
2. Souteyrand G, Valladier M, Amabile N, Derimay F, Harbaoui B, Leddet P, et al. Diagnosis and Management of Spontaneously Recanalized Coronary Thrombus Guided by Optical Coherence Tomography—Lessons From the French "Lotus Root" Registry. Circ J. 2018;82(3):783-90.
3. Pyxaras SA, Tu S, Barbato E, Barbati G, Di Serafino L, De Vroey F, et al. Quantitative angiography and optical coherence tomography for the functional assessment of nonobstructive coronary stenoses: comparison with fractional flow reserve. Am Heart J. 2013;166(6):1010-8.
4. Kim Y, Jeong MH, Kim MC, Sim DS, Hong YJ, Kim JH, et al. Multivessel Disease With Recanalized Thrombus—Etiologic Insights From Optical Coherence Tomography. Circ J. 2019;83(3):688.
5. Yang DH, Kang SJ, Kim YH, Kang JW, Ahn JM, Park DW, et al. Recanalization of organized thrombi demonstrated by coronary CT angiography compared with OCT. JACC: Cardiovascular Imaging. 2016;9(7):887-90.

CASE 1

OCT-guided percutaneous coronary intervention (PCI) of recanalized thrombus of left anterior descending (LAD) and PCI of left circumflex (LCX).

CLINICAL HISTORY

A 67-year-old male presented with established inferior wall myocardial infarction (MI), postinfarct angina, and breathlessness. Electrocardiogram (ECG)-evolved inferior wall MI. 2D Echo-RWMA+ (regional wall motion abnormality), hypokinesia of inferior and posterior wall, moderate left ventricular (LV) systolic dysfunction, ejection fraction (EF)—40%.

Coronary angiography (CAG)-left main coronary artery (LMCA)—normal, LAD—proximal to mid 90% ambiguous lesion (possible dissection/recanalized thrombus/calcification), LCX—proximal 80% lesion, right coronary artery (RCA)—proximal total occlusion, distal vessel filling retrogradely **(Figs. 1A to C)**.

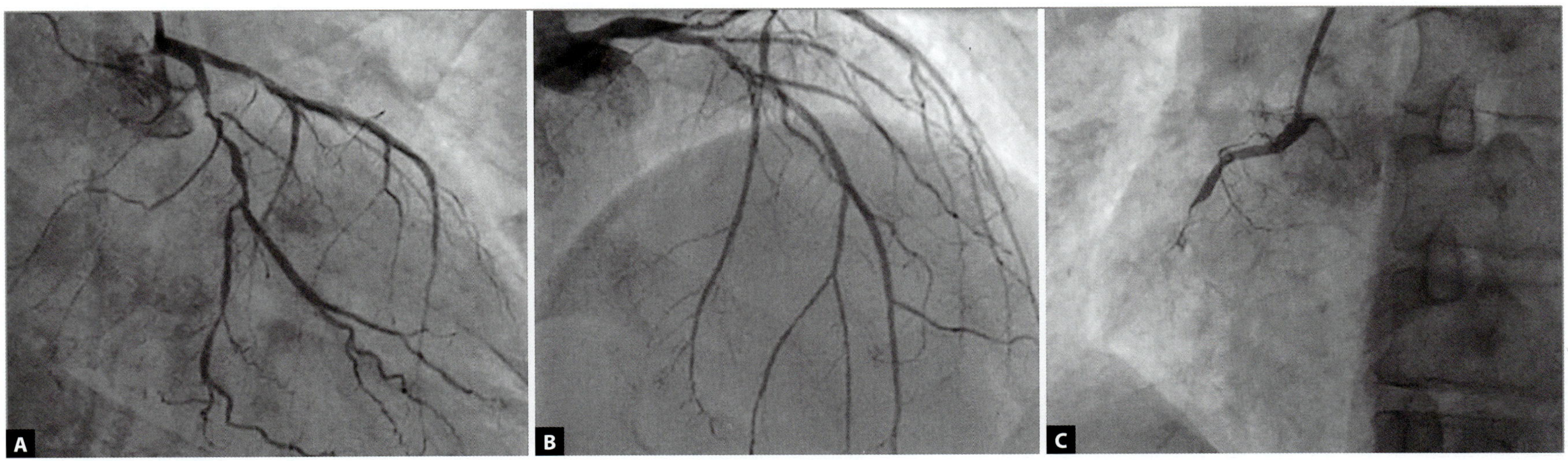

Figs. 1A to C

PROCEDURE

PCI of RCA: Right radial route, using 6 Fr Judkins right (JR) 3.5 guiding catheter, RCA lesion crossed with 0.014″ Sion blue wire; predilatation with 1.5 × 10 mm Tazuna, and 2.0 × 12 mm Mini Trek balloons; distal RCA stenting done with 2.75 × 33 mm Xience Xpedition stent [drug-eluting stent (DES)]; proximal RCA overlapping stenting done with 3.0 × 38 mm Xience Xpedition stent (DES), postprocedure angio view showed well-implanted stents with TIMI-III (thrombolysis in myocardial infarction III) flow without any dissection **(Figs. 1D to F)**.

PCI of LAD: Right radial route, using 6 Fr XB 3.5 guided catheter, 0.014″ Sion blue wire was placed in LAD. Pre-OCT study to assess ambiguous lesion of LAD to decide the plan of management. OCT showed recanalized thrombus-A honeycomb-like structure with multiple channels of various sizes, separated by highly backscattering septa **(Fig. 2)** and distal landing zone minimum lumen area (MLA)—2.8 mm^2, minimum lumen diameter (MLD)—1.9 mm, mid portion of the lesion recanalized thrombus, proximal landing zone MLA—3.8 mm^2, length of the lesion—29.8 mm **(Fig. 3)**.

Predilatation done with 1.25 × 10 mm, 1.5 × 10 mm, 2.5 × 10 mm Tazuna balloons; stenting done with 2.75 × 35 mm Orsiro stent (DES); Postdilatation done with 3.0 × 12 mm NC Trek balloon. Poststenting OCT showed well-apposed and well-expanded stent struts with no edge dissection **(Figs. 4 and 5)**. Postprocedure angio view showed well-implanted stents with TIMI-III flow without any dissection.

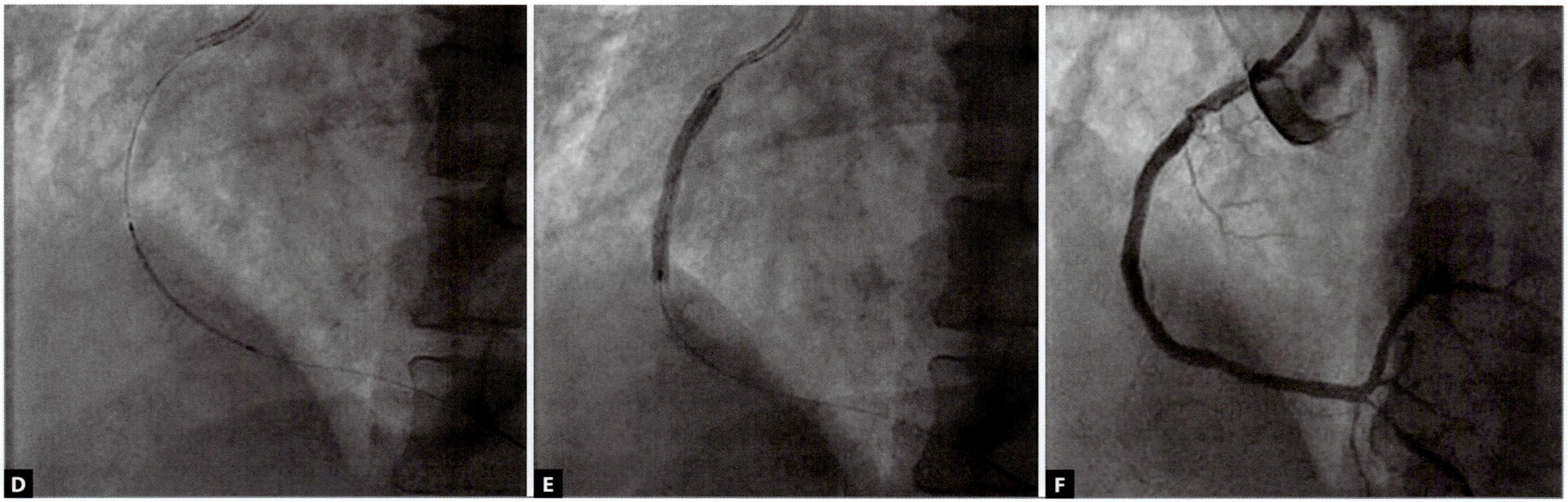

Figs. 1D to F

Figs. 1A to F: Coronary angiogram (A to C), stenting of proximal and distal right coronary artery (RCA) (D to F).

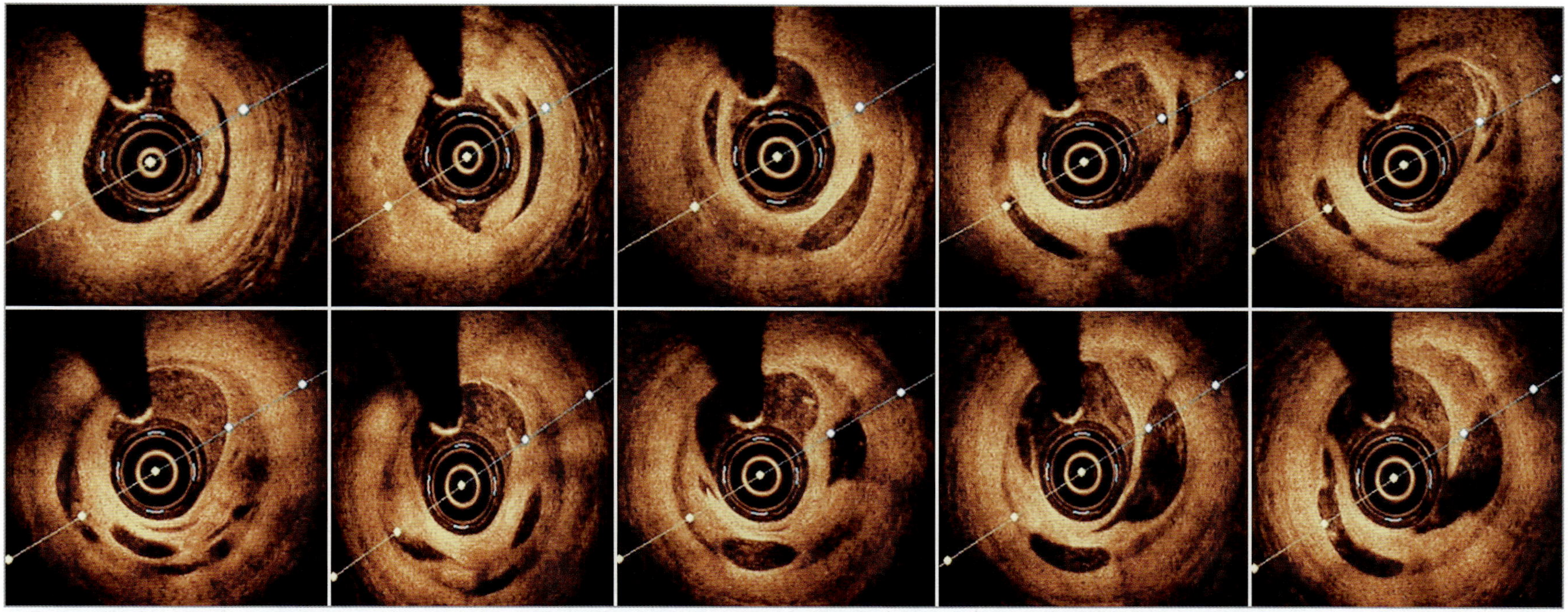

Fig. 2: Optical coherence tomography (OCT) showed recanalized thrombus—a honeycomb-like structure with multiple channels of various sizes, separated by highly backscattering septa.

PCI of LCX: Right radial route, 6 Fr XB 3.5 guided catheter, LCX lesion was crossed with 0.014″ Versaturn wire.

Pre-OCT analysis: Thick narrowing fibrotic plaque **(Fig. 6)**.

Predilatation done with 1.5 × 10 mm, 2.5 × 10 mm Tazuna balloon; stenting done with 2.75 × 38 mm Xience Xpedition stent **(Fig. 7A)**; poststenting OCT showed well-apposed and well-expanded stent struts with no edge dissections **(Fig. 8)**. Postprocedure angio view showed well-implanted stents with TIMI-III flow without any dissection **(Fig. 7B)**. Patient was discharged on third postprocedure in a stable status.

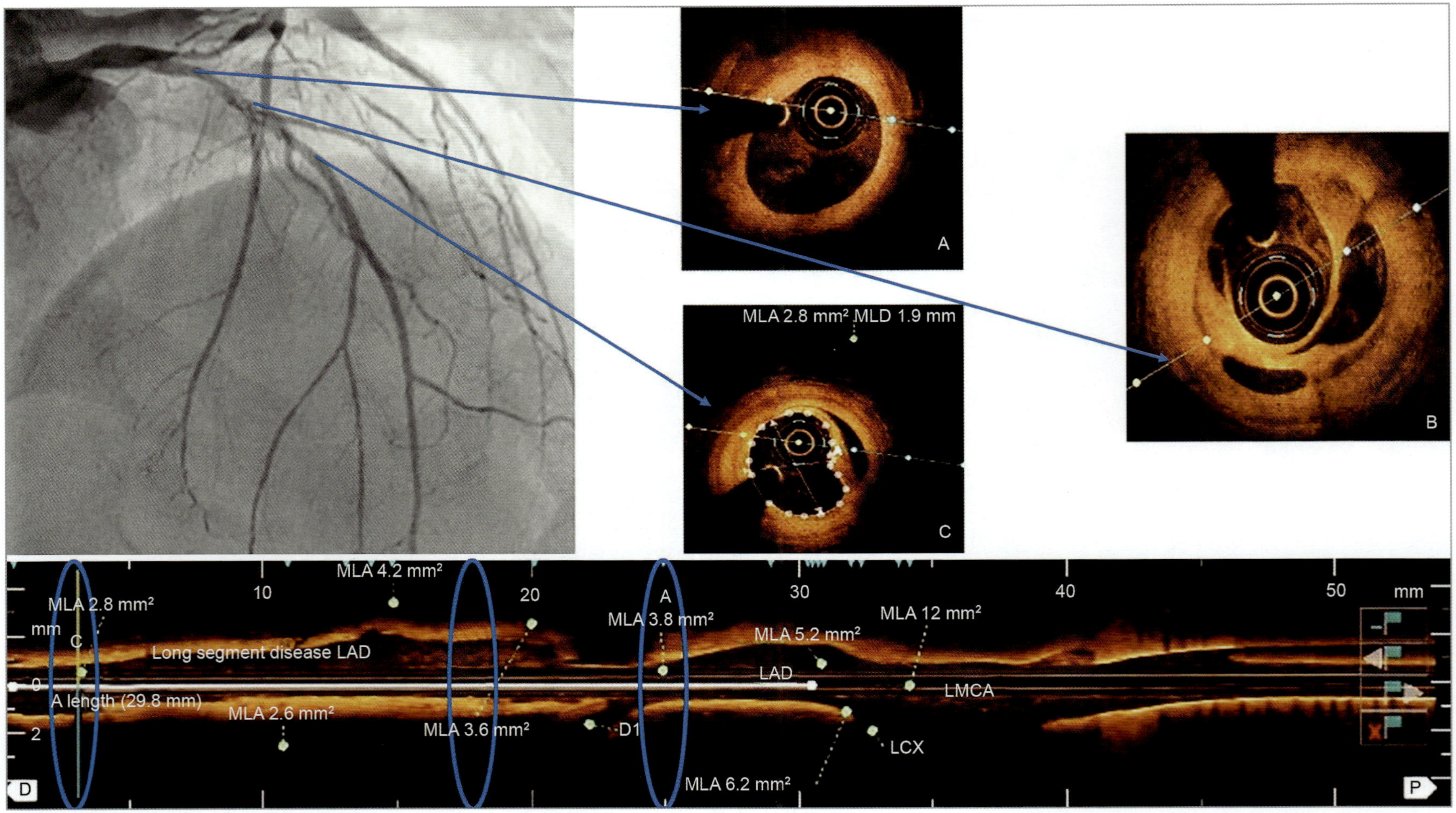

Fig. 3: Prestenting optical coherence tomography (OCT) assessment for device selection. (LAD: left anterior descending; LMCA: left main coronary artery; LCX: left circumflex; MLA: minimum lumen area; MLD: minimum lumen diameter)

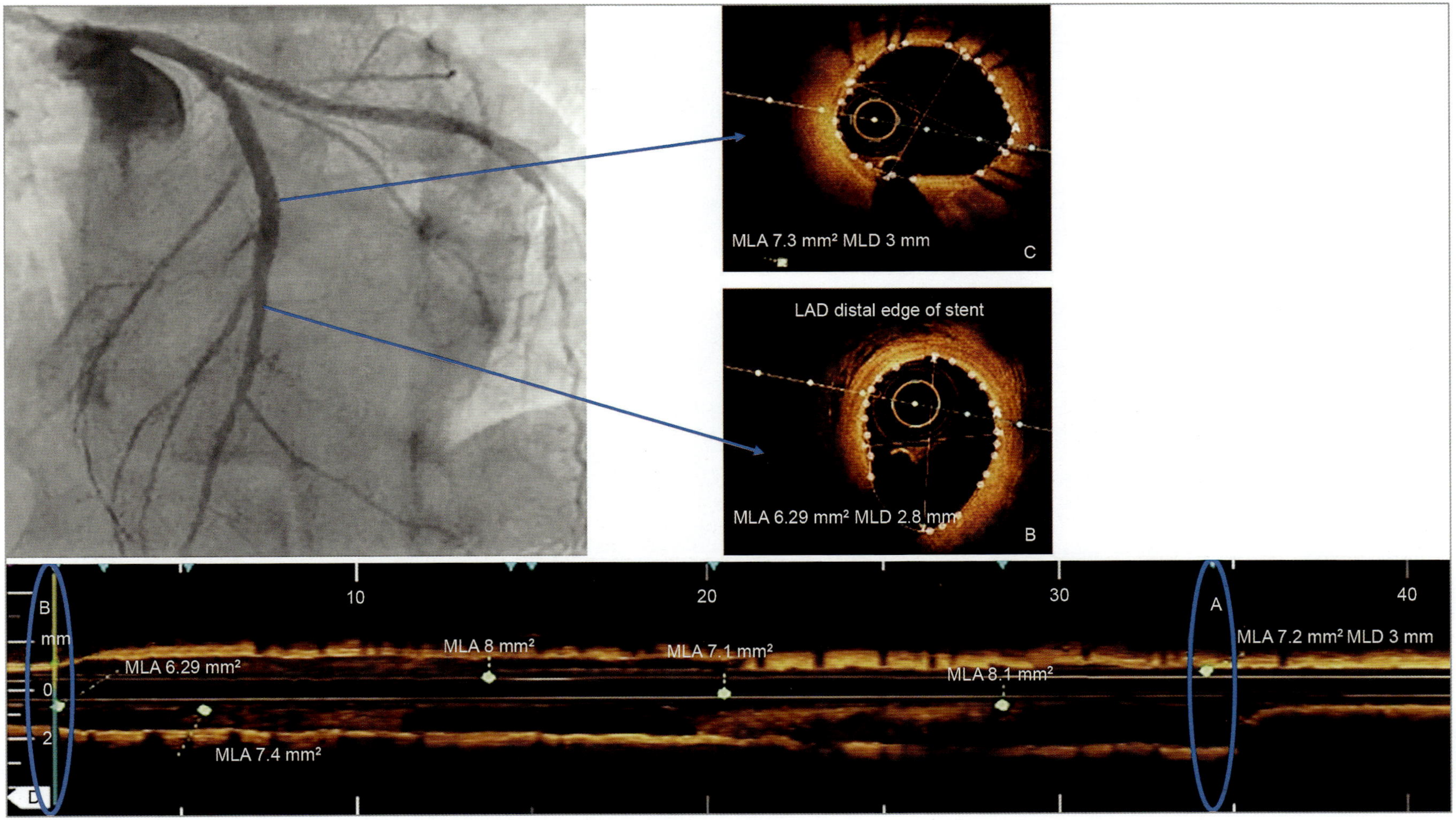

Fig. 4: Poststenting optical coherence tomography (OCT) assessment showed well-apposed and expanded stent struts at distal half with no medial edge dissection. (LAD: left anterior descending; LCX: left circumflex; MLA: minimum lumen area; MLD: minimum lumen diameter)

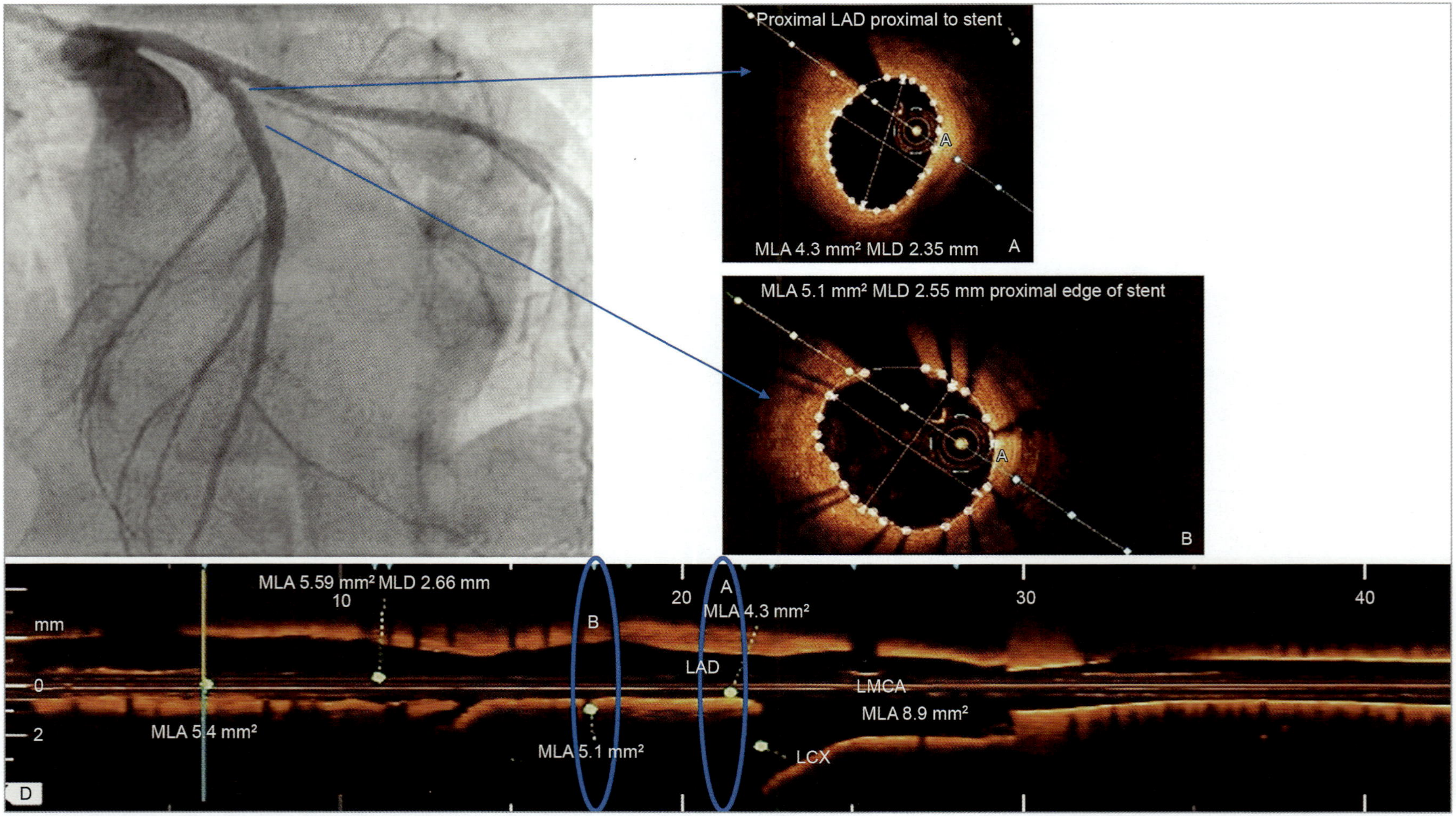

Fig. 5: Poststenting optical coherence tomography (OCT) assessment showed well-apposed and expanded stent struts at proximal half with no medial edge dissection. (LAD: left anterior descending; LCX: left circumflex; MLA: minimum lumen area; MLD: minimum lumen diameter)

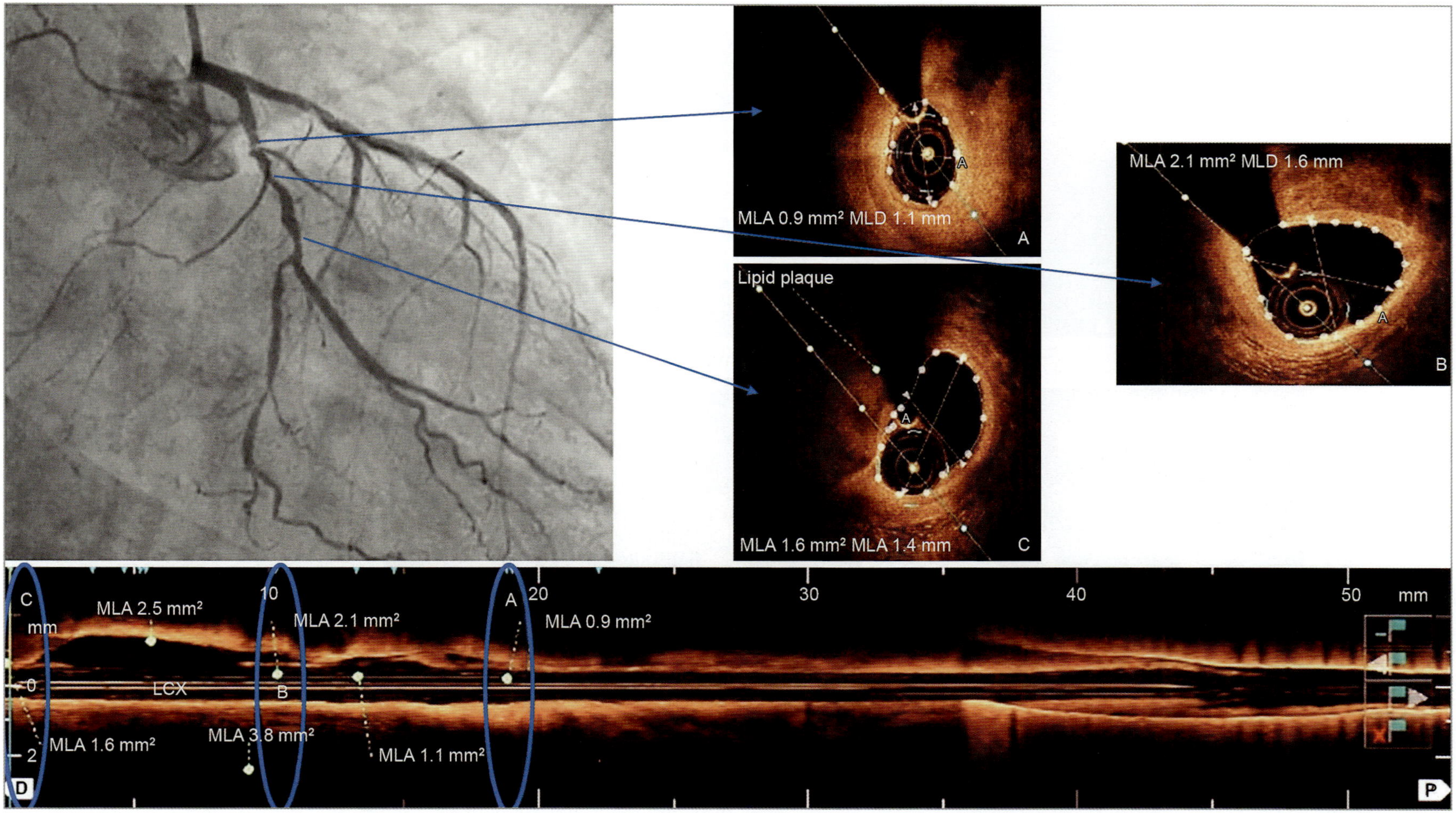

Fig. 6: Pre-OCT (optical coherence tomography) analysis: Thick narrowing fibrotic plaque. (LCX: left circumflex; MLA: minimum lumen area; MLD: minimum lumen diameter)

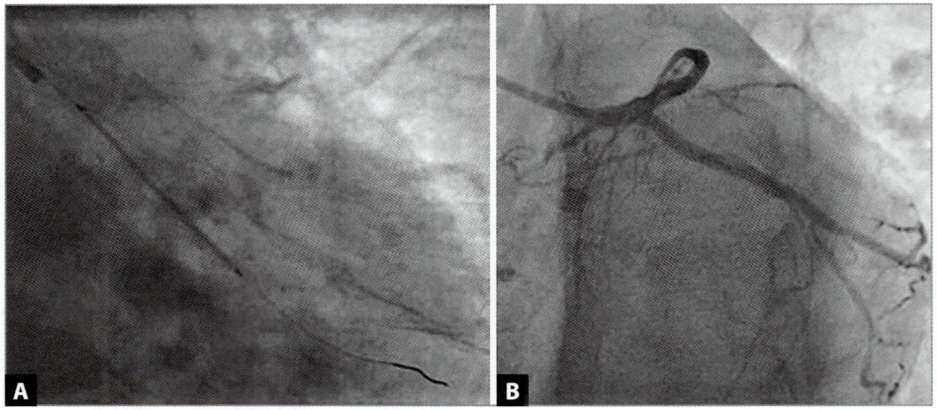

Figs. 7A and B: Stenting and final result.

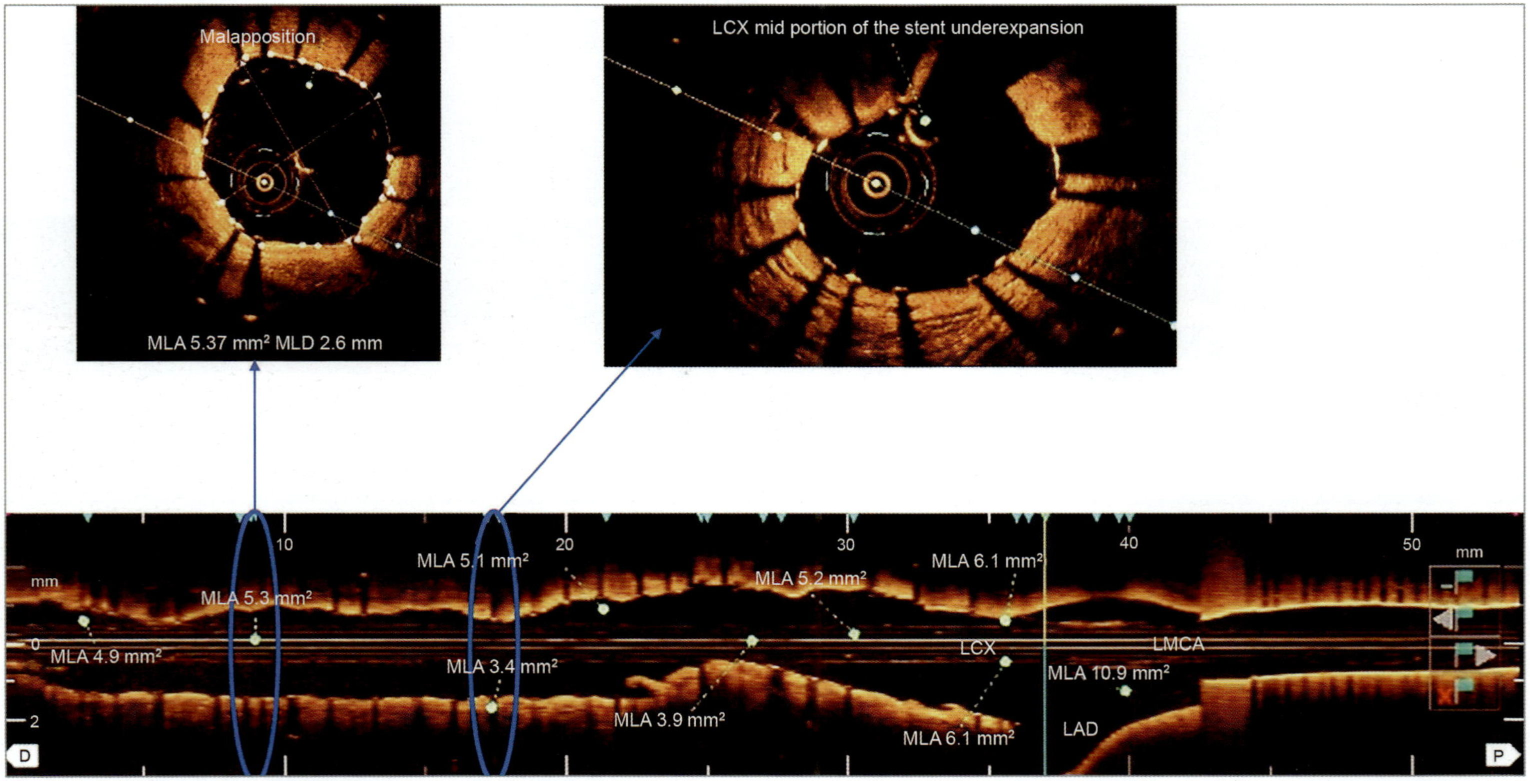

Fig. 8: Poststenting OCT (optical coherence tomography) showed well-apposed and well-expanded stent struts with no edge dissections. (LAD: left anterior descending; LCX: left circumflex; LMCA: left main coronary artery; MLA: minimum lumen area)

CASE 2

OCT assessment of ambiguous lesion of LAD with anterior-NSTEMI (non-ST segment elevation myocardial infarction).

CLINICAL HISTORY

A 36-year-old male presented with anterior-NSTEMI, and chest pain associated with breathlessness. ECG-T-inversions in anterior leads. 2D Echo-RWMA in LAD territory, moderate LV dysfunction, EF—38%; CAG—right radial approach LMCA—normal, ambiguous lesion of proximal LAD lesion suggestive of dissection/recanalized thrombus/calcific lesion; diagonal—normal, LCX—normal, RCA—normal **(Figs. 9A and B)**.

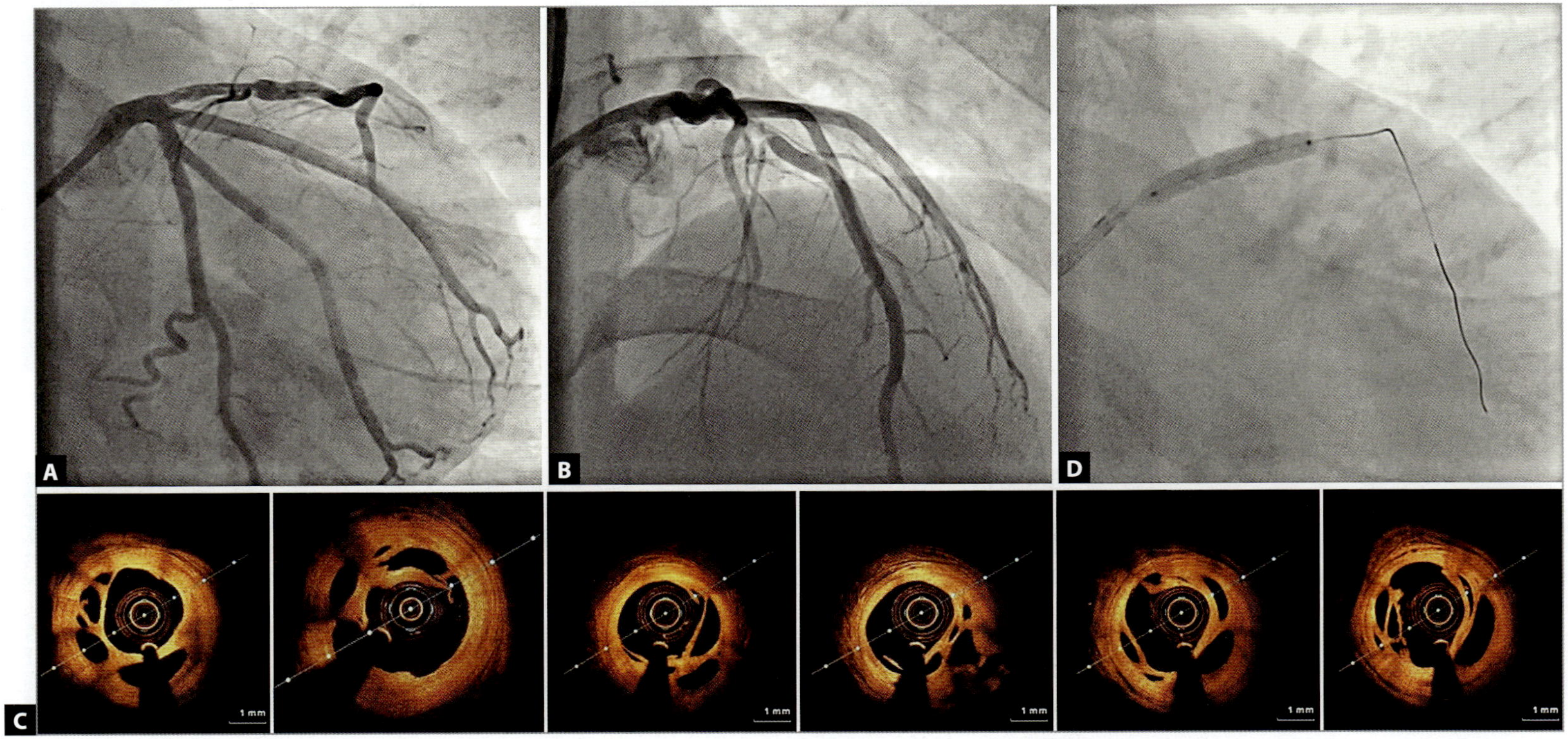

Figs. 9A to D: (A and B) Coronary angiogram; (C) a honeycomb-like structure with multiple channels of various sizes, separated by highly backscattering septa; (D) angioplasty.

PROCEDURE

Right radial route, 6 Fr EBU 3.5 guiding catheter; LAD lesion was crossed with 0.014" Sion blue wire, predilated with 2.0 × 10 mm Tazuna balloon. Pre-OCT study showed recanalized thrombus-A honeycomb-like structure with multiple channels of various sizes, separated by highly backscattering septa **(Fig. 9C)**; distal landing zone MLA—8.6 mm^2, MLD—3.3 mm, mid portion of the lesion recanalized thrombus, proximal landing zone MLA—5.4 mm^2, MLD—2.6 mm, total length of the lesion 23.1 mm **(Fig. 10)**. LAD lesion was stented with 3.5 × 24 mm Biomime stent **(Fig. 9D)**. Poststenting OCT showed well-apposed and well-expanded stent struts with no edge dissections **(Fig. 11)**. Postprocedure angio view showed well-implanted stents with TIMI-III flow without any dissection. Patient was discharged on third postprocedure in a stable status.

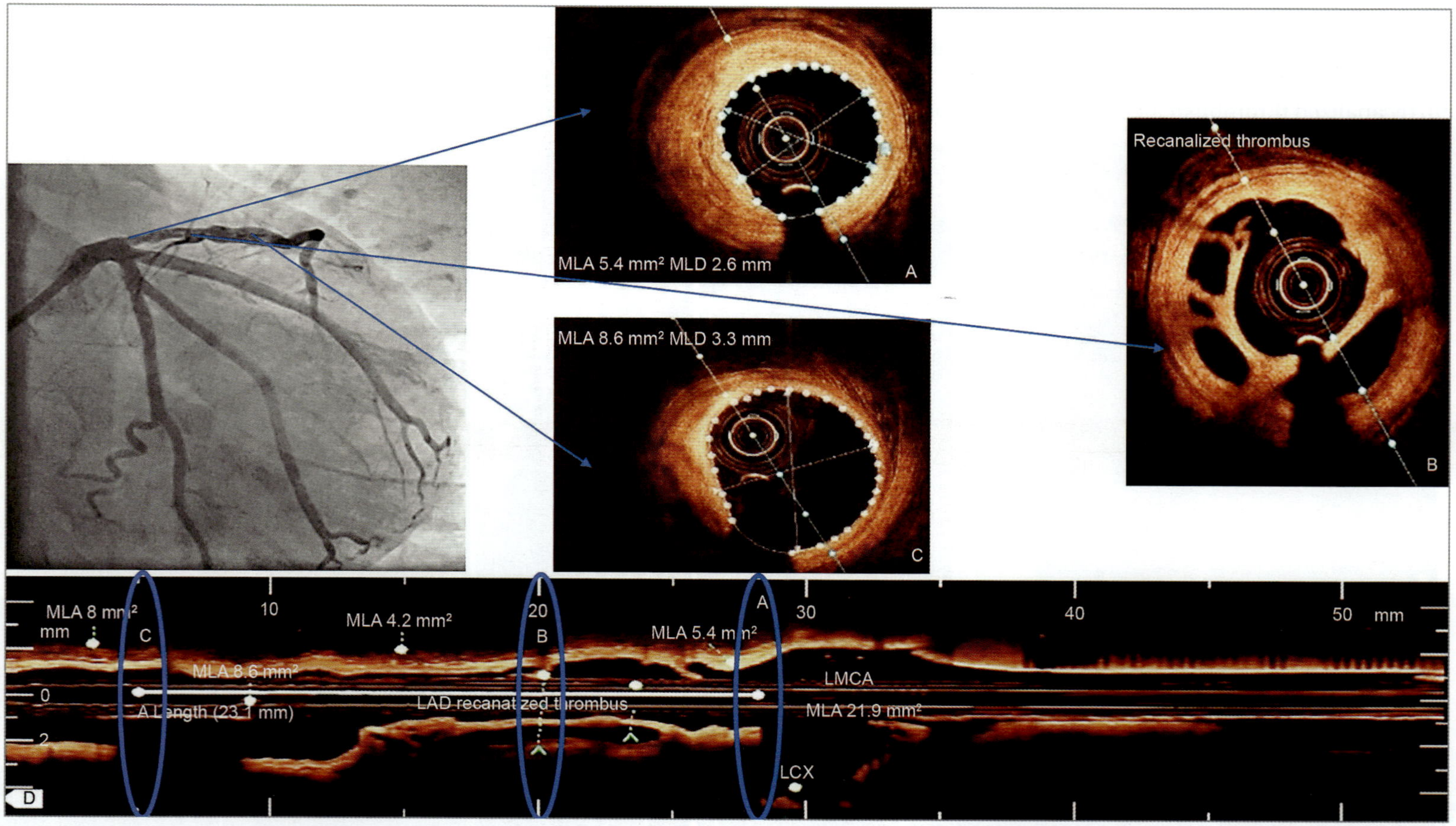

Fig. 10: Prestenting OCT (optical coherence tomography) analysis for device selection and plaque morphology. (LAD: left anterior descending; LCX: left circumflex; LMCA: left main coronary artery; MLA: minimum lumen area)

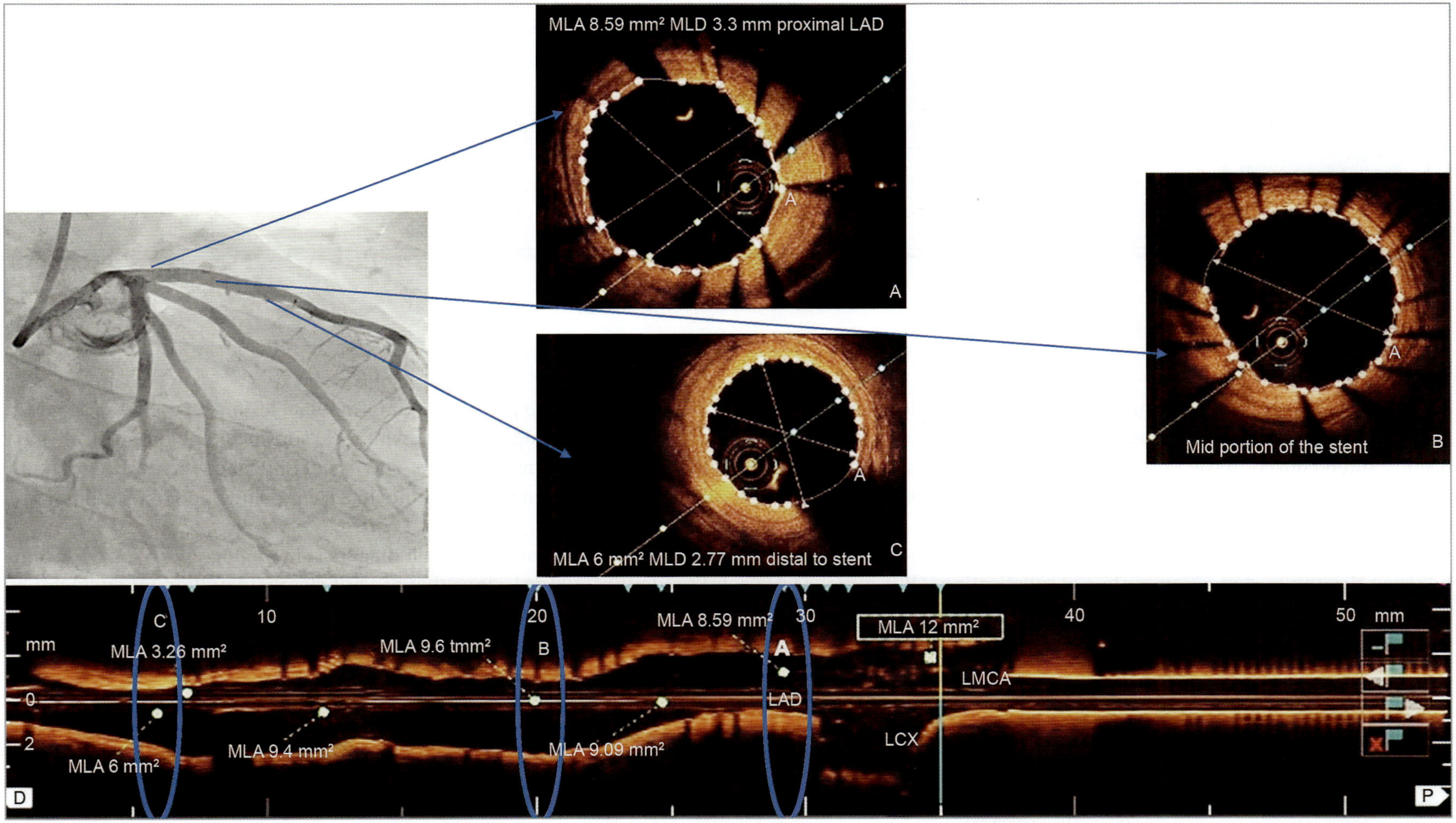

Fig. 11: Poststenting OCT (optical coherence tomography) showed well-apposed and well-expanded stent struts with no edge dissections. (LAD: left anterior descending; LCX: left circumflex; LMCA: left main coronary artery; MLA: minimum lumen area; MLD: minimum lumen diameter)

CHAPTER 14

Ambiguous Lesions

INTRODUCTION

Sometimes it is very difficult to make angiographic diagnosis due to improper visualization in the presence of intermediate lesions of uncertain severity, very short lesions, pre- or postaneurysmal lesions, ostial or left main stenosis, disease at branching sites, sites with focal spasm, or angiographically hazy lesions, often caused in the presence of thrombus or calcifications due to ambiguous nature of angio image. The use of optical coherence tomography (OCT) is very helpful for proper diagnosis due to clear visualization of the luminal structure and dimensions due to a clear delineation of the lumen wall interface.[1]

OCT can identify the presence or absence of plaque (e.g., in coronary spasm) and allows for differential diagnosis in angiographic "hazy" lesions between thrombus, dissection, or heavy calcification. OCT is also very useful to identify culprit lesions that are not clearly identified on angiography [e.g., thrombosed or ruptured lesions in patient with acute coronary syndrome (ACS) and angiographically mild lesions or in the presence of multivessel disease].[2]

Pre-percutaneous coronary intervention (PCI):

- Assessment of culprit lesion in ACS—evaluation for plaque rupture or thrombus in patients without angiographically evident culprit lesion
- Evaluation of lesions with angiographic haziness—differential diagnosis between thrombus, dissection, heavy calcification
- Determination about presence or absence of plaque (coronary spasm)
- Recanalized thrombus
- Spontaneous coronary artery dissection (SCAD)

Post-PCI:

- Tissue prolapse
- Edge dissections
- Thrombus
- Intramural/extramural hematomas
- Coronary spasm
- Myocardial bridging.

REFERENCES

1. Prati F, Regar E, Mintz GS, Arbustini E, Di Mario C, Jang IK, et al. Expert review document on methodology, terminology, and clinical applications of optical coherence tomography: physical principles, methodology of image acquisition, and clinical application for assessment of coronary arteries and atherosclerosis. Eur Heart J. 2010;31(4):401-15.
2. Regar E, van Ditzhuijzen N, van der Sijde J, Ligthart J, Witberg K, van Soest G, et al. Identifying stable coronary plaques with OCT technology. Contin Cardiol Educ. 2016;2(2):77-88.

CASE 1

Ambiguous lesion (thrombus)—assessment of haziness at the proximal edge of the stent during PCI of LAD (left anterior descending).

CLINICAL HISTORY

A 44-year-old male presented with acute STEMI (ST segment elevation myocardial infarction) of anterior wall with Window period (WP)—48 hours); is known diabetic with history of chest pain associated with profuse sweating of 48 hours' duration. Investigations: random blood sugar (RBS)—116 mg/dL, blood urea—40 mg/dL, serum creatinine—0.95 mg/dL, estimated glomerular filtration rate (eGFR)—97. Electrocardiogram (ECG)-ST elevation in anterior leads, 2D Echo-RWMA+ (regional wall motion abnormality) LAD territory, moderate left ventricular (LV) dysfunction, ejection fraction (EF)—40%. Coronary angiography (CAG)-left main coronary artery (LMCA)—normal, LAD—proximal total occlusion, left circumflex (LCX) and right coronary artery (RCA)—normal **(Figs. 1A and B)**.

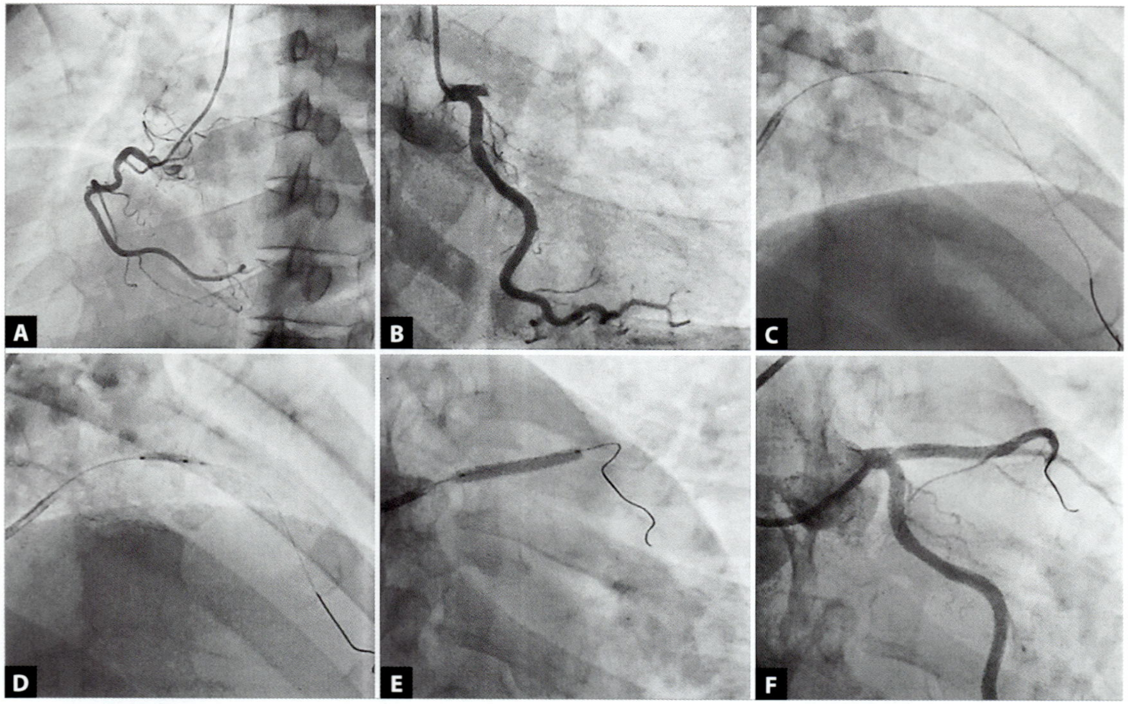

Figs. 1A to F: Coronary angiogram (A and B), predilatation (C and D), and stenting (E and F).

PROCEDURE

Right radial approach (RRA)—route, 6 Fr EBU 3.5 guiding catheter, totally occluded LAD lesion was crossed with 0.014″ Sion blue wire. Predilatation with 1.5 × 10 mm, 2.25 × 10 mm Tazuna balloon; proximal LAD stenting with 3.0 × 24 mm Ultimaster stent. Poststenting angio showed radiolucent ambiguous lesion proximal to the stent with possible thrombus/dissection/tissue prolapse **(Figs. 1C to F)**. OCT was used to assess ambiguous lesion to guide further intervention which revealed large thrombus in ostial LAD proximal to stent **(Fig. 2)**.

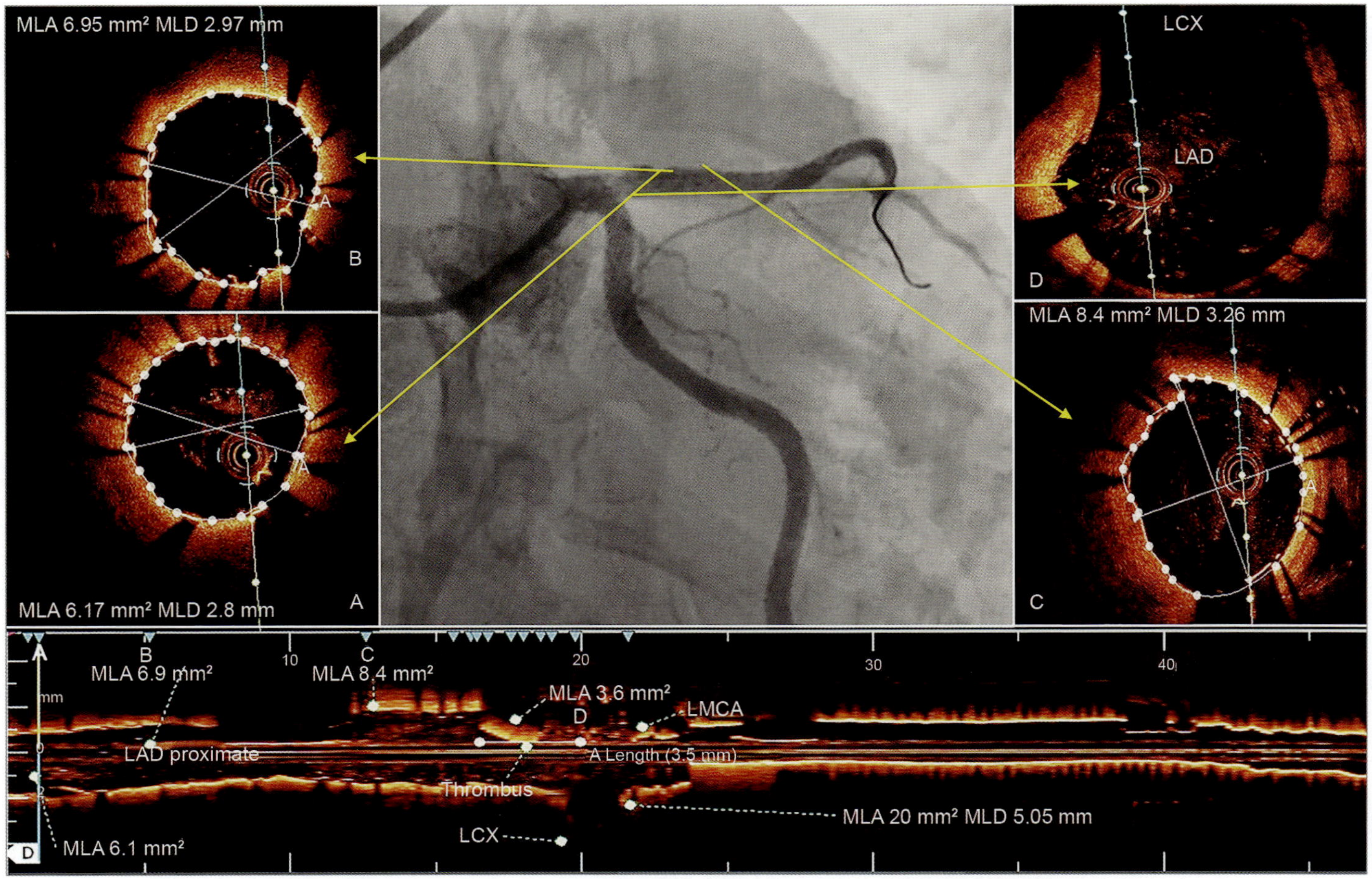

Fig. 2: Poststenting optical coherence tomography (OCT) assessment. (LAD: left anterior descending; LCX: left circumflex; LMCA: left main coronary artery; MLA: minimal lumen area; MLD: minimum lumen diameter)

Uncovered portion of proximal LAD 2.5 mm, malapposition with thrombus proximal edge of stent 3.0 × 24 mm, minimum lumen area (MLA)—9.79 mm^2, minimum lumen diameter (MLD)—3.52 mm, minimal stent area (MSA)—7.25 mm^2, minimal stent diameter (MSD)—3 mm, stent under expansion—25% **(Fig. 3)**.

Percentage of thrombus to MLA—60%, MLA—11 mm^2, red thrombus area—4.4 mm^2.

Length of the uncovered portion of LAD-LM (left main) bifurcation to proximal edge of LAD stent—3.5 mm **(Fig. 4)**.

Ostial LAD stenting done with 3.5 × 09 mm Orsiro stent. Postprocedure angio showed well-deployed stents with good TIMI-III (thrombolysis in myocardial infarction III) flow without any dissection **(Figs. 5A to D)**. Patient was discharged on third postprocedure in a stable status.

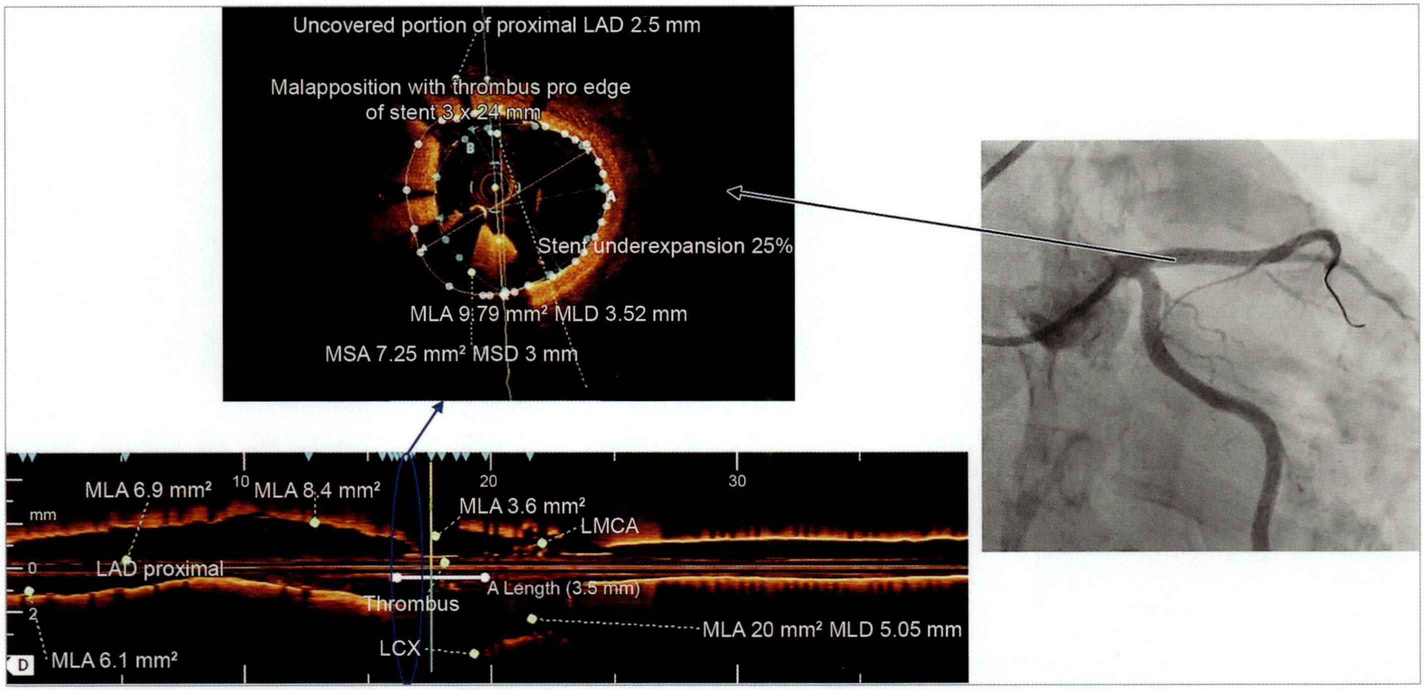

Fig. 3: Identifying under-expansion, malapposition and uncovered portion of proximal LAD. (LCX: left circumflex; LMCA: left main coronary artery; MLA: minimal lumen area; MSA: minimal stent area; MSD: minimal stent diameter)

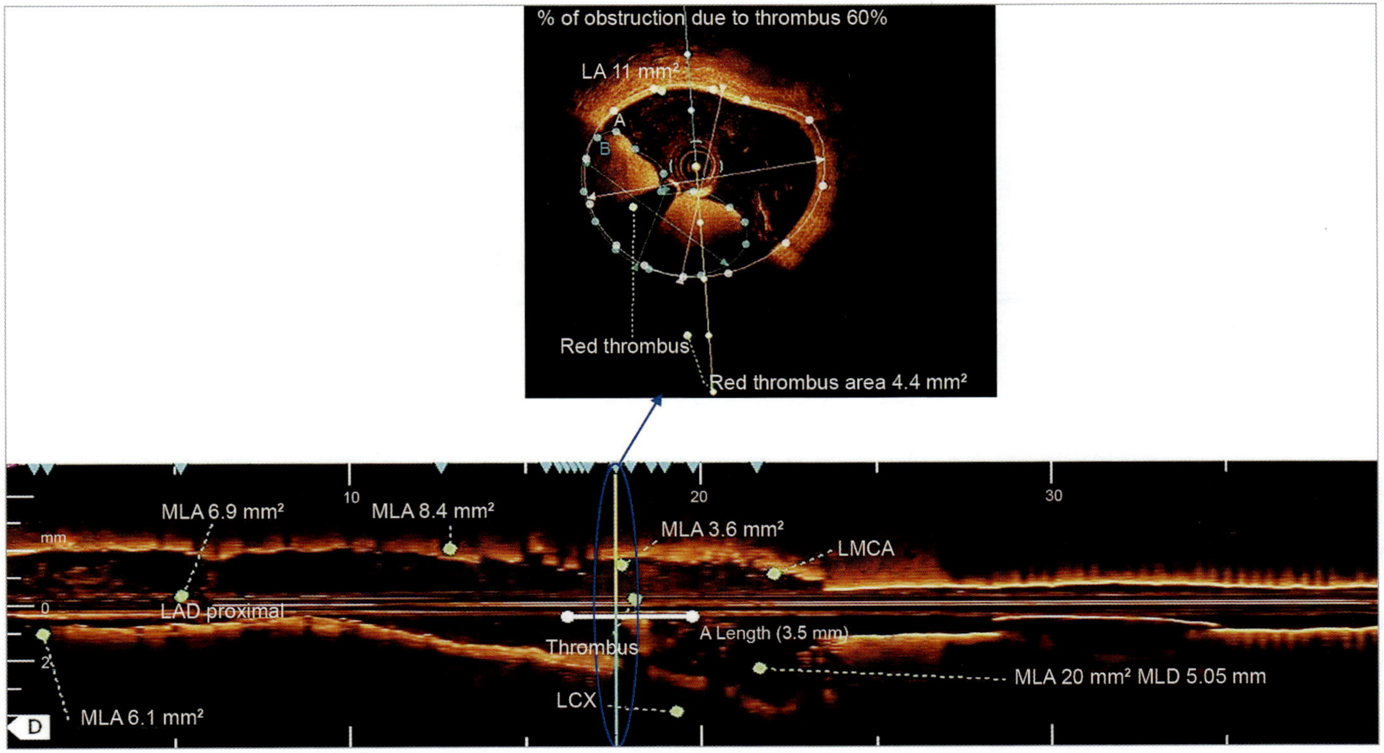

Fig. 4: Identifying thrombus burden by optical coherence tomography (OCT).
(LA: lumen area; LAD: left anterior descending; LCX: left circumflex; LMCA: left main coronary artery; MLA: minimal lumen area)

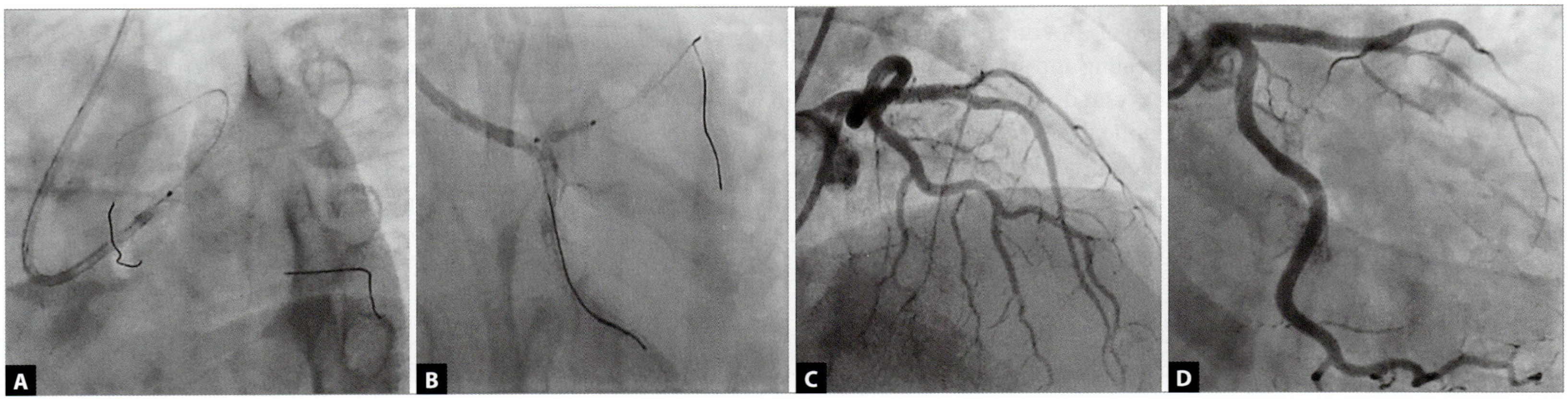

Figs. 5A to D: Postdilatation and final result.

CHAPTER 15

Evaluation of Coronary Artery Aneurysm

DEFINITION

Coronary artery aneurysms (CAA) are described as aberrant dilatations of a coronary artery segment >1.5 times or 50% greater than that of the adjacent normal vessel.[1]

The incidence ranges from 0.3% to 5.3%.

ETIOLOGY AND INTRODUCTION

- Atherosclerosis
- Vasculitis
- Congenital aneurysms
- Tissue disorders
- Inflammatory disorders
- Post-drug-eluting stent (DES) implantation.

The exact pathogenesis and development of CAA due to DES is not known but may be due to: (1) in some patients, the antiproliferative effect of the DES may lead to CAA by inhibiting neointimal healing and endothelialization; (2) a hypersensitivity inflammatory reaction to DES metal/polymer/drug leading to aneurysmal formation;[2] (3) mycotic aneurysm due to infection at the site of DES implantation.

Intravascular ultrasound (IVUS) and optical coherence tomography (OCT) are more useful compared to angiography in assessing dimensions of aneurysm and its neck, and in making differential diagnosis of aneurysm, assessing the exact location and origin of aneurysm in relation to DES and coronary artery. OCT is useful for selecting proper stent size to cover entire aneurysmal sac with good landing zones. Post-PCI (percutaneous coronary intervention), OCT is helpful in assessing proper expansion, edge dissection, and any malapposition at the edges which are useful in predicting acute and long-term outcomes.

MANAGEMENT OF CORONARY ANEURYSM

- PCI with covered stent to exclude aneurysmal sac from main lumen which is an alternative mode of treatment to surgical approach.[3]
- Surgical treatment indicated in patients with multiple coronary aneurysms/coronary aneurysm involving major vessels proximally particularly aneurysms of mycotic nature and post-PCI recurrent aneurysms.

Examples of CAA are shown in **Figures 1 and 2**.

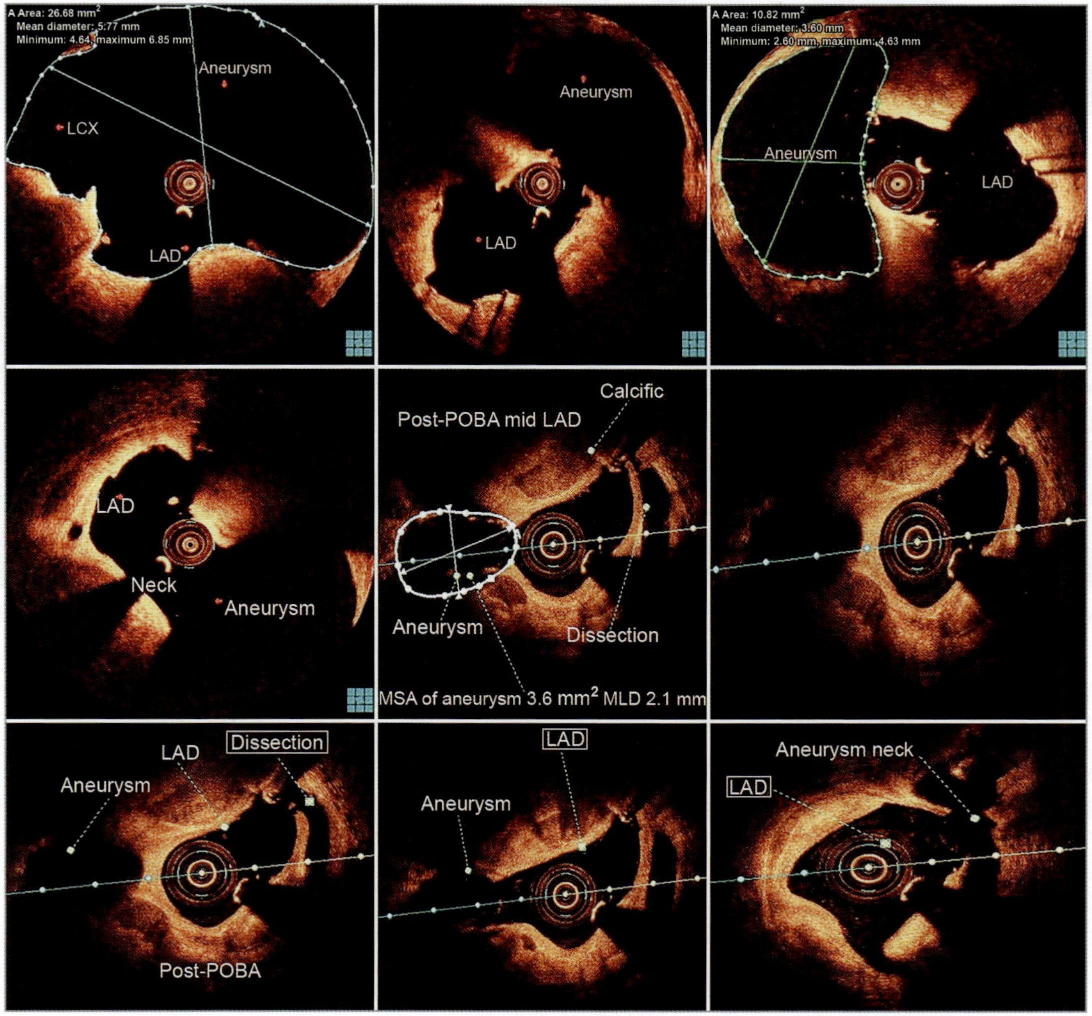

Fig. 1: Coronary artery aneurysms—Case 1. (LAD: left anterior descending; LCX: left circumflex; MLD: minimal lumen diameter; MSA: mean stent area; POBA: plain old balloon angioplasty)

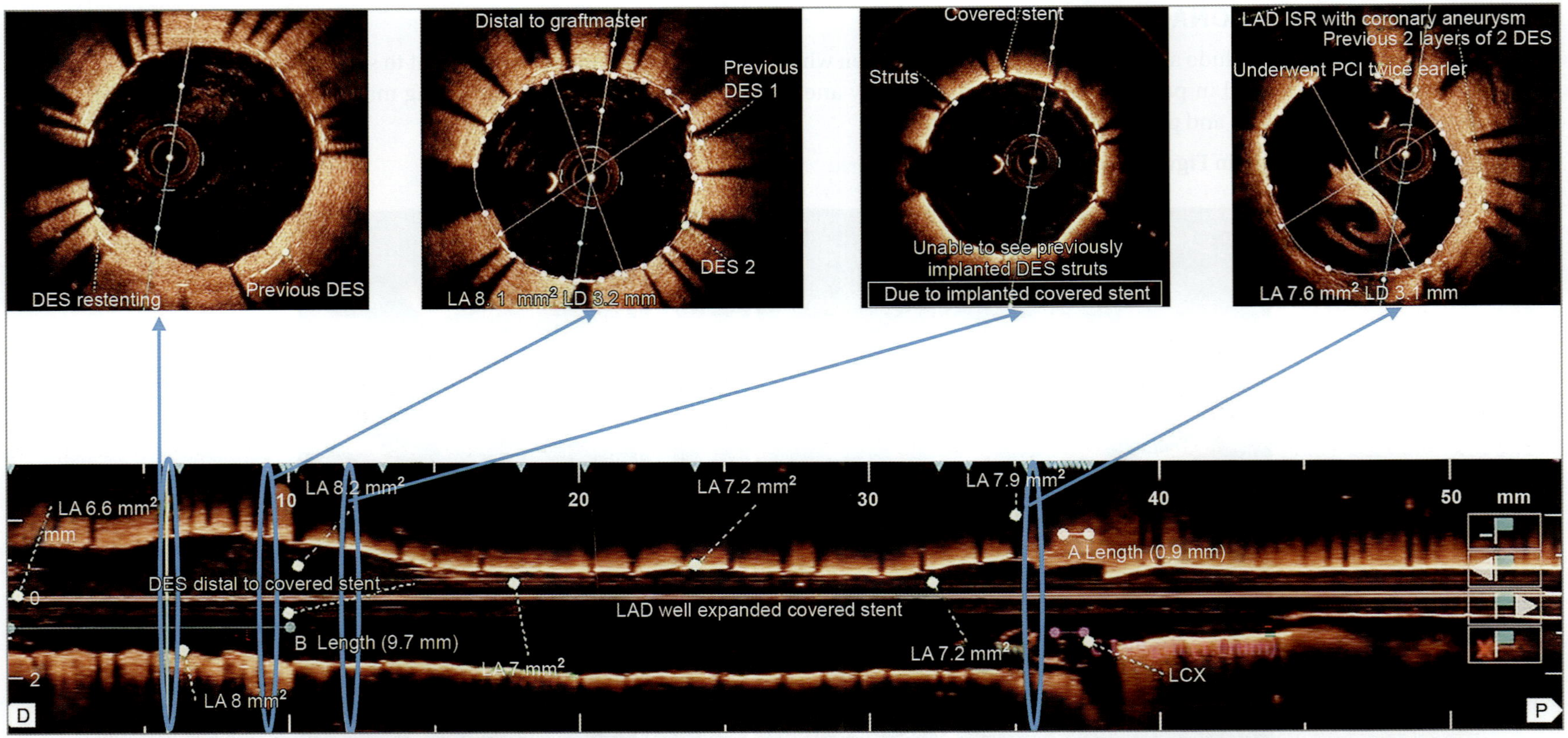

Fig. 2: Coronary artery aneurysms—Case 2. (DES: drug-eluting stent; ISR: in-stent restenosis; LA: lumen area; LAD: left anterior descending; LCX: left circumflex)

REFERENCES

1. Dionne A, Ibrahim R, Gebhard C, Bakloul M, Selly JB, Leye M, et al. Coronary wall structural changes in patients with Kawasaki disease: new insights from optical coherence tomography (OCT). J Am Heart Assoc. 2015;4(5):e001939.
2. Mukku VK, Cai Q, Barbagelata A, Conti VR, Fujise K. Very late development of coronary artery aneurysm with total occlusion following sirolimus-eluting stent implantation. Int J Angiol. 2012;21(04):229-32.
3. Bajaj S, Parikh R, Hamdan A, Bikkina M. Covered-stent treatment of coronary aneurysm after drug-eluting stent placement: case report and literature review. Tex Heart Inst J. 2010;37(4):449-54.

CASE 1

PCI of calcified left anterior descending (LAD) with coronary aneurysm.

CLINICAL HISTORY

A 55-year-old male known hypertensive, diabetic, and ex-smoker presented with unstable angina (USA), recent onset of angina of 2 months' duration. ECG–LVH (electrocardiogram–left ventricular hypertrophy) with anterior lateral ST depression and T-inversions. 2D Echo-No RWMA (regional wall motion abnormality), normal left ventricular (LV)/right ventricular (RV) function, ejection fraction (EF)—76%. Coronary angiography (CAG)-left main coronary artery (LMCA)—borderline lesion, mid LAD 90% calcific bifurcation lesion at origin of D1, right coronary artery (RCA)—mild disease **(Figs. 3A to C)**.

Pre-PCI angio showed LMCA spasm which was treated with intracoronary injection nitroglycerin (NTG) and nikoran. Post-NTG angio showed borderline lesion of LMCA. Pre-PCI OCT was done to assess plaque morphology, severity of lesion, selection landing zones, and device diameter and length assessment of LMCA disease whether stenting of left main is required or not.

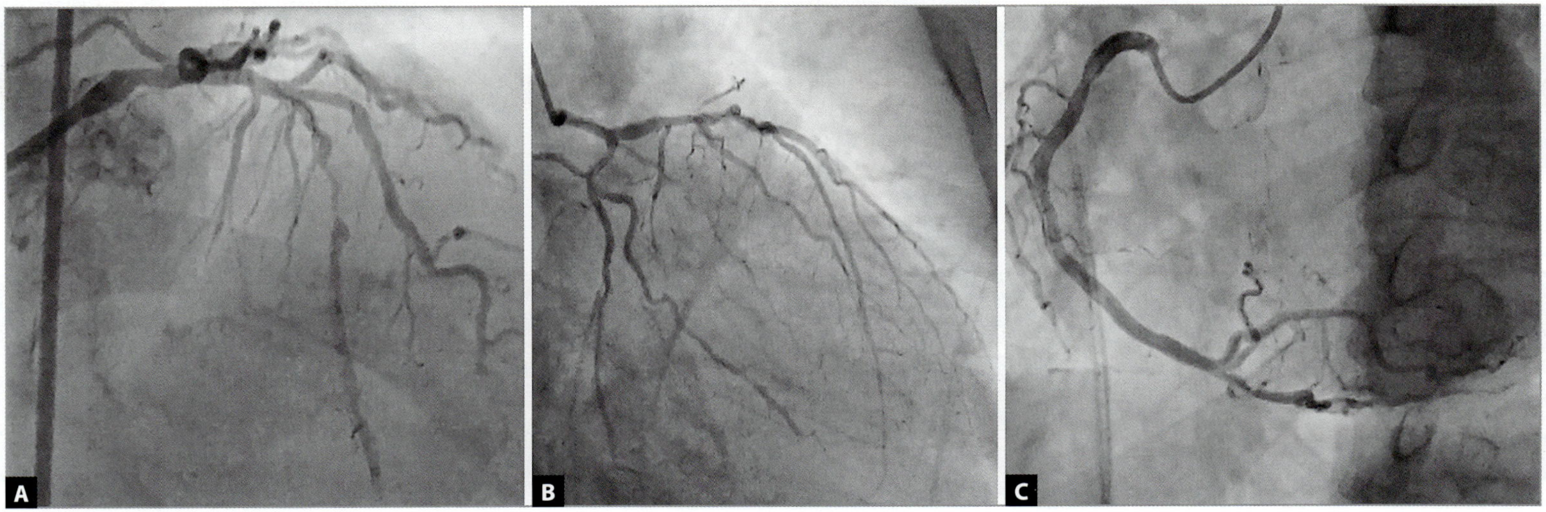

Figs. 3A to C: Coronary angiogram.

PROCEDURE

Right femoral artery (RFA) route, 7 Fr EBU 3.5 guiding catheter, LAD wired with 0.014″ Sion blue wire and D1 wired with 0.014″ Rinato wire.

Pre-OCT analysis: Distal LAD fibrolipid plaque with minimal lumen area (MLA)—5.4 mm^2, minimal lumen diameter (MLD)—2.6 mm, post-POBA (plain old balloon angioplasty) dissection of tight mid LAD lesion with calcified nodule (CN) with fibrocalcific plaque, aneurysm, proximal LAD MLA—8.7 mm^2, MLD—3.3 mm **(Figs. 4 to 6)**, LMCA MLA >9 mm^2 hence PCI of LMCA differed **(Fig. 7)**.

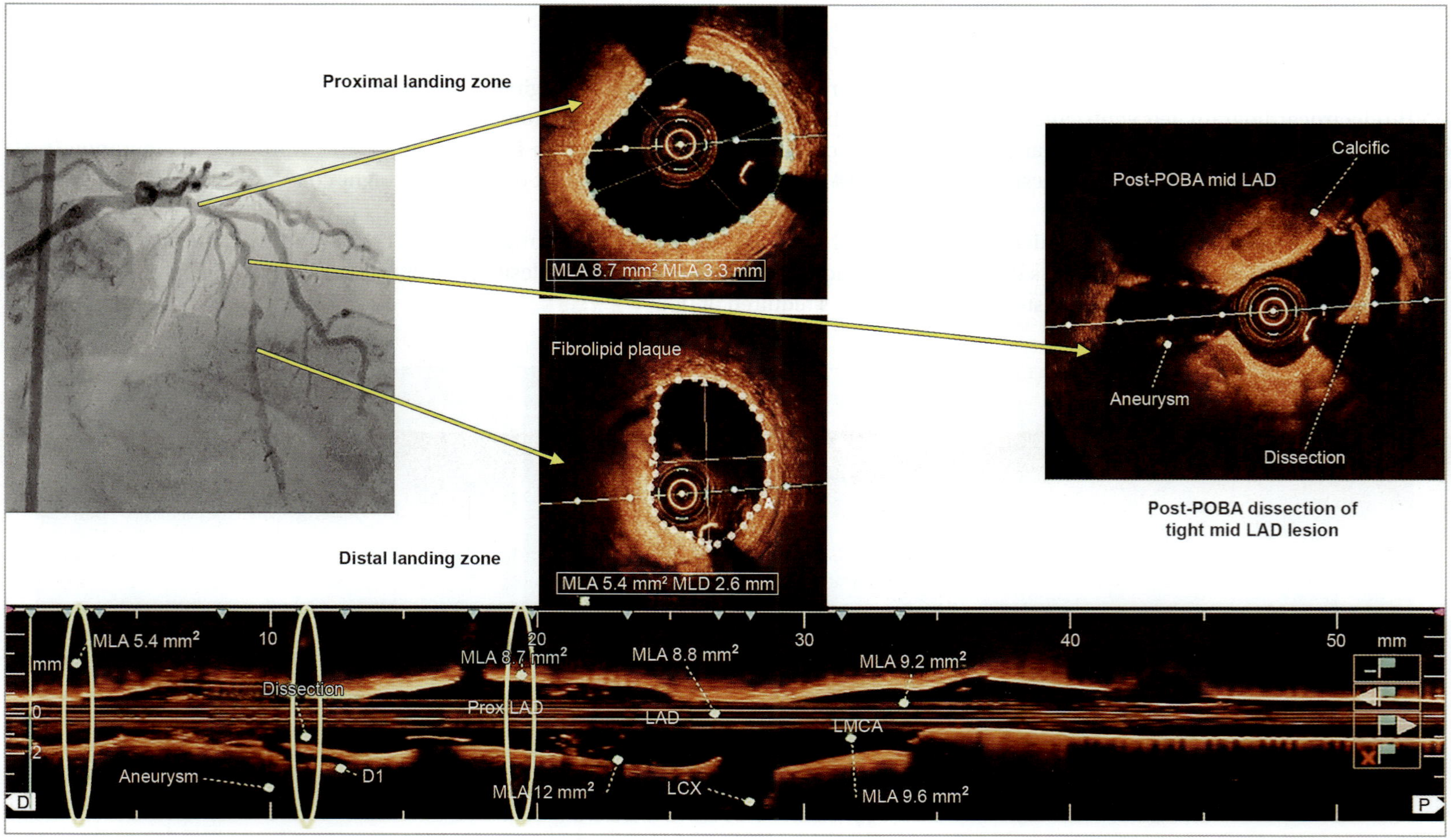

Fig. 4: Pre-stenting optical coherence tomography (OCT) assessment for device selection. (DES: drug-eluting stent; LAD: left anterior descending; LCX: left circumflex; LMCA: left main coronary artery; MLA: minimal lumen area; MLD: minimal lumen diameter)

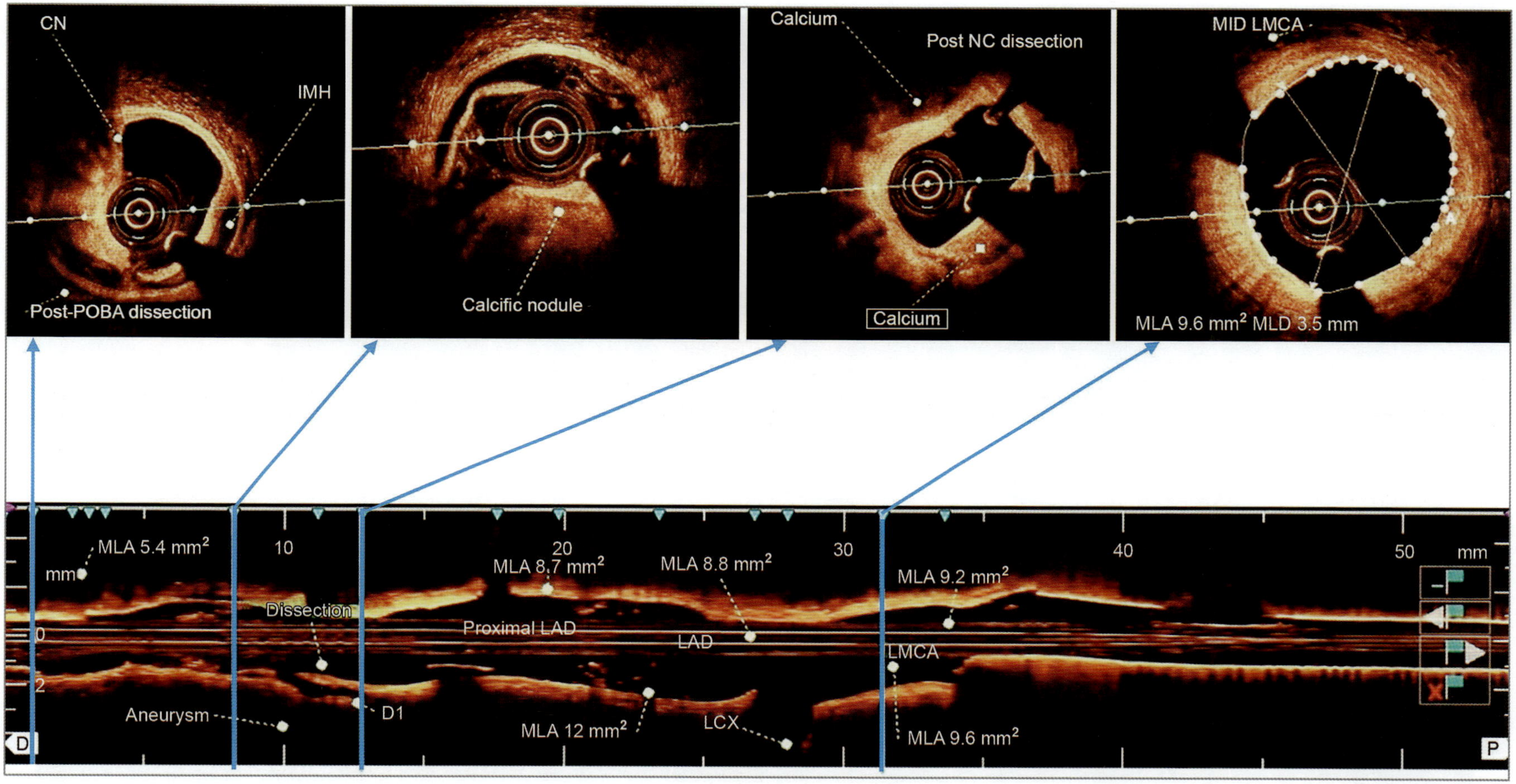

Fig. 5: Pre-stenting optical coherence tomography (OCT) assessment of plaque morphology. (CN: calcified nodule; IMH: intramural hematoma; LAD: left anterior descending; LCX: left circumflex; LMCA: left main coronary artery; MLA: minimal lumen area; MLD: minimal lumen diameter; POBA: plain old balloon angioplasty; NC: noncompliant)

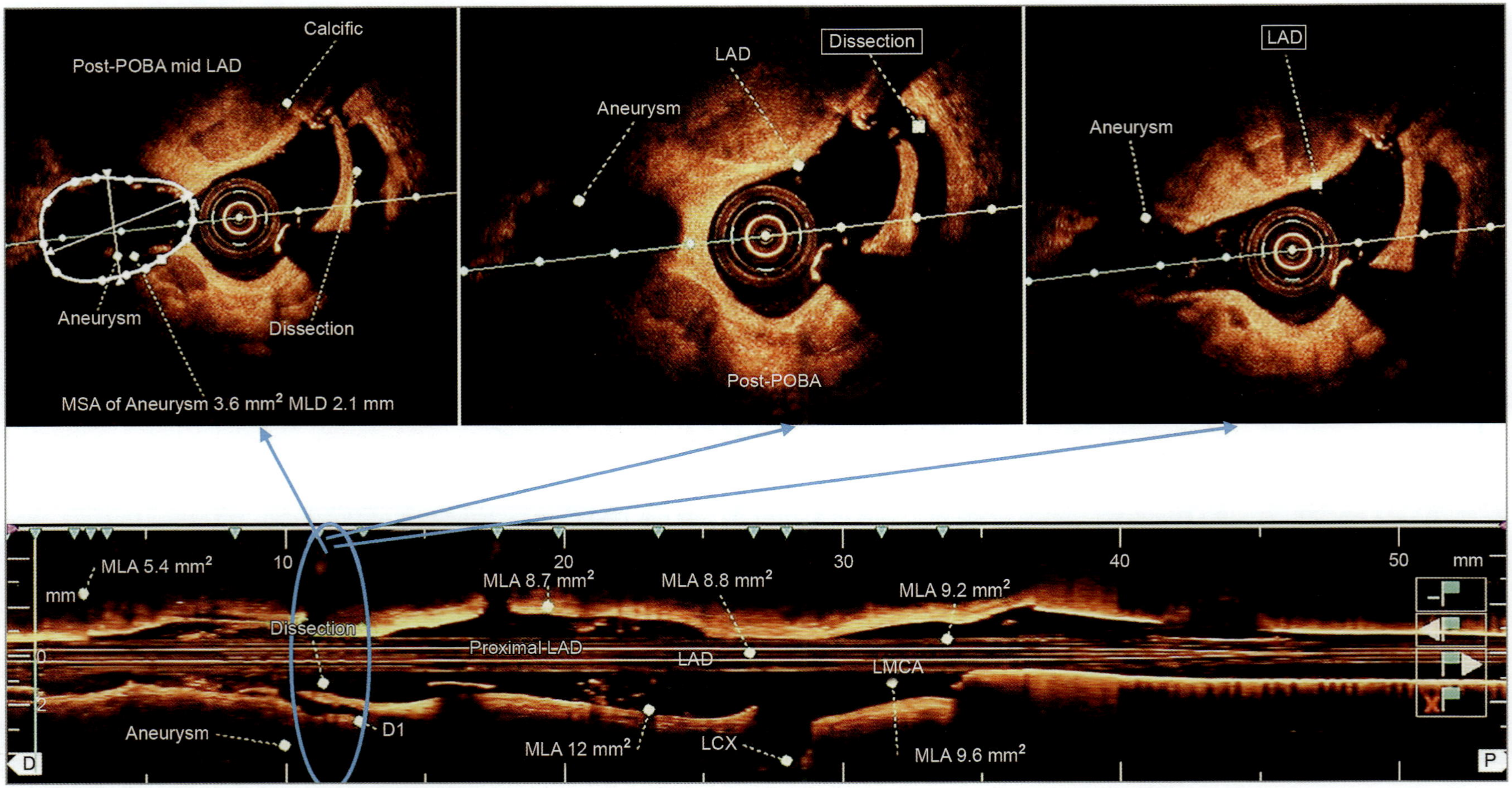

Fig. 6: Coronary aneurysms by optical coherence tomography (OCT). (LAD: left anterior descending; LCX: left circumflex; LMCA: left main coronary artery; MLA: minimal lumen area; POBA: plain old balloon angioplasty)

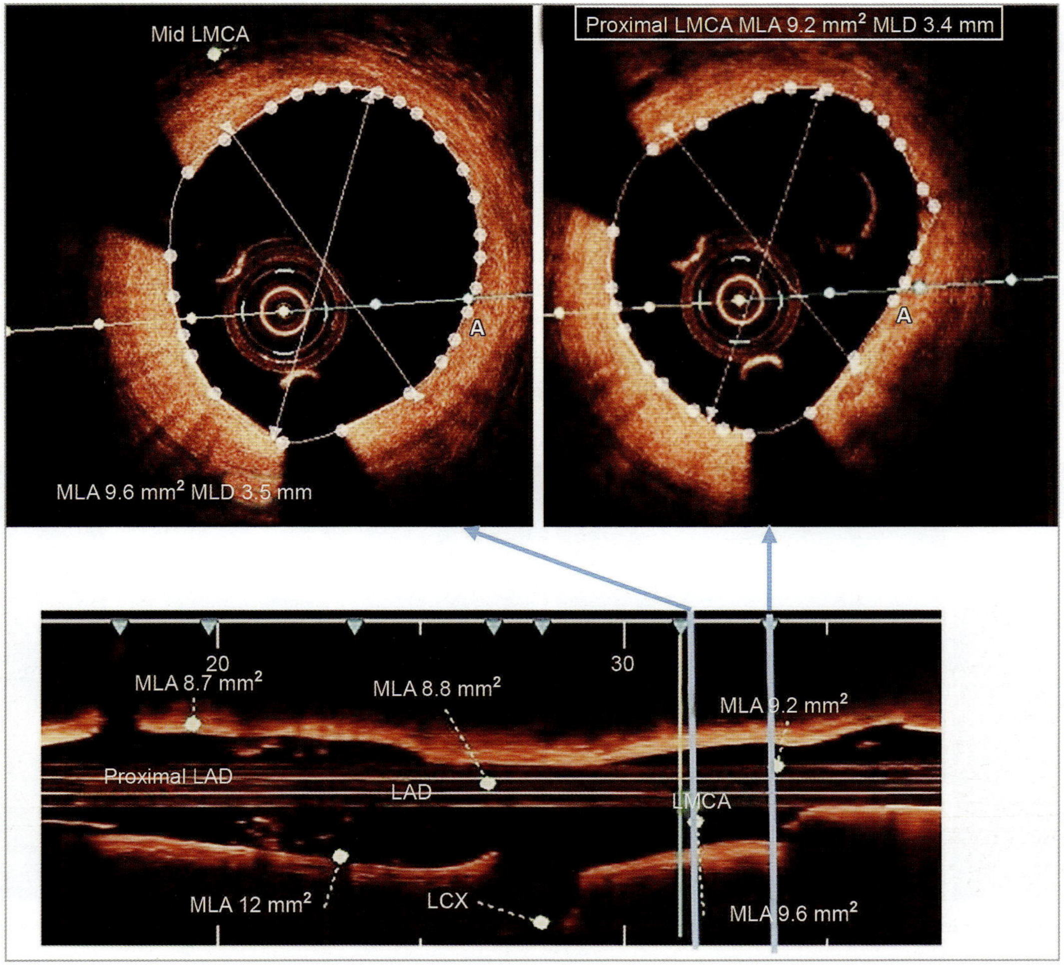

Fig. 7: Left main coronary artery (LMCA) assessment by optical coherence tomography (OCT). (LAD: left anterior descending; LCX: left circumflex; LMCA: left main coronary artery; MLA: minimal lumen area; MLD: minimal lumen diameter)

Left anterior descending predilated with 1.0 × 10 mm Sapphire, 1.5 × 10 mm Tazuna, 2.0 × 12 mm Trek, and 2.5 × 15 mm NC Trek Balloons, subsequently tried to place 3.0 × 33 mm Xience Xpedition stent (DES) but could not cross the lesion. Hence, mid LAD stenting was done with 3.0 × 33 mm Xience Xpedition stent (DES) with 6 Fr GuideLiner support. Postdilatation done with 3.5 × 15 mm NC Trek balloon. Check angiogram revealed D1 compromised. POBA to D1 done with 2.0 × 08 mm Trek balloon. Postdilatation of LAD with 3.5 × 15 mm NC Trek balloon **(Figs. 8A to D)**. Distal landing zone MLA—6.6 mm^2, MLD—2.9 mm, proximal edge of stent MLA—7.8 mm^2, MLD—3 mm, and LMCA MLA—8.6 mm^2, MLD—3.3 mm. Proximal edge dissection length—3 mm, width—0.4 mm, 60°, nonflow-limiting, hence managed conservatively **(Figs. 9 to 11)**. Postprocedure angio views showed well-implanted stents with TIMI-III flow without any dissection. Patient was discharged on third postprocedure day in a stable status.

Optical coherence tomography showed no significant luminal narrowing of left main (LM) (9.6 mm^2). Hence, LMCA stenting avoided. Thick fibro-calcific lesion required adequate high pressure noncompliant (NC) inflations for adequate expansion and apposition. Significant calcium in the proximal landing zone which resulted in proximal edge dissection, managed conservatively due to nonflow-limiting dissection. GuideLiner was required for the placement of stent due to severely calcified lesion. Despite high pressure inflations, CN is usually associated with irregular expansion. But aim for achieving good luminal area with adequate expansion of the stent for better long-term outcomes.

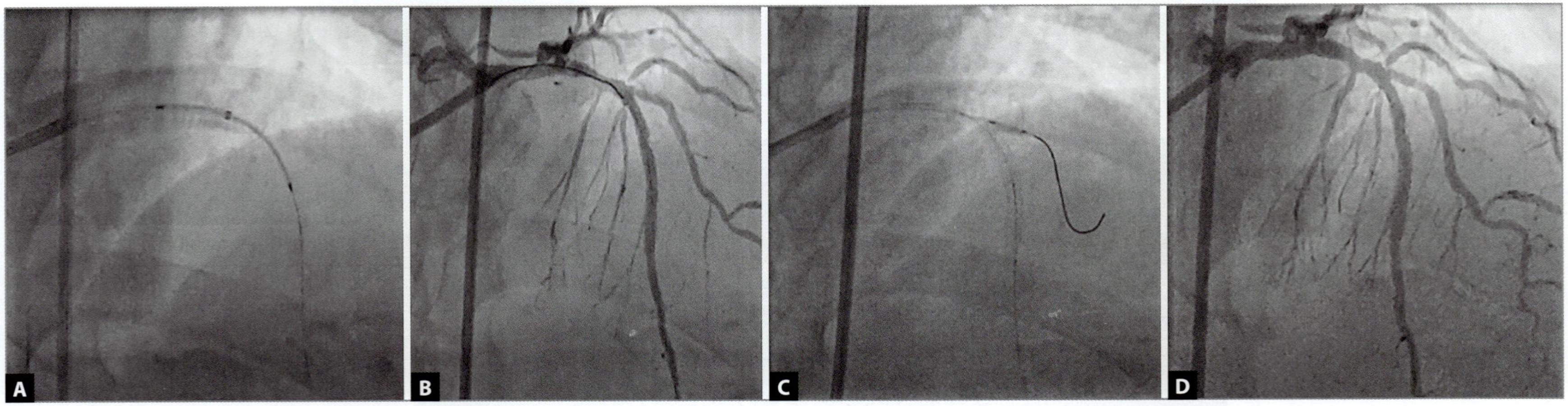

Figs. 8A to D: Left anterior descending (LAD) stenting, check angio POBA (plain old balloon angioplasty) to D1 and final result.

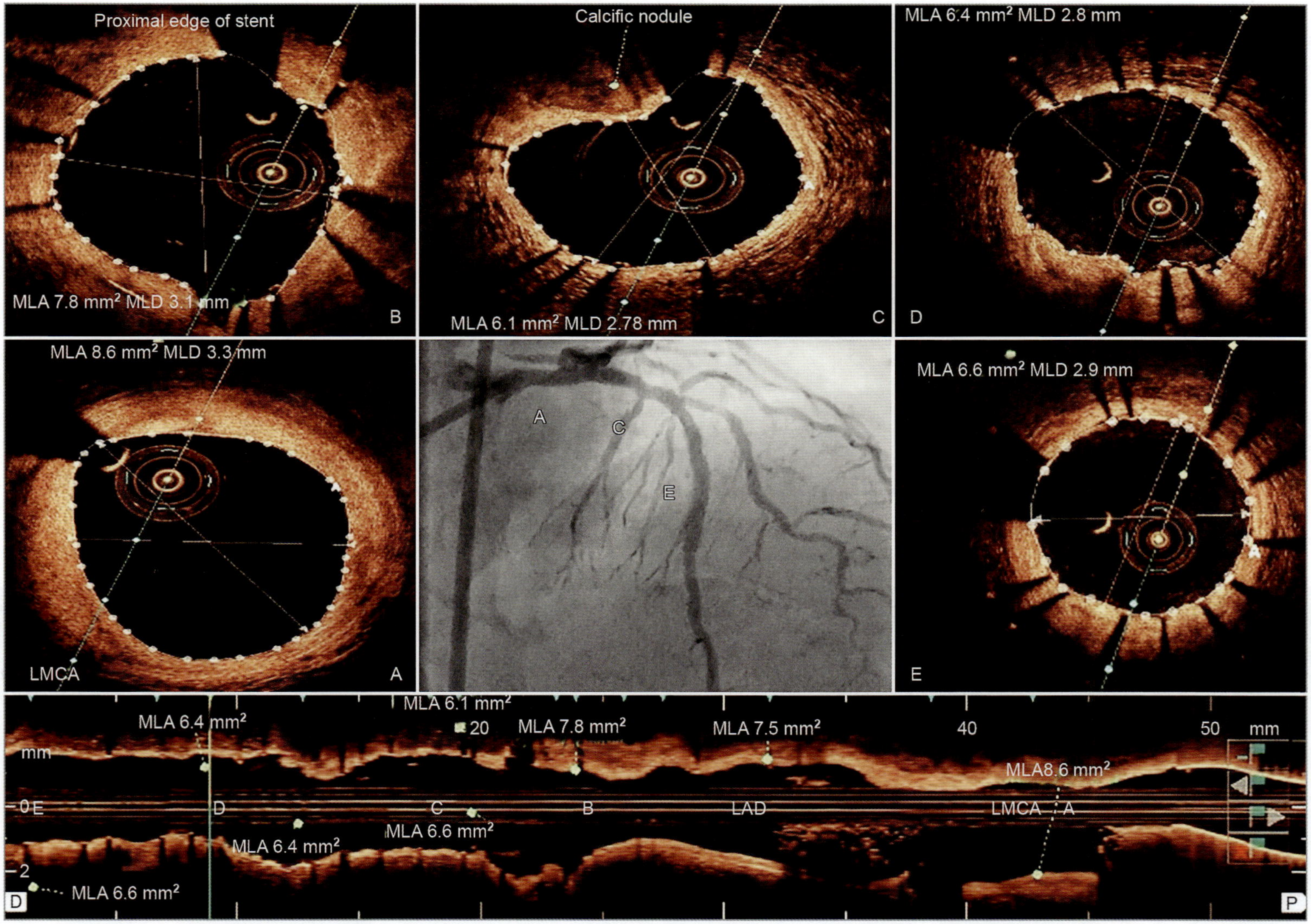

Fig. 9: Poststenting optical coherence tomography (OCT) assessment showed well-expanded and apposed stent struts. (LAD: left anterior descending; LMCA: left main coronary artery; MLA: minimal lumen area; MLD: minimal lumen diameter)

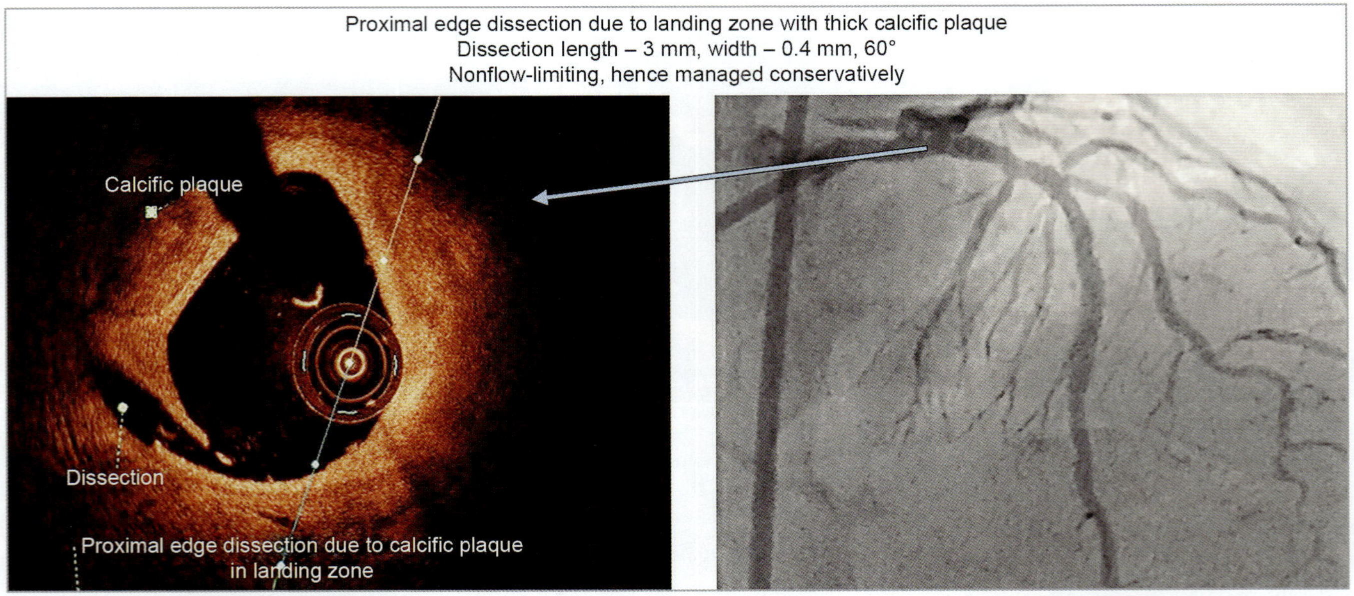

Fig. 10: Post-OCT (optical coherence tomography) showed proximal edge dissection which is nonflow-limiting.

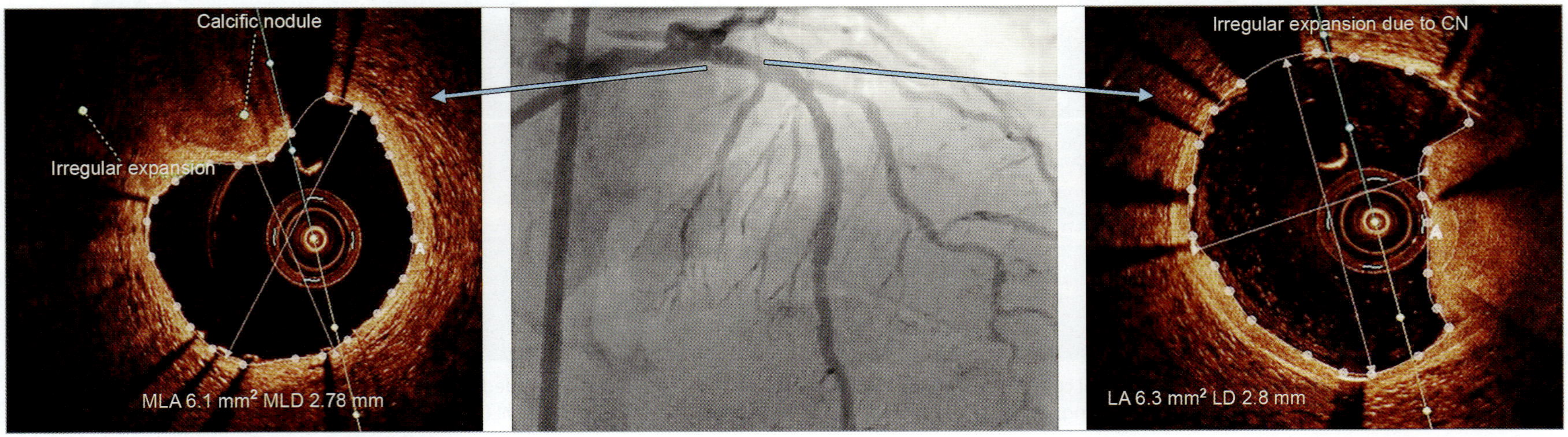

Fig. 11: Asymmetrical stent expansion due to calcific nodule (CN). (LA: lumen area; MLA: minimal lumen area; LD: lumen diameter; MLD: minimal lumen diameter)

CASE 2

OCT assessment of post-covered stenting proximal LAD for DES-induced aneurysm.

CLINICAL HISTORY

A 47-year-old male, known hypertensive, diabetic, presented with coronary artery disease (CAD)—unstable angina, chest pain associated with shortness of breath. He had history of PCI of LAD with DES in 2015. Investigations: random blood sugar (RBS)—148 mg/dL, blood urea—18 mg/dL, serum creatinine—0.68 mg/dL, estimated glomerular filtration rate (eGFR)—114, troponin I—0.02. CAG-LMCA—normal, LAD—proximal stent severe in-stent restenosis (ISR) with aneurysm, LCX and RCA normal **(Fig. 12A)**.

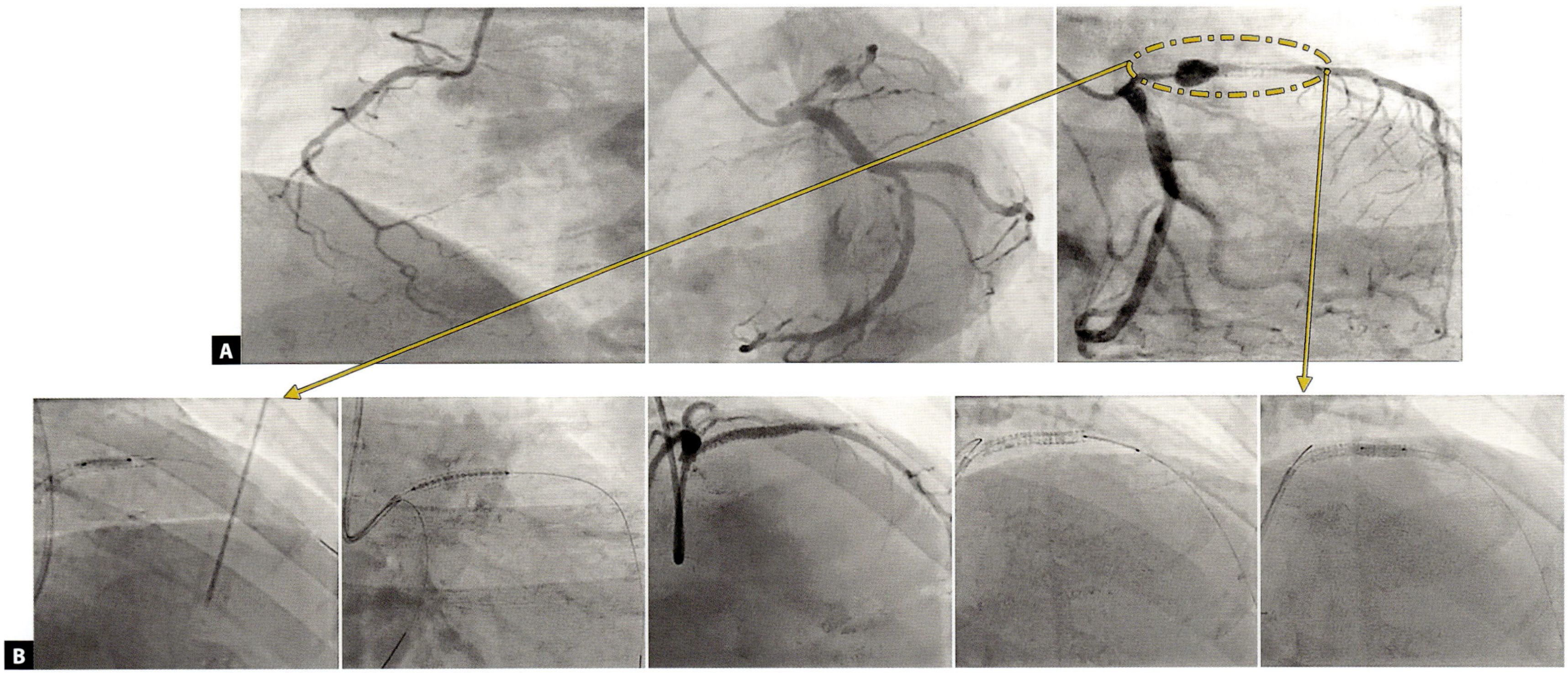

Figs. 12 A and B: (A) Coronary angiogram; (B) coronary angioplasty of aneurysmal portion and open surgical repair (OSR) segment.

PROCEDURE

Route—right radial approach (RRA), 6 Fr XB 3.5 guiding catheter, LAD lesion crossed with 014″ Sion blue wire which was predilated with 2.5 × 12 mm Apollo balloon and 3.0 × 20 mm Magic Touch drug-eluting balloon. Preprocedure IVUS showed severe ISR with aneurysm in proximal LAD which was stented with 2.8 × 26 mm Graftmaster stent, distal LAD stenting with 2.75 × 13 mm Orsiro stent and postdilated with 3.5 × 12 mm NC Trek balloon **(Fig. 12B)**.

Post-OCT showed distal portion of the covered stent (Graft Master) MLA—6.6 mm^2, MLD—2.9 mm with well-expanded **(Fig. 13)**. Mid portion of the covered stent with MLA—7.2 mm^2, MLD—3 mm, proximal portion of the covered stent MLA—7.9 mm^2, MLD—3.2 mm **(Fig. 14)**. LAD ostial dissection with nonflow-limiting <3 mm **(Fig. 15)**.

Post-OCT LAD ostial dissection with nonflow-limiting <3 mm, well-apposed and expanded stent struts, with no evidence of aneurysm **(Fig. 16)**. Postprocedure angio view showed well-implanted stents with TIMI-III flow without any dissection. Patient was discharged on third postprocedure in a stable status.

Patient was readmitted 1 month later for severe angina, repeat angio showed severe critical stenosis of distal LMCA, underwent emergency coronary artery bypass grafting (CABG) with excision of LAD aneurysm, removal of stent graft **(Figs. 17A to C)**, and stents with proximal ligation of LAD, left internal mammary artery (LIMA) to LAD and saphenous vein graft (SVG) to obtuse marginal (OM). Patient is under follow-up for the past 1 year without any cardiovascular (CV) symptoms.

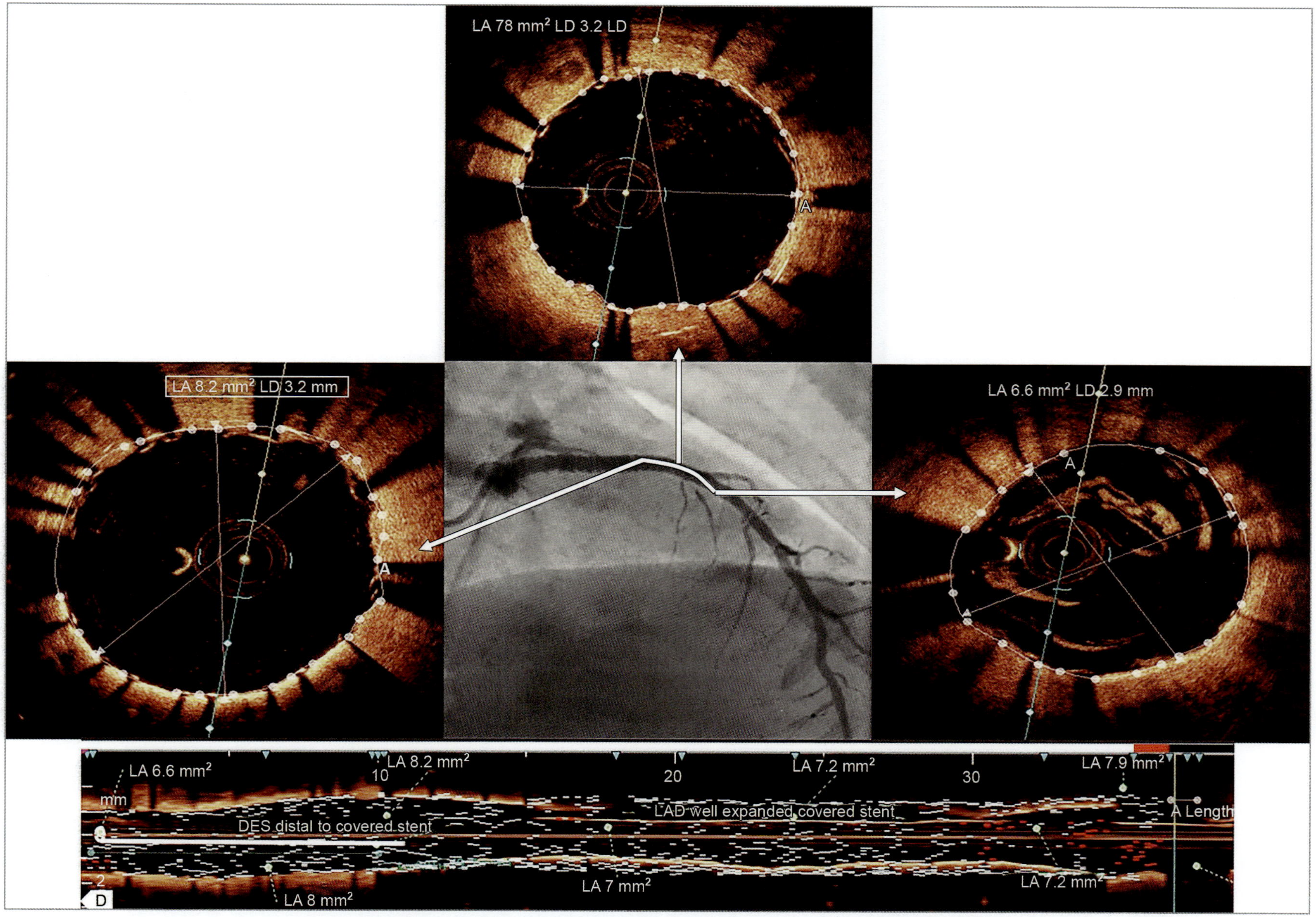

Fig. 13: Post-optical coherence tomography (OCT) showed distal portion of the cover stent. (DES: drug-eluting stent; LA: lumen area; LAD: left anterior descending; LD: lumen diameter)

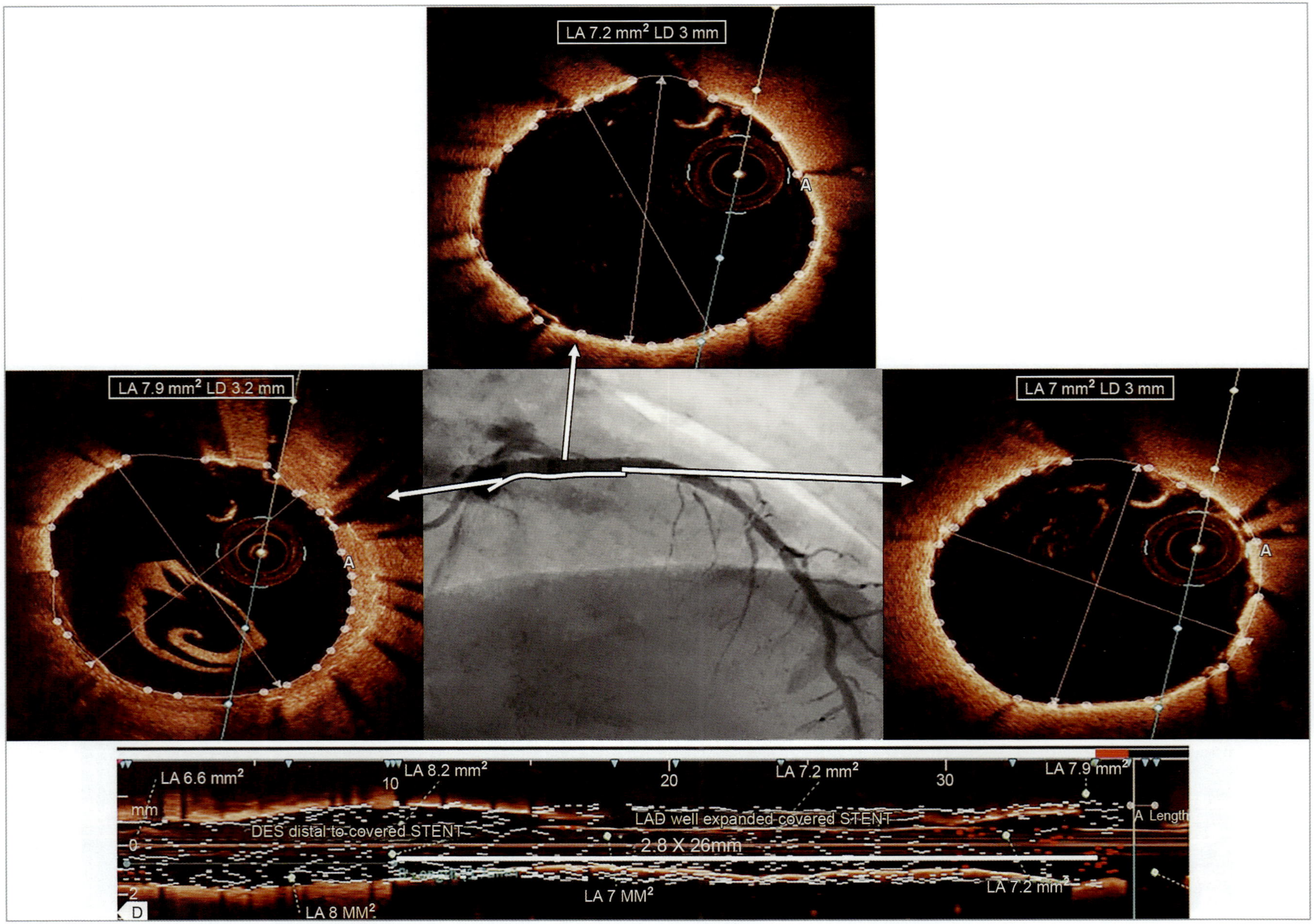

Fig. 14: Post-optical coherence tomography (OCT) showed proximal portion of the cover stent. (DES: drug-eluting stent; LA: lumen area; LAD: left anterior descending; LD: lumen diameter)

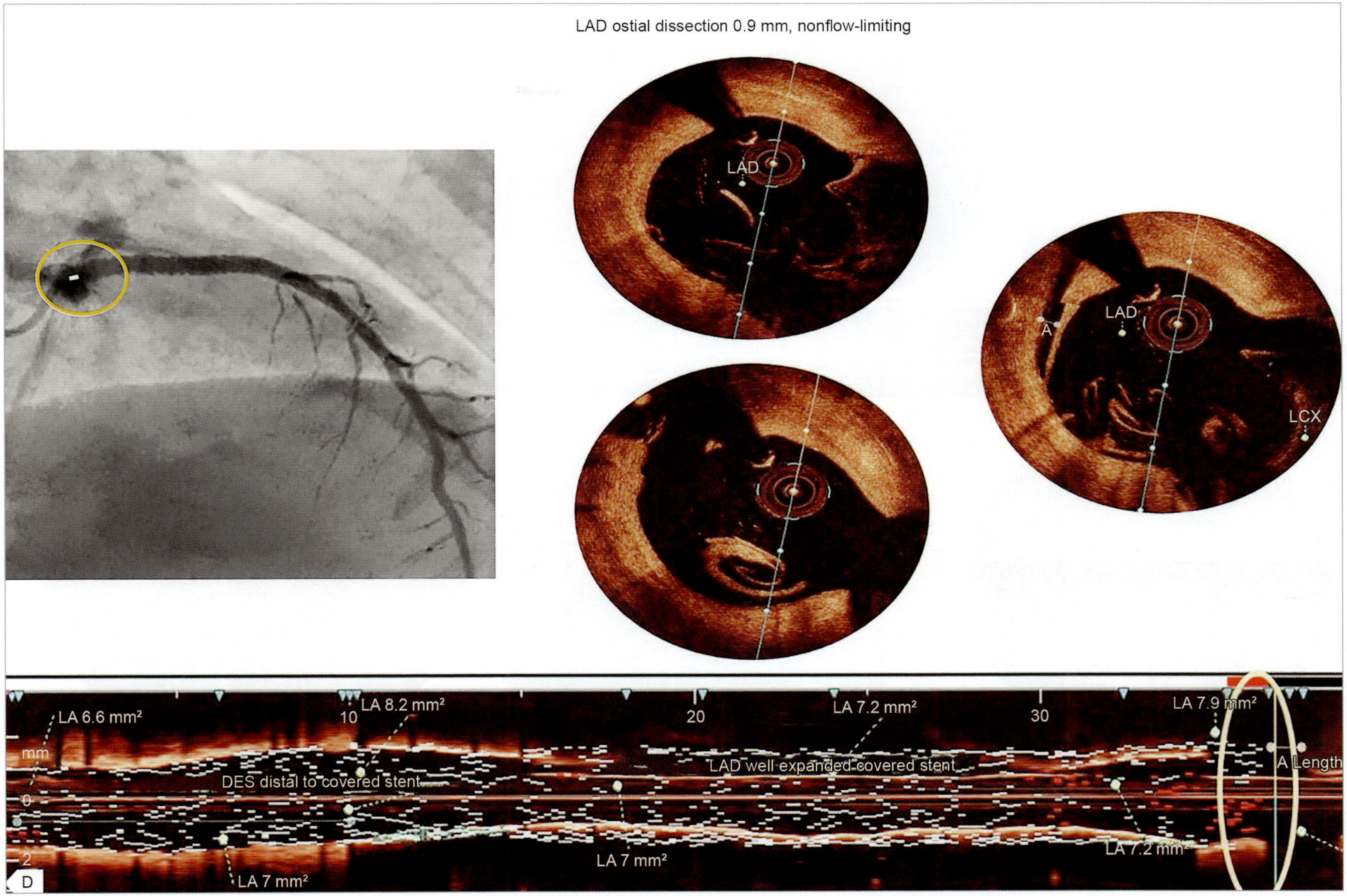

Fig. 15: Left anterior descending (LAD) ostial dissection with nonflow-limiting length: 3 mm, width: 4 mm. (DES: drug-eluting stent; LA: lumen area)

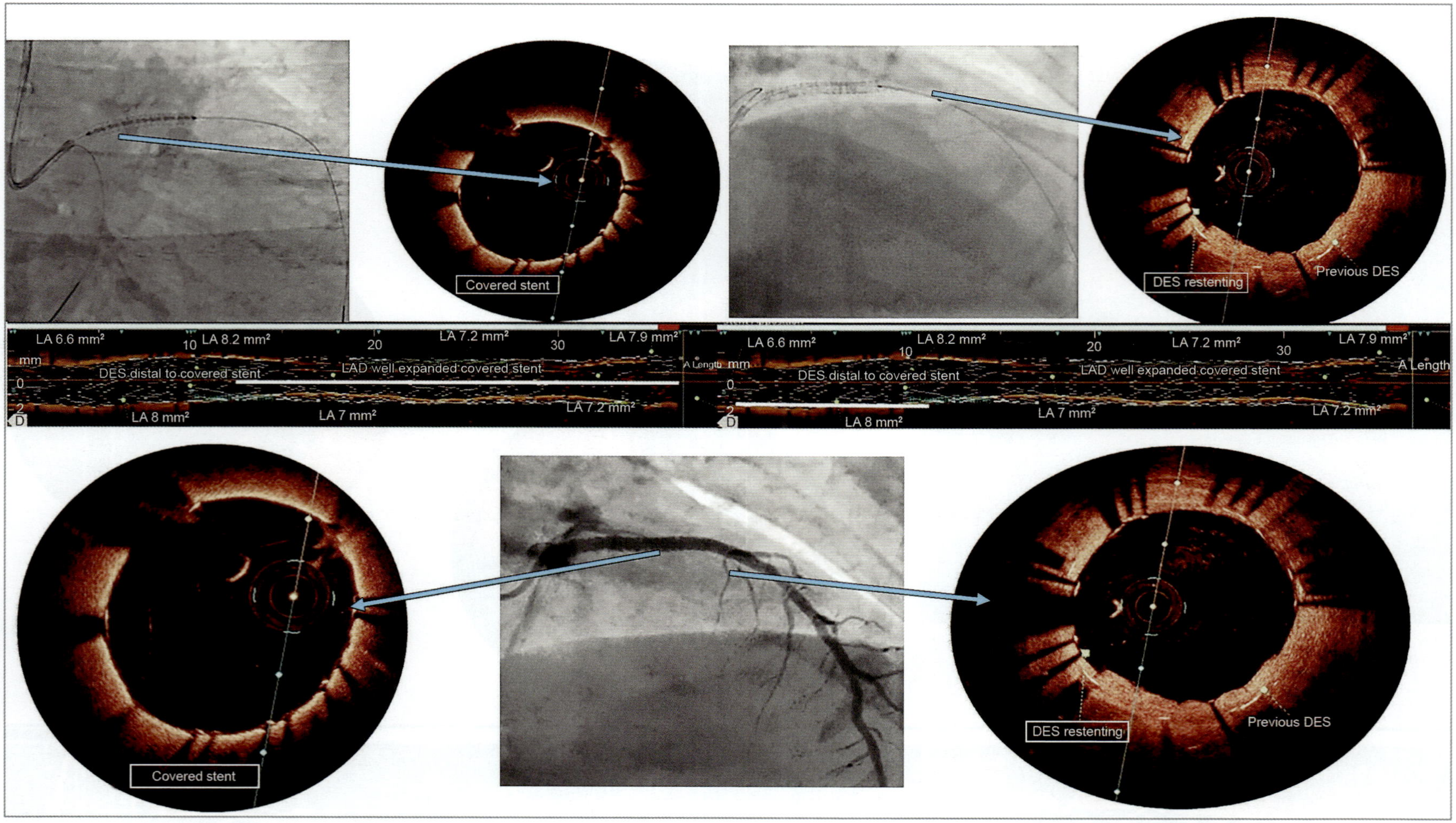

Fig. 16: Post-optical coherence tomography (OCT) showed, well-apposed and expanded stent struts, with no evidence of aneurysm. (DES: drug-eluting stent; LA: lumen area; LAD: left anterior descending)

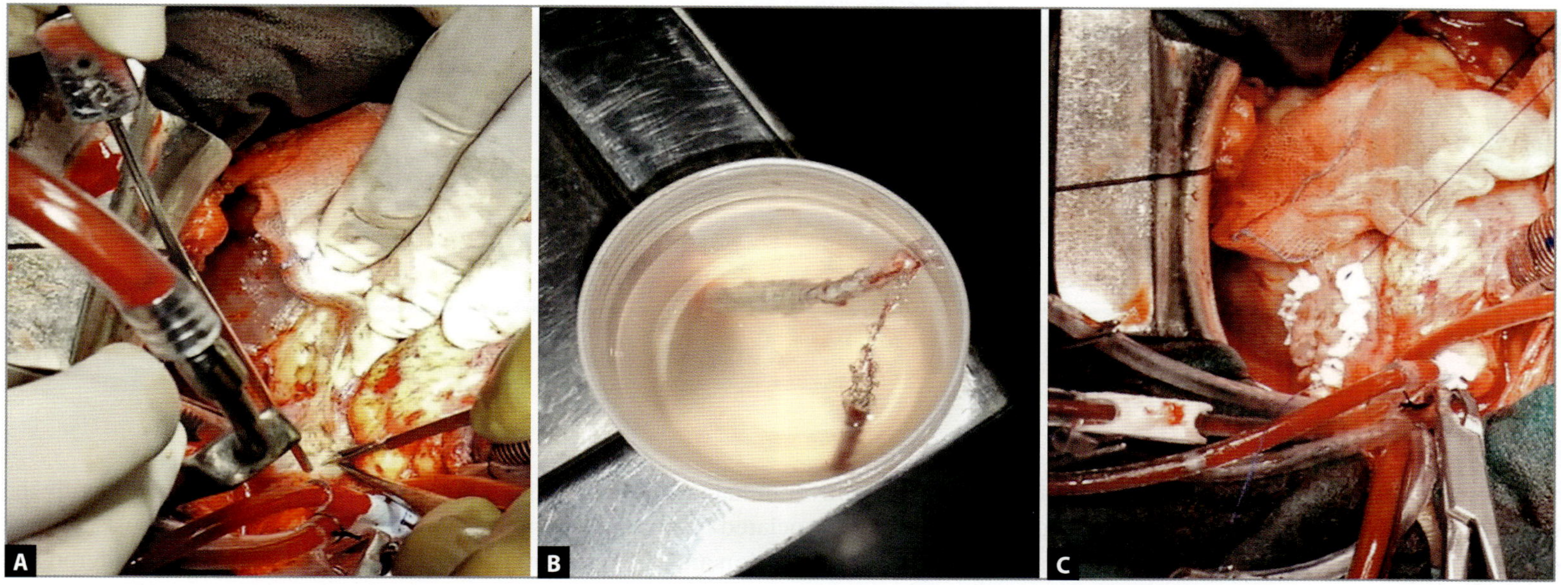

Figs. 17A to C: Removed stent from the aneurysm segment after coronary artery bypass grafting (CABG).

CHAPTER 16

Stent Fracture

Rajesh M Dave

INTRODUCTION

Many times, it would be difficult to diagnose stent fracture (SF) with conventional imaging modalities. Subclinical SF occurs more frequently than those reported cases. Early detection and treatment of SF crucial due to the associated high risk of in-stent restenosis (IRS), stent thrombosis, and aneurysm formation. Pressure during stent deployment and aggressive balloon postdilation and the resultant damage to the stent strut are considered risk factors for the development of SFs; risk factors for SF-right coronary artery (RCA), vessel tortuosity, and the sharp angle of the hinge motion of vessels, longer and overlapped stents, may increase metal fatigue during a cardiac cycle and lead to SF. Although the lack of circumferential struts on 2-dimensional (2D) Optical coherence tomography (OCT) has been previously regarded as SF, this criterion should not be applied to confirm SF with open-cell platforms. Transverse OCT, an intact closed-cell design stent produced circumferential strut images, open-cell stents showed various strut patterns, depending on the position and inclination of a cross-sectional cut. Enhanced stent imaging (ESI) to suggest SF after stent implantation, a suspicion that may be confirmed by 3-dimensional (3D) OCT.[1]

DIAGNOSIS OF STENT FRACTURE

- Magnified fluoroscopic/stent boost images may show partial or complete separation with displacement of the stent segment.
- OCT 2D/3D—lack of circumferential struts in a stented segment.
- Longitudinal optical coherence tomographic images may show multiple SFs with gaps.

Three-dimensional OCT confirms diagnosis of SF in majority of cases particularly in cases where fluoro images are doubtful **(Fig. 1)**.[2]

- Usefulness of optical coherence tomography imaging for diagnosis of in-stent restenosis due to a stent fracture and morphological assessment **(Figs. 2A to D)**.
- *Optical coherence tomography-guided treatment of multiple stent fracture in patients with overlapping drug-eluting stents (DES):*
    - Coronary angiography (CAG) shows intraluminal haziness (arrow) at the mid portion of the previous RCA stent without significant IRS. Magnified fluoroscopic images showed suspicious complete separation with displacement of the previous DES overlapping site. **Figures 3A to F** show each site of axial optical coherence images. Longitudinal optical coherence tomographic images showed multiple SFs with four gaps. 3D reconstructed

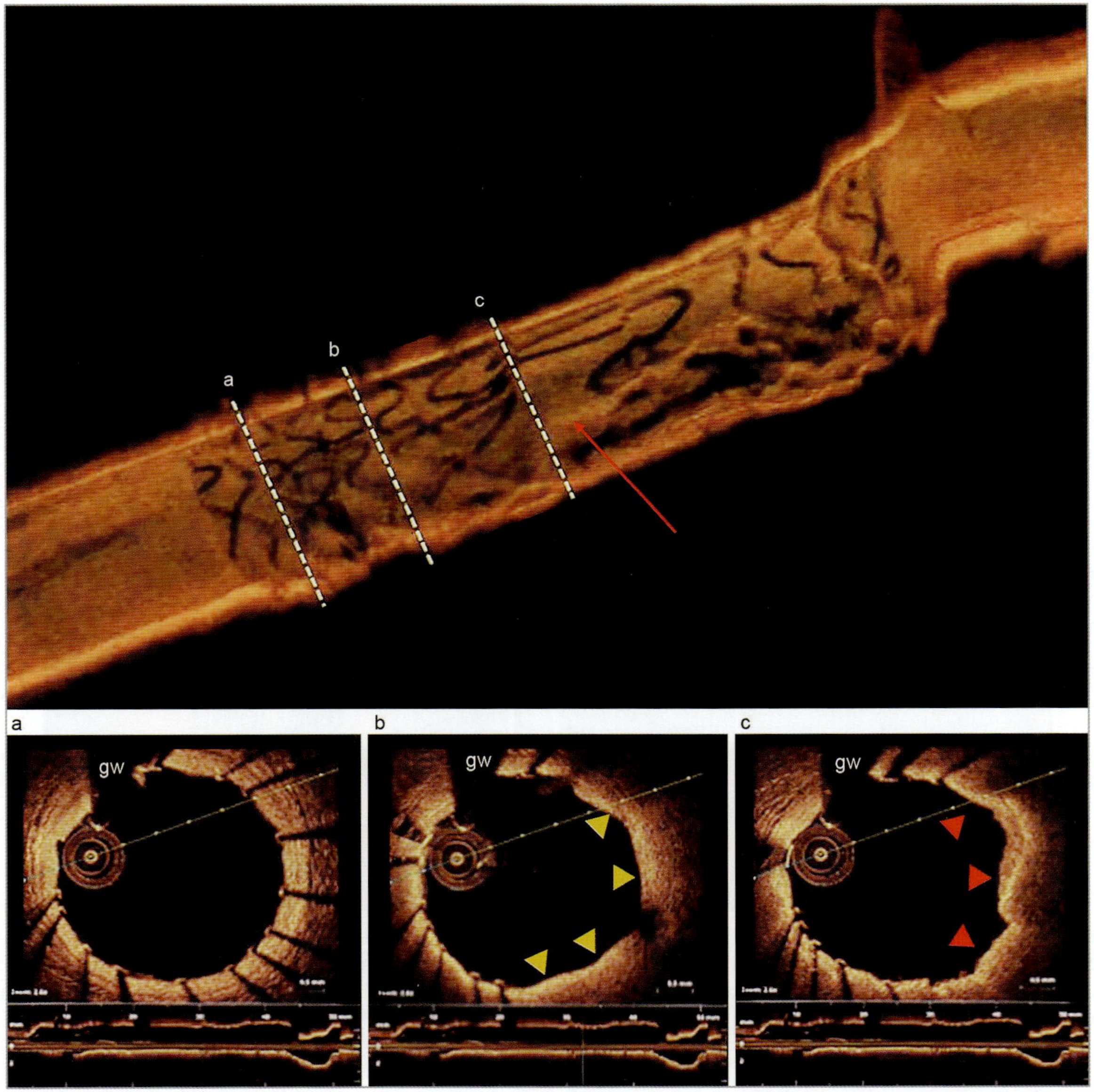

Fig. 1: Usefulness of three-dimensional optical coherence tomography (3D OCT) to diagnose a noncircumferential open-cell stent fracture. 3D OCT reconstruction showing a relatively large area without metal scaffolding due to links breakage (red arrow); yellow lines correspond to 2D cross sections in a, b, and c—(a) circumferential stent struts; (b) lack of circumferential struts (yellow arrowheads) on 2D OCT, corresponding on 3D OCT (line b) to a normal gap, without links breakage, between stent crowns due to open-cell design; and (c) lack of circumferential struts (red arrowheads) clearly confirmed as a fracture on 3D OCT (line c).

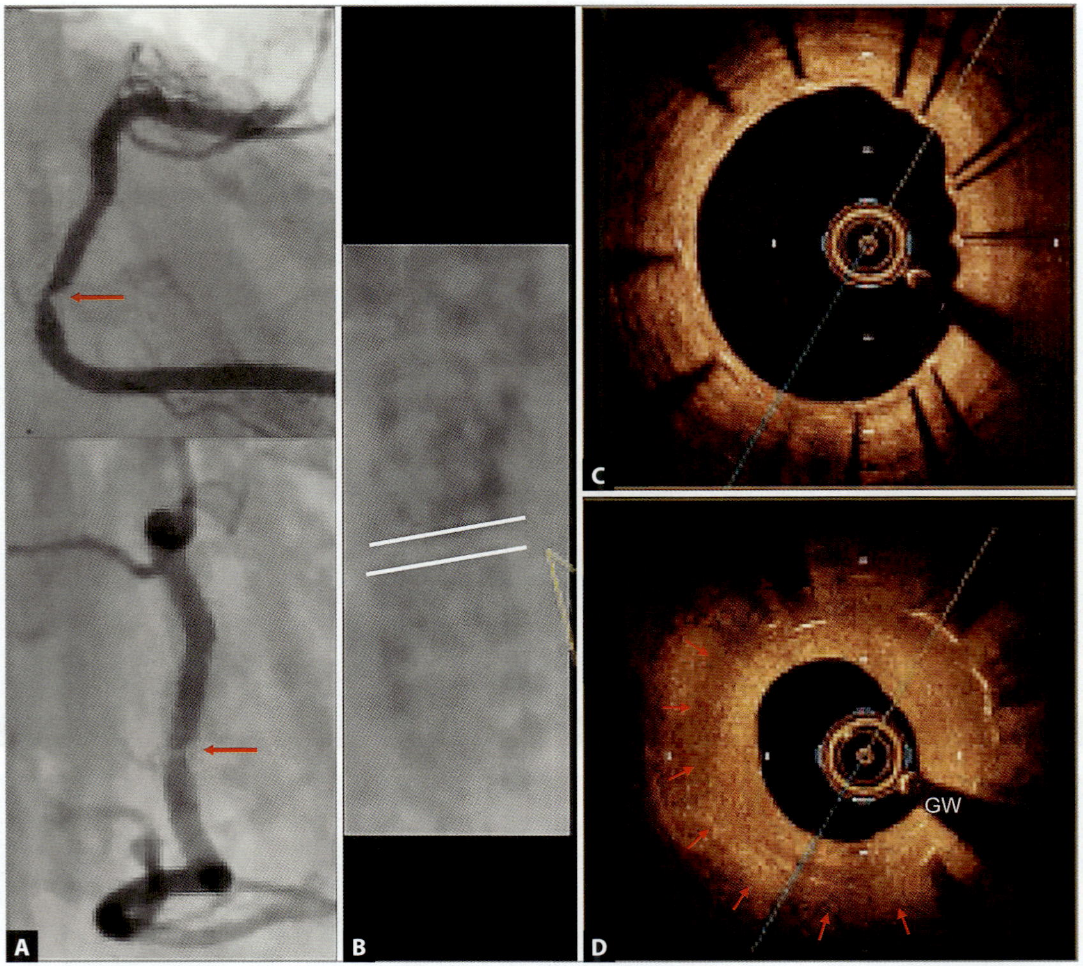

Figs. 2A to D: Usefulness of optical coherence tomography (OCT) imaging for diagnosis of in-stent restenosis due to a stent fracture and morphological assessment. (A) Coronary angiogram illustrating in-stent restenosis in the right coronary artery; (B) The stent fracture as seen on the coronary angiogram; (C) Two-dimensional cross-sectional OCT revealed circumferentially covered stent struts and a guidewire artifact (GW); (D) two-dimensional cross-sectional OCT indicating the lack of stent struts (red arrow) and homogeneous neointima pattern.

stent strut images clearly demonstrated multiple SF with four gaps (arrows). 3D reconstructed images showed that the guidewire was clearly inside the whole fractured stents. After 4.0 × 18-mm Onyx (Medtronic, Minneapolis, MN, USA) implantation, the final angiogram revealed good distal flow without any residual stenosis or dissection **(Figs. 3A to F)**.

- Focal ISR generally treated with angioplasty, whereas diffuse ISR is usually treated with repeat DES **(Flowchart 1)**.

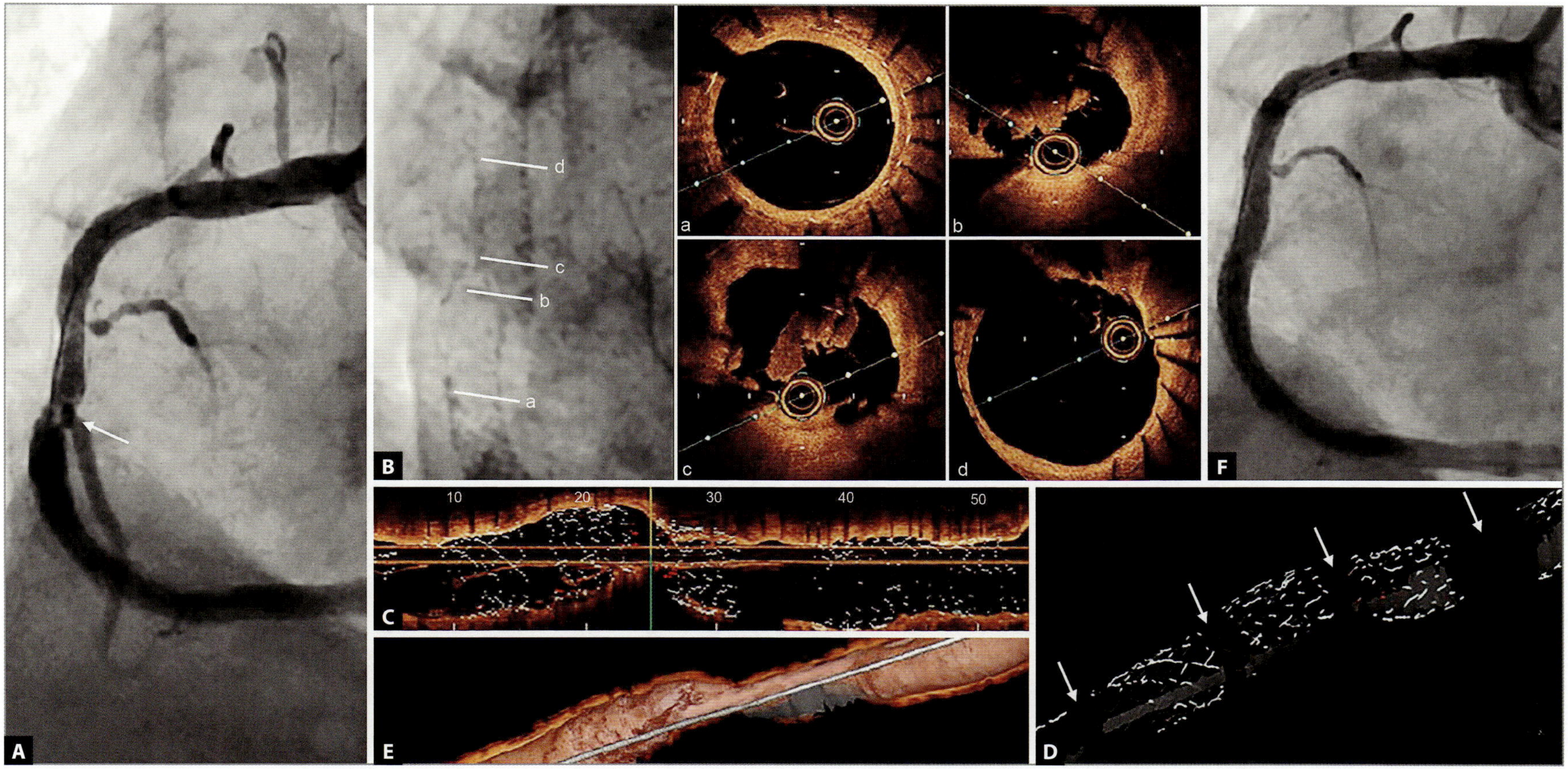

Figs. 3A to F: Optical coherence tomography (OCT)-guided treatment of multiple stent fracture in patients with overlapping drug-eluting stent (DES).

Flowchart 1: Stent fracture (SF).

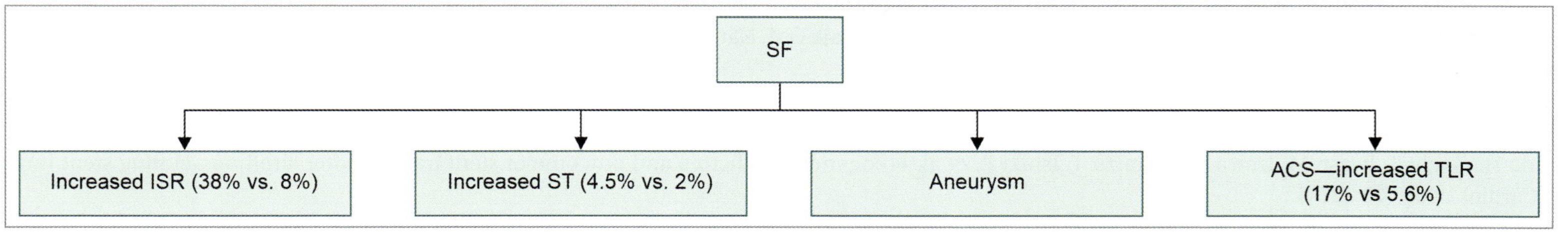

(ACS: acute coronary syndrome; ISR: in-stent restenosis; ST: stent thrombosis; TLR: target lesion revascularization)

PROCEDURE

Discussion

There has been increasing awareness of stent fracture (SF) as a potential complication of drug-eluting stent (DES) implant.

There are reports of SF as a potential cause of stent restenosis and thrombosis, which can lead to adverse clinical outcome such as recurrent angina, myocardial infarction (MI) and death.

Although, reported incidence of stent fracture varies between 1 and 8%,[3] an autopsy study has reported incidence as high as 29%. High-grade V stent Fracture was associated with significant pathology.[4]

Predictors of stent fracture are stent overexpansion, stent overlap, long stents, and stent conformability.[5-7]

There are anatomical and pathological factors such as tortuous highly angulated artery/lesion, change in vessel angulation poststent implant, complexity of lesion such as chronic total occlusion and right coronary artery (RCA) location.[3,7-10]

The timing of occurrence of stent fracture is poorly understood and as early as 3 days' poststent fracture has been reported.[11]

There are reported cases of coronary aneurysm with SF as well.[3,12]

In a study by Kashiwagi et al.,[13] Optical coherence tomography was used to detect SF and absence of stent strut was the most common feature.

SF represents important entity with clinical presentation ranging from asymptomatic to angina, MI and even death. Factors such as RCA, long overlapping stents, complexity of lesion, angulation as seen in our patient are all associated with increased prevalence of SF. With high resolution imaging modalities such as OCT, recognition of this frequently underreported entity will become more common.

REFERENCES

1. Francaviglia B, Capranzano P, Gargiulo G, Longo G, Tamburino CI, Ohno Y, et al. Usefulness of 3D OCT to diagnose a noncircumferential open-cell stent fracture. JACC Cardiovasc Imaging. 2016;9(2):210-1.
2. Lee JH, Kim U. Optical coherence tomography-guided treatment of multiple stent fracture in patients with overlapping drug-eluting stents. Korean Circ J. 2018;48(11):1030.
3. Sianos G, Hofma S, Ligthart JM, Saia F, Hoye A, Lemos PA, et al. Stent fracture and restenosis in the drug-eluting stent era. Catheter Cardiovasc Interv. 2004;61:11-6.
4. Nakazawa G, Finn AV, Vorpahl M, Ladich E, Kutys R, Balazs I, et al. Incidence and predictors of drug-eluting stent fracture in human coronary artery a pathologic analysis. J Am Coll Cardiol. 2009;54:1924-31.
5. Chhatriwalla AK, Unzek S, Kapadia SR. Recurrent Stent Fracture in the Right Coronary Artery. Clin Cardiol. 2010;33:E70-2.
6. Ramegowda RT, Chikkaswamy SB, Bharatha A, Radhakrishna J, Krishnanaik GM, Nanjappa MC, et al. Circumferential Stent Fracture. Novel detection and treatment with the use of stent boost. Tex Heart Inst J. 2012;39:431-4.
7. Surmely JF, Kinoshita Y, Dash D, Matsubara T, Terashima M, Ehara M, et al. Stent strut Fracture-Induced restenosis in a bifurcation lesion treated with the crush stenting technique. Circ J. 2006;70:936-8.
8. Umeda H, Gochi T, Iwase M, Izawa H, Shimizu T, Ishiki R, et al. Frequency, predictors and outcome of stent fracture after sirolimus-eluting stent implantation. Int J Cardiol. 2009;133:321-6.
9. Canan T, Lee MS. Drug-eluting stent fracture: Incidence, contributing factors, and clinical implications. Catheter Cardiovasc Interv. 2010;75:237-45.

10. Kandzari DE, Rao SV, Moses JW, Dzavik V, Strauss BH, Kutryk MJ, et al. Clinical and angiographic outcomes with sirolimus-eluting stents in total coronary occlusions: The across/tosca-4 (approaches to chronic occlusions with sirolimus-eluting stents/total occlusion study of coronary arteries-4) trial. JACC Cardiovasc Interv. 2009;2:97-110.
11. Smaldone C, Bacà M, Niccoli G. A case if early drug-eluting stent fracture. J Invasive Cardiol. 2010;22:E186-8.
12. Alexopoulos D, Xanthopoulou I. Coronary Stent Fracture: How Frequent It Is? Does It Matter? Hellenic J Cardiol. 2011;52:1-5.
13. Kashiwagi M, Tanaka A, Kitabata H, Ino Y, Tsujioka H, Komukai K, et al. OCT-Verified neointimal hyperplasia is increased at fracture site in drug-eluting stents. JACC Cardivasc Imaging. 2010;5:230-6.

CASE 1

Optical Coherence Tomography Imaging for Detection of Stent Fracture.

Rajesh M Dave

CLINICAL HISTORY

Patient is an 82-year-old male with history of hyperlipidemia, hypertension, and diet control diabetes who was admitted to an outlaying facility with Canadian Class III angina pectoris. He underwent cardiac catheterization which revealed heavily calcified subtotal occlusion of proximal RCA **(Fig. 4A)** and minimal disease in left coronary arteries. His ejection fracture was normal. He was then referred for RCA intervention at our facility. In this case, 7FJR4 Guide Catheter was utilized and intravascular ultrasound (IVUS) examination was attempted. However, due to heavy calcification, IVUS catheter did not cross the lesion. Rotational atherectomy was now performed using 1.25 mm as well as 1.5 mm rotablator burrs **(Fig. 4B)**. After rotational atherectomy, IVUS examination was able to be performed **(Fig. 4C)**. The proximal RCA was treated using 3.5 mm × 33 mm Xience Sierra™ (Abbott Vascular–Santa Clara, CA) **(Fig. 4D)** and mid segment was treated using 3.0 mm × 38 mm Synergy™ (Boston Scientific Corporation–Marlborough, MA) DES. Proximal RCA was post dilated to 4 mm with noncompliant balloon. Final good result was achieved **(Fig. 4E)** and patient was discharged next day on dual antiplatelet therapy.

Approximately 1-week later patient again experienced severe angina and was admitted to an outlying facility. Due to ongoing intermittent chest discomfort, he was transferred back to my facility for repeat coronary angiography. Repeat coronary angiography did not reveal any new left coronary system stenoses; however, 70% eccentric lesion was observed in proximal RCA at the side of previously placed DES **(Fig. 5A)**. To identify the etiology of this lesion, we elected to perform OCT of RCA. OCT of proximal RCA revealed SF in proximal RCA **(Fig. 5B)**. This area was now treated with 4 mm × 30 mm synergy DES **(Fig. 5C)**. This stent was post-dilated to 4.5-mm diameter balloon. Repeat angiography and OCT demonstrated excellent result **(Fig. 5D)**. Patient at 30 days' follow-up remained asymptomatic and active.

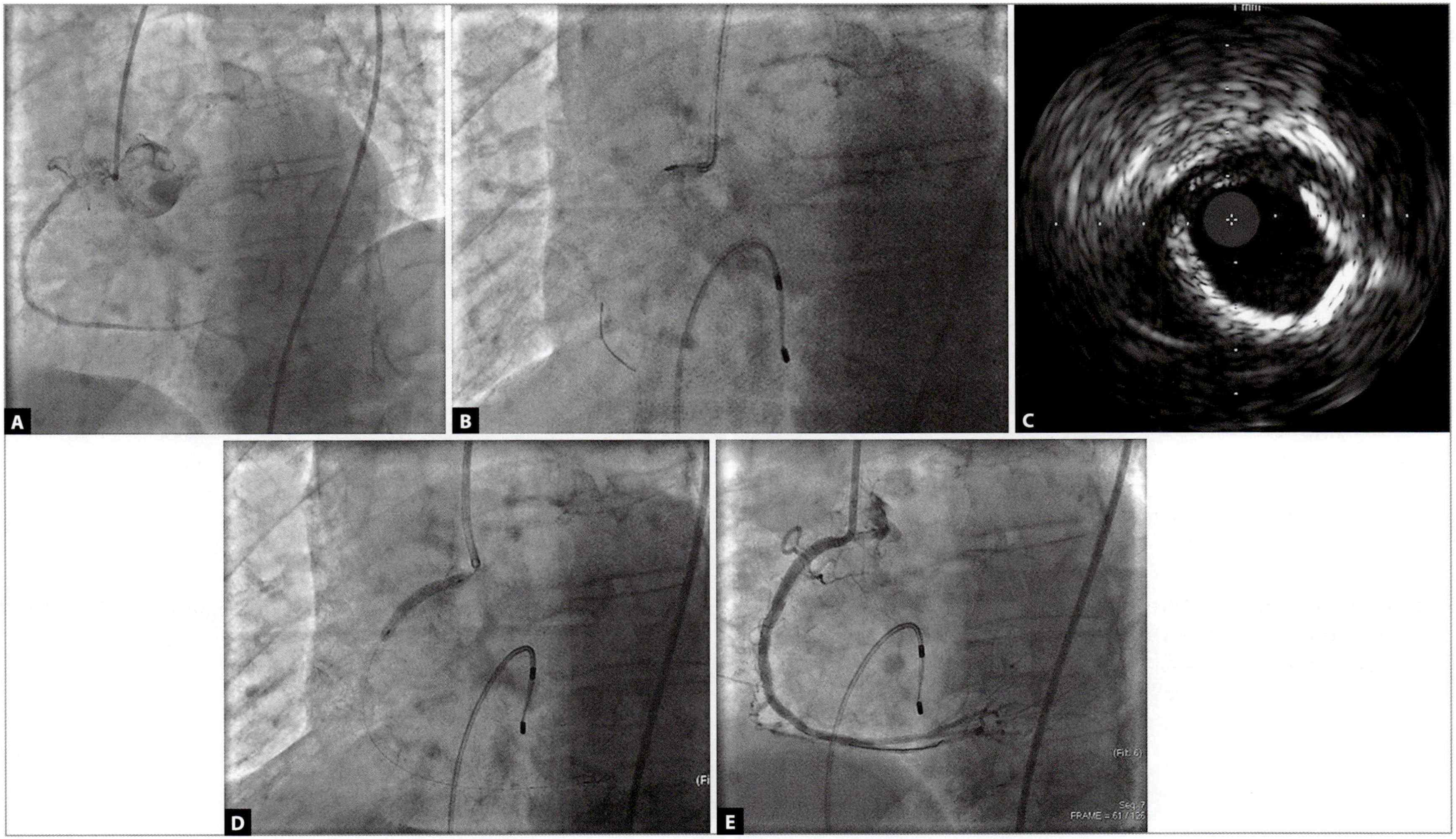

Figs. 4A to E: Intravascular ultrasound (IVUS) and ROTA stenting of right coronary artery (RCA) vessel.

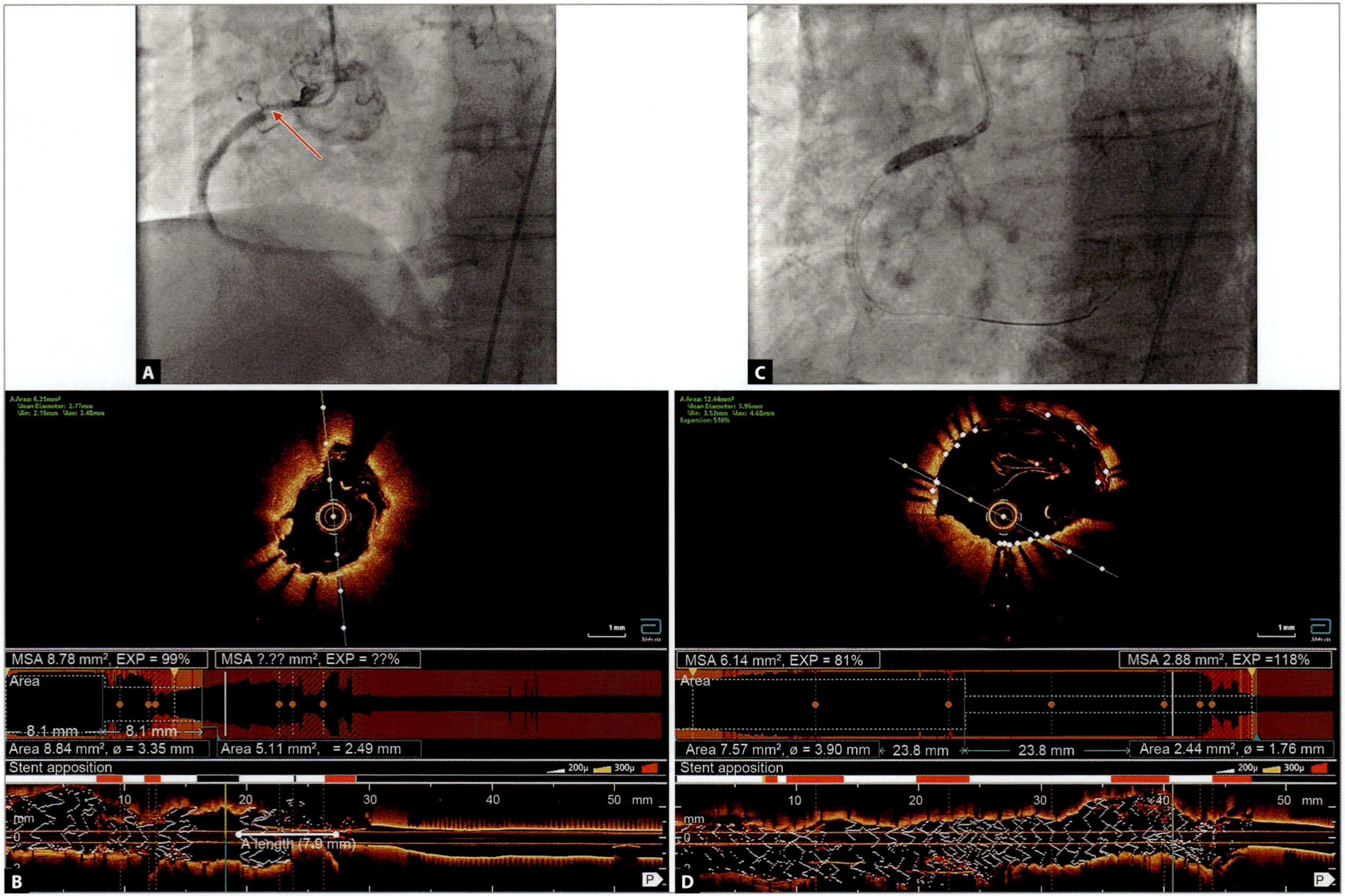

Figs. 5A to D: Detection of stent fracture by angiographically and Optical coherence tomography (OCT), covered with additional stent and final OCT assessment.

CASE 2

Optical coherence tomography (OCT) assessment of bioresorbable vascular scaffold (BVS) stent fracture.

CLINICAL HISTORY

A 62-year-old male known hypertensive and diabetic presented with unstable angina of 3 days' duration. Investigations: ECG—Normal, 2D echo—normal with ejection fraction (EF)—62%. Treadmill test (TMT) positive for inducible ischemia, and routine blood investigations were in the normal range. CAG-proximal left circumflex (LCX) 70% lesion, proximal left anterior descending (LAD) 80% bifurcation lesion, distal LAD 80–90% lesion **(Figs. 6A and B)**.

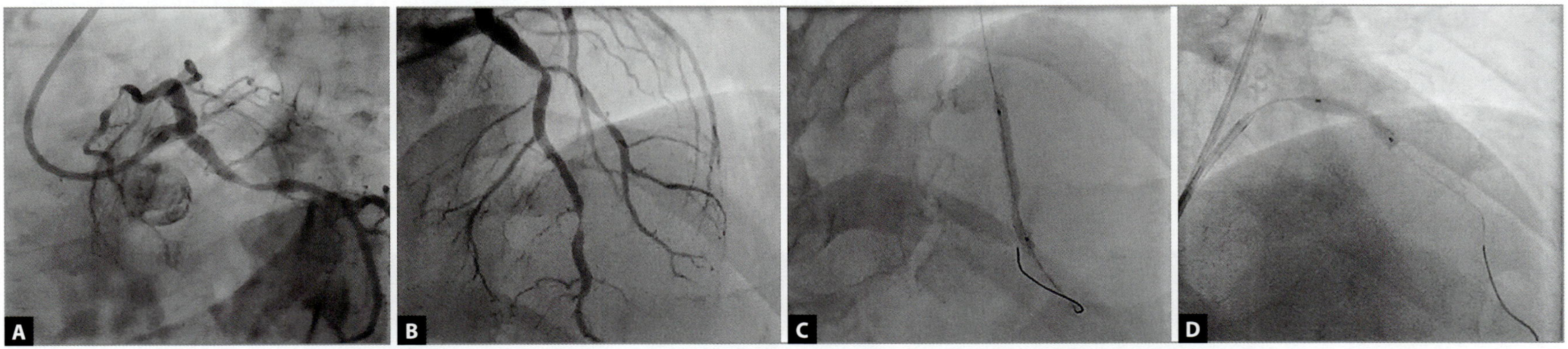

Figs. 6A to D: Coronary angiogram, proximal, and distal left anterior descending (LAD) angioplasty.

PROCEDURE

RFA—route, XB 3.06 Fr guiding catheter, after placing 0.014 Rinato wire in LAD, predilated with 2.25 × 10 mm Tazuna, 2.75 × 15 mm NC Trek, 2.5 × 14 mm Falcon, and 3 × 10 mm Hiryu NC balloons. Plaque modification of proximal LAD lesion was done with 2.5 × 10 m cutting balloon. Distal LAD stenting done with 2.5 × 28 mm Absorb stent and postdilated with 2.75 × 15 mm NC Trek balloon. Proximal LAD stenting was done with 3.5 × 18 mm Absorb stent and postdilated with 4.0 × 8 mm NC trek balloon due to residual lesion **(Fig. 6C and D)**.

Poststent OCT study was done to assess bioresorbable vascular scaffold (BVS) status due to high pressure postdilation of 3.5 × 18 mm BVS with 4.0 × 8 mm NC which might result in BVS fracture even though angiographically no significant evidence of BVS fracture/dissection with thrombolysis in myocardial infarction III (TIMI-III) grade flow. OCT revealed fracture of absorb stent with multiple fractured struts within the lumen with dehiscence of scaffold **(Figs. 7 to 9A and B)**.

Hence, proximal LAD lesion restenting was done with 3.5 × 26 mm resolute integrity stent (DES) covering beyond proximal and distal edges of BVS to avoid scaffold thrombosis and ISR. Postdilation was done with 4.0 × 8 mm NC Trek balloon. Final result was good with TIM-3 flow and no complications **(Figs. 9C and D)**.

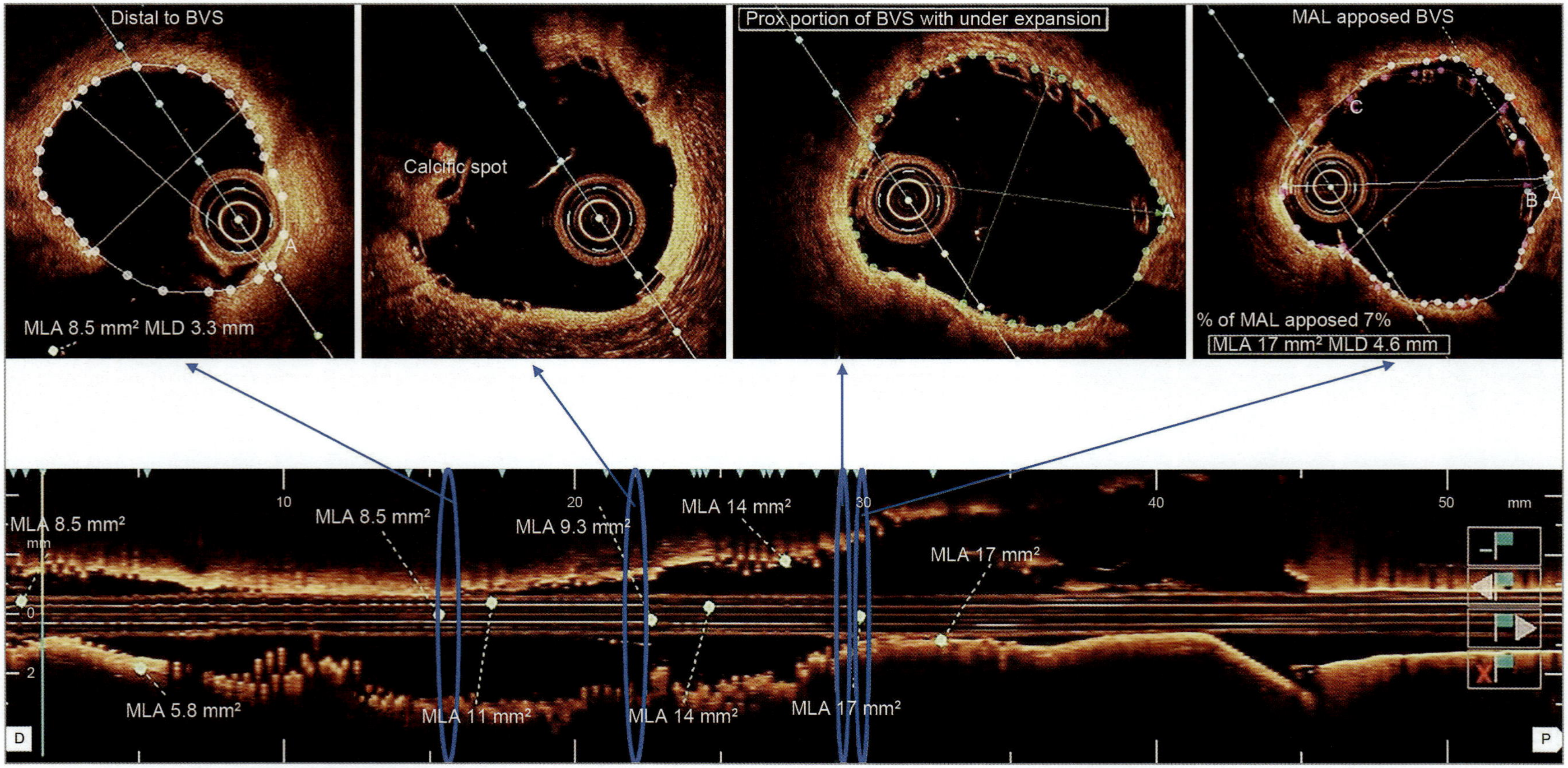

Fig. 7: Poststenting OCT assessment of LAD vessel which showed underexpansion and malapposition at proximal portion. (LAD: left anterior descending; MLA: minimal lumen area; OCT: optical coherence tomography)

High pressure inflation of BVS sometimes may lead to scaffold fracture. BVS fracture cannot be detected by routine angiographic views but intravascular imaging like IVUS, OCT detects very clearly. Undetected BVS fracture can lead to scaffold thrombosis and ISR which are associated with high major adverse cardiovascular events (MACE) rate. BVS scaffold fracture can be managed by restenting with DES. Patient has been under follow-up for the past 5 years without any CV symptoms.

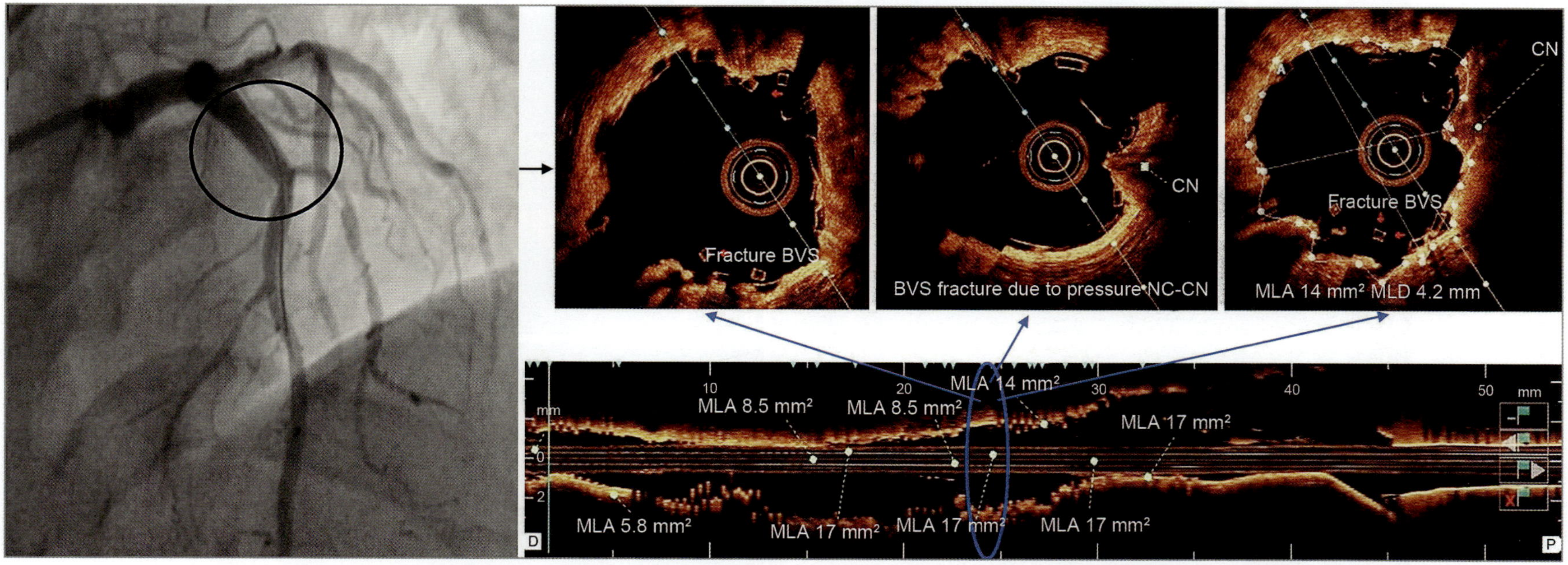

Fig. 8: Detection of BVS fractures by OCT at proximal portion of the proximal BVS. (BVS: bioresorbable vascular scaffold; MLA: minimal lumen area; OCT: optical coherence tomography)

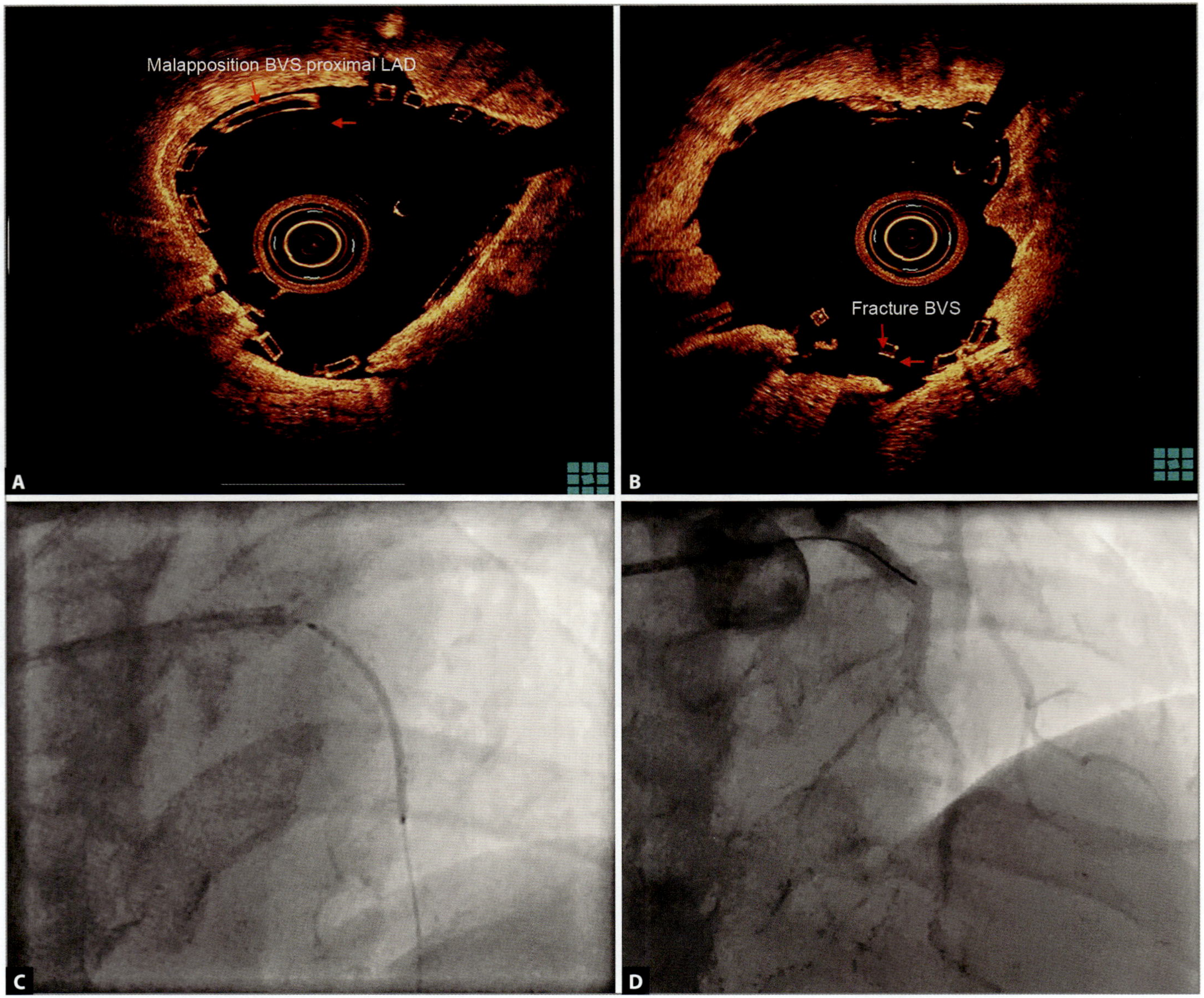

Figs. 9A to D: Malapposition and fracture of BVS covered with additional DES and final result.
(BVS: bioresorbable vascular scaffold; DES: drug-eluting stent)

CASE 3

Assessment of provisional stenting of left main coronary artery (LMCA) bifurcation in acute coronary syndrome (ACS)—stent fracture.

CLINICAL HISTORY

A 79-year-old female known hypertensive, S/P thrombolytic therapy (TLT) with streptokinase (STK) presented with complaints of chest pain, CAD – ACS – IW + PWMI, mild LV dysfunction. O/I Hb—10.8 g/dL, S.Cr—0.79 mg/dL, Trop-I-1.1 pg/mL. CAG—triple vessel disease with mild lesion of distal LMCA, mid LAD 70% stenosis, proximal LCX 80% stenosis, proximal obtuse marginal (OM) 90% lesion, mid RCA total occlusion, posterior descending artery (PDA), and PLVB filling retrogradely from left system **(Figs. 10A to C)**.

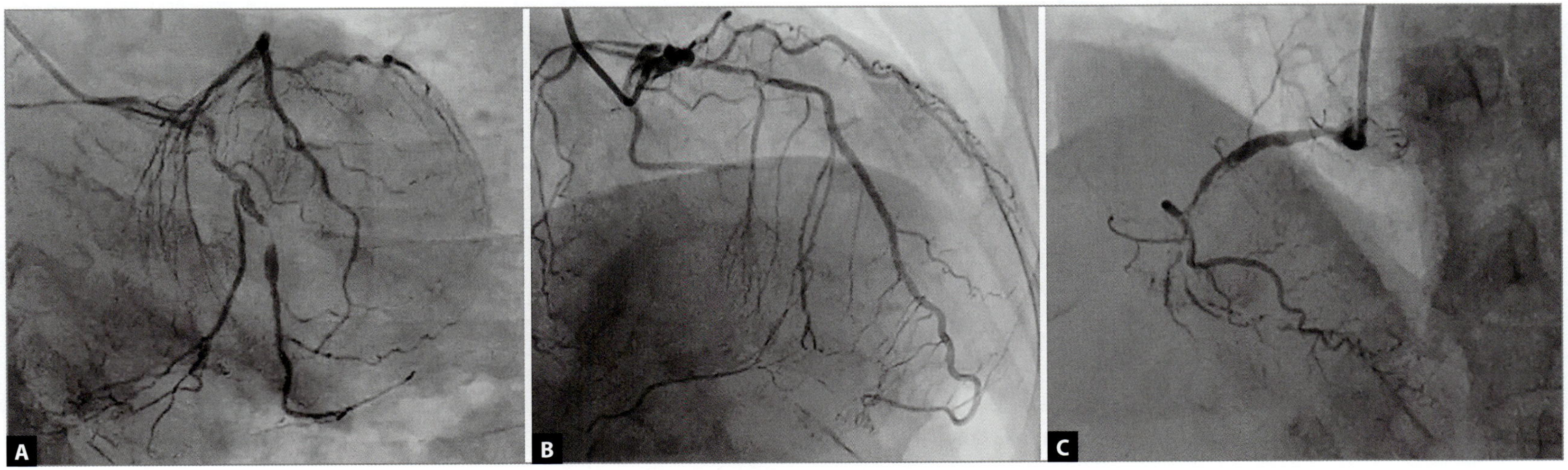

Figs. 10A to C: Coronary angiogram.

PROCEDURE

The RCA engaged with JR 3.5–6 Fr guiding catheter, RCA lesion was crossed with 0.014″ Fielder-XT Wire using microcatheter support. Predilated with 1.25 × 10 mm and 2.0 × 15 mm Tazuna balloon. Then proximal RCA stenting was done with 2.25 × 38 mm and mid RCA with 2.25 × 18 mm Onyx stent. Postdilated with balloon 2.25 × 18 mm up to 18 atms. Final result was good with TIMI-III flow with no complications **(Figs. 11A to F)**.

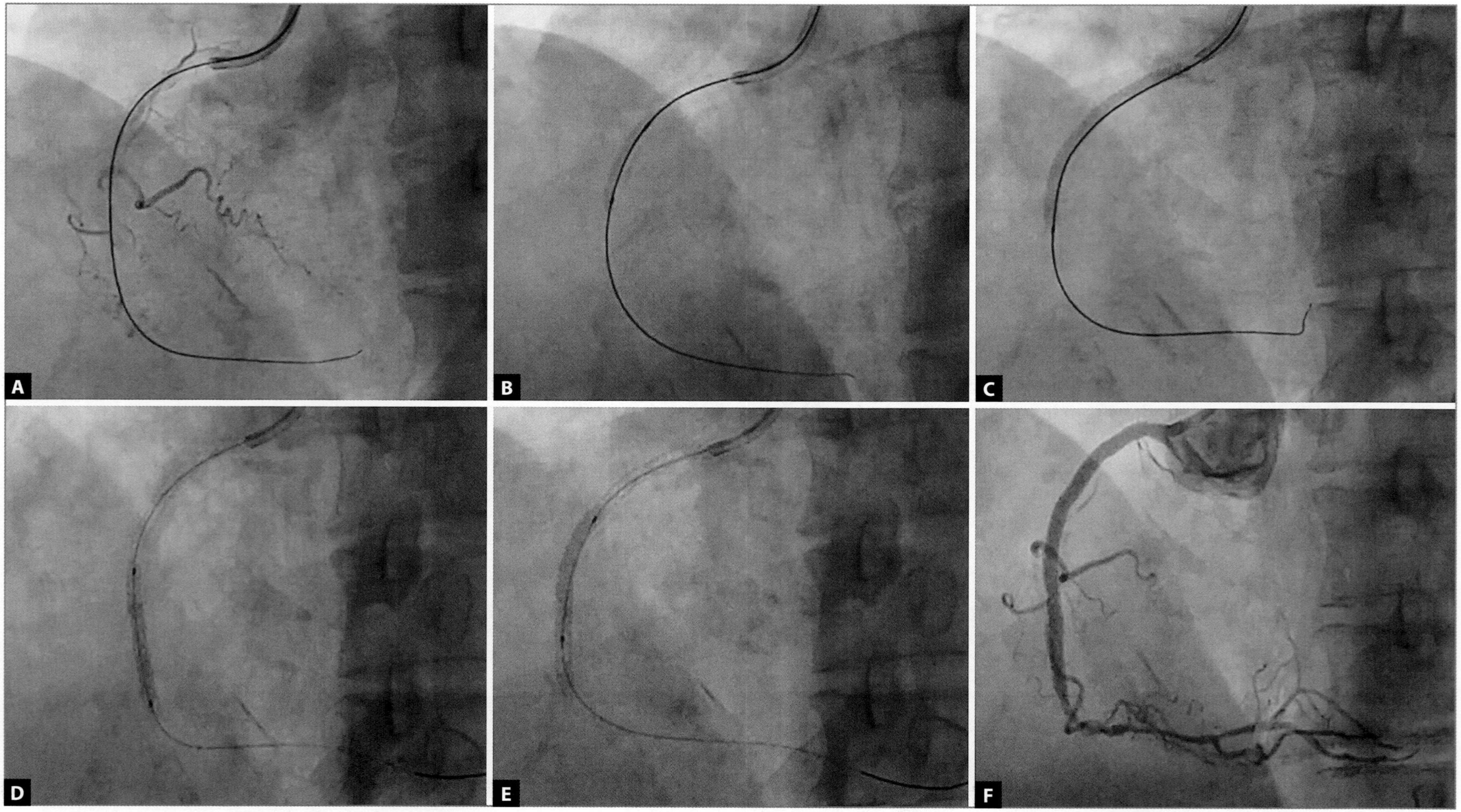

Figs. 11A to F: Coronary angioplasty of right coronary artery (RCA) vessel.

Pre-PCI assessment OCT of LMCA-LAD showed fibrocalcific plaque in distal LMCA and Proximal LAD **(Figs. 12A and B)**.

The LMCA engaged with EBU 3.5–7 Fr guiding catheter, LCX lesion was crossed with 0.014″ Fielder FC wire with fine cross microcatheter support. Predilated with 1.25 × 10 mm, 1.5 × 10 mm and 2.0 × 10 mm Tazuna balloons. Then with the GuideLiner support distal LCX stenting done with 2.5 × 22 mm Resolute Onyx Stent and proximal LCX with 3.0 × 12 mm Resolute Onyx stent. Postdilated with 3 mm NC balloon up to 14 atms. The final result was good with TIMI-III flow with no complications **(Figs. 13A to F)**.

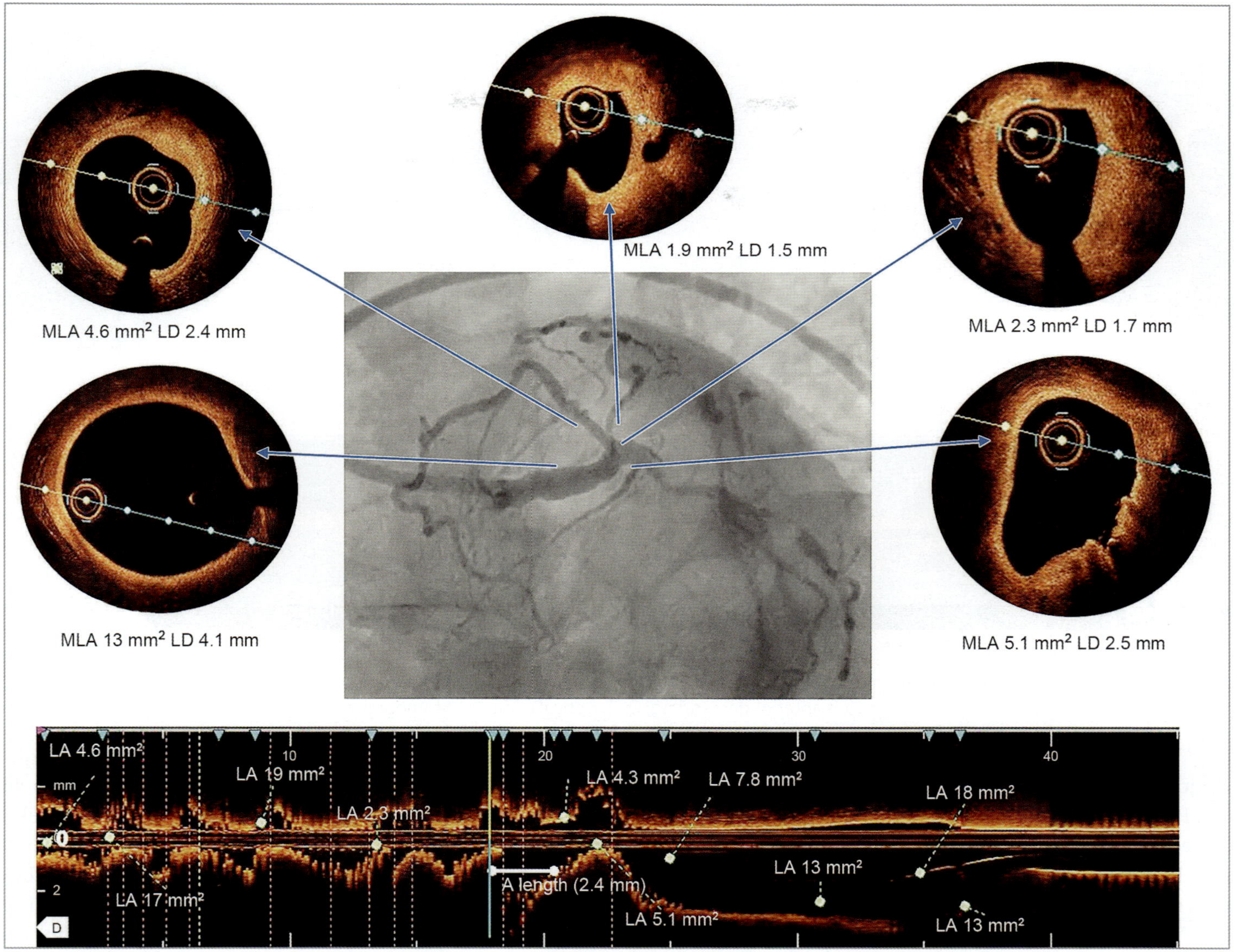
MLA 4.6 mm² LD 2.4 mm
MLA 1.9 mm² LD 1.5 mm
MLA 2.3 mm² LD 1.7 mm
MLA 13 mm² LD 4.1 mm
MLA 5.1 mm² LD 2.5 mm
LA 4.6 mm²
mm
LA 19 mm²
LA 2.3 mm²
LA 17 mm²
LA 4.3 mm²
LA 7.8 mm²
LA 18 mm²
LA 13 mm²
LA 5.1 mm²
LA 13 mm²
A length (2.4 mm)
10
20
30
40
2
D

Fig. 12A

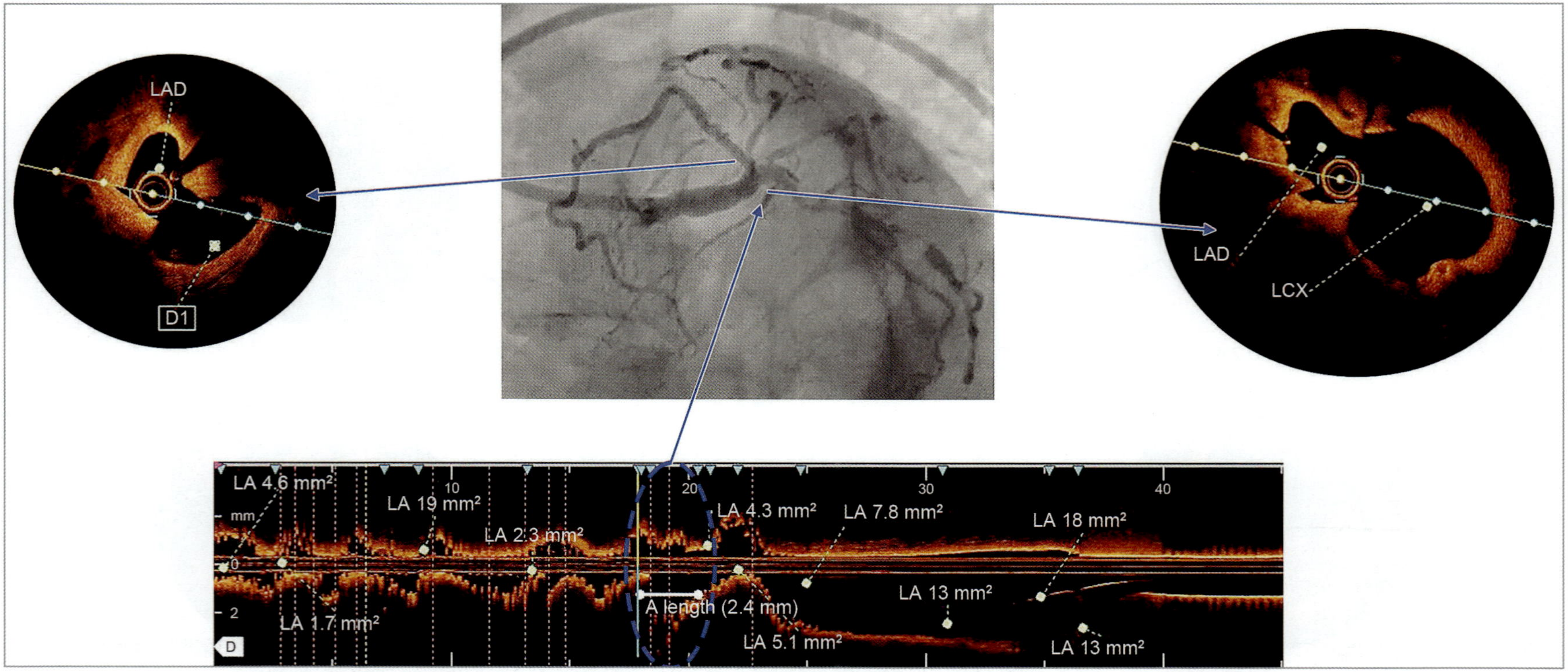

Fig. 12B

Figs. 12A and B: (A) Prestenting of LAD OCT assessment for devise selection and (B) showing narrowing at bifurcation zones. (LAD: left anterior descending; OCT: optical coherence tomography)

The LAD lesion was crossed with 0.014″ Sion Blue wire, predilated with 2.0 × 10 mm Tazuna balloon, stenting of LAD with 2.75 × 48 mm Xience Xpedition Stent. POT of LMCA was done with 4.5 × 12 mm NC Trek balloon up to 14 atms and LAD postdilated with 3.0 × 12 mm NC Trek balloon up to 16 atms. LCX wire recrossed through stent struts dilated with 2.0 × 10 mm Tazuna balloon. Kissing balloon dilation done with 3.0 × 12 mm NC Trek balloon in LAD and 3.0 × 12 mm NC Trek balloon in LCX up to 14 atms **(Figs. 14A to H)**. Poststenting OCT showed well-expanded stent struts in LMCA and LAD malapposition is seen in proximal LCX with fracture of few struts **(Figs. 15A and B)**. Second kissing balloon inflation done with 3.5 × 12 mm NC Trek balloon in LAD and 3.5 × 12 mm NC Trek balloon up to 12 atms. The final result was good with TIMI-III flow with no complications **(Figs. 16A to E)**.

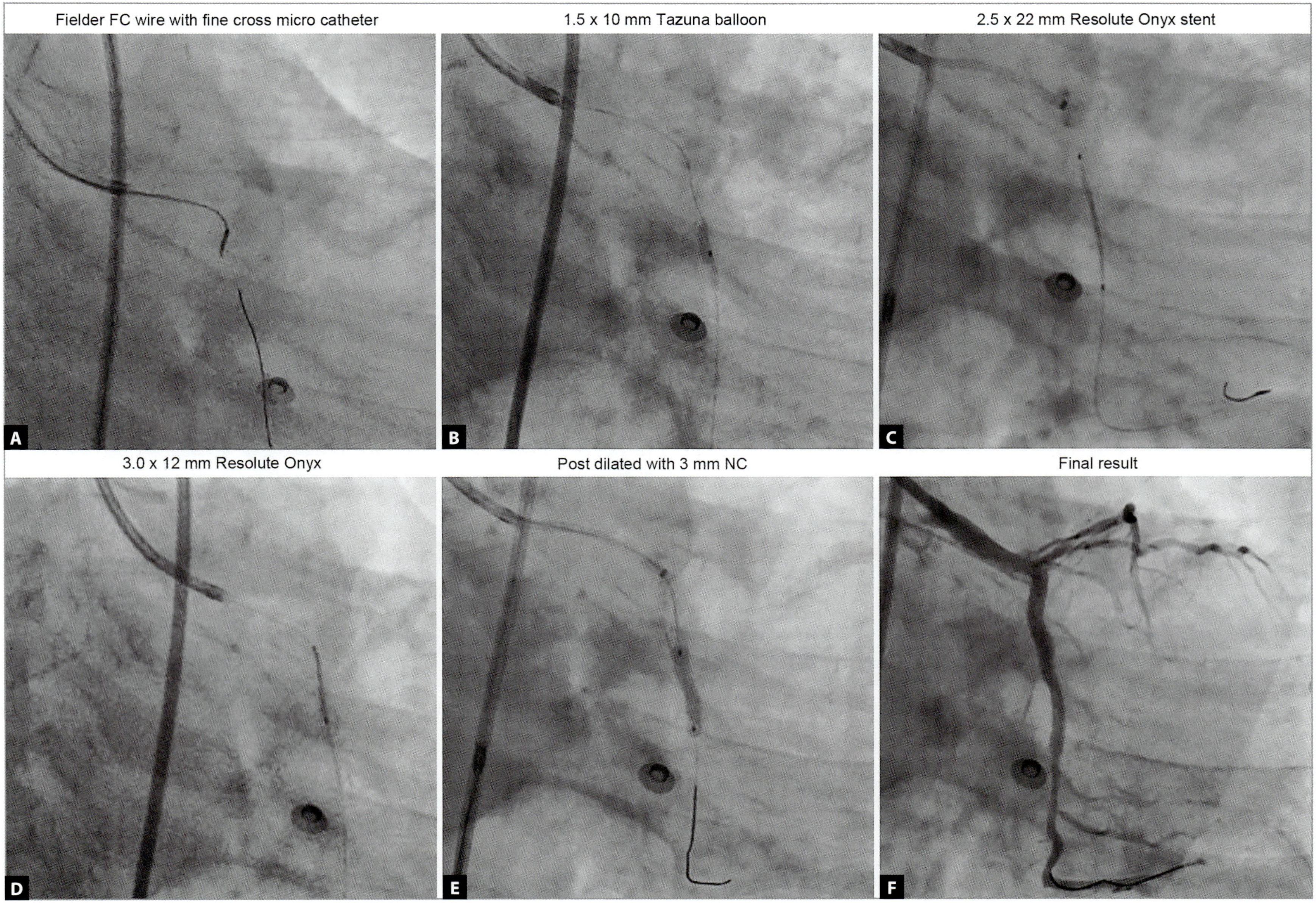

Figs. 13A to F: Coronary angioplasty of left circumflex (LCX) with GuideLiner and microcatheter support.

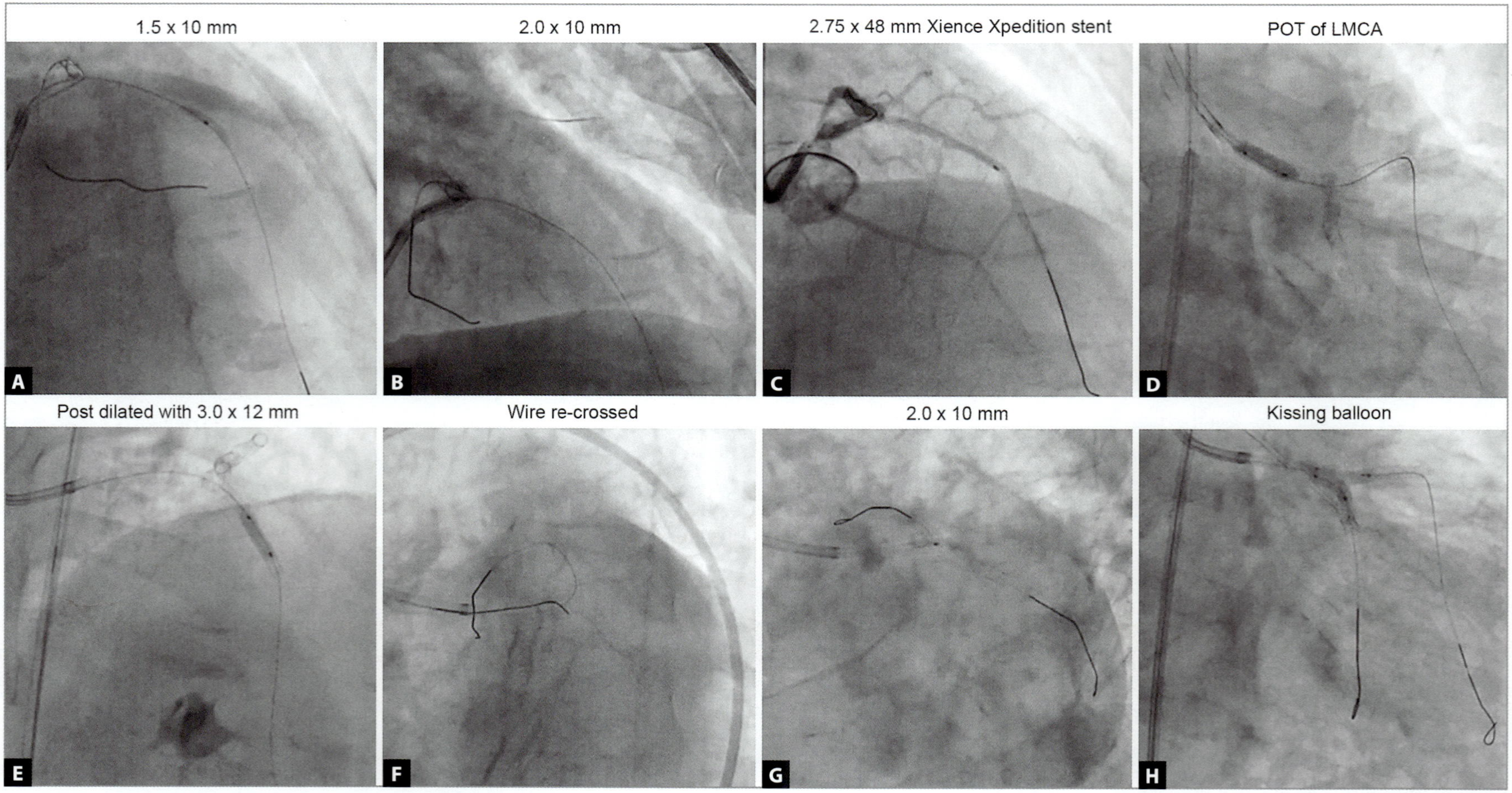

Fig. 14A to H: Coronary angioplasty of left anterior descending (LAD).

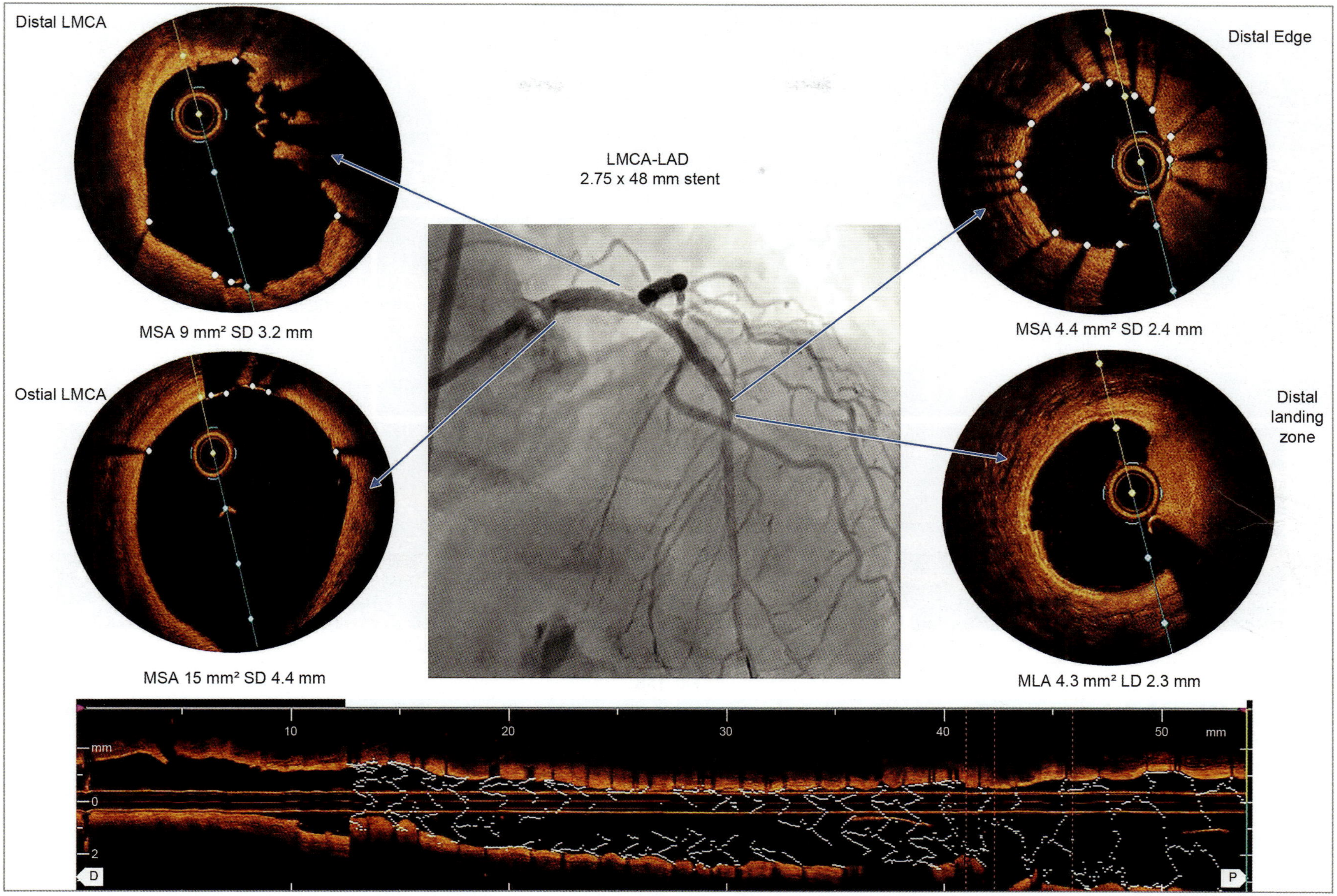
Distal LMCA
MSA 9 mm² SD 3.2 mm
Ostial LMCA
MSA 15 mm² SD 4.4 mm
LMCA-LAD
2.75 x 48 mm stent
Distal Edge
MSA 4.4 mm² SD 2.4 mm
Distal
landing
zone
MLA 4.3 mm² LD 2.3 mm
10
20
30
40
50
mm
0
2
D
P

Fig. 15A

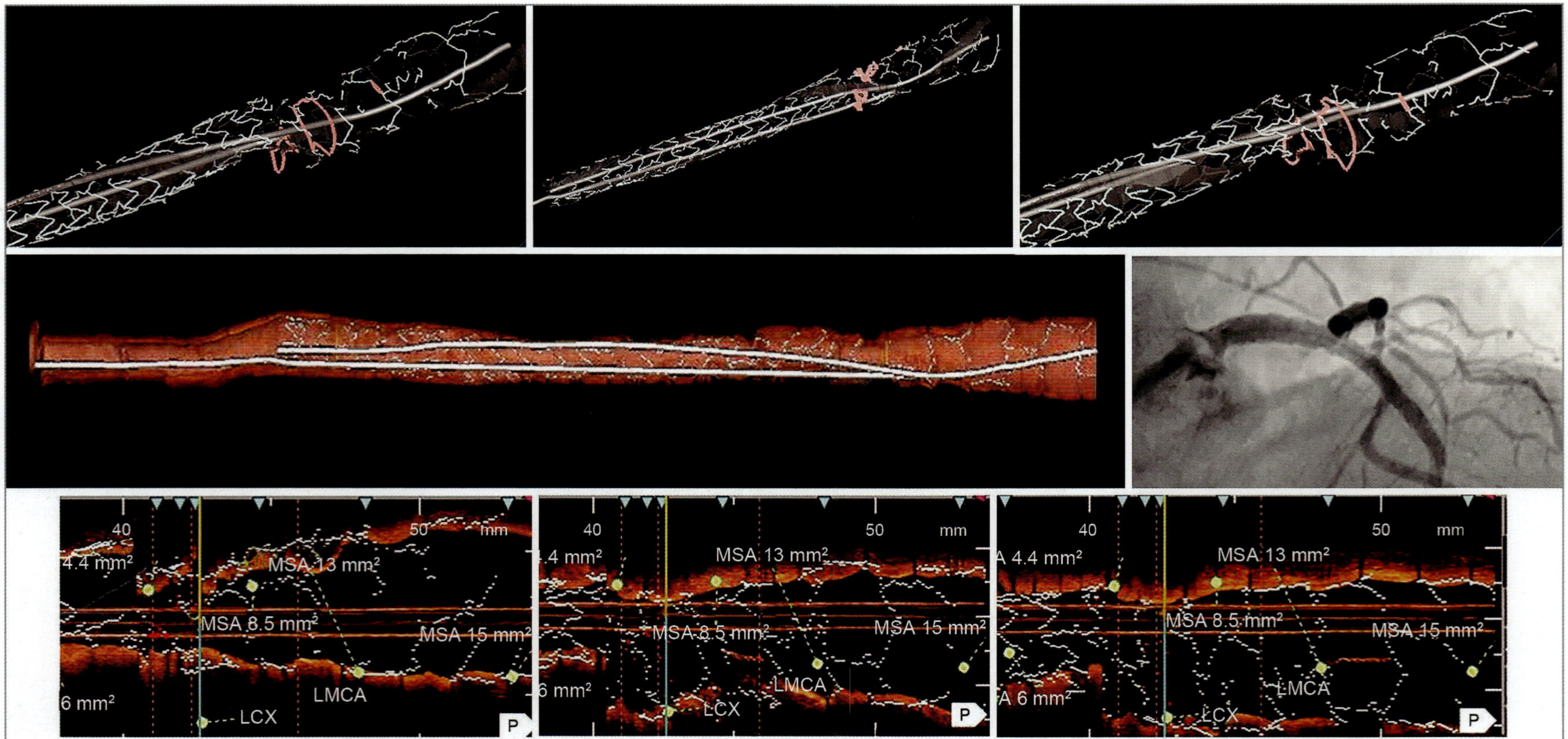

Stent fracture in distal LMCA which is non flow limiting, hence another stenting differed

Fig. 15B

Figs. 15A and B: (A) Poststenting OCT assessment for analysis of expansion, apposition and edge dissections. (B) Finding of stent fracture at LMCA bifurcation which is non flow limiting. (LAD: left anterior descending; LMCA: left main coronary artery; MLA: minimal luminal area; MSA: minimal stent area)

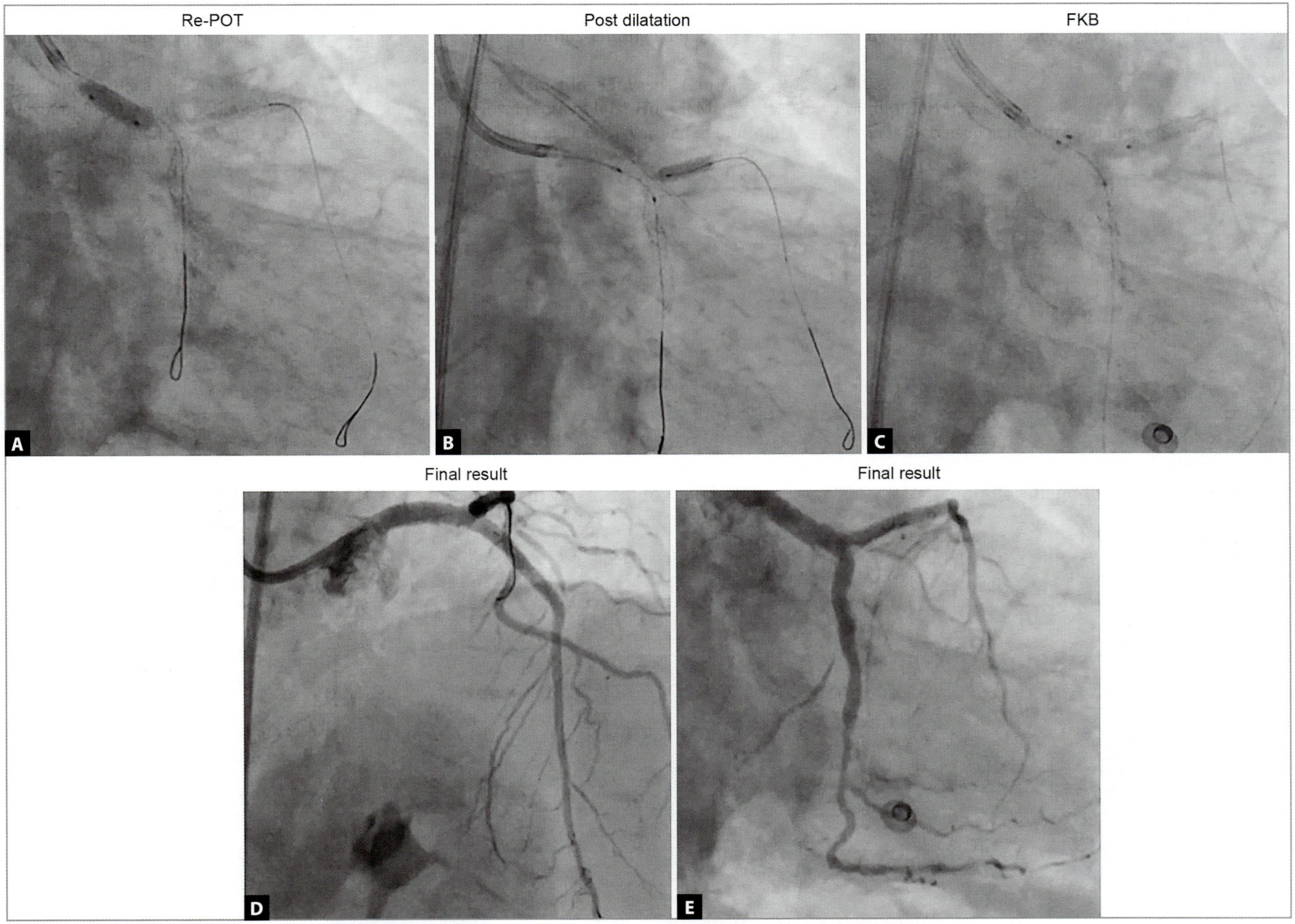

Figs. 16A to E: (A) Re-POT of LMCA, (B) postdilation of LAD, (C) final kissing balloon, and (D and E) final result which showed TIMI III flow. (LMCA: left main coronary artery; POT: proximal optimization technique; TIMI-III: thrombolysis in myocardial infarction III)

CHAPTER 17

Myocardial Bridging

INTRODUCTION

Myocardial bridging (MB) is a clinical condition when segment of a major epicardial coronary artery goes intramurally through the myocardium beneath the muscle bridge[1] which is visible on angiography as narrowing during systolic phase with normal or normal appearance in diastole due to milking effect of coronary by the myocardial compression. Although majority of the patients with MB are asymptomatic and carry good prognosis, still some patients present with acute coronary syndrome (ACS) or sudden events due to arrhythmias.

Possible mechanisms of the development of the MB responsible for coronary artery disease, and favorable treatments based on the causes are shown in **Flowchart 1**.

Flowchart 1: Intravascular ultrasound (IVUS) shows myocardial bridging with a variable degree of compression that persists into diastole, with the classical appearance of an echolucent—"half-moon phenomenon," seen only between the bridged coronary segment and epicardial tissue throughout the cardiac cycle.[2,3]

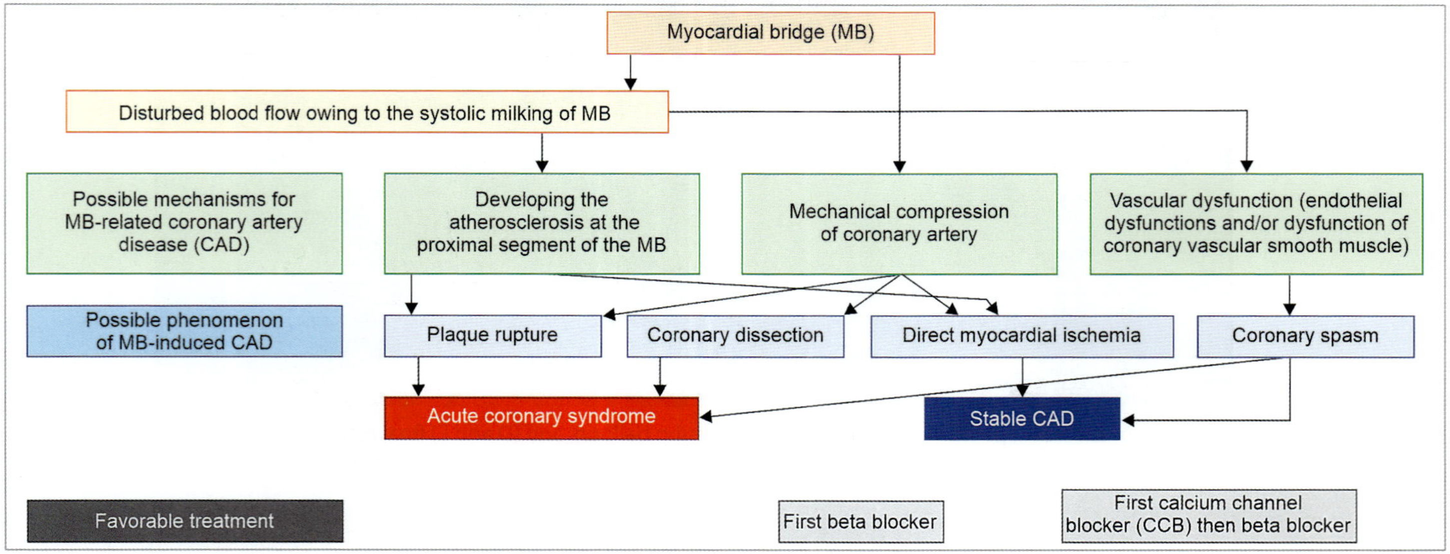

OCT IN ASSESSMENT OF MYOCARDIAL BRIDGING (FIGS. 1A AND B)

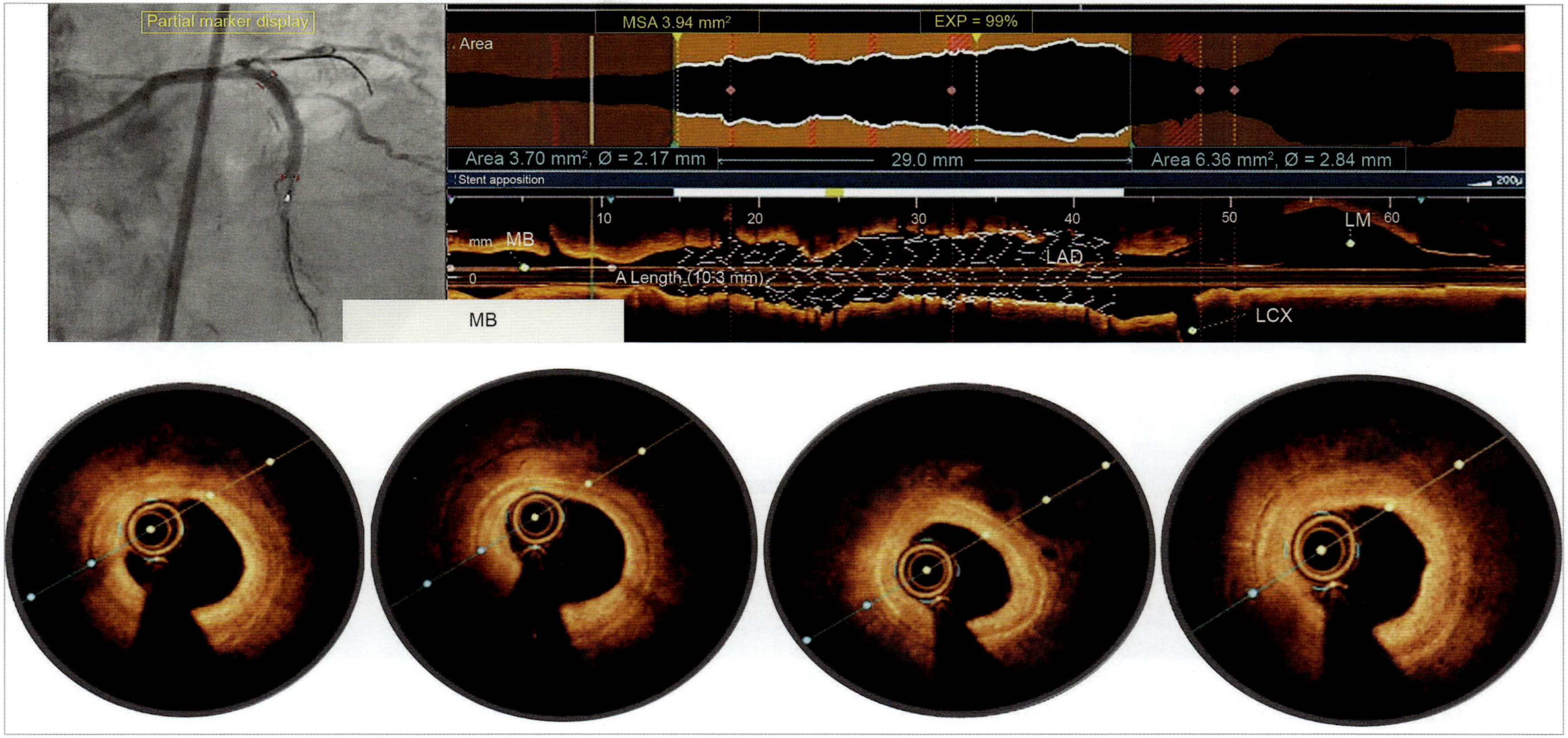

Fig. 1A

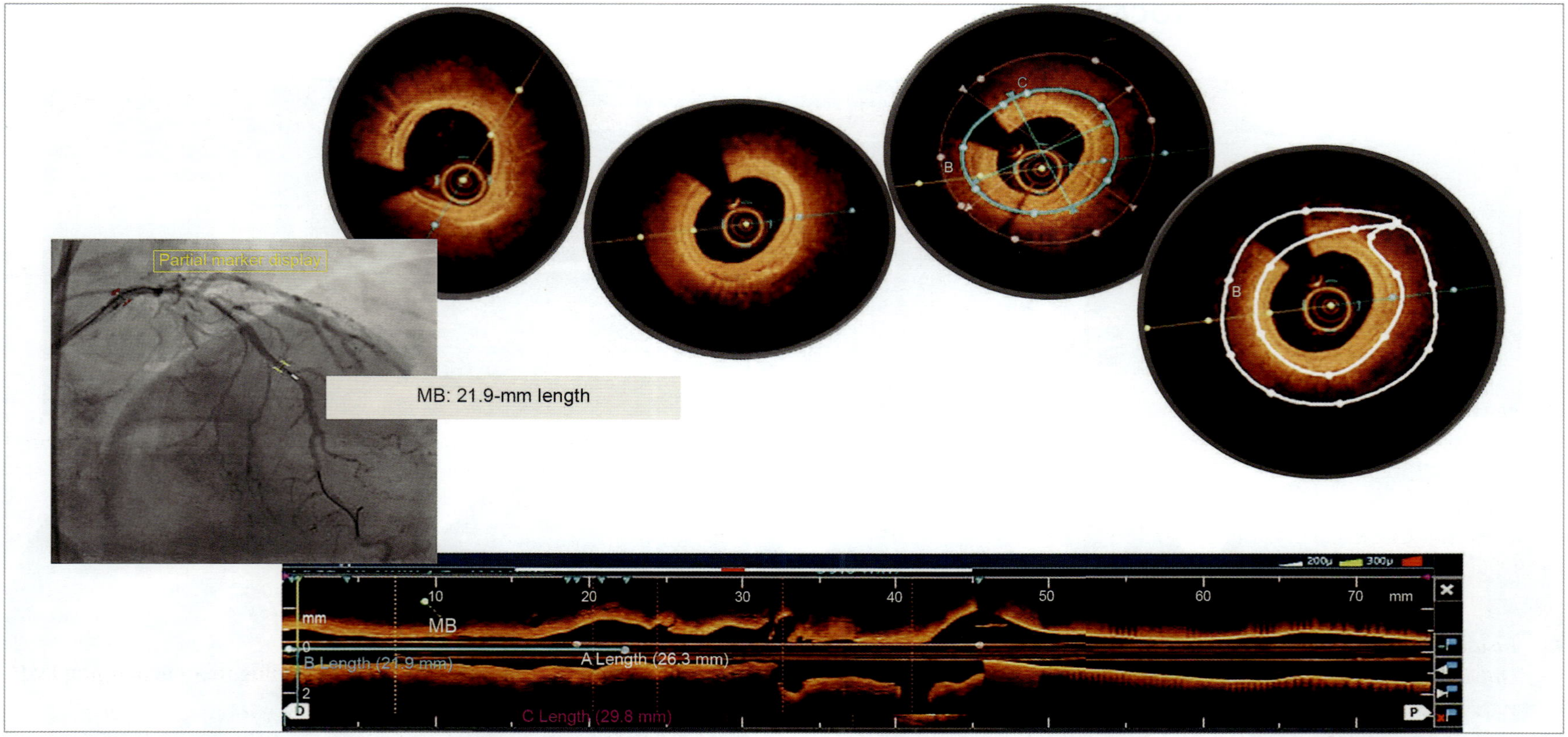

Fig. 1B

Figs. 1A and B: Myocardial bridging (MB) showed in two different cases. (LAD: left anterior descending; LCX: left circumflex; LM: left main; MSA: minimal stent area)

MANAGEMENT STRATEGY FOR LAD–MB

Flow diagram shows proposed management strategy of MB of the LAD (left anterior descending) on the basis of the presence of clinical symptoms and/or objective signs of ischemia.

REFERENCES

1. Daoud EM, Wafa AA. Does isolated myocardial bridge really interfere with coronary blood flow? Egypt Heart J. 2013;65(2):65-70.
2. Tarantini G, Migliore F, Cademartiri F, Fraccaro C, Iliceto S. Left anterior descending artery myocardial bridging: a clinical approach. J Am Coll Cardiol. 2016;68(25):2887-99.
3. Ye Z, Lai Y, Mintz GS, Yao Y, Tang J, Luo Y, et al. Fusiform Appearance of Myocardial Bridging Detected by OCT. JACC Cardiovasc Imaging. 2016;9(7):892-4.

CHAPTER 18

Spontaneous Coronary Artery Dissection

INTRODUCTION

Spontaneous coronary artery dissection (SCAD) is defined as a nontraumatic and noniatrogenic separation of the coronary arterial wall by intramural hemorrhage (IMH) and the resultant creation of a false lumen. The dissection plane can occur at the intimal medial or medial adventitial interface and need not have intimal dissection flap. IMH can occlude compromise the true vessel lumen leading to myocardial infarction (MI).

Spontaneous coronary artery dissection can present with various clinical symptoms and signs like acute coronary syndrome (ACS), arrhythmias, cardiogenic shock, and sudden death **(Fig. 1)**.

Possible mechanisms of SCAD:

- *"Inside-out" mechanism:* A "tear" in the endothelium-intima layer allows blood to accumulate in the media.
- *"Outside-in" mechanism:* Possibly due to consisting of microvessel rupture that occurs within the vessel wall **(Fig. 2)** leading to an expanding IMH, creating a false lumen.

Increased pressure in the false lumen, leads to compression of the true lumen, and the intima-media membrane may rupture, resulting in decompression of false lumen pressure and equalization of pressure between true and false lumens.

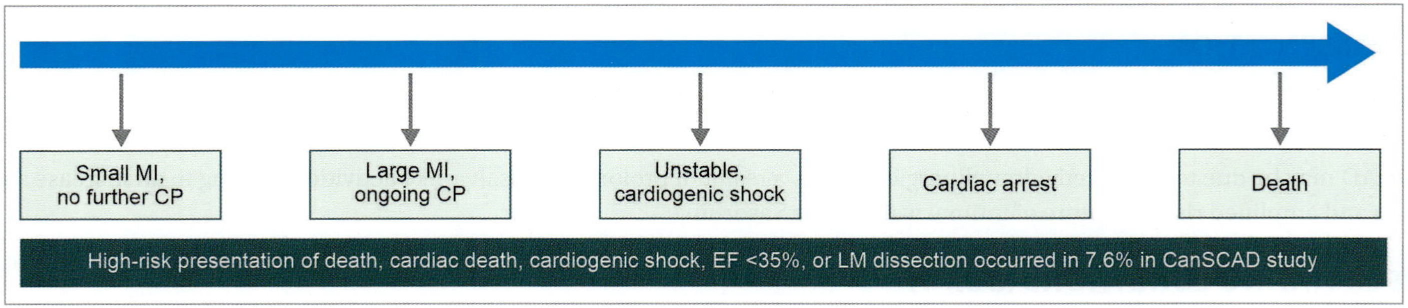

Fig. 1: Spectrum of spontaneous coronary artery dissection (SCAD) presentation. (CP: chest pain; CanSCAD: Canadian SCAD; EF: ejection fraction; LM: left main; MI: myocardial infarction)

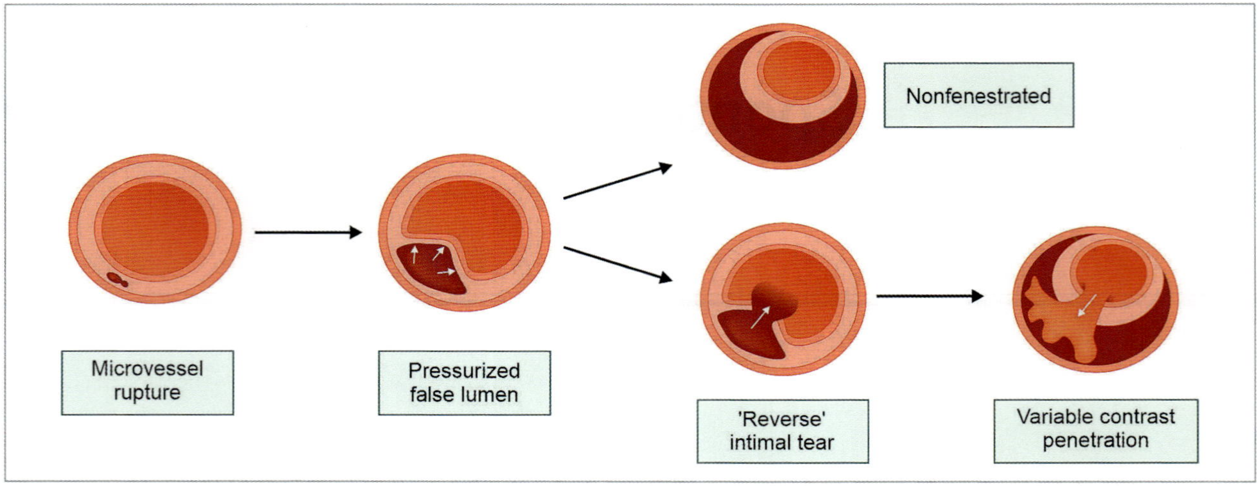

Fig. 2: Outside–in hypothesis.

BOX 1: SCAD-precipitating conditions.

Nonatherosclerotic conditions: Fibromuscular dysplasia (FMD), pregnancy, chronic use of hormonal therapy

Chronic inflammatory diseases: Polyarteritis nodosa, Crohn's disease, ulcerative colitis, sarcoidosis, Churg–Strauss syndrome, Wegener's, granulomatosis, rheumatoid arthritis, giant cell arteritis, celiac disease (vasculitis)

Connective tissue disorders: Ehlers–Danlos syndrome, systemic lupus erythematosus, Marfan syndrome, cystic medial necrosis, alpha-1 antitrypsin deficiency, polycystic kidney disease, significantly to the development of spontaneous coronary artery dissection (SCAD) (alteration of the elastic fibers composition of coronary wall)

Stressful events: Intense physical exercise, sympathetic–mimetic substances

CLINICAL PRESENTATION

Spontaneous coronary artery dissection may present with complete absence of symptoms to ACS, cardiogenic shock, cardiac arrest, or sudden cardiac death **(Box 1)**.

Pathogenesis: SCAD may be due to increased adrenalinergic drive as a result of prolonged Valsalva-like activities, leading to an increase sheer stress in of coronary arteries and amplified risk of rupture of intimal wall or vasa vasorum.[1]

SCAD-PRECIPITATING CONDITIONS (BOX 1)

Conventionally, SCAD is diagnosed when coronary angiogram (CAG) confirms findings of dissection or a diffuse narrowing lesion. However, several cases show unclear findings; therefore, it is difficult to accurately diagnose this disease using only CAG as a diagnostic tool.

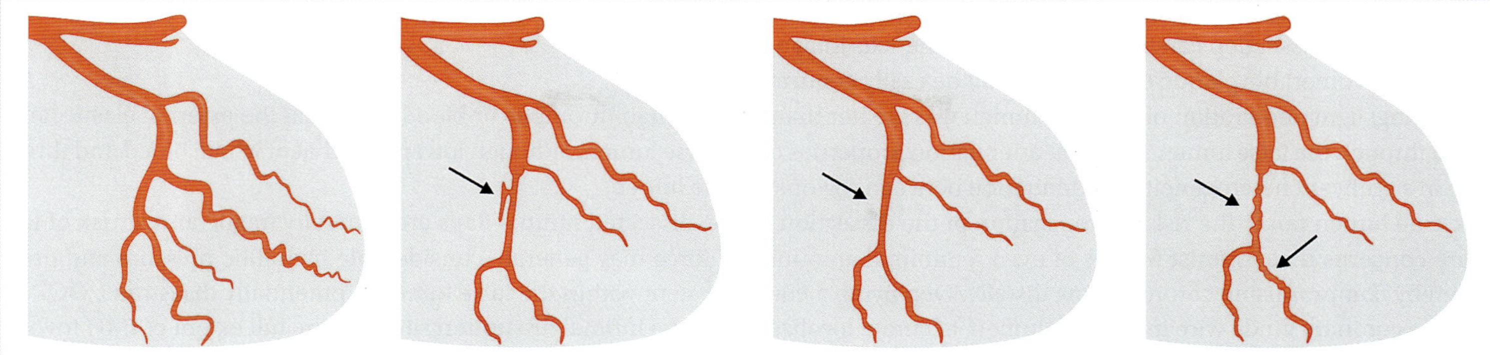

Fig. 3: Distinctive angiographic patterns to improve the diagnostic accuracy of spontaneous coronary artery dissection (SCAD).

Pathognomonic angiographic appearances may include multiple radiolucent lines, false lumen, contrast staining, and late contrast clearing. All of which are consistent with intimal tear.[2]

Saw proposed three distinctive angiographic patterns to improve the diagnostic accuracy of SCAD **(Fig. 3)**.

1. *Type 1:* Evident arterial wall stain has the characteristically described angiographic appearance and easily detected on CAG <30% of the patients with SCAD.
2. *Type 2 (67% of cases):* Angio shows widespread and long stenosis (typically >20 mm) limited either to the area of IMH (type 2A) or involving the coronary in toto (type 2B). It involves predominantly the mid to distal coronary segments with subtle but abrupt change in vessel caliber, significantly higher involvement of left anterior descendent (70–75% of cases) followed by the right coronary artery (20% of cases). Coronary artery spasm should be ruled out by giving intracoronary injection nitroglycerine before making a diagnosis of SCAD.
3. *Type 3:* Mimic atherosclerosis, stenosis on CAG, and is virtually impossible to diagnose without the adjunctive use of intracoronary imaging. It may have suggestive features such as long length, hazy or linear stenosis, and an absence of atherosclerotic changes in the other coronary arteries.

Type 2 and 3 SCAD are easily missed using conventional angiography.

Optical coherence tomography (OCT) useful in comprehensive visualization and assessment of coronary anatomy and pathology. OCT has proved to be an invaluable imaging modality in guiding the diagnosis of patients with suspected SCAD. It facilitates the visualization of IHM, double lumen, dissection flap at the intimal-media interface, which are readily defined on OCT. Alfonso and colleagues reported the largest prospective series of SCAD with OCT. The characteristic double lumen was seen in all cases, however only 3 of 11 had a distinct intimal flap or entry point, with the remainder showing IMH only without intimal flap. OCT also allows for detailed assessment and identification of the precise origin of intimal disruption, the length of affected vessel, thickness and distribution of dissection flap, magnitude of luminal compromise, side branch involvement, and associated thrombus formation.

Optical coherence tomography useful for diagnosis of SCAD:

- Lesions between the tunica intima and media can be accurately visualized.
- The boundary between the true and false lumen is clearly and distinctly noted.

- Presence/absence of thrombus occluding the false lumen can be assessed.
- The entire length of a dissection can be visualized in a long-axis image.
- The presence of a vulnerable plaque or thrombus can be easily confirmed.

On OCT imaging, light penetration of the false lumen was greater than that through thrombus or blood, such that the external elastic lamina (EEL) is often visualized through the false lumen. The light attenuation properties of the false lumen, although lower than that of whole blood and thrombi, are still high, resulting in significant heterogeneity of attenuation between regions of false lumen.

Wiring the true lumen poses the risk of propagation of the dissection plane, dissected intimal flaps are generally fragile and at risk of further extensions, there are concerns that contrast flushes of even a minimal amount and force may generate considerable hydraulic pressure and propagate axial dissection, thereby compromising coronary flow distally. Deploying a coronary stent within the false lumen is potentially disastrous. OCT confirms the positioning of the coronary guide wire in the true lumen, accurate localization of the intimal disruption site, and the full extent of IMH involved, thereby facilitating stent sizing and deployment. Adequate apposition of deployed stent struts is readily assessed using OCT, and this is important to avoid late stent thrombosis related to malapposition. This risk can be increased with acquired malapposition following resorption of the IMH with dissection healing.

When compared with OCT, IVUS is inferior in identifying intimal tears.

Optical coherence tomography was superior to IVUS in the recognition of intimal ruptures and intraluminal thrombi. The presence of a false lumen and IMH was well-elucidated by OCT, but their full extent could not be determined because of shadowing interference and inadequate penetration. This was easily overcome by concomitant use of IVUS which provided complete vessel visualization with the assessment of significantly longer diseased segment and larger false lumen areas. IVUS provides useful pictures of the underlying substrate, even in patients without antegrade coronary flow and in those with an occlusive intracoronary thrombus.[3]

Optical coherence tomography can show clearly intimal tear with entry and exit points, true lumen, false lumen, and sometimes organized thrombus in the false lumen due to its high-resolution images compared to IVUS **(Fig. 4)**.

SCAD MANAGEMENT

If patient is asymptomatic without any hemodynamic imbalance, conservative medical management is the best option. Revascularization is indicated if ongoing cardiovascular symptom or cardiogenic shock is present. Percutaneous coronary intervention (PCI) should be considered in patients with localized proximal dissections in large vessel associated with ongoing ischemia or reduced TIMI (thrombolysis in myocardial infarction) flow. PCI can be performed by using new-generation drug-eluting stents (DES) and cutting balloon to decompress false lumen. PCI success rate 64–91%, high complication rate (iatrogenic dissection, extension of dissection, stent thrombosis, etc.). Oversized stent or aggressive dilatation with oversized balloon may lead to propagation of the dissection or perforation. Direct stenting may be preferable to predilatation when possible and the stent placement can be guided by OCT. In recent cohort of 168 patients, 33 underwent PCI, which was unsuccessful in 12 cases (36%). Of those cases with successful or partially successful PCI, 57% had extension of dissection, and 6%, 24%, 12% had subsequent stent thrombosis, restenosis, or required coronary artery bypass graft, respectively. Overall, the number of PCIs with a durable, successful result was a meagre 30%.[4]

Coronary artery bypass graft should be reserved for patients with left main or multivessel proximal large-vessel dissection, especially in the setting of hemodynamic compromise particularly when PCI is not feasible or has failed. However, graft patency failure after the resolution of the IMH and restoration of native coronary flow has been reported, presumably caused by competitive flow in the native arteries.

Routine long-term therapy with aspirin and a beta blocker is advised. Routine thrombolytic therapy should be differed due to potential expansion and extension of IMH leading to sudden clinical deterioration of patients with SCAD.[5]

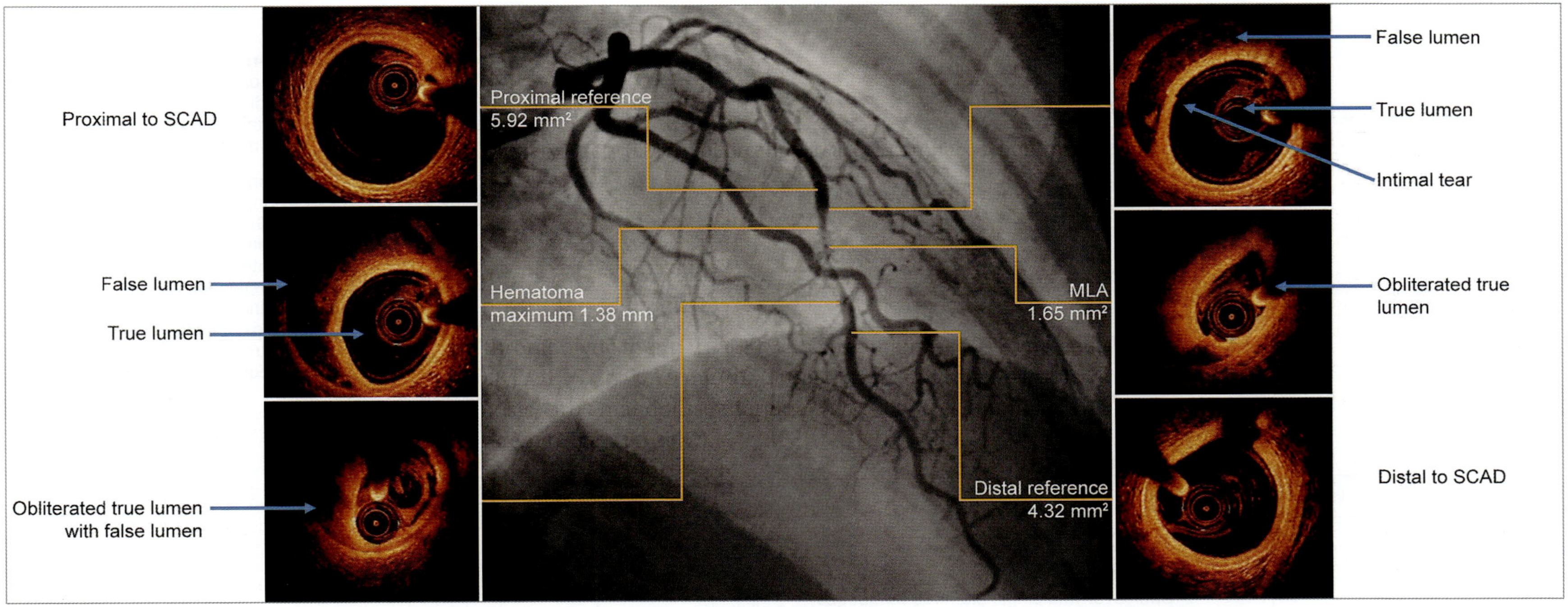

Fig. 4: Optical coherence tomography (OCT) assessment of spontaneous coronary artery dissection (SCAD) showing intimal tear and true and false lumen. (MLA: minimal lumen area)

Indicators for conservative treatment:

- Reserved thrombolysis in myocardial infarction (TIMI 2–3) blood flow
- The presence of a thrombus occluding the false lumen
- Confirmation that there is no entry tear of the dissection
- The absence of a thrombus in the true lumen
- OCT is inappropriate if contrast pooling is seen on angiography because of the risk of expanding the dissection cavity secondary to the injection of contrast medium. It remains a very useful diagnostic technique in cases in which at least TIMI 2–3 blood flow is reserved.
- Avoid where the diagnosis of SCAD is clear at angiography and conservative management is practical.
- OCT identifies the position of the guidewire whether it is in true or false lumen prior to balloon dilatation and stenting.

Davlouros et al. reported that OCT was used to confirm the spontaneous healing of SCAD within 4 months. Alfonso et al. also reported the SCAD spontaneously disappeared in 7 of 13 patients during 6 years of follow-up. With the exact mechanism underlying the spontaneous resolution of SCAD, it has been hypothesized that thrombus formation in the false lumen occludes the false lumen and causes fibrosis between the two dissected layers in cases with aortic dissection. It is presumed that the intramural hematoma found in the false lumen is gradually absorbed due to some unknown mechanism, and finally, the inner membrane and media are reorganized with the restoration of the normal three-layer structure of blood vessels.[2]

The SCAD-PCI algorithm is given in the **Figure 5** for better understanding.

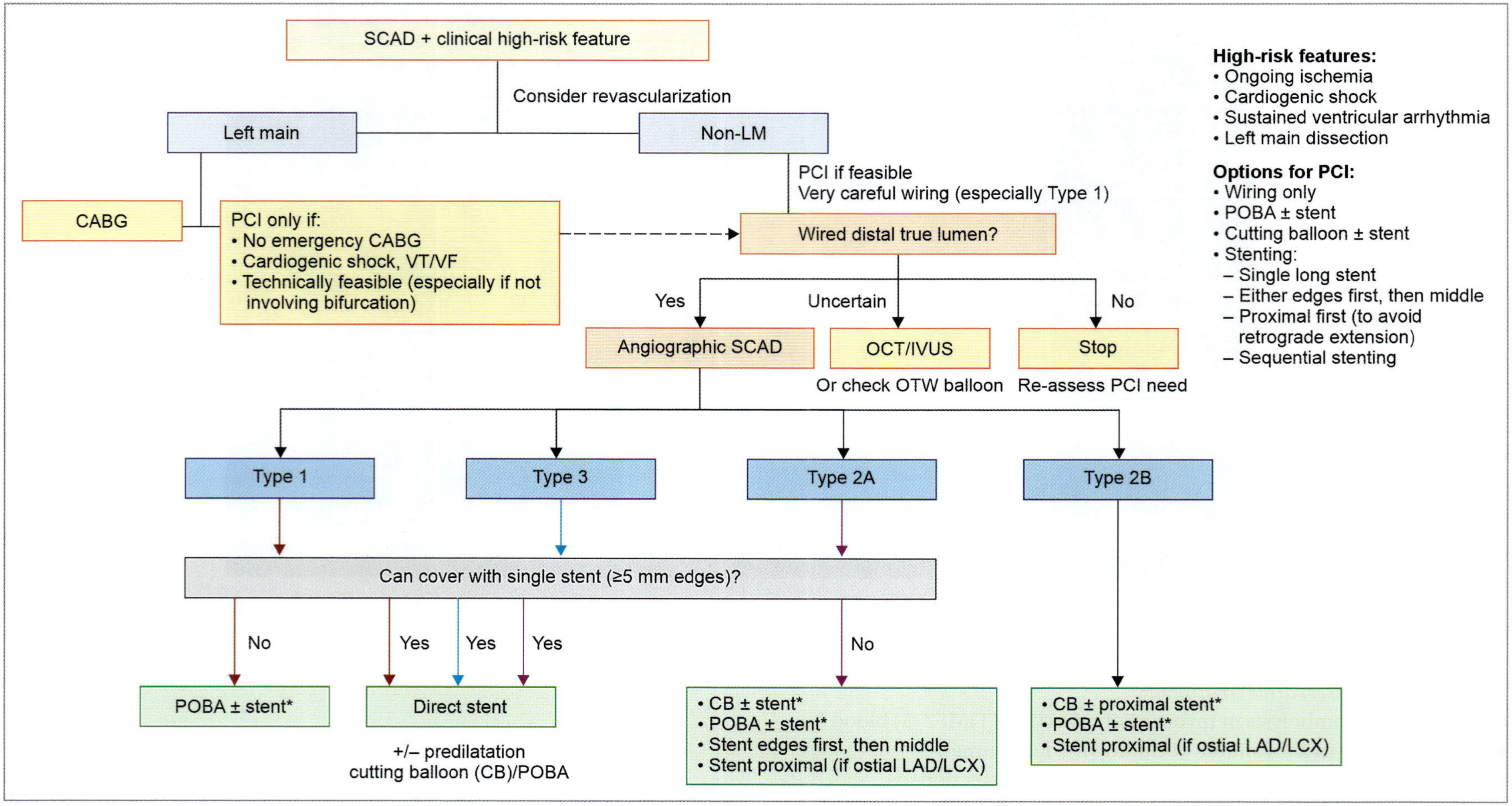

Fig. 5: Spontaneous coronary artery dissection (SCAD)–percutaneous coronary intervention (PCI) algorithm. (CABG: coronary artery bypass graft; IVUS: intravascular ultrasound; LAD: left anterior descending; LCX: left circumflex; OCT: optical coherence tomography; OTW: over-the-wire; POBA: plain old balloon angioplasty; VF: ventricular fibrillation; VT: ventricular tachycardia)

*Can avoid stenting especially if normal flow + no residual dissection.

REFERENCES

1. Sivam S, Yozghatlian V, Dentice R, McGrady M, Moriarty C, Di Michiel J, et al. Spontaneous coronary artery dissection associated with coughing. J Cyst Fibros. 2014;13(2):235-7.
2. Kanda T, Tawarahara K, Matsukura G, Matsunari M, Takabayashi R, Tamura J, et al. The diagnosis of spontaneous coronary artery dissection by optical coherence tomography. Intern Med. 2018;57(4):523-6.
3. Alfonso F, Bastante T, Cuesta J, Rodríguez D, Benedicto A, Rivero F. Spontaneous coronary artery dissection: novel insights on diagnosis and management. Cardiovasc Diagn Ther. 2015;5(2):133-40.
4. Saw J, Humphries K, Aymong E, Sedlak T, Prakash R, Starovoytov A, et al. Spontaneous coronary artery dissection: clinical outcomes and risk of recurrence. J Am Coll Cardiol. 2017;70(9):1148-58.
5. Pepe M, Cecere A, Napodano M, Ciccone MM, Bartolomucci F, Navarese EP, et al. How to approach a spontaneous coronary artery dissection: an up-to-date. Interv Cardiol J. 2017;3(1):3.

CHAPTER 19

Ectatic Coronary Arteries

CASE 1

Optical coherence tomography (OCT) assessment of percutaneous coronary intervention (PCI) of recanalized thrombus and ectatic left circumflex (LCX).

CLINICAL HISTORY

A 52-year-old male, known hypertensive, presented with evolved interior wall (IW) + posterior wall myocardial infarction (PWMI) (late presentation) Window period (WP) > 24 hours, epigastric burning sensation, orthopnea due to acute pulmonary edema as a result of acute severe mitral regurgitation (MR).

On examination (O/E): Pulse rate (PR)—110 beats/min, blood pressure (BP)—110/70 mm Hg, peripheral oxygen saturation (SPO_2)—85% on right atrium (RA), heart—S^1+, S^2+, $S3^{+}$, $S4^0$, 2/6 pansystolic murmur in mitral area, lungs: bilateral basal crepitation. Investigations: hemoglobin (Hb)—13.6 g%, serum creatinine—1.1 mg/dL, blood urea—29 mg/dL, random blood sugar (RBS)—114 mg/dL. Electrocardiogram (ECG)—evolved IW + PWMI, 2D Echo—regional wall motion abnormality (RWMA) in right coronary artery (RCA) territory, hypokinetic basal IW and posterior wall, mild left ventricular (LV) dysfunction, severe MR, trivial tricuspid regurgitation (TR)/mild pulmonary arterial hypertension (PAH), ejection fraction (EF)—45%.

Angio showed triple-vessel disease with left main coronary artery (LMCA)—normal, left anterior descending (LAD)—mid short segment ambiguous lesion, high thrombus burden containing lesion of LCX (dominant), RCA—nondominant mild disease **(Figs. 1A to D)**.

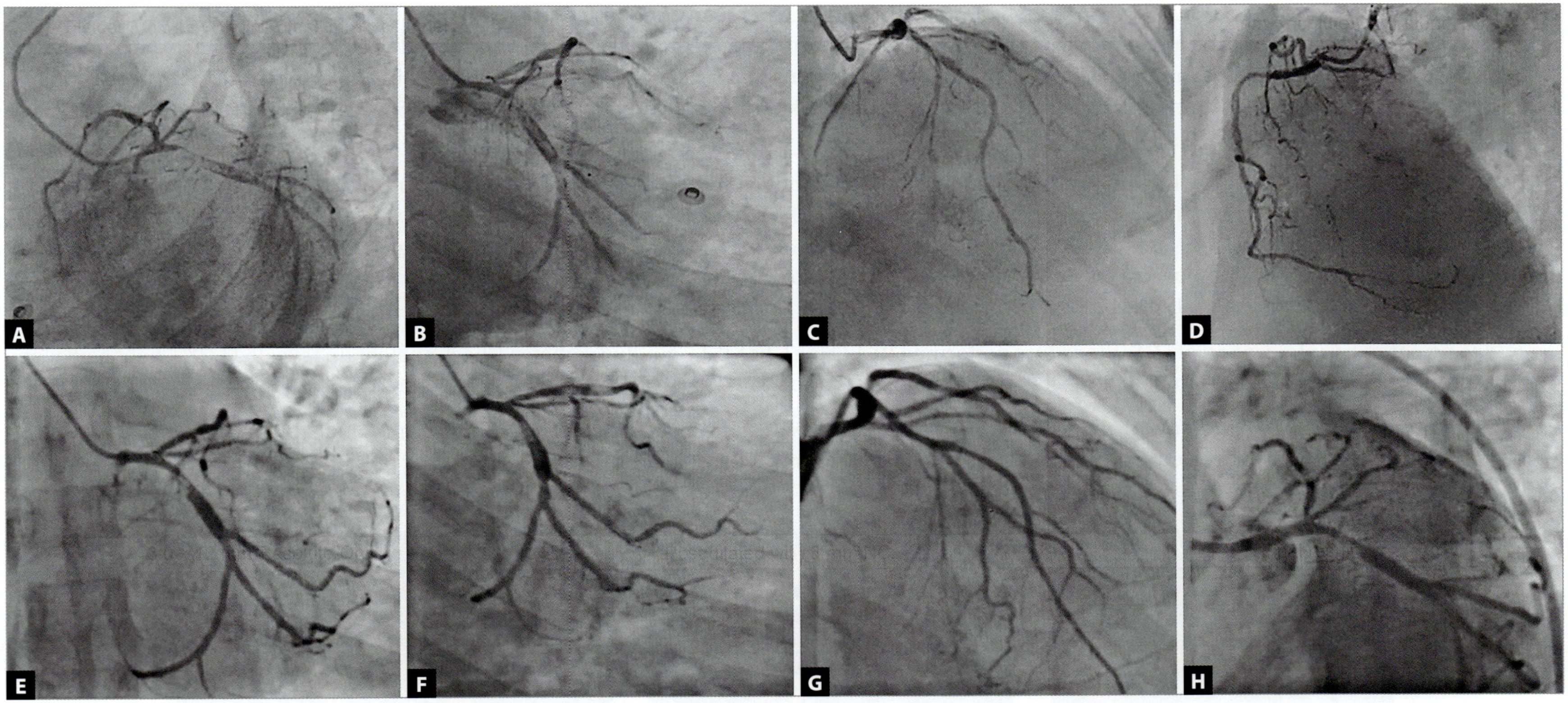

Figs. 1A to H: (A to D) Coronary angiogram; (E and F) Post-thrombolytic therapy (TLT) angiogram; (G and H) 30 days later angiogram.

PROCEDURE

In view of massive thrombotic burden, PCI with stenting was differed, intracoronary (IC) thrombolytic therapy [Inj. tenecteplase (TNK) 10 mg and integrilin 10-mL bolus] was given and intravenous (IV) integrilin infusion continued for another 24 hours. Clinical status markedly improved over a period of 48 hours with relief of pulmonary edema and angina. Three days later repeat angio showed decreased thrombotic burden of LCX lesion with distal TIMI III (thrombolysis in myocardial infarction III) flow **(Figs. 1E and F)**.

Patient was managed with medications and discharged on seventh day, and advised to continue anticoagulation treatment for 30 days. Thallium assessment was done prior to repeat angio which showed totally viable LAD and RCA, significantly viable myocardium in LCX territory. Check angio after 1 month showed LAD—short-segment ambiguous lesion, LCX—tight narrowing with 70–80% lesion, markedly reduced MR. OCT was planned to assess the severity of LAD lesion and to decide management strategy—PCI versus CABG **(Figs. 1G and H)**.

Percutaneous coronary intervention of LAD: Procedure performed through right femoral artery (RFA) using 6 Fr XB 3.5 guiding catheter. Coronary angiogram (CAG) revealed mid short segment ambiguous lesion, initially tried with Sion and Fielder XT but could not cross the lesion, acute total occlusion of LAD happened while attempting to cross ambiguous lesion leading to sudden onset of severe chest pain, ST elevation in anterior leads with hypotension and severe sweating. After multiple attempts finally lesion was crossed with Gaia I wire, predilatation was done with 2.5 × 15 mm Mini Trek balloon.

Pre-OCT analysis: Pre-OCT distal LAD red thrombus, LAD/D1 bifurcation—recanalized thrombus **(Figs. 2A to D)**.

Pre-OCT showed LAD to LMCA which showed distal LMCA fibrotic plaque minimal lumen area (MLA)—6.2 mm^2, minimal lumen diameter (MLD)—2.2 mm, mid LMCA MLA—11 mm^2, MLD—3.75 mm, ostium LAD MLA—3.9 mm^2, MLD—2.2 mm **(Figs. 3A to D)**.

Left anterior descending stenting done with 3.0 × 28 mm Xience Xpedition stent [drug-eluting stent (DES)] **(Figs. 4A)**.

Post-OCT study showed well-apposed stent struts, no dissection, and no edge dissection.

Post-OCT of LAD showed ostium LAD MLA—6.5 mm^2, MLD—2.87 mm, distal portion of stent MLA—6.2 mm^2, MLD—2.8 mm **(Figs. 5A to D)**.

Percutaneous coronary intervention of LCX: Procedure performed RFA using 6 Fr XB 3.5 guiding catheter. Check angiogram revealed LCX—tight narrowing with 70–80% lesion, Sion blue wire crossed the lesion. Predilatation was done with 2.5 × 08 mm Mini Trek balloon.

Pre-OCT analysis: LCX to LMCA showed tight narrowing with 70%–80% lesion, distal to LCX/OM (obtuse marginal) bifurcation MLA—4.5 mm^2, MLD—2.38 mm, proximal to LCX/OM ectatic vessel with MLA—14.2 mm^2, MLD—4.26 mm, distal portion of proximal LCX lesion MLA—3.4 mm^2,

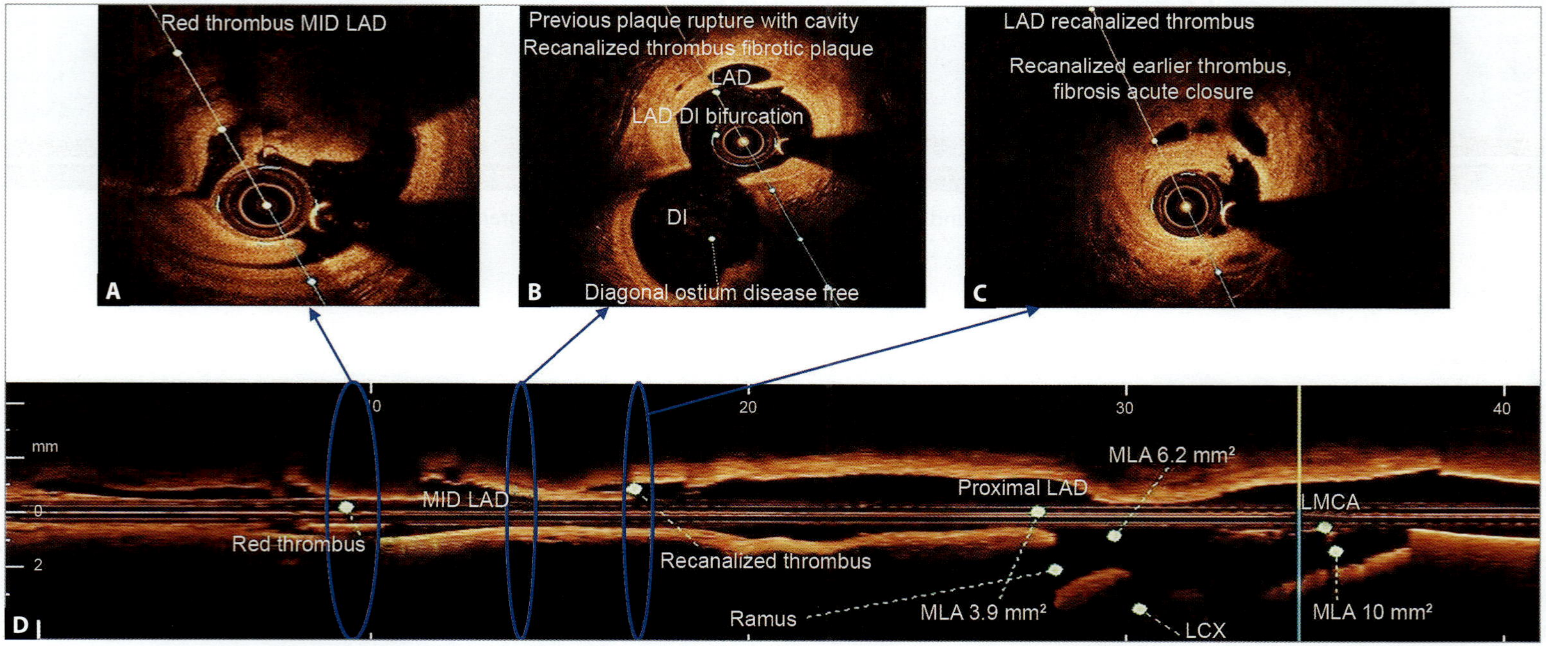

Figs. 2A to D: Pre-OCT distal LAD red thrombus, LAD/D1 bifurcation—recanalized thrombus. (LAD: left anterior descending; LCX: left circumflex; LMCA: left main coronary artery; MLA: minimal lumen area)

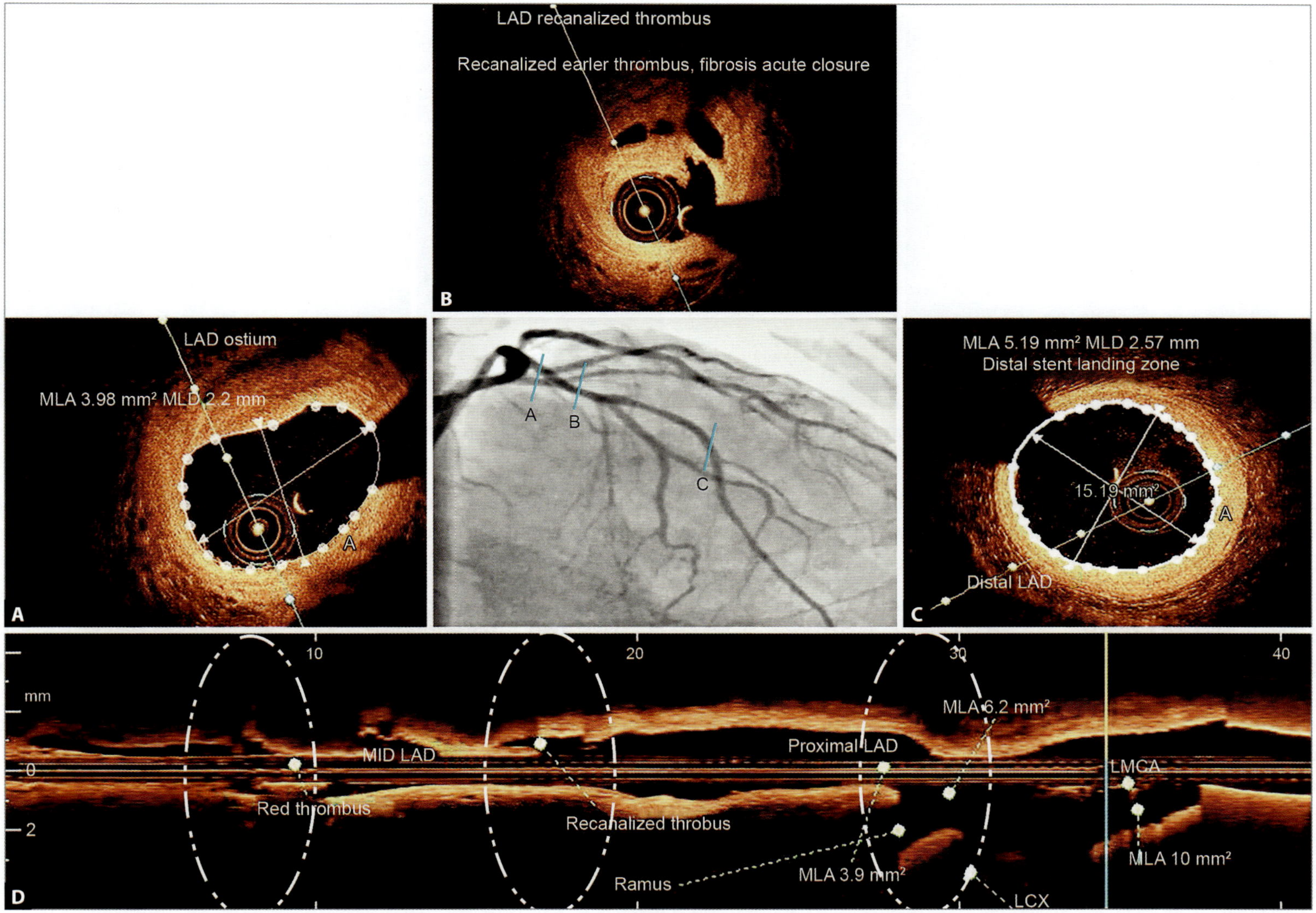

Figs. 3A to D: Pre-OCT assessment of plaque morphology and device selection. (LAD: left anterior descending; LCX: left circumflex; LMCA: left main coronary artery; MLA: minimal lumen area; MLD: minimal lumen diameter)

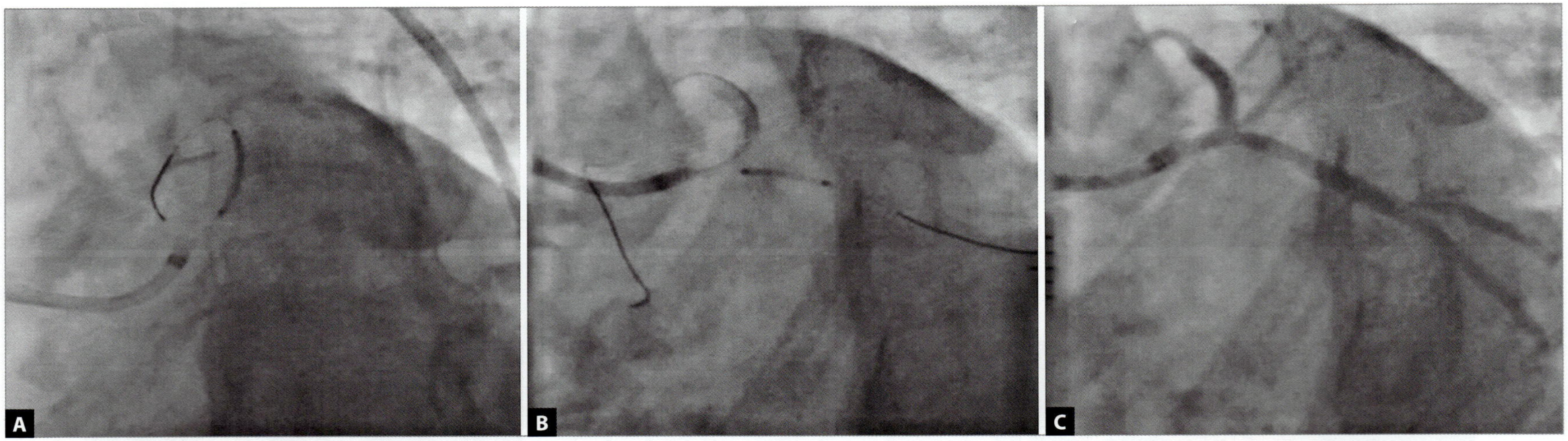

Figs. 4A to C: (A) Coronary angioplasty of left anterior descending (LAD); (B and C) Coronary angioplasty of left circumflex (LCX).

MLD—2.08 mm, tight recanalized thrombus proximal LCX with MLA—2.1 mm^2, MLD—1.6 mm, ostium of LCX MLA—6.2 mm^2, MLD—2.8 mm. Total length of the narrowed proximal segment of LCX [from left main (LM) bifurcation ectatic segment of LCX] was 11.2 mm **(Figs. 6A and B)**.

LCX lesion stenting done with 3 × 12 mm Xience Xpedition stent and final result **(Figs. 4B and C)**.

Post-OCT analysis: Post-OCT LCX to LMCA showed distal just at LCX/OM bifurcation MLA—2.86 mm^2, MLD—1.88 mm, LCX ostium MLA—5.94 mm^2, MLD—2.75 mm **(Figs. 7A to D)**.

Postprocedure angio view showed well-implanted stents with TIMI-III flow without any dissection. Patient was discharged on third postprocedure in a stable status.

Optical coherence tomography is very useful in choosing proper landing zones by assessing luminal areas of different segments of coronary artery with significant size mismatch, and choosing proper device size. OCT assesses plaque morphology and helps in identifying any need for plaque modification strategy. Image-guided optimization PCI with covering significantly diseased segment improves acute and long-term outcomes.

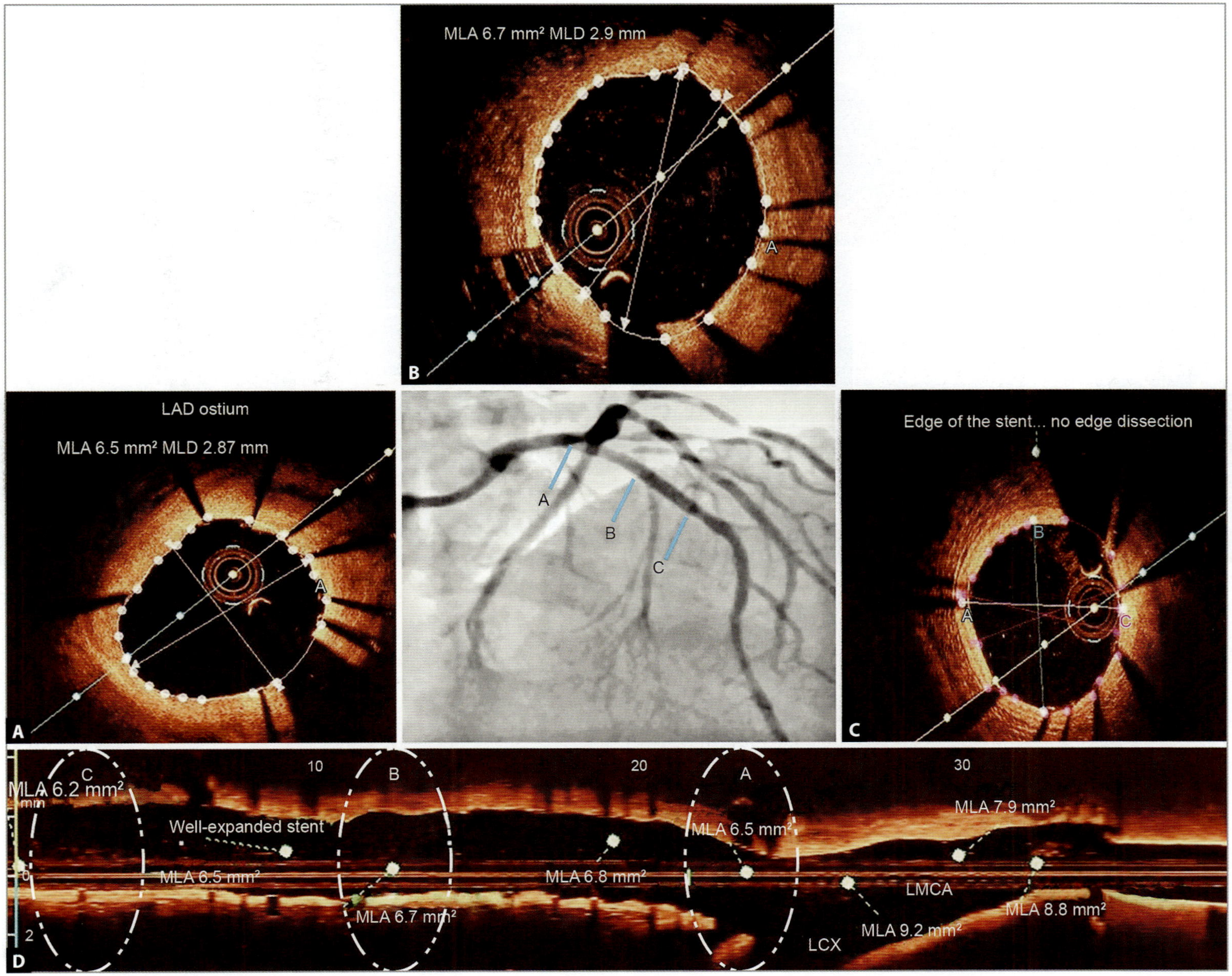

Figs. 5A to D: Post-OCT of left anterior descending (LAD) showed well-expanded, no edge dissection, and no tissue prolapse. (LCX: left circumflex; LMCA: left main coronary artery; MLA: minimal lumen area; MLD: minimal lumen diameter)

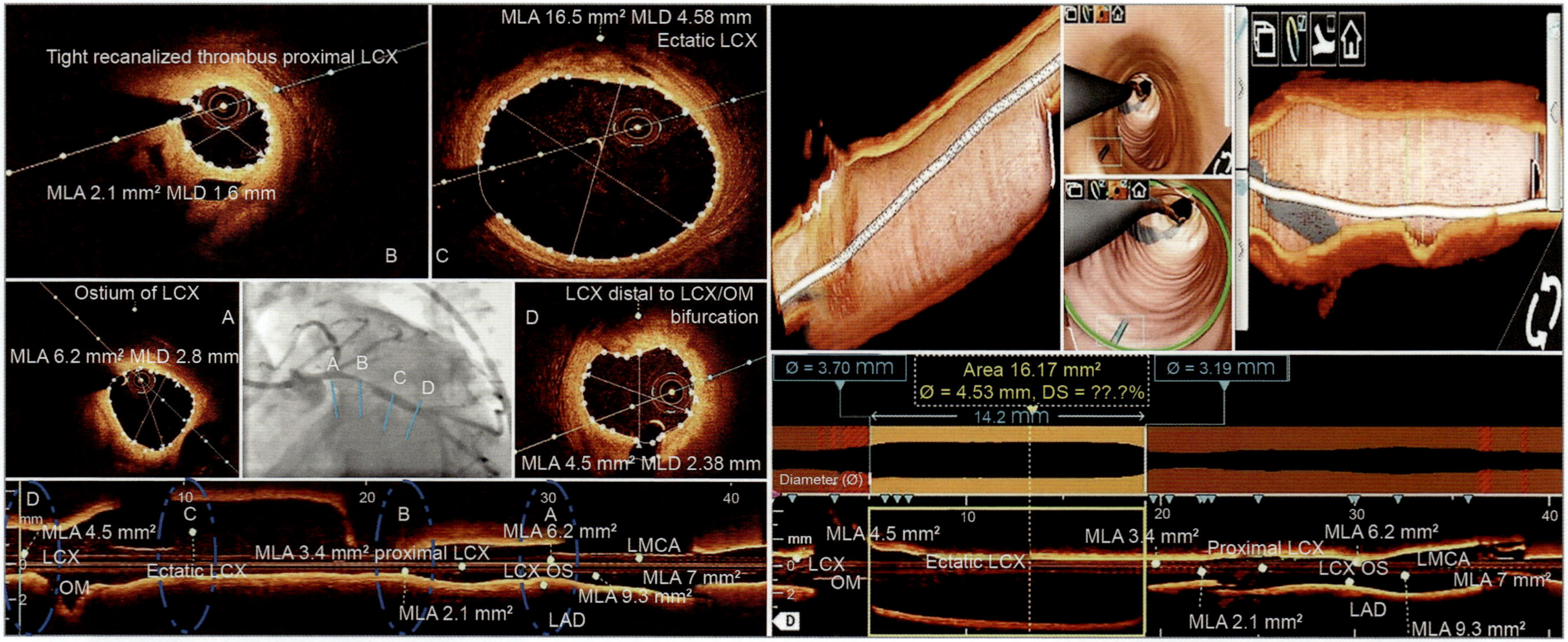
Tight recanalized thrombus proximal LCX
MLA 2.1 mm² MLD 1.6 mm
B
MLA 16.5 mm² MLD 4.58 mm
Ectatic LCX
C
Ostium of LCX
A
MLA 6.2 mm² MLD 2.8 mm
A B C D
LCX distal to LCX/OM bifurcation
D
MLA 4.5 mm² MLD 2.38 mm
D
C
B
A
mm
MLA 4.5 mm²
LCX
OM
Ectatic LCX
MLA 3.4 mm² proximal LCX
MLA 2.1 mm²
MLA 6.2 mm²
LCX OS
LAD
LMCA
MLA 7 mm²
MLA 9.3 mm²
Ø = 3.70 mm
Area 16.17 mm²
Ø = 4.53 mm, DS = ??.?%
Ø = 3.19 mm
14.2 mm
Diameter (Ø)
MLA 4.5 mm²
LCX
OM
Ectatic LCX
MLA 3.4 mm²
Proximal LCX
MLA 6.2 mm²
LCX OS
LMCA
MLA 7 mm²
LAD
MLA 2.1 mm²
MLA 9.3 mm²

Fig. 6A

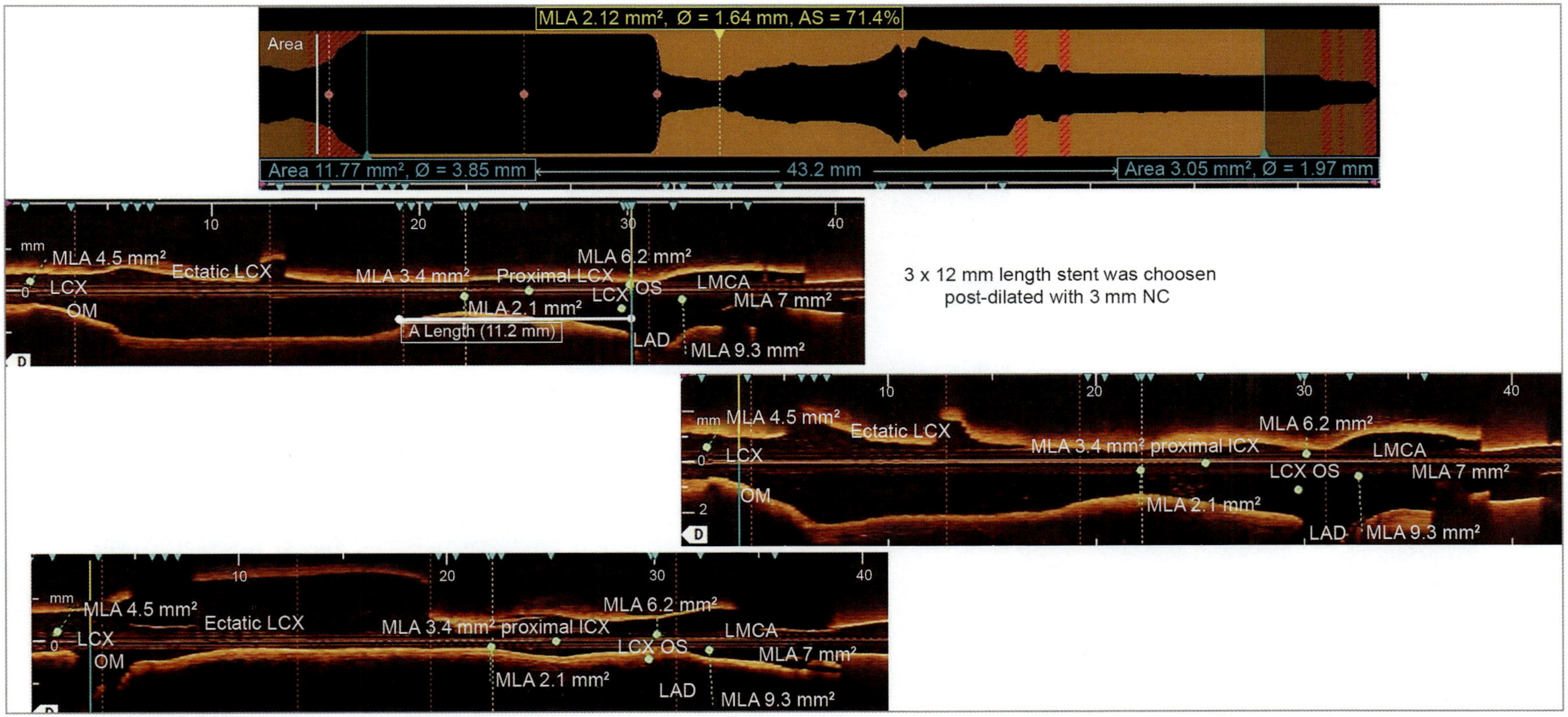

Fig. 6B

Figs. 6A and B: (A) Prestent OCT of left circumflex (LCX) showed morphology of left main (LM)–LCX segment; (B) Device selection. (LAD: left anterior descending; LMCA: left main coronary artery; MLA: minimal lumen area; MLD: minimal lumen diameter; NC: noncompliant; OM: obtuse marginal; OS: ostium)

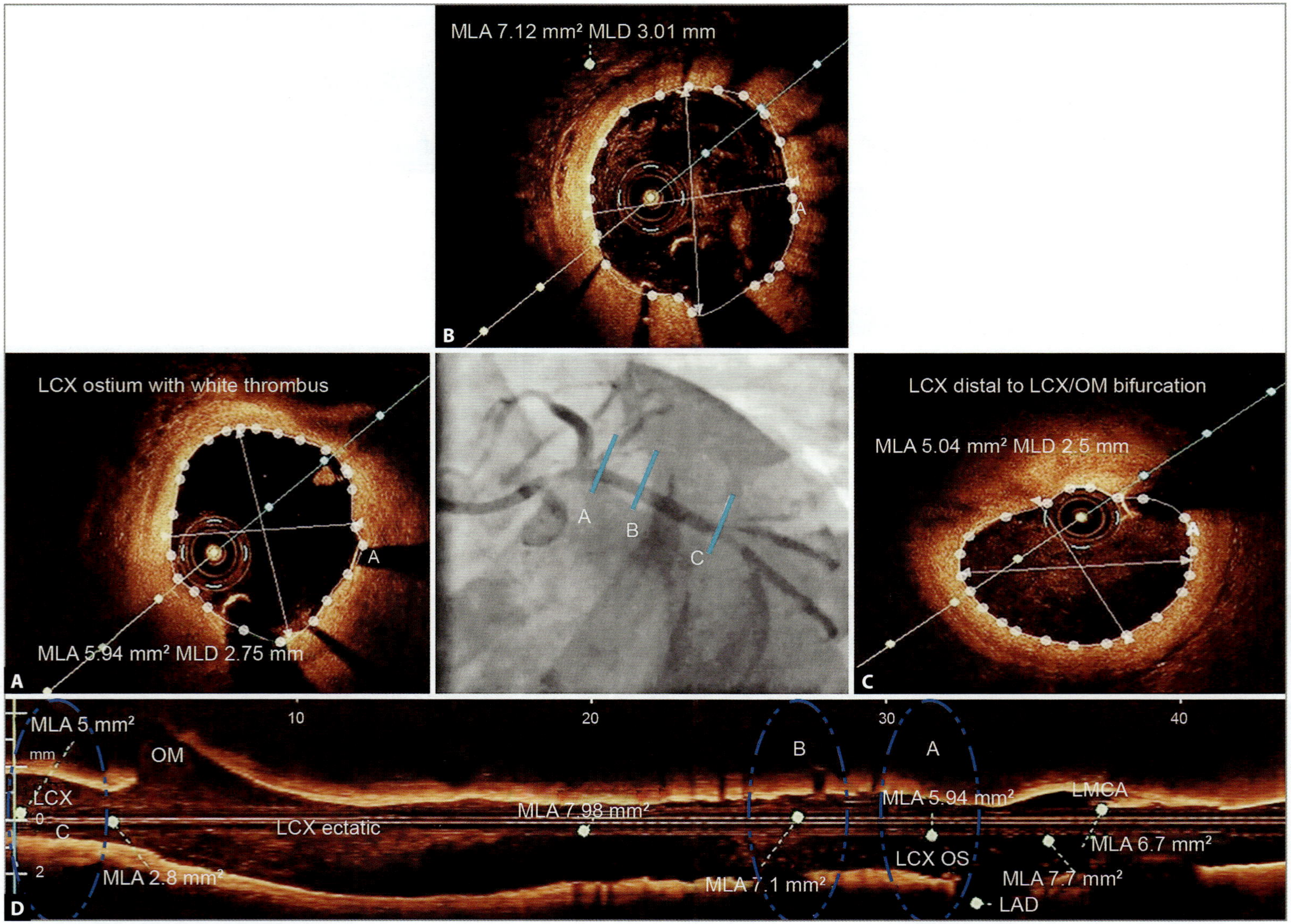

Figs. 7A to D: Poststent OCT analysis of left circumflex (LCX) vessel. (LAD: left anterior descending; LMCA: left main coronary artery; MLA: minimal lumen area; MLD: minimal lumen diameter; OS: ostium)

CASE 2

OCT assessment of borderline distal LMCA, ostioproximal LAD lesions with ectasia during PCI of LAD.

CLINICAL HISTORY

A 63-year-old male, known hypertensive, diabetic, presented with recent anterior wall MI treated with thrombolytic therapy (STK) referred for postinfarct angina. Hb—14.3 g/dL, blood urea—25 mg/dL, serum creatinine—0.92 mg/dL, estimated glomerular filtration rate (eGFR)—88 mL/min, pro brain natriuretic peptide (BNP)—1,639 pg/mL, ECG—anterior wall STEMI (ST elevation myocardial infarction), 2D Echo-RWMA in LAD territory, mild LV function (EF—41%). CAG-LMCA—ostioproximal lesion, ostial LAD—proximal ectatic followed by mid 80% lesion, LCX—normal, RCA—proximal and mid 60% lesion **(Figs. 8A to D)**.

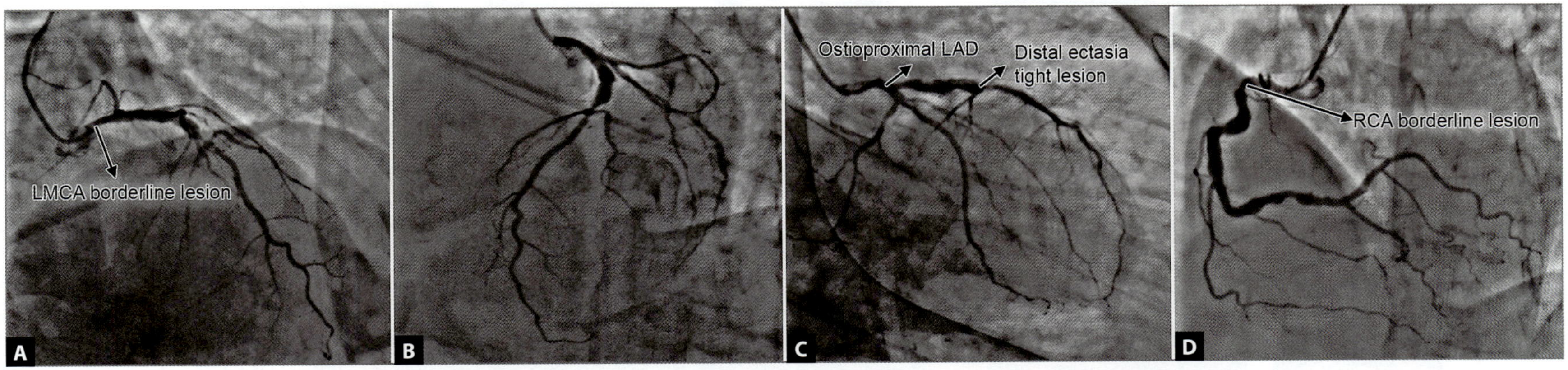

Figs. 8A to D: Coronary angiogram. (LAD: left anterior descending; LMCA: left main coronary artery; RCA: right coronary artery)

PROCEDURE

Route—RFA, using 6 Fr EBU 3.5 guiding catheter, LAD wired with 0.014 × 190 cm" Turntrac wire, D1 crossed with 0.014" BMW wire. Predilatation done with 2.0 × 10 mm Tazuna balloon.

Optical coherence tomography was planned to assess the severity of lesion, plaque morphology, to decide device length due to tandem lesions involving ostioproximal segment of LM, ostial LAD, tight lesion after ectatic segment of proximal LAD to decide following strategies:

- To cover entire length of the lesion extending from ostial LM to lesion after ectatic segment of proximal LAD
- To cover proximal and distal lesions of proximal LAD including the ectatic segment
- Focal stenting of tight lesion after ectatic segment of proximal LAD

Decision of PCI was based on MLA of LM, ostial LAD, ectatic segment, and tight lesion of LAD just after ectatic segment **(Figs. 9A to D)**.

- LMCA MLA 7.1 mm^2—insignificant LM lesion, hence LM stent differed
- MLA measure by OCT is significantly smaller than by IVUS, OCT MLA being 10–15% lower than IVUS MLA **(Fig. 9E)**
- Ostial LAD 4.4 mm^2—insignificant lesion, hence ostial LAD stent differed
- Critical lesion MLA after ectatic segment—1.6 mm^2 (post-POBA with 2 mm Tazuna), hence stenting of critical lesion was planned.

Mid-LAD stenting done with 3.0 × 18 mm Resolute Onyx stent. Postdilatation done with 3.5 × 12 mm NC Trek balloon. Post-OCT showed well-apposed stent struts, no edge dissection, and no residual thrombus **(Figs. 10A to E)**.

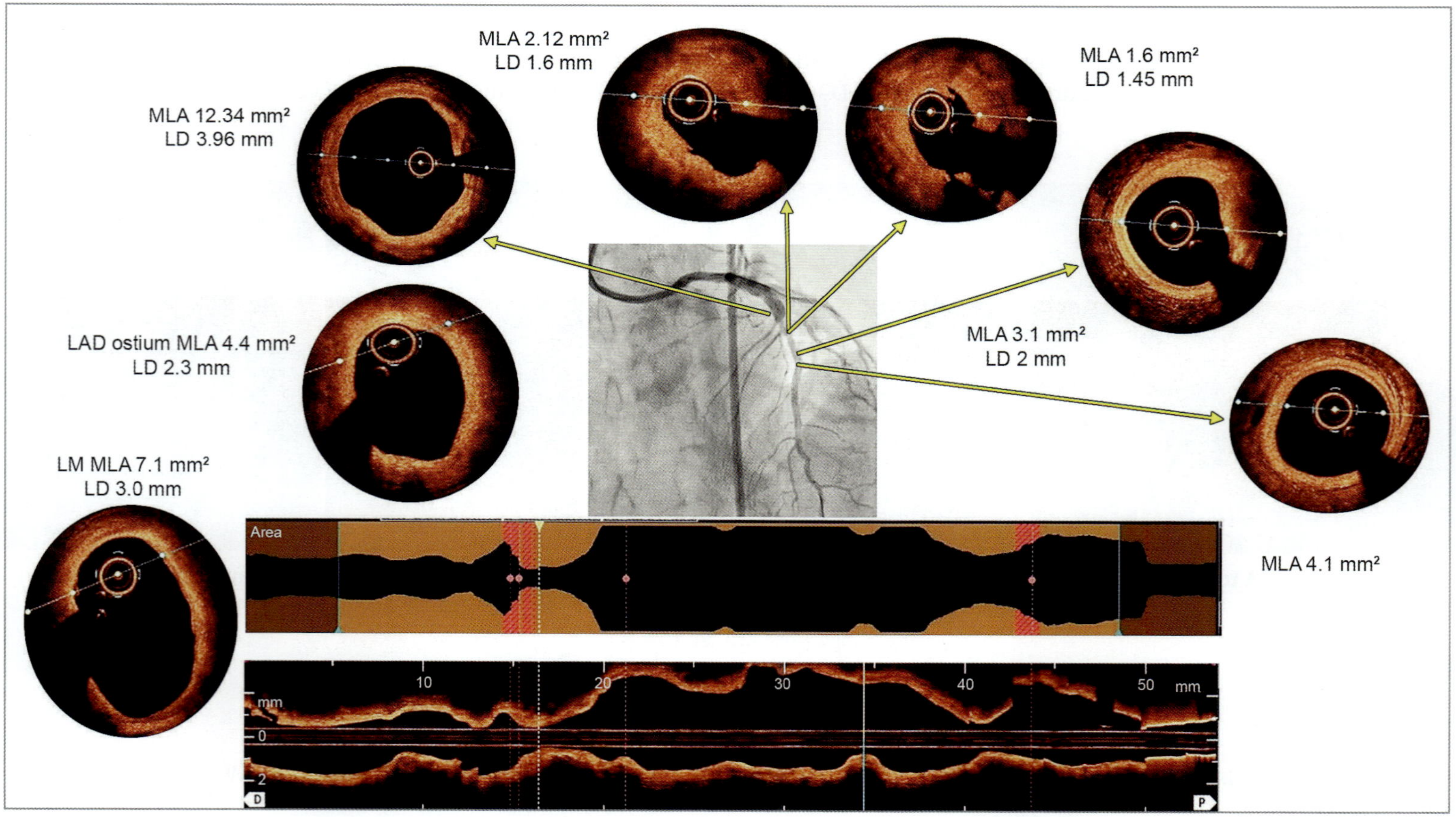

Fig. 9A

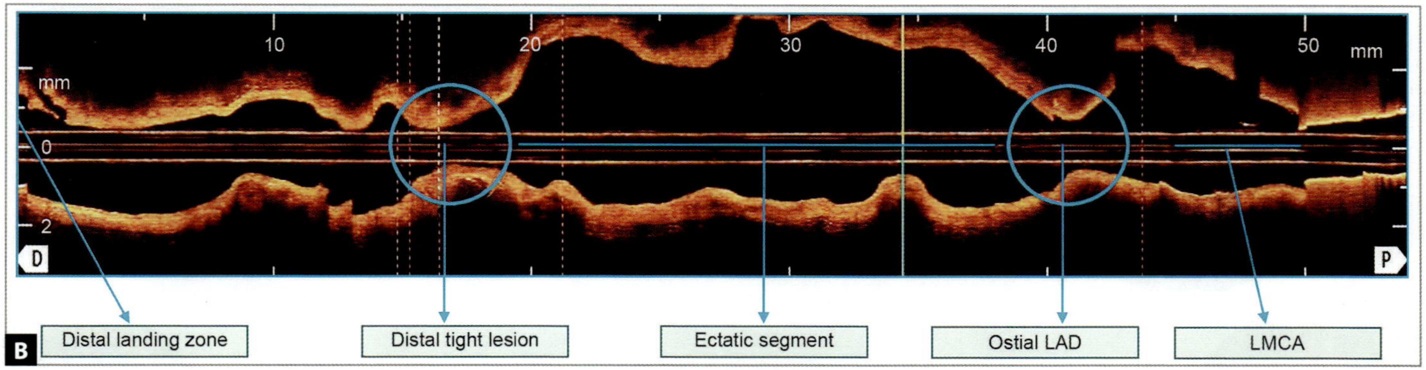

10
20
30
40
50
mm
mm
0
2
D
P
Distal landing zone
Distal tight lesion
Ectatic segment
Ostial LAD
LMCA
B

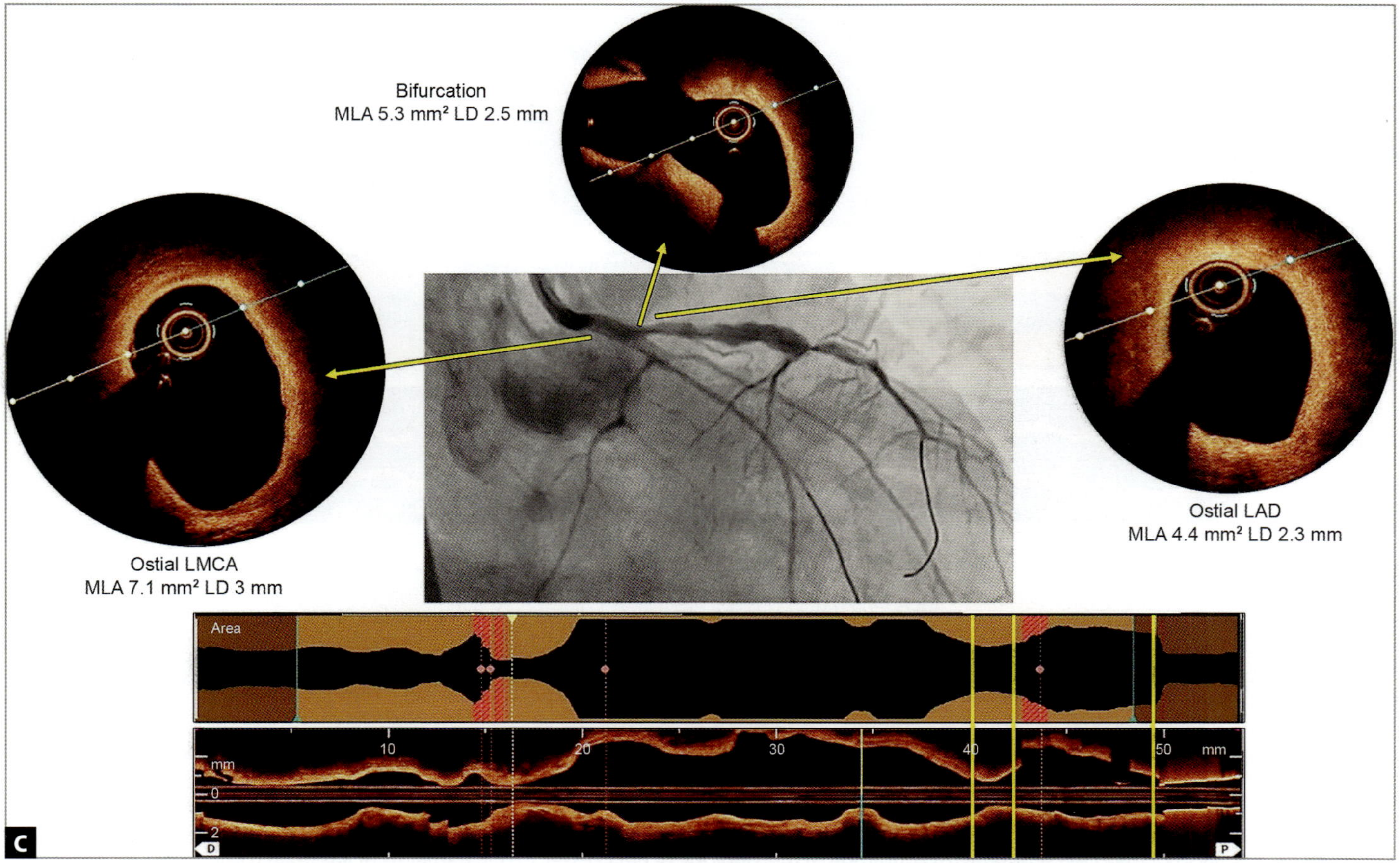

Bifurcation
MLA 5.3 mm² LD 2.5 mm
Ostial LMCA
MLA 7.1 mm² LD 3 mm
Ostial LAD
MLA 4.4 mm² LD 2.3 mm
Area
C

Figs. 9B and C

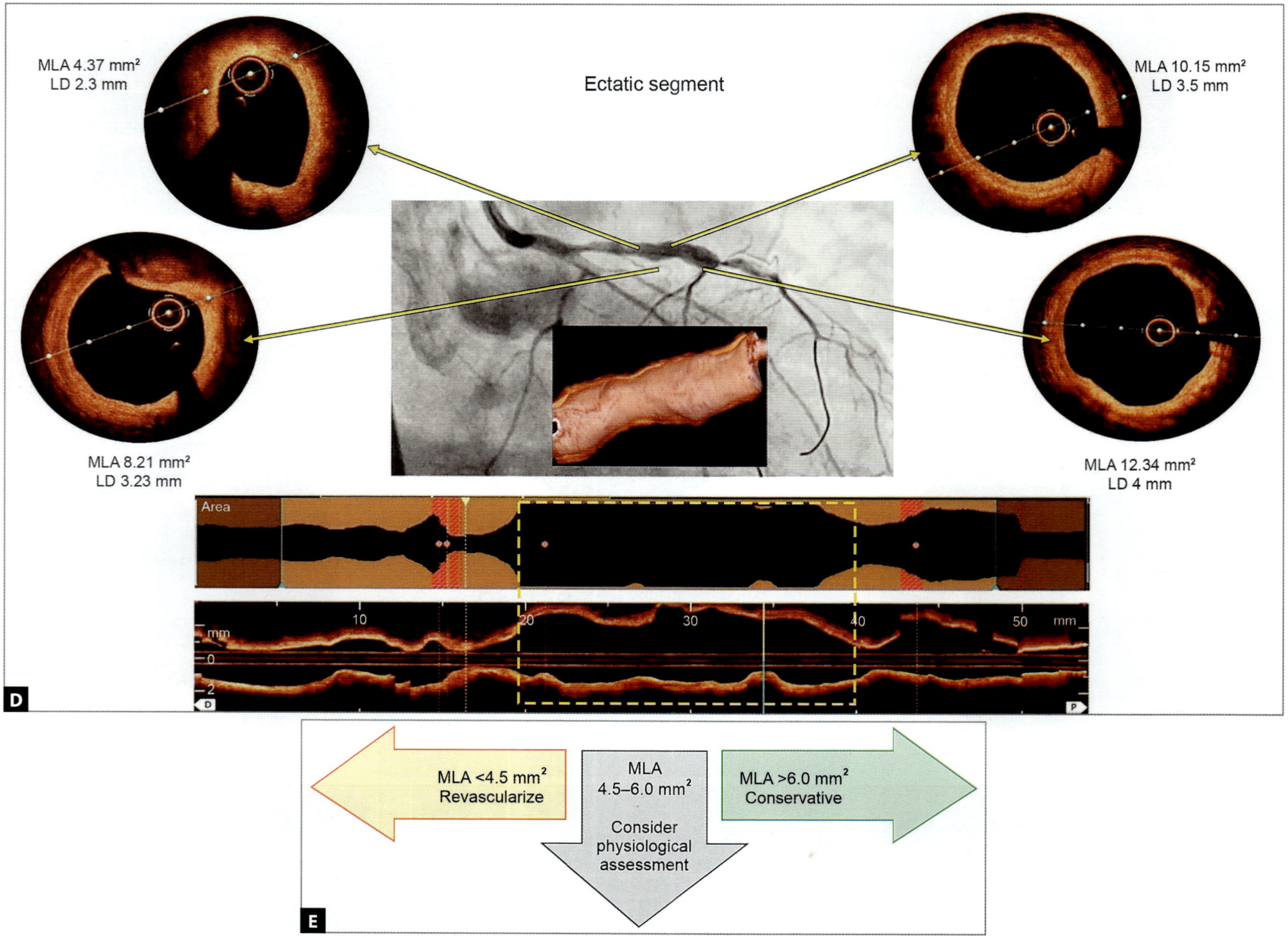

Figs. 9D and E

Figs. 9A to E: (A) Prestent OCT analysis of mid-LAD segment; (B) Longitudinal morphology of LAD vessel; (C) OCT analysis of left main (LM)–ostial LAD segment; (D) OCT analysis of ectatic segment; (E) Criteria of selection of stent for left main coronary artery (LMCA). (MLA: minimal lumen area; LAD: left anterior descending) segment; LD: lumen diameter)

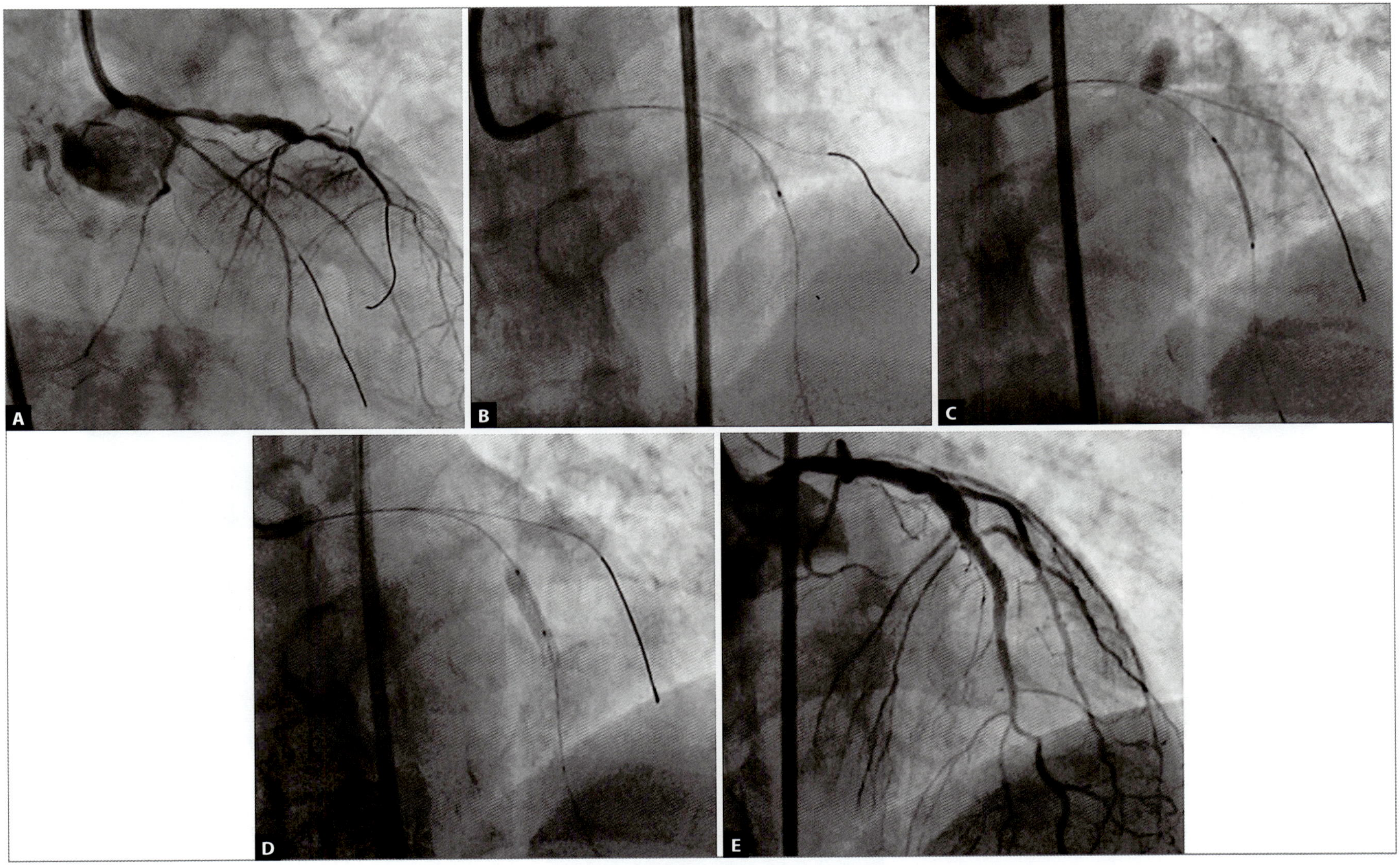

Figs. 10A to E: Coronary angioplasty of left anterior descending (LAD) vessel. (A) 0.014 × 190 cm″ Turntrac wire, D1 crossed with 0.014″ BMW wire; (B) Predilatation done with 2.0 × 10 mm Tazuna balloon; (C) Mid-LAD stenting done with 3.0 × 18 mm Resolute Onyx stent; (D) Postdilatation done with 3.5 × 12 mm NC Trek balloon, (E) Final result.

Post-OCT assessment: OCT was done to assess LMCA, LAD ostioproximal lesion, ectatic segment, and critical narrowing just after ectasia to decide stenting of only distal segment or to stent LM to ostioproximal segment of LAD and distal lesion **(Figs. 11A and B)**.

Fractional flow reserve (FFR) at baseline was 0.95, after IC-NTG (nitroglycerin) 100 µg 0.91 **(Fig. 12A)**, with IV adenosine for 2 minutes, FFR value 0.87 **(Fig. 12B)**, hence LM and ostial LAD stenting was deferred. FFR of RCA baseline 0.98 with NTG 0.95 **(Fig. 12C)**. Post-stenting FFR was negative which indicated insignificant LMCA, and ostioproximal lesion of LAD, hence stenting was deferred.

Postprocedure angio view showed well-implanted stents with TIMI-III flow without any dissection. Patient was discharged on third postprocedure in a stable status.

Post-OCT analysis ***(Figs. 11A and B):***

Fractional flow reserve and OCT was used to assess severity of distal LMCA and ostial LAD lesions to decide precise placement of properly sized stent to cover the significant ischemia contributing lesions. OCT and FFR confirmed that lesion situated distal to the ectatic segment of LAD was significant, hence stenting of only this lesion was done. Imaging helped in choosing short-length stent and avoiding unnecessary covering of insignificant lesions.

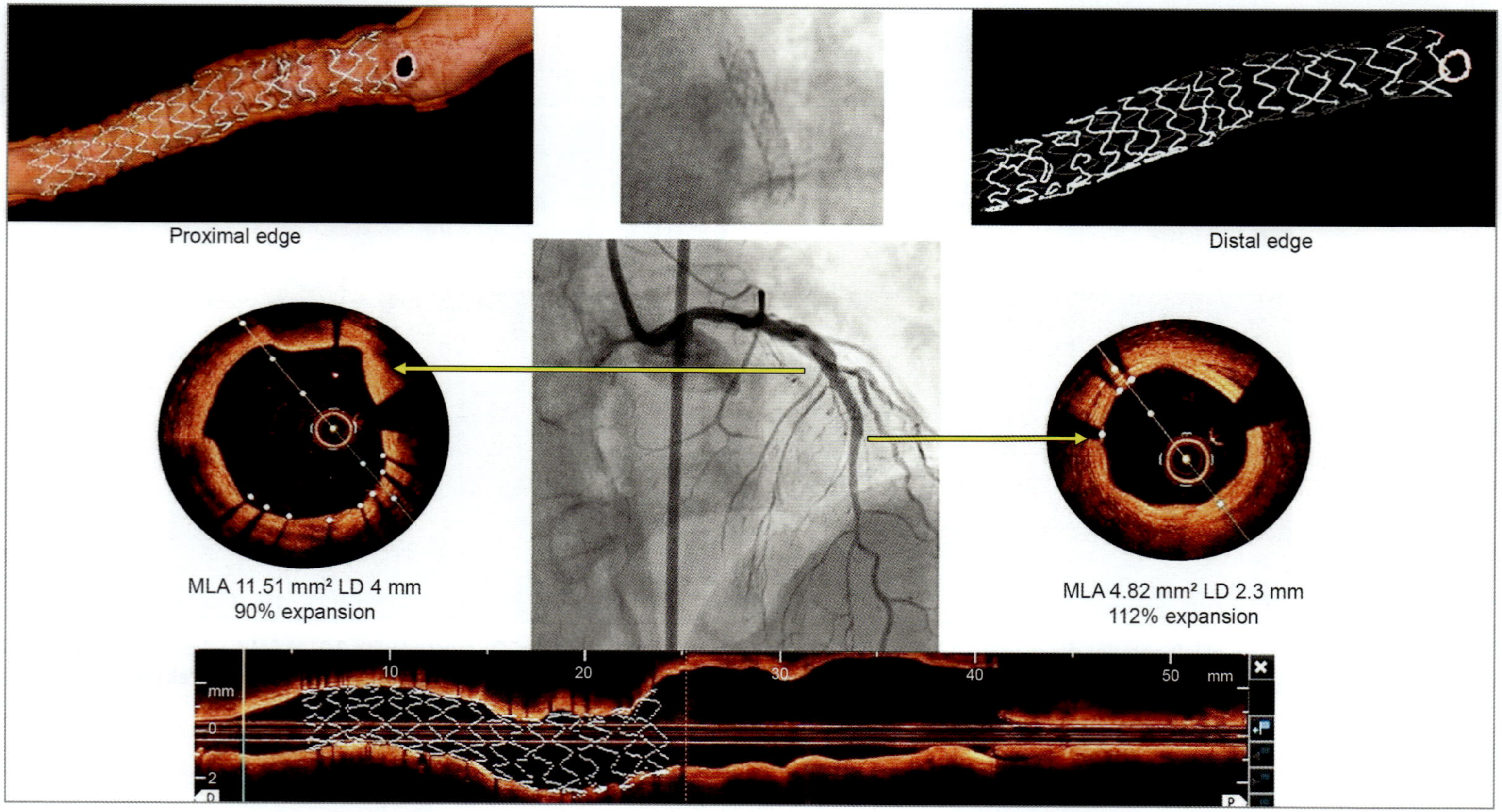

Fig. 11A

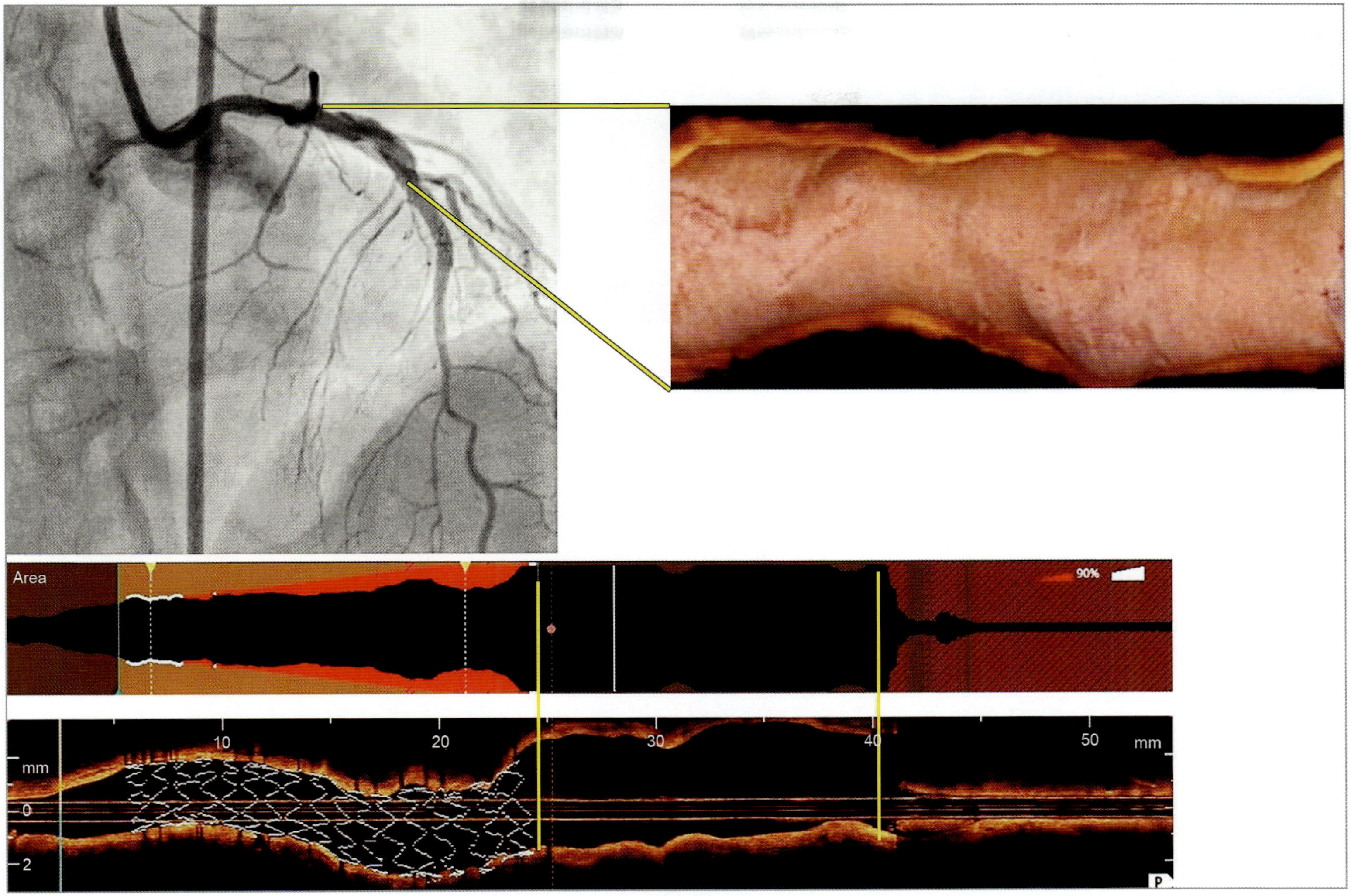

Fig. 11B

Figs. 11A and B: (A) Poststent OCT analysis of left anterior descending (LAD) showed well-expanded, no edge dissection, and no tissue prolapse; (B) Poststent ectatic segment of LAD.

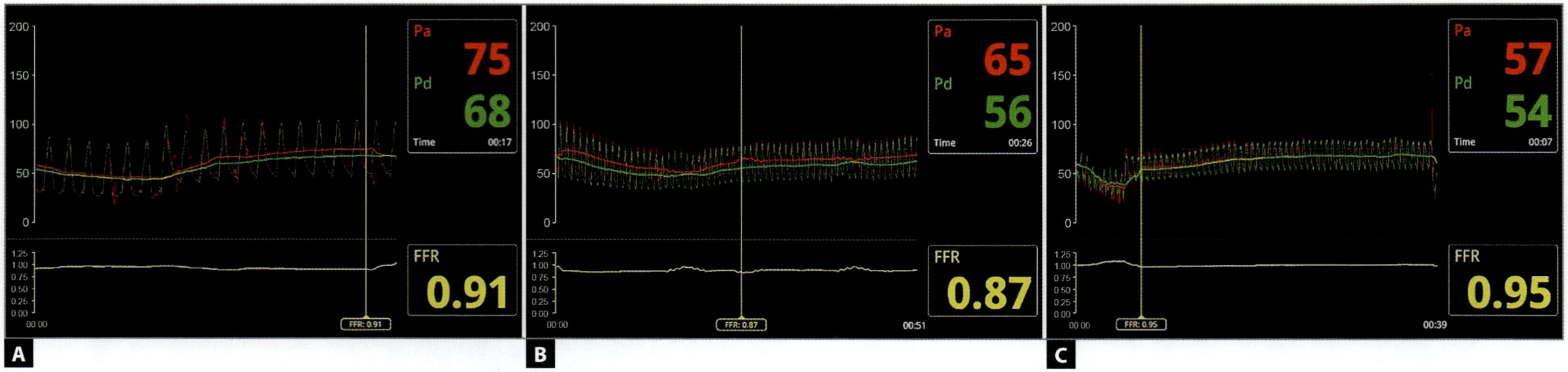

Figs. 12A to C: Fractional flow reserve (FFR) study of left main (LM)—left anterior descending (LAD) segment before ectatic segment.

CHAPTER

20 Percutaneous Coronary Intervention of Diffuse Long Segment Lesions

CASE 1

Percutaneous coronary intervention (PCI) of diffusely diseased long segment left anterior descending (LAD).

CLINICAL HISTORY

A 51-year-old male known hypertensive presented with coronary artery disease (CAD)—unstable angina, severe chest pain radiating to back, electrocardiogram (ECG)—normal, 2D echo—no regional wall motion abnormalities (RWMA), concentric left ventricular hypertrophy (LVH), normal LV function, and ejection fraction (EF)—65%. Aortogram was done to rule out aortic dissection which was normal.

Investigations: Random blood sugar (RBS)—99 mg/dL, blood urea—20 mg/dL, serum creatinine (S. Cr)—0.94 mg/dL, estimated glomerular filtration rate (eGFR)—95.

Coronary angiography left main coronary artery (CAG-LMCA)—normal, left anterior descending (LAD)—proximal 90% eccentric lesion. Mid 80% lesion, distal diffuse disease. Left circumflex (LCX)—normal, right coronary artery (RCA)—mid mild disease. Distal 70–80% lesion, posterior descending artery (PDA)—long segment 80–90% lesion **(Figs. 1A to C)**.

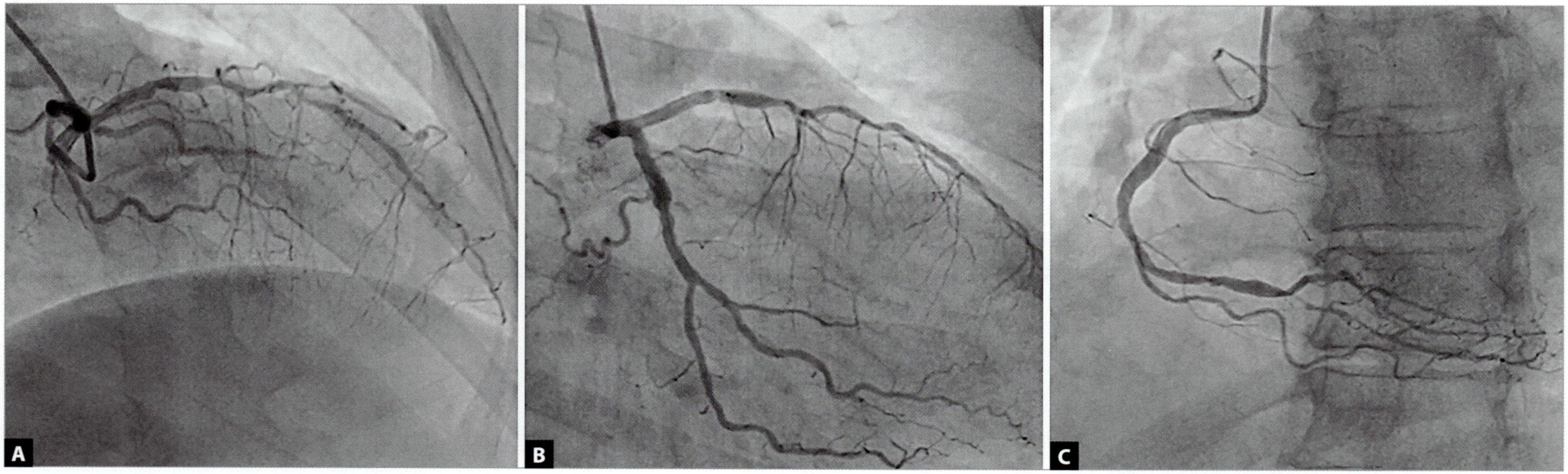

Figs. 1A to C: *Coronary angiogram:* (A) LAD; (B) LCX; (C) RCA. (Significant disease of proximal to mid LAD and PDA).

PROCEDURE

Percutaneous Coronary Intervention of Left Anterior Descending

Route—right radial approach (RRA), using 6 Fr XB 3.5 guiding catheter, LAD lesion which was crossed with 0.014″ Sion Blue wire.

Left Anterior Descending Preoptical Coherence Tomography Analysis

Preoptical coherence tomography (OCT) showed proximal landing zone of LAD minimal lumen area (MLA)—8.3 mm^2, minimal lumen diameter (MLD)—3.25 mm, MLA with thick fibrolipid plaque, MLA 1.36 mm^2, LD 1.26 mm, distal landing zone of LAD MLA—2.7 mm^2, MLD—1.8 mm **(Fig. 2)**.

Pre-OCT showed fibrolipid plaque with MLA—1.27 mm^2, MLD—1.2 mm **(Figs. 3 and 4)**.

Distal LAD direct stenting done with 2.5 × 30 mm Resolute Onyx Stent. Proximal LAD stenting was tried with 3.0 × 30 mm Resolute Onyx, but could not crossed the lesion, finally stented with GuideLiner support and postdilated with 2.5 × 12 mm NC Trek balloon **(Figs. 5A to E)**.

Post-OCT showed proximal edge of drug-eluting stent (DES) MLA—8.3 mm^2, MLD—3.25 mm, distal edge of DES MLA—8.3 mm^2, MLD—3.25 mm, ostium of LAD proximal to the stent with MLA 4.7 mm^2, and MLD—2.4 mm.

Post-OCT showed proximal edge of DES MLA—8.3 mm^2, MLD—3.25 mm, distal edge of DES MLA—8.3 mm^2, and MLD—3.25 mm **(Fig. 6)**.

Post-OCT showed well expanded and apposed stent struts, without any edge dissection, ostium of LAD 4.7 mm^2, MLD—2.4 mm, tissue prolapse with MLA—8.45 mm^2, MLD—3.3 mm **(Fig. 7)**.

Postprocedure Angio view showed well-implanted stents with thrombolysis in myocardial infarction III (TIMI-III) flow without any dissection.

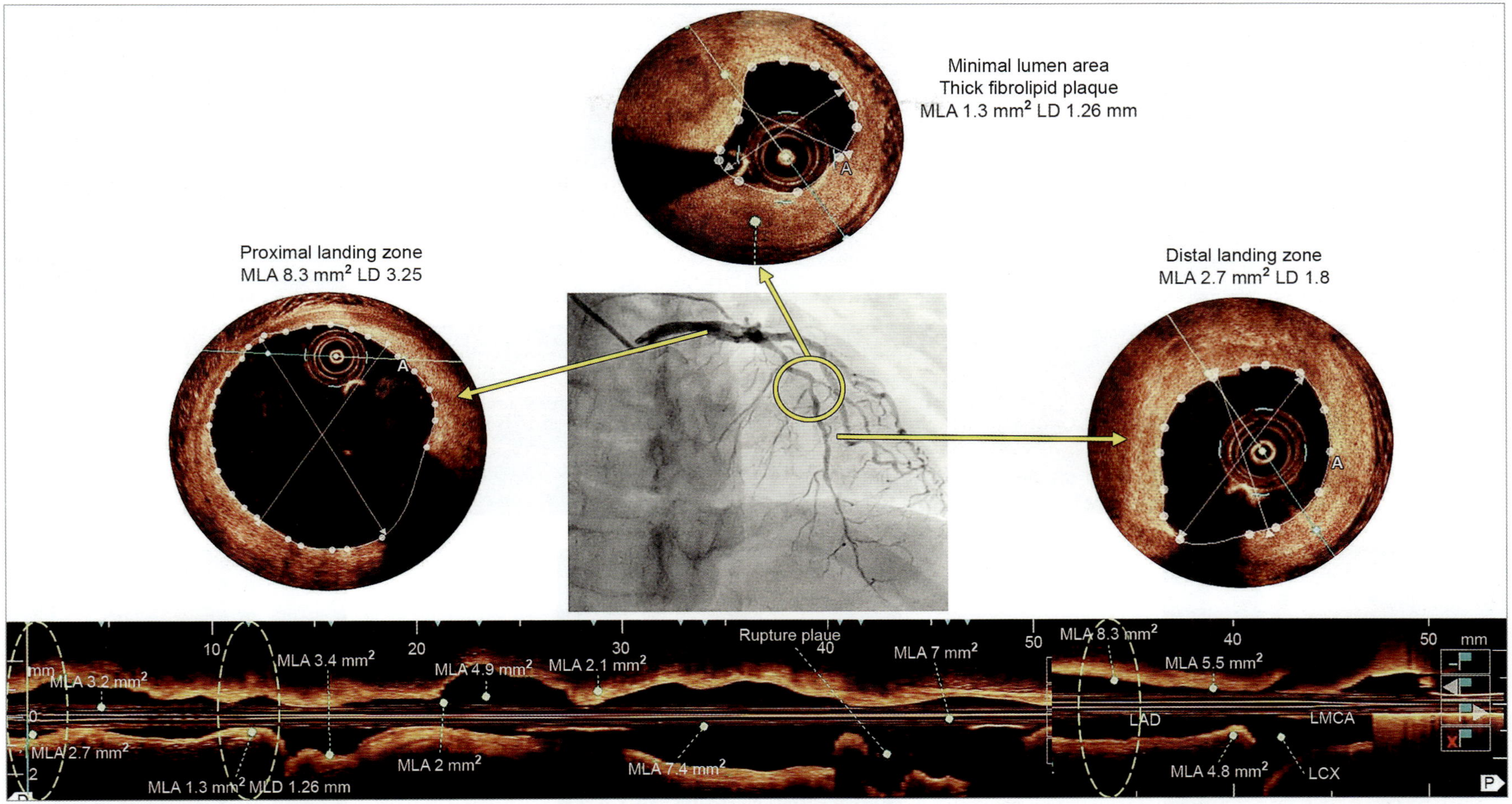

Fig. 2: Prestenting OCT assessment for device selection. (LAD: left anterior descending; LD: luminal diameter; MLA: minimal luminal area; MLD: minimal lumen diameter; OCT: optical coherence tomography)

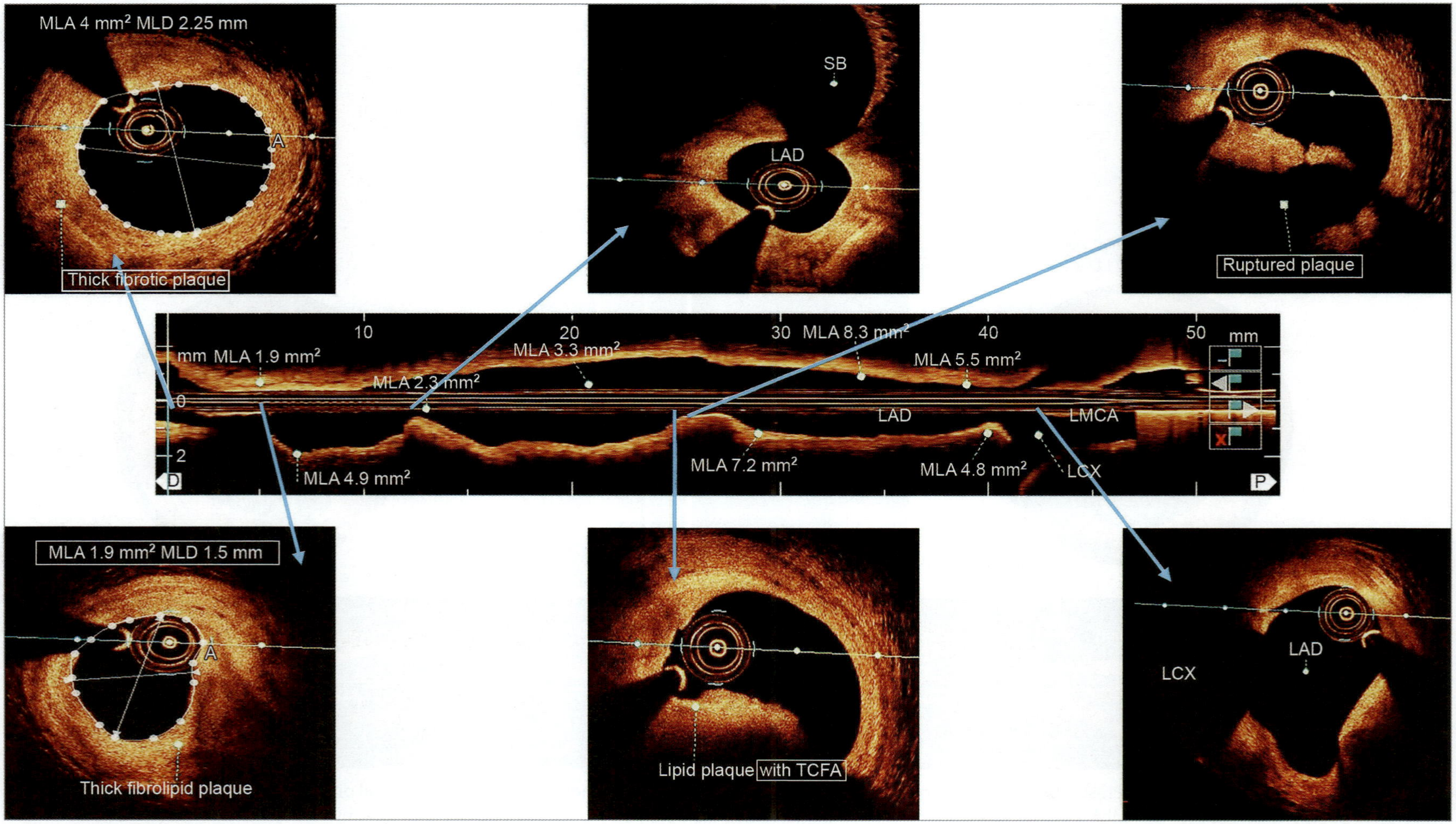

Fig. 3: Prestenting OCT assessment for plaque morphology. (LAD: left anterior descending; LMCA: left main coronary artery; MLA: minimal luminal area; MLD: minimal lumen diameter; TCFA: thin-cap fibroatheroma; OCT: optical coherence tomography)

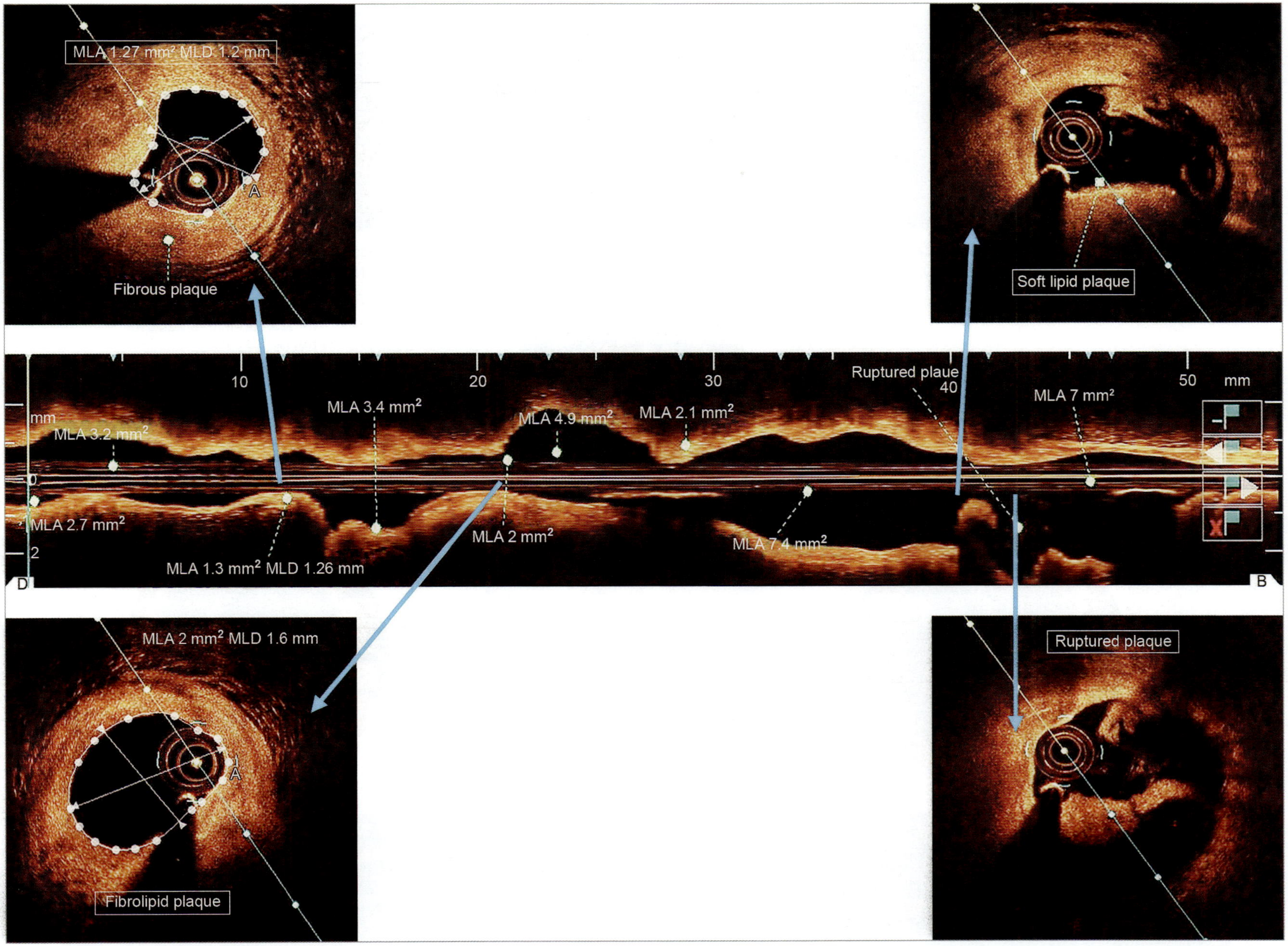

Fig. 4: Prestenting OCT assessment for plaque morphology. (MLA: minimal luminal area; MLD: minimal lumen diameter)

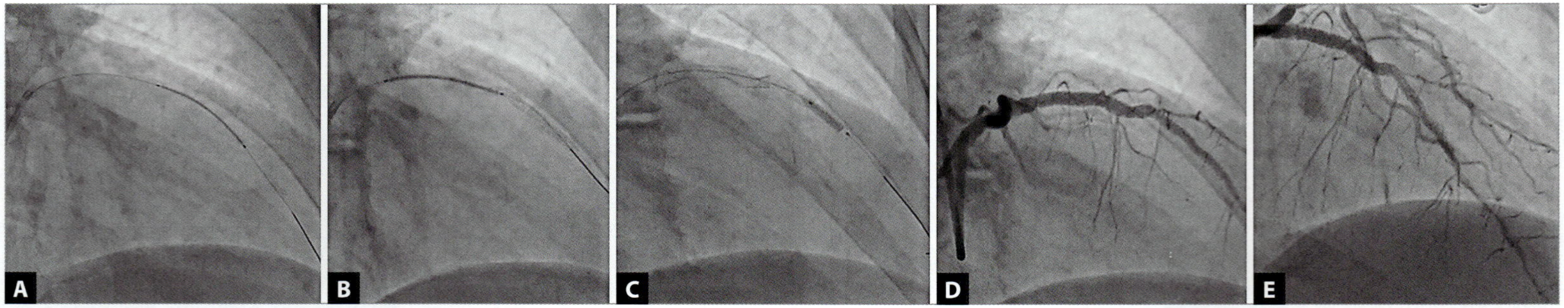

Figs. 5A to E: Coronary angioplasty. (A) Distal left anterior descending (LAD) direct stenting done with 2.5 × 30 mm Resolute Onyx Stent; (B) proximal LAD stenting done with 3.0 × 30 mm Resolute Onyx Stent with GuideLiner support; (C) Postdilatation done with 2.5 × 12 mm NC Trek balloon; (D and E) final result.

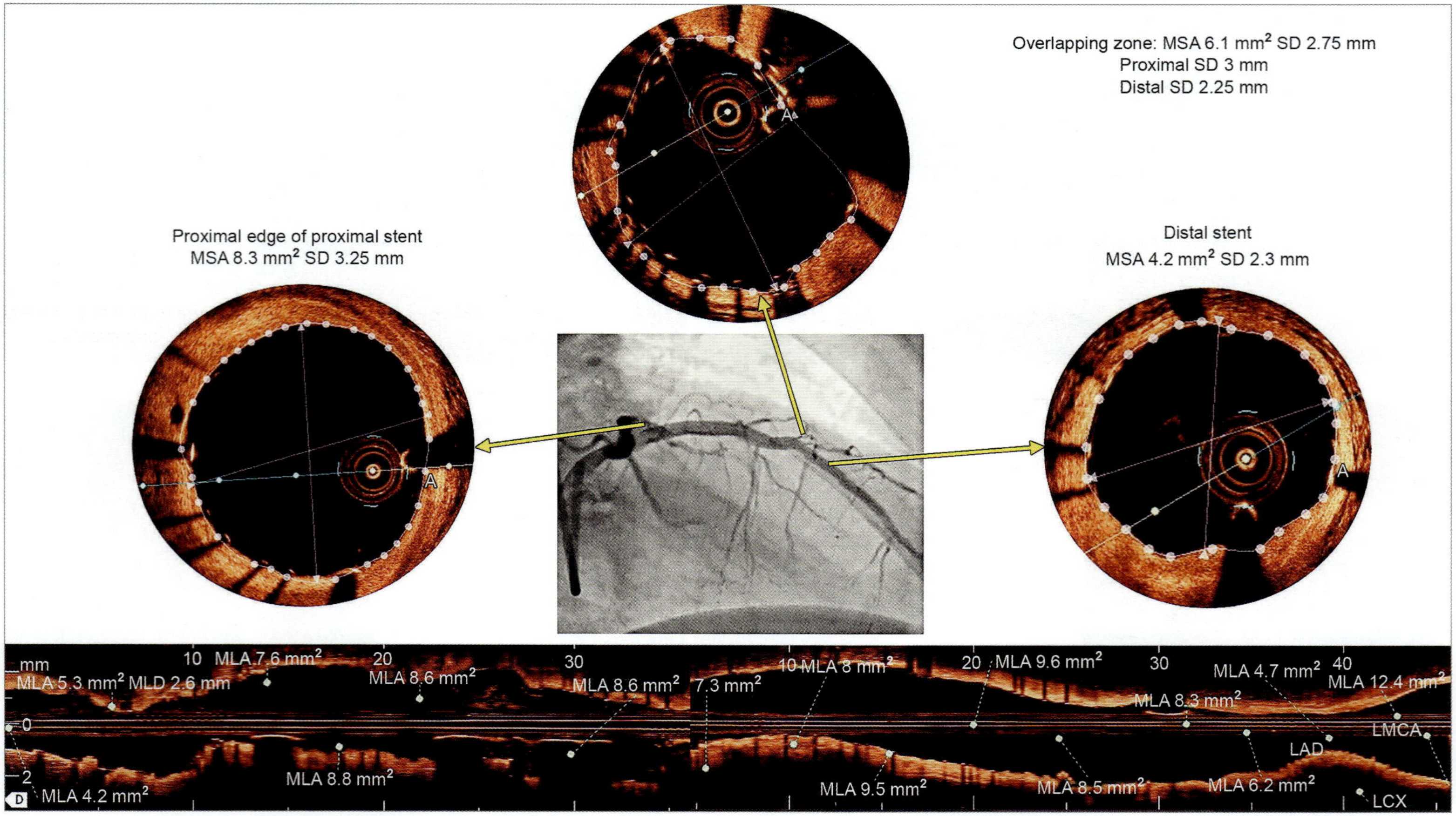

Fig. 6: Poststenting OCT assessment of MAX. (LAD: left anterior descending; LMCA: left main coronary artery; MLA: minimal luminal area; MSA: minimal stent area; OCT: optical coherence tomography)

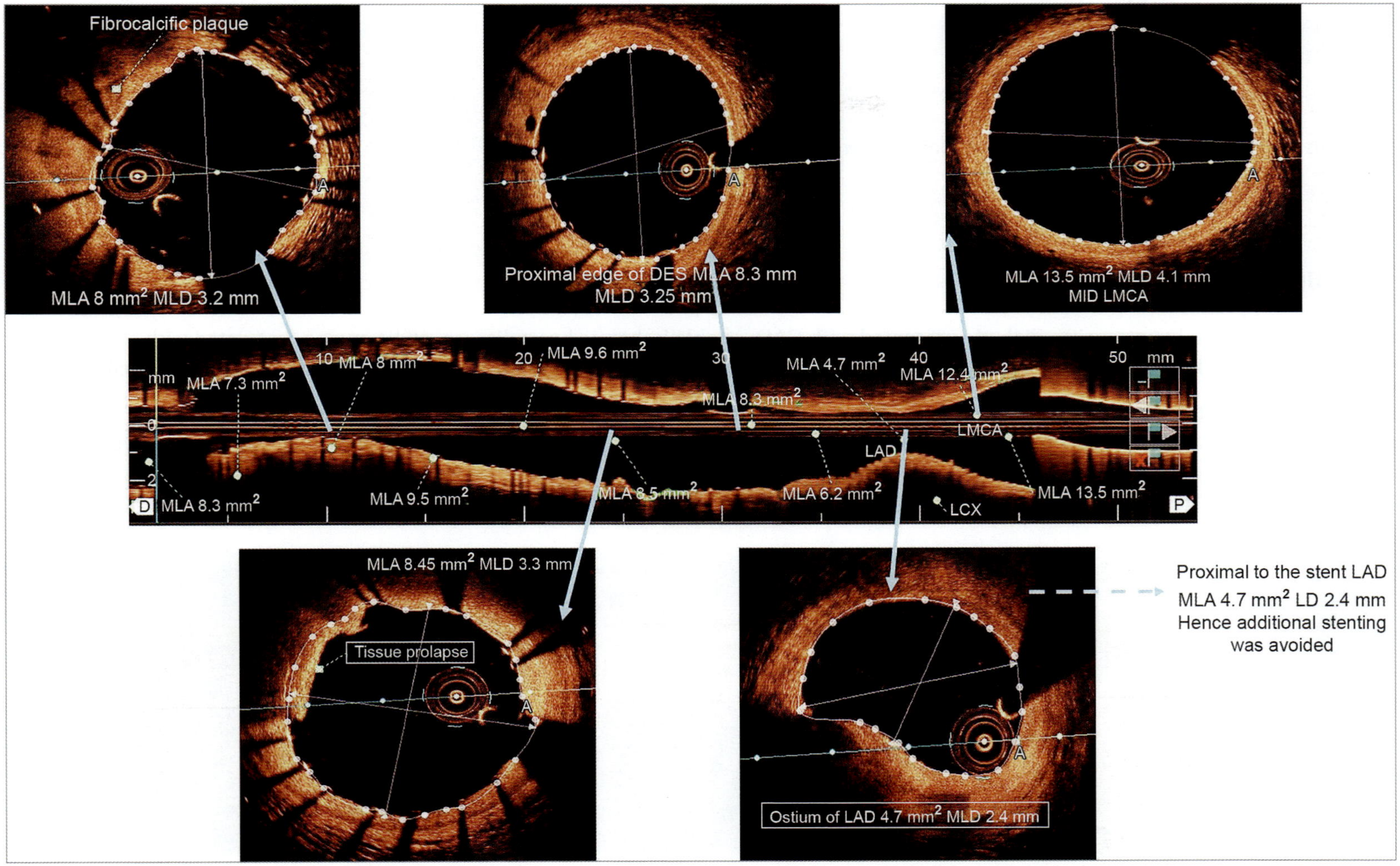

Fig. 7: Poststenting OCT assessment revealed plaque burden proximal to the proximal stent. (LAD: left anterior descending; LMCA: left main coronary artery; MLA: minimal luminal area; MSA: minimal stent area; OCT: optical coherence tomography)

CASE 2

Percutaneous coronary intervention (PCI) of diffuse long segment of right coronary artery (RCA)

CLINICAL HISTORY

A 53-year-old male known hypertensive, diabetic presented with CAD—stable ischemic heart disease, effort angina associated with shortness of breath (SOB) for the past 2 months, and 2D Echo—no RWMA, good LV function, and EF—62%. Treadmill test (TMT) showed positive for inducible ischemia.

Investigations: Hb—12.6 g/dL, S.Cr—0.79 mg/dL, eGFR—103 mL/min, and RBS—114 mg/dL.

Coronary angiography-LMCA—normal, LAD—mid 60-70% lesion, LCX—proximal 90% lesion, and RCA—proximal to distal long segment 80% lesion **(Figs. 8A to C)**.

Fractional flow reserve (FFR) to LAD showed insignificant lesion, LCX showed significant lesion (adenosine-0.76) **(Fig. 8D)**.

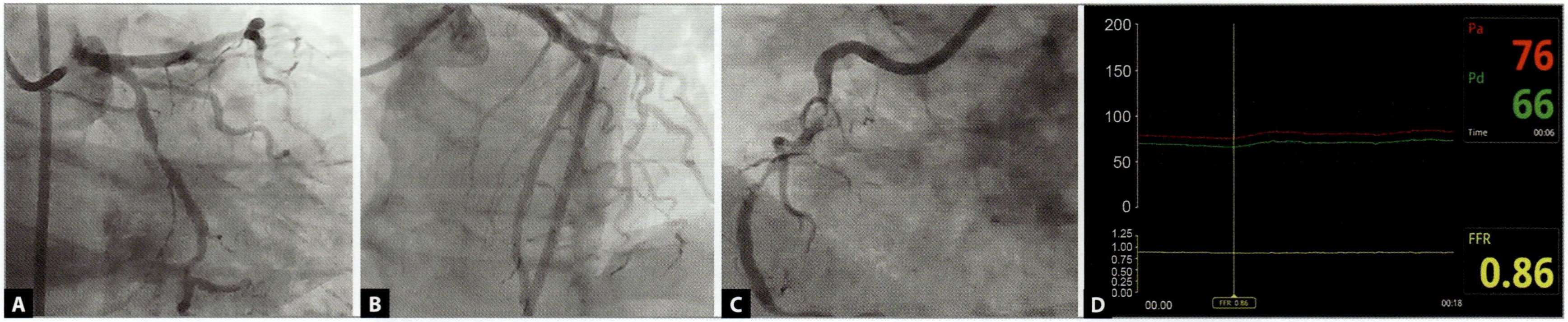

Figs. 8A to D: Coronary angiogram and FFR study of LAD vessel (–ve FFR of LAD). (FFR: fractional flow reserve; LAD: left anterior descending)

PROCEDURE

Percutaneous Coronary Intervention of Right Coronary Artery

Route—right femoral artery (RFA), using 7 Fr JR 3.5 guiding catheter, RCA lesion was crossed with 0.014″ BMW wire and predilated with 2.0 × 10 mm Tazuna balloon.

Pre-OCT showed proximal to distal long segment fibrocalcific lesion **(Figs. 9A to C)**.

Distal RCA stenting done with 2.75 × 33 mm Xience Xpedition Stent, and proximal RCA stenting done with 3.5 × 38 mm Xience Xpedition Stent **(Figs. 10A to E)**.

Post-OCT showed well expanded with no edge dissection and malapposition of distal RCA stent which was corrected with 3.0 × 12 mm NC Apollo balloon **(Figs. 11A to C)**. The final result was good with TIMI-III flow.

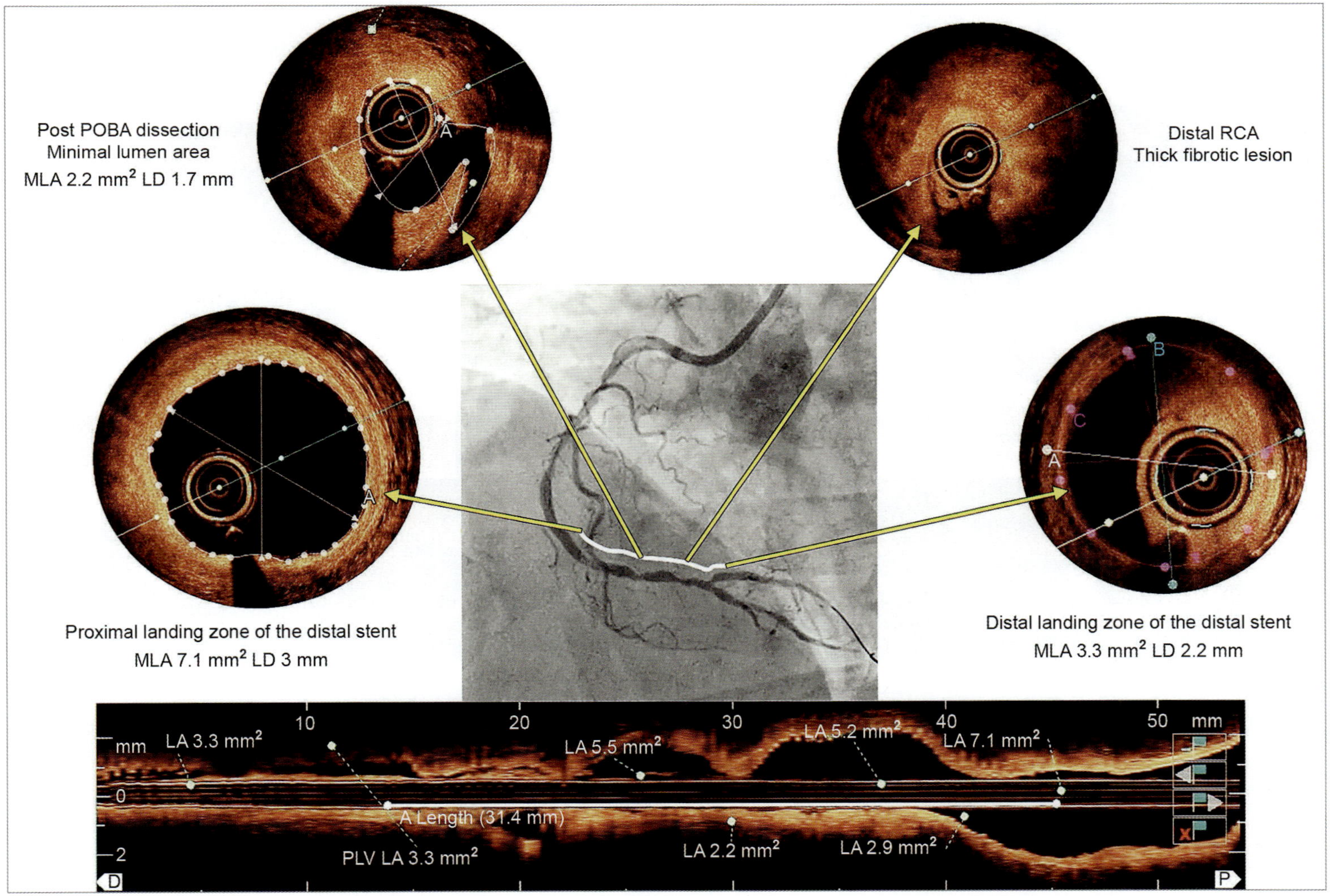

Fig. 9A

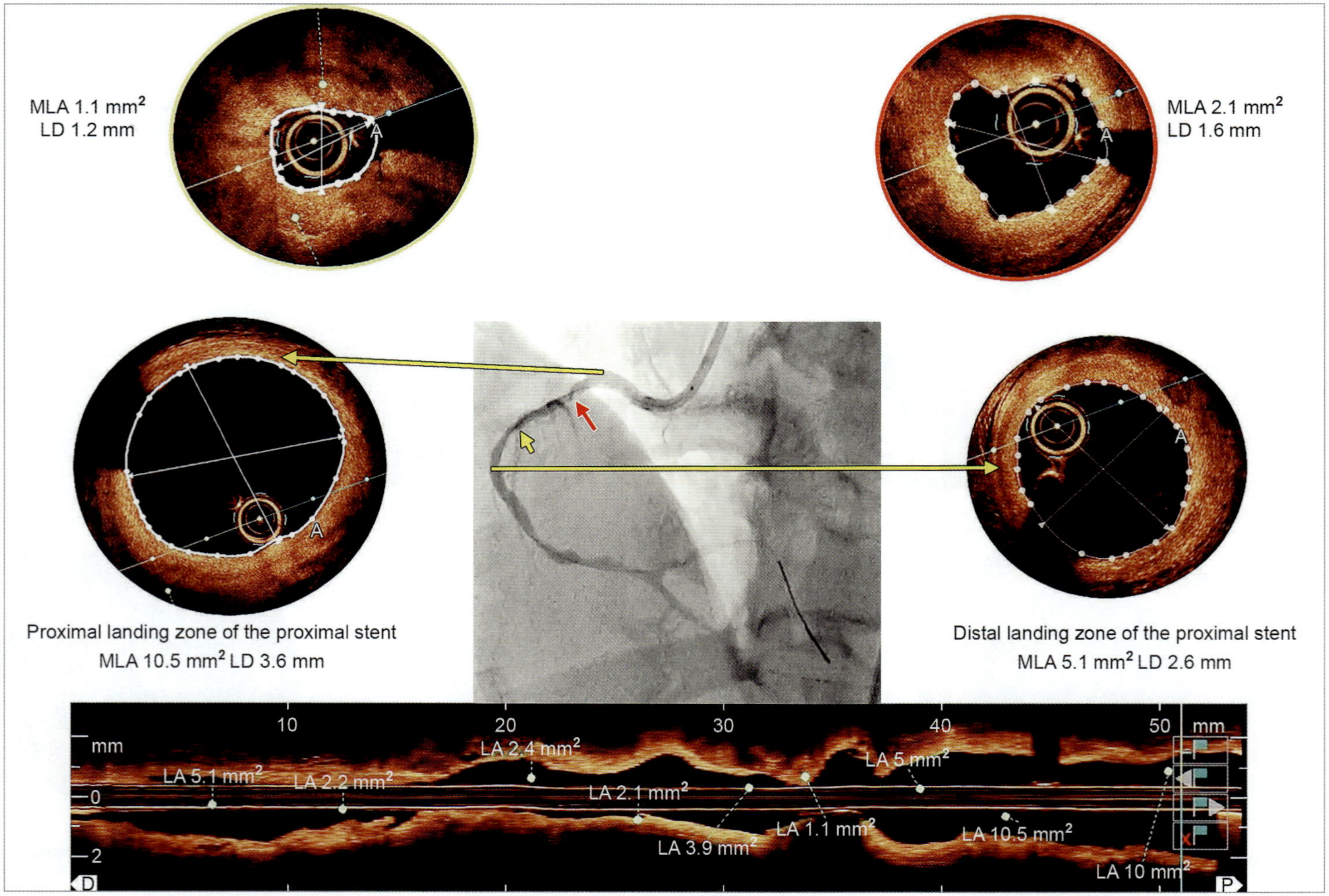

MLA 1.1 mm²
LD 1.2 mm
MLA 2.1 mm²
LD 1.6 mm
Proximal landing zone of the proximal stent
MLA 10.5 mm² LD 3.6 mm
Distal landing zone of the proximal stent
MLA 5.1 mm² LD 2.6 mm
mm
10
20
30
40
50
LA 2.4 mm²
LA 5.1 mm²
LA 2.2 mm²
LA 2.1 mm²
LA 5 mm²
LA 1.1 mm²
LA 3.9 mm²
LA 10.5 mm²
LA 10 mm²
D
P

Fig. 9B

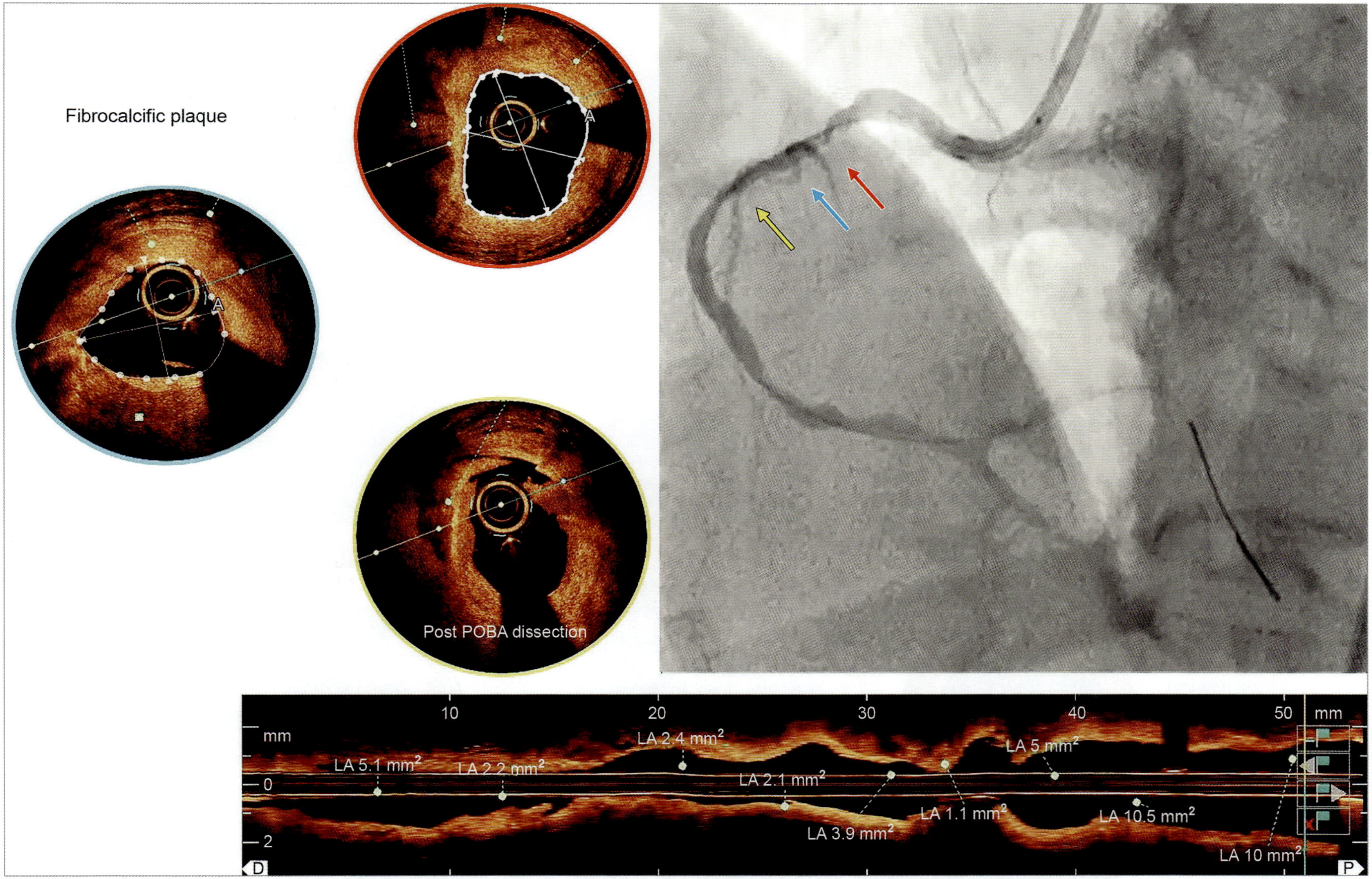

Fig. 9C

Figs. 9A to C: (A) Prestenting OCT assessment of distal RCA segment for device selection; (B) Prestenting OCT assessment of proximal RCA segment for device selection; (C) Prestenting OCT assessment of proximal RCA segment for plaque morphology. (LD: luminal diameter; MLA: minimal luminal area; OCT: optical coherence tomography; POBA: plain old balloon angioplasty; RCA: right coronary artery)

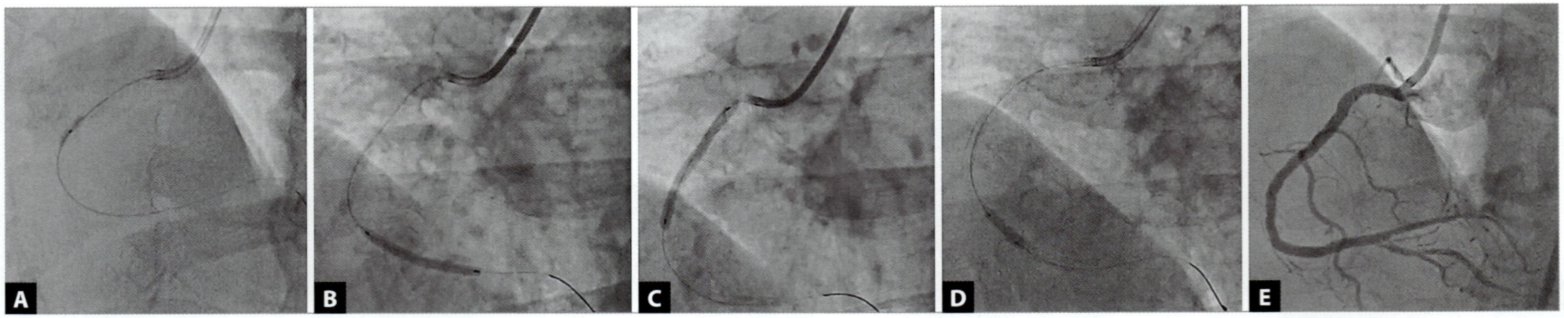

Figs. 10A to E: Coronary angioplasty of proximal and distal segments of RCA. (A) Predilatation done with 2.0 × 10 mm Tazuna balloon; (B) Distal RCA stenting done with 2.75 × 33 mm Xience Xpedition Stent; (C) Proximal RCA stenting done with 3.5 × 38 mm Xience Xpedition Stent; (D) Post-dilatation done with 3.0 × 12 mm NC Apollo balloon; (E) Final result. (LD: luminal diameter; MLA: minimal luminal area; RCA: right coronary artery)

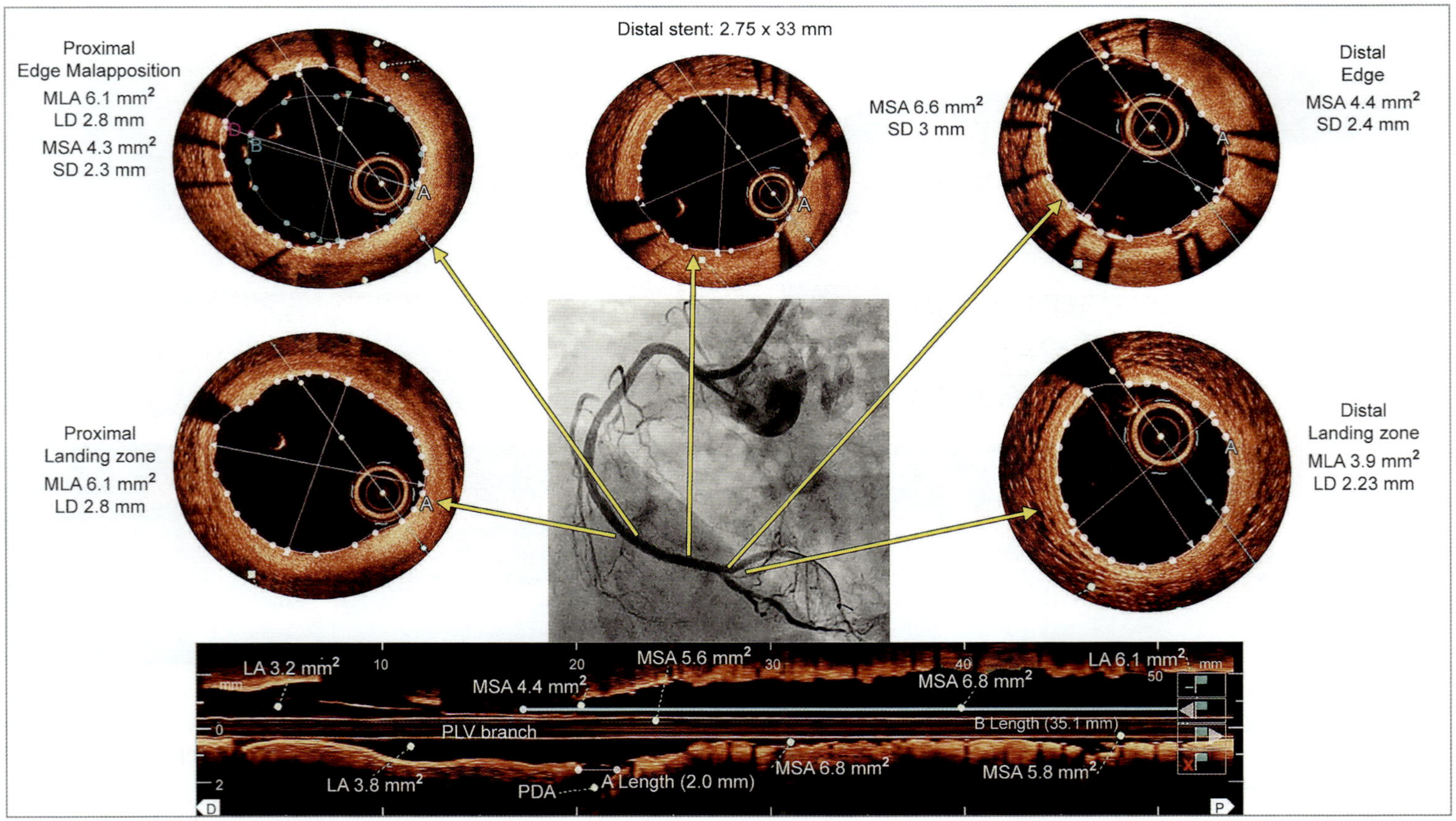

Fig. 11A

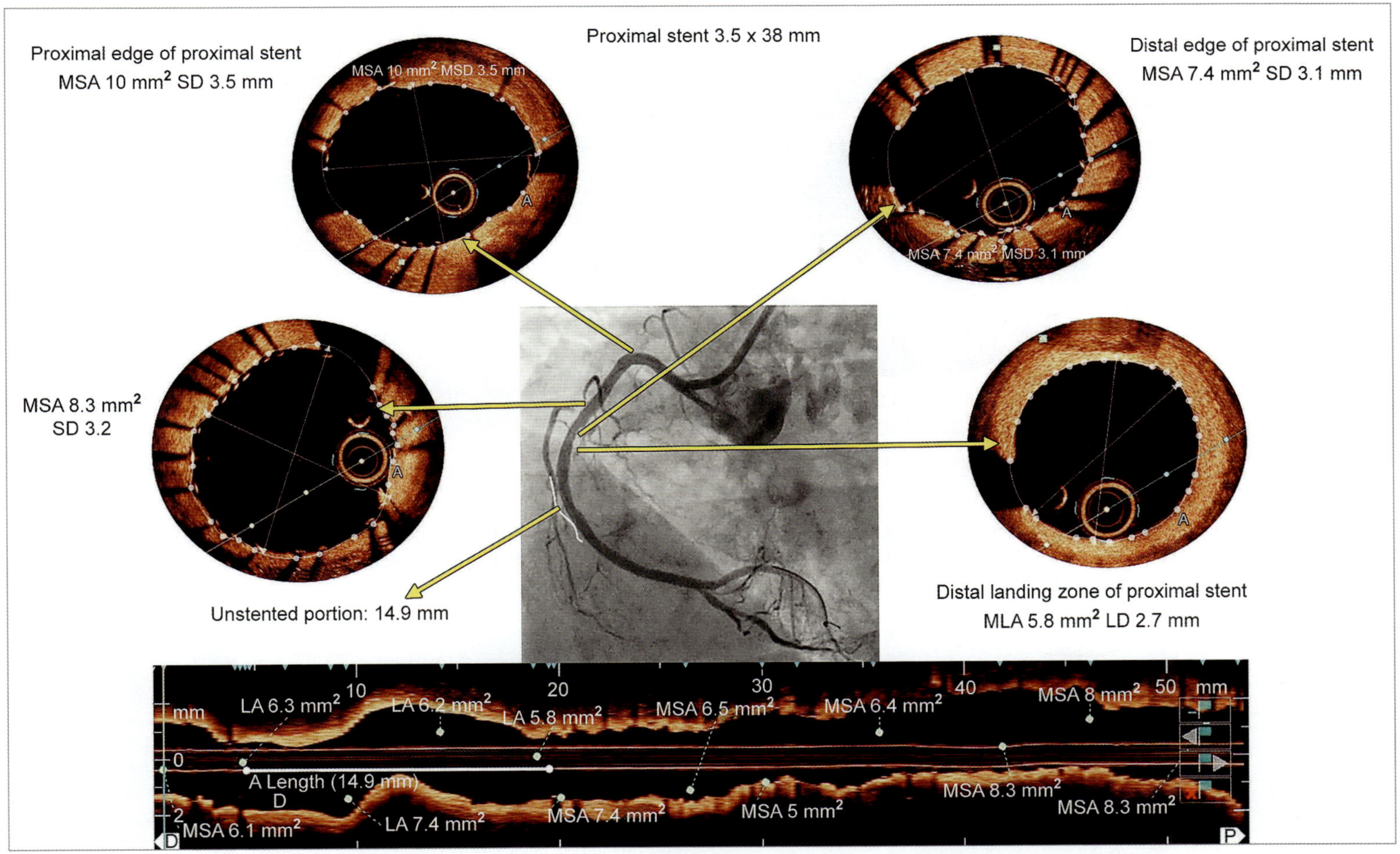
Proximal stent 3.5 x 38 mm
Proximal edge of proximal stent
MSA 10 mm² SD 3.5 mm
MSA 10 mm² MSD 3.5 mm
Distal edge of proximal stent
MSA 7.4 mm² SD 3.1 mm
MSA 7.4 mm² MSD 3.1 mm
MSA 8.3 mm²
SD 3.2
Unstented portion: 14.9 mm
Distal landing zone of proximal stent
MLA 5.8 mm² LD 2.7 mm
LA 6.3 mm²
LA 6.2 mm²
LA 5.8 mm²
MSA 6.5 mm²
MSA 6.4 mm²
MSA 8 mm²
A Length (14.9 mm)
MSA 6.1 mm²
LA 7.4 mm²
MSA 7.4 mm²
MSA 5 mm²
MSA 8.3 mm²
MSA 8.3 mm²

Fig. 11B

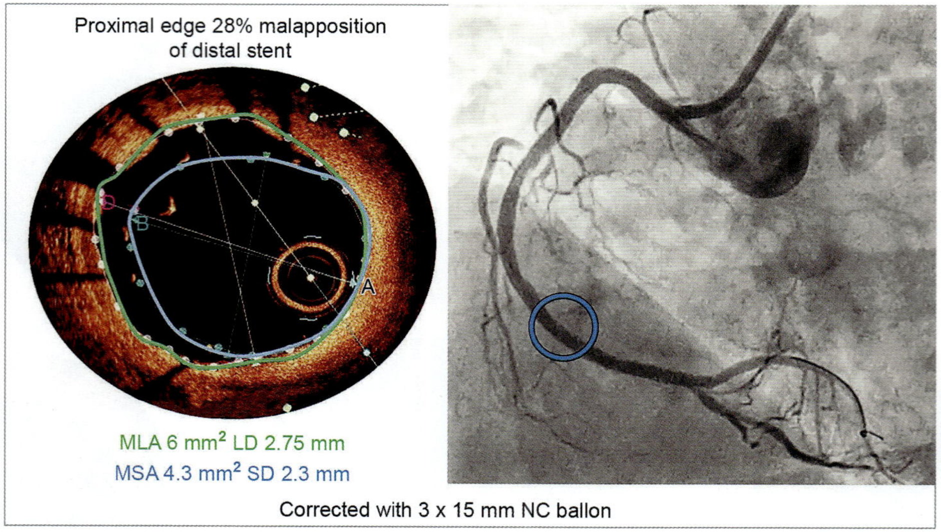

Fig. 11C

Figs. 11A to C: (A) Poststenting OCT assessment of distal RCA stent showed proximal edge malapposition with well expanded and no medial edge dissections; (B) Poststenting OCT assessment of proximal RCA stent showed well-apposed and well-expanded stent struts with no medial edge dissections; (C) Proximal edge of distal stent malapposed portion which is corrected with NC balloon. (LD: luminal diameter; MLA: minimal luminal area; MSA: minimal stent area)

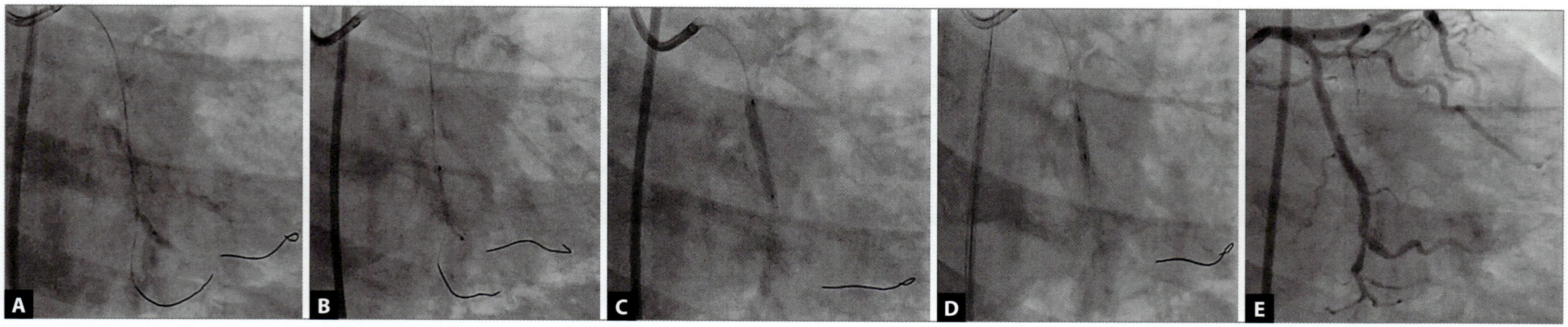

Figs. 12A to E: Coronary angioplasty of left circumflex segment.

Percutaneous Coronary Intervention of Left Circumflex

Route—RFA, 7 Fr EBU 3.5 guiding catheter, LCX lesion was crossed with 0.014″ BMW wire and obtuse marginal (OM) crossed with 0.014″ run through wire. Predilated with 1.5 × 10 mm Tazuna balloon, LCX to OM stenting done with 2.25 × 18 mm Xience Xpedition Stent. Proximal LCX stenting done with 3.0 × 23 mm Xience Xpedition stent. Postdilated with 2.5 × 10 mm Tazuna balloon and 3 × 10 mm NC. Postprocedure Angio view showed well-implanted stents with TIMI-III flow without any dissection **(Figs. 12A to E)**. Patient was discharged on third postprocedure in a stable status.

CASE 3

Percutaneous coronary intervention (PCI) of diffuse fibro calcific long segment of left anterior descending (LAD)-anterior non-ST-elevation myocardial infarction (NSTEMI).

CLINICAL HISTORY

A 54-year-old male known hypertensive, diabetic presented with anterior-NSTEMI, chest pain associated with SOB of 1 day duration. 2D Echo—no RWMA, normal LV function, and EF—64%.

Investigations: Trop I—16 ng/mL, N-terminal pro-brain natriuretic peptide (NT-Pro BNP)—1,222 pg/mL, S.Cr—0.9 mg/dL, eGFR—87 mL/min, blood urea—29 mg/dL, and RBS—263 mg/dL.

Coronary angiography-LMCA—normal, LAD—proximal 70% lesion, mid total thrombotic occlusion, LCX—distal 90% lesion, RCA—mild disease **(Figs. 13A to E)**.

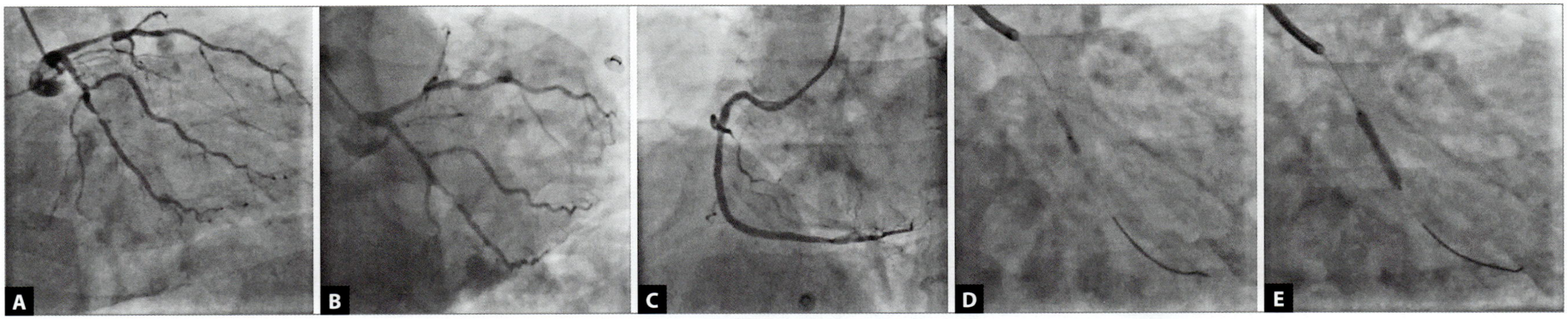

Figs. 13A to E: Coronary angiogram, predilatation, and stenting of left circumflex lesion.

PROCEDURE

Percutaneous Coronary Intervention of Left Circumflex

Route—RFA, 6 Fr-3.5 XB guiding catheter, LCX lesion was crossed with 0.014″ run through wire, predilated with 2.0 × 10 mm Tazuna balloon, LCX stented with 2.75 × 18 mm Resolute Onyx Stent **(Figs. 13A to E)** and postdilated with 3.5 × 12 mm NC Trek balloon. Check Angio showed good TIMI-III flow.

Percutaneous Coronary Intervention of Left Anterior Descending

Route—RFA, 6 Fr EBU 3.5 guiding catheter, totally occluded LAD lesion was crossed with 0.014″ run through wire, D1 wired with 0.014″ Sion Blue wire, predilated with 2.0 × 10 mm Tazuna balloon.

Pre-OCT showed fibrotic plaque in proximal LAD **(Figs. 14A to E)**.

Distal LAD stenting done with 2.25 × 26 mm Resolute Onyx Stent, proximal LAD stenting done with 3.0 × 38 mm Resolute Onyx Stent. Postdilatation done with 3.5 × 12 mm NC Trek balloon **(Figs. 15A to F)**.

Poststenting OCT showed well apposed and expanded stent struts, and no edge dissection **(Figs. 16A and B)**.

Postprocedure Angio view showed well-implanted stents with TIMI-III flow without any dissection.

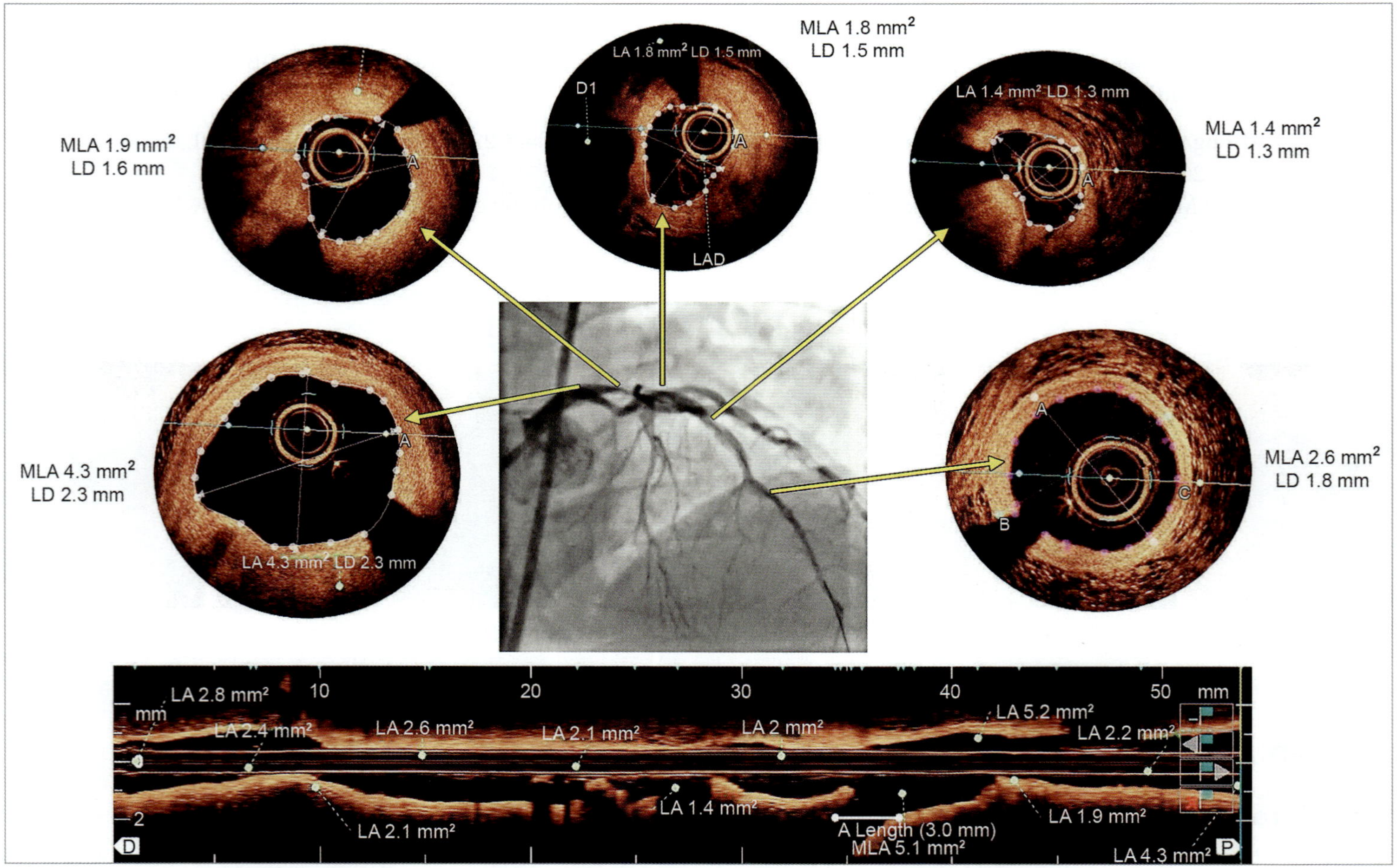

Fig. 14A

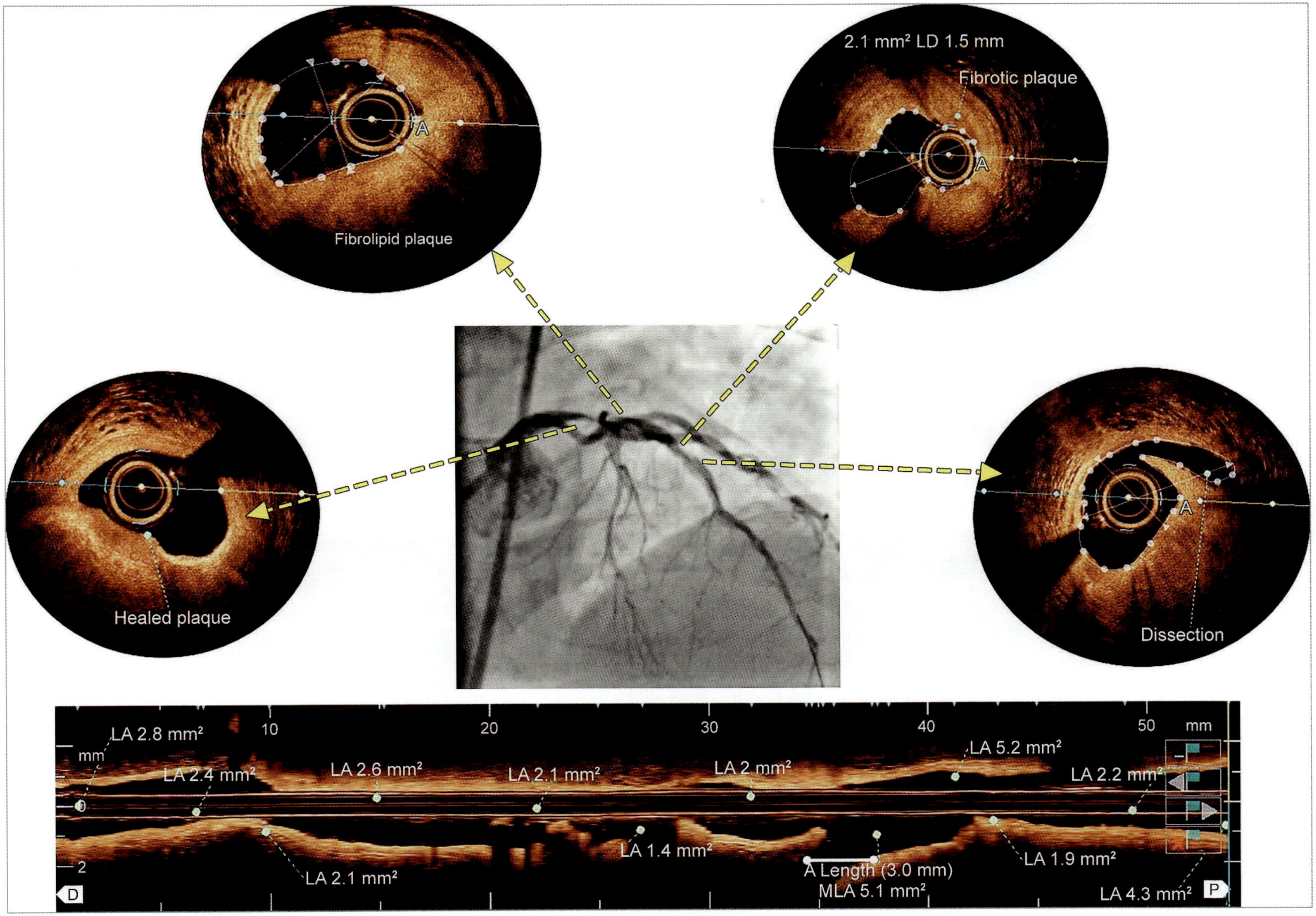
2.1 mm² LD 1.5 mm
Fibrotic plaque
Fibrolipid plaque
Healed plaque
Dissection
LA 2.8 mm²
LA 2.4 mm²
LA 2.6 mm²
LA 2.1 mm²
LA 2 mm²
LA 5.2 mm²
LA 2.2 mm²
LA 2.1 mm²
LA 1.4 mm²
A Length (3.0 mm)
MLA 5.1 mm²
LA 1.9 mm²
LA 4.3 mm²
mm
D
P

Fig. 14B

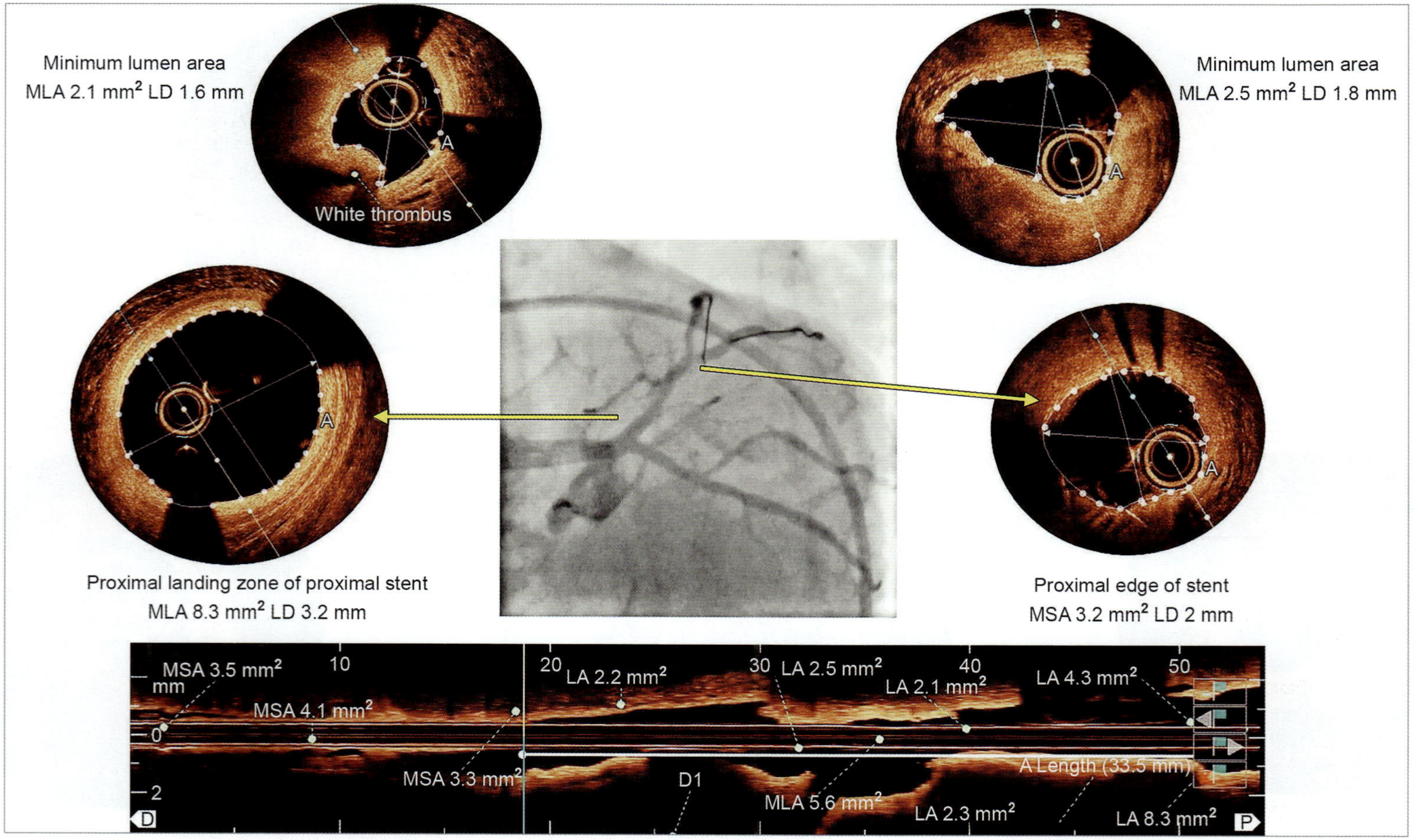

Minimum lumen area
MLA 2.1 mm2 LD 1.6 mm
White thrombus
Minimum lumen area
MLA 2.5 mm2 LD 1.8 mm
Proximal landing zone of proximal stent
MLA 8.3 mm2 LD 3.2 mm
Proximal edge of stent
MSA 3.2 mm2 LD 2 mm
MSA 3.5 mm2
MSA 4.1 mm2
MSA 3.3 mm2
LA 2.2 mm2
LA 2.5 mm2
LA 2.1 mm2
LA 4.3 mm2
MLA 5.6 mm2
LA 2.3 mm2
LA 8.3 mm2
A Length (33.5 mm)
D1
D
P

Fig. 14C

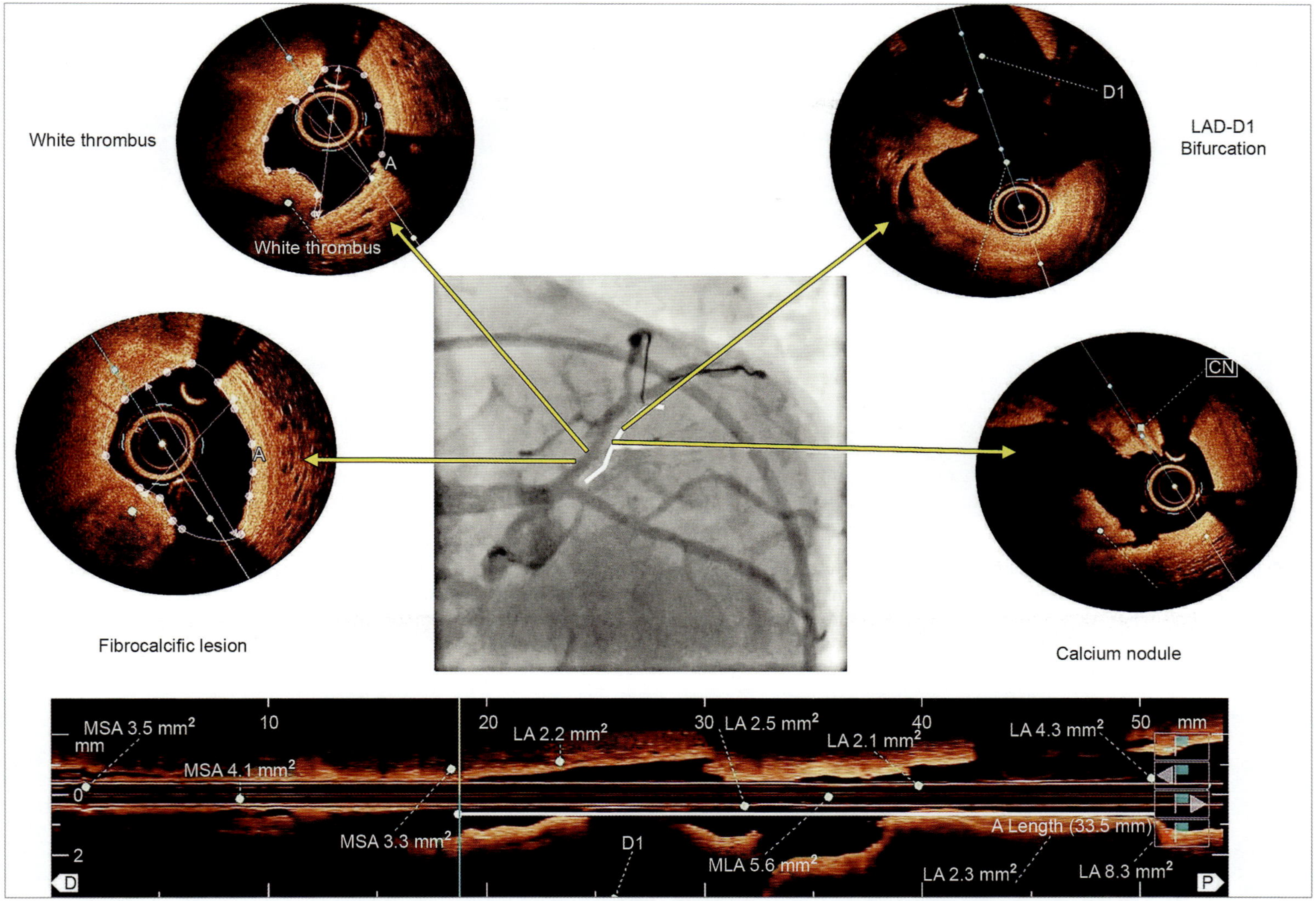

White thrombus
A
White thrombus
D1
LAD-D1
Bifurcation
CN
A
Fibrocalcific lesion
Calcium nodule
MSA 3.5 mm²
mm
10
20
LA 2.2 mm²
30
LA 2.5 mm²
40
LA 2.1 mm²
LA 4.3 mm²
50
mm
MSA 4.1 mm²
0
MSA 3.3 mm²
D1
MLA 5.6 mm²
A Length (33.5 mm)
2
LA 2.3 mm²
LA 8.3 mm²
D
P

Fig. 14D

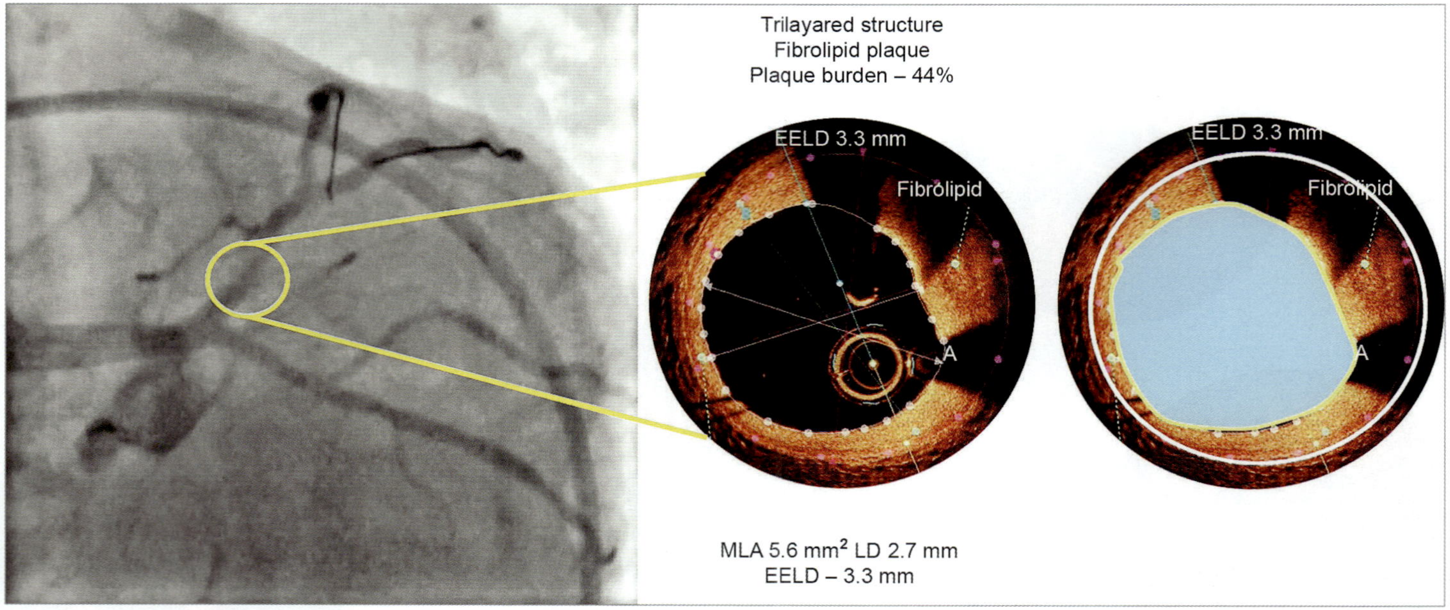

Fig. 14E

Figs. 14A to E: (A) Prestenting OCT analysis of LAD disease segment; (B) Prestenting OCT analysis for plaque morphology; (C) Prestenting OCT analysis for device selection; (D) Prestenting OCT analysis showed mixed plaque in LAD segment; (E) Trilayered structure of LAD lesion showed fibrolipid plaque with plaque burden 44%. (LAD: left anterior descending; LD: luminal diameter; MLA: minimal luminal area; MSA: minimal stent area; OCT: optical coherence tomography)

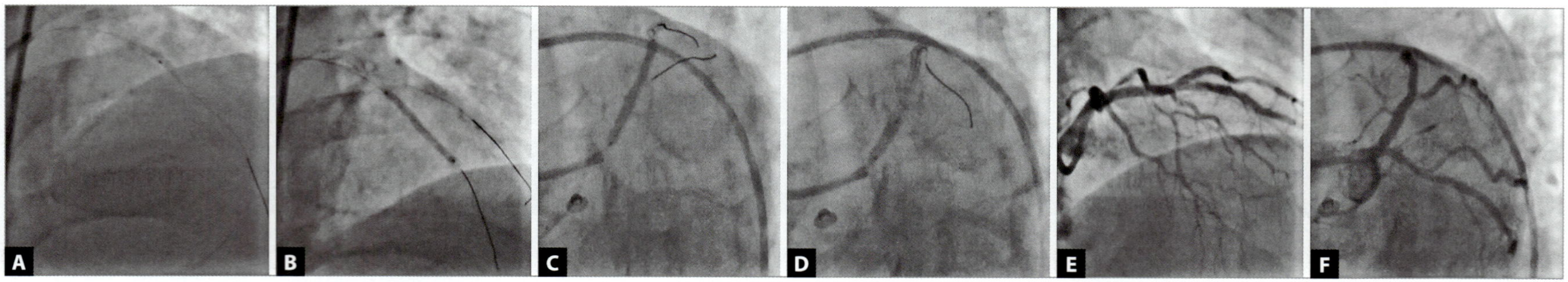

Figs. 15A to F: Coronary angioplasty of left anterior descending vessel and final result.

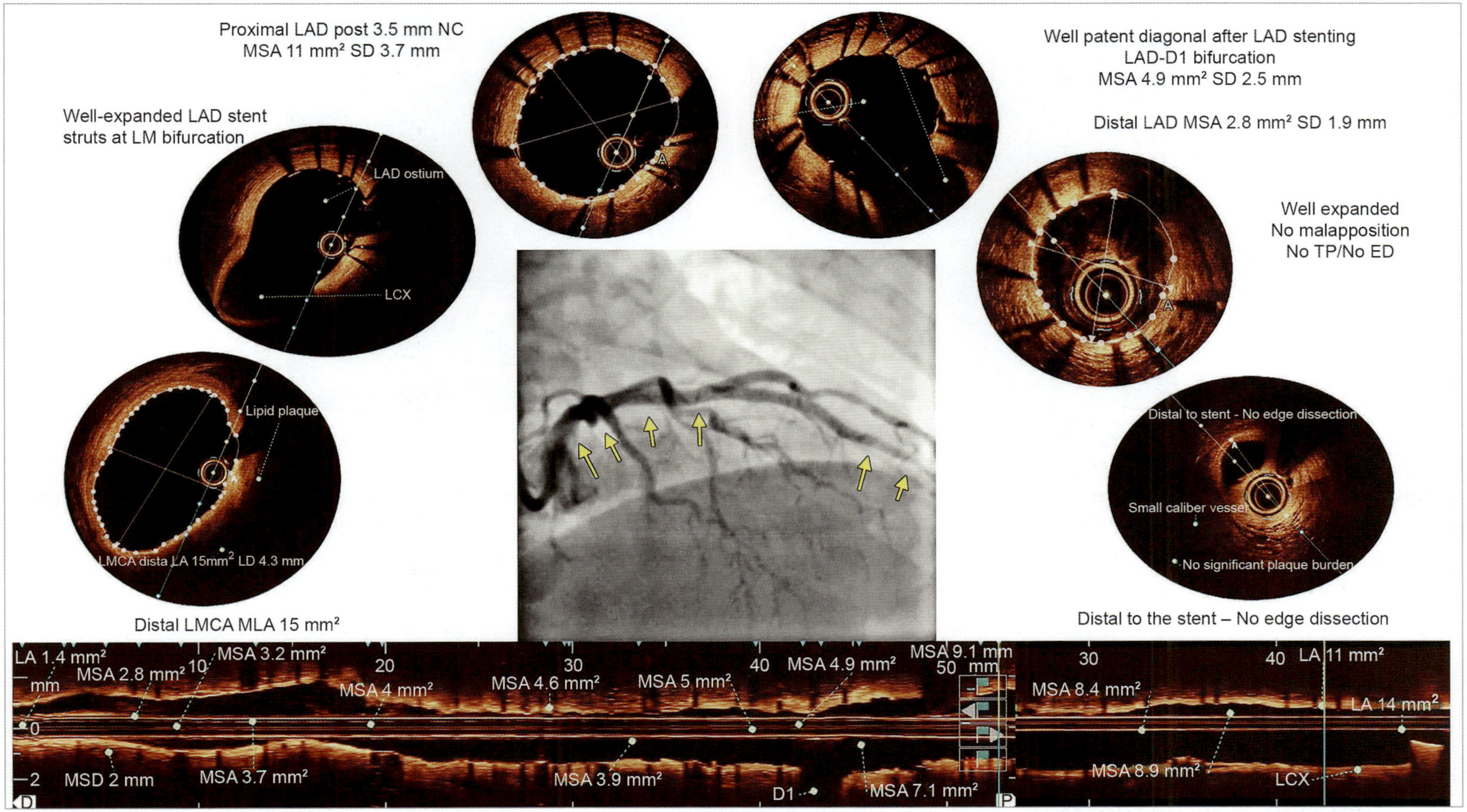
Proximal LAD post 3.5 mm NC
MSA 11 mm² SD 3.7 mm
Well-expanded LAD stent struts at LM bifurcation
LAD ostium
LCX
Lipid plaque
LMCA dista LA 15mm² LD 4.3 mm
Distal LMCA MLA 15 mm²
Well patent diagonal after LAD stenting
LAD-D1 bifurcation
MSA 4.9 mm² SD 2.5 mm
Distal LAD MSA 2.8 mm² SD 1.9 mm
Well expanded
No malapposition
No TP/No ED
Distal to stent - No edge dissection
Small caliber vessel
No significant plaque burden
Distal to the stent – No edge dissection
LA 1.4 mm²
MSA 2.8 mm²
MSA 3.2 mm²
MSD 2 mm
MSA 3.7 mm²
MSA 4 mm²
MSA 4.6 mm²
MSA 3.9 mm²
MSA 5 mm²
MSA 4.9 mm²
D1
MSA 7.1 mm²
MSA 9.1 mm
MSA 8.4 mm²
MSA 8.9 mm²
LA 11 mm²
LA 14 mm²
LCX

Fig. 16A

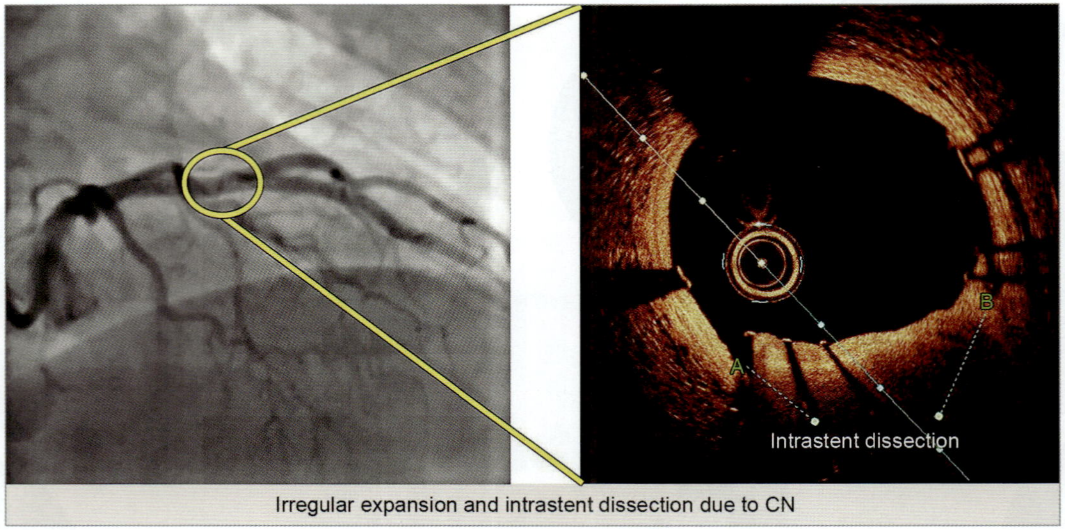

Fig. 16B

Figs. 16A and B: (A) Poststenting OCT analysis showed well apposed and expanded stent struts with no medial edge dissections; (B) Irregular expansion and intrastent dissection due to calcific nodule which is nonflow limiting. (LAD: left anterior descending; MLA: minimal luminal area; OCT: optical coherence tomography)

CASE 4

Usefulness of optical coherence tomography for diffusely long segment of Left Anterior Descending

CLINICAL HISTORY

A 60-year-old male known hypertensive, diabetic presented with unstable angina, left side chest pain associated with SOB and sweating, 2D Echo—no RWMA, good LV function with EF—69%.

Investigations: Hb—12.8 g/dL, S.Cr—0.80 mg/dL, eGFR—104 L/min, CAG-LMCA—Normal, LAD—mid LAD 70-80% disease, LCX—ostioproximal LCX mild disease, RCA—distal RCA 95% lesion **(Figs. 17A and B)**.

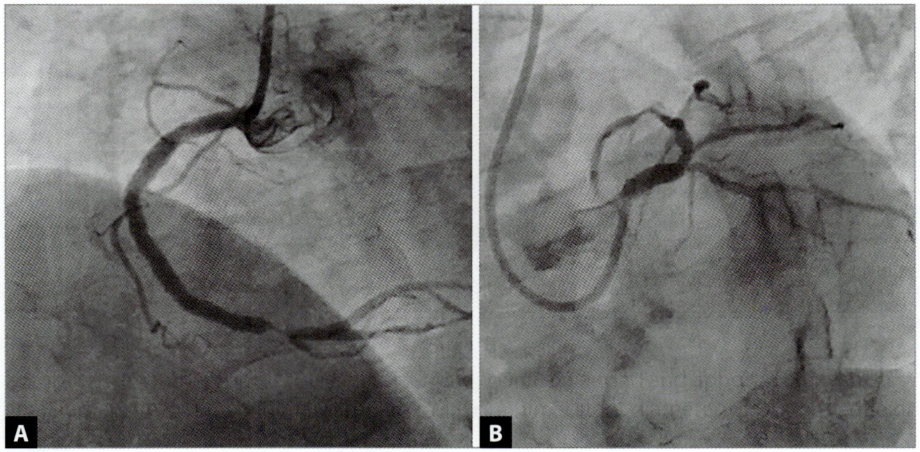

Figs. 17A and B: Coronary angiogram.

PROCEDURE

PCI of Left Anterior Descending

Route—RRA, 6 Fr EBU 3.5 guiding catheter, LAD lesion was crossed with 0.014″ run through wire, predilated with 2.0 × 10 mm Tazuna balloon. Pre-OCT showed fibrotic plaque from distal to proximal LAD **(Figs. 18A and B)**. Distal LAD stenting done with 2.5 × 38 mm Resolute Onyx Stent, proximal to mid

LAD stenting done with 3.0 × 26 mm Resolute Onyx Stent. Postdilatation done with 2.75 × 12 mm NC Trek balloon and proximal LAD with 3.5 × 12 mm NC Trek balloon **(Fig. 19)**. Postprocedure OCT study showed well-apposed and well-expanded stent struts, no residual stenosis and no thrombosis **(Figs. 20A and B)**. Postprocedure Angio views showed well-implanted stents with TIMI-III flow without any dissection. Patient was discharged on third postprocedure day in a stable status.

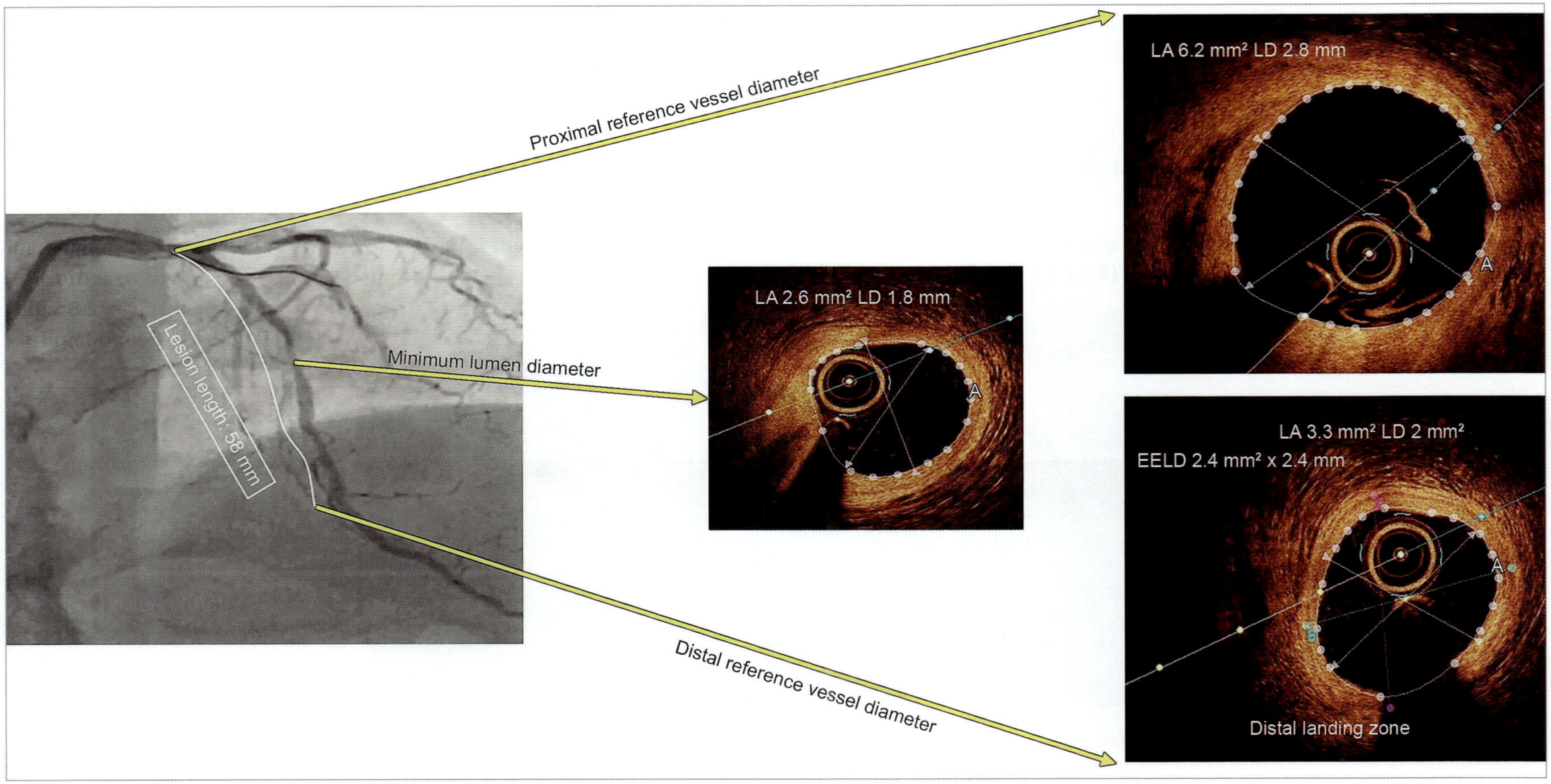

Fig. 18A

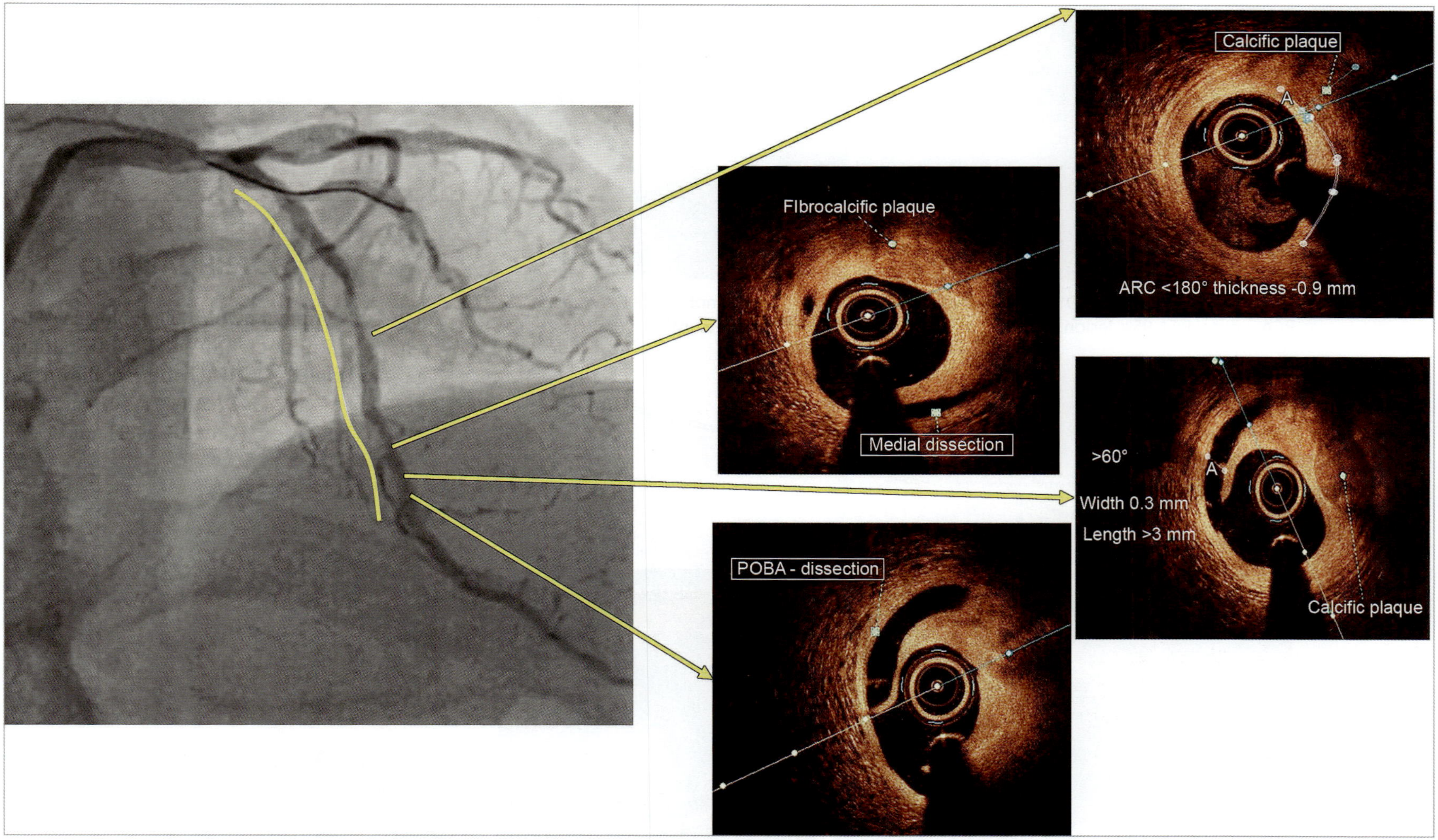

Fig. 18B

Figs. 18A and B: Prestenting optical coherence tomography (OCT) analysis—(A) for device selection and (B) for plaque morphology.

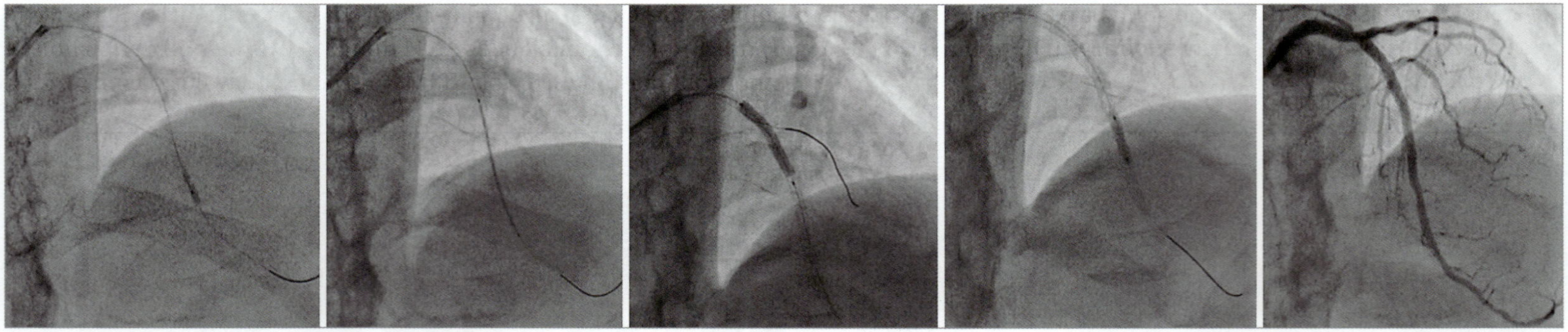

Fig. 19: Coronary angioplasty of LAD segment. Coronary angiography: LMCA—normal, LAD—mid LAD 70–80% disease, LCX—ostioproximal LCX mild disease, RCA—distal RCA 95% lesion. (LAD: left anterior descending; LCX: left circumflex; LMCA: left main coronary artery; RCA: right coronary artery)

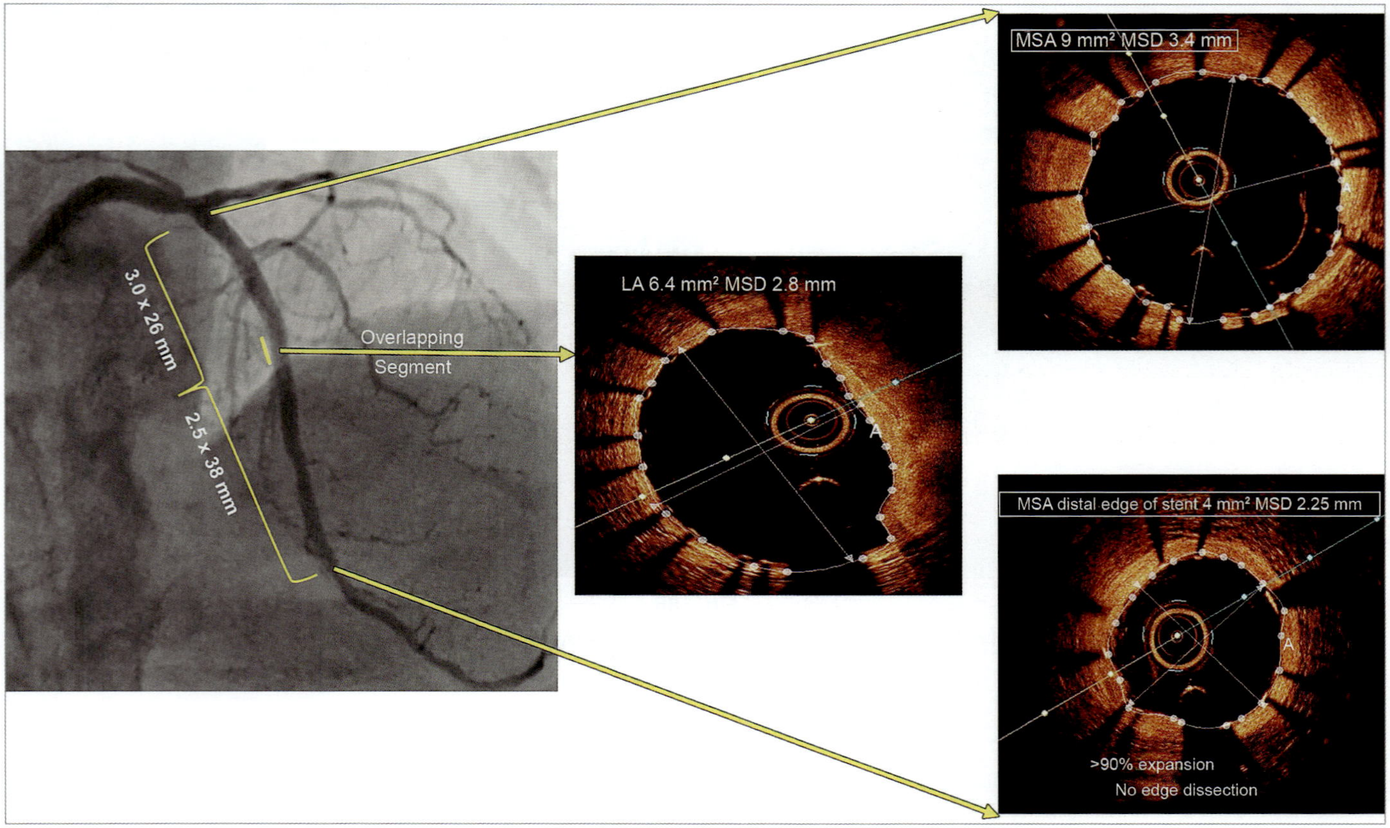

Fig. 20A

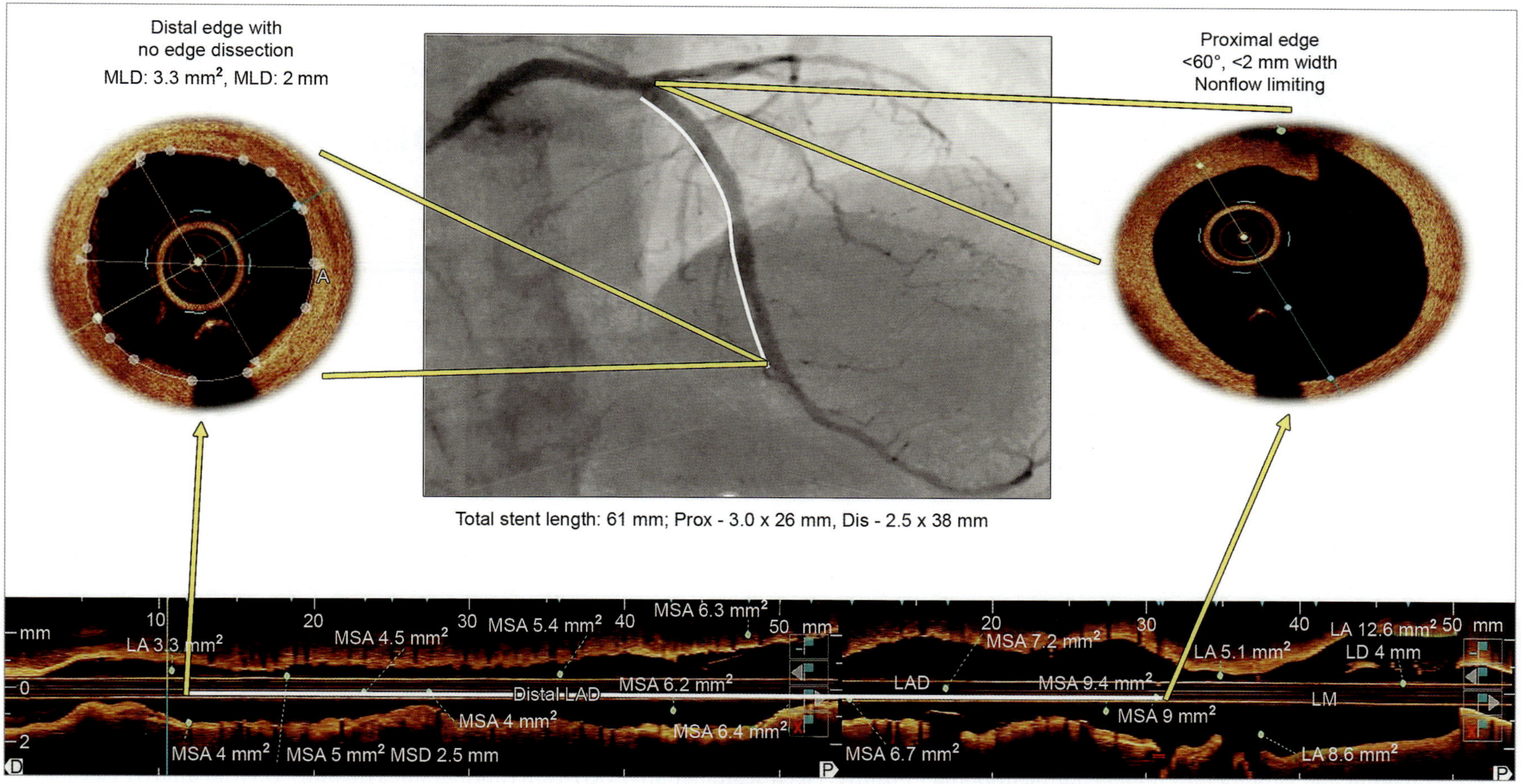

Fig. 20B

Figs. 20A and B: Poststent OCT assessment of LAD showed well expanded and apposed stent struts with no medial edge dissections. (LAD: left anterior descending; MSA: minimal stent area; MSD: minimal stent diameter)

CHAPTER

21 Multivessel Percutaneous Coronary Intervention

CASE 1

Optical coherence tomography (OCT)-guided triple-vessel stenting with biovascular scaffold (BVS).

CLINICAL HISTORY

A 42-year-old male, known diabetic, smoker with strong family history of (H/o) coronary artery disease (CAD), admitted for one episode of severe retrosternal burning pain lasting for 24 hours associated with exertional shortness of breath (SOB) class-III since 2 days, H/o bronchial asthma since 15 years on bronchodilator therapy under control, troponin I-positive, electrocardiogram (ECG)-NSR (normal sinus rhythm), QS with mild ST elevation in lead I, and augmented vector left (AVL), mild ST-elevation in V5 and V6, R/S ratio more than 1 in V1 with T upright [lateral and true post MI (myocardial infarction)], 2D Echo—hypokinetic basal inferior and lateral wall, ejection fraction (EF)—55%. Coronary angiogram (CAG) through right radial route, left main coronary artery (LMCA)—normal, left anterior descending (LAD) type-III vessel; diffuse severe long segment disease from proximal LAD to proximal portion of distal LAD, left circumflex (LCX)—co-dominant, total occlusion of obtuse marginal (OM) branch. Right coronary artery (RCA)—dominant, long segment disease of proximal and mid-RCA with area of 70%–80% narrowing **(Fig. 1)**. In view of severe triple-vessel disease option of coronary artery bypass grafting (CABG) versus multivessel percutaneous coronary intervention (PCI) was given. OCT-guided BVS stenting of triple-vessel disease was planned.

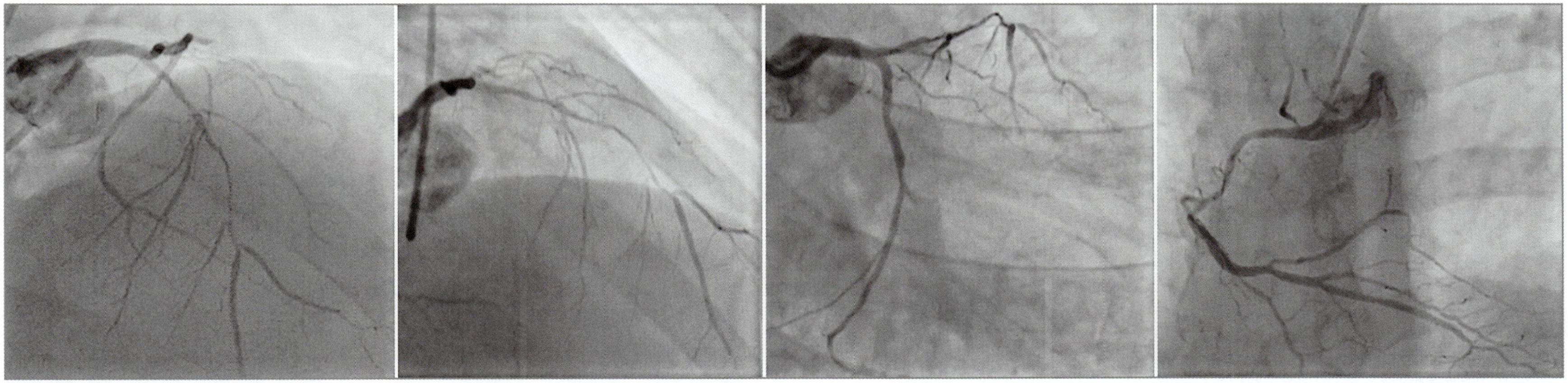

Fig. 1: Coronary angiogram.

PROCEDURE

PCI of LAD: Right femoral artery (RFA) route, 6 Fr 3.5 XB guiding catheter, 0.014″ Sion blue wire placed in LAD, predilatation done with 1.5 × 12 mm Mini Trek balloon. Pre-OCT—minimal lumen area 1.8 mm^2 with fibrotic plaque **(Figs. 2 and 3)**. Predilatation with 2.5 × 12 mm Trek balloon, mid to distal LAD stenting done with 2.5 × 28 mm Absorb stent (BVS) at 14–16 atm. Proximal to mid LAD overlapping stenting done with 3.0 × 28 mm Absorb stent (BVS) at 14 atm. Postdilatation done with 2.75 × 14 mm NC trek balloon, proximal stent postdilatation done with 3.0 × 12 mm NC Trek balloon, distal stent postdilatation done with 3.0 × 15 mm NC Trek balloon **(Fig. 4)**. Poststenting OCT study showed mild edge dissection, stent struts well-opposed and no residual stenosis **(Figs. 5A to C)**. The final result was good with TIMI III (thrombolysis in myocardial infarction III) flow.

PCI of LCX: 0.014″ Rinato wire was placed in OM1 and 0.014″ Sion blue wire was placed in distal LCX. Predilatations were carried out with 1.5 × 12 mm, 1.5 × 15 mm Mini Trek and 2.5 × 15 mm Trek balloon, faced difficulty in crossing stent due to entangled wires of LCX and OM hence 0.014″ Sion blue wire removed from distal LCX, finally BVS was placed with deep respirations without any buddy wire technique. LCX to OM stenting done with 2.5 × 28 mm Absorb stent (BVS) at 10 atm for 30 seconds **(Fig. 6)**. Postdilatation done with 3.0 × 15 mm NC Trek balloon. OCT study showed well-apposed stents struts and well-preserved LCX and OM bifurcation site without any edge dissection/thrombosis **(Figs. 7A and B)**.

PCI of RCA: 6 Fr 3.5 JR guiding catheter, 0.014″ Sion blue wire placed in RCA, predilatation done with 2.75 × 14 mm NC Falcon balloon. Stenting of mid RCA done with 3.5 × 28 mm Absorb stent (BVS) at 14–16 atm, proximal RCA overlapping stenting done with 3.5 × 18 mm Absorb stent (BVS) at 18 atm **(Fig. 8)**. Postdilatation done with 3.5 × 12 mm NC Trek balloon. OCT study showed well-apposed stent struts **(Figs. 9A and B)**. Final result was good with TIMI-III flow. Patient was discharged on fourth postprocedure day in stable status. Five days after discharge patient was readmitted for check angio due to two to three episodes of retrosternal burning sensations which revealed well patent stents with good TIMI-III flow. Patient was advised to continue dual antiplatelet therapy (DAPT), statin therapy with additional proton-pump inhibitor (PPI) drugs. After 3 years' follow-up computed tomography (CT) angio showed well patent BVS stents **(Figs. 10A and B)**.

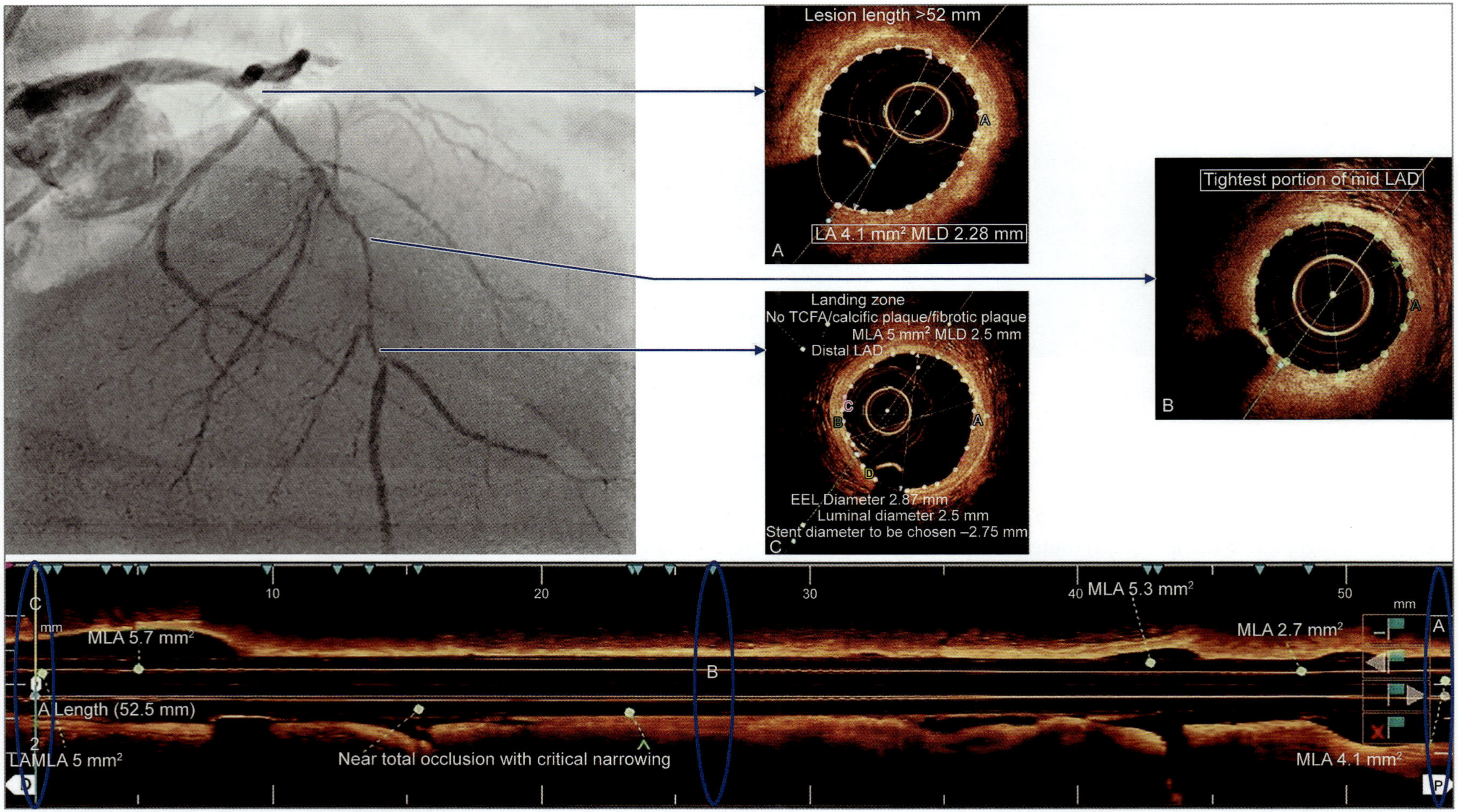

Fig. 2: Prestent optical coherence tomography (OCT) analysis for device selection. (EEL: external elastic lamina; LA: lumen area; LAD: left anterior descending; MLA: minimal lumen area; MLD: minimal lumen diameter; TCFA: thin-cap fibroatheroma)

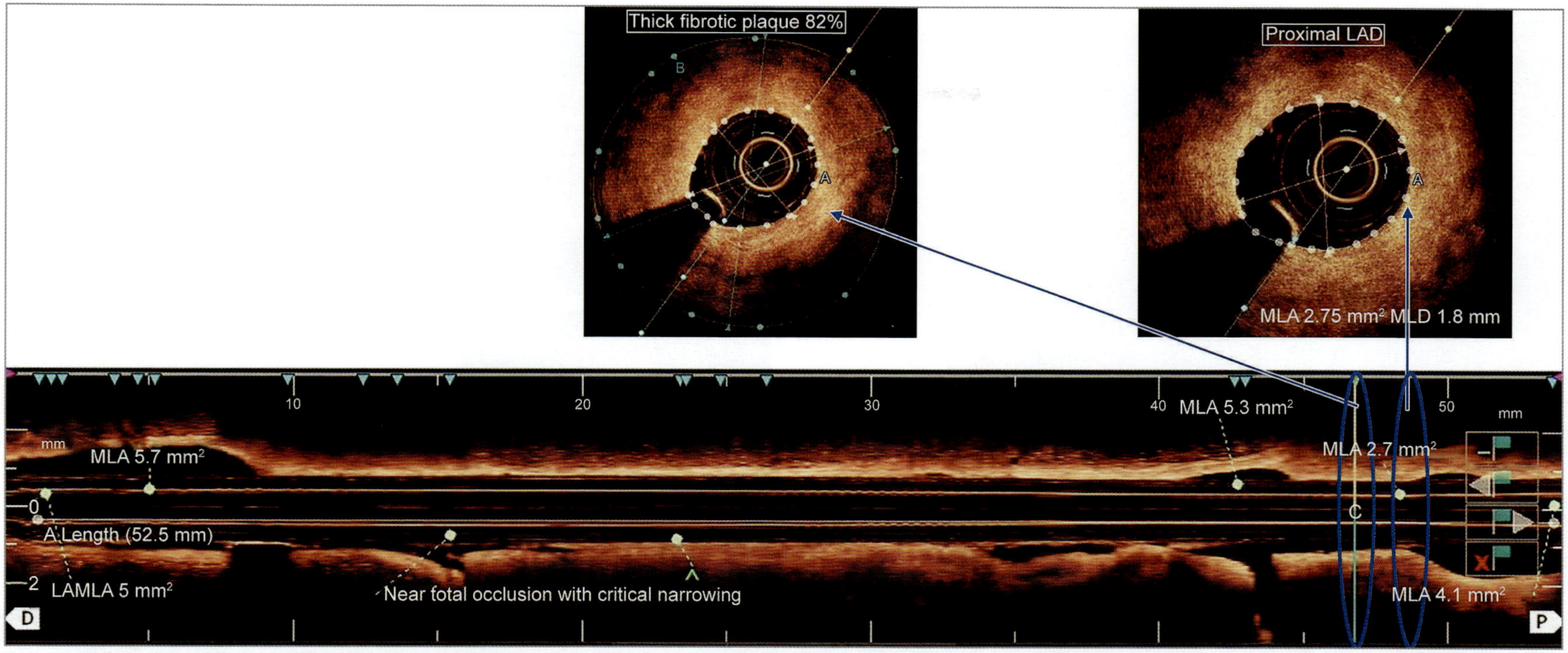

Fig. 3: Plaque morphology. (LAD: left anterior descending; MLA: minimal lumen area)

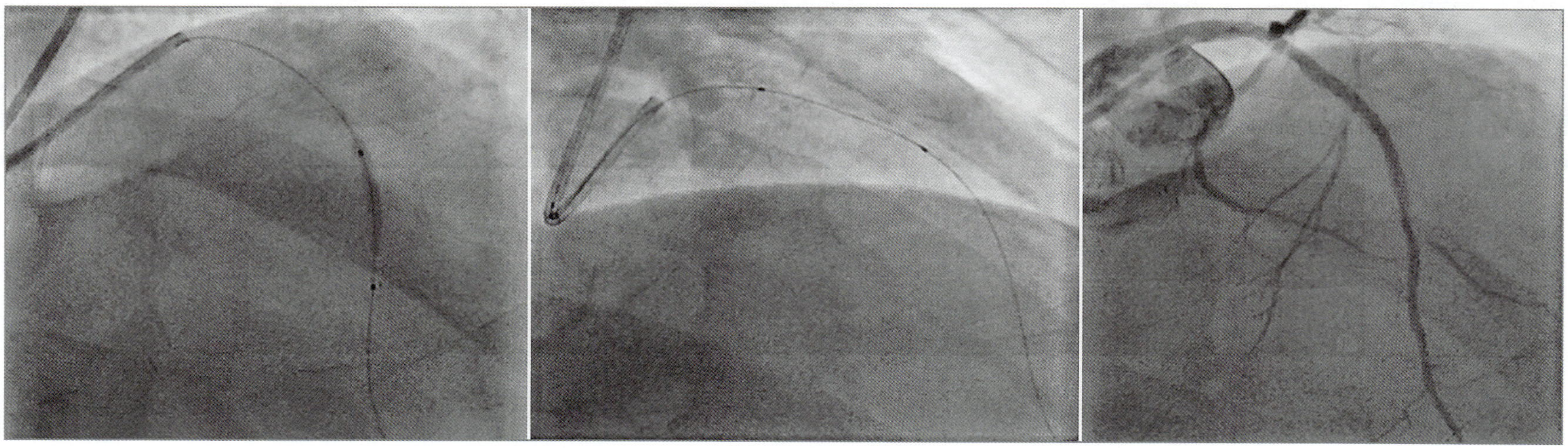

Fig. 4: Coronary angioplasty for left anterior descending (LAD) lesion.

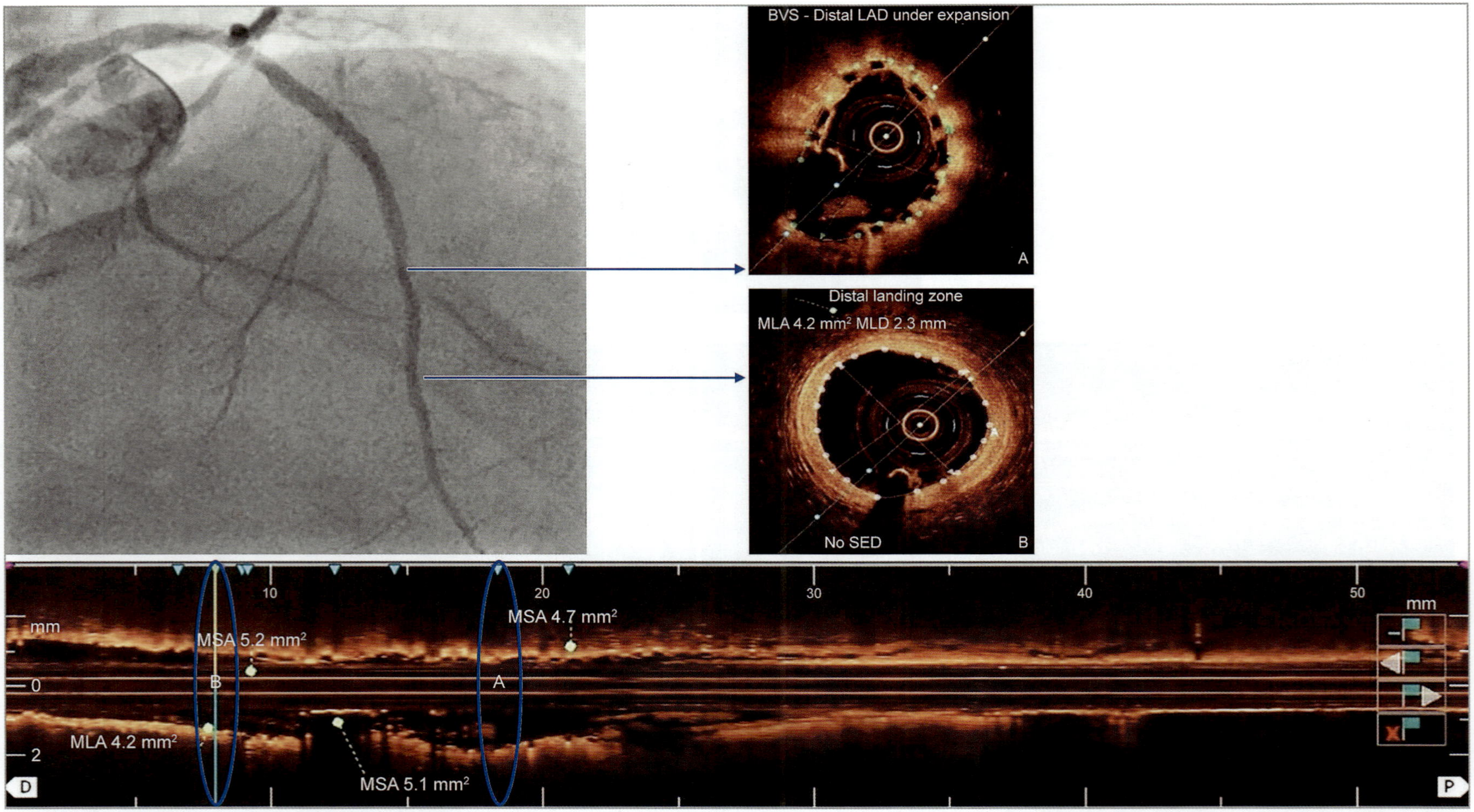
BVS - Distal LAD under expansion
A
Distal landing zone
MLA 4.2 mm² MLD 2.3 mm
No SED
B
10
20
30
40
50
mm
mm
MSA 4.7 mm²
MSA 5.2 mm²
0
B
A
MLA 4.2 mm²
2
MSA 5.1 mm²
D
P

Fig. 5A

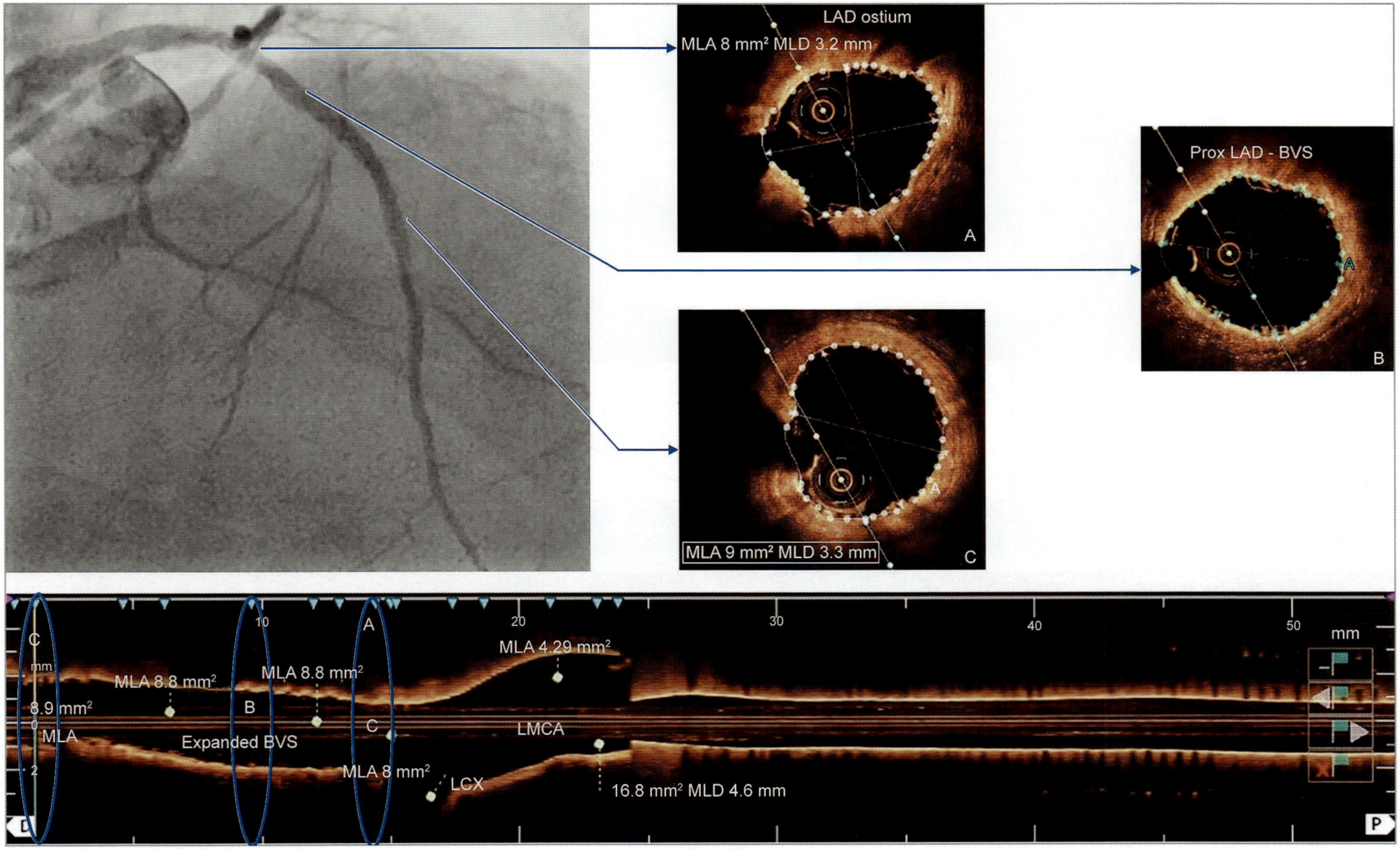
LAD ostium
MLA 8 mm² MLD 3.2 mm
A
Prox LAD - BVS
B
MLA 9 mm² MLD 3.3 mm
C
MLA 4.29 mm²
MLA 8.8 mm²
MLA 8.8 mm²
8.9 mm²
MLA
Expanded BVS
LMCA
MLA 8 mm²
LCX
16.8 mm² MLD 4.6 mm
mm
10
20
30
40
50
D
P

Fig. 5B

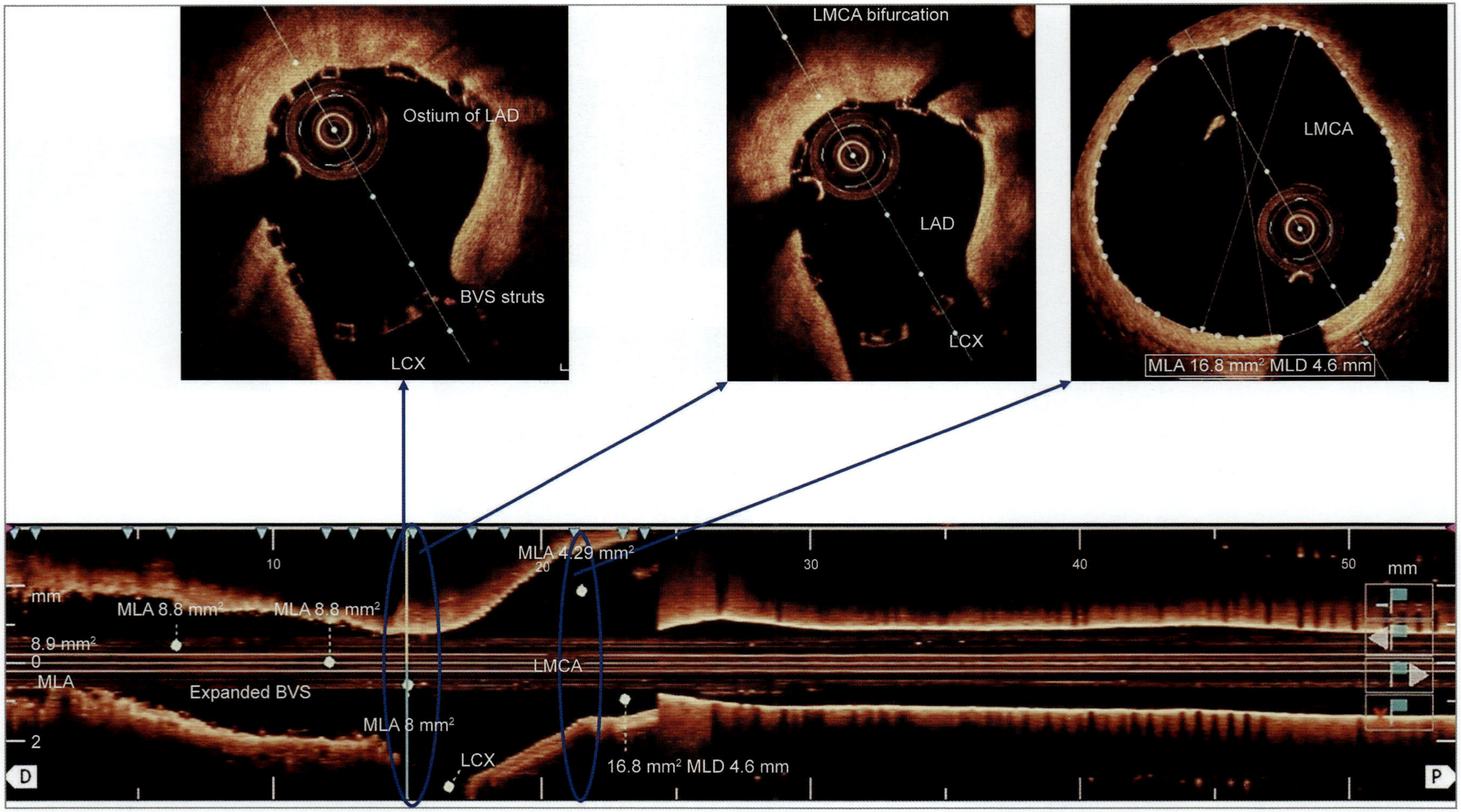

Fig. 5C

Figs. 5A to C: Poststent optical coherence tomography (OCT) analysis showed (A) Well-expanded and apposed stent struts with no medial edge dissections; (B) Assessment of LM–LAD (left main–left anterior descending) lesion; (C) Post BVS stenting OCT showing no residual stenosis across the LM bifurcation; (MLA: minimal lumen area; MSA: minimal stent area)

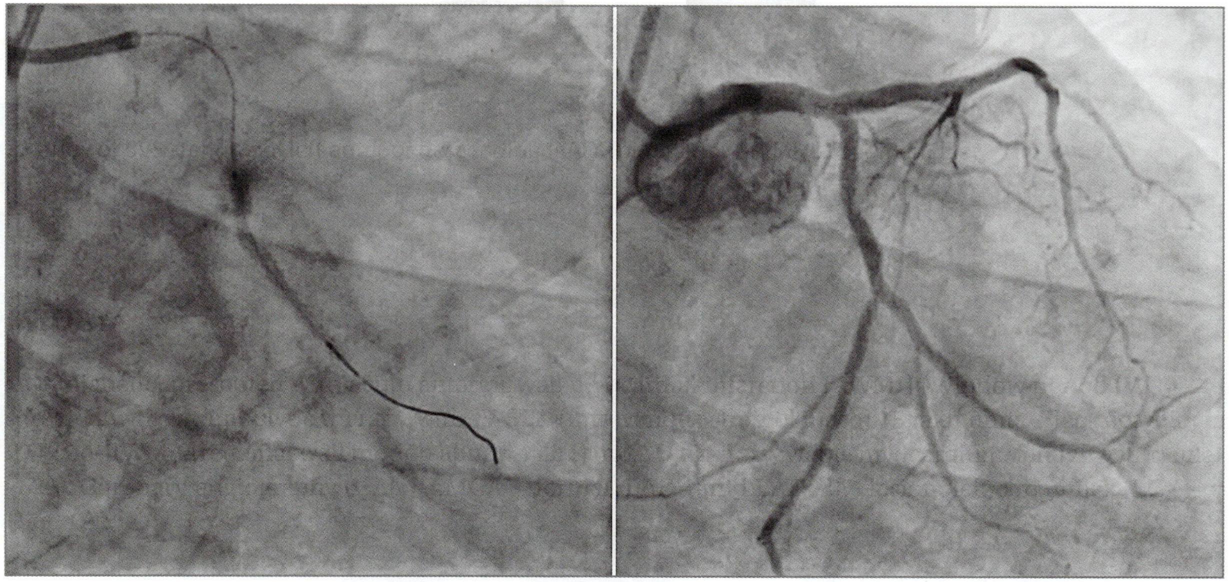

Fig. 6: Coronary angioplasty of left circumflex (LCX) lesion.

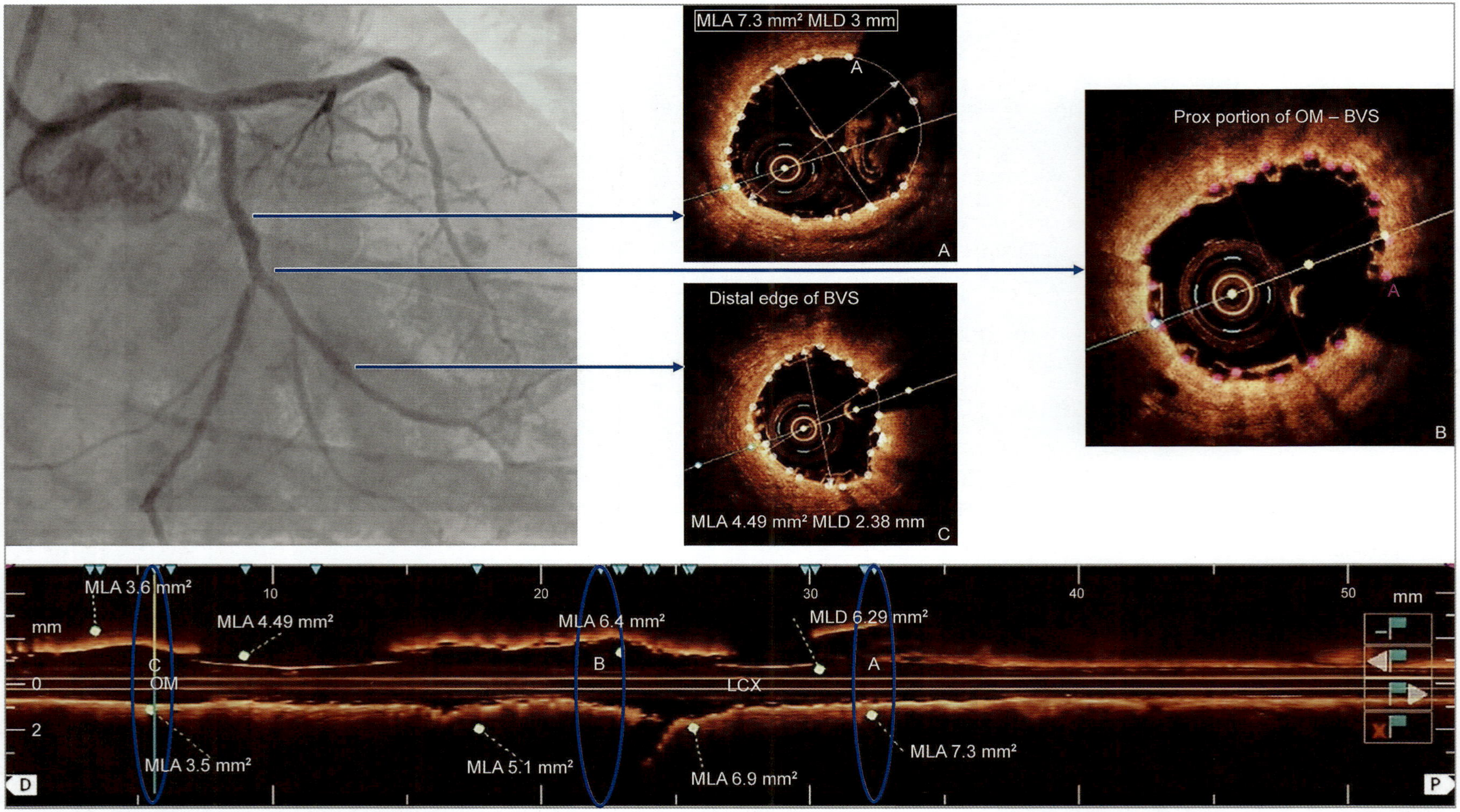
MLA 7.3 mm² MLD 3 mm
A
Prox portion of OM – BVS
B
Distal edge of BVS
MLA 4.49 mm² MLD 2.38 mm
C
MLA 3.6 mm²
MLA 4.49 mm²
MLA 6.4 mm²
MLD 6.29 mm²
MLA 3.5 mm²
MLA 5.1 mm²
MLA 6.9 mm²
MLA 7.3 mm²
OM
LCX
mm
D
P

Fig. 7A

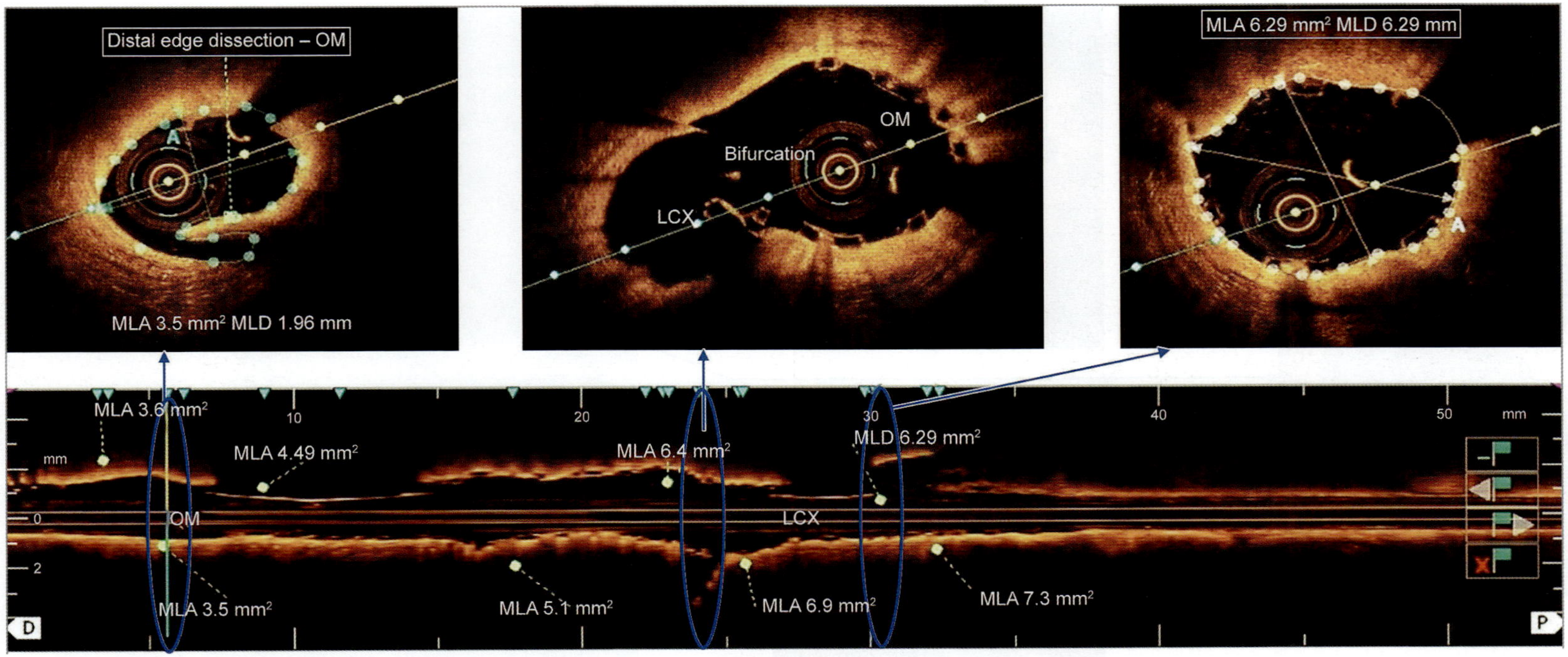

Fig. 7B

Figs. 7A and B: Poststenting optical coherence tomography (OCT) analysis showed well-expanded and apposed stent struts with no medial edge dissections. (BVS: biovascular scaffold; LCX: left circumflex; OM: obtuse marginal; MLA: minimal lumen area; MLD: minimal lumen diameter)

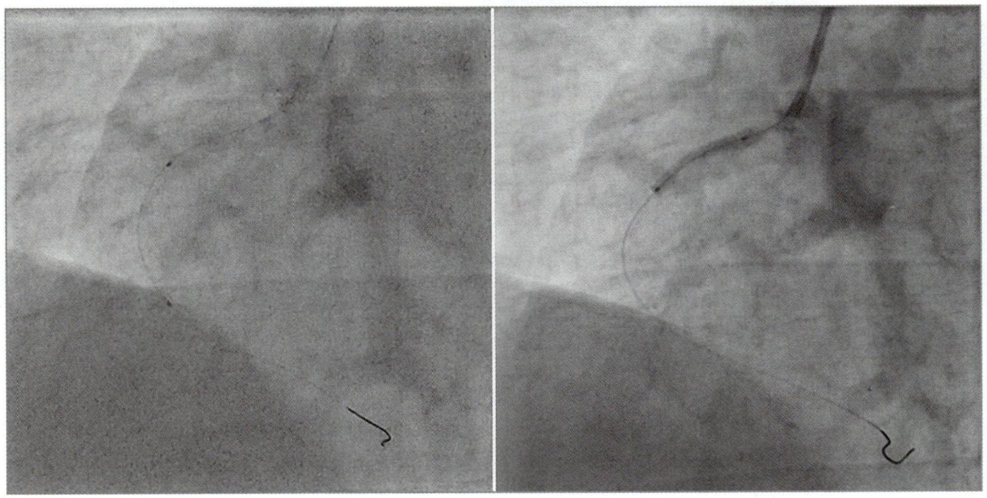

Fig. 8: Coronary angioplasty of right coronary artery (RCA) lesion.

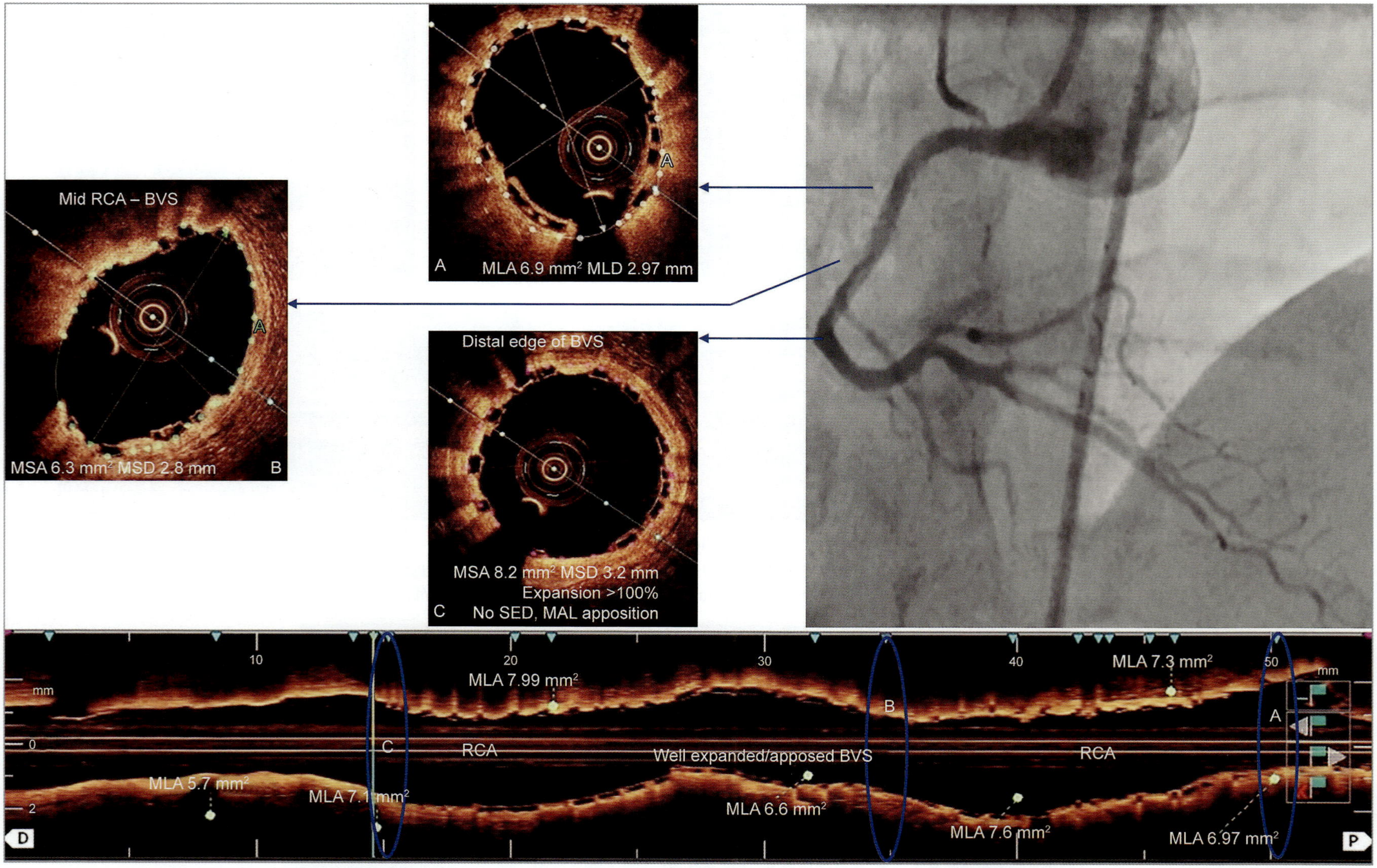
A MLA 6.9 mm² MLD 2.97 mm
Mid RCA – BVS
MSA 6.3 mm² MSD 2.8 mm
B
Distal edge of BVS
MSA 8.2 mm² MSD 3.2 mm
Expansion >100%
C No SED, MAL apposition
MLA 7.99 mm²
MLA 7.3 mm²
RCA
Well expanded/apposed BVS
RCA
MLA 5.7 mm²
MLA 7.1 mm²
MLA 6.6 mm²
MLA 7.6 mm²
MLA 6.97 mm²
D
P

Fig. 9A

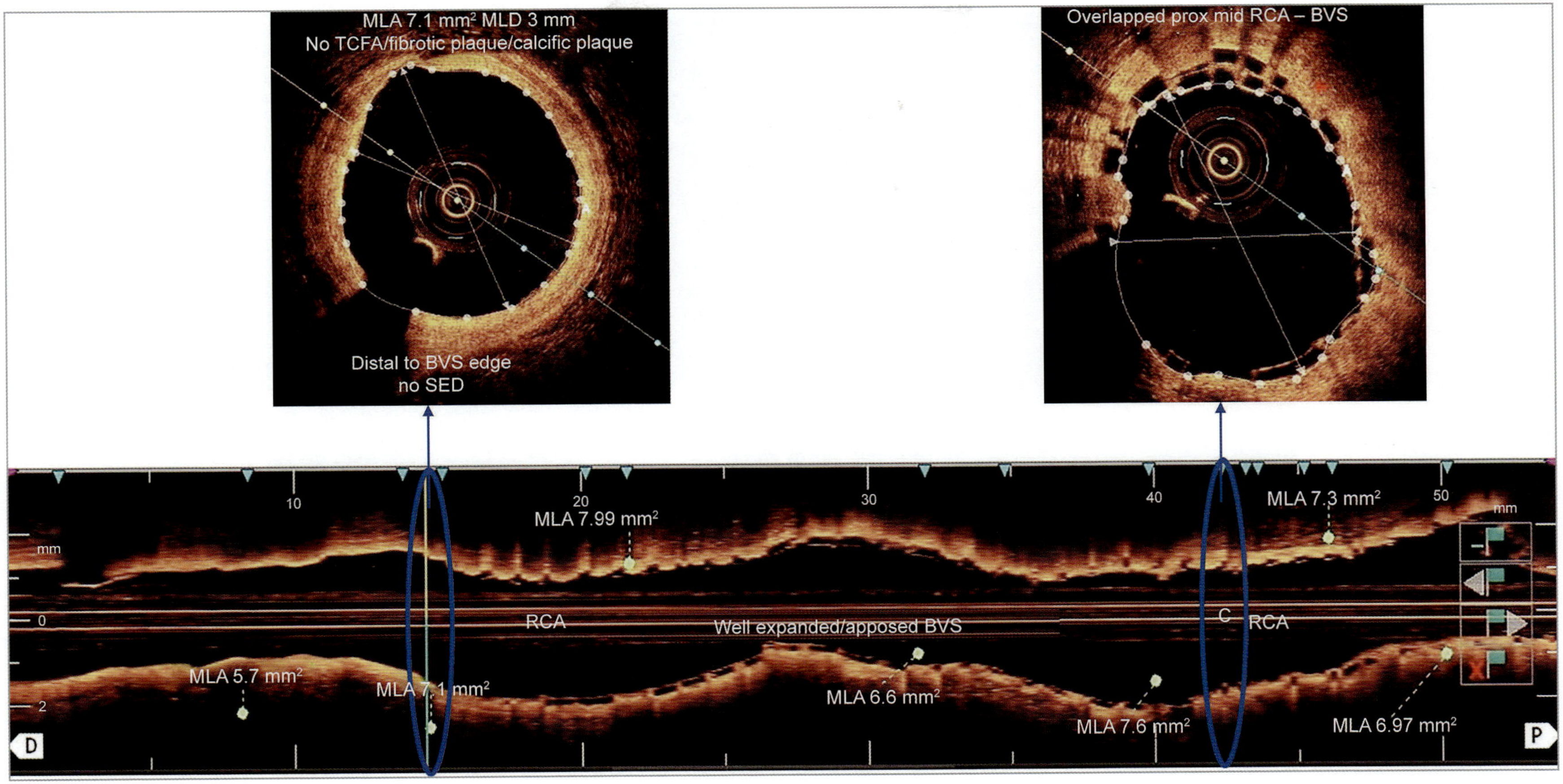

Fig. 9B

Figs. 9A and B: Poststent optical coherence tomography (OCT) analysis showed well expanded and apposed stent struts with no medial edge dissections. (BVS: biovascular scaffold; MLA: minimal lumen area; MSA: minimal stent area; MSD: minimal stent diameter; SED: stent edge dissection; RCA: right coronary artery)

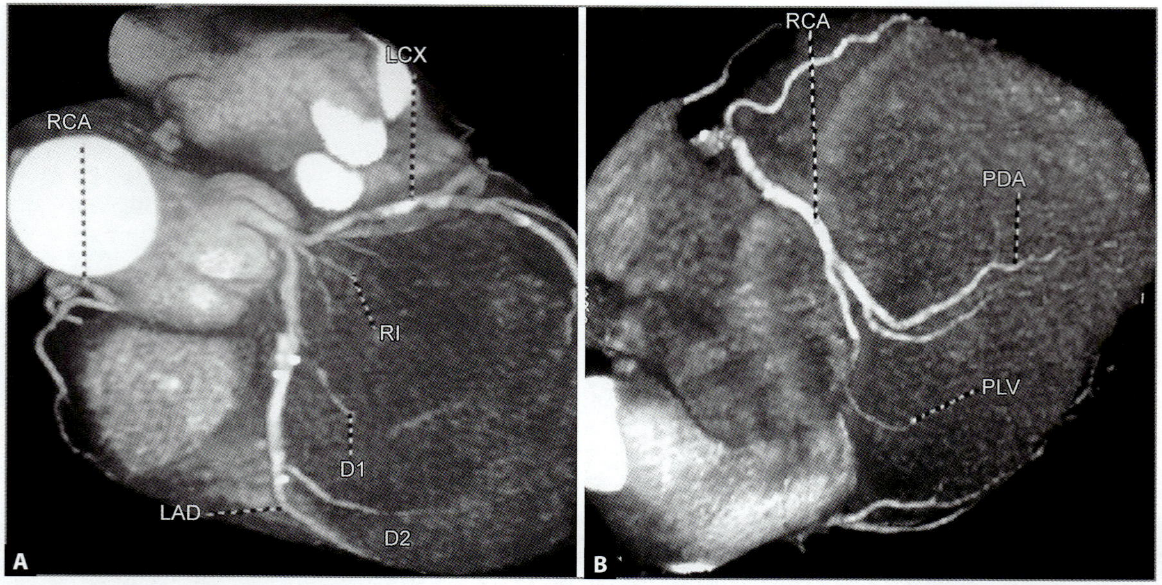

Figs. 10A and B: A 3-year follow-up computed tomography (CT); coronary angio showed well patent biovascular scaffold (BVS) stents. (LAD: left anterior descending; LCX: left circumflex; PDA: posterior descending artery; PLV: posterior left ventricular artery; RCA: right coronary artery)

CASE 2

Usefulness of OCT in acute coronary syndrome (ACS) with transradial triple-vessel drug-eluting stent (DES) stenting.

CLINICAL HISTORY

A 60-year-old male, known case of diabetes mellitus (DM) and hypertension (HTN), admitted with history of chest pain. 2D Echo—no RWMA (regional wall motion abnormality), good left ventricular (LV) function. CAG showed 70% stenosis of proximal LAD, 90% stenosis of mid LAD bifurcation lesion, 80% long segment stenosis from proximal to distal LCX, 90% stenosis of proximal RCA, 70–80% stenosis of distal RCA **(Fig. 11)**. Advised CABG/multivessel PCI with heart team approach. PCI of multivessel stenting was done due to willingness for multivessel PCI with plaque modification using rotablation/intravascular lithotripsy (IVL) under image guidance.

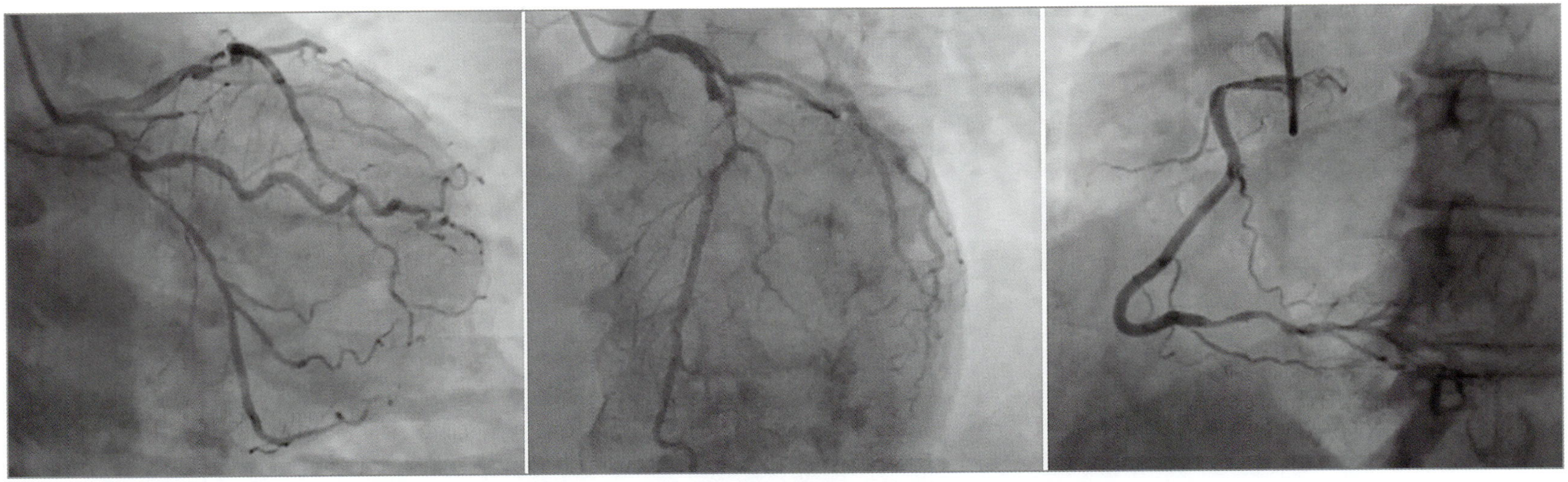

Fig. 11: Coronary angiogram.

PROCEDURE

Left main coronary artery engaged with EBU 3.5–6 Fr guiding catheter, LAD lesion crossed with 0.014" Runthrough wire and LCX crossed with BMW wire. Predilatation done with 2.0 × 15 mm Tazuna balloon. Presenting OCT was done which revealed no significant calcium-requiring plaque modification, calcium arc <180°, <5 mm length noted, hence plaque modification was differed **(Figs. 12A and B)**. Then stenting done with 2.75 × 38 mm Xience Xpedition stent. Postdilatation done with 3 × 15 mm NC Apollo balloon up to 18 atm **(Fig. 13)**. Poststenting OCT was done which showed well-opposed stent struts **(Fig. 14)**. The final result was good with TIMI III flow with no complications.

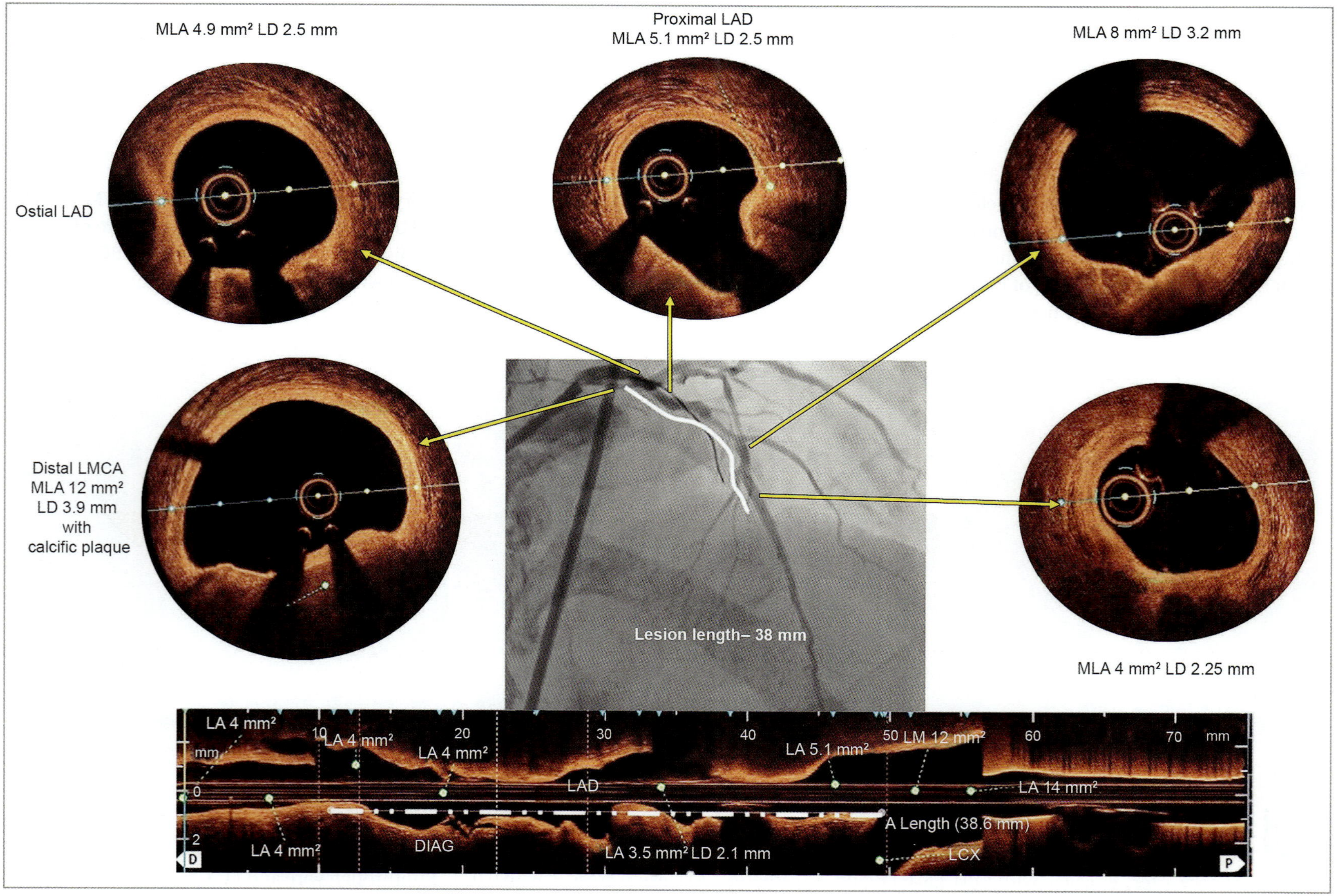

Fig. 12A

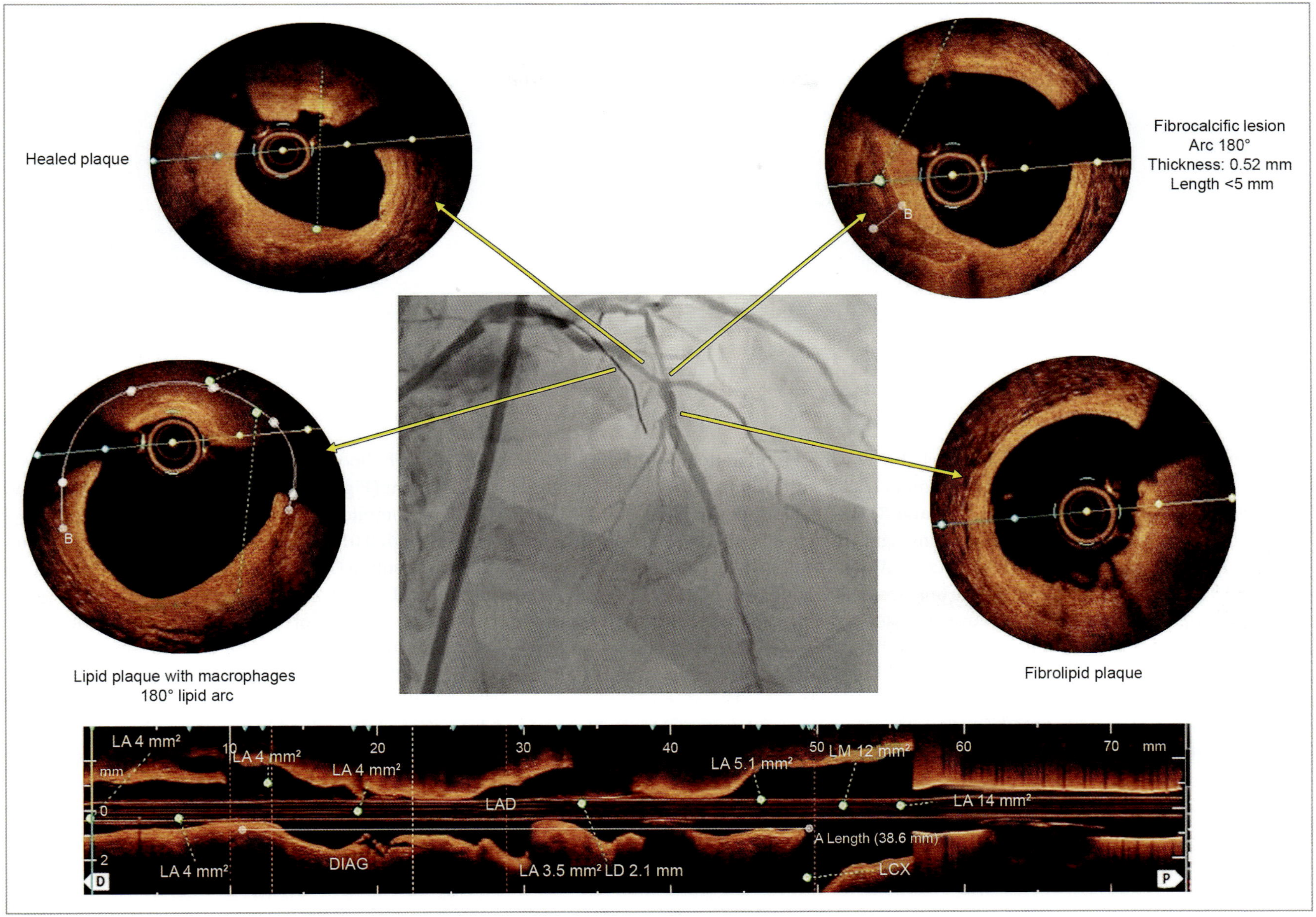

Fig. 12B

Figs. 12A and B: Prestenting optical coherence tomography (OCT) of left anterior descending (LAD) lesion for (A) Device selection and (B) Plaque morphology. (LA: lumen area; LCX: left circumflex; LD: lumen diameter; MLA: minimal lumen area)

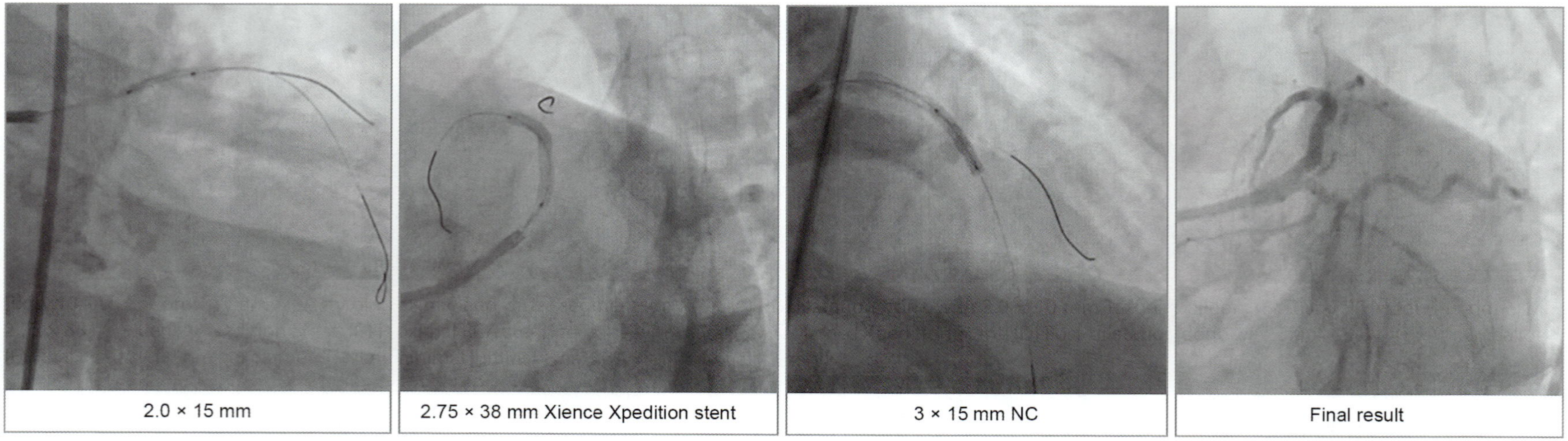

Fig. 13: Coronary angioplasty of left anterior descending (LAD) lesion.

Left circumflex lesion crossed with 0.014″ BMW wire. Predilatation done with 2.0 × 15 mm Tazuna balloon. Then distal LCX stenting done with 2.25 × 26 mm Resolute Onyx stent. Then proximal LCX stenting done with 2.5 × 18 mm Resolute Onyx stent **(Fig. 15)**. Poststenting OCT was done which showed well-opposed stent struts **(Figs. 16A and B)**. The final result was good with TIMI III flow with no complications.

Right coronary artery engaged with Judkins right (JR) 3.5–6 Fr guiding catheter, RCA lesion crossed with 0.014″ Runthrough wire. Predilatation done with 2.0 × 15 mm Tazuna balloon. Then distal RCA stenting done with Guideliner support 2.5 × 18 mm Resolute Onyx stent. Proximal RCA stenting done with 3.0 × 18 mm Resolute Onyx stent. The final result was good with TIMI-III flow with no complications **(Fig. 17)**.

Optical coherence tomography was used to assess calcium expansion index of proximal LAD with angio evidence of calcified lesion which may require rotablation/IVL for plaque modification OCT did not show significant calcium despite flouro evidence of moderate calcium. Assessment of LAD-D1 bifurcation lesion for side branch (SB) closure and to choose single vs. two stent technique, OCT revealed SB plaque burden was less, SB–CT angle, SB angle and blood pressure (BP)–CT length were favorable for provisional stenting with low predictability of SB closure. Hence, two-stent technique was avoided due to more favorable MACE (major adverse cardiovascular events) rate with provisional stenting compared to two-stent technique. Poststenting LCX optimization was done with OCT to identify and rectify post-PCI–DES predictors due to stenting of long-segment lesion for providing better short- and long-term outcomes.

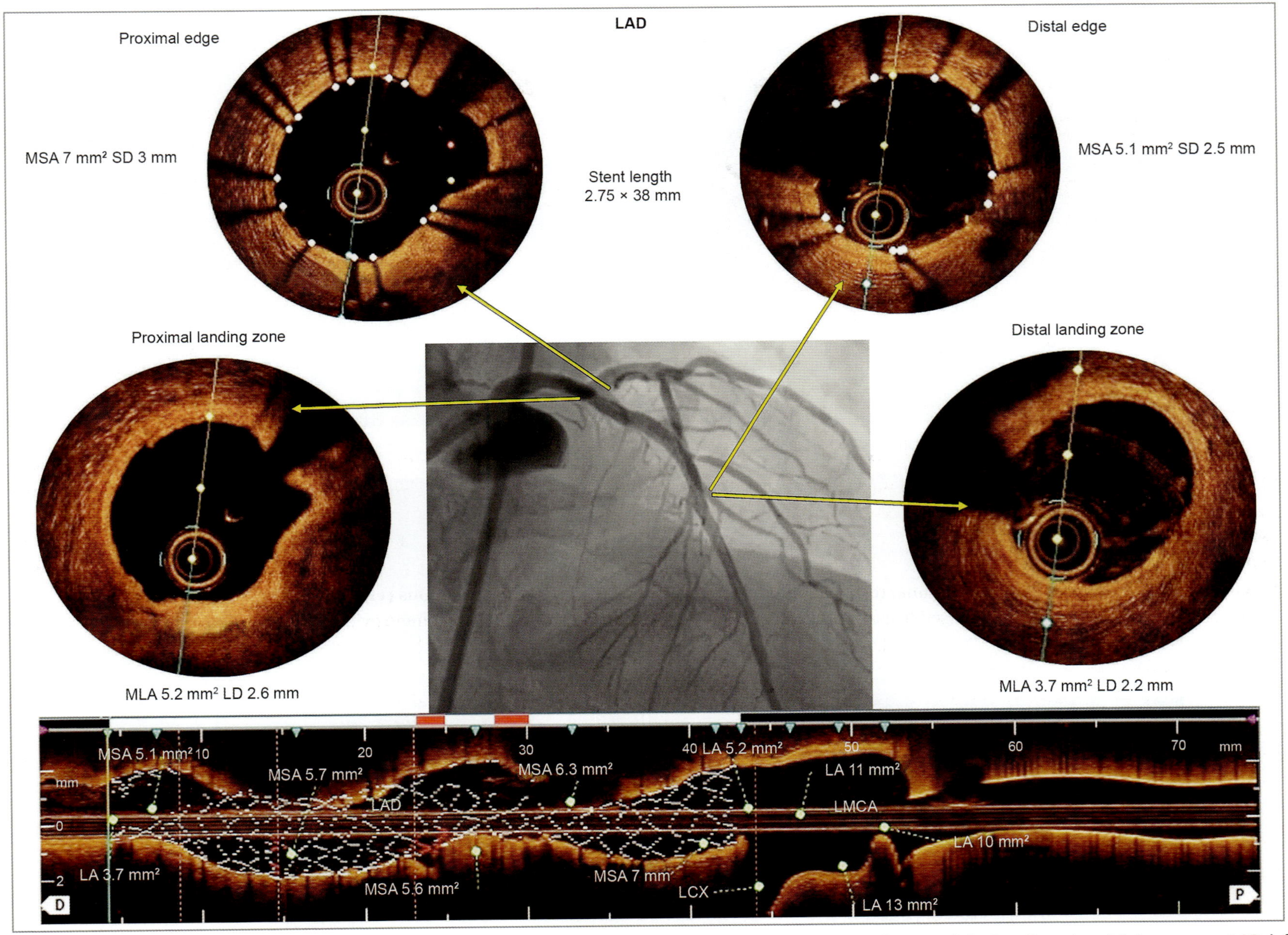

Fig. 14: Poststent optical coherence tomography (OCT) analysis showed well-expanded and apposed stent struts with no medial edge dissection. (LA: lumen area; LAD: left anterior descending; LCX: left circumflex; LD: lumen diameter; LMCA: left main coronary artery; MLA: minimal lumen area; MSA: minimal stent area; SD: stent diameter)

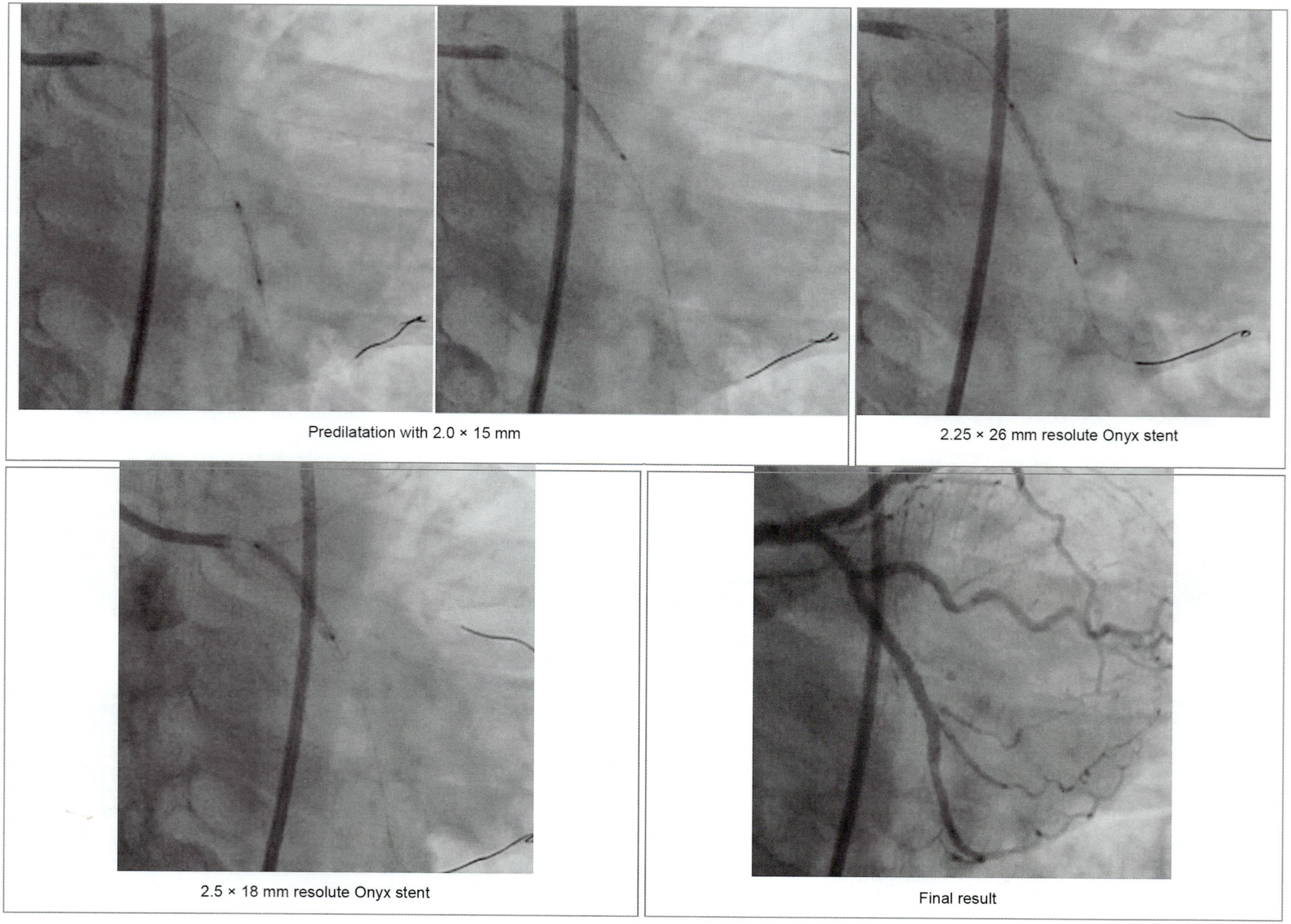

Fig. 15: Stenting of left circumflex (LCX) lesion.

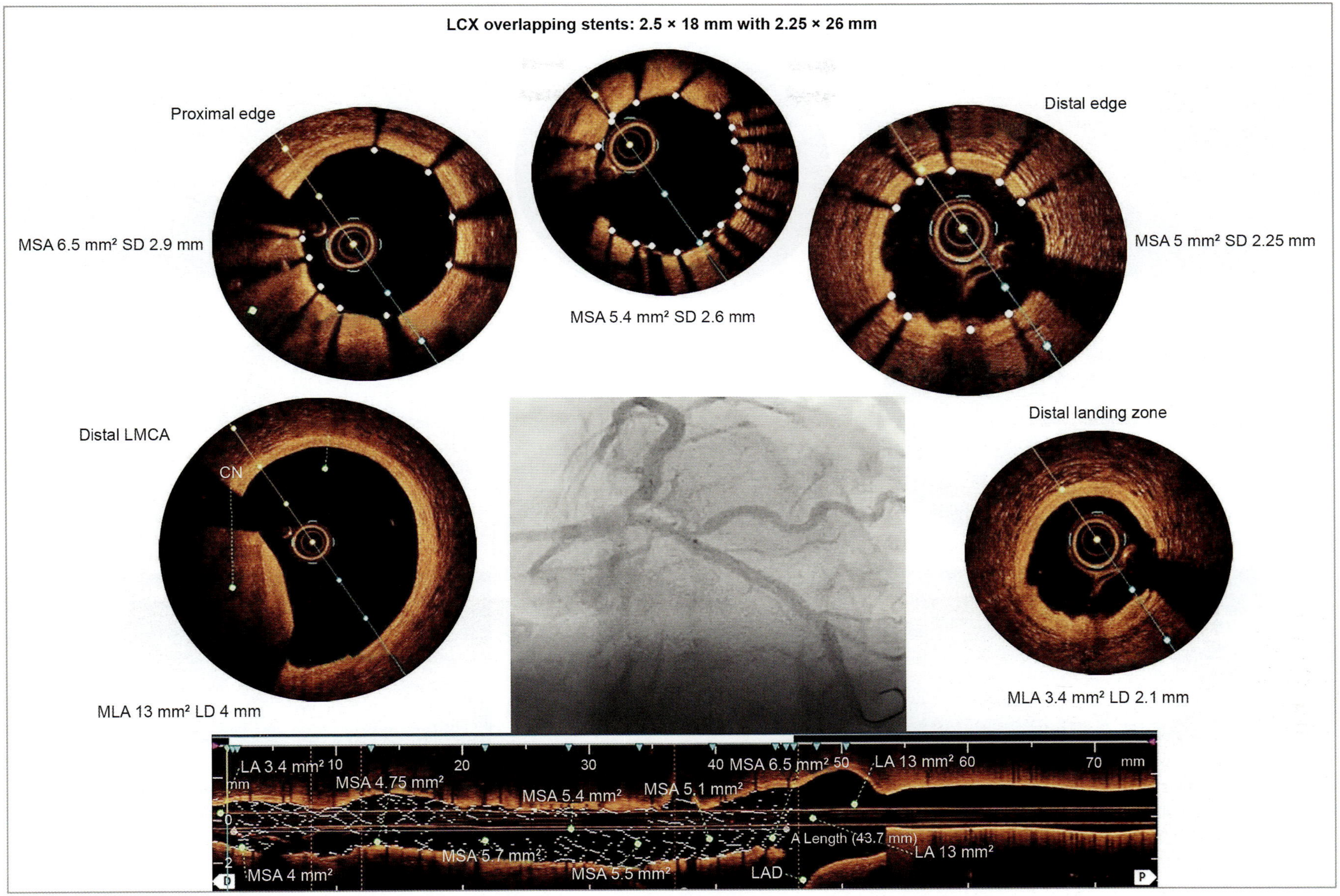
LCX overlapping stents: 2.5 × 18 mm with 2.25 × 26 mm
Proximal edge
MSA 6.5 mm² SD 2.9 mm
MSA 5.4 mm² SD 2.6 mm
Distal edge
MSA 5 mm² SD 2.25 mm
Distal LMCA
CN
MLA 13 mm² LD 4 mm
Distal landing zone
MLA 3.4 mm² LD 2.1 mm
LA 3.4 mm²
MSA 4.75 mm²
MSA 5.4 mm²
MSA 5.1 mm²
MSA 6.5 mm²
LA 13 mm²
MSA 4 mm²
MSA 5.7 mm²
MSA 5.5 mm²
LAD
Length (43.7 mm)
LA 13 mm²
D
P

Fig. 16A

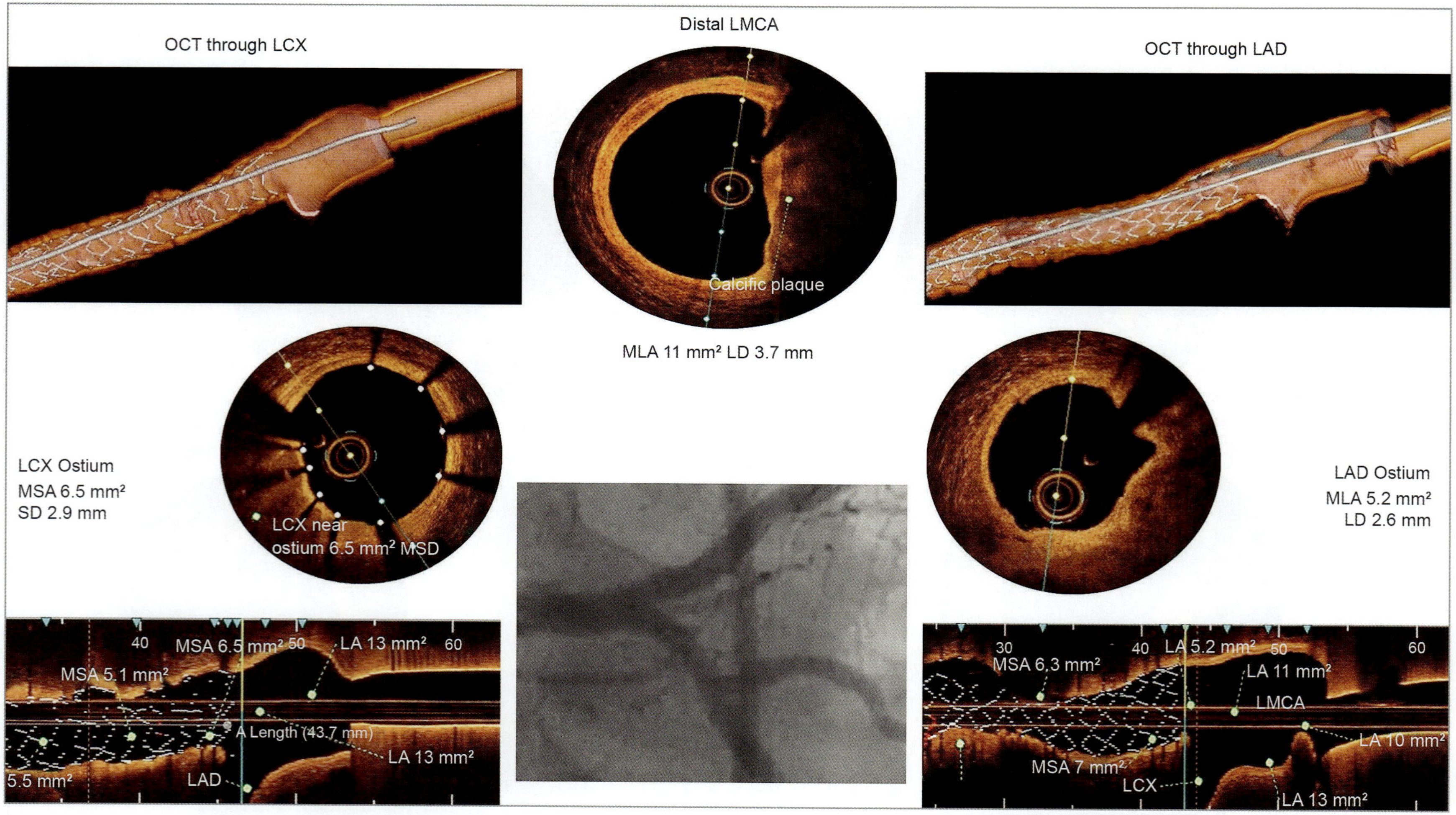

Fig. 16B

Figs. 16A and B: Poststent optical coherence tomography (OCT) of left circumflex (LCX) showed (A) well-expanded and apposed stent struts with no medial edge dissection; (B) poststent OCT analysis of left main (LM), ostial left anterior descending (LAD) and ostial LCX lesions. (LA: lumen area; LAD: left anterior descending; LCX: left circumflex; LD: lumen diameter; LMCA: left main coronary artery; MLA: minimal lumen area; MSA: minimal stent area)

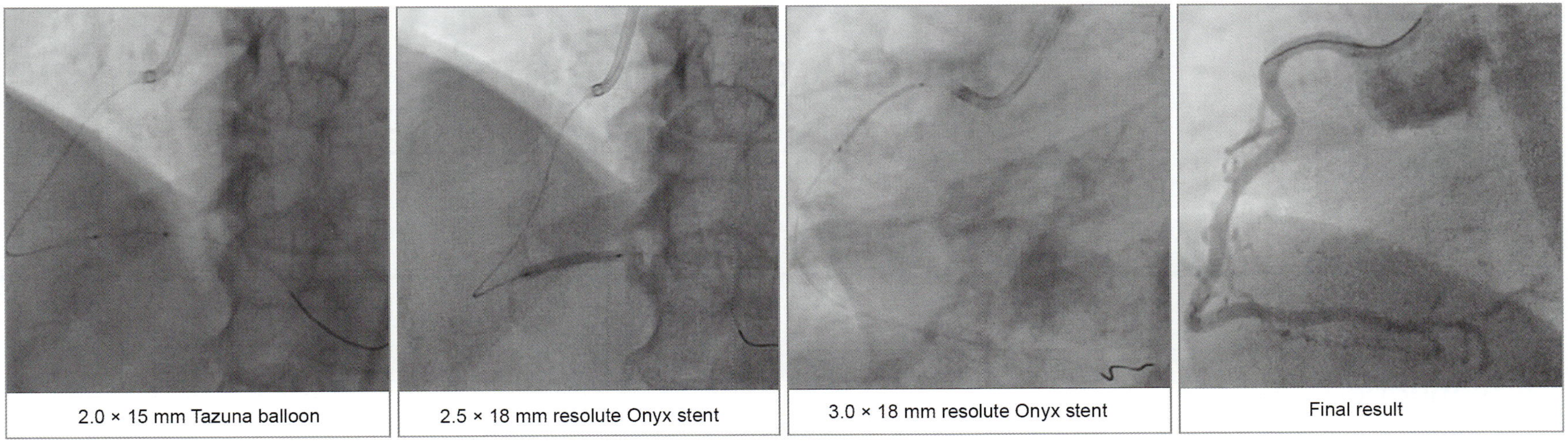

Fig. 17: Coronary angioplasty of right coronary artery (RCA) lesion.

CHAPTER 22

Optical Coherence Tomography Follow-up Biovascular Scaffold Cases

INTRODUCTION

Biovascular scaffold (BVS) follow-up optical coherence tomography (OCT) imaging mainly to assess disappearance of due to degradation of polylactic acid polymer. On OCT imaging 4–5 years of follow-up imaging of BVS segment shows classic appearance of "golden tube" and sometimes footprints of degraded scaffold struts.

CASE 1

Five-year OCT follow-up study of BVS stenting of left anterior descending (LAD) for anterior STEMI (ST segment elevation myocardial infarction).

CLINICAL HISTORY

A 52-year-old male, known diabetic, presented with acute anterior wall myocardial infarction (AWMI) (Window period (WP)—4 hours), persistent pain with high ST elevations treated with thrombolytic therapy with IV-STK (intravenous streptokinase) 15 lakh units. Electrocardiogram (ECG)-ST elevation in anterolateral leads, 2D Echo-RWMA (regional wall motion abnormality) in LAD territory, viable myocardium, fair left ventricular (LV) systolic function, ejection fraction (EF)—52%. Coronary angiography (CAG)-LMCA—normal, LAD—mid LAD 90% lesion, left circumflex (LCX)—normal, right coronary artery (RCA)—normal **(Fig. 1A)**.

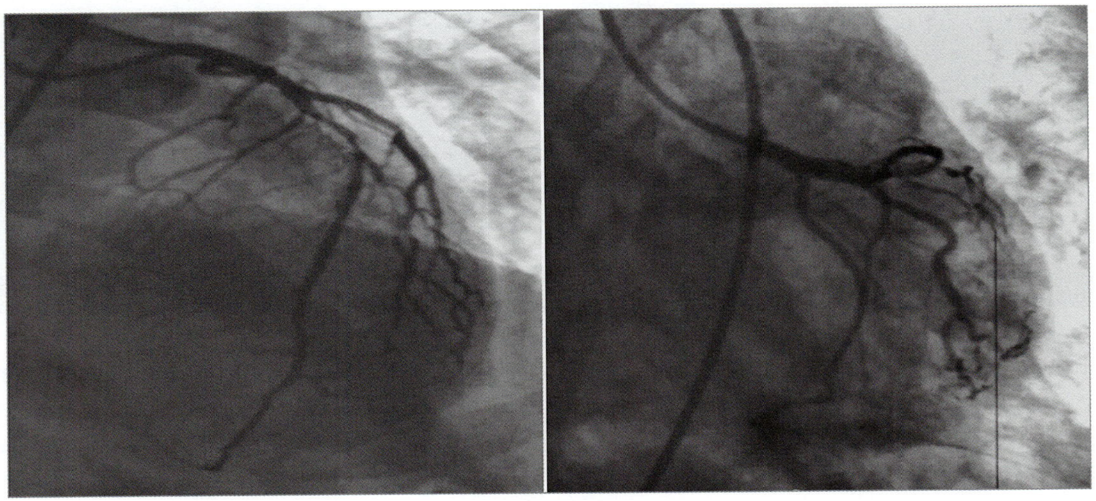

Fig. 1A

PROCEDURE

Route—right femoral artery (RFA), using 6 Fr XB 3.5 guiding catheter, angiogram revealed mid LAD 90% lesion which was crossed with 0.014″ Sion blue wire, predilated with 2.0 × 12 mm balloon, mid LAD stenting done with 3.0 × 28 mm BVS, and postdilated with 2.75 × 12 mm NC balloon. Check angiogram showed good TIMI III (thrombolysis in myocardial infarction III) flow **(Fig. 1B)**. Patient was discharged on fourth postprocedure day in a hemodynamically stable condition.

After 5 years of follow-up, check angiogram showed good TIMI-III flow **(Figs. 2A to D)** and OCT showed total disappearance of BVS with footprints in few cross-sectional images (golden tube appearance), minimal lumen area (MLA)—4.1 mm^2, minimal lumen diameter (MLD)—2.2 mm, LAD ostium MLA—10 mm^2, MLD—3.7 mm **(Figs. 3A and B)**.

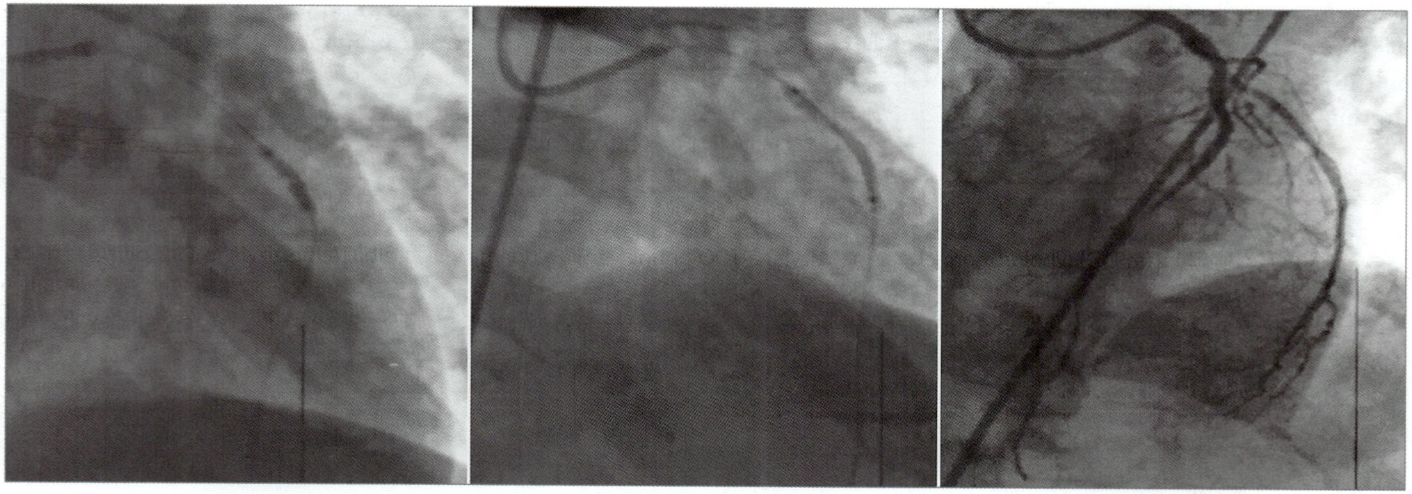

Fig. 1B

Figs. 1A and B: (A) Coronary angiogram; (B) percutaneous coronary intervention (PCI) with biovascular scaffold (BVS).

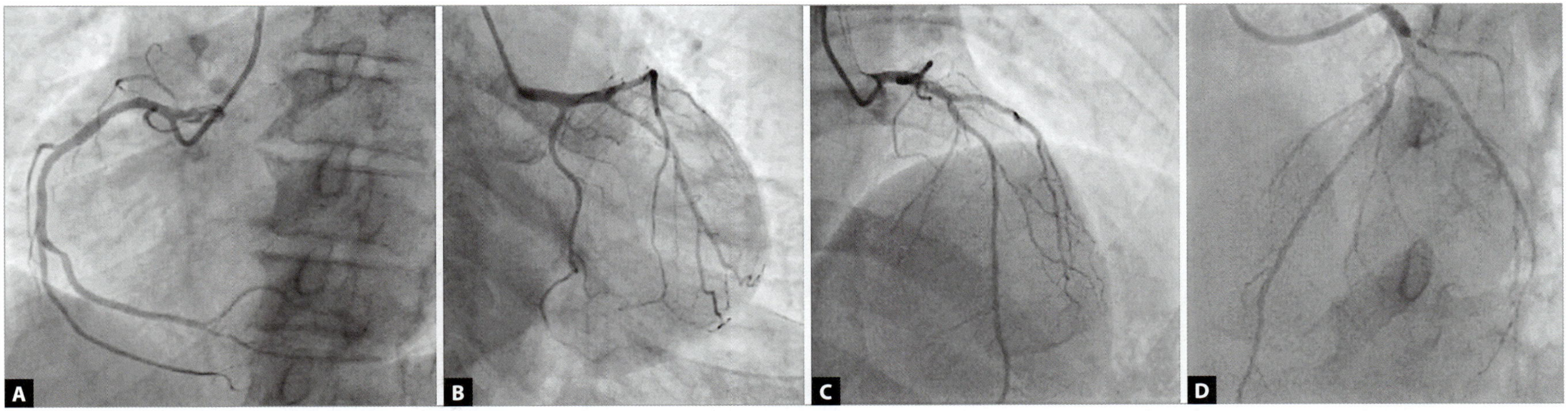

Figs. 2A to D: Five years later follow-up coronary angiogram showed patent stent.

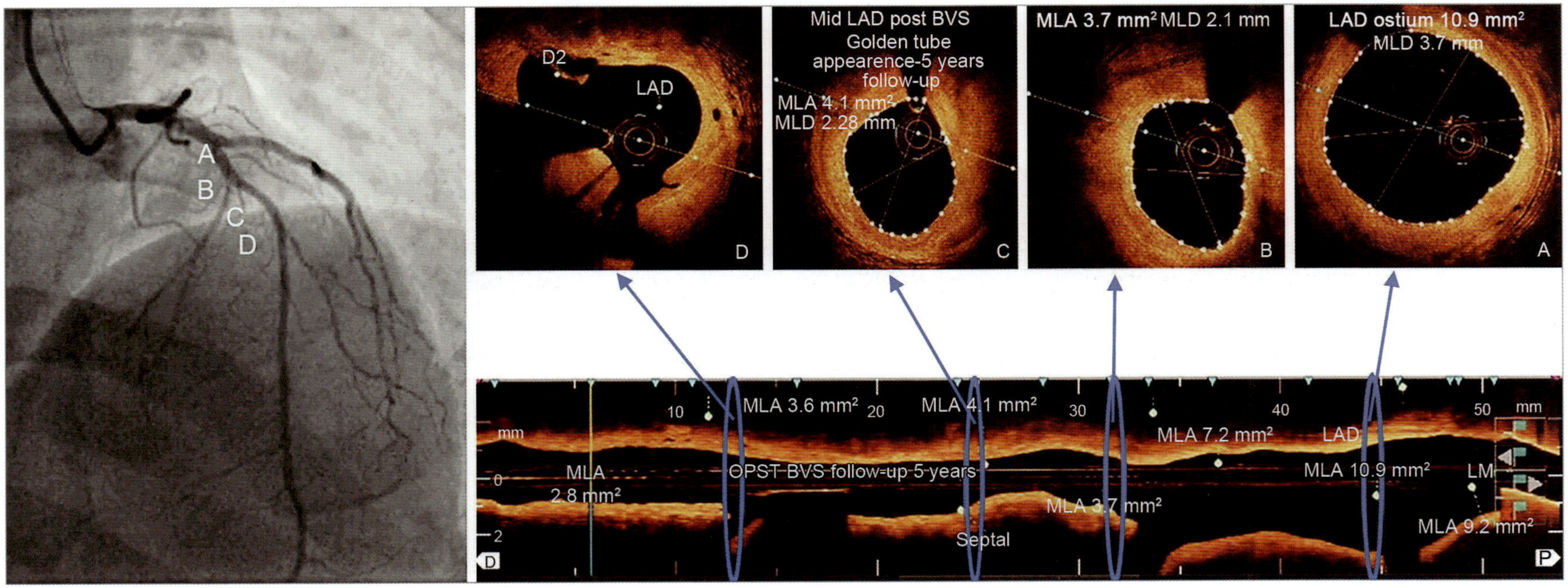

Fig. 3A

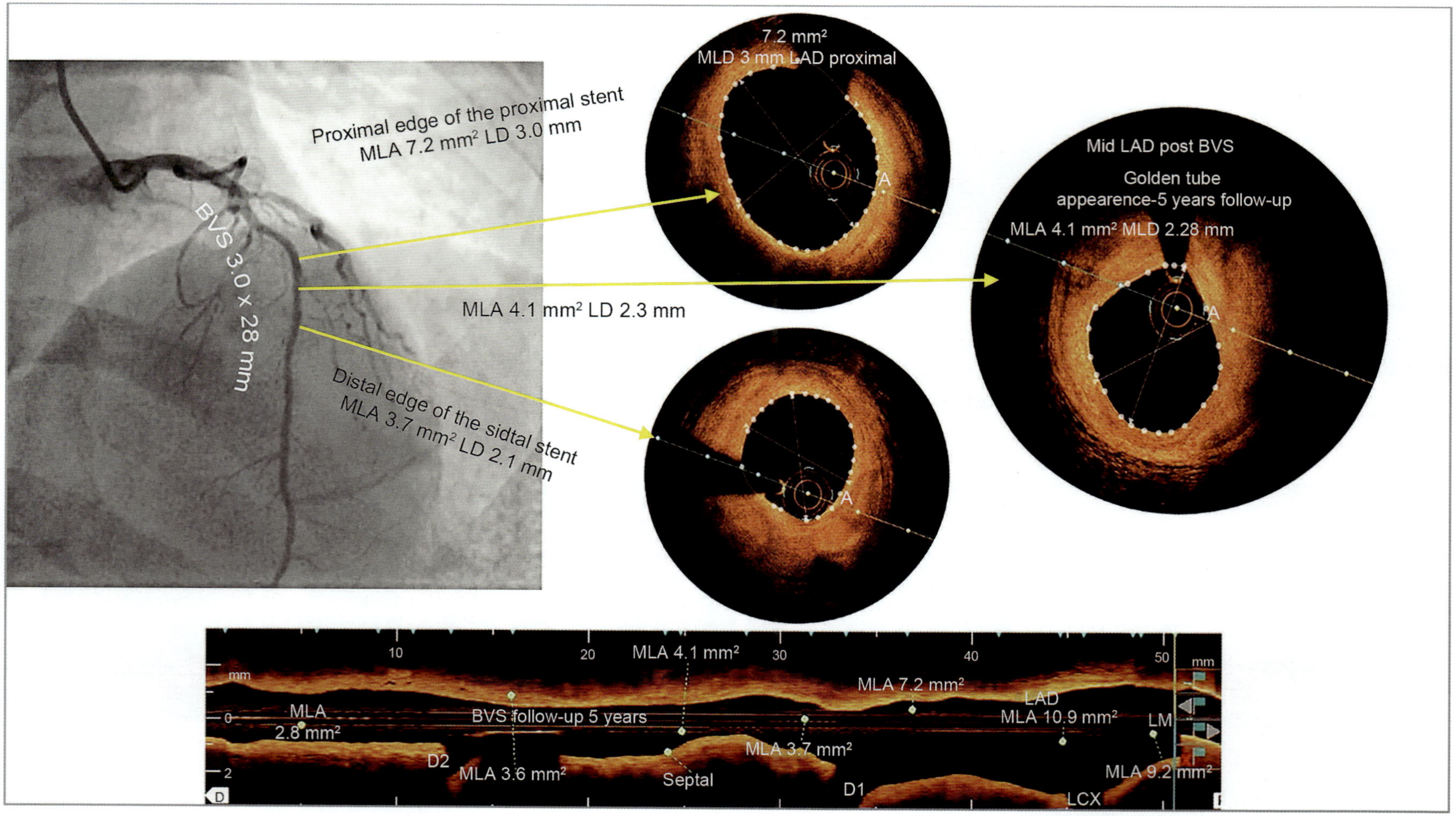

Fig. 3B

Figs. 3A and B: Follow-up optical coherence tomography (OCT) analysis for biovascular scaffold (BVS).
(LAD: left anterior descending; LCX: left circumflex; LD: lumen diameter; LM: left main; MLA: minimal lumen area)

CASE 2

Four-year' OCT follow-up study of BVS stenting of LAD and RCA.

CLINICAL HISTORY

A 56-year-old male, who is diabetic and with severe dyslipidemia, was admitted for 4-year BVS follow-up study. Previously underwent 1-BVS stenting of LAD and 2-BVS to RCA with positive treadmill test (TMT) with effort angina.

Previous PCI details (4 years back): CAG-A-LAD—proximal LAD 80% lesion, LCX—proximal 70%–80% disease, B-RCA—proximal RCA 80% lesion, and mid 90% lesion **(Fig. 4)**.

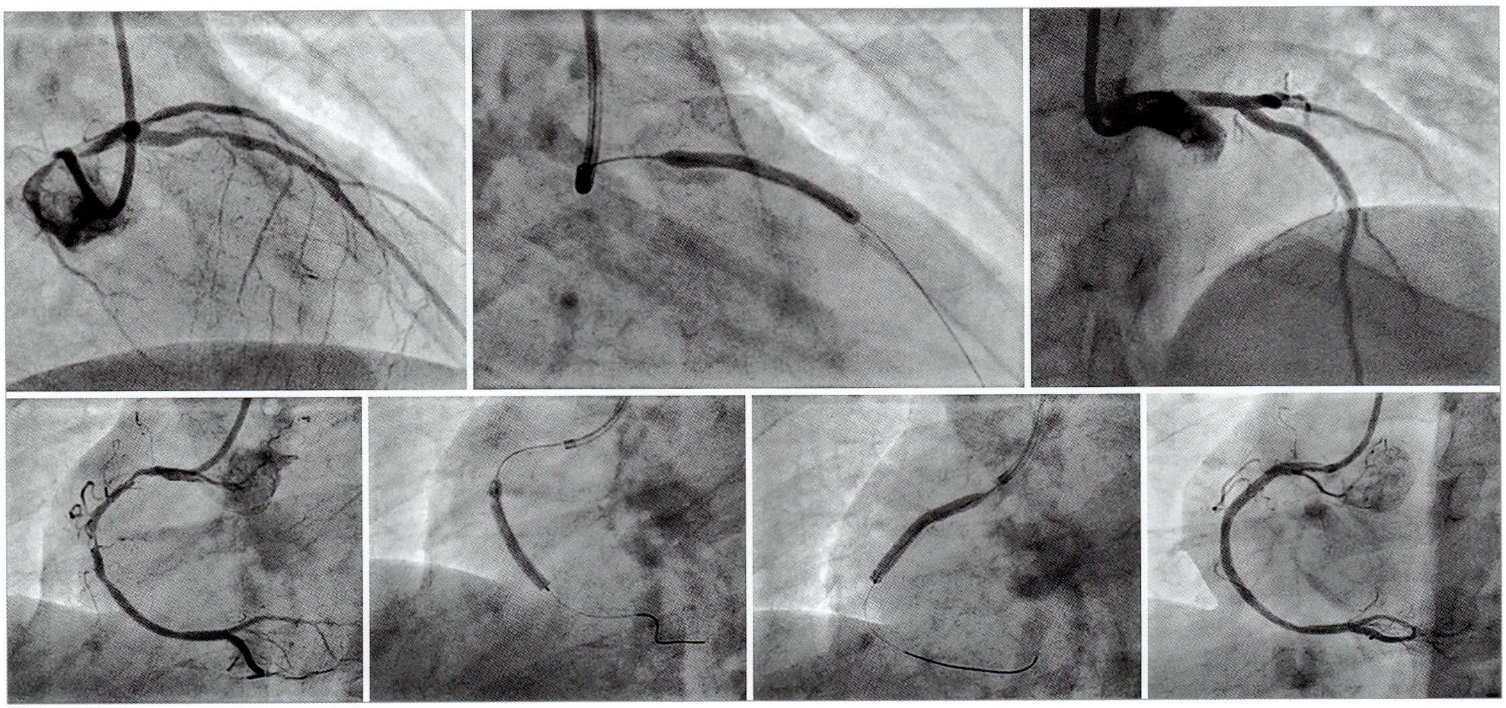

Fig. 4: Coronary angiogram and angioplasty for left anterior descending (LAD) and right coronary artery (RCA) with biovascular scaffold (BVS).

PROCEDURE

Proximal LAD stenting with 3.0 × 28 mm BVS stent, mid RCA stenting done with 3.0 × 28 mm BVS stent. Proximal RCA overlapping stenting done with 3.5 × 28 mm BVS stent **(Fig. 4)**.

After 4 years follow-up check angiogram showed good TIMI-III flow **(Figs. 5A to C)**.

Four-year follow-up OCT study of RCA—disappeared BVS struts with footprints in the area of previous BVS overlap zone of RCA **(Figs. 6A to D)**.

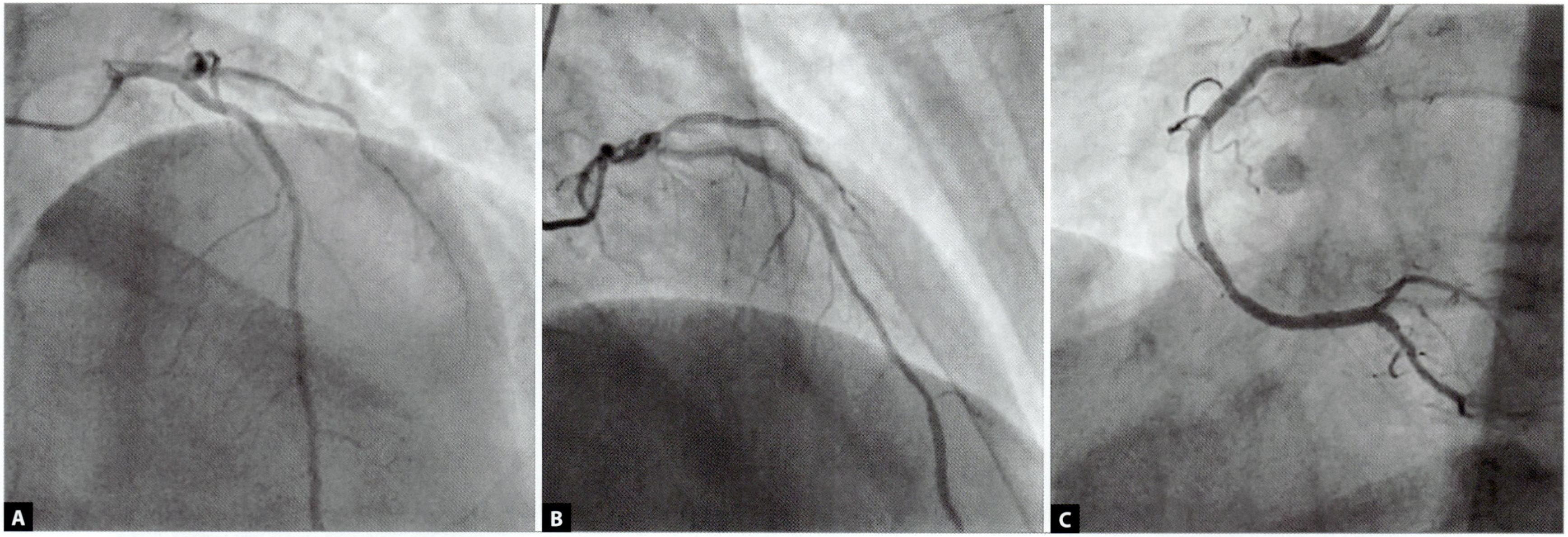

Figs. 5A to C: Four years later follow-up coronary angiogram showed patents stents in left anterior descending (LAD) and right coronary artery (RCA).

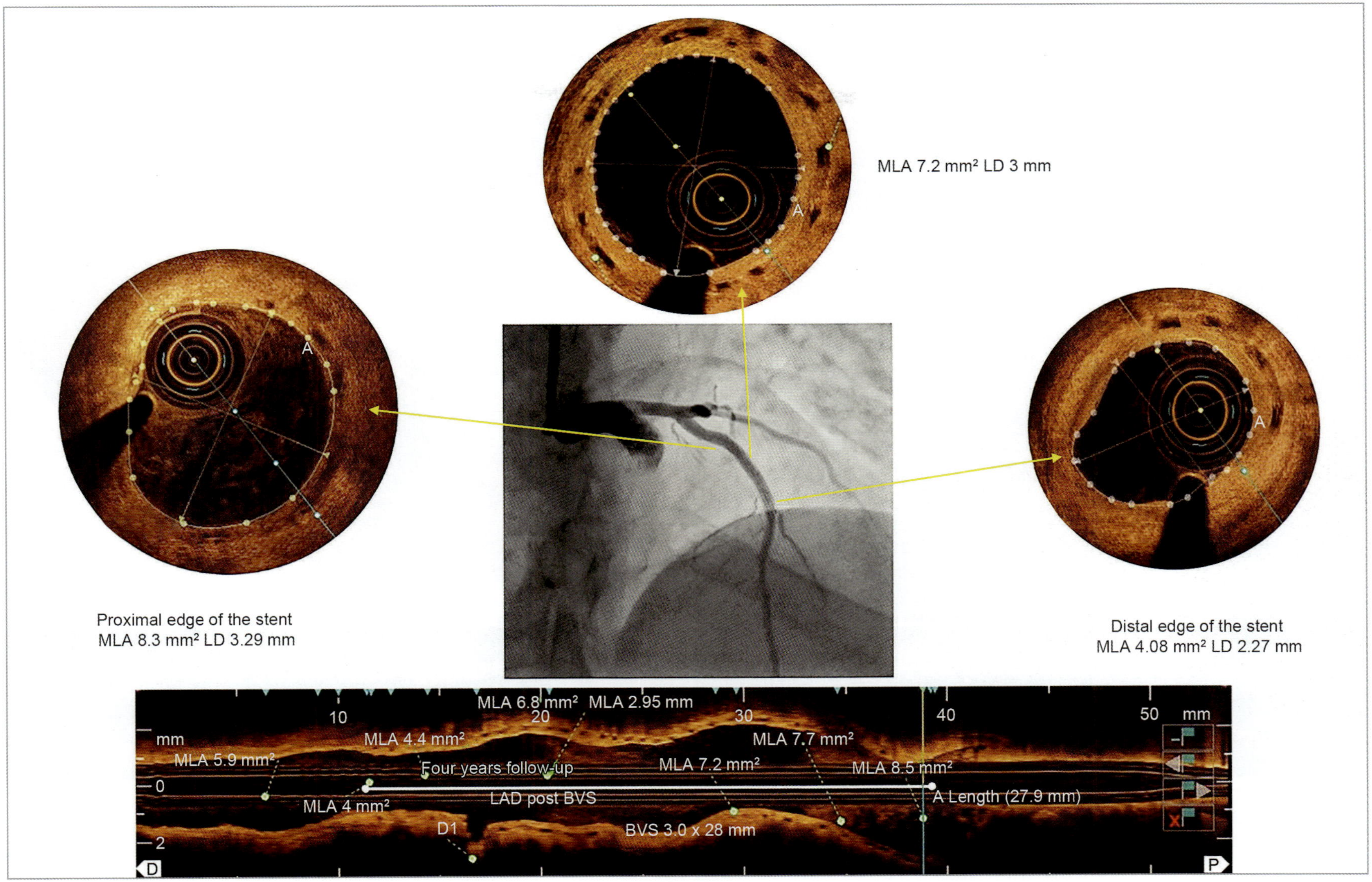
MLA 7.2 mm² LD 3 mm
Proximal edge of the stent
MLA 8.3 mm² LD 3.29 mm
Distal edge of the stent
MLA 4.08 mm² LD 2.27 mm
MLA 6.8 mm² MLA 2.95 mm
MLA 4.4 mm²
MLA 5.9 mm²
Four years follow-up
MLA 7.7 mm²
MLA 7.2 mm²
MLA 8.5 mm²
MLA 4 mm²
LAD post BVS
A Length (27.9 mm)
D1
BVS 3.0 x 28 mm
mm
10
20
30
40
50
mm
0
2
D
P

Fig. 6A

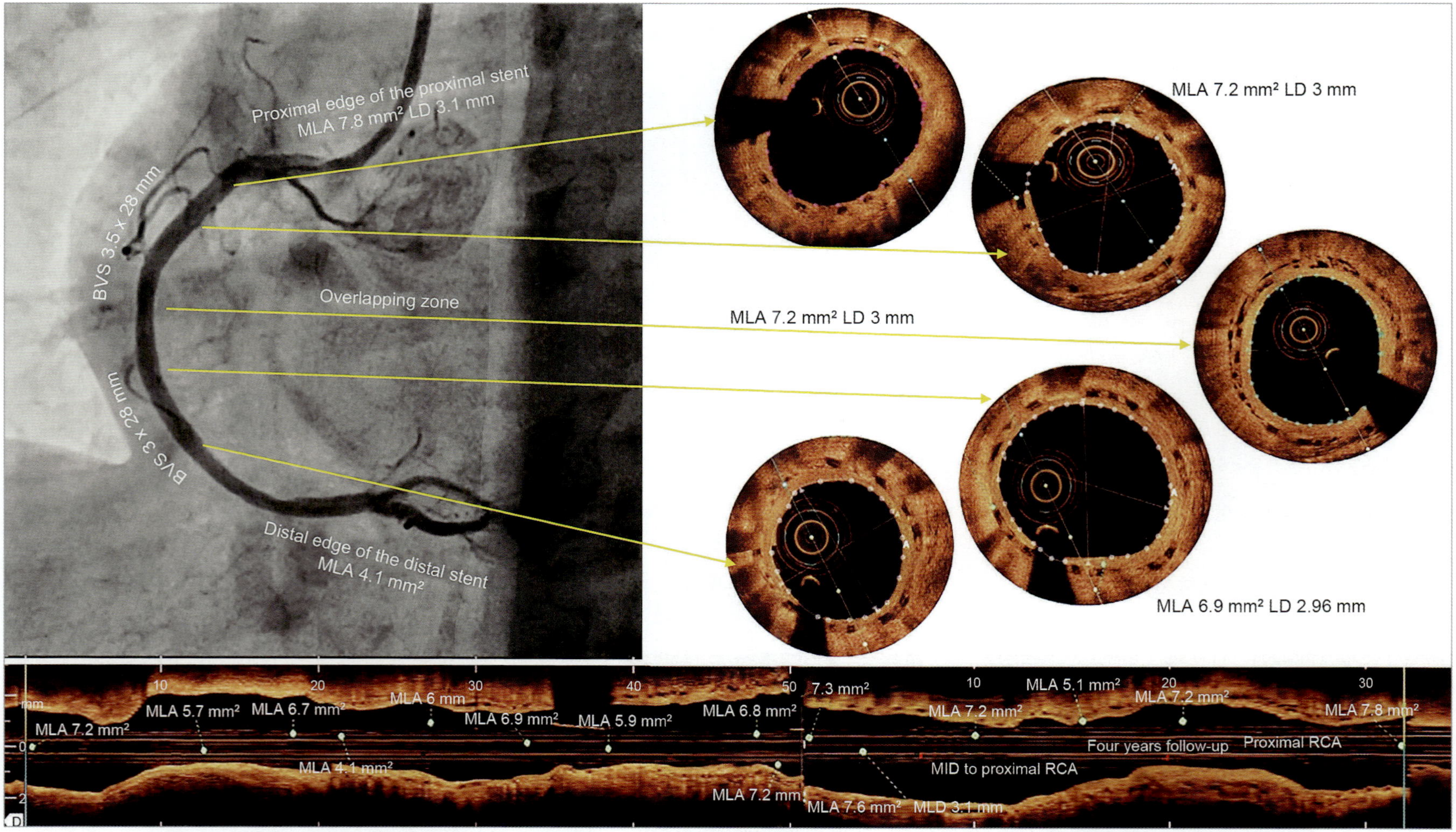
Proximal edge of the proximal stent
MLA 7.8 mm² LD 3.1 mm
BVS 3.5 x 28 mm
Overlapping zone
BVS 3 x 28 mm
Distal edge of the distal stent
MLA 4.1 mm²
MLA 7.2 mm² LD 3 mm
MLA 7.2 mm² LD 3 mm
MLA 6.9 mm² LD 2.96 mm
MLA 7.2 mm²
MLA 5.7 mm²
MLA 6.7 mm²
MLA 4.1 mm²
MLA 6 mm
MLA 6.9 mm²
MLA 5.9 mm²
MLA 6.8 mm²
MLA 7.2 mm
7.3 mm²
MLA 7.2 mm²
MLA 5.1 mm²
MLA 7.2 mm²
MLA 7.8 mm²
Four years follow-up
Proximal RCA
MID to proximal RCA
MLA 7.6 mm² MLD 3.1 mm

Fig. 6B

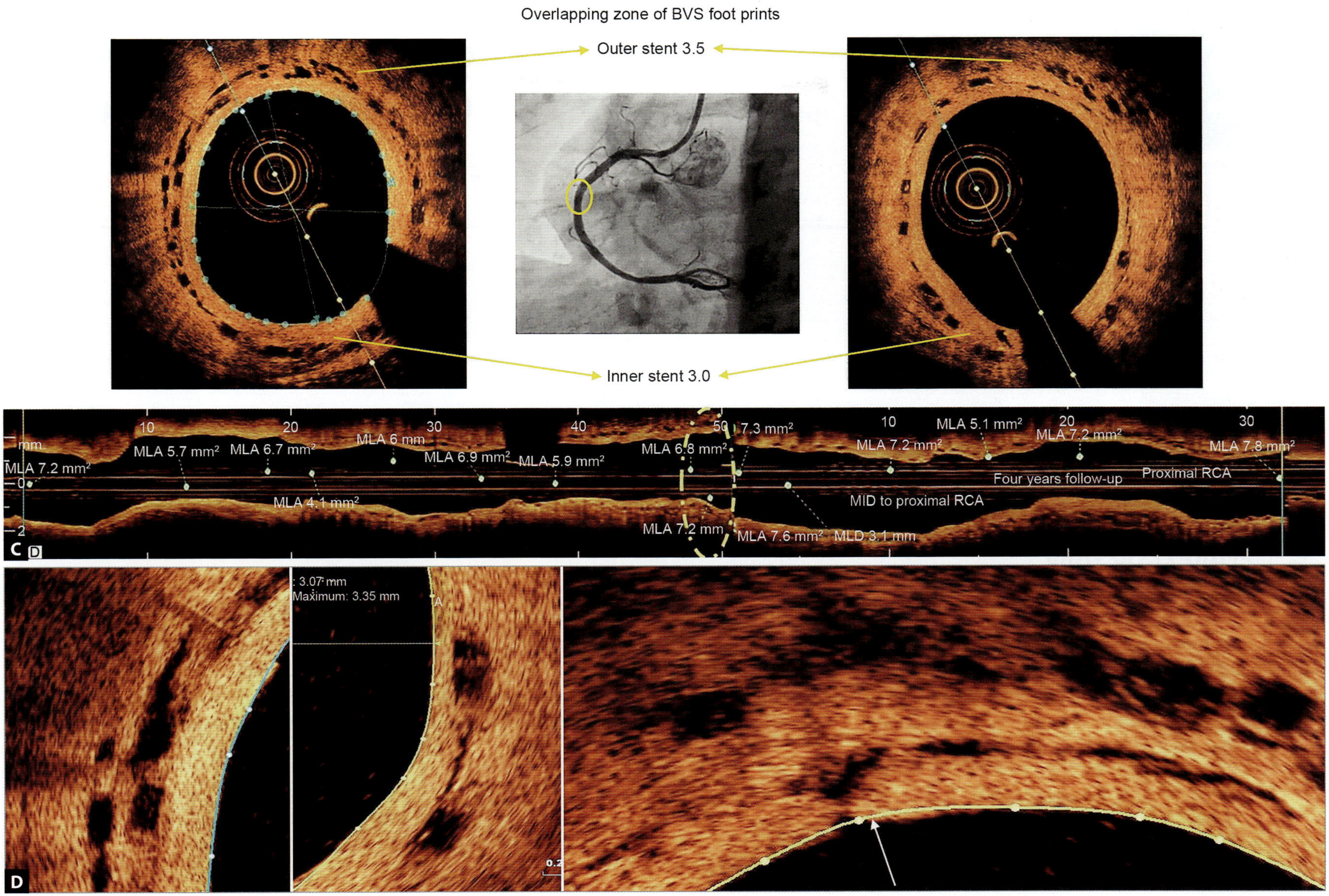

Figs. 6C and D

Figs. 6A to D: (A) Four years late follow-up optical coherence tomography (OCT) analysis showed golden tube appearance in left anterior descending (LAD); (B) 4 years' late follow-up OCT analysis showed golden tube appearance in right coronary artery (RCA); (C) footprints of biovascular scaffolds (BVS) after 4 years at overlapping zone; (D) footprints of BVS. (LD: lumen diameter; MLA: minimal lumen area)

CHAPTER 23

Percutaneous Coronary Intervention of Chronic Total Occlusion

CASE 1

Percutaneous coronary intervention (PCI) of left anterior descending (LAD)—recent anterior wall myocardial infraction (AWMI) with total occlusion of LAD.

CLINICAL HISTORY

A 66-year-old male, known diabetic, presented with evolved anterior wall STEMI (ST segment elevation myocardial infarction) with postinfarct angina. 2D Echo—hypokinetic distal interventricular septum (IVS), apex, anterior wall, RWMA (regional wall motion abnormality) in LAD territory, moderate left ventricular (LV) systolic dysfunction, ejection fraction (EF)—38%. Investigations: hemoglobin (Hb)—14 g/dL, serum creatinine—1.0 mg/dL, estimated glomerular filtration rate (eGFR)—70 mL/min, blood urea—36 mg/dL, random blood sugar (RBS)—218 mg/dL, NT-pro BNP—7,028 pg/mL.

Coronary angiography-left main coronary artery (CAG-LMCA)—normal, LAD—proximal total thrombotic occlusion, left circumflex (LCX)—normal, right coronary artery (RCA)—normal **(Fig. 1)**.

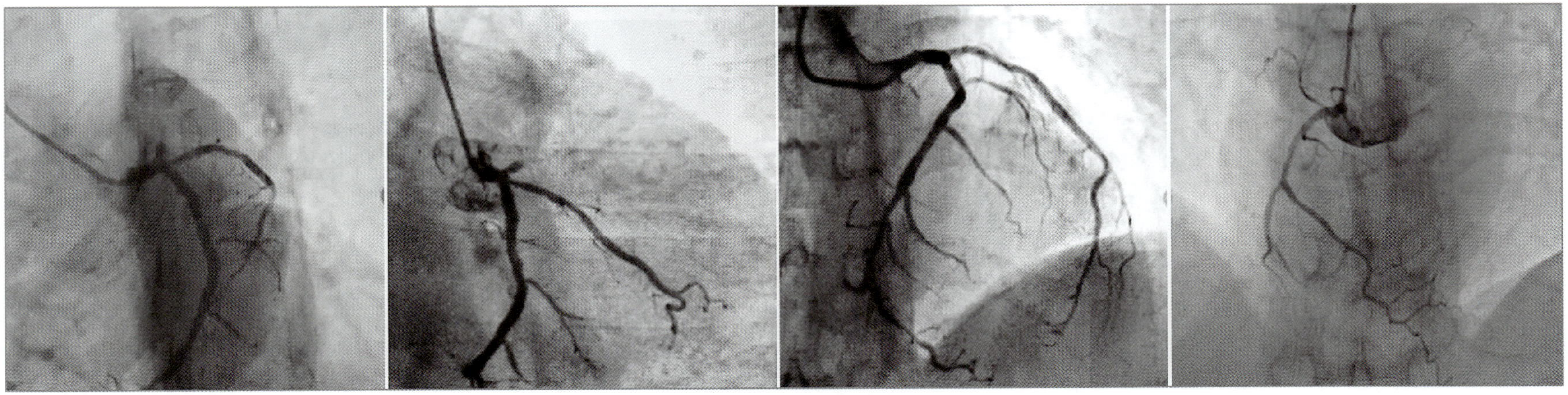

Fig. 1: Coronary angiogram.

PROCEDURE

Right radial approach (RRA)—route, 6 Fr EBU 3.5 guiding catheter, left anterior descending (LAD) crossed with 0.014″ Runthrough wire, 0.014″ Sion blue wire passes using microcatheter support. Predilatation done with 2.5 × 15 mm Tazuna balloon.

Post-plain old balloon angioplasty (POBA) optical coherence tomography (OCT) showed fibrocalcific plaque extending from proximal to mid LAD **(Figs. 2A to D)**.

Proximal LAD stenting done with 2.75 × 38 mm Xience Xpedition stent. Distal LAD stenting done with 2.5 × 28 mm Xience Xpedition stent. Proximal LAD postdilatation done with 3.0 × 15 mm NC Trek balloon and distal LAD postdilatation done with 2.5 × 15 mm NC Trek balloon **(Figs. 3A to F)**.

Post-OCT study of LAD showed well-expanded and apposed stent struts with no medial edge dissections **(Fig. 4A)**, post-OCT study of overlapping segment **(Fig. 4B)**.

Post-OCT study was done which showed underexpansion in mid LAD due to calcific lesion **(Fig. 5)**.

Postdilated with OPN noncompliant (NC) 2.5 × 10 mm balloon dilatation done up to 40 atm with GuideLiner support. Postprocedure angio view showed well-implanted stents with TIMI-III (thrombolysis in myocardial infarction III) flow without any dissection. Patient was discharged on third postprocedure day in a stable status.

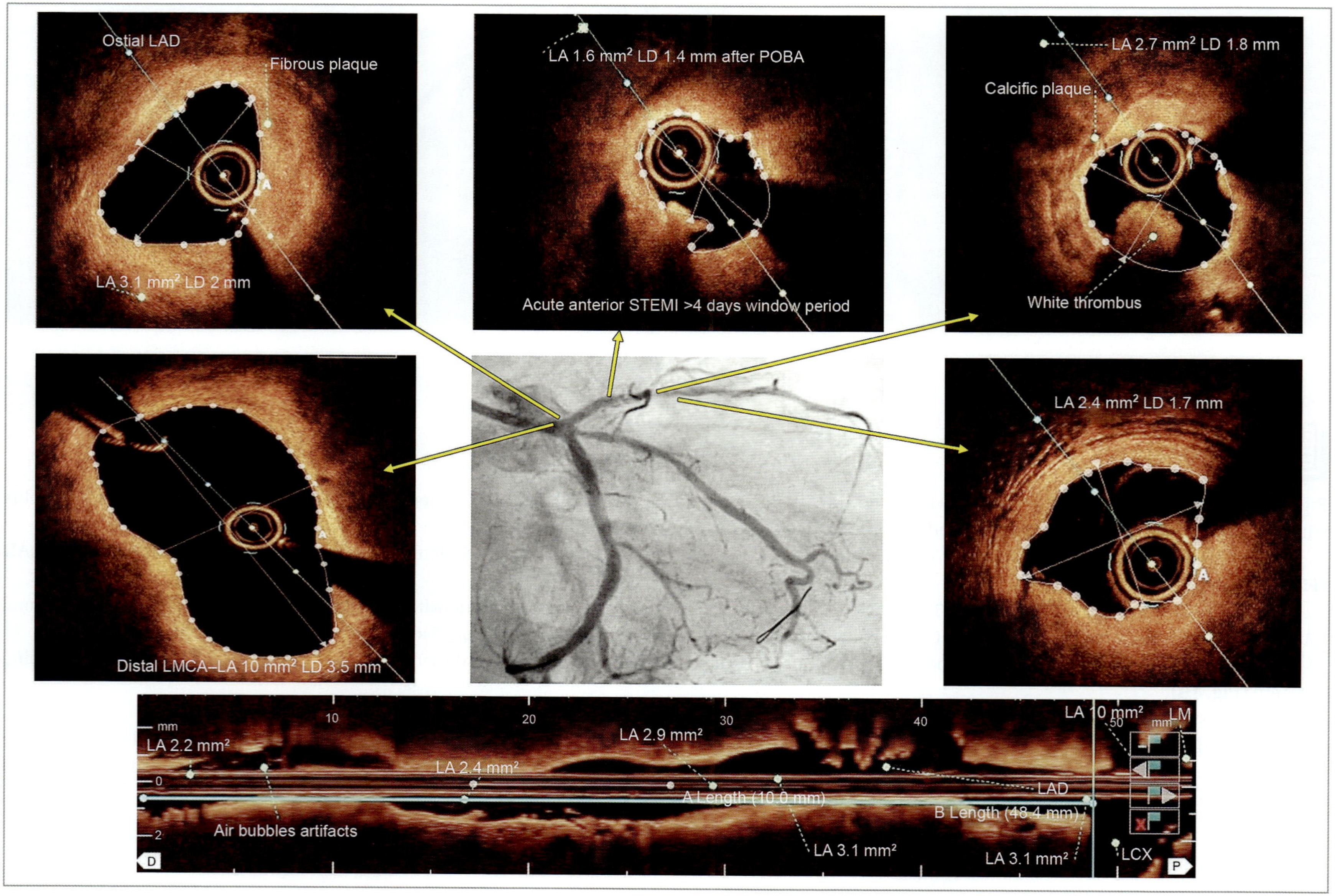
Ostial LAD
Fibrous plaque
LA 3.1 mm² LD 2 mm
LA 1.6 mm² LD 1.4 mm after POBA
Acute anterior STEMI >4 days window period
LA 2.7 mm² LD 1.8 mm
Calcific plaque
White thrombus
Distal LMCA–LA 10 mm² LD 3.5 mm
LA 2.4 mm² LD 1.7 mm
LA 2.2 mm²
LA 2.4 mm²
LA 2.9 mm²
A Length (10.0 mm)
B Length (48.4 mm)
Air bubbles artifacts
LA 3.1 mm²
LA 3.1 mm²
LA 10 mm²
LM
LAD
LCX

Fig. 2A

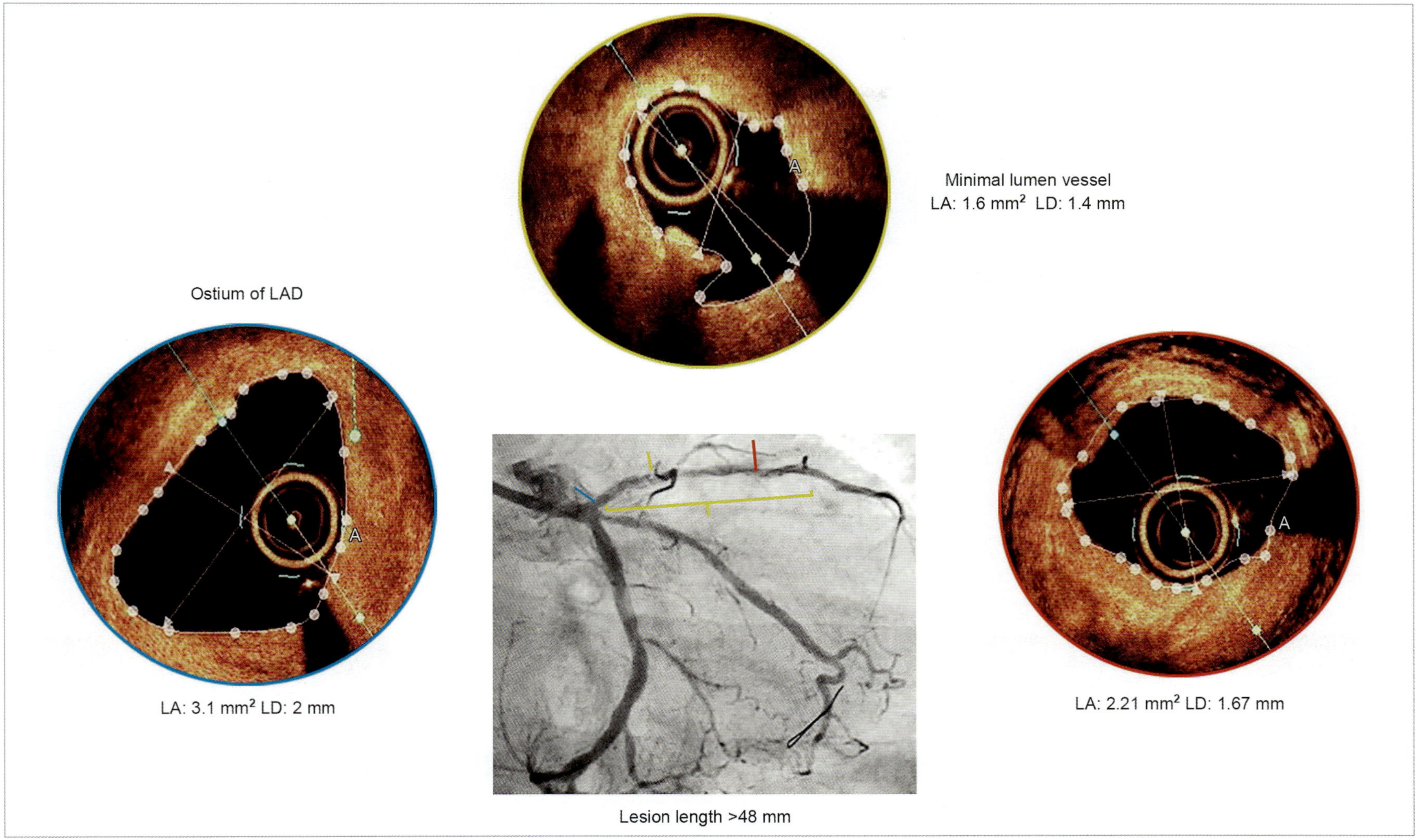
Minimal lumen vessel
LA: 1.6 mm² LD: 1.4 mm
Ostium of LAD
LA: 3.1 mm² LD: 2 mm
LA: 2.21 mm² LD: 1.67 mm
Lesion length >48 mm

Fig. 2B

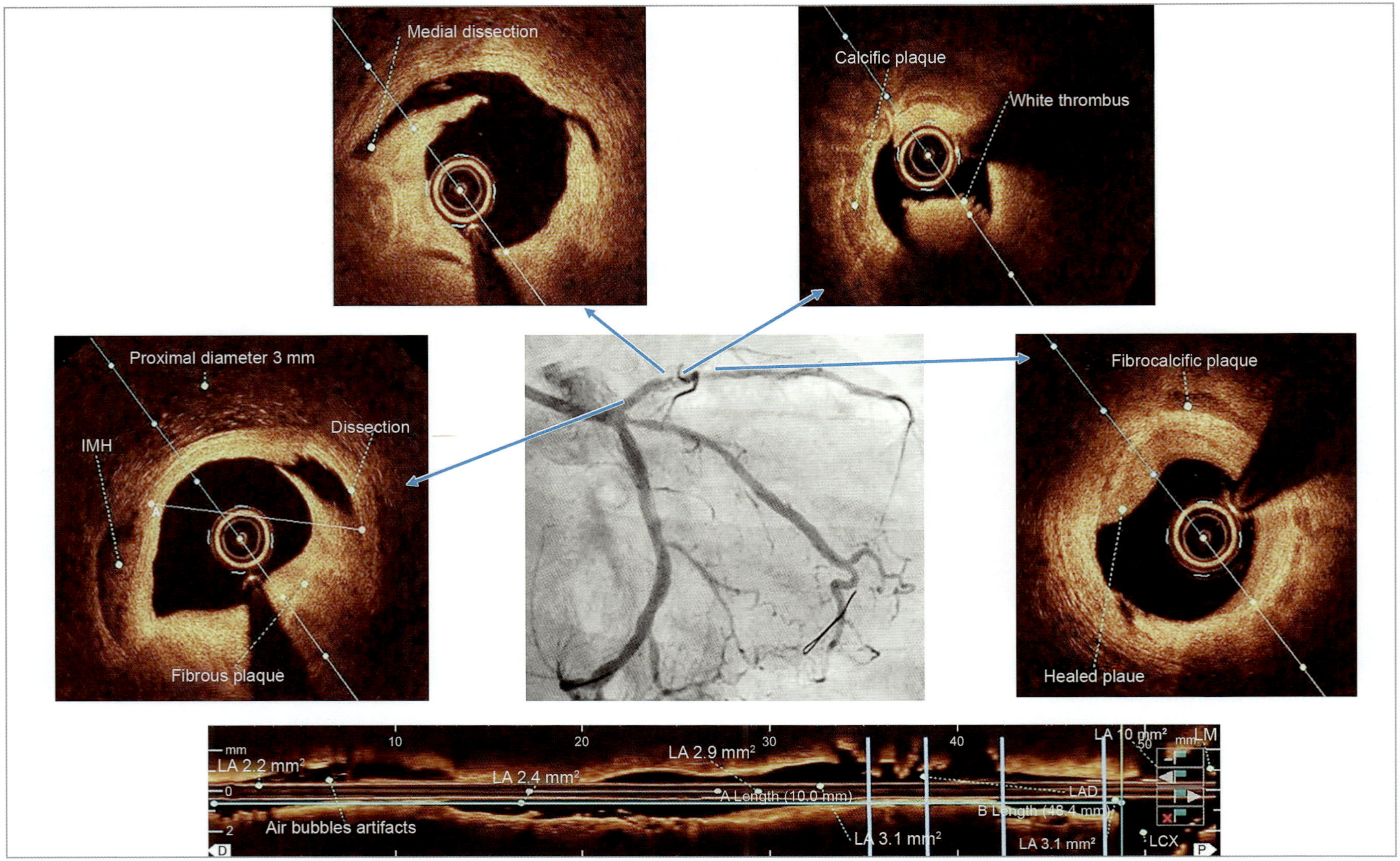
Medial dissection
Calcific plaque
White thrombus
Proximal diameter 3 mm
Dissection
IMH
Fibrous plaque
Fibrocalcific plaque
Healed plaue
LA 2.2 mm²
LA 2.4 mm²
LA 2.9 mm²
LA 3.1 mm²
LA 3.1 mm²
Air bubbles artifacts
A Length (10.0 mm)
B Length (48.4 mm)
LAD
LM
LCX

Fig. 2C

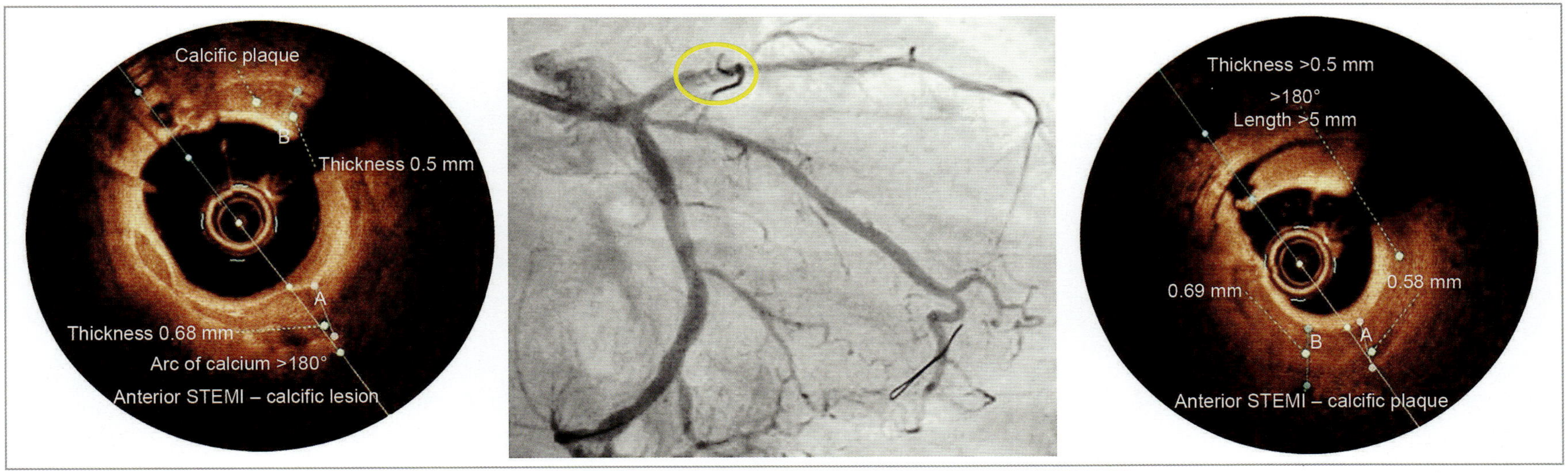

Fig. 2D

Figs. 2A to D: (A) Prestenting optical coherence tomography (OCT) assessment of left anterior descending (LAD); (B) Analysis for devise selection; (C) Plaque morphology; (D) Calcific plaque in STEMI (ST segment elevation myocardial infarction) (IMH: intramural hematoma; LA: lumen area; LD: lumen diameter)

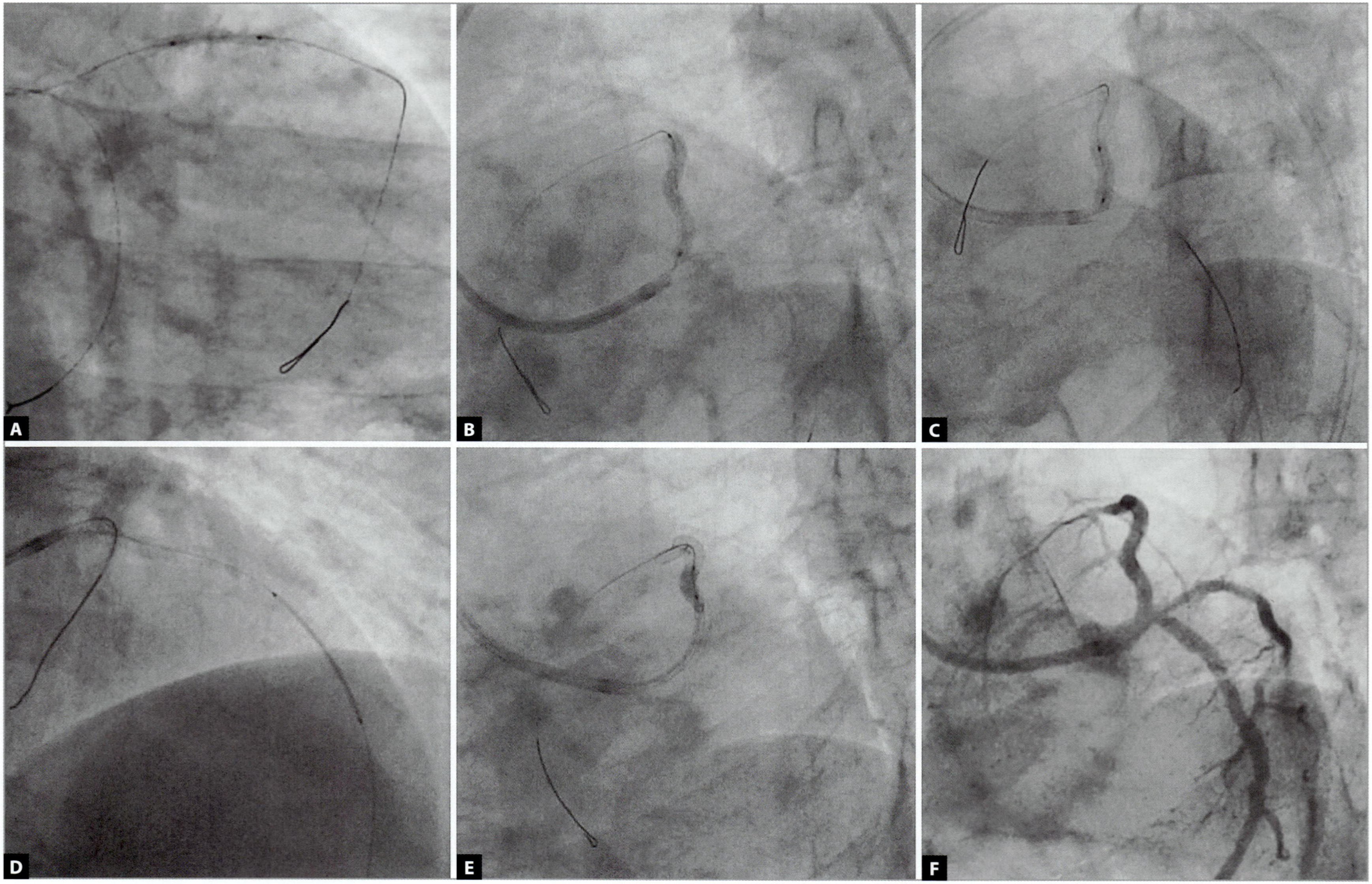

Figs. 3A to F: Coronary angioplasty. (A) Predilatation done with 2.5 × 15 mm Tazuna balloon; (B) Proximal left anterior descending (LAD) stenting done with 2.75 × 38 mm Xience Xpedition stent; (C) Proximal LAD postdilatation done with 3.0 × 15 mm NC Trek balloon; (D) Distal LAD stenting done with 2.5 × 28 mm Xience Xpedition stent; (E) Proximal LAD postdilatation done with 3.0 × 15 mm NC Trek balloon and distal LAD postdilatation done with 2.5 × 15 mm NC Trek balloon; (F) Final result.

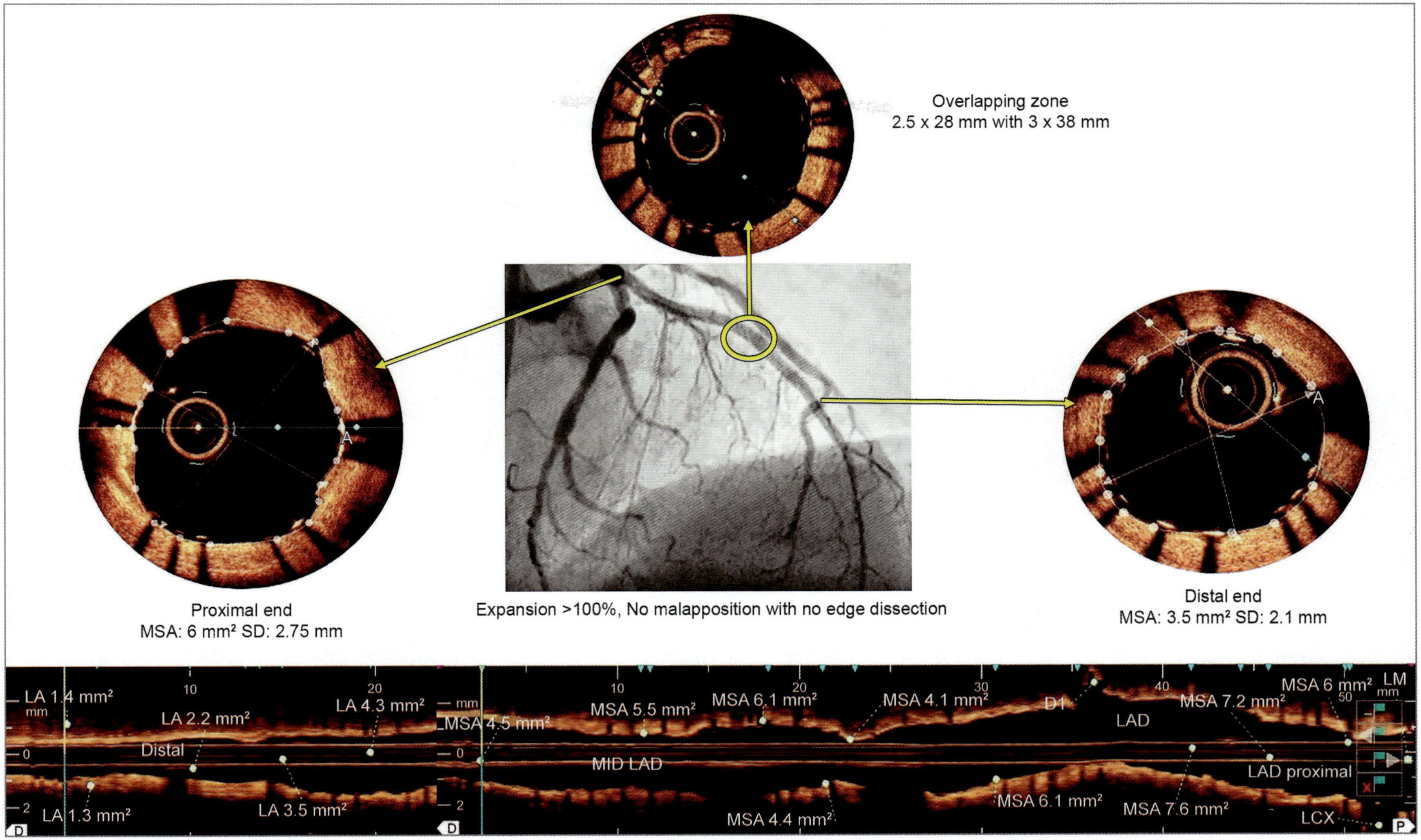
Overlapping zone
2.5 x 28 mm with 3 x 38 mm
Proximal end
MSA: 6 mm² SD: 2.75 mm
Expansion >100%, No malapposition with no edge dissection
Distal end
MSA: 3.5 mm² SD: 2.1 mm
LA 1.4 mm²
LA 2.2 mm²
LA 4.3 mm²
Distal
LA 1.3 mm²
LA 3.5 mm²
MSA 4.5 mm²
MSA 5.5 mm²
MSA 6.1 mm²
MSA 4.1 mm²
D1
LAD
MSA 7.2 mm²
MSA 6 mm²
LM
MID LAD
LAD proximal
MSA 4.4 mm²
MSA 6.1 mm²
MSA 7.6 mm²
LCX

Fig. 4A

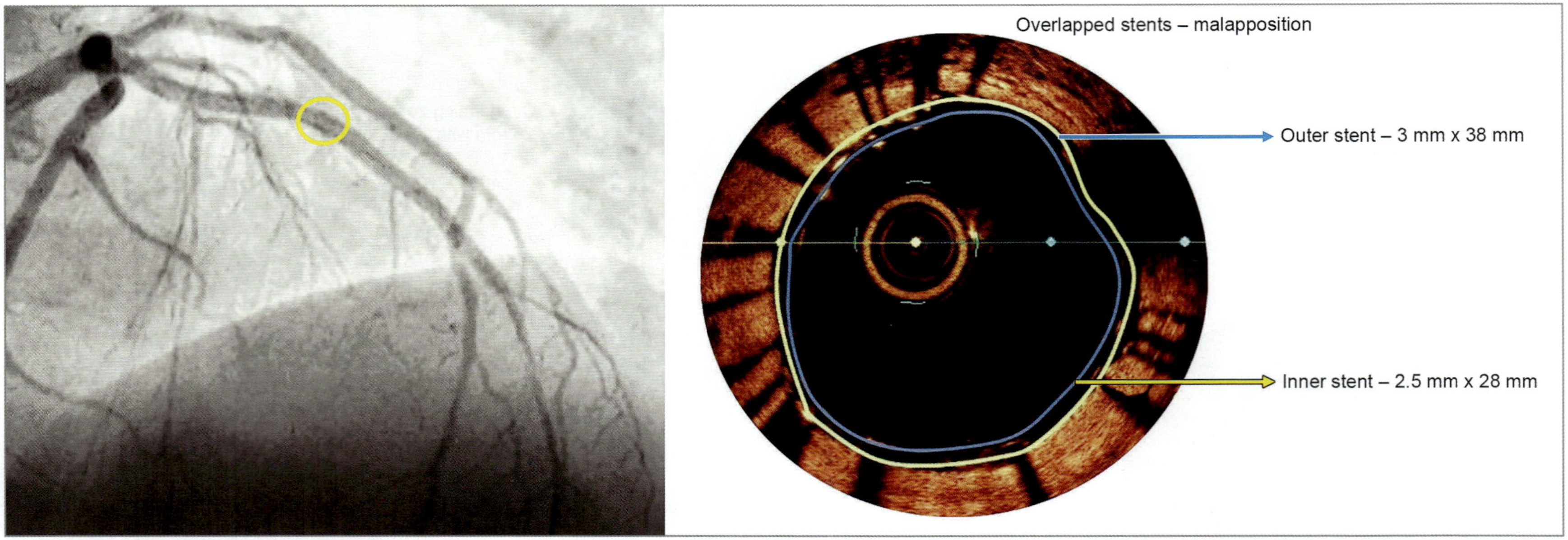

Fig. 4B

Figs. 4A and B: Poststent optical coherence tomography (OCT) analysis showed (A) well-apposed stent struts with no medial edge dissections; (B) overlapping segment. (LA: lumen area; LAD: left anterior descending; LM: left main; MSA: minimal stent area; MSD: minimal stent diameter; SD: stent diameter)

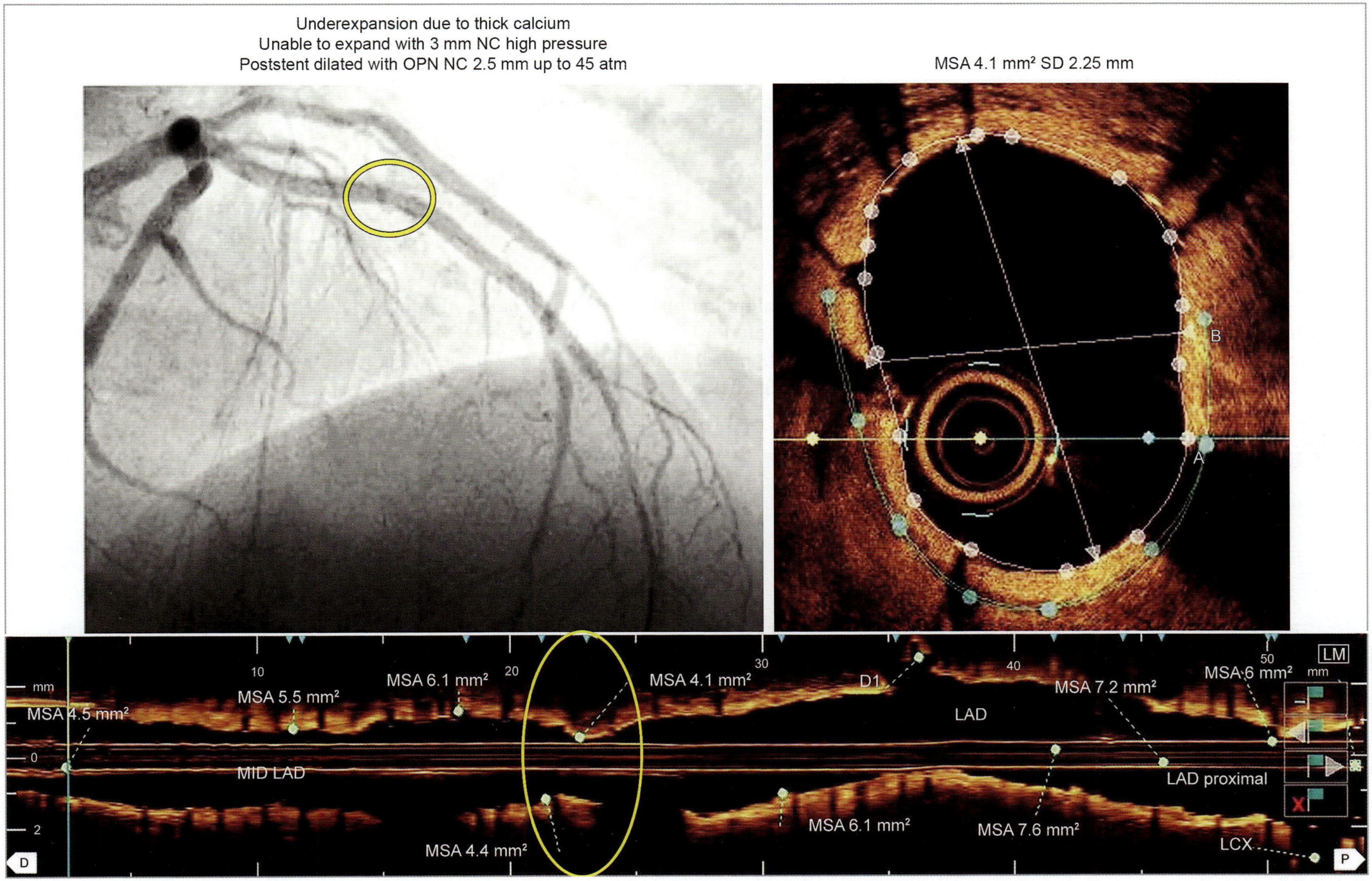

Fig. 5: Underexpansion segment of left anterior descending (LAD) which was corrected with NC. (LA: lumen area; LAD: left anterior descending; LCX: left circumflex; LM: left main; MSA: minimal stent area; SD: stent diameter)

CASE 2

OCT assessment of PCI of total occlusion of RCA.

CLINICAL HISTORY

A 54-year-old male presented with acute inferior wall myocardial infarction (IWMI), chest pain radiating to left arm associated with sudden onset of shortness of breath. Electrocardiogram (ECG)-ST elevation in inferior leads with T inversions. 2D Echo—RWMA in RCA territory, mild LV systolic dysfunction, ejection fraction (EF)—50%. Investigations: RBS—113 mg/dL, blood urea—19 mg/dL, serum creatinine—0.82 mg/dL, eGFR—100. CAG-LMCA, LAD, and LCX—normal, RCA—proximal total occlusion **(Fig. 6)**.

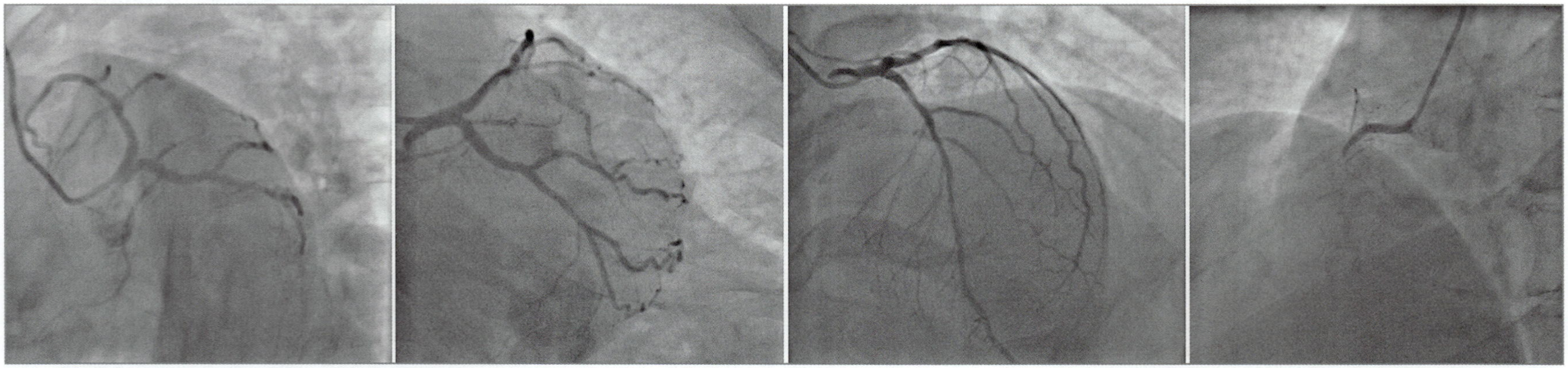

Fig. 6: Coronary angiogram.

PROCEDURE

Route—RRA, 6 Fr Judkins right (JR) 3.5 guiding catheter, lesion crossed with 0.014″ Sion blue wire, predilatation with 2.0 × 10 mm Tazuna balloon.

Pre-OCT study showed proximal RCA thrombotic occlusion with fibrocalcific plaque with minimal lumen area (MLA)—2.1 mm^2, minimal lumen diameter (MLD)—1.6 mm, proximal RCA MLA—8.27 mm^2, MLD—3 mm **(Fig. 7)**.

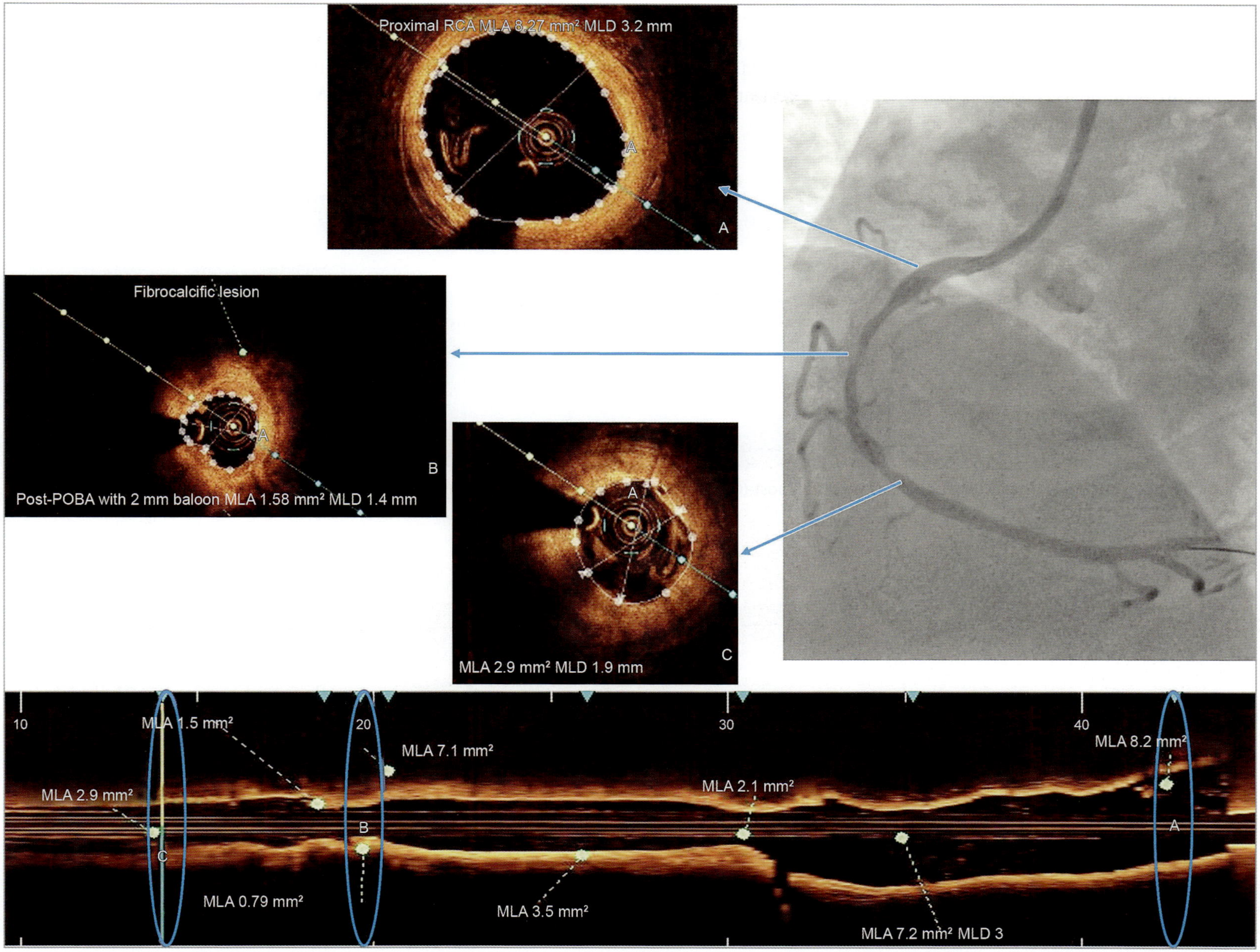

Fig. 7: Prestent optical coherence tomography (OCT) analysis of right coronary artery (RCA) lesion plaque morphology and devise selection. (MLA: minimal lumen area; MLD: minimal lumen diameter; POBA: plain old balloon angioplasty)

Right coronary artery stenting done with 3.5 × 40 mm Yukon Choice Elite stent. Postdilatation done with 3.5 × 12 mm NC Trek balloon **(Fig. 8)**. Postprocedure OCT showed distal to the stent-significant discrete stenosis and which was covered with 3.0 × 16 mm Yukon Choice Elite stent **(Fig. 9)**. After postdilatation OCT showed proximal edge of RCA stent MLA—9.1 mm^2, distal landing zone-MLA—6.6 mm^2, well-apposed stent struts, no residual stenosis, and no thrombosis **(Figs. 10A and B)**. Postprocedure angio view showed well-implanted stents with TIMI-III flow without any dissection. Patient was discharged on third postprocedure in a stable status.

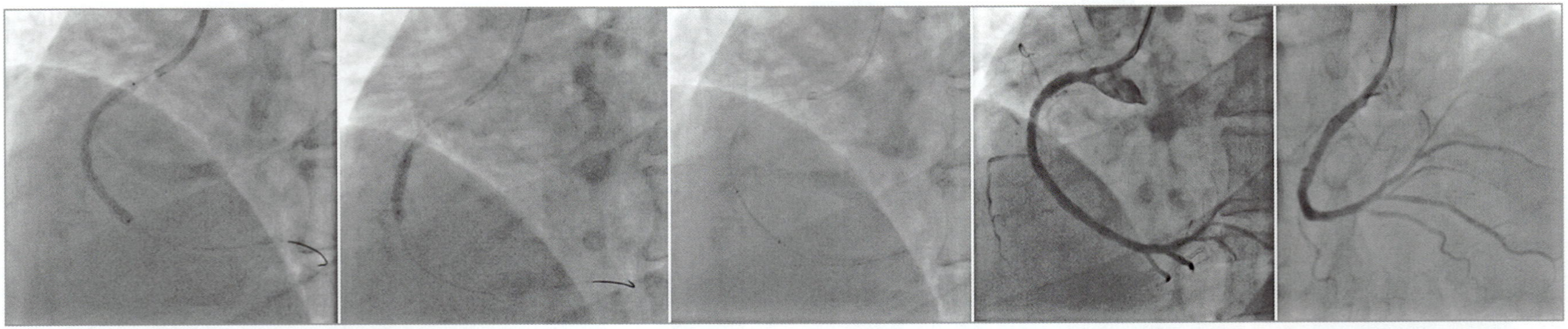

Fig. 8: Coronary angioplasty of proximal and distal [post-(OCT) optical coherence tomography stenting] segments of right coronary artery (RCA).

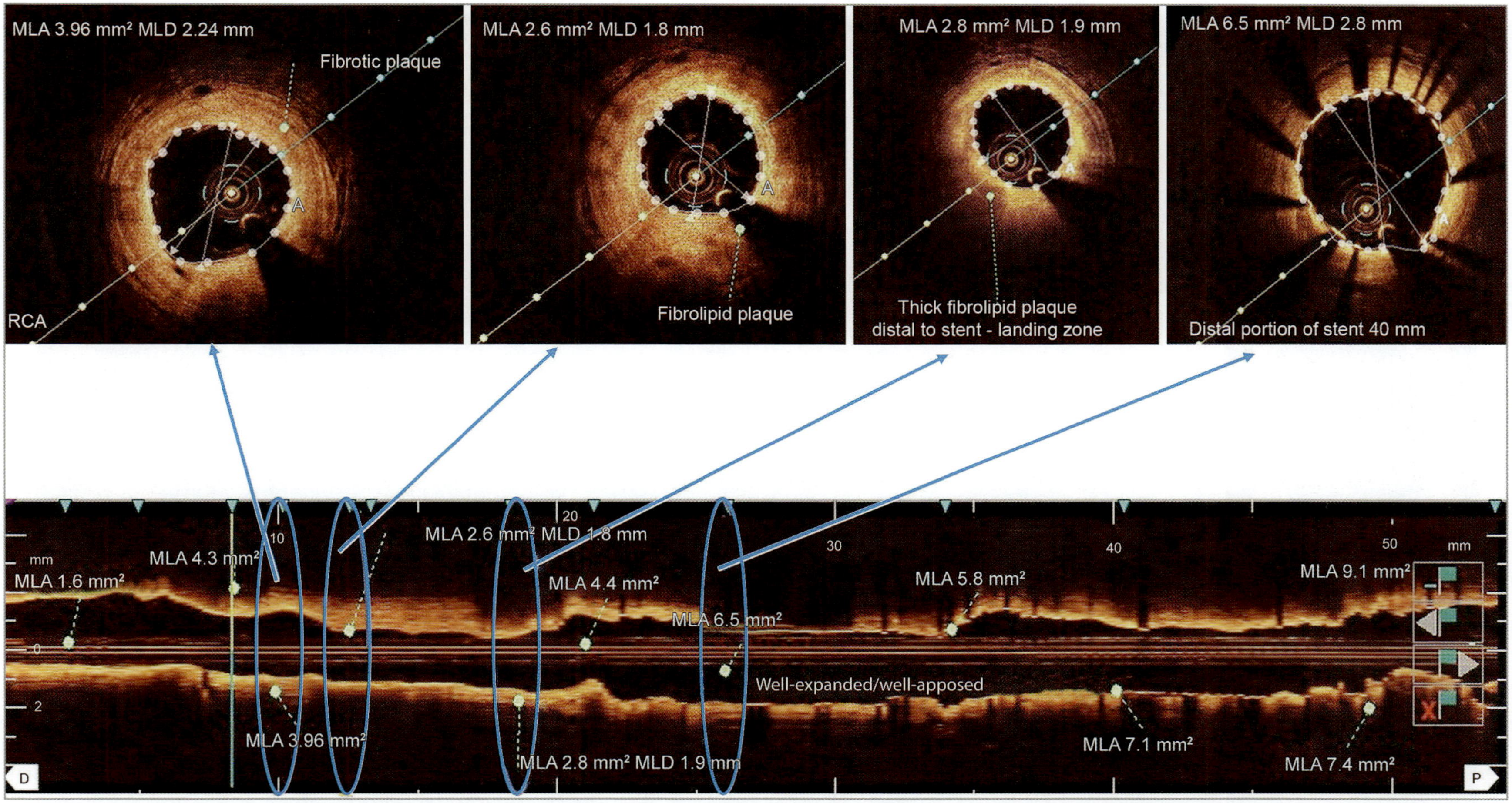

Fig. 9: Postproximal stent optical coherence tomography (OCT) analysis showed distal thick fibrolipid plaque from distal landing zone of proximal stent which was covered with additional stent.

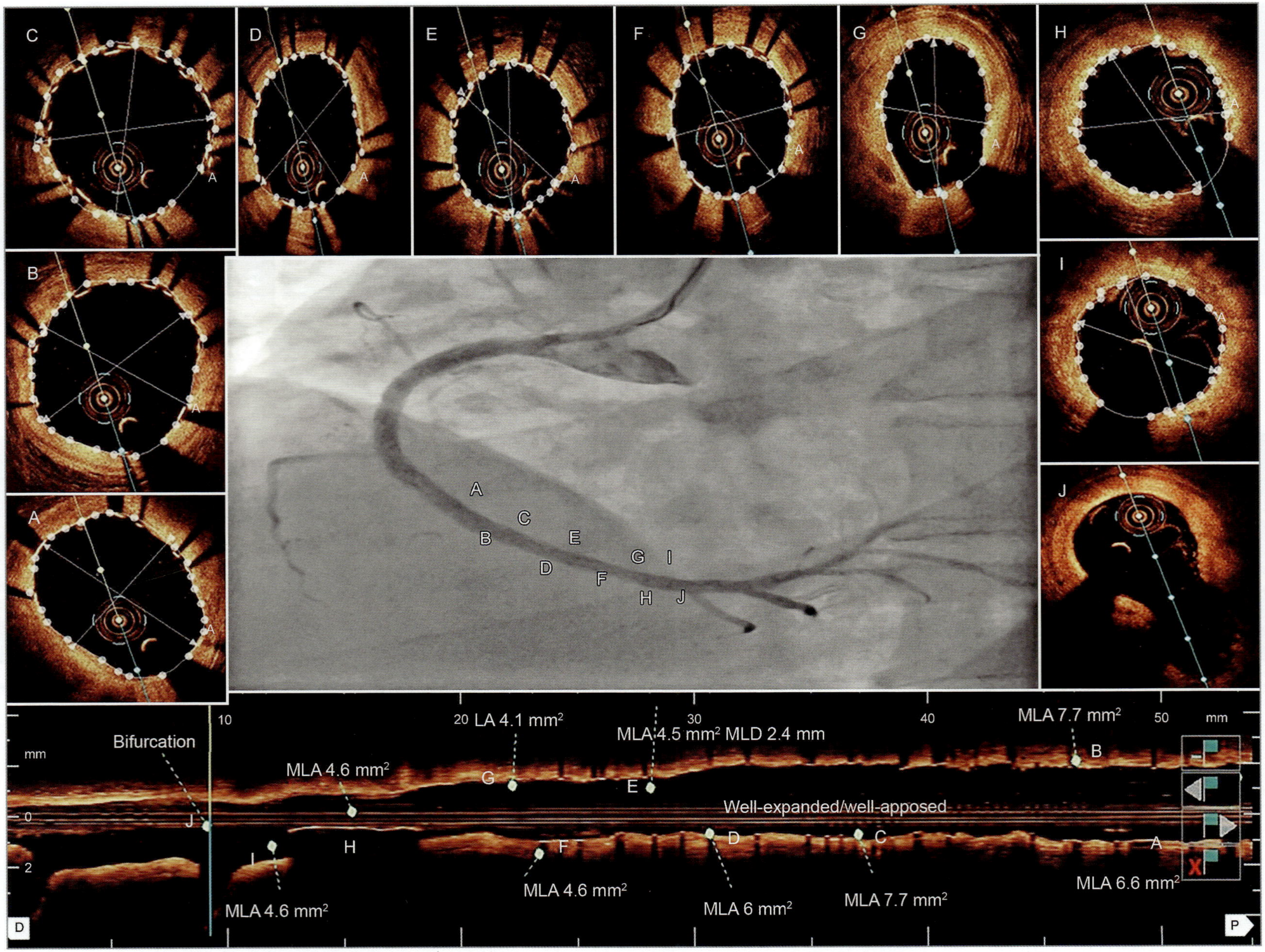

C
D
E
F
G
H
B
I
A
J
A
C
B
E
D
G
I
F
H
J
10
20
30
40
50
mm
LA 4.1 mm²
MLA 4.5 mm² MLD 2.4 mm
MLA 7.7 mm²
Bifurcation
MLA 4.6 mm²
Well-expanded/well-apposed
MLA 4.6 mm²
MLA 4.6 mm²
MLA 6 mm²
MLA 7.7 mm²
MLA 6.6 mm²
D
P

Fig. 10A

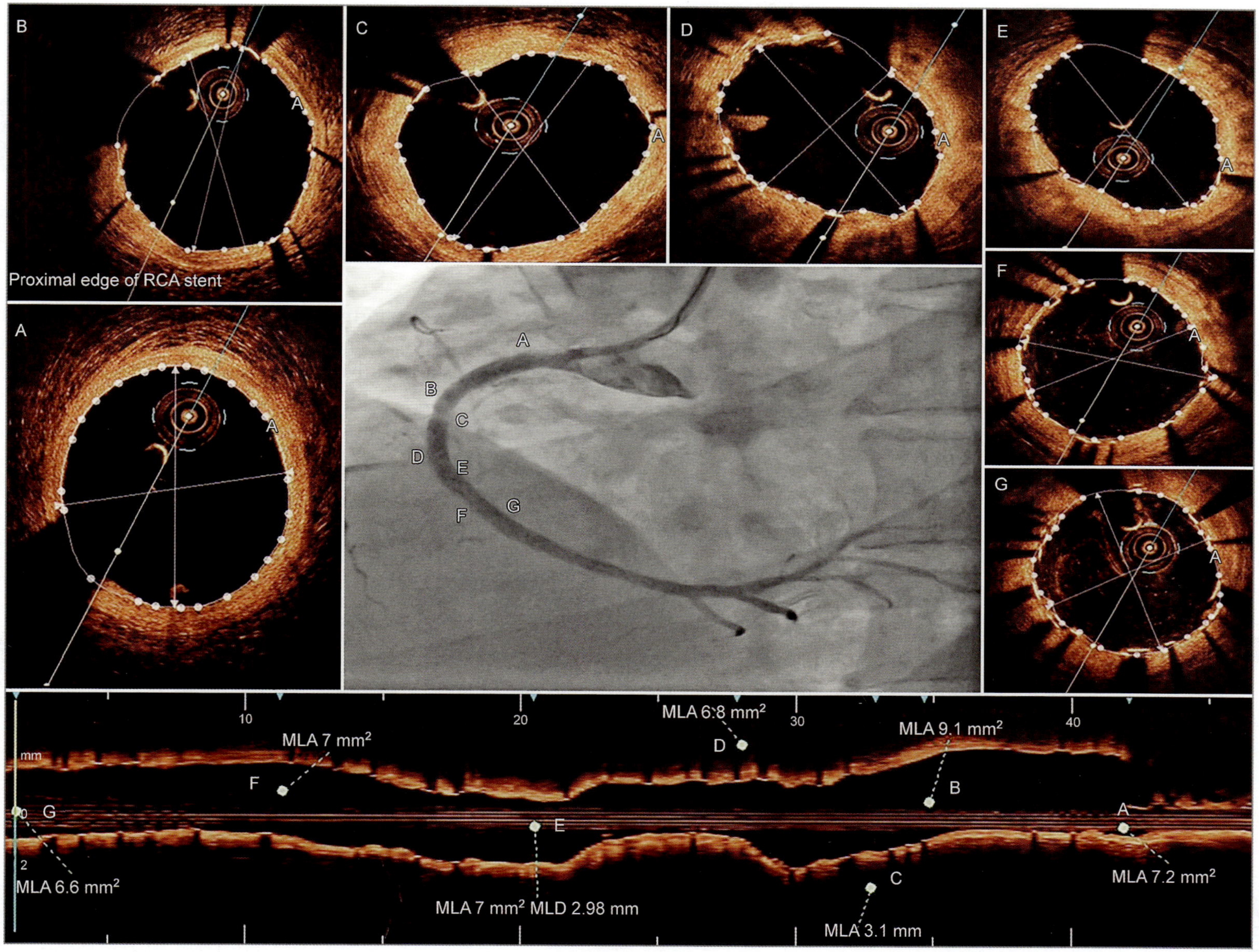

Fig. 10B

Figs. 10A and B: (A) Poststent optical coherence tomography (OCT) analysis of distal right coronary artery (RCA) showed well-expanded and apposed stent struts with no medial edge dissection; (B) Poststent OCT analysis of proximal RCA showed well-expanded and apposed stent struts with no medial edge dissection. (MLA: minimal lumen are; MLD: minimal lumen diameter)

CASE 3

Assessment of retrograde wire entry by OCT in CTO of LAD segment.

CLINICAL HISTORY

A 64-year-old male, known hypertensive, with old AWMI presented with chest pain associated with shortness of breath. Investigations: Hb—14.5 g/dL, serum creatinine—1 mg/dL, blood urea—23 mg/dL, RBS—112 mg/dL. ECG—old AWMI, 2D Echo—hypokinetic inferior wall, normal LV systolic function, EF—50%. CAG-LMCA—normal, LAD-CTO of LAD, LCX—mild ostial narrowing, RCA—proximal 90%, and distal 80% lesions **(Fig. 11)**.

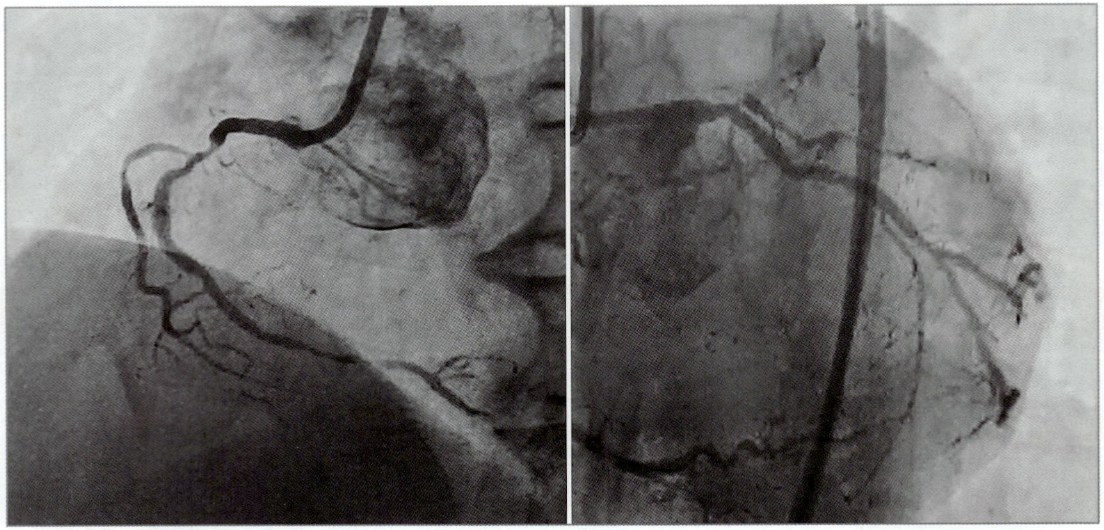

Fig. 11: Coronary angiogram.

PROCEDURE

PCI of LAD: Right femoral artery (RFA)—route, 7 Fr, Amplatz left (AL) 1 guiding catheter in RCA and 7 Fr XB 3.5 guiding catheter, 0.014″ Runthrough wire was passed through RCA with Finecross microcatheter support. Runthrough wire exchanged with Sion blue wire and crossed through septal collaterals with Finecross microcatheter support, and wire externalized into left guiding catheter with 2.0 × 15 mm balloon occlusion in the catheter. Sion blue wire exchanged with RG3 wire externalized through left guiding catheter. Proximal LAD predilatation done with 2.0 × 10 mm Tazuna balloon. Runthrough wire passed into antegradely into LAD and Sion blue wire in LCX. Predilatation done with 2.5 × 10 mm Tazuna balloon.

Post-POBA OCT study of LAD after retrograde wire access—long segment tight fibrotic long-length lesion with large dissection at the LAD origin from LMCA **(Fig. 12)**, distal portion of the lesion with MLA—2.4 mm^2, MLD—1.7 mm, fibrotic plaque with MLA—3.6 mm^2, MLD—2.1 mm, LCX ostium with MLA—3.5 mm^2, MLD—2 mm **(Fig. 13)**.

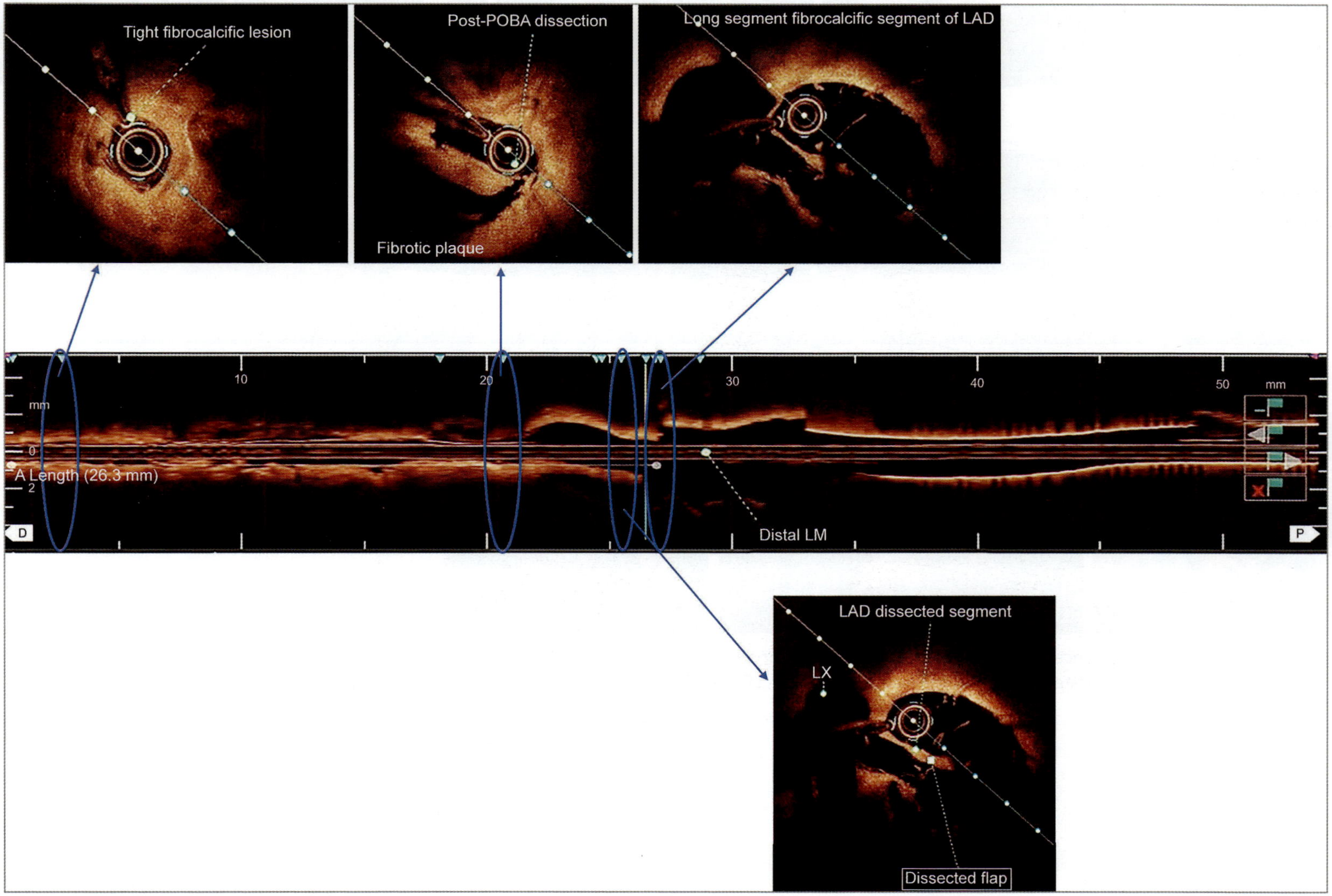

Fig. 12: Prestent optical coherence tomography (OCT) assessment for plaque morphology. (LAD: left anterior descending; LM: left main; POBA: plain old balloon angioplasty)

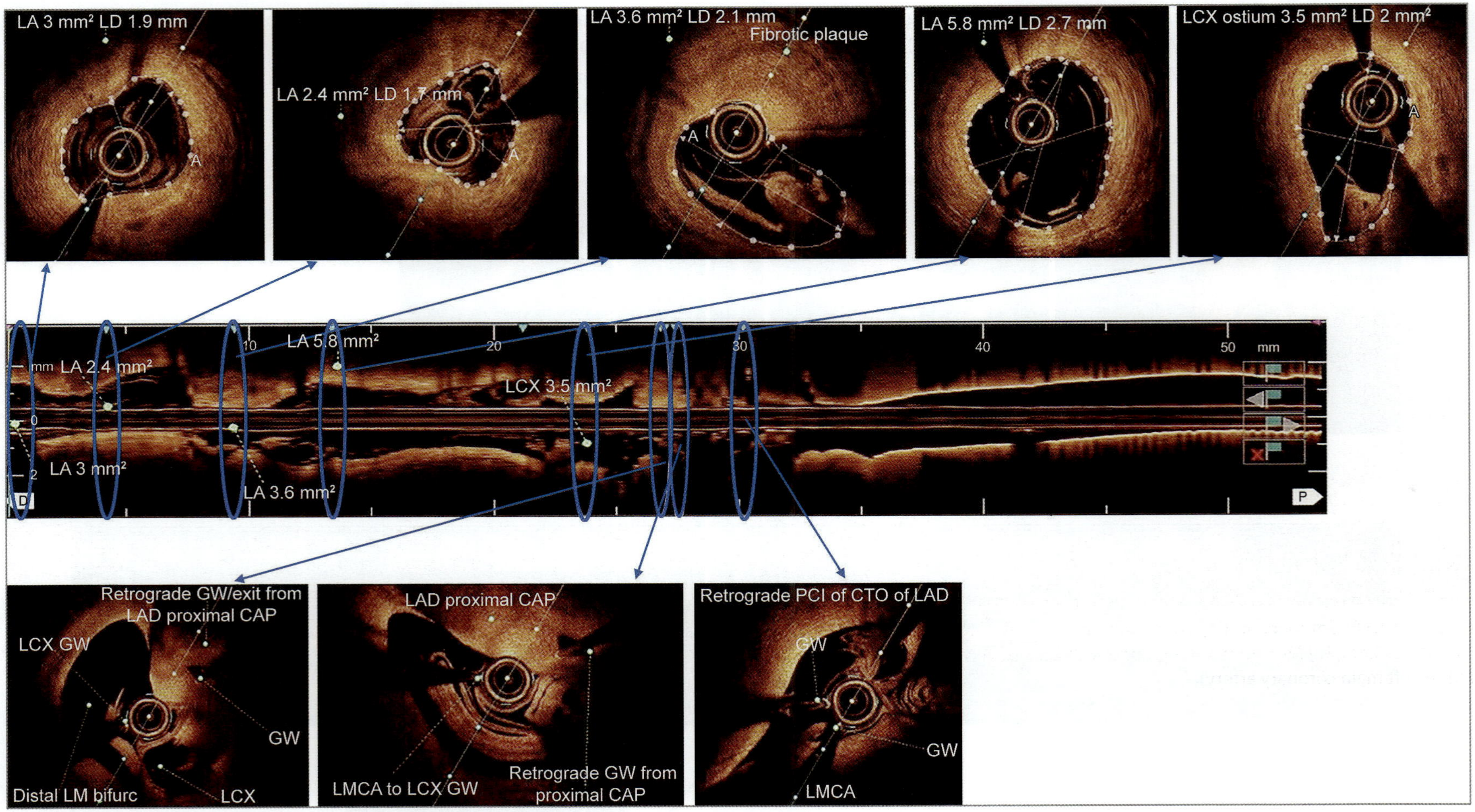

Fig. 13: Prestent optical coherence tomography (OCT) assessment for devise selection. (CTO: chronic total occlusion; LAD: left anterior descending; LA: lumen area; LD: lumen diameter; LMCA: left main coronary artery; LCX: left circumflex; GW: guidewire; PCI: percutaneous coronary intervention)

Pre-OCT showed post-POBA long segment tight fibrotic lesion of LAD, lesion length 26.3 mm **(Fig. 12)**.

Pre-OCT showed distal portion of the lesion with MLA—2.4 mm^2, MLD—1.7 mm, fibrotic plaque with MLA—3.6 mm^2, MLD—2.1 mm, LCX ostium with MLA—3.5 mm^2, MLD—2 mm **(Fig. 13)**.

Proximal LAD stenting done with 3.5 × 24 mm Ultimaster stent. LMCA to LAD stenting done with 4.0 × 18 mm Ultimaster stent. Mid LAD stenting done with 2.5 × 33 mm Ultimaster stent. After LMCA to LAD stenting sudden acute closure of LCX with hypotension and chest pain, emergency recrossing of LCX with pilot guidewire through LMCA to LAD stent struts with and dilated with 2.5 × 12 mm Tazuna balloon and 3.0 × 15 mm balloon with restoration of LCX blood flow LMCA to LCX. Intravascular ultrasound (IVUS) showed plaque in ostial LCX. LMCA to LAD IVUS showed well-expanded stent in proximal and mid LAD. Postdilatation done with 3.0 × 15 mm balloon. Intracoronary 10 mL of Gp IIb/IIIa infusion was given. Postprocedure angio view showed well-implanted stents with TIMI-III flow without any dissection **(Figs. 14A to E)**. Patient was discharged on third postprocedure in a stable status.

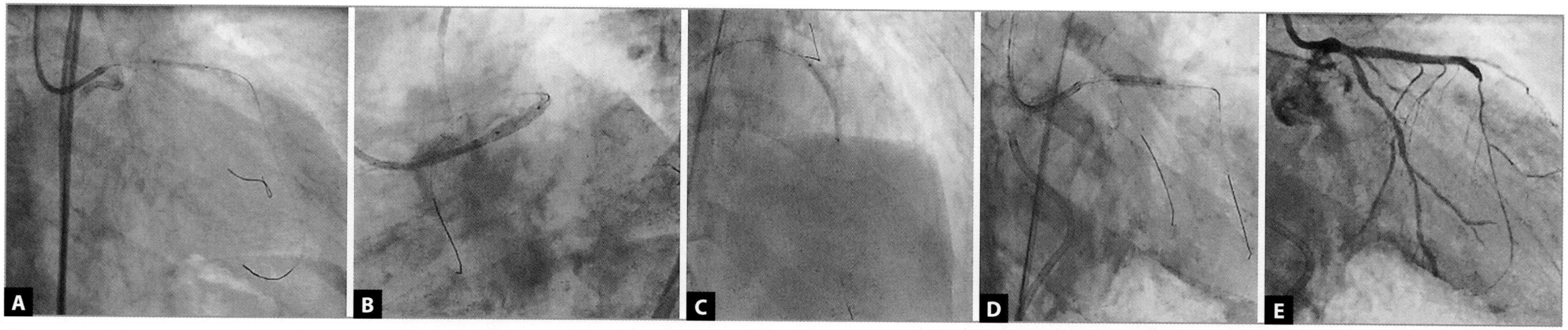

Figs. 14A to E: Coronary angioplasty and final result. (A) Proximal LAD stenting done with 3.5 × 24 mm Ultimaster stent; (B) LMCA to LAD stenting done with 4.0 × 18 mm Ultimaster stent; (C) Mid LAD stenting done with 2.5 × 33 mm Ultimaster stent; (D) Postdilatation done with 3.0 × 15 mm balloon; (E) Final result. (LAD: left anterior descending; LMCA: left main coronary artery)

CASE 4

PCI of CTO of RCA.

CLINICAL HISTORY

A 58-year-old male, known hypertensive, diabetic, smoker, and ethanolic, presented with chest pain associated with shortness of breath (SOB) class II. ECG showed anterior NSTEMI. 2D Echo—RWMA in inferior territory, mild LV dysfunction with EF—40%, previous CAG report showed two-vessel disease, underwent PCI with stenting of LAD, failed attempt of CTO of RCA in peripheral center and referred here for PCI of CTO of RCA. Initial plan was to do antegrade approach, otherwise retrograde strategy **(Fig. 15)**.

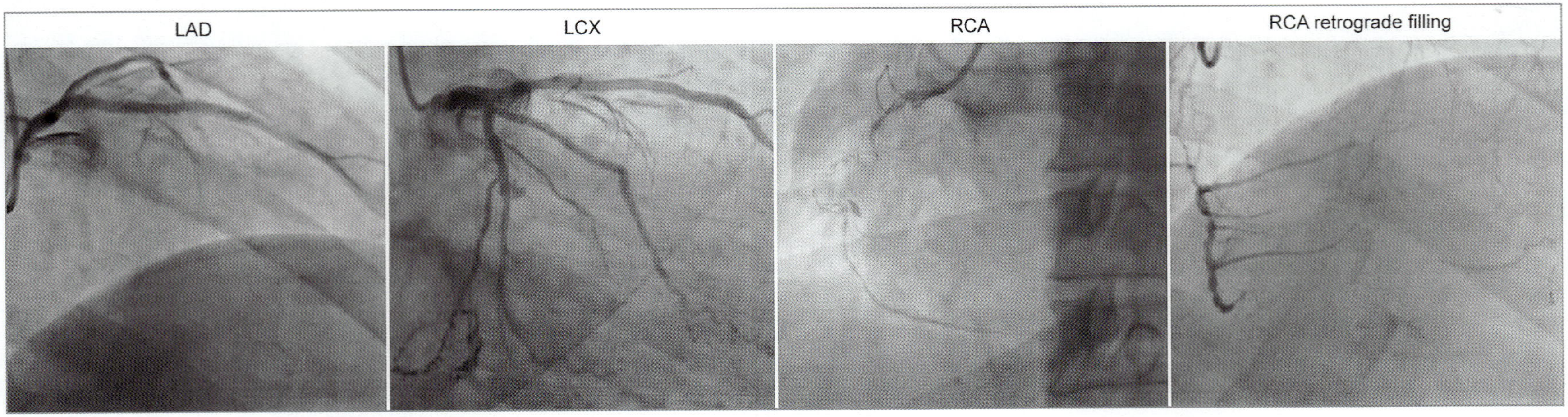

Fig. 15: Coronary angiogram. (LAD: left anterior descending; LCX: left circumflex; RCA: right coronary artery)

PROCEDURE

Procedure performed through right femoral artery using 7 Fr sheath, 6 Fr JR, and left femoral artery using 6 Fr sheath, 5 Fr JL guiding catheter, check angiogram revealed mid RCA 100% occluded. Initially tried with 0.014″ Sion blue, Fielder FC wires using microcatheter but could not cross the lesion despite multiple attempts with different wires, finally lesion was crossed with Gaia II wire with Finecross microcatheter support. Predilatation done with 1.5 × 10 mm Tazuna, 2.5 × 15 mm, 2.5 × 08 mm Trek balloons, and 2.75 × 08 mm, 3.0 × 08 mm NC Trek balloons.

Pre-OCT analysis: OCT showed diffused long-segment fibrocalcific lesion **(Figs. 16A and B)**.

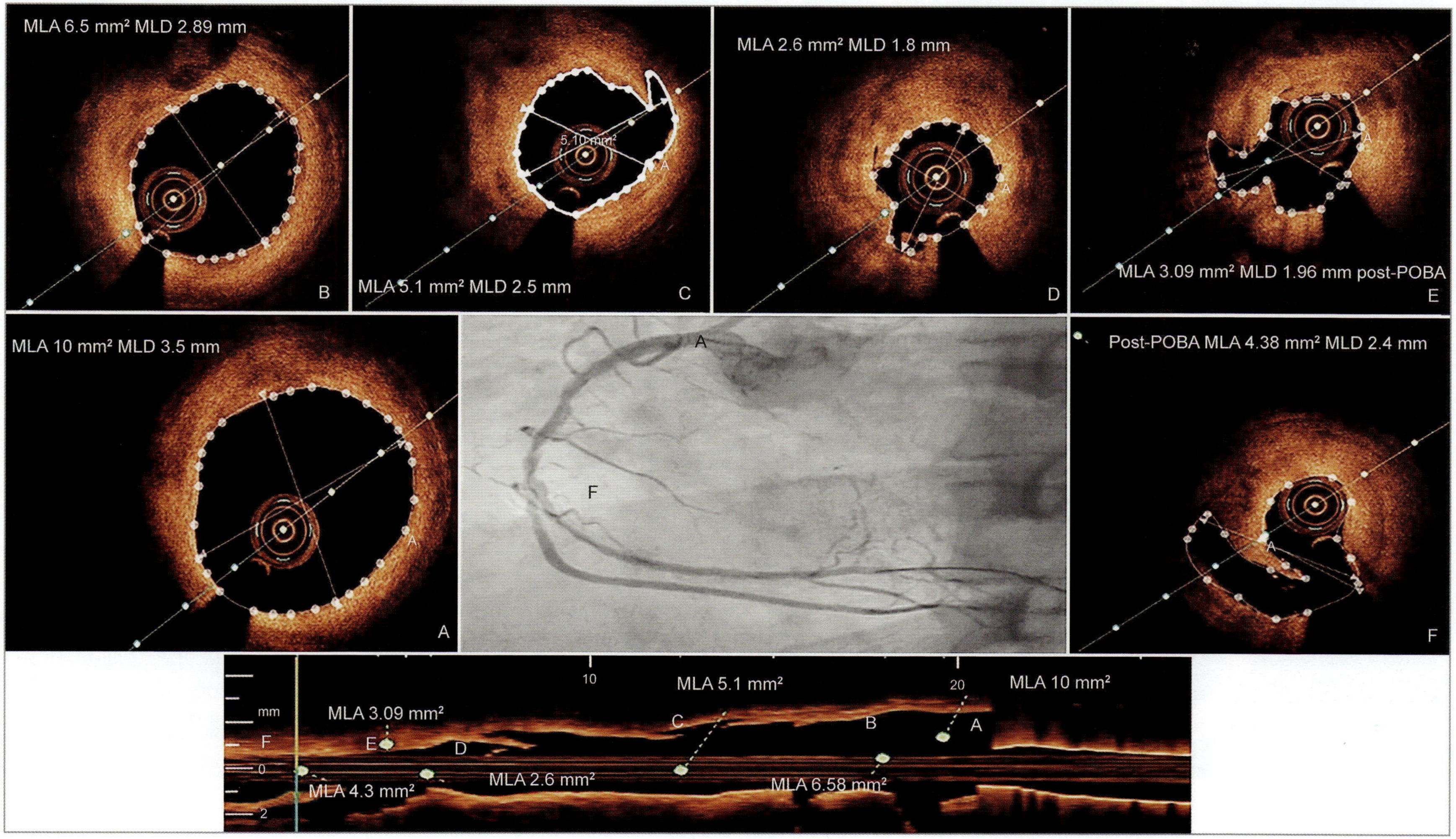

Fig. 16A

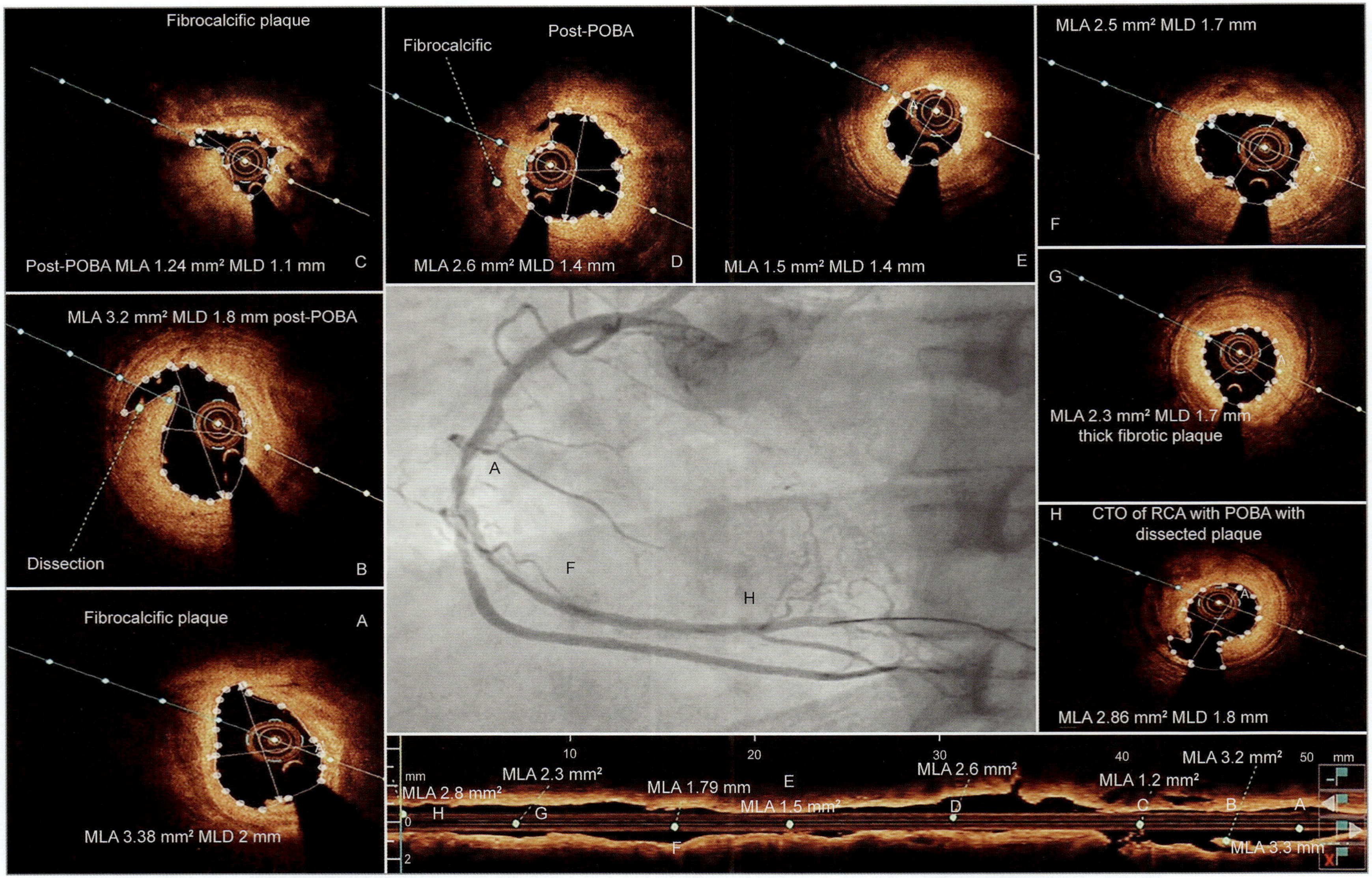

Fig. 16B

Figs. 16A and B: Prestent optical coherence tomography (OCT) analysis of (A) proximal right coronary artery (RCA); (B) distal RCA. (MLA: minimal lumen area; MLD: minimal lumen diameter; POBA: plain old balloon angioplasty)

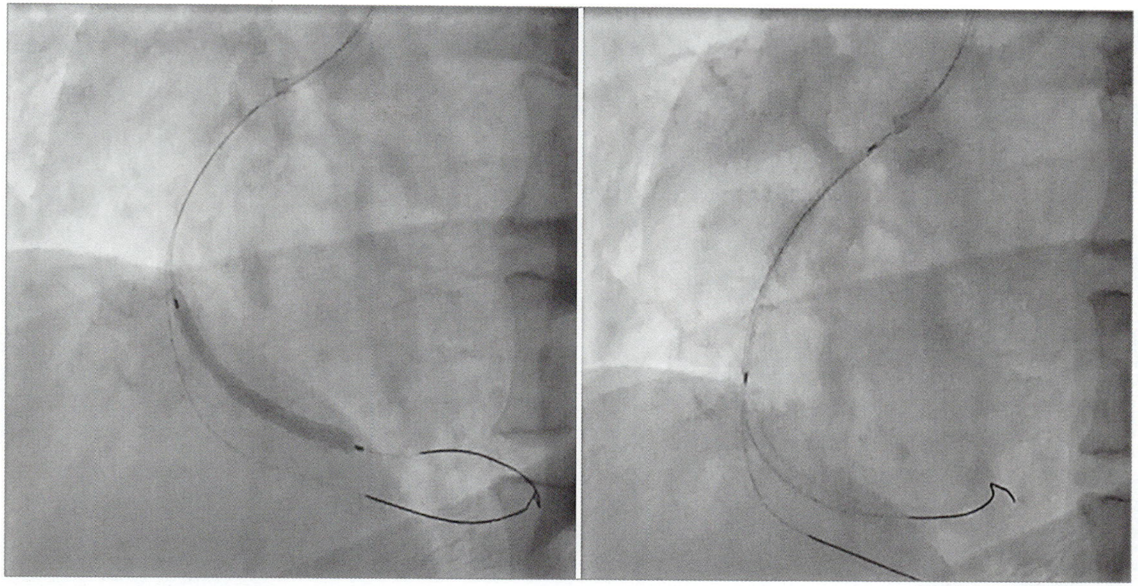

Fig. 17: Coronary angioplasty of proximal and distal right coronary artery (RCA).

Distal RCA stenting done with 2.75 × 38 mm Xience Xpedition stent [drug-eluting stent (DES)]. Proximal RCA stenting done with 3.5 × 38 mm Xience Xpedition stent (DES) **(Fig. 17)**.

Post-OCT analysis: Well-apposed and well-expanded stent struts without any edge dissections **(Fig. 18)**.

Postdilatation done with 3.75 × 12 mm NC Trek balloon. Postprocedure angio view showed well-implanted stents with TIMI-III flow without any dissection. Patient was discharged on third postprocedure in a stable status.

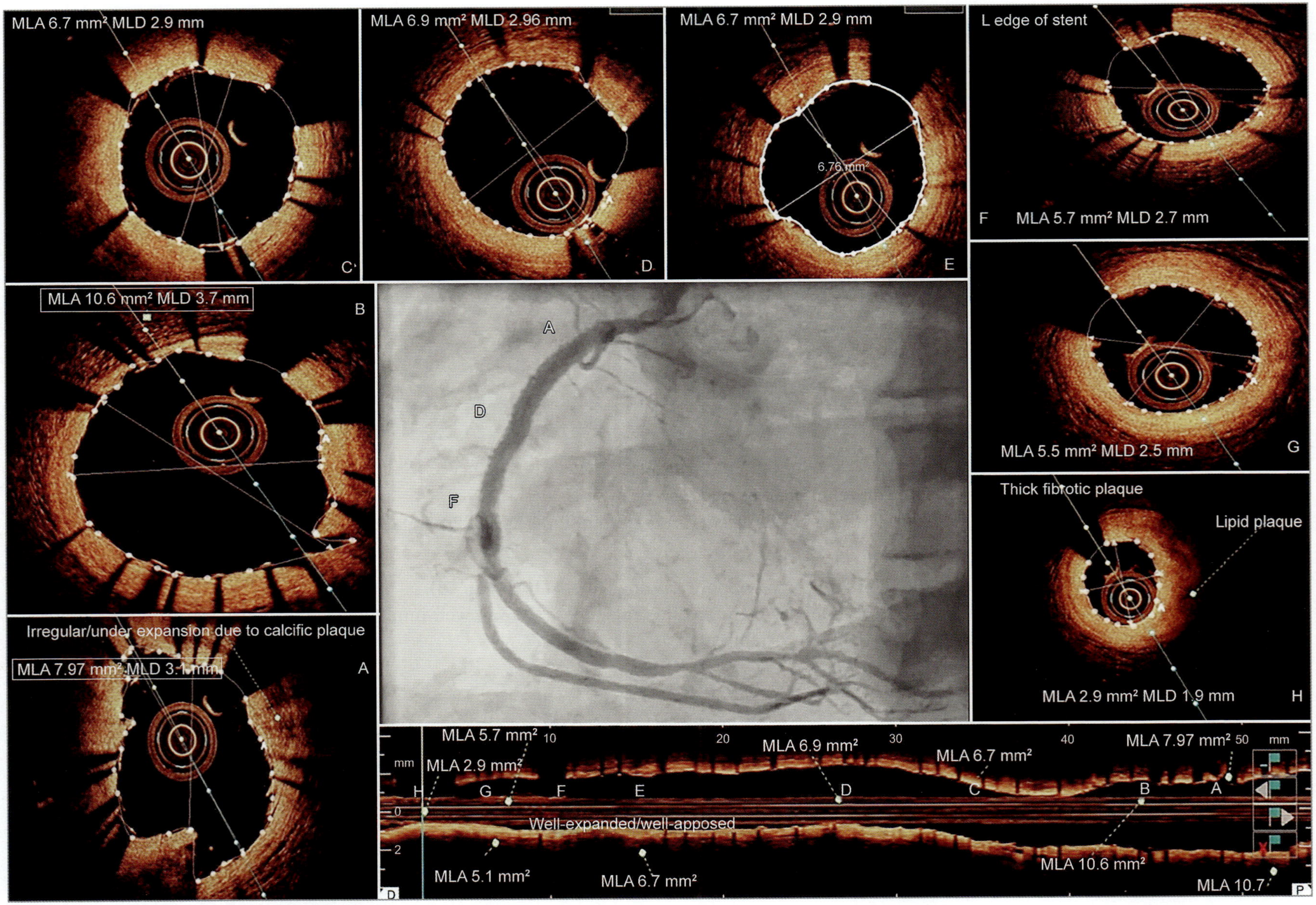

Fig. 18: Poststent OCT analysis showed well-expanded and apposed stent struts with no medial edge dissections. (MLA: minimal lumen area; MLD: minimal lumen diameter)

CHAPTER 24

Air Embolism

CASE 1

Air embolism during optical coherence tomography (OCT)-guided percutaneous coronary intervention (PCI) of left anterior descending (LAD).

CLINICAL HISTORY

A 69-year-old male, known hypertensive and diabetic, presented with stable ischemic heart disease, effort angina associated with shortness of breath (SOB). 2D Echo—No RWMA (regional wall motion abnormality), normal left ventricular (LV) function, ejection fraction (EF)—62%.

Investigations: random blood sugar (RBS)—156 mg/dL, blood urea—21 mg/dL, serum creatinine—1.17 mg/dL, estimated glomerular filtration rate (eGFR)—63. Coronary angiogram (CAG)-LMCA (left main coronary artery)—normal, LAD—mid 90% lesion, left circumflex (LCX)—normal, right coronary artery (RCA)—normal **(Fig. 1)**.

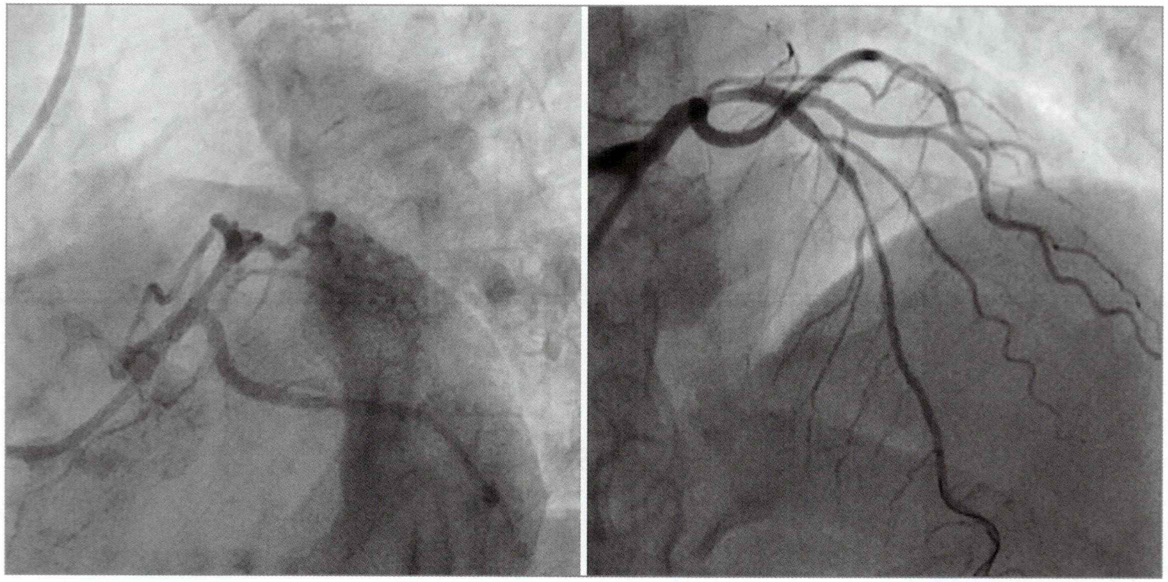

Fig. 1: Coronary angiogram.

PROCEDURE

Route—right radial approach (RRA), 6 Fr XB 3.5 guiding catheter, 0.014″ Sion blue wire placed in LAD, 0.014″ BMW wire placed in LCX **(Fig. 1)**. OCT revealed critical fibrotic lesion with proximal landing zone minimal lumen area (MLA)—6.8 mm^2, minimal lumen diameter (MLD)—2.9 mm, and distal landing zone-MLA—2.8 mm^2, MLD—1.9 mm **(Fig. 2)**.

Predilated with 2.5 × 12 mm NC Trek balloon, LAD stented with 2.75 × 40 mm Orsiro stent and postdilated with 3.0 × 15 mm NC Trek balloon **(Figs. 3A to C)**.

Post-OCT—proximal minimal stent area (MSA)—8 mm^2, minimal stent diameter (MSD)—3.2 mm, distal MSA—4.5 mm^2, MSD—2.4 mm, proximal portion of the stent postdilated with 3.0 × 15 mm NC at 18 atm, well-covered mild intrastent dissection and well-expanded and apposed stent struts with no edge dissection **(Fig. 4A)**.

Patient developed air embolism during OCT procedure **(Fig. 4B)**, angio showed decreased coronary flow with contrast stasis associated with bradycardia, hypotension, and chest pain which was cleared with repeated coughing, aspiration of air and blood through guide catheter, and atropine injection **(Fig. 3D)**.

Postprocedure angio view showed well-implanted stents with TIMI-III (thrombolysis in myocardial infarction III) flow without any dissection **(Fig. 3E)**.

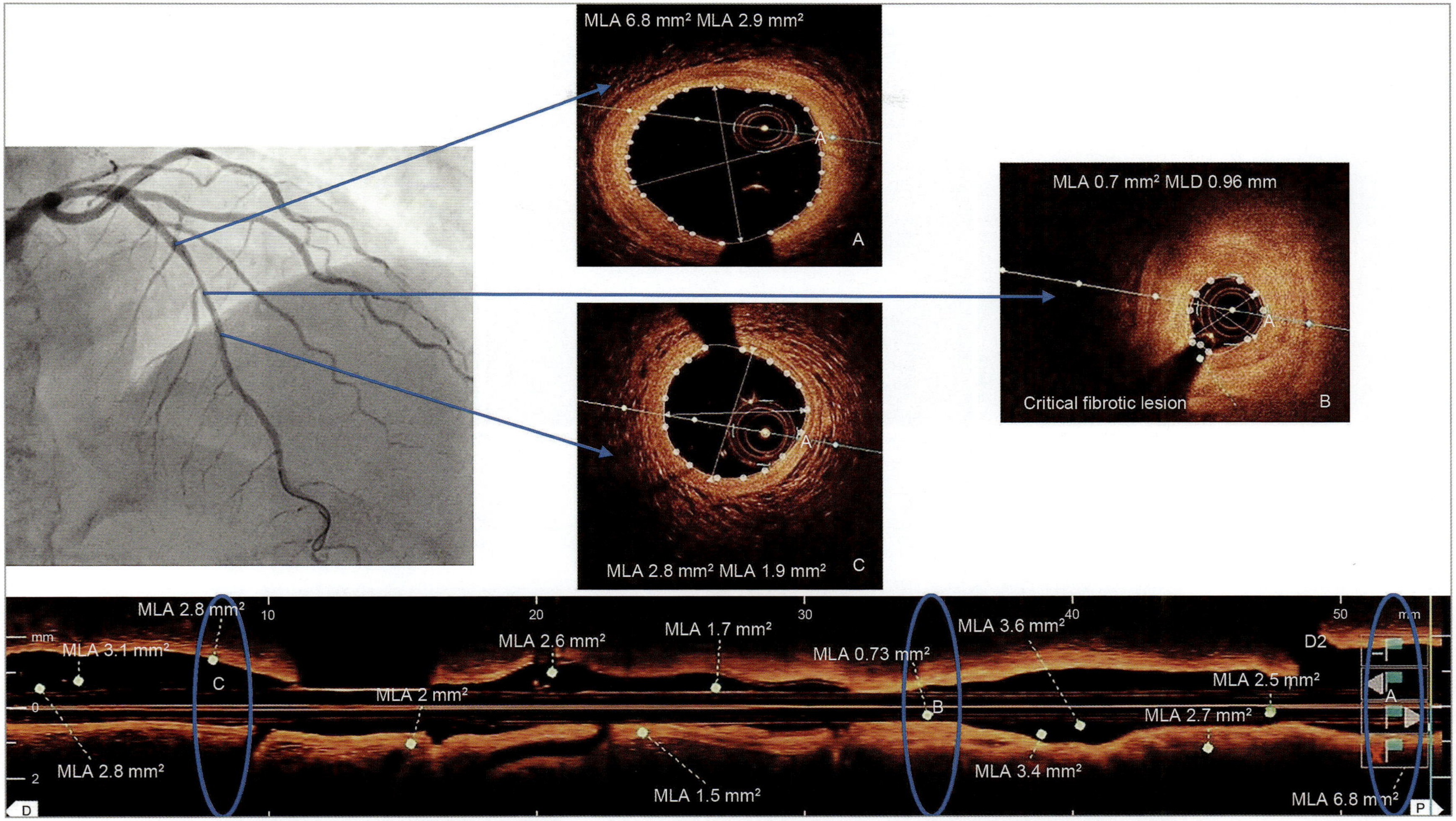

Fig. 2: Prestenting OCT (optical coherence tomography) analysis for device selection and plaque morphology. (MLA: minimal lumen area; MLD: minimal lumen diameter)

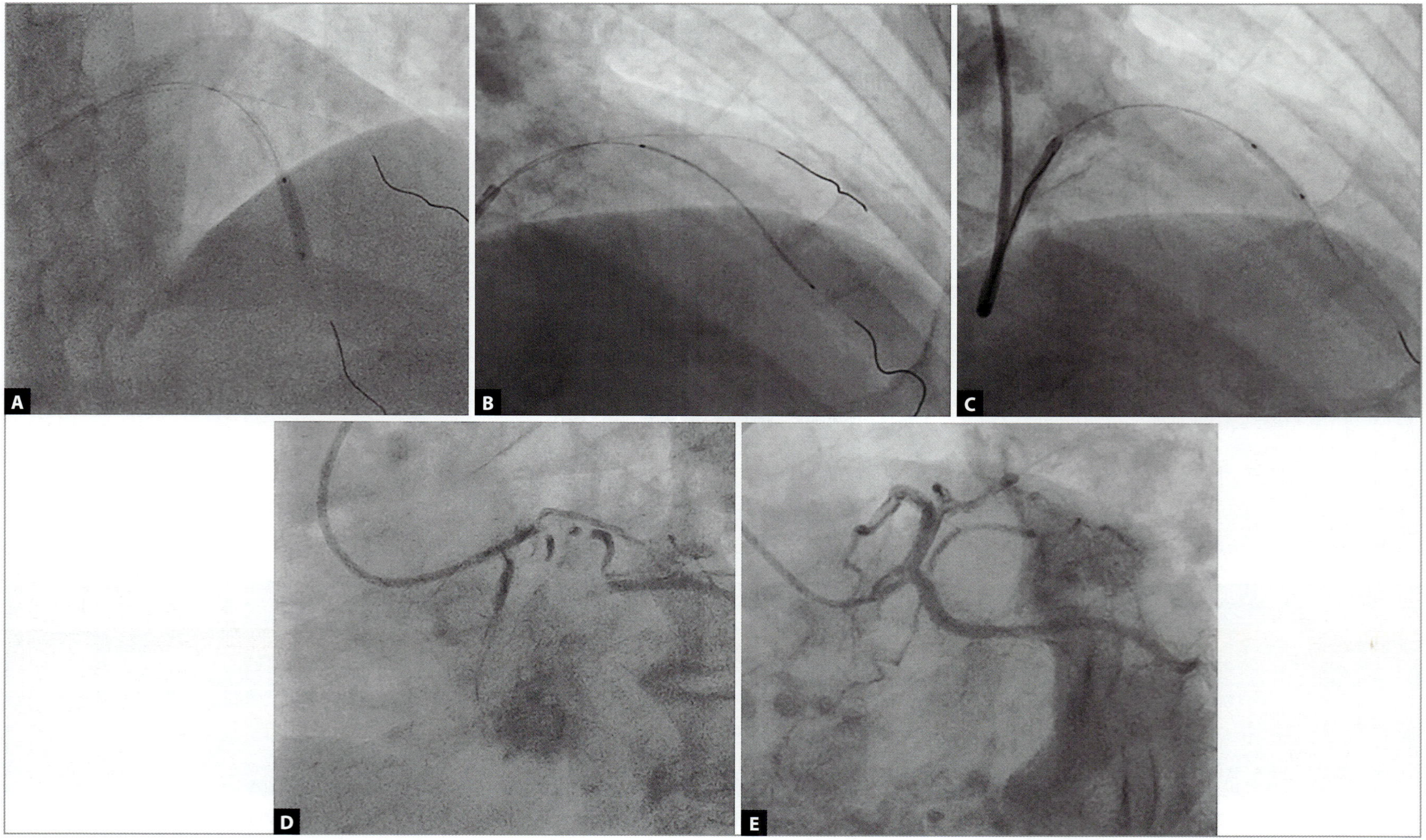

Figs. 3A to E: (A) Predilatation; (B) stenting; (C) postdilatation; (D) decreased coronary flow poststenting optical coherence tomography (OCT); (E) final result.

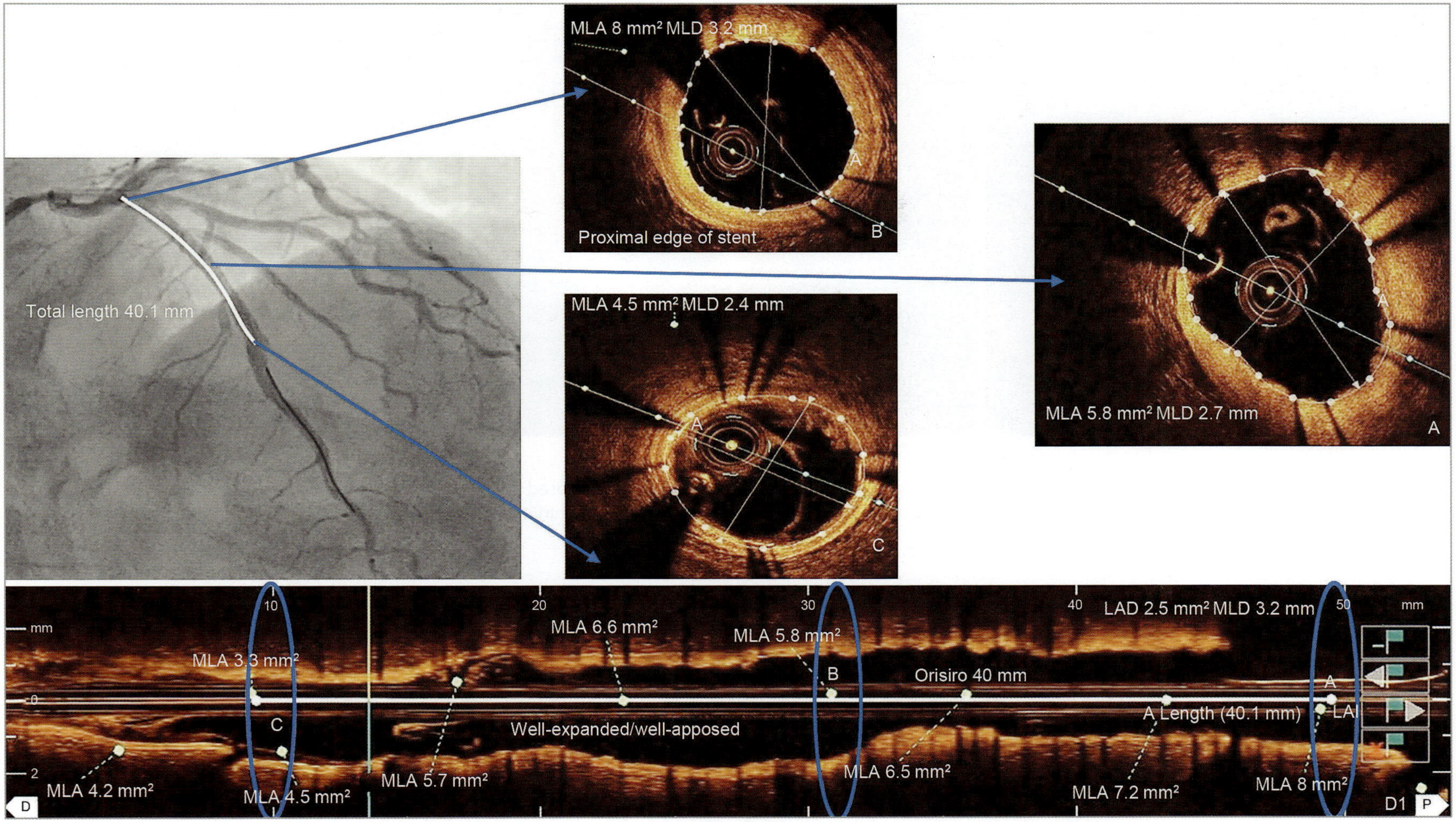
MLA 8 mm² MLD 3.2 mm
Proximal edge of stent
A
B
Total length 40.1 mm
MLA 4.5 mm² MLD 2.4 mm
A
C
MLA 5.8 mm² MLD 2.7 mm
A
LAD 2.5 mm² MLD 3.2 mm
MLA 3.3 mm²
MLA 6.6 mm²
MLA 5.8 mm²
Orisiro 40 mm
Well-expanded/well-apposed
Length (40.1 mm)
MLA 4.2 mm²
MLA 4.5 mm²
MLA 5.7 mm²
MLA 6.5 mm²
MLA 7.2 mm²
MLA 8 mm²

Fig. 4A

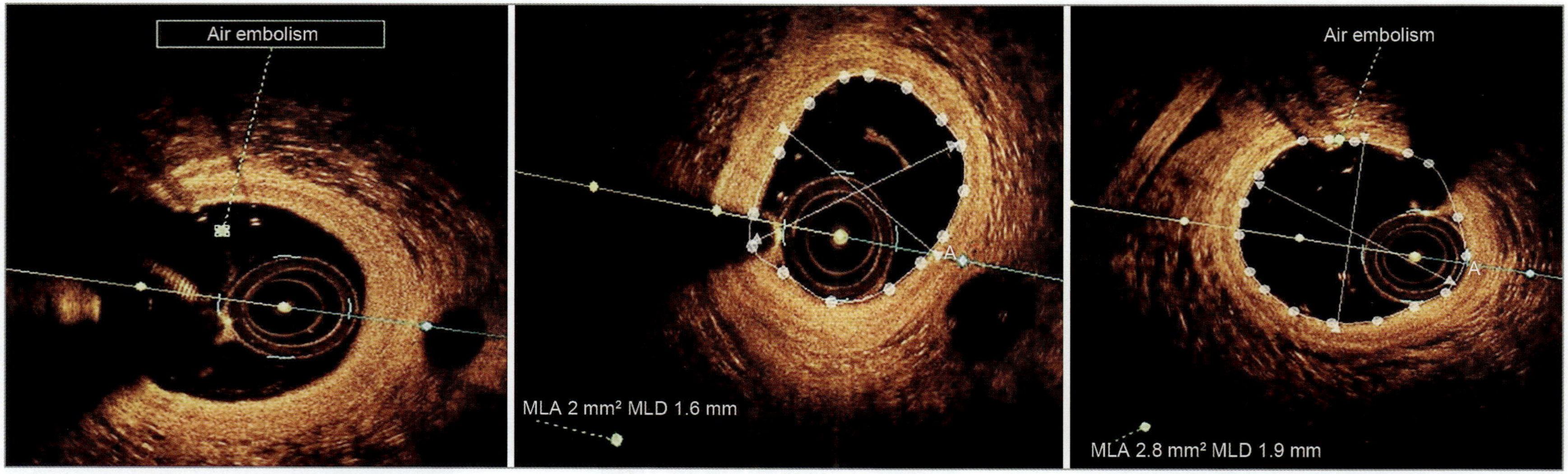

Fig. 4B

Figs. 4A and B: (A) Poststent OCT (optical coherence tomography) showed well-expanded and apposed stent struts; (B) air embolism caused due to air bubbles. (LAD: left anterior descending; MLA: minimal lumen area; MLD: minimal lumen diameter)

CHAPTER 25

Post Coronary Artery Bypass Graft Angioplasty

CASE 1

Post bypass graft drug-eluting balloon (DEB) + drug-eluting stent (DES) strategy.

CLINICAL HISTORY

A 62-year-old male, known hypertensive, and diabetic presented with chest pain associated with breathlessness. Coronary artery bypass graft (CABG) [LIMA to LAD (left internal mammary artery to left anterior descending artery), saphenous vein graft (SVG) to RAMUS and SVG to right coronary artery (RCA)] was done in 2005. Post-percutaneous coronary intervention (PCI) of SVG to RAMUS in 2017 **(Fig. 1)**. On examination PR—86, BP—110/70, SPO_2—98%, heart—S^1+, S^2+, $S3^0$, $S4^0$, lungs—clear. Investigations: hemoglobin (Hb)—11.5 g%, serum creatinine—1.1 mg/dL, blood urea—16 mg/dL, random blood sugar (RBS)—121 mg/dL, human immunodeficiency virus (HIV), hepatitis B surface antigen (HBsAg), hepatitis C virus (HCV)—negative. Electrocardiogram (ECG) showed non-ST elevation myocardial infarction. 2D Echo—mild left ventricular (LV) dysfunction, ejection fraction (EF)—45%. Computed tomography (CT) aortogram showed mild atheromatous changes in the distal abdominal aorta. Coronary angiography (CAG)—right femoral artery approach—5 LMCA—distal 90% lesion, LAD—ostial total occlusion, left circumflex (LCX)—diffuse 60-70% lesion, obtuse marginal (OMs)—diffuse disease, right coronary artery (RCA)—proximal total occlusion, graft angio-LIMA to LAD—patent, distal graft 80% lesion. SVG to posterior descending artery (PDA)—mild lesion, SVG to RAMUS—proximal 90% in-stent restenosis (ISR), mid 70% ISR **(Fig. 2)**.

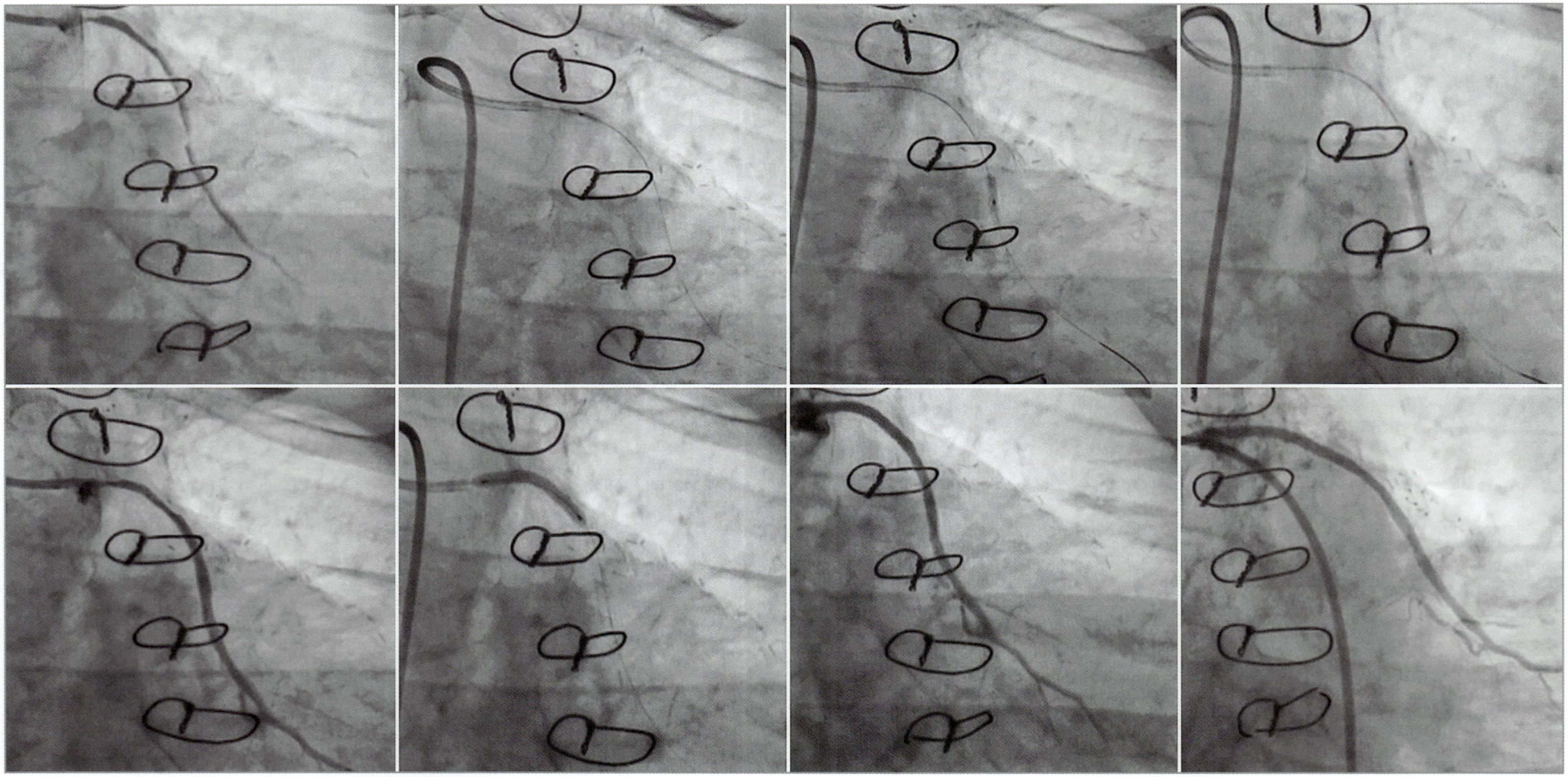

Fig. 1: Coronary angiogram and angioplasty of saphenous vein graft (SVG) to RAMUS.

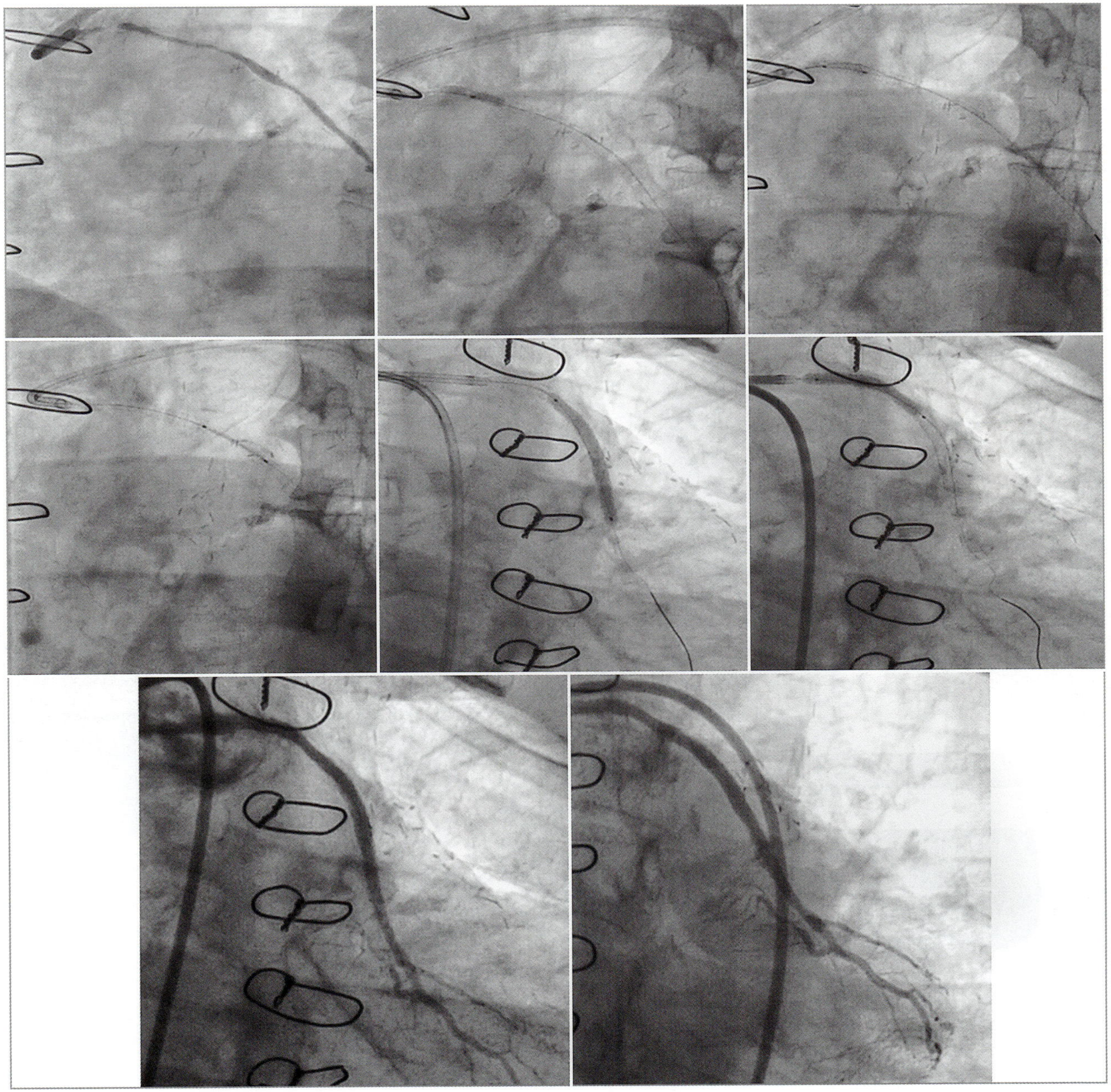

Fig. 2: 1 year later in-stent restenosis (ISR) in saphenous vein graft (SVG)–RAMUS stent and coronary angioplasty.

PROCEDURE

Procedure performed through right femoral artery using AR 2 guiding catheter, check angiogram revealed SVG to OM proximal 80–90% ISR, mid 70% ISR which was crossed with 0.014 × 190 cm" Sion blue wire, predilatation with 2.0 × 10 mm Tazuna balloon and 2.5 × 10 mm Scoreflex cutting balloon **(Fig. 2)**. Subsequently stented with 3.0 × 15 mm Orsiro stent (DES) and DEB inflation was done with 3.5 × 40 mm Magic touch balloon at 14 atm for 1 minute and redilatation done with same balloon up to 16 atm for 1 minute. Ostioproximal SVG graft DEB was done with 3.5 × 35 mm Magic Touch balloon up to 16 atm for 1 minute **(Fig. 2)**. Post-cutting OCT (optical coherence tomography) study showed well-expanded and apposed stent struts with no edge dissections and issue prolapse of 22% with minimal lumen area (MLA)—3.47 mm^2 **(Figs. 3A to C)**. Postprocedure angio view showed well-implanted stents with TIMI III (thrombolysis in myocardial infarction III) flow without any dissection **(Fig. 2)**.

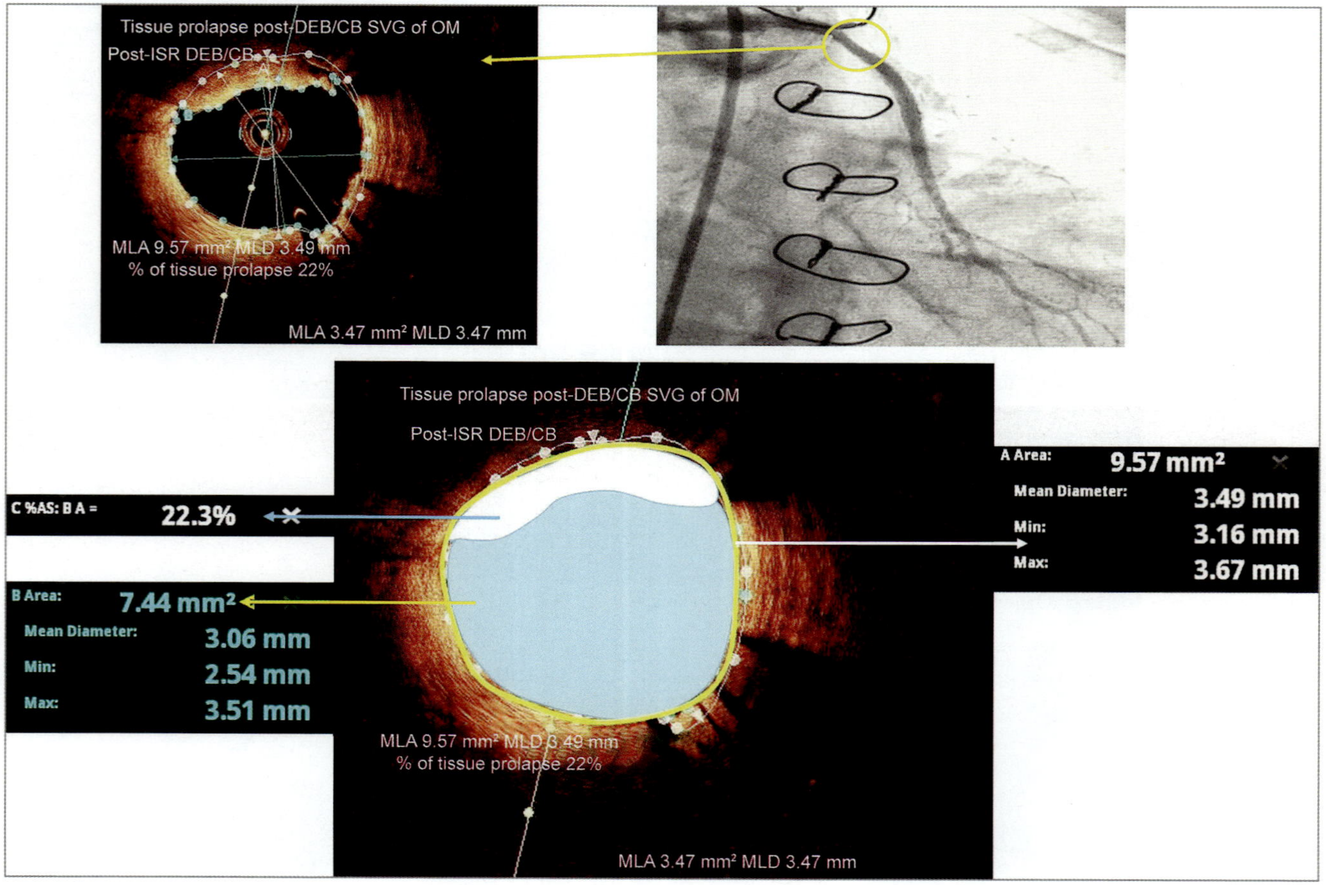

Fig. 3A

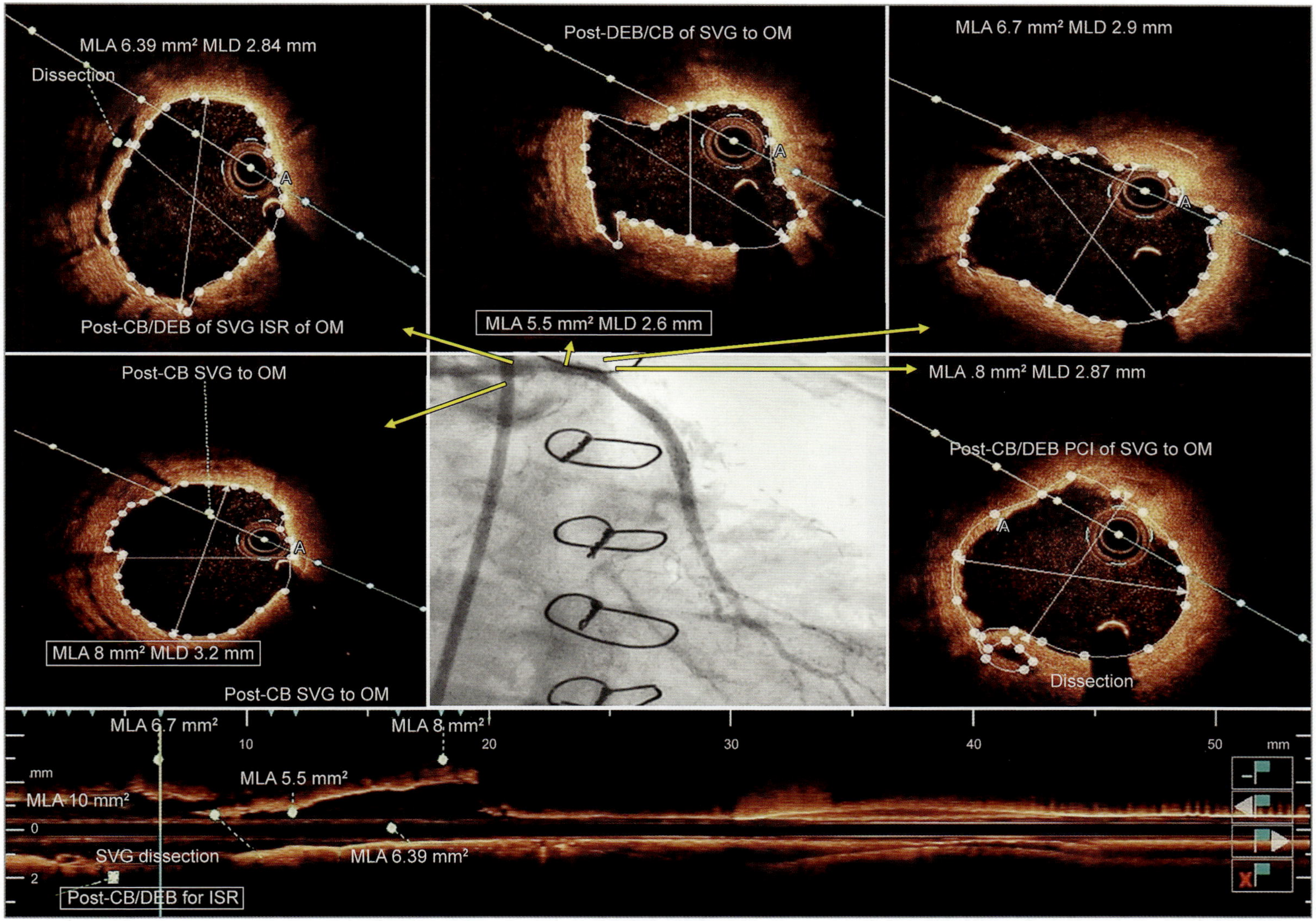
MLA 6.39 mm² MLD 2.84 mm
Dissection
Post-CB/DEB of SVG ISR of OM
Post-DEB/CB of SVG to OM
MLA 5.5 mm² MLD 2.6 mm
MLA 6.7 mm² MLD 2.9 mm
MLA .8 mm² MLD 2.87 mm
Post-CB SVG to OM
MLA 8 mm² MLD 3.2 mm
Post-CB SVG to OM
Post-CB/DEB PCI of SVG to OM
Dissection
MLA 6.7 mm²
MLA 8 mm²
MLA 5.5 mm²
MLA 10 mm²
SVG dissection
MLA 6.39 mm²
Post-CB/DEB for ISR
10
20
30
40
50
mm
0
2

Fig. 3B

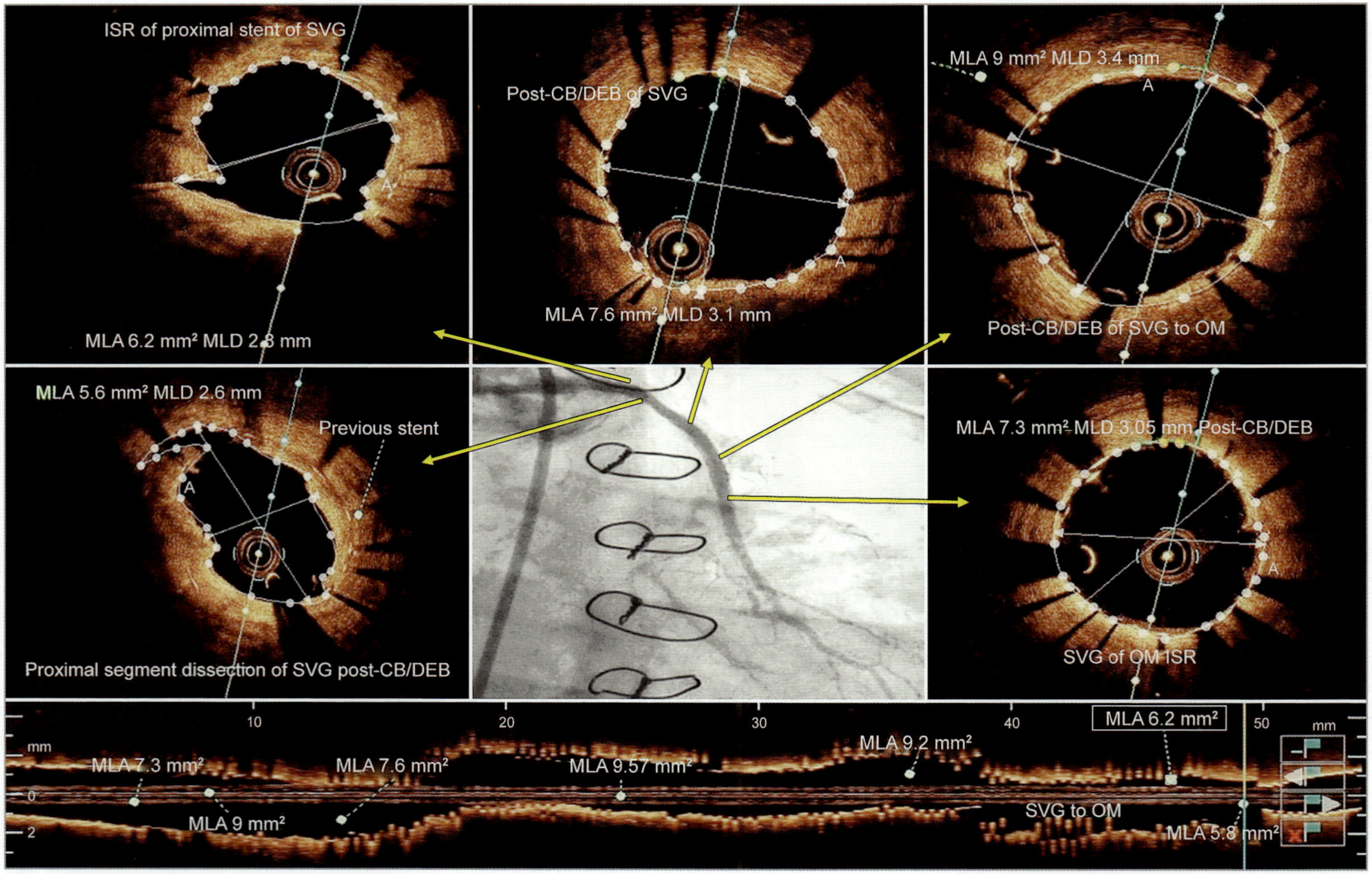

Fig. 3C

Figs. 3A to C: (A) Poststenting optical coherence tomography (OCT) showed tissue prolapse which is nonflow-limiting; (B) Poststenting OCT analysis of proximal portion; (C) Poststenting OCT analysis of distal segment. (CB: cutting balloon; DEB: drug-eluting balloon; ISR: in-stent restenosis; MLA: minimal lumen area; MLD: minimal lumen diameter; OM: obtuse marginal; PCI: percutaneous coronary intervention; SVG: saphenous vein graft)

CASE 2

Post CABG PCI of SVG.

CLINICAL HISTORY

A 55-year-old male, known diabetic with chronic kidney disease (CKD), underwent CABG in 2014, presented with coronary artery disease (CAD)—unstable angina, recent angina, and effort shortness of breath (SOB), 2D echo: RWMA+ (regional wall motion abnormality), moderate LV dysfunction with EF: 40%, severe mitral regurgitation (MR). CAG: CAD—native triple vessel disease, total occlusion of LIMA—D1 and RAMUS, patent right internal mammary artery (RIMA) to LAD, patent SVG to RCA, large posterolateral ventricular branch (PLVB) with 70% lesion. Investigations: Hb—9.3 g/dL, RBS—146 mg/dL, serum creatinine—1.25 mg/dL, estimated glomerular filtration rate (eGFR)—64 mL/min.

PROCEDURE

Saphenous vein graft to RCA engaged with Judkins right (JR) 3.5–7 Fr guiding catheter, distal RCA 90% lesion was crossed with 0.014 × 190 cm″ BMW wire.

Pre-stenting OCT showed fibrocalcific plaque in PLVB **(Figs. 4A and B)**.

Predilated with 2.5 × 10 mm Tazuna balloon, stented with 2.5 × 38 mm Resolute Onyx stent and postdilated with 3.0 × 15 mm NC Trek balloon **(Fig. 5)**.

Poststenting OCT was done which showed well-expanded and apposed stent struts with no edge dissections **(Figs. 6A and B)**.

The final result was good with TIMI III flow with no complications.

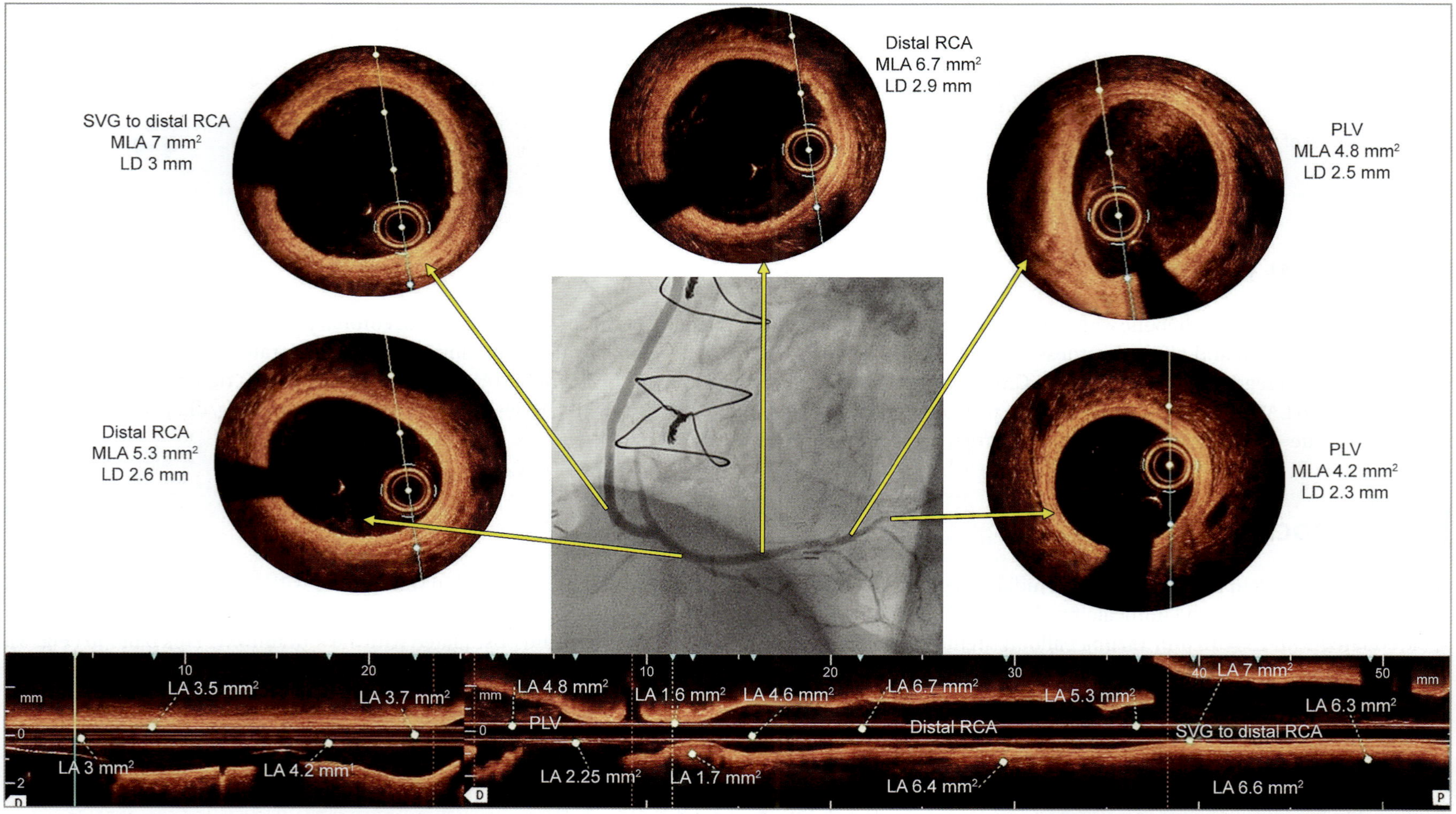
SVG to distal RCA
MLA 7 mm²
LD 3 mm
Distal RCA
MLA 6.7 mm²
LD 2.9 mm
PLV
MLA 4.8 mm²
LD 2.5 mm
Distal RCA
MLA 5.3 mm²
LD 2.6 mm
PLV
MLA 4.2 mm²
LD 2.3 mm
LA 3.5 mm²
LA 3.7 mm²
LA 3 mm²
LA 4.2 mm²
LA 4.8 mm²
PLV
LA 1.6 mm²
LA 4.6 mm²
LA 6.7 mm²
Distal RCA
LA 5.3 mm²
LA 7 mm²
LA 6.3 mm²
SVG to distal RCA
LA 2.25 mm²
LA 1.7 mm²
LA 6.4 mm²
LA 6.6 mm²

Fig. 4A

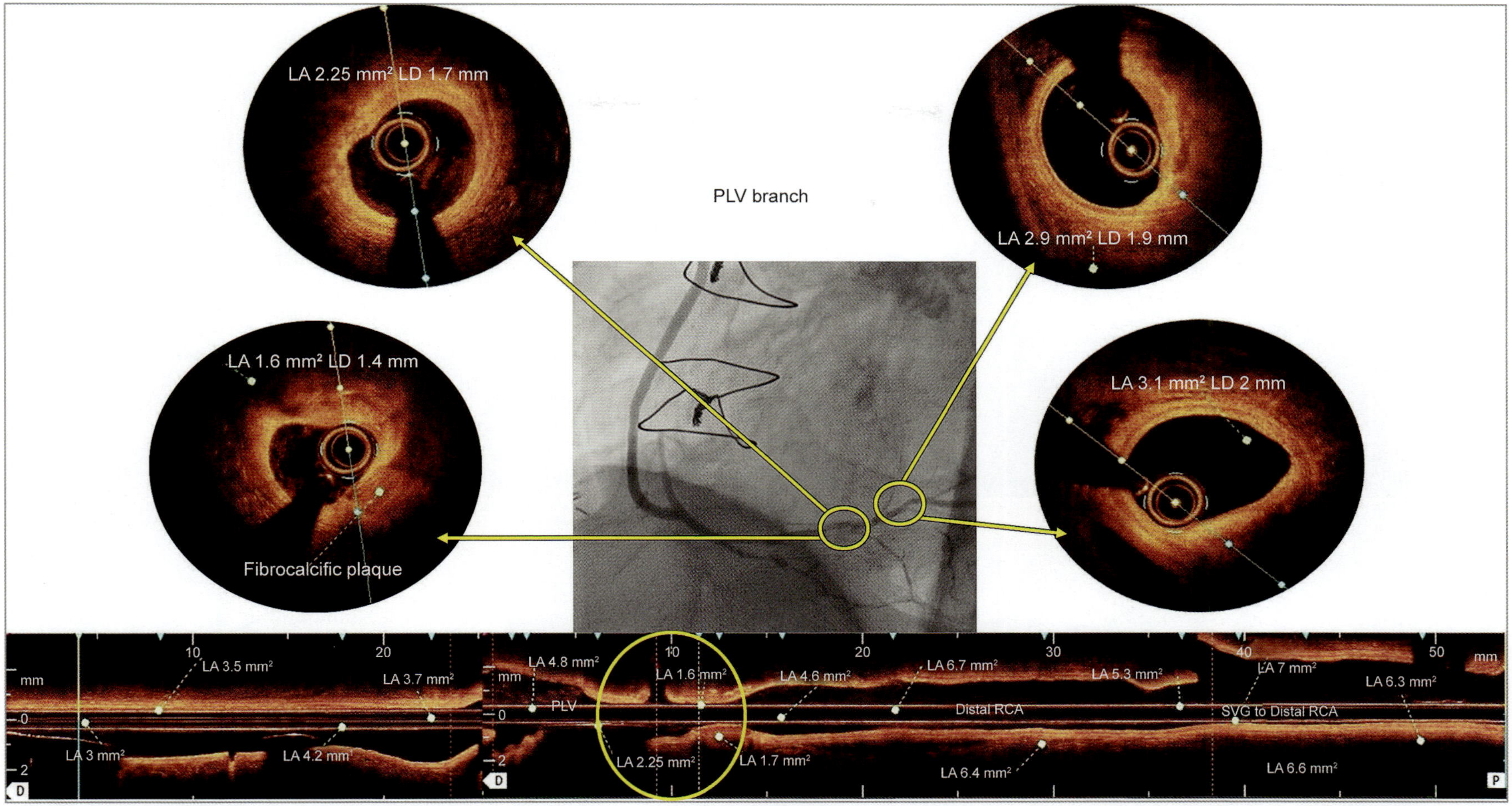

Fig. 4B

Figs. 4A and B: (A) Presenting optical coherence tomography (OCT) analysis for device selection; (B) Plaque morphology in posterolateral ventricular (PLV) branch by OCT. (LD: lumen diameter; MLA: minimal lumen area; SVG: saphenous vein graft; RCA: right coronary artery)

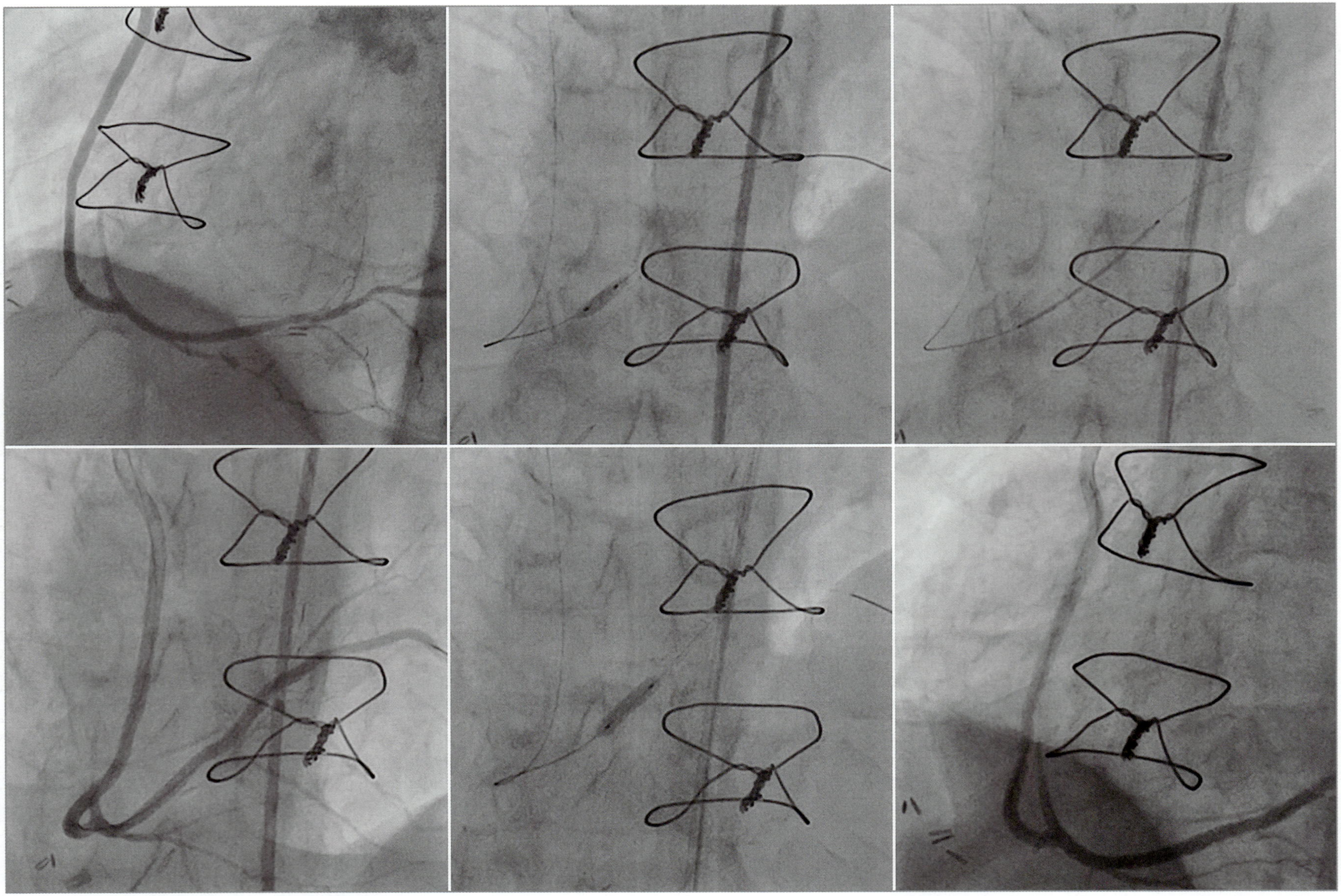

Fig. 5: Coronary angioplasty through saphenous vein graft (SVG) to right coronary artery (RCA)/posterolateral ventricular (PLV) branch.

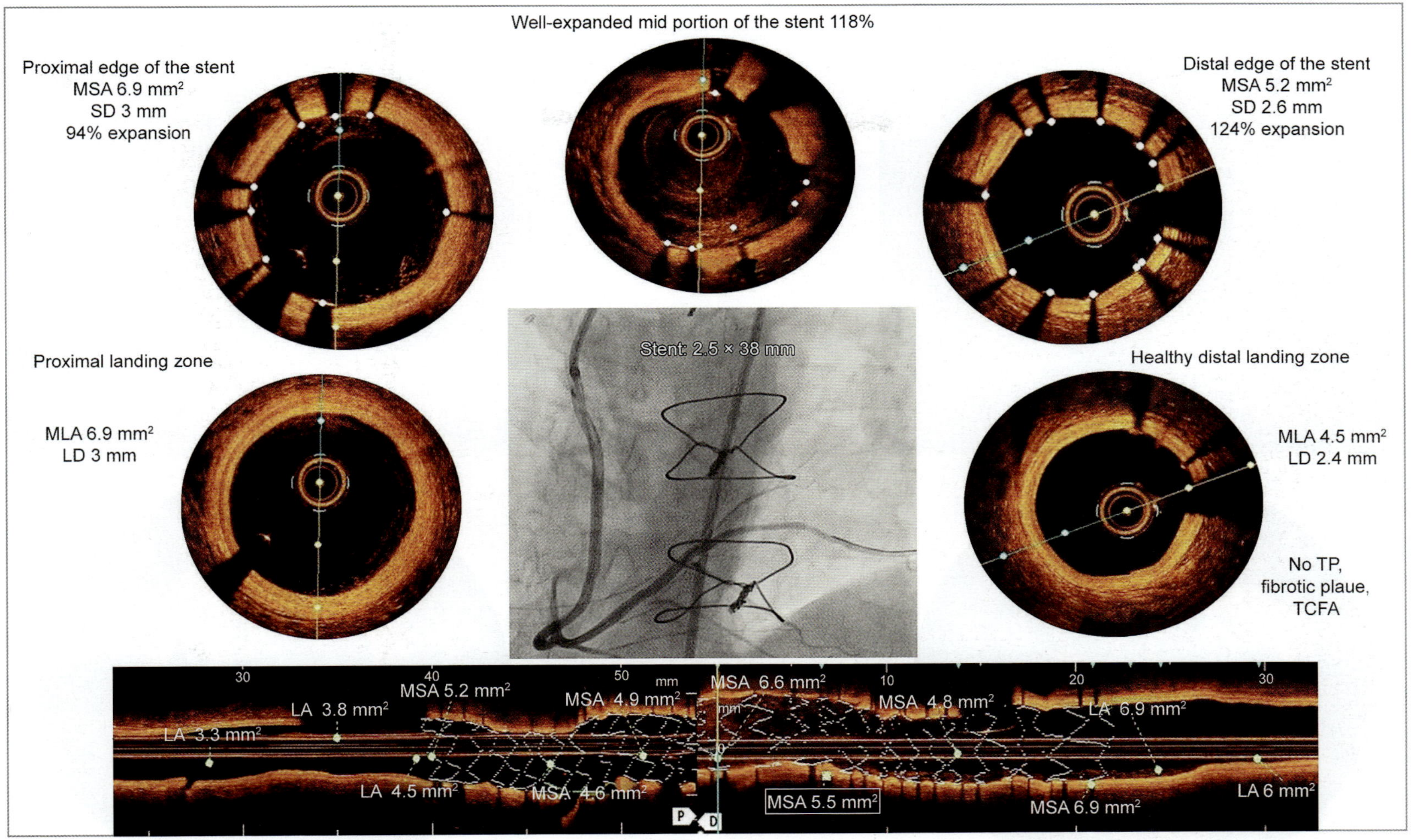

Well-expanded mid portion of the stent 118%
Proximal edge of the stent
MSA 6.9 mm²
SD 3 mm
94% expansion
Distal edge of the stent
MSA 5.2 mm²
SD 2.6 mm
124% expansion
Proximal landing zone
MLA 6.9 mm²
LD 3 mm
Stent: 2.5 × 38 mm
Healthy distal landing zone
MLA 4.5 mm²
LD 2.4 mm
No TP,
fibrotic plaue,
TCFA
MSA 5.2 mm²
LA 3.8 mm²
LA 3.3 mm²
MSA 4.9 mm²
MSA 6.6 mm²
MSA 4.8 mm²
LA 6.9 mm²
LA 4.5 mm²
MSA 4.6 mm²
MSA 5.5 mm²
MSA 6.9 mm²
LA 6 mm²

Fig. 6A

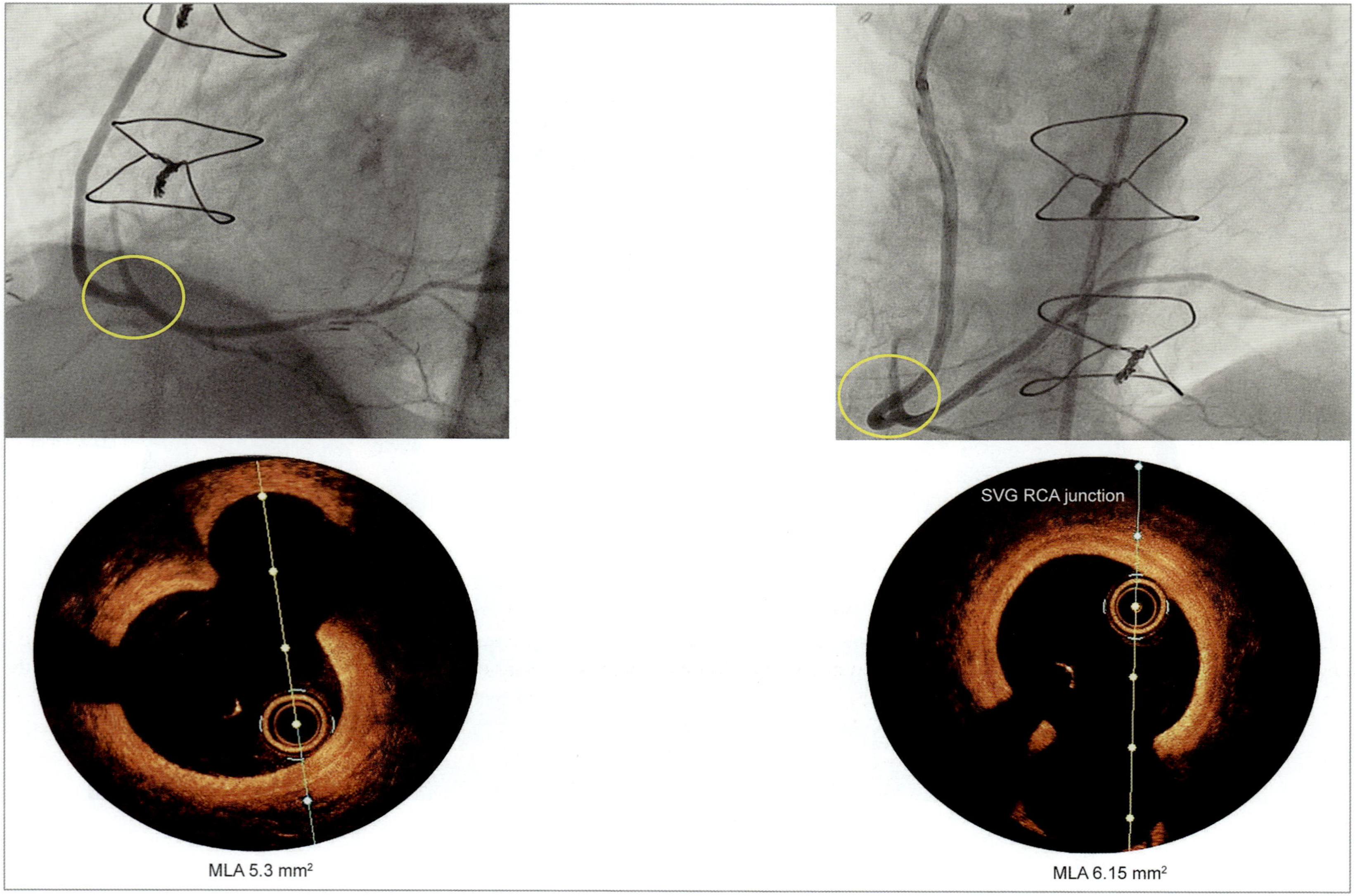

Fig. 6B

Figs. 6A and B: (A) Poststenting optical coherence tomography (OCT) analysis showed well-expanded and apposed stent struts with no medial edge dissection; (B) OCT (pre and post) assessment at anastomosis region. (LD: lumen diameter; MLA: minimal lumen area; MSA: minimal stent area; RCA: right coronary artery; SD: stent diameter; SVG: saphenous vein graft; TCFA: thin-cap fibroatheroma; TP: tissue prolapse)

CHAPTER 26

Optical Coherence Tomography Assessment of Intramural Hematoma during Left Main Percutaneous Coronary Intervention

INTRODUCTION

Intramural hematoma (IMH) is defined as an accumulation of blood within the medial space, displacing the internal elastic membrane inward and the external elastic membrane outward with or without identifiable entry and exit points [American College of Cardiology (ACC) Task Force on Clinical Expert Consensus Documents report].[1] The incidence of IMH after percutaneous coronary intervention (PCI) was 6.7% and these are associated with a dissection into the media with extension into the medial space of contiguous normal arterial segments where blood accumulated because of a lack of reentry and hematoma formation and expansion seem to require a normal segment or arc of arterial wall. Because the "diseased" media is more scarred, it may prevent propagation of the medial dissection. IMH commonly occurs in de novo lesions and diabetics and tendency develops in patients with less advanced coronary artery disease (CAD). During PCI, usual location of dissection is at the junction of the thinnest plaque and adjacent normal arterial wall. Similarly, after stent implantation, dissection occurs at the edge of a stent that is the transition point between the rigid stent and unstented reference segment.[2] It is associated with increased acute [non-Q-wave myocardial infarction (MI) and need for repeat revascularization within 1 month] and long-term events (death and need for repeat revascularization at 1 year). Although there is no clear consensus on management of multivessel IMH, the key principal of reestablishing coronary flow in the setting of ongoing ischemia to establish coronary flow as early as possible to mitigate symptoms and signs of ischemia. We are highlighting the importance of usefulness of optical coherence tomography (OCT) during PCI with case-based examples with useful tips and tricks to manage such cases in day-to-day clinical practice.

CASE 1

OCT-guided stenting of triple vessel disease.

CLINICAL HISTORY

A 64-year-old male, a known diabetic and hypertensive, presented with exertional breathlessness of Class 2–3 with recent worsening for 5 months and he was referred for further management of CAD—triple vessel disease (TVD).

Investigations: Electrocardiography (ECG) showed normal sinus rhythm, first-degree arteroventricular block, two-dimensional (2D) echo showed no regional wall motion abnormality (RWMA), ejection fraction (EF) 60%, serum creatinine (S Cr) 1.1 mg/dL, estimated glomerular filtration rate (eGFR) 81 mL/min/1.73 m^2, and hemoglobin (Hb) 12 gm% **(Figs. 1A to D)**.

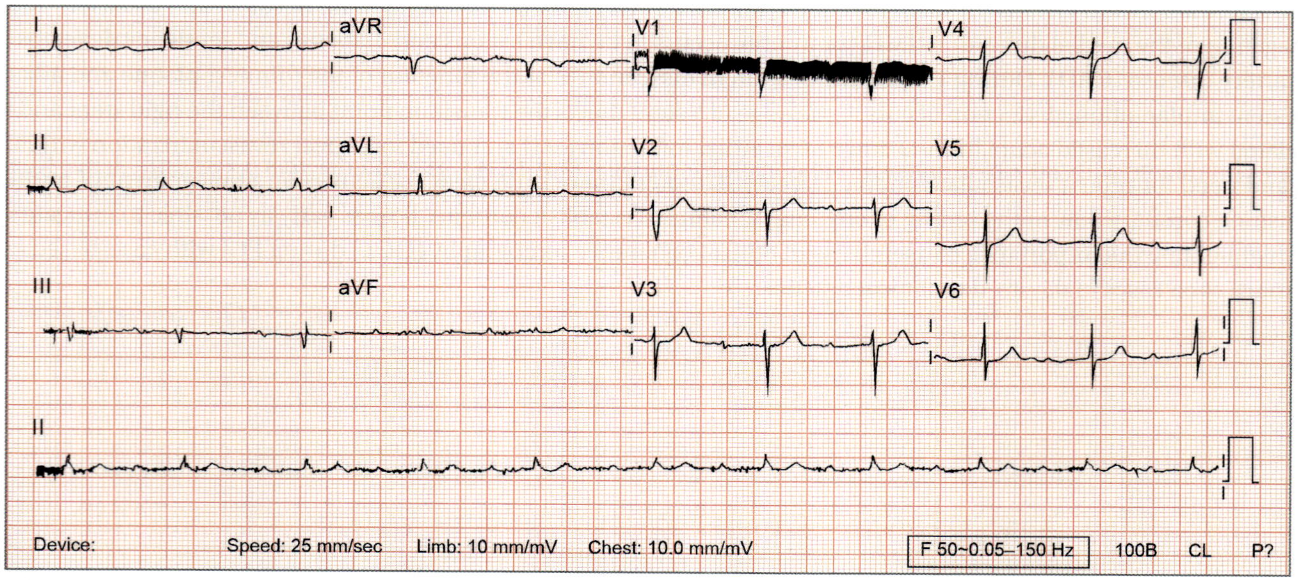

Fig. 1A

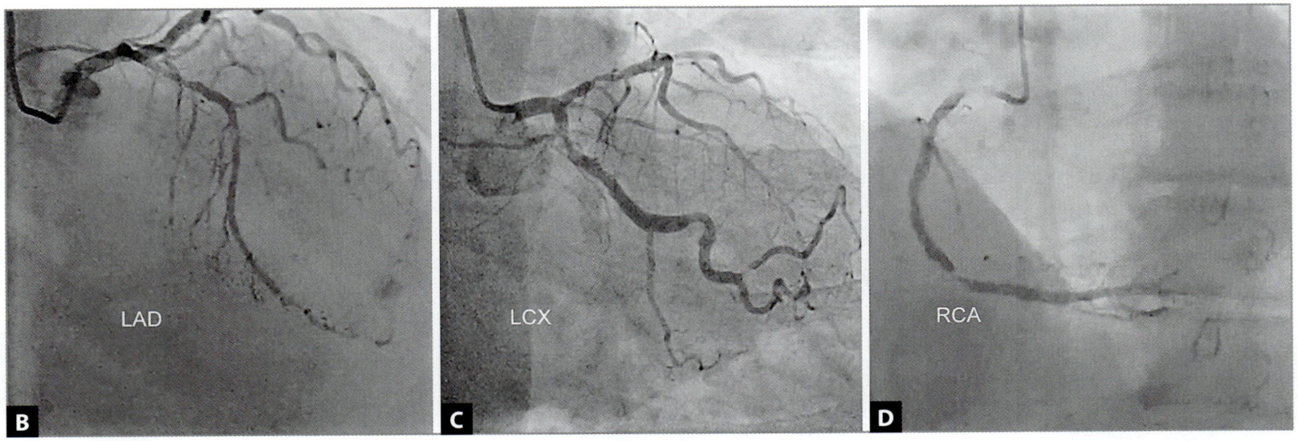

Figs. 1B to D

Figs. 1A to D: (A) ECG, CAG; (B) LAD; (C) LCX; (D) RCA. (ECG: electrocardiography; CAG: coronary angiography; LAD: left anterior descending; LCX: left circumflex; RCA: right coronary artery)

PROCEDURE

After obtaining informed consent, multivessel PCI was planned due to peak coronavirus disease 2019 (COVID-19) pandemic and nonavailability of surgical staff and surgical intensive care beds. Initially, PCI of right coronary artery (RCA) was done using 7 Fr Judkin's right (JR) guide and wired with Runthrough, lesion was predilated with 2.0 × 10 mm Ryurei balloon. Subsequently, mid-RCA was stented with 3.5 × 33 mm Xience Xpedition and proximal RCA was stented with 3.5 × 38 mm Xience Xpedition with 2–3 mm overlap of both stents. Later, distal stent was postdilated with 4.0 × 15 mm and proximal stent was dilated with 4.5 × 15 mm noncompliant (NC) balloons. Poststent angio views showed excellent end result without any complications.

Percutaneous coronary intervention of left main coronary artery (LMCA) to left artery descending (LAD) and left circumflex (LCX)—LMCA was engaged with 7 Fr EBU guide and LAD was wired with 0.14 BMW wire. Preprocedure OCT run showed fibrocalcific long-segment disease of the ostioproximal and mid-LAD **(Figs. 2 and 3)**.

Initially, proximal- and mid-LAD segments were dilated with 2.0 × 10 mm Tazuna balloon. Subsequently, it was dilated with 2.5 × 15 mm OPN NC balloon inflations at 35 atm due to unyielding proximal LAD lesion with Tazuna balloon. Post-OPN NC check angio showed contrast staining at the ostium of the LAD, which was possibly due to dissection of ostioproximal LAD with IMH extension to LCX **(Fig. 4)**.

Subsequently, mid-LAD was stented with 2.75 × 38 mm Xience Xpedition and LCX was wired with 0.014″ Runthrough wire before stenting of LMCA—LAD segment with 3.5 × 38 mm Xience Xpedition stent and proximal optimization technique (POT) of LMCA was performed with 4.5 × 08 mm NC Trek balloon, postdilatation of LAD stent was done with 3.0 × 12 mm NC Trek balloon. Later, LCX was recrossed with Fielder FC wire through stent struts **(Fig. 4)**. Poststenting study of OCT of LAD showed well-expanded and well-apposed stent struts with no medial edge dissections **(Fig. 5)**.

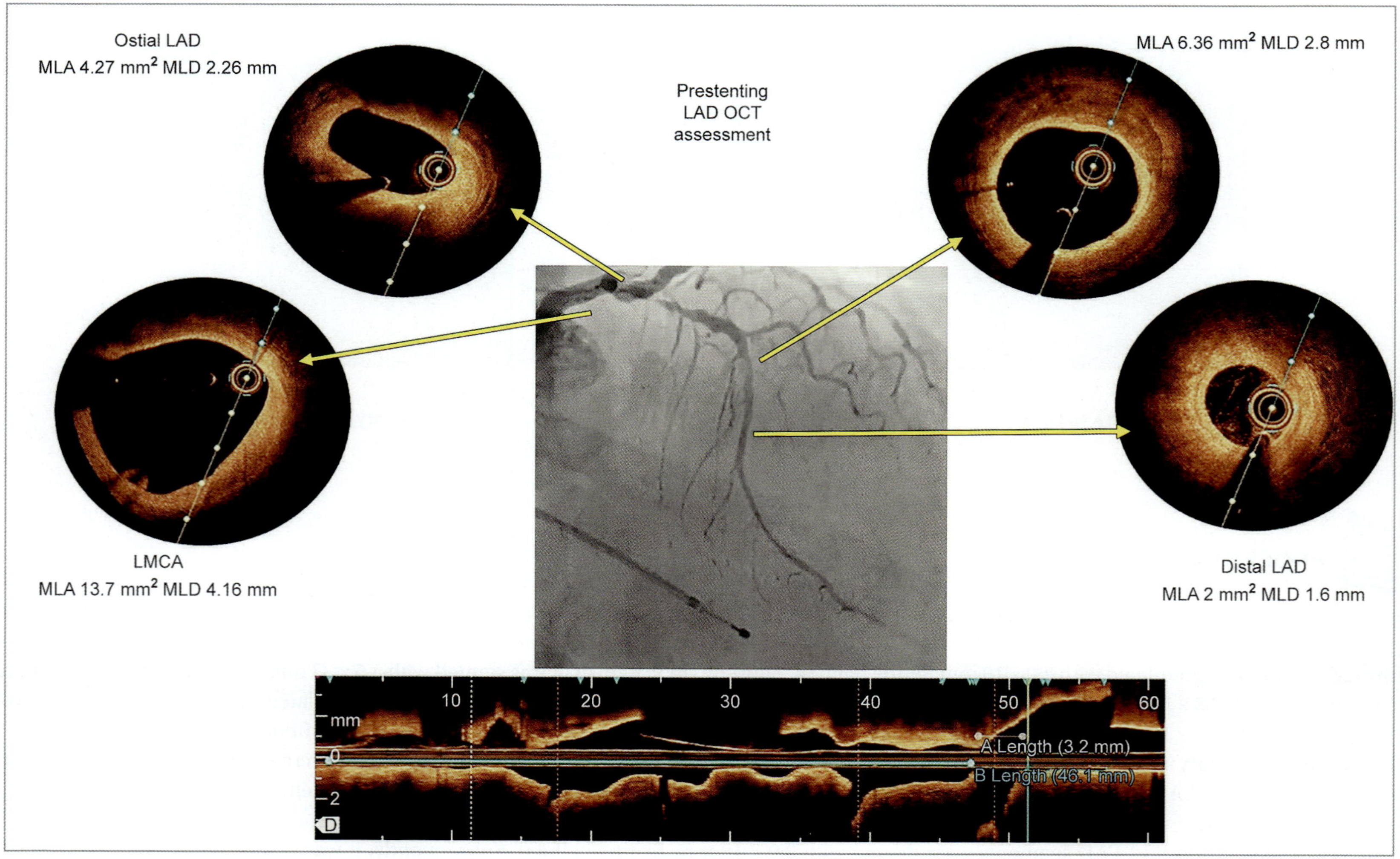

Fig. 2: Prestenting LAD OCT assessment. (LAD: left anterior descending; LMCA: left main coronary artery; MLA: minimal lumen area; MLD: minimal lumen diameter; OCT: optical coherence tomography)

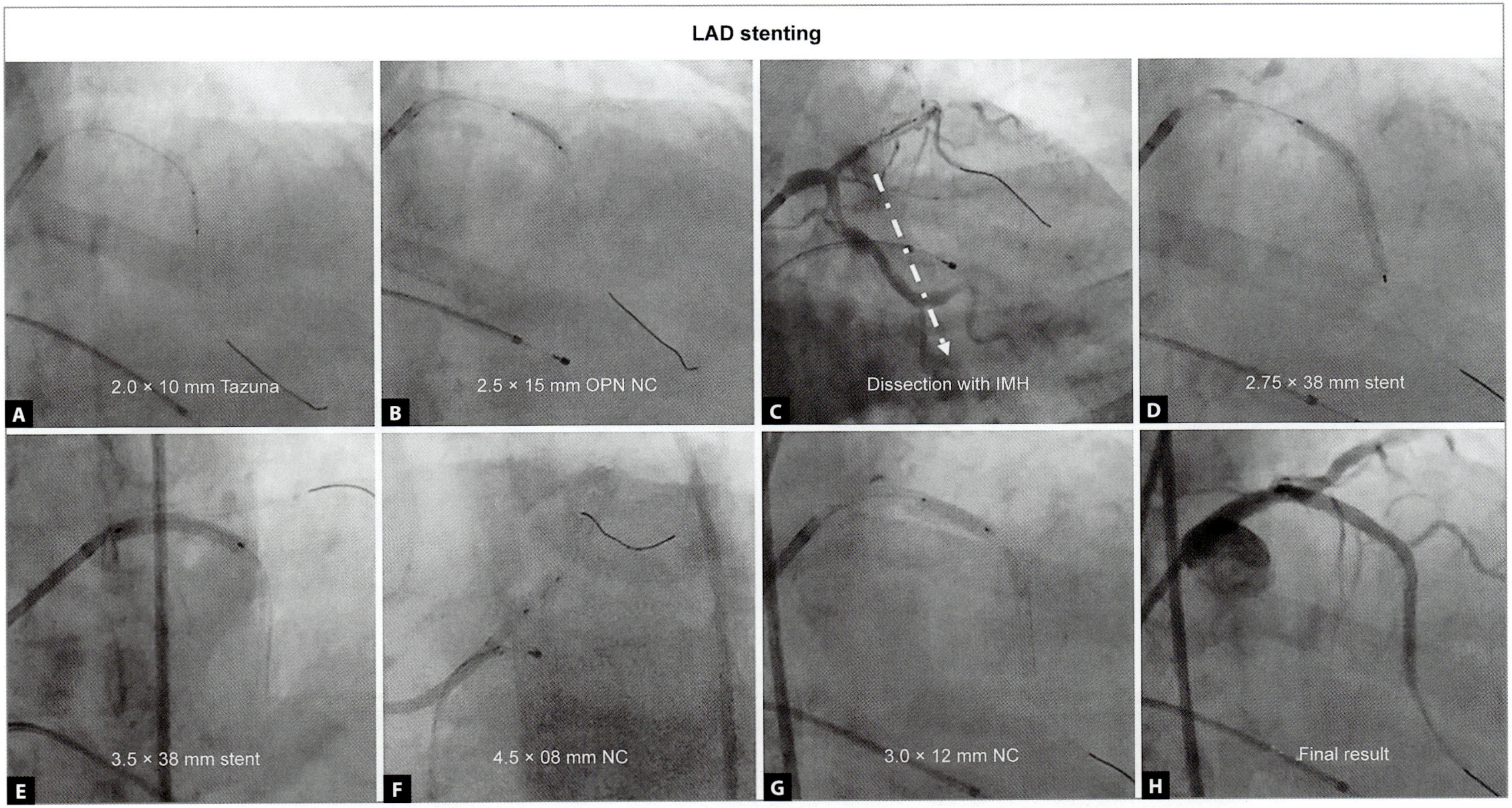

Figs. 3A to H: Angioplasty of LAD. (IMH: intramural hematoma; LAD: left anterior descending; NC: noncompliant)

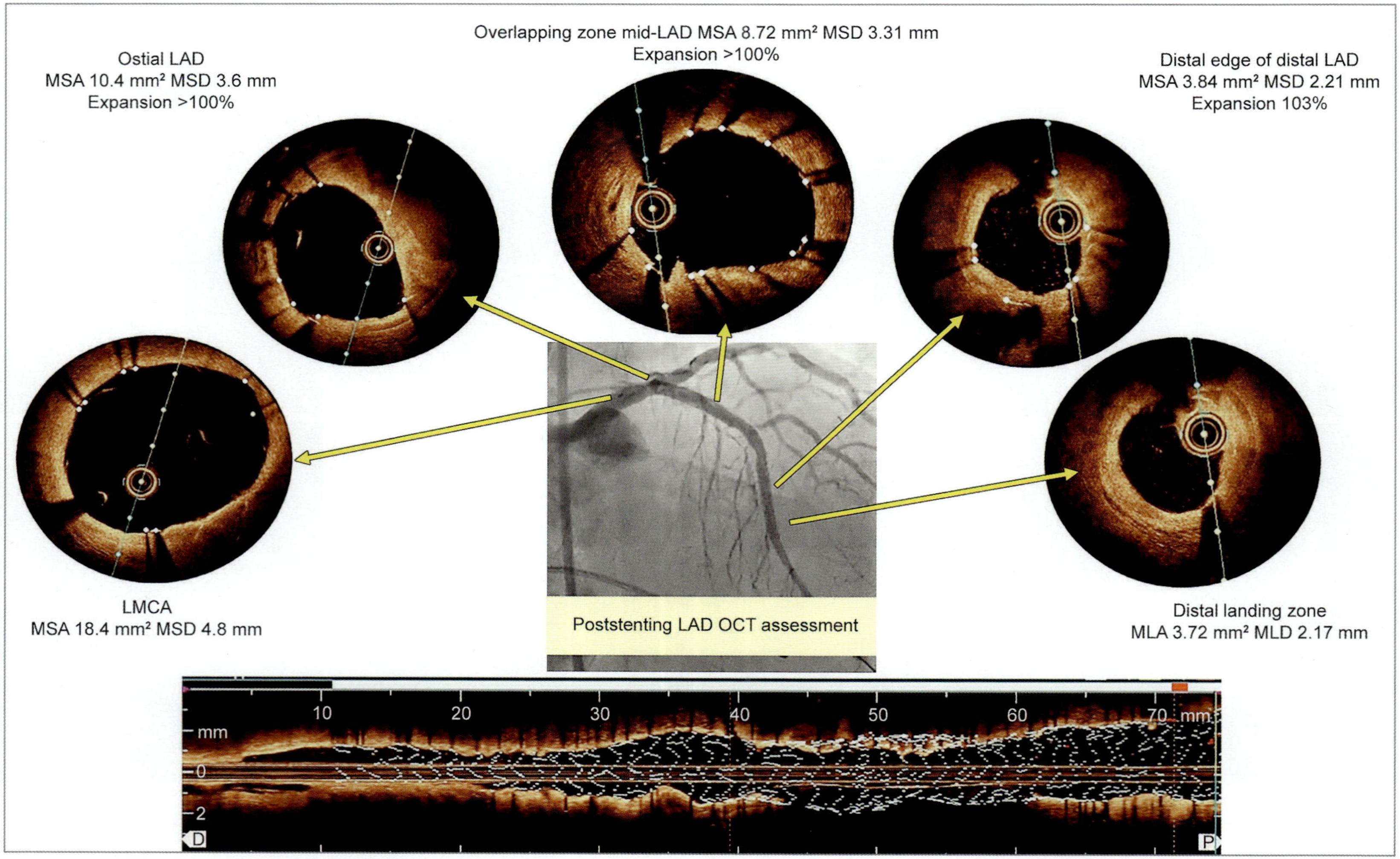

Fig. 4: Poststenting LAD OCT assessment. (LAD: left anterior descending; LMCA: left main coronary artery; MLA: minimal lumen area; MLD: minimal lumen diameter; MSA: minimal stent area; MSD: minimal stent diameter; OCT: optical coherence tomography)

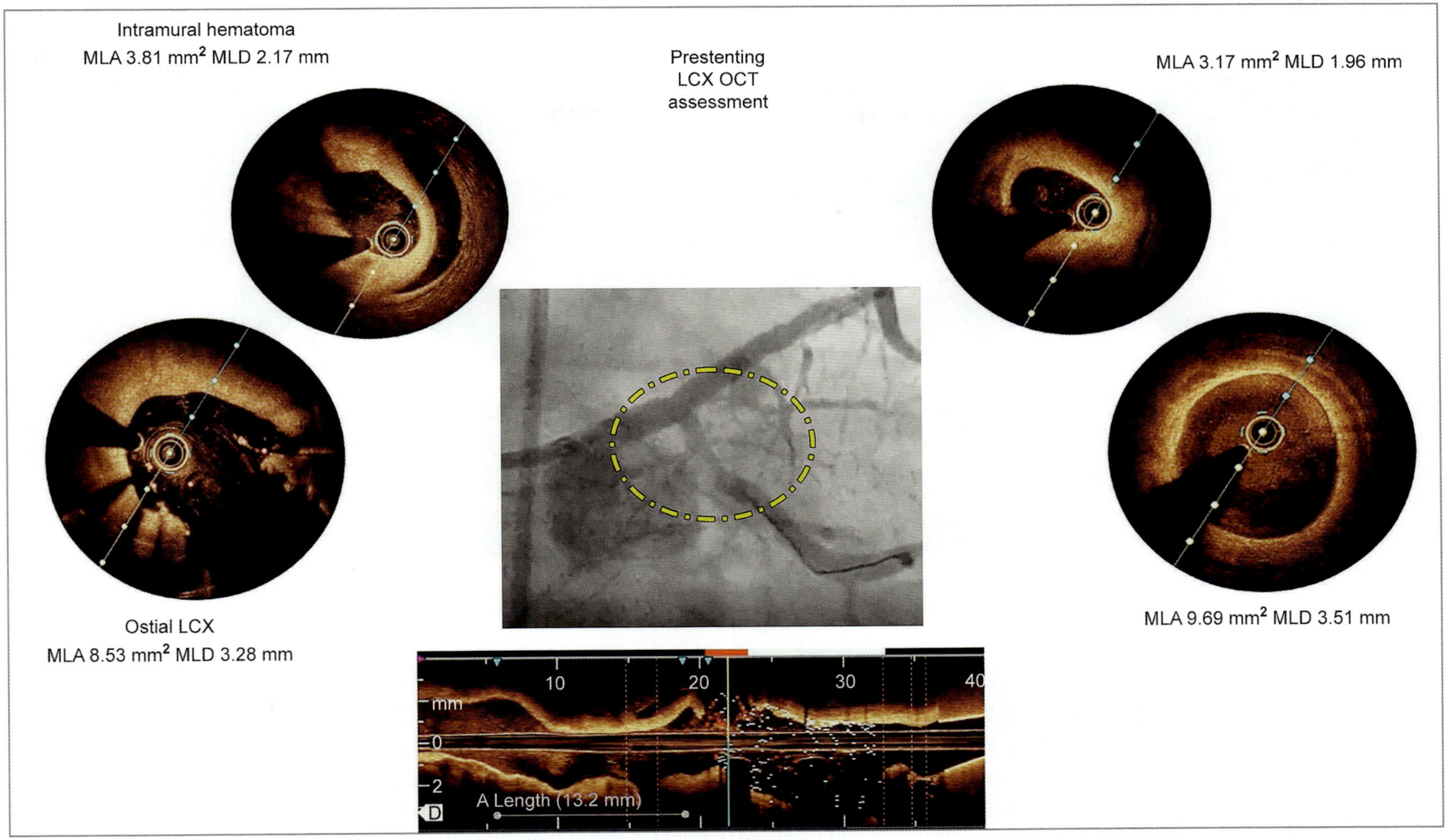

Fig. 5: Prestenting LCX OCT assessment. (LCX: left circumflex; MLA: minimal lumen area; MLD: minimal lumen diameter; OCT: optical coherence tomography)

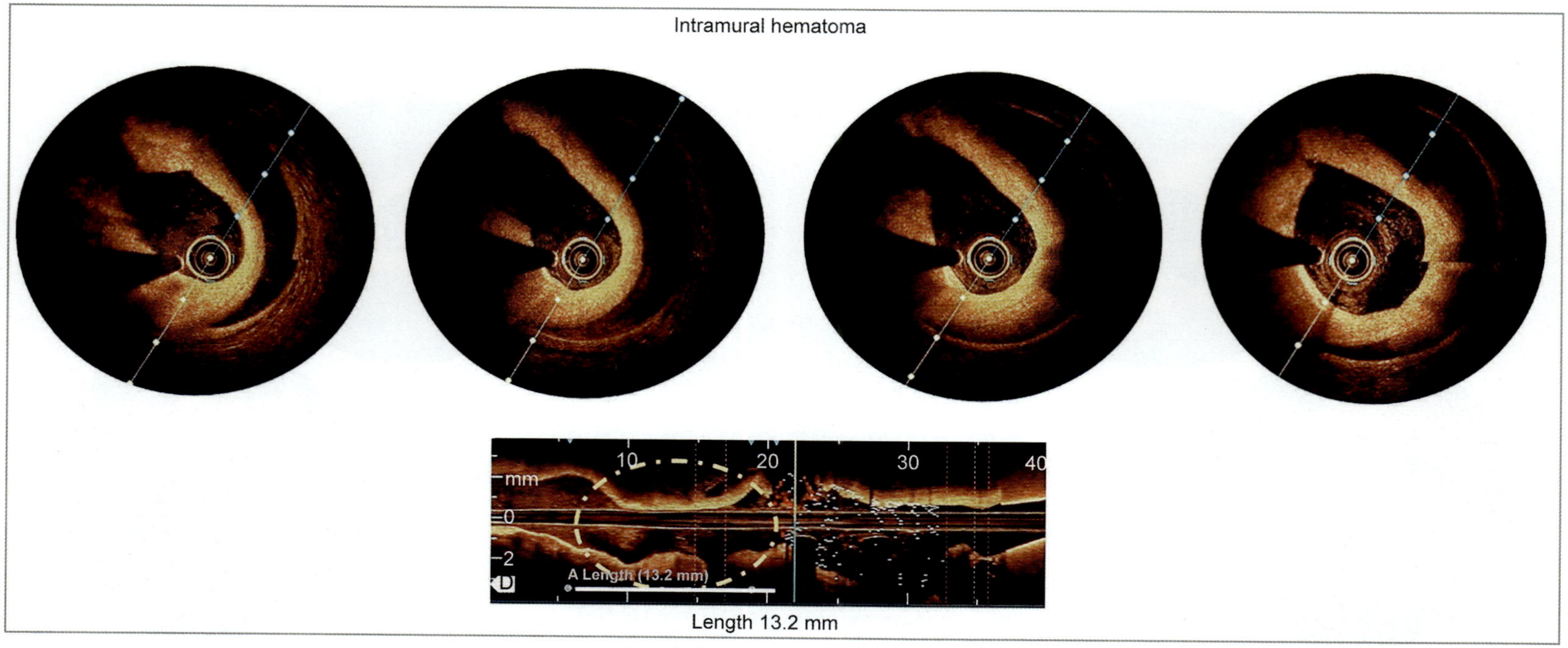

Fig. 6: Intramural hematoma in left main coronary artery (LMCA).

But OCT run of LCX showed fibrous plaque in proximal LCX with extension of IMH compromising luminal area of ostioproximal LCX **(Figs. 6 and 7)** and stent struts across the ostium of LCX opened with 3.0 × 12 mm NC Trek balloon **(Figs. 8A to H)**.

Then, LCX stenting was done by 3.5 × 23 mm Xience Xpedition (T-TAP technique) by using Guideliner support. Final kissing balloon (FKB) of LM was done with 3.0 × 12 mm NC Trek balloon in LAD and 3.5 × 23 mm stent balloon in LCX, re-POT of LM was done with 4.5 × 08 mm NC Trek balloon. Post-FKB angio showed decreased flow of major obtuse marginal (OM) possibly due to spasm/dissection and it was dilated with 1.5 × 10 mm and 2.0 × 10 mm Tazuna balloon to improve antegrade flow of LCX, which resulted in slight increase in the LCX distal flow. Next day, check angio showed markedly improved OM flow and well-patent stents **(Figs. 9A to D)**.

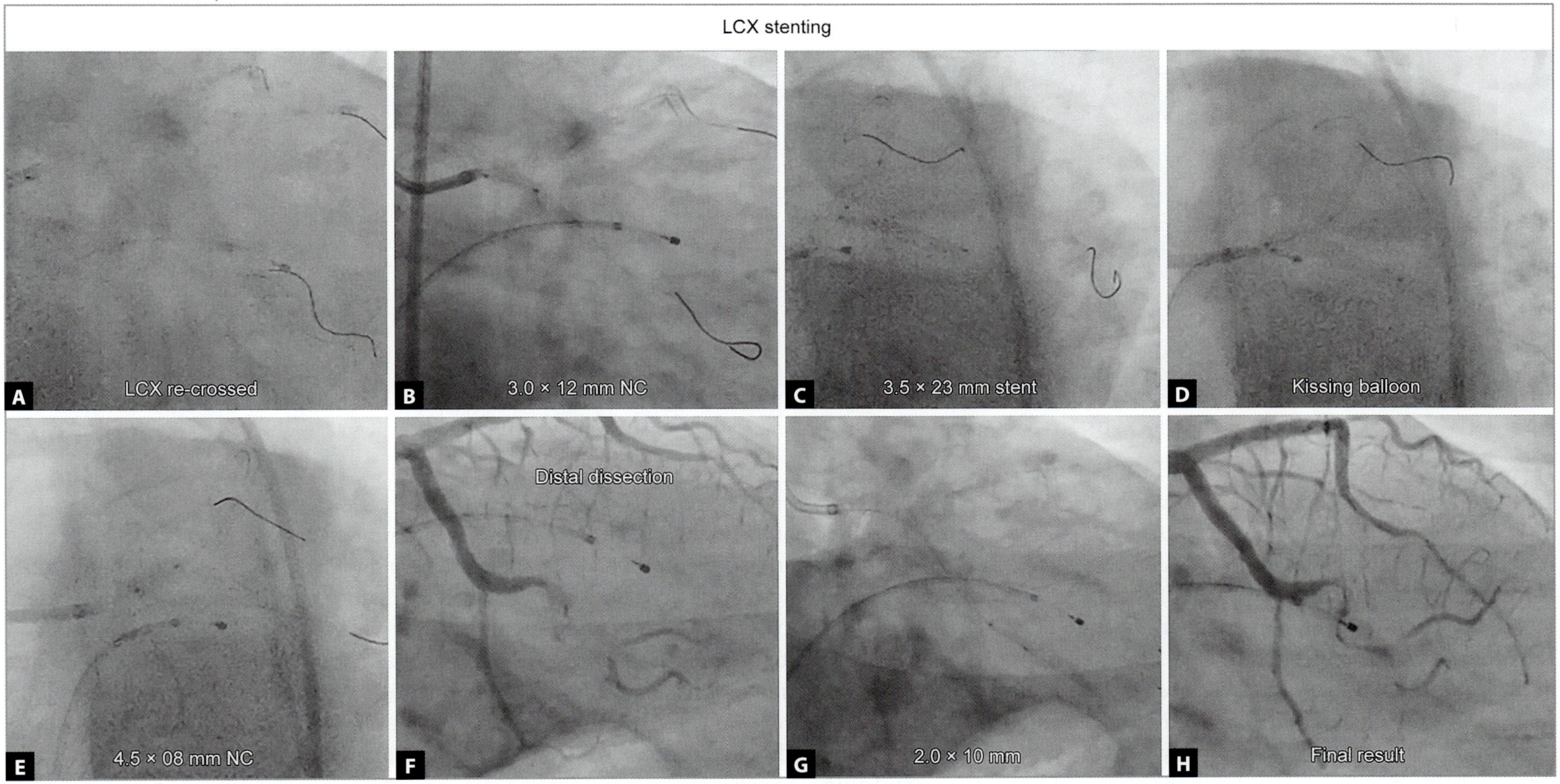

Figs. 8A to H: Angioplasty of left circumflex (LCX). (NC: noncompliant)

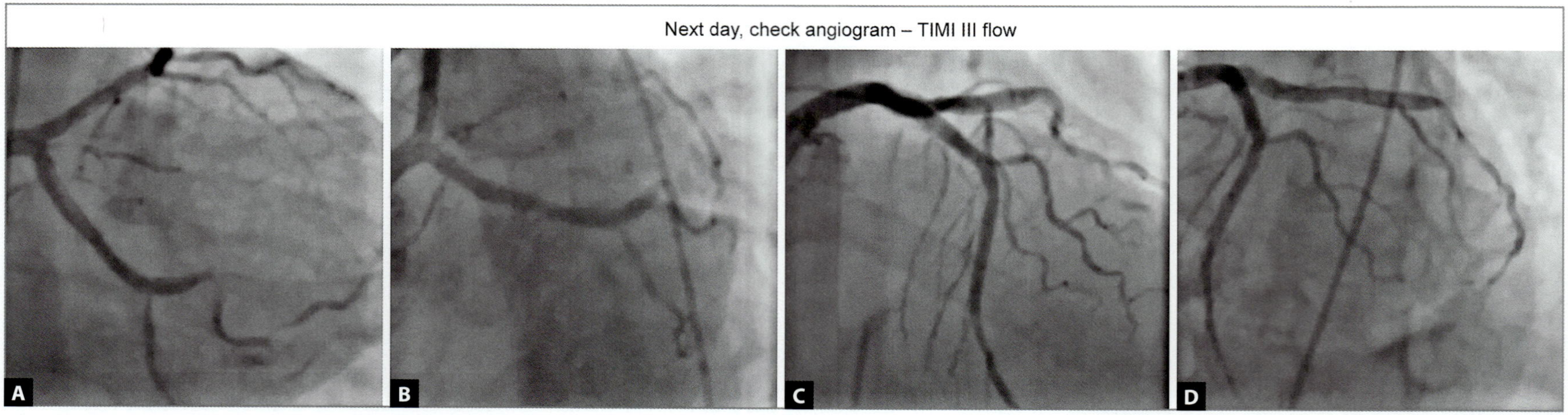

Figs. 9A to D: Next day, check angiogram—thrombolysis in myocardial infarction III (TIMI III) flow.

Sometimes, PCI of moderate-to-severe fibrocalcific lesion with high-pressure balloon inflations of NC/OPN NC balloons might lead to dissection with IMH extension either proximally or distally. During PCI procedure, if any of the following findings is observed, immediate steps for additional stenting or relief of intramural hematoma tension by evacuating it with cutting/scoring balloon dilatations are to be considered: (1) Flow-limiting dissections/IMH with decreased coronary flow, (2) symptoms and signs of ongoing ischemia, (3) evidence of ischemia on ECG, and (4) compromised luminal areas on intravascular imaging. Careful attention should be paid to early identification and rectification of these issues while applying high-pressure balloon inflations prior to stenting and these could be minimized by scoring/cutting balloons which would reduce chances of development and spreading of dissections/IMH by making controlled dissections of severely fibrocalcific lesions. Pre-PCI plaque modification with adequately sized rotablation (ROTA)/orbital atherectomy (OA)/intravascular lithotripsy (IVL) devices is useful when lesions are not yielding even with cutting or scoring balloons. Angiographically hazy lesions are very difficult to diagnose and it may be due to dissection/IMH/thrombus/calcific lesion/reanalyzed thrombus. OCT imaging helps in differentiating various causes of hazy lesions and guides in selecting appropriate PCI strategies. This case illustrates extension of IMH from ostioproximal LAD dissection to distal LM and ostioproximal segment of LCX which was managed with additional stenting to cover IMH with compromised luminal area of LCX with ischemic symptoms.

CASE 2

Intramural hematoma of left main (LM).

CLINICAL HISTORY

A 63-year-old male, a known hypertensive with complaints of classical effort angina with positive treadmill test (TMT) for inducible ischemia admitted for evaluation and further management of CAD—stable ischemic heart disease (SIHD).

Investigations: 2D echo—no RWMA with good left ventricular (LV) function, EF 60%, Hb 13.4 g/dL, random blood sugar (RBS) 126 mg/dL, S Cr 0.79 mg/dL, eGFR 96 mL/min. Coronary angiography (CAG)-LMCA—normal, LAD—proximal 70% lesion, LCX—normal, RCA—mid-total occlusion.

Percutaneous coronary intervention of RCA—it was engaged with AL1 6 Fr guiding catheter and lesion was crossed with 0.014″ Fielder XT wire using fine cross microcatheter support, which was exchanged with 0.014″ BMW wire. RCA lesion was predilated with 2.0 × 15 mm Tazuna and OCT run was obtained to assess morphology, length, and diameter (MLD) medial edge dissection, apposition, and expansion (MAX). Morphology showed long-segment lesion with fibrolipid with areas of fibrocalcific plaque, lesion length was 33 mm, distal external elastic luminal diameter (EELD) was 3.6 × 3.8 mm, proximal EELD 3.6 × 3.7 mm, and device selected was 3 × 38 mm stent. Proximal-to-mid RCA stenting was done with 3.0 × 38 mm Resolute Onyx stent and postdilated with 3.5 × 12 mm NC Trek balloon. Post-OCT showed well-expanded and apposed stent struts with no medial distal edge dissection. Poststenting angio showed uncovered ostioproximal portion of RCA which was covered with 3.5 × 08 mm Resolute Onyx and postdilated with 3.5 × 12 mm NC. Final result was good with thrombolysis in myocardial infarction III (TIMI III) flow.

PROCEDURE

Percutaneous coronary intervention of LAD—LMCA was engaged with EBU 3.5–6 Fr guiding catheter, LAD lesion was crossed with 0.014″ Sion Blue wire. Pre-PCI OCT run showed lipid-rich plaque—180° arc with macrophages and fibrous plaque with cholesterol crystals and occasional areas showing fibrous plaque with calcific plaque of <90° **(Fig. 10)**. Lesion length 42 mm, diameter—proximal EELD 3.5 mm and distal EELD 3.4 × 2.9 mm **(Fig. 11)**.

Proximal stenting done with 3.5 × 30 mm Resolute Onyx stent just sparing the ostium of the LAD, distal LAD stenting was done with 3.0 × 15 mm Resolute Onyx and postdilated with 3.5 × 12 mm NC Trek balloon **(Fig. 12)**. Poststent angio views showed mild haziness with mild narrowing distal LM and ostium of LAD stent. OCT was done for optimization of PCI and need for extension of additional stent to LM to LAD, it showed well-expanded and apposed stent struts with no distal edge dissection **(Fig. 13)**, but small proximal edge dissection with IMH of ostium of LAD extending to distal LM **(Figs. 14 and 15)**.

In view of well-expanded stent with good luminal area and no significant compromise of distal LM and ostial LAD, it was treated conservatively without any additional stenting of LM. Final result was good with TIMI III flow.

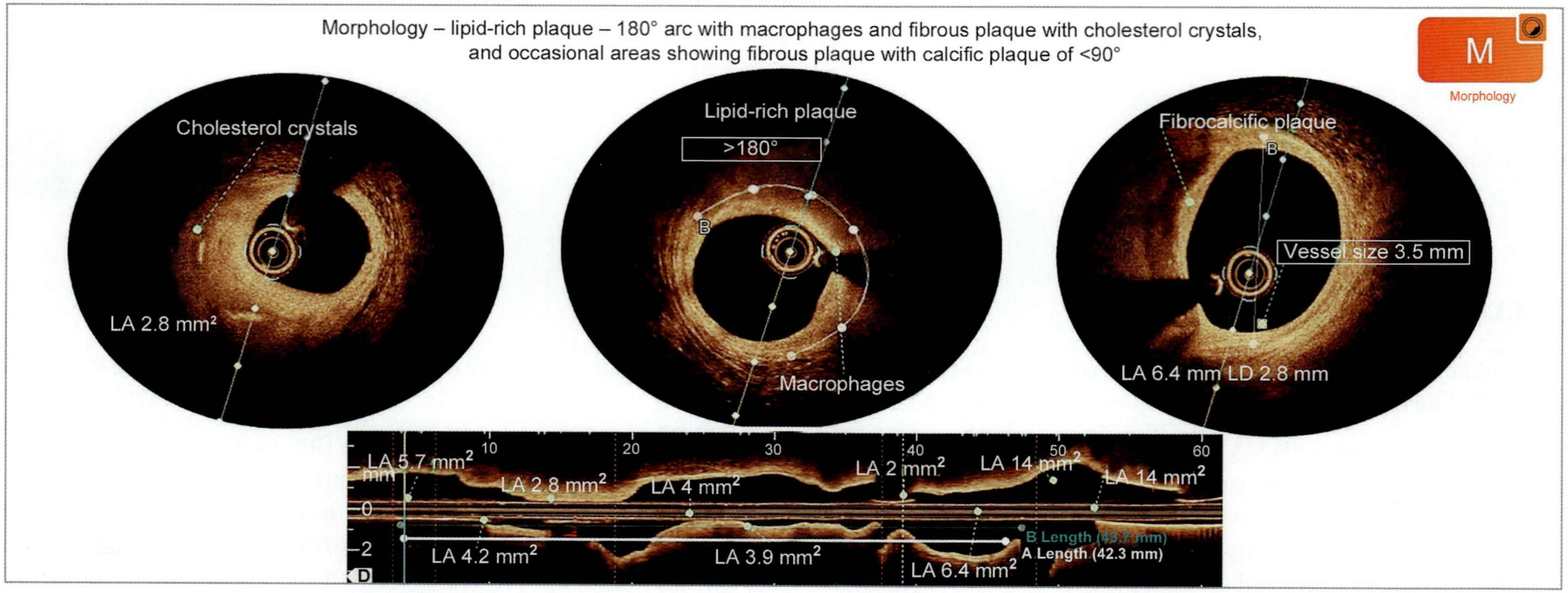

Fig. 10: OCT assessment for MLD. (LA: lumen area; LAD: left anterior descending; MLA: minimal lumen area; LD: lumen diameter; MLD: morphology, length, and diameter; OCT: optical coherence tomography)

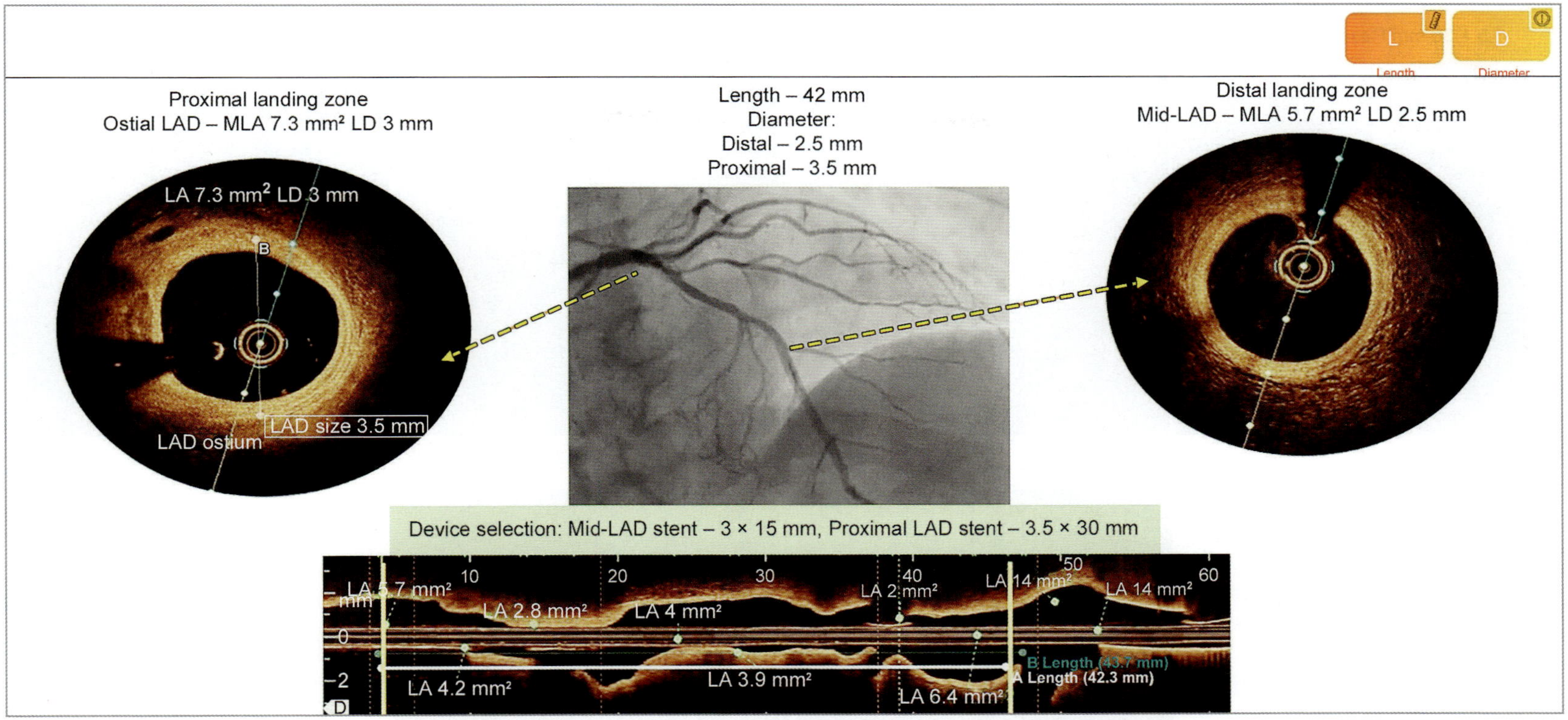

Fig. 11: OCT assessment for MLD. (LA: lumen area; LAD: left anterior descending; MLA: minimal lumen area; LD: lumen diameter; MLD: morphology, length, and diameter; OCT: optical coherence tomography)

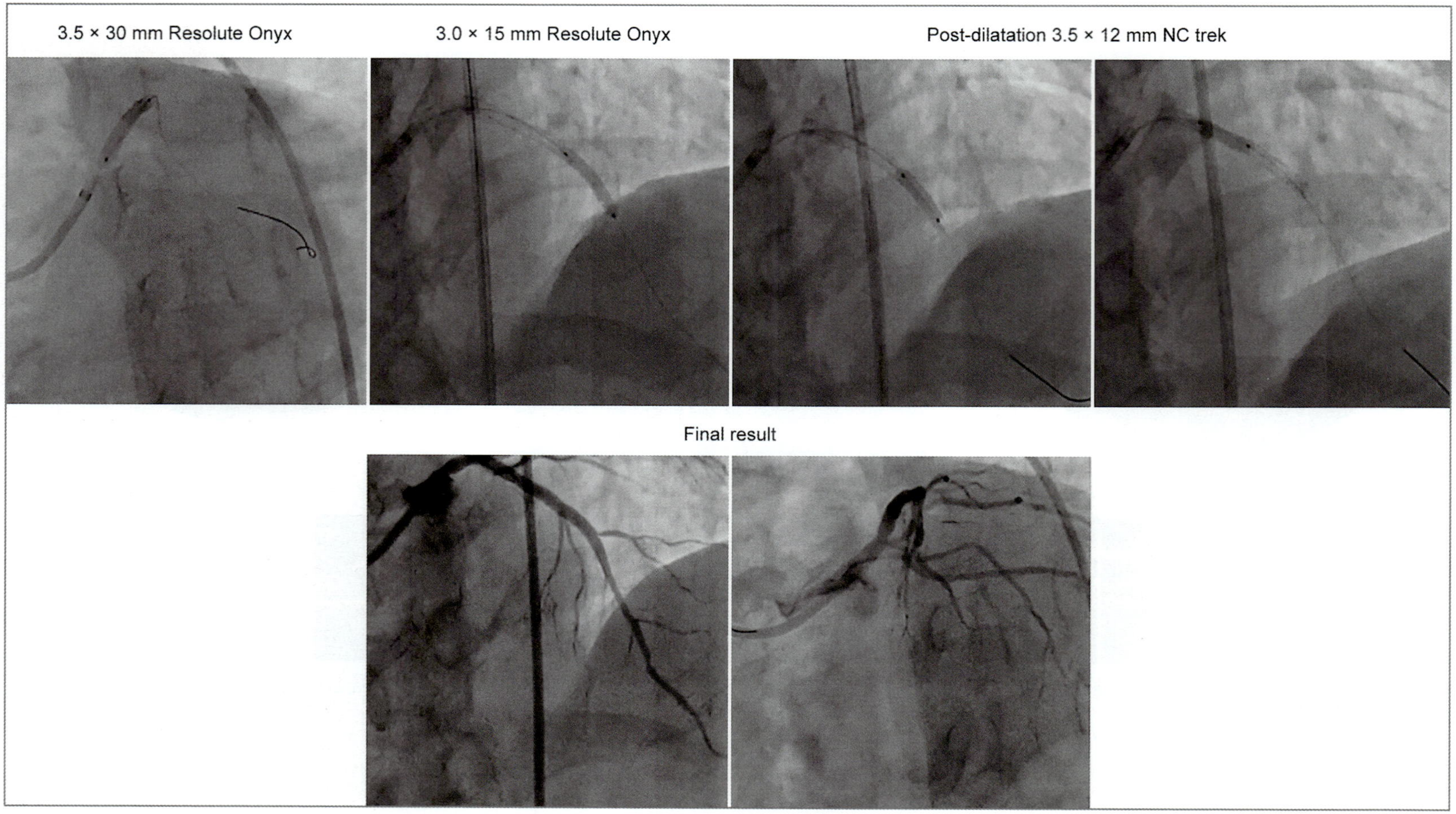

Fig. 12: Angioplasty of left anterior descending (LAD).

Post-OCT clearly distinguishes IMH from other causes of ambiguous lesions due to its high-resolution images about its extent longitudinally and circumferentially. IMH needs treatment with additional stenting or scoring with cutting balloon prior to stenting which is required if any compromise in lumen, decreased antegrade flow, and presence of symptoms or is hemodynamically unstable.

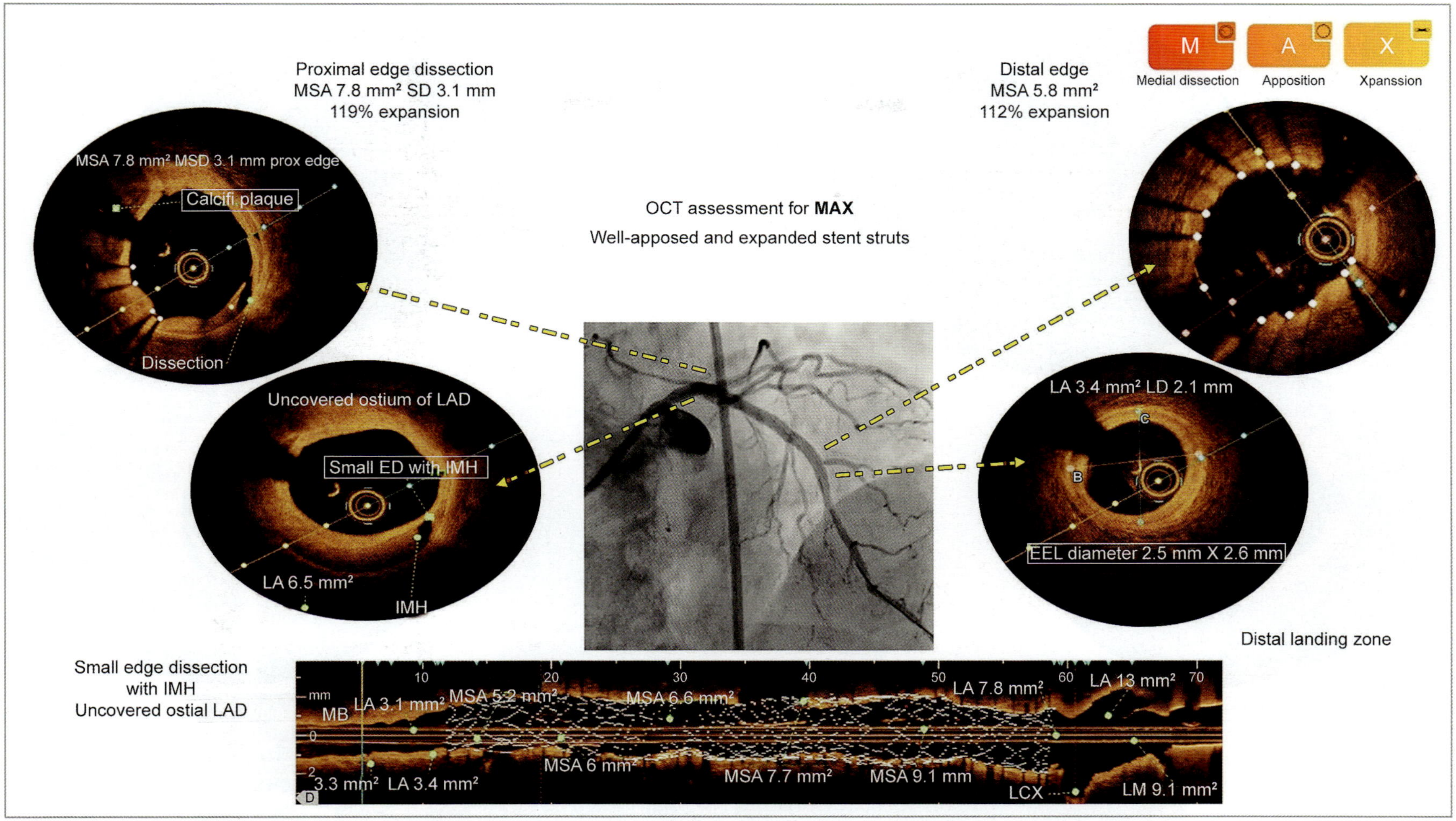

Fig. 13: Poststenting OCT assessment for MAX (EELD: external elastic luminal diameter; IMH: intramural hematoma; LA: lumen area; LAD: left anterior descending; LD: lumen diameter; MSA: minimal stent area; OCT: optical coherence tomography)

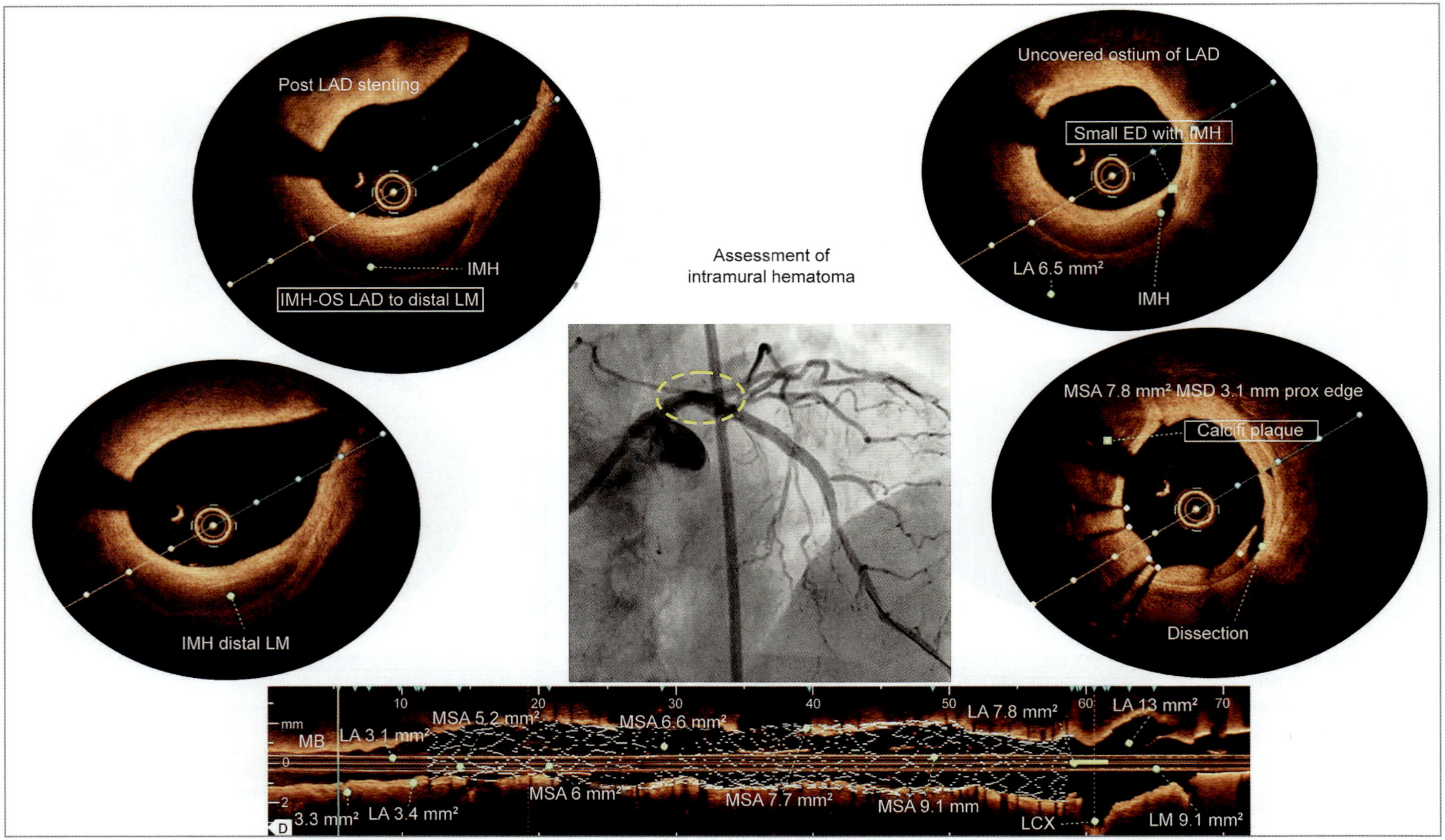

Fig. 14: Assessment of IMH. (IMH: intramural hematoma; LA: lumen area; LAD: left anterior descending; LCX: left circumflex; MSA: minimal stent area)

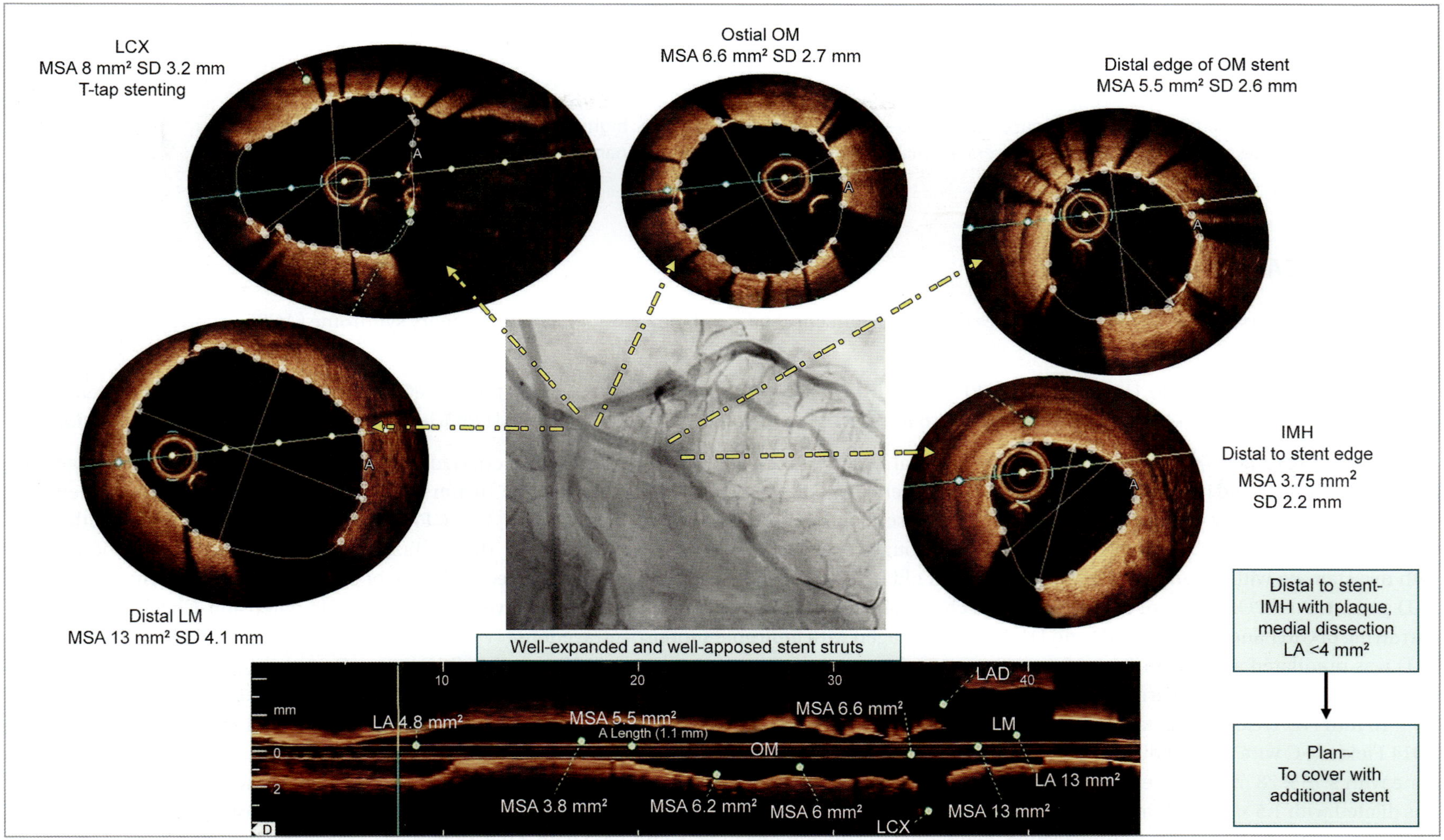

Fig. 15: Well-expanded and well-apposed stent struts. (IMH: intramural hematoma; MSA: minimal stent area; LA: left atrium; LCX: left circumflex; LM: left main; OM: obtuse marginal)

CASE 3

Intravascular OCT-guided PCI of ostioproximal calcified LAD—HD IVUS and OCT. (HD IVUS: high-definition intravascular ultrasound; LAD: left anterior descending; OCT: optical coherence tomography; PCI: percutaneous coronary intervention)

CLINICAL HISTORY

A 42-year-old male patient with no comorbidities presented with chest pain of 1-day duration, acute coronary syndrome (ACS)—evolved inferior wall MI (IWMI).

Investigations: 2D echo—mild LV dysfunction, EF 42%, Hb 14.2 g/dL, RBS 131 mg/dL, S Cr 0.95 mg/dL, eGFR 98 min/mL, C-reactive protein (CRP) 94.4 mg/L, and D-dimer 1,743 ng/mL. CAG—TVD with normal LM, mid-LAD 80% lesion, major-OM1 90% lesion, and proximal RCA total occlusion.

Percutaneous coronary intervention of RCA: Right radial access (RRA)—JR 3.5—6 Fr, lesion was crossed with 0.014″ BMW wire and predilated with 2.0 × 10 mm Tazuna and it was stented with 2.5 × 38 mm Xience Xpedition stent, postdilated with 3.0 × 10 mm NC Trek, and final angio images showed good result with TIMI III flow without any complications. Subsequently, PCI of LAD was done with EBU 3.5—6 Fr guide, LAD lesion was crossed with 0.014″ Sion Blue wire, and D1 was crossed with 0.014″ Runthrough wire. Lesion was predilated with 2.0 × 10 mm Tazuna, which resulted in dissection of LAD with dye staining without any extravasation. Pre-plain old balloon angioplasty (POBA) views showed OM1 free of plaque and no narrowing of proximal LAD and D1. Post-POBA patient developed severe chest pain, ST elevations in anterolateral leads, severe sweating, and hypotension. Check angio showed narrowing of OM1 and proximal LAD and D1; he was managed with inotropic support, intravenous (IV) fluids, and noninvasive ventilation (NIV) support. LAD was predilated again with 2.5 × 10 mm Tazuna and it was stented with 3.0 × 38 mm Xience Xpedition stent. Poststent check angio showed well-implanted stent, with mild narrowing of proximal LAD and significant narrowing of proximal D1 and OM1. Postdilatation of LAD stent was done with 3.5 × 10 mm NC Trek. Postdilatation check angio showed worsening of OM1 and D1 ostioproximal lesions and emergency wiring of OM1 was done with 0.014 Fielder FC wire and predilatations of OM were carried out with 2.5 × 10 mm angiosculpt to evacuate IMH. Subsequently, LMCA–OM stenting was done with 2.75 × 28 mm Xience Xpedition stent and POT of LMCA was done with 4.5 × 08 mm NC. Post-POT check angio showed pinching of D1 which was dilated with 1.5 × 10 mm Tazuna and proximal LAD was predilated with 3.0 × 12 mm NC Trek. Then LAD was recrossed through LCA-OM stent struts which were opened with 1.5 × 10 mm Tazuna. Sequential postdilatations of LCX and LAD with 3.0 × 12 mm NC Trek were done due to repeated failed attempts to perform FKB due to difficulty in passing two NC balloons simultaneously through 6 Fr guide catheter. Proximal LAD stenting was done 3.5 × 15 mm Xience Xpedition stent with minimal protrusion of stent into the distal LMCA using T-TAP stent strategy. Postdilatation of LAD stent was done with 3.5 NC and re-POT of LM was done with 4.5 NC. Finally, procedure was changed to right femoral route due to radial spasm for final FKB. LCA was engaged with JL 3.5–7 Fr, FKB was done with 3.0 × 12 mm in OM and 3.5 × 12 mm NC Trek in LAD at 12 and 16 atm and final POT of LMCA was done with 5.0 × 8 mm NC Apollo. Poststent OCT of LAD showed well-expanded, well-apposed stent struts **(Fig. 16)** and intravascular ultrasound (IVUS) study was done to study ostium of LMCA stent which showed well-expanded, well-apposed stent struts **(Fig. 17)**. Poststenting OCT of LCX-OM showed well-expanded, well-apposed stent struts **(Fig. 18)**, with distal medial edge dissection and IMH with plaque burden, causing luminal area of <4 mm^2, which was covered with additional stent using 2.5 × 15 mm Xience Xpedition; final angio showed excellent result with TIMI III flow with no complications.

Iatrogenic procedural dissection of the LAD is sometimes associated with development and extension of an IMH, proximally involving LM and LCX arteries and distally resulting in ACS with life-threatening angina, arrhythmia, acute pulmonary edema, and sudden cardiovascular collapse due to compromised flow of LAD and LCX. Our case developed extension of IMH to ostium of LAD, distal LM, and ostium of LCX which was treated with provisional stenting of LM to OM with T-TAP stenting of LAD, and OCT guidance was used for optimization of PCI result.

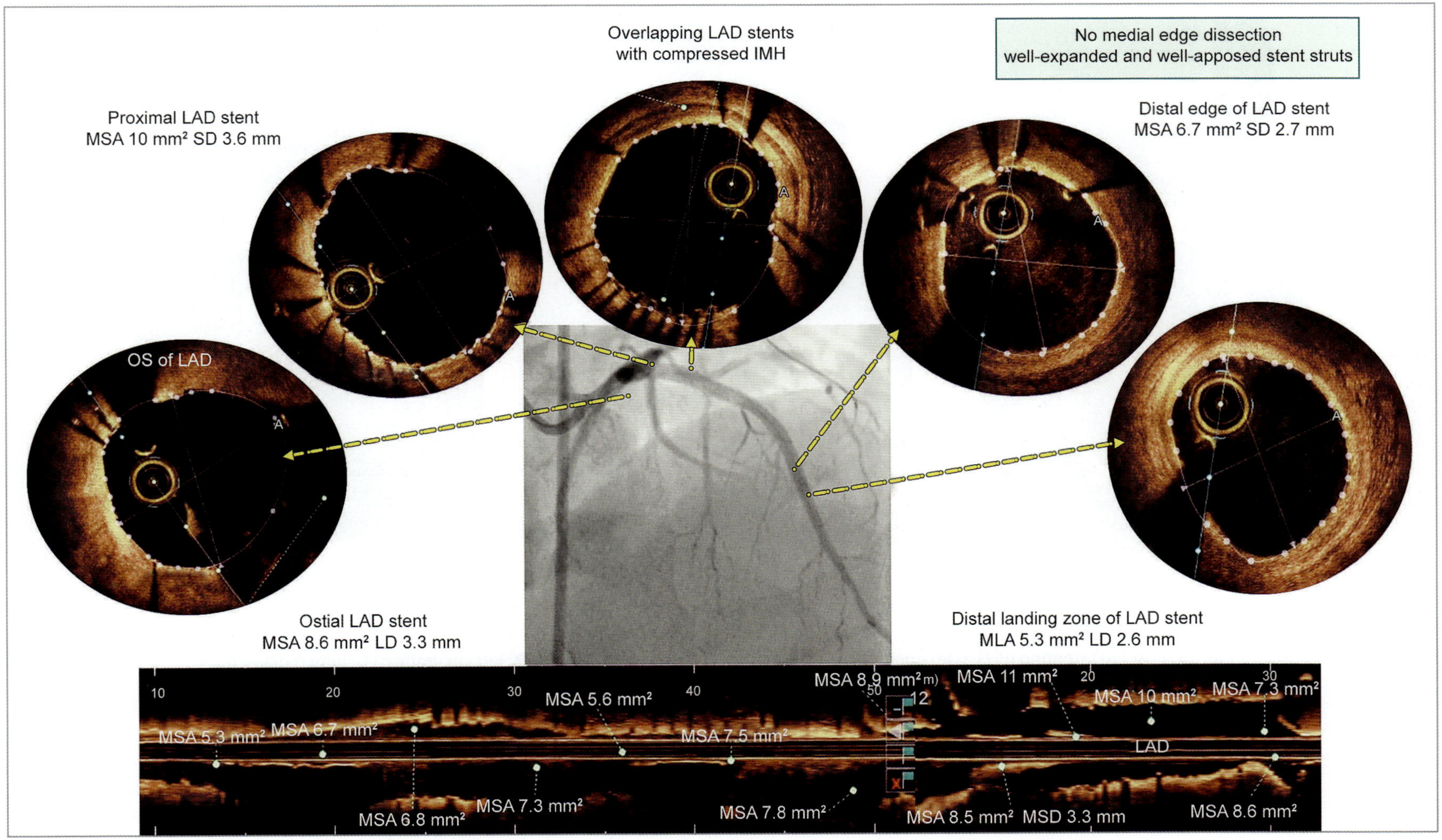

Fig. 16: Post LAD stenting OCT assessment for MAX. (IMH: intramural hematoma; LAD: left anterior descending; LD: lumen diameter; MSA: minimal stent area)

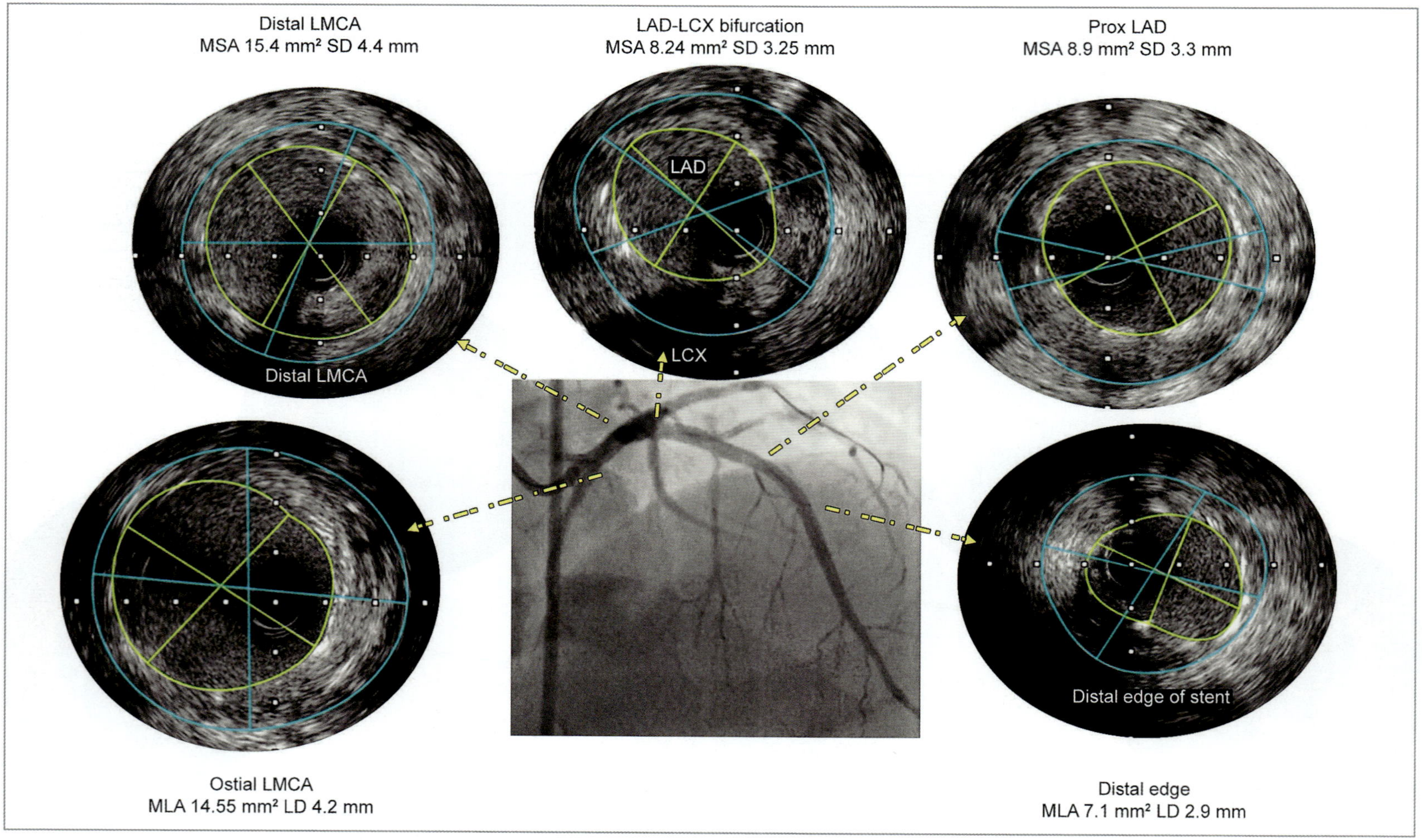

Fig. 17: Post LAD stenting IVUS assessment for MAX. (LAD: left anterior descending; LCX: left circumflex; LD: lumen diameter; LMCA: left main coronary artery; MLA: minimal lumen area; MSA: minimal stent area)

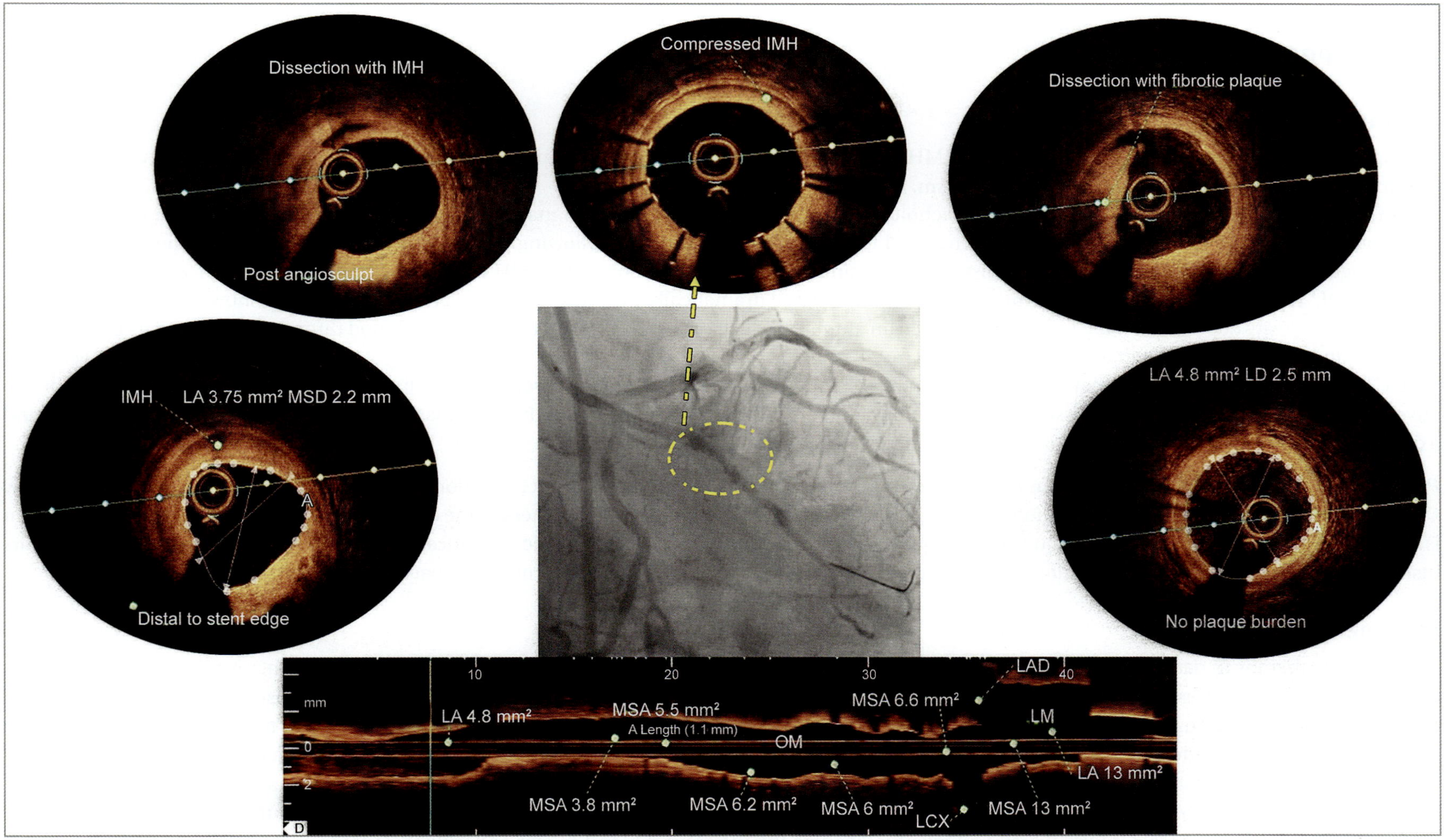

Fig. 18: Post LCX-OM stenting OCT assessment for IMH. (IMH: intramural hematoma; LA: lumen area; LCX: left circumflex; LD: lumen diameter; MSA: minimal stent area)

PROCEDURE

Diagnosis

Angiography—the angiographic appearance of an IMH may vary widely, about one third of patients having no significant abnormality and 10% may present with the appearance of a new stenosis or spasm.[3]

IVUS—IMH is visible as a homogenous, hyperechoic, and crescent-shaped area. IVUS may show evidence of flow from the true lumen into the hematoma and is evident in only 50% of the patients, and features of IMH include the following:[4] (1) An entry site of dissection plane into the media, (2) propagation of the IMH that is more often distal than proximal, and (3) propagation of the IMH into more normal segments or arcs of arterial wall. Yamada et al.[5] reported that the backscatter intensity of blood increased dramatically with stagnant flow. van der Heiden et al.[6] showed that the increase in backscatter intensity depended on red cell aggregation. In an animal model, Fowlkes et al.[7] showed that whole-blood thrombus increased its echogenicity over time and that this was related to the fibrin content.

OCT—IMH appears as a low-signal area with low-light attenuation usually located at the level of the media tunica and demarcated externally by the adventitia,[4] showing an entry site of dissection plane into the media, extent of propagation of the IMH that is longitudinally (distal and proximal), and axially into less diseased or normal segments or arcs of arterial wall.

Prevention of IMH during PCI: A meticulous catheterization technique should be used to prevent formation of IMH.[8] This includes utilizing appropriately sized and shaped catheters without deep intubation of the vessel, avoidance of noncoaxial alignment of the catheter, not injecting if the pressure waveform is dampened or at an atherosclerotic plaque, and adequate plaque modification of severe fibrotic or fibrocalcific lesions with scoring or cutting balloons instead of initial high-pressure NC predilatations, particularly in the presence of less diseased or normal adjacent segments.

Management

Thrombolytic therapy in patients with coronary dissections and IMHs is not recommended due to the possibility of extension, resulting in poor prognosis and management strategies include additional stenting, reentry with a stiff chronic total occlusion (CTO) guidewire and also intimal fenestrations with either a cutting or a scoring balloon and an additional stenting of IMH carries a risk of further spreading the hematoma more distally.[9] Manipulating techniques with a stiff guidewire is sometimes challenging and requires additional skill to wire-induced complications like dissection, perforation, and further expansion of hematoma. It can be treated effectively by creating reentry points of microfenestrations in the intima by using cutting or scoring balloon which requires a balloon–artery size ratio of 1:1 with a target of inflating the balloon with a nominal pressure at the site of the distal edge of the stent to minimize the vessel injury, which will eventually allow the intramural blood to exit and induce decompression of the medial space with successive resolution of the luminal stenosis. In addition, minimal vessel trauma will ensure smooth healing of the vessel wall without the need for further stent deployment. Sumiyoshi et al.[10] thus illustrate a technique to effectively reestablish distal flow in dissections complicated by severe compressive hematomas, minimizing the need for extensive stenting beyond the original dissection site.

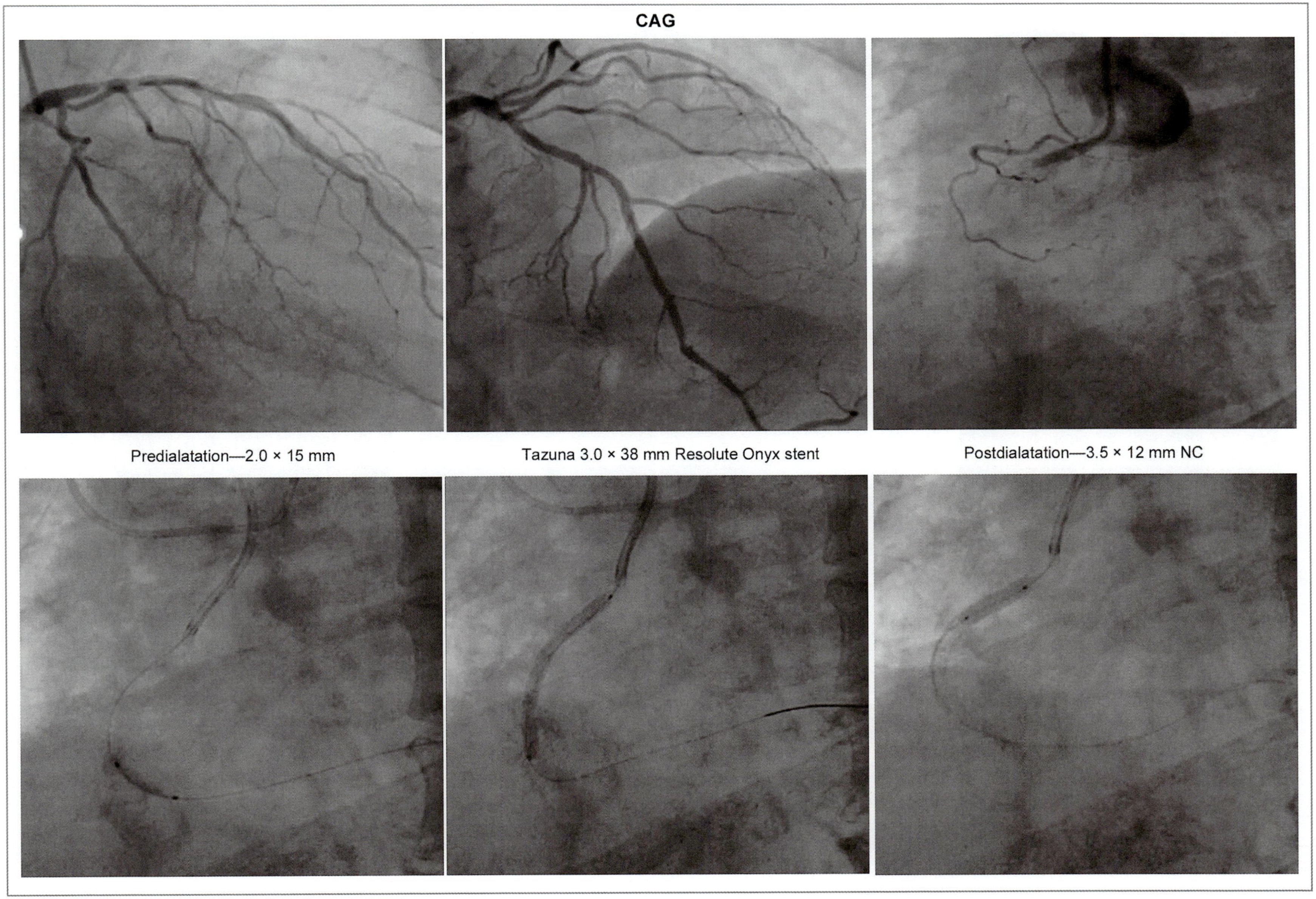

Fig. 19: Coronary angiogram showed LAD, LCX, and RCA; coronary angioplasty of RCA vessel. (LAD: left anterior descending; LCX: left circumflex; NC: noncompliant; RCA: right coronary artery)

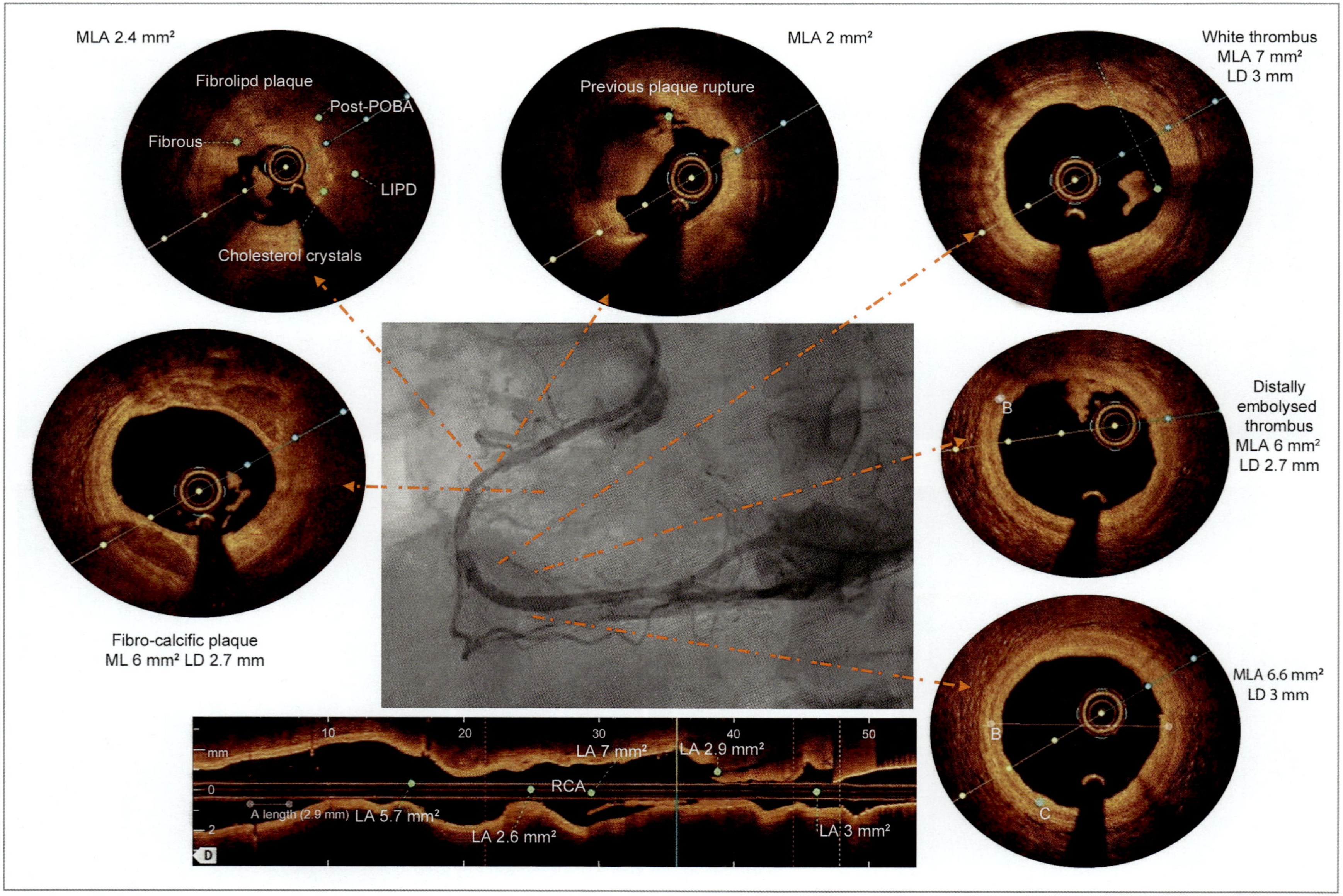
MLA 2.4 mm²
Fibrolipd plaque
Post-POBA
Fibrous
LIPD
Cholesterol crystals
MLA 2 mm²
Previous plaque rupture
White thrombus
MLA 7 mm²
LD 3 mm
Distally
embolysed
thrombus
MLA 6 mm²
LD 2.7 mm
Fibro-calcific plaque
ML 6 mm² LD 2.7 mm
MLA 6.6 mm²
LD 3 mm
B
C
mm
LA 7 mm²
LA 2.9 mm²
RCA
A length (2.9 mm)
LA 5.7 mm²
LA 2.6 mm²
LA 3 mm²
D

Fig. 20A

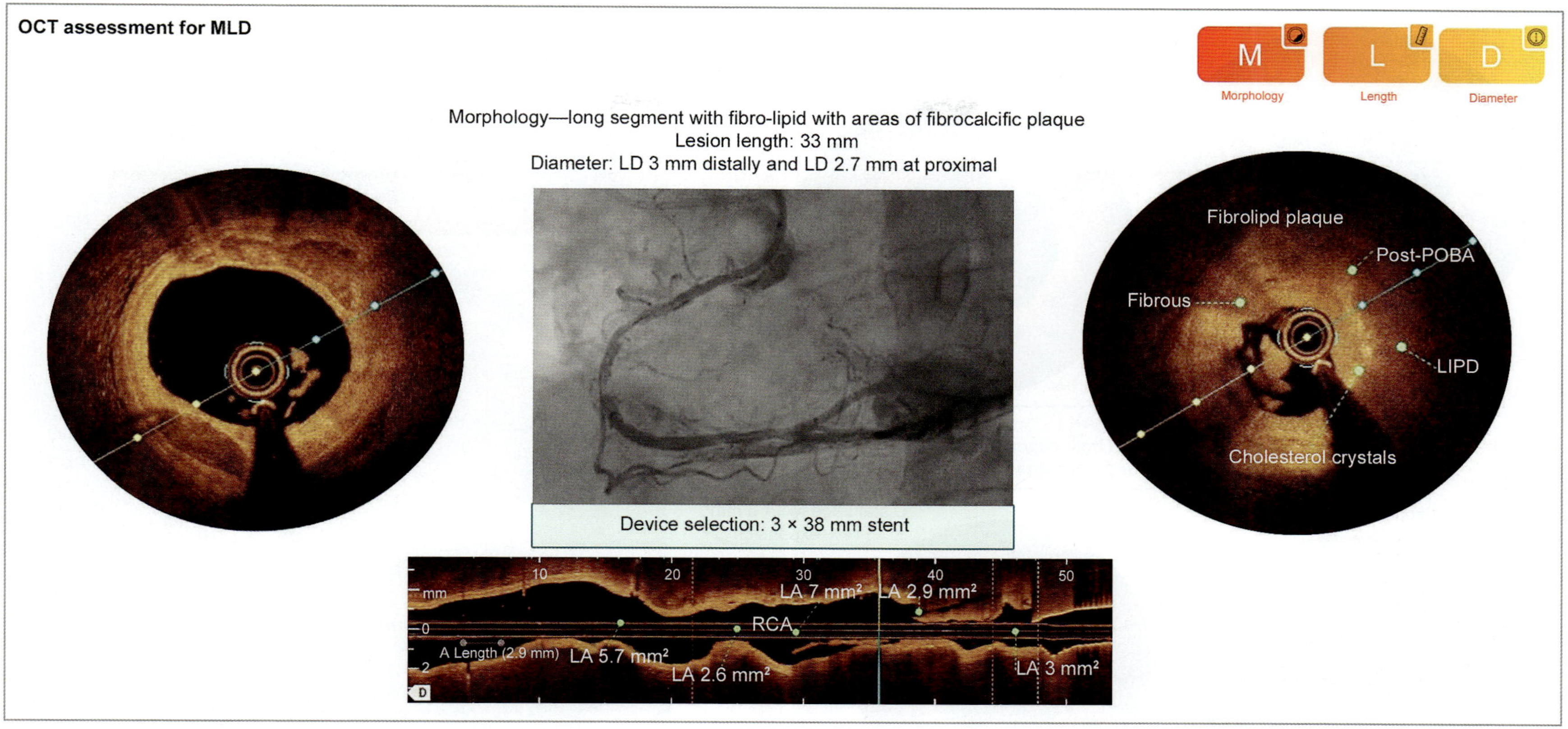

Fig. 20B

Figs. 20A and B: Pre-PCI OCT assessment of RCA (A) for plaque morphology, (B) device selection. (LA: lumen area; LD: lumen diameter; MLA: minimal lumen area; OCT: optical coherence tomography; PCI: percutaneous coronary intervention; POBA: plain old balloon angioplasty; RCA: right coronary artery)

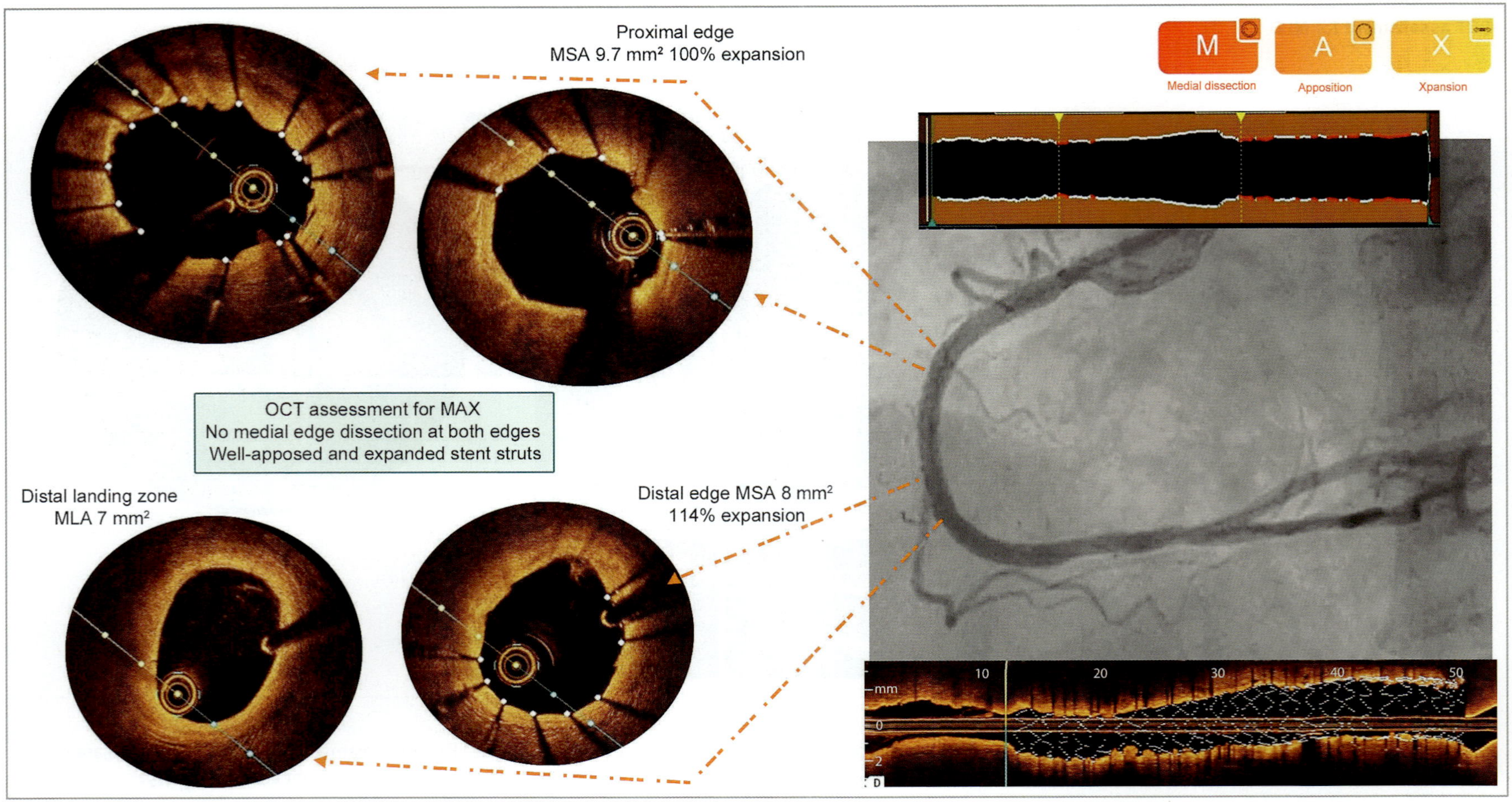

Fig. 21: Post-PCI OCT assessment of RCA showed well-expanded and apposed stent struts with no medial edge dissections. (OCT: optical coherence tomography; PCI: percutaneous coronary intervention; RCA: right coronary artery)

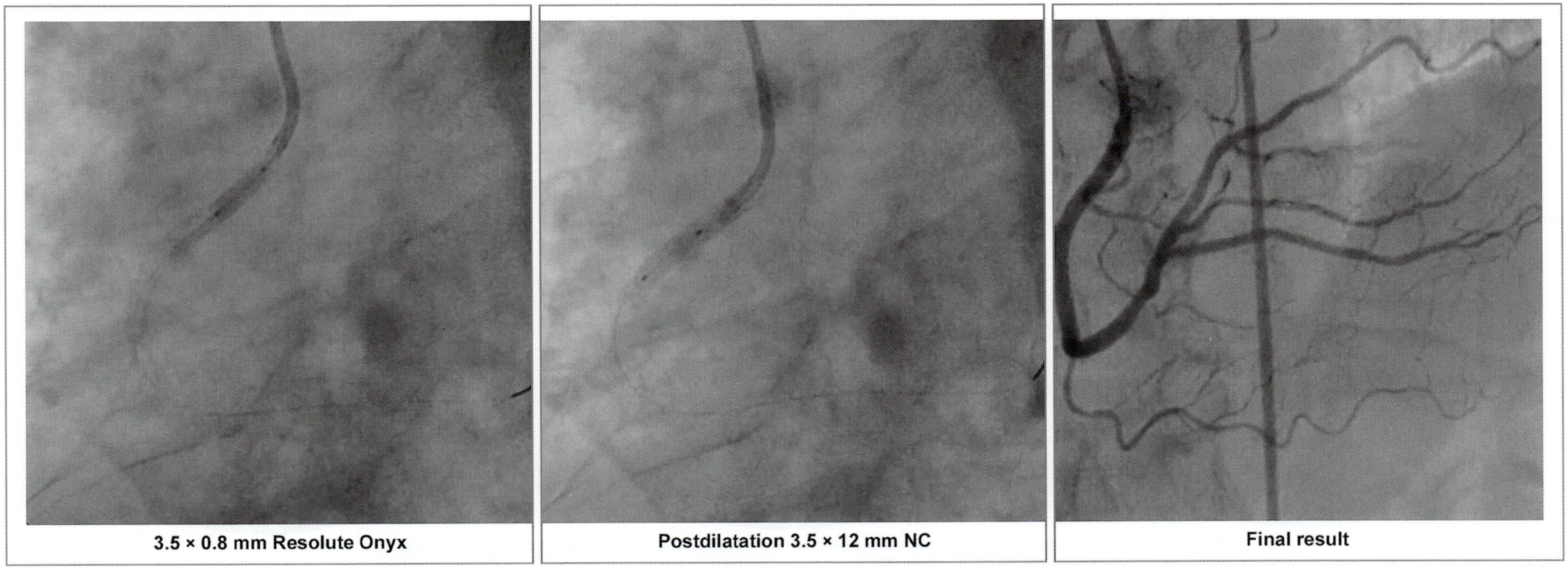

Fig. 22: Ostial right coronary artery (RCA) stenting, postdilatation, and final result of RCA vessel.

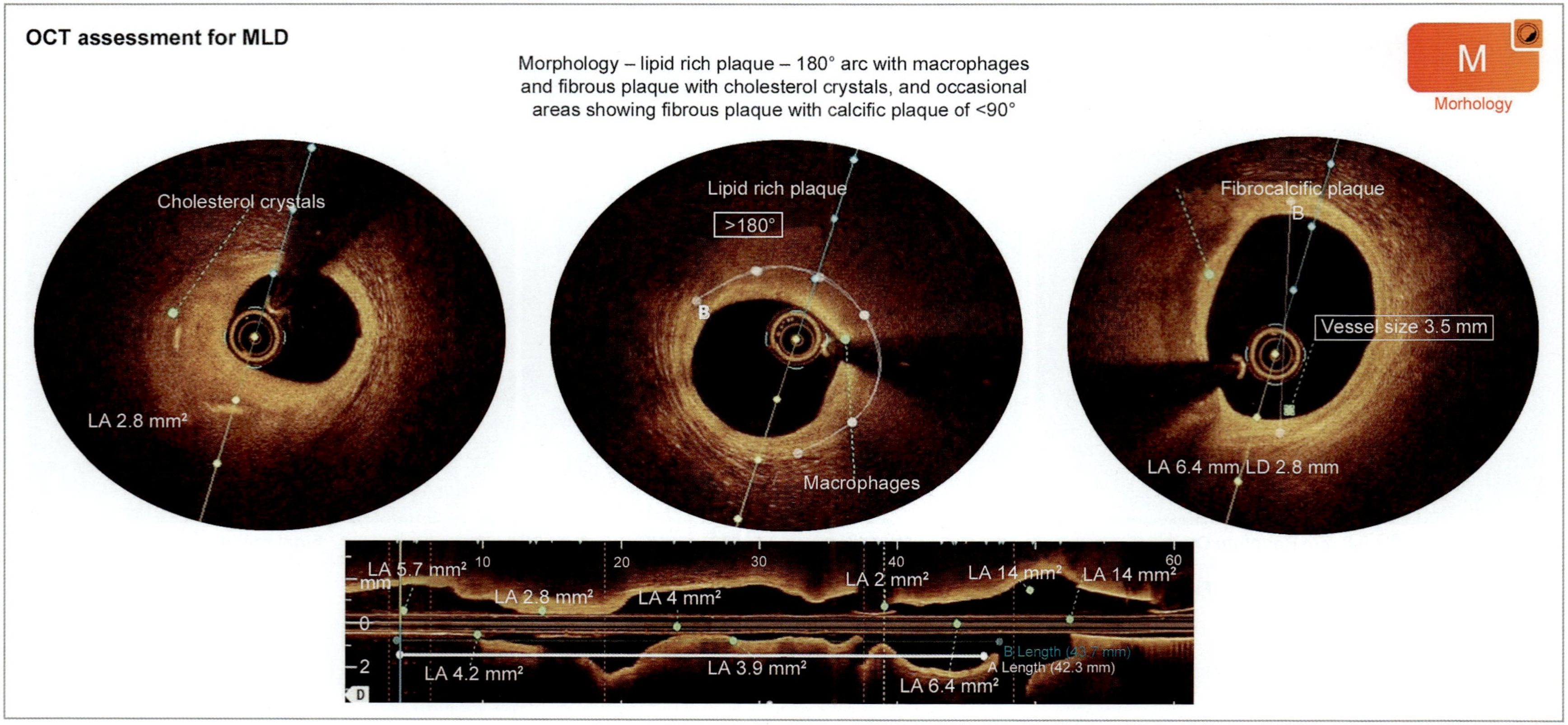
OCT assessment for MLD
Morphology – lipid rich plaque – 180° arc with macrophages and fibrous plaque with cholesterol crystals, and occasional areas showing fibrous plaque with calcific plaque of <90°
M
Morhology
Cholesterol crystals
LA 2.8 mm²
Lipid rich plaque
>180°
B
Macrophages
Fibrocalcific plaque
B
Vessel size 3.5 mm
LA 6.4 mm/LD 2.8 mm
LA 5.7 mm²
LA 2.8 mm²
LA 4 mm²
LA 2 mm²
LA 14 mm²
LA 14 mm²
LA 4.2 mm²
LA 3.9 mm²
LA 6.4 mm²
A Length (42.3 mm)

Fig. 23A

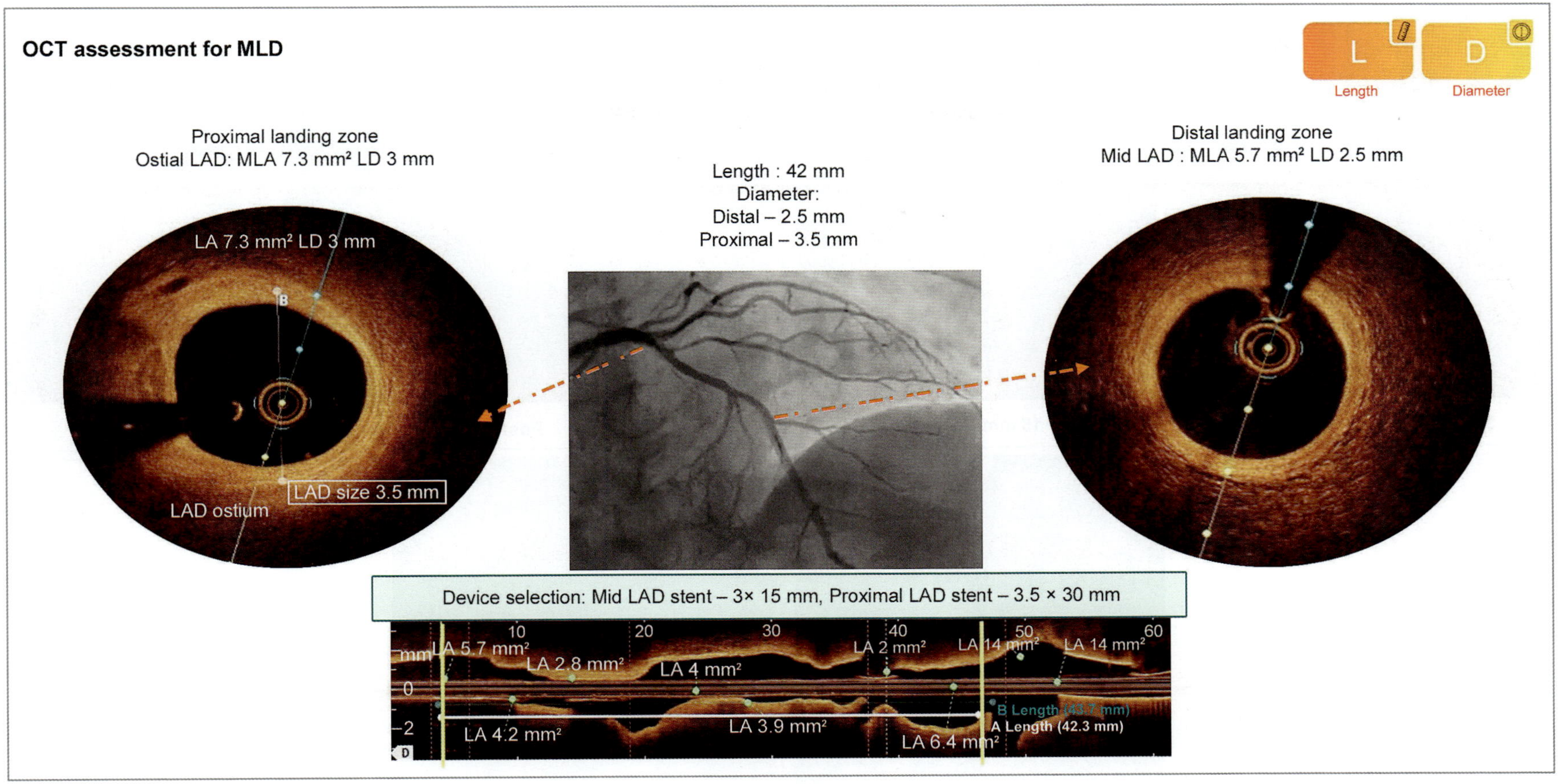

Fig. 23B

Figs. 23A and B: Pre-PCI OCT assessment of LAD (A) for plaque morphology and (B) device selection. (LA: lumen area; LAD: left anterior descending; LD: lumen diameter; OCT: optical coherence tomography; PCI: percutaneous coronary intervention)

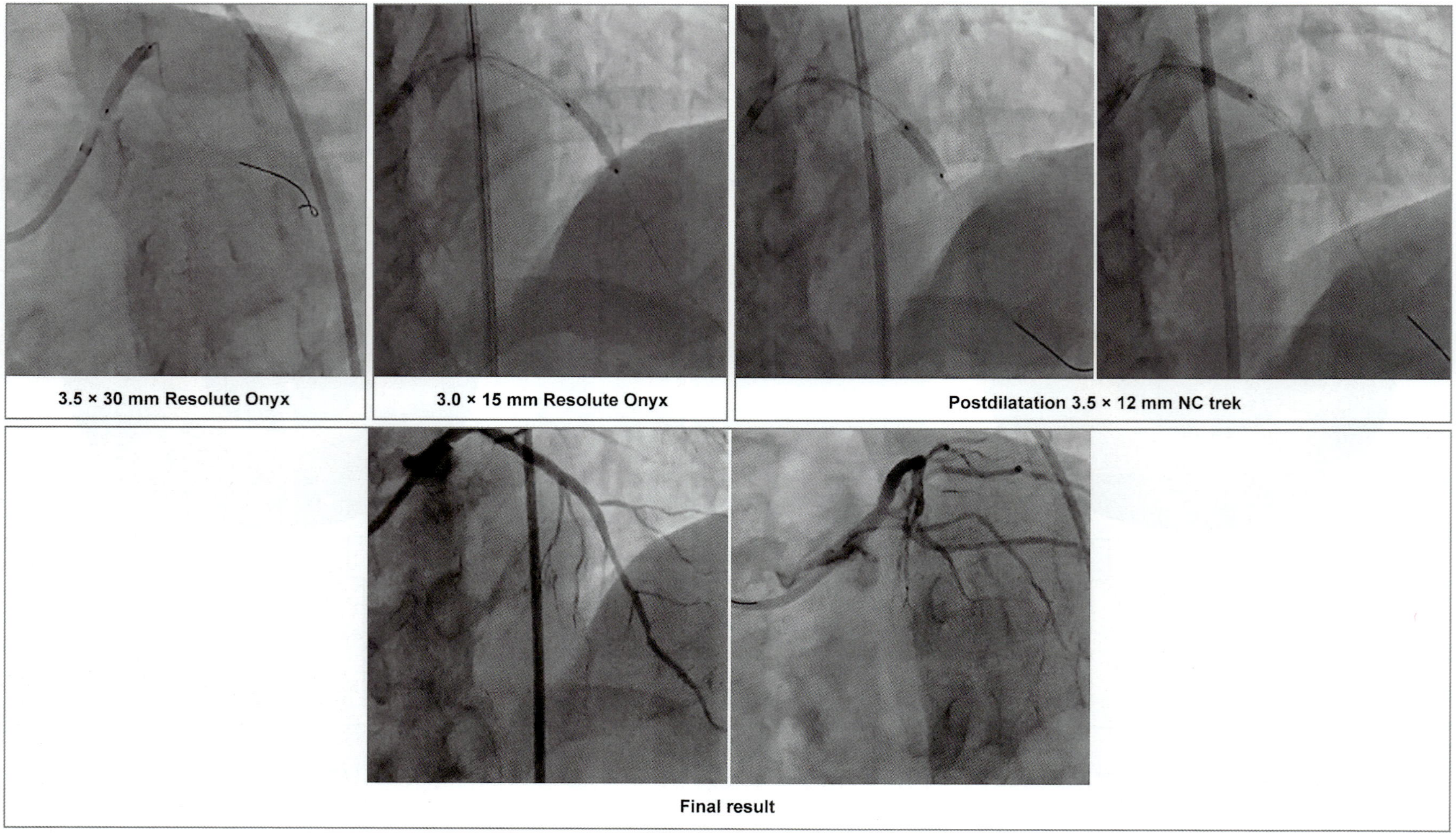

Fig. 24: Coronary angioplasty of left anterior descending (LAD) vessel. (NC: noncompliant)

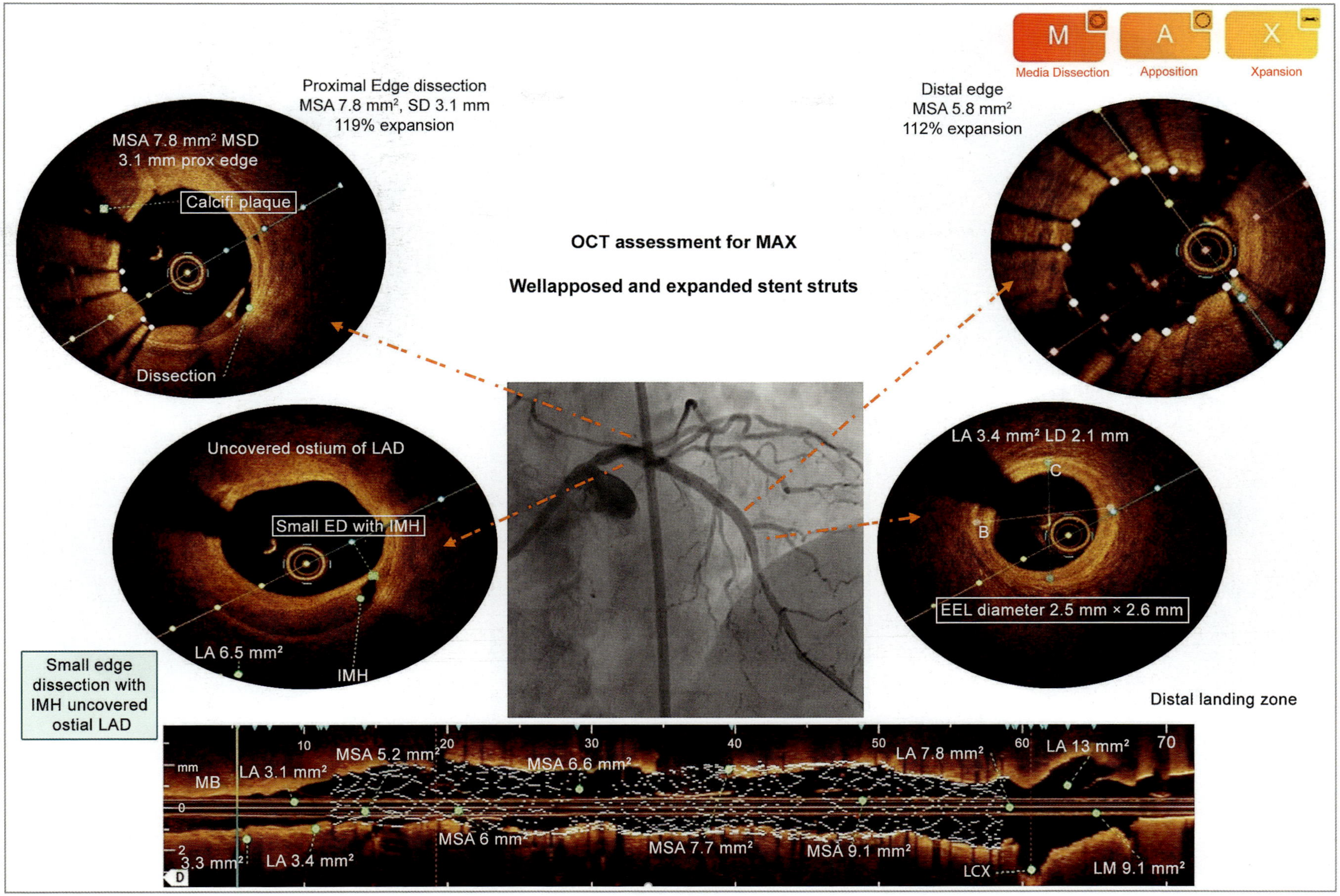
M
A
X
Media Dissection
Apposition
Xpansion
Proximal Edge dissection
MSA 7.8 mm², SD 3.1 mm
119% expansion
MSA 7.8 mm² MSD
3.1 mm prox edge
Calcifi plaque
Dissection
OCT assessment for MAX
Wellapposed and expanded stent struts
Distal edge
MSA 5.8 mm²
112% expansion
Uncovered ostium of LAD
Small ED with IMH
LA 6.5 mm²
IMH
LA 3.4 mm² LD 2.1 mm
C
B
EEL diameter 2.5 mm × 2.6 mm
Small edge dissection with IMH uncovered ostial LAD
Distal landing zone
MB
LA 3.1 mm²
MSA 5.2 mm²
MSA 6.6 mm²
LA 7.8 mm²
LA 13 mm²
3.3 mm²
LA 3.4 mm²
MSA 6 mm²
MSA 7.7 mm²
MSA 9.1 mm²
LCX
LM 9.1 mm²

Fig. 25A

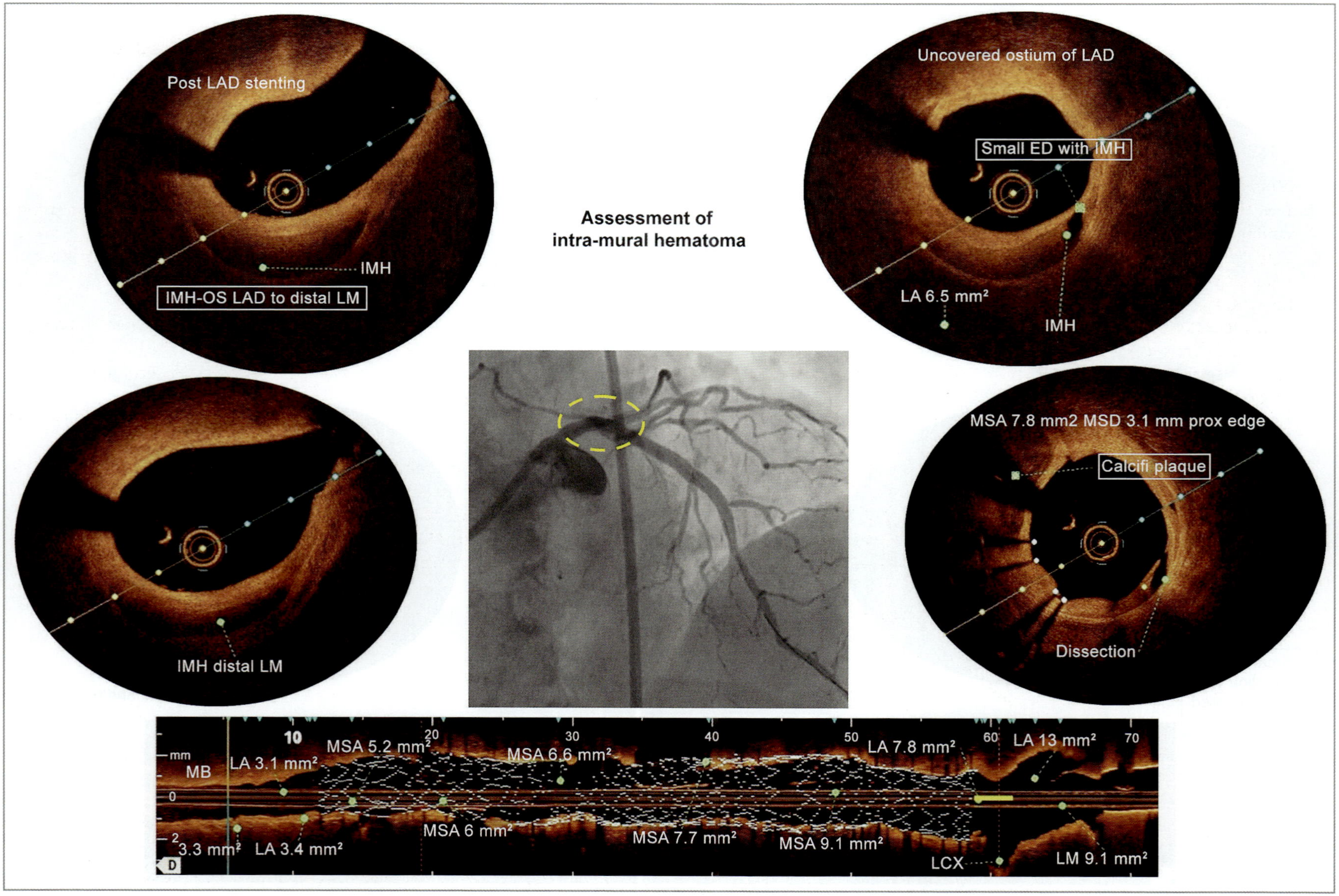

Fig. 25B

Figs. 25A and B: Post-PCI OCT assessment of LAD vessel showed (A) well-expanded and apposed stent struts in distal half; (B) well-expanded and apposed stent struts with medial edge dissection with intramural hematoma (IMH). (LA: lumen area; LAD: left anterior descending; LCX: left circumflex; LM: left main; MSA: minimal stent area; OCT: optical coherence tomography; PCI: percutaneous coronary intervention; SD: stent diameter)

CONCLUSION

Although there is no clear consensus on management of multivessel IMH, the key principle of reestablishing coronary flow in the setting of ongoing ischemia is to establish coronary flow as early as possible to mitigate symptoms and signs of ischemia. The proper management of coronary IMH optimal treatment strategy depends on the site of hematoma, number of affected vessels, the reduction in coronary blood flow, and hemodynamic status.

REFERENCES

1. Moidy M, Al Kindi F. Coronary intramural hematoma: challenges in diagnosis and management. Heart Views. 2019;20(1):17-20.
2. Noh HJ, Choi JH, Song YB, Jo HC, Yang JH, Kim SM, et al. Intravascular ultrasound-guided troubleshooting in a large hematoma treated with fenestration using a cutting balloon. Korean Circ J. 2009;39(4):171-4.
3. Maehara A, Mintz GS, Bui AB, Castagna MT, Walter OR, Pappas C, et al. Incidence, morphology, angiographic findings, and outcomes of intramural hematomas after percutaneous coronary interventions: an intravascular ultrasound study. Circulation. 2002;105(17):2037-42.
4. Song JK. Diagnosis of aortic intramural haematoma. Heart. 2004;90(4):368-71.
5. Yamada EG, Fitzgerald PJ, Sudhir K, Hargrave VK, Yock PG. Intravascular ultrasound imaging of blood: the effect of hematocrit and flow on backscatter. J Am Soc Echocardiogr. 1992;5(4):385-92.
6. van der Heiden MS, de Kroon MG, Bom N, Borst C. Ultrasound backscatter at 30 MHz from human blood: influence of rouleau size affected by blood modification and shear rate. Ultrasound Med Biol. 1995;21(6):817-26.
7. Fowlkes JB, Strieter RM, Downing LJ, Brown SL, Saluja A, Salles-Cunha S, et al. Ultrasound echogenicity in experimental venous thrombosis. Ultrasound Med Biol. 1998;24(8):1175-82.
8. Basta M. Iatrogenic intramural hematoma of the ascending aorta complicating inadvertent arterial cannulation during central venous catheter placement. A case report and review of the literature. Ann Card Anaesth. 2020;23(4):502.
9. Koh JS, Jeong YH, Yoon SE, Park JR, Park Y, Hwang SJ, et al. A case of spontaneous coronary artery dissection healed by medical treatment: serial findings of coronary angiography, intravascular ultrasound and multi-detector computed tomography. Korean Circ J. 2011;41(6):346-8.
10. Sumiyoshi A, Okamura A, Iwamoto M, Nagai H, Yamasaki T, Tanaka T, et al. Aspiration after sealing the entrance by stenting is a promising method to treat subintimal hematoma. Case Rep. 2021;3(3):380-4.

CHAPTER 27

Artifacts

GUIDEWIRE SHADOW

An artifact that is caused by the guidewire. The guidewire shadow will completely mask the underlying tissue and stents **(Fig. 1)**.[1,2]

GHOST LINES

Ghost lines appear as circular features in the optical coherence tomography (OCT) image **(Figs. 2A to C)**.[3]

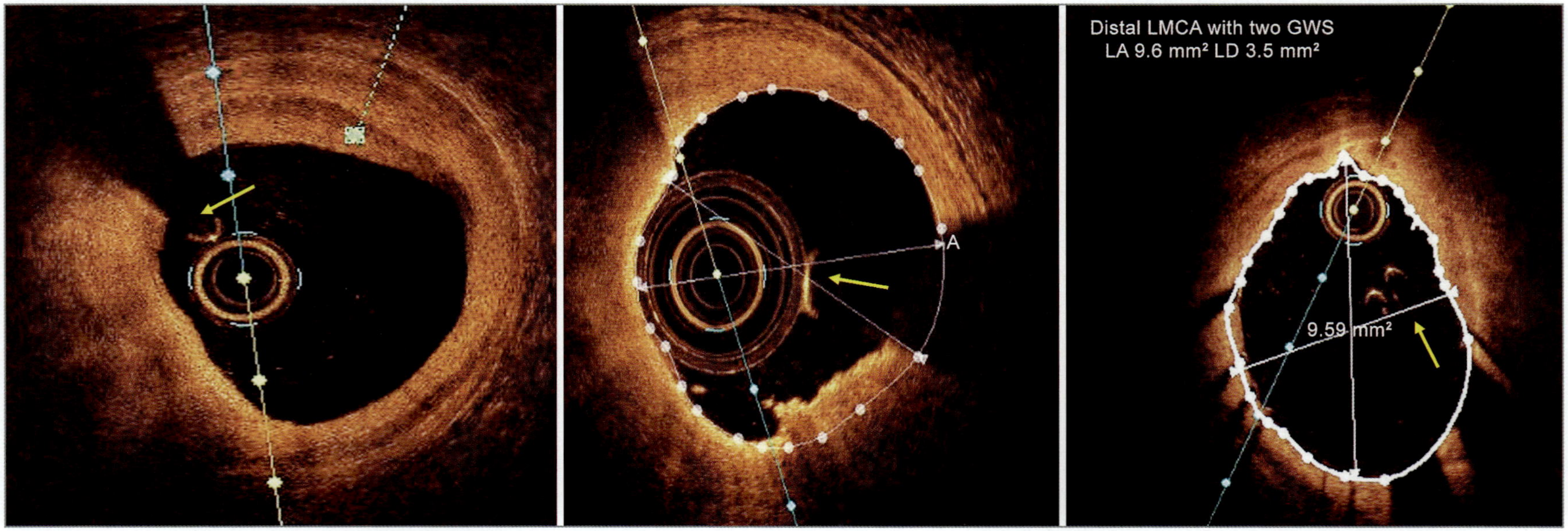

Fig. 1: Guidewire shadow (GWS). (LA: lumen area; LD: lumen diameter; LMCA: left main coronary artery)

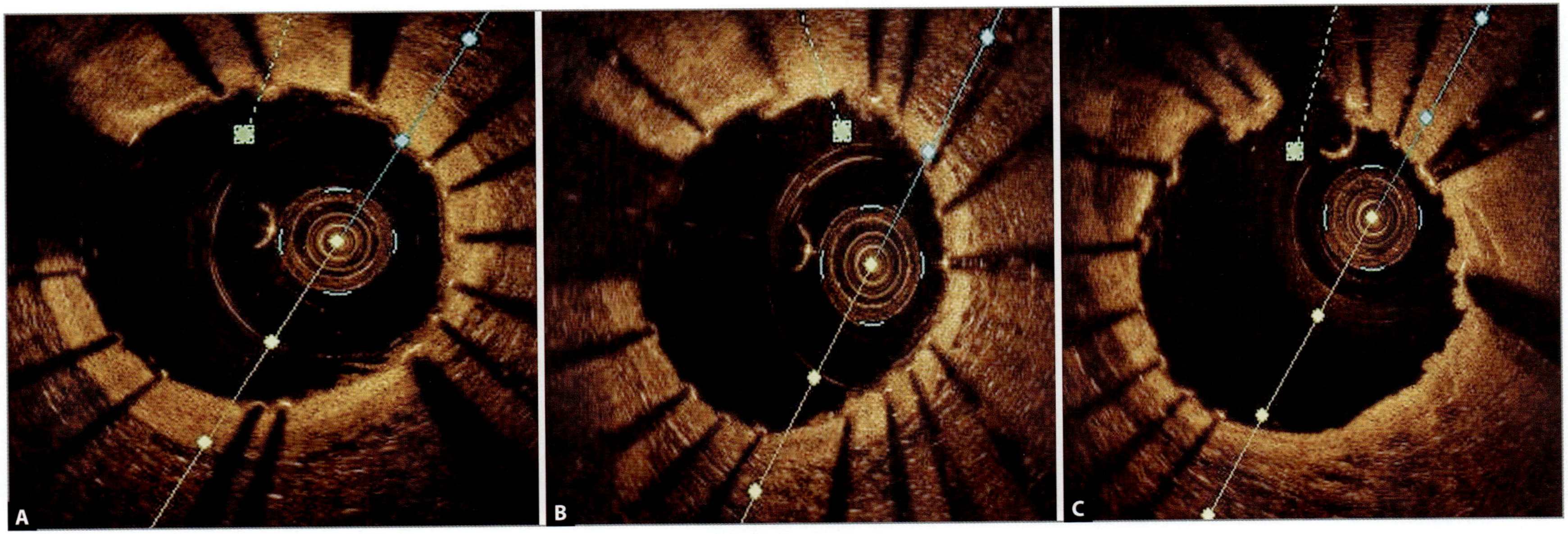

Figs. 2A to C: Ghost lines.

RESIDUAL BLOOD FROM INCOMPLETE LUMEN FLUSHING

Improper clearance of blood from the vessel lumen due to inadequate injection force and speed of the contrast at the time of OCT image acquisition lead to artifacts that are seen as signal-rich areas instead of a transparent lumen completely free of OCT signal **(Figs. 3A to C)**.[4]

THROMBUS

Red cell thrombus produces high backscatter on surface with high attenuation due to red blood cell (RBC) shadow and tissue or structures cannot see red thrombus beyond and it is difficult to assess the depth of red thrombus due to this shadow effect. White thrombus characterized by high backscatter, low attenuation, and possible to tissue or structures beyond thrombus **(Fig. 4)**.[5]

GAS BUBBLES

Gas bubbles appear as a distinct region of brightness inside the catheter and diminished signal in the part of the OCT image in the path of the disrupted region of the catheter. These are due to inadequate flushing of imaging catheter before inserting the OCT catheter **(Fig. 5)**.[4]

METALLIC AND BIODEGRADABLE STENTS

Metal stents cause shadows behind each strut which appear like a single leading-edge feature that casts a single expanding broad shadow over the arterial wall beginning with the width of the stent strut **(Fig. 6)**.[4]

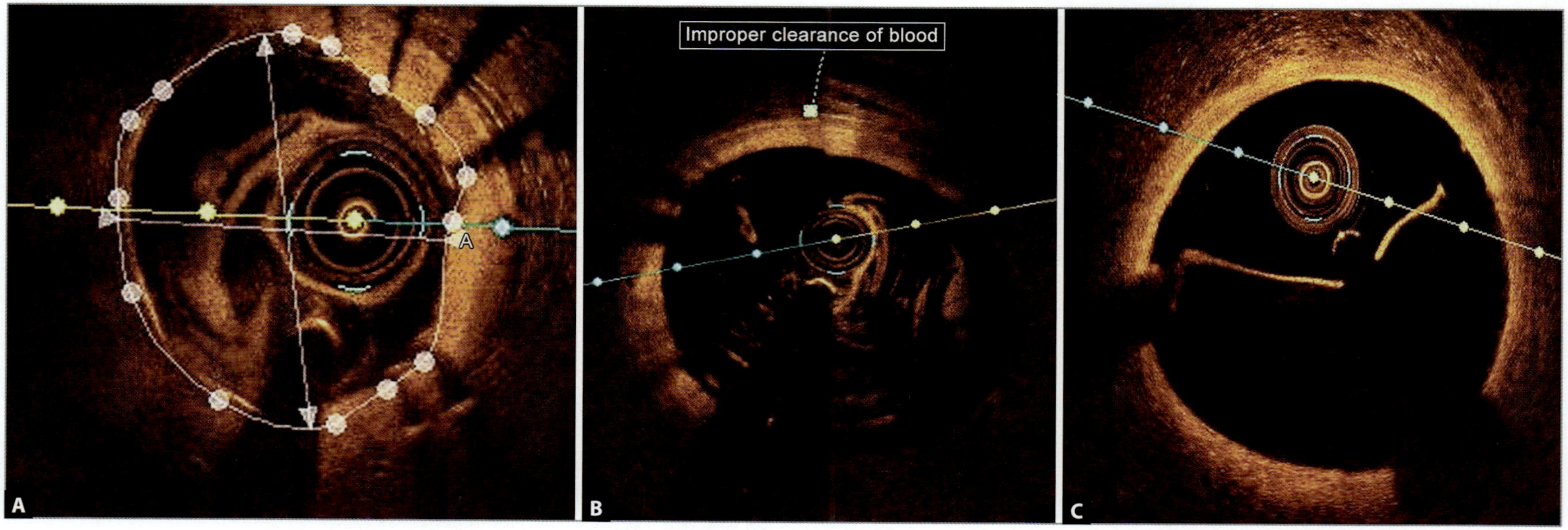

Figs. 3A to C: Residual blood from incomplete lumen flushing.

SUPERFICIAL SHADOWING BY MACROPHAGES

Attenuation of light by macrophage accumulations can cause shadows that appear falsely as an underlying lipid pool or necrotic core **(Fig. 7)**.[5]

NONUNIFORM ROTATIONAL DEFORMITY

Nonuniform rotational deformity is a consequence of mechanical catheter systems that arises from binding of the drive cable or rotating optical components during image acquisition.

It occurs as a result of binding of the driving cable or rotating optical components during image acquisition.

It appears like geometric distortion in the image that masks the structures in that part of the circumference **(Fig. 8)**.[6]

FOLDOVER ARTIFACT

Foldover artifact is observed when the vessel diameter is too large for the field of view of the imaging catheter **(Fig. 9)**.[5]

TANGENTIAL LIGHT DROPOUT

Tangential light dropout artifact may be confused with the appearance of a thin-capped fibroatheroma and superficial accumulation of macrophages **(Fig. 10)**.

When the catheter is located near the vessel wall, the OCT beam can be directed almost parallel to the tissue surface which can produce signal poor image below the luminal surface.

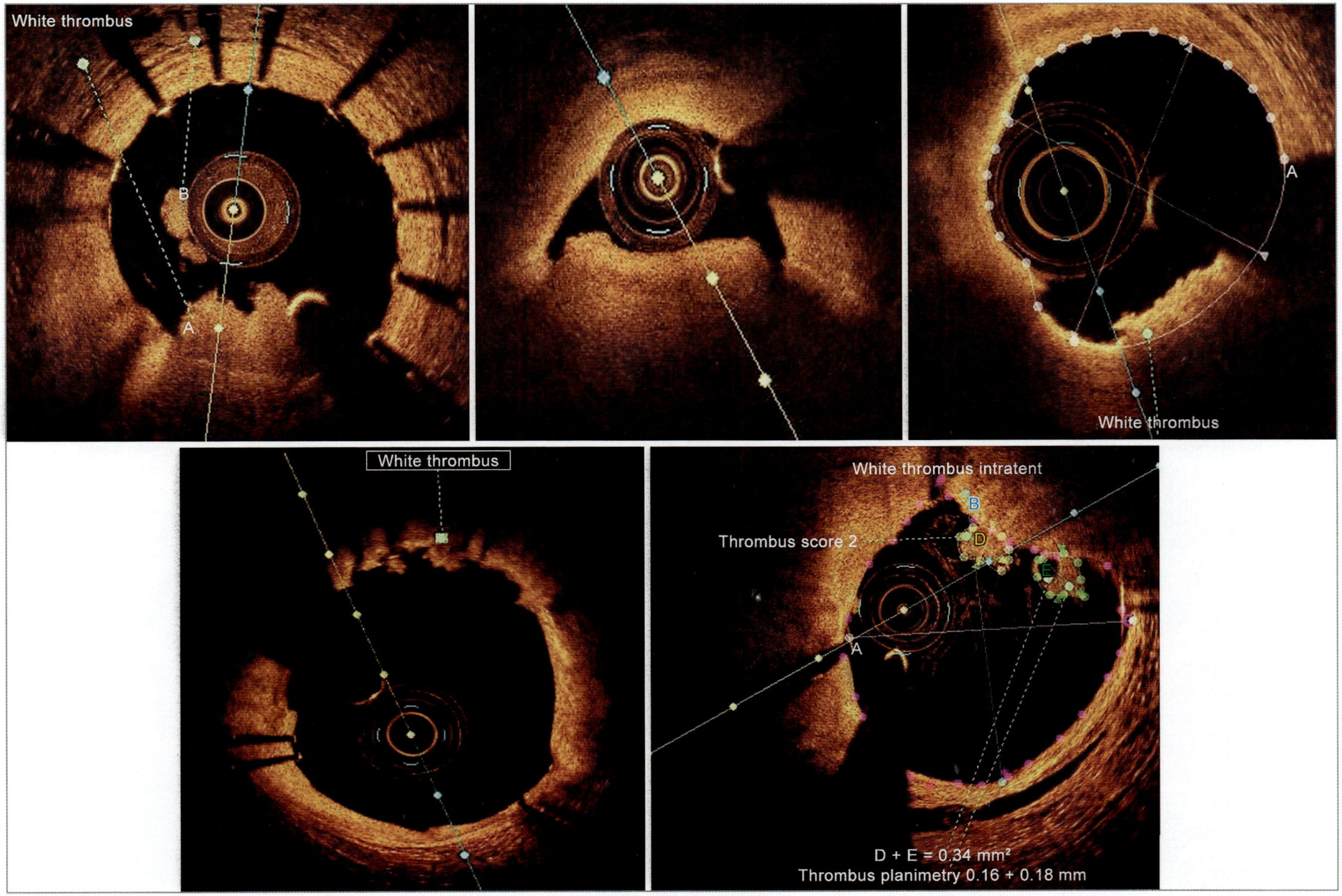

Fig. 4: Thrombus.

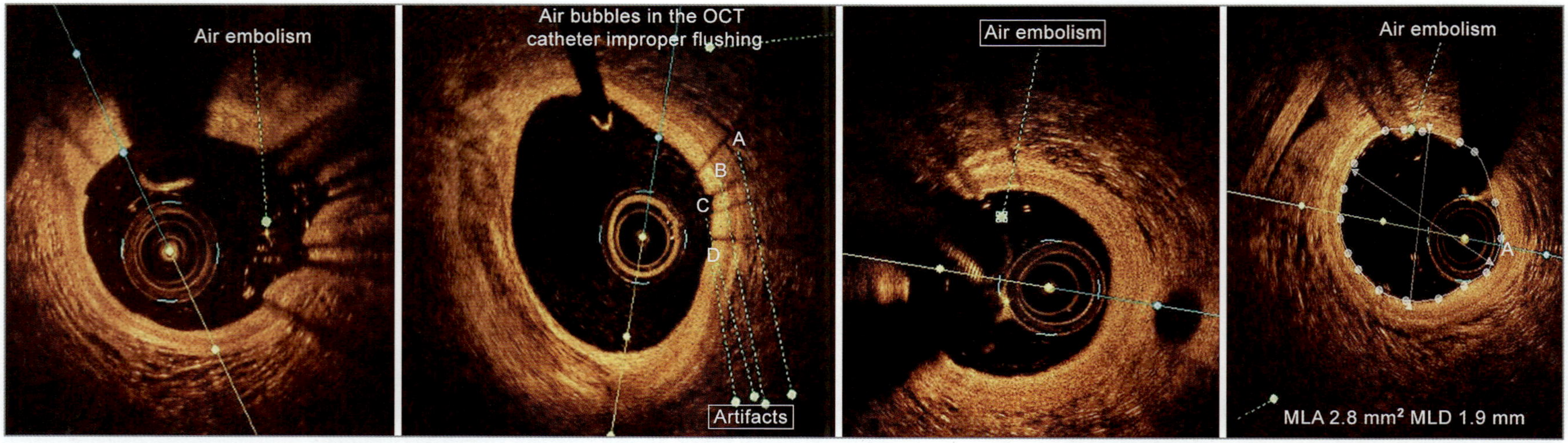

Fig. 5: Gas bubbles.

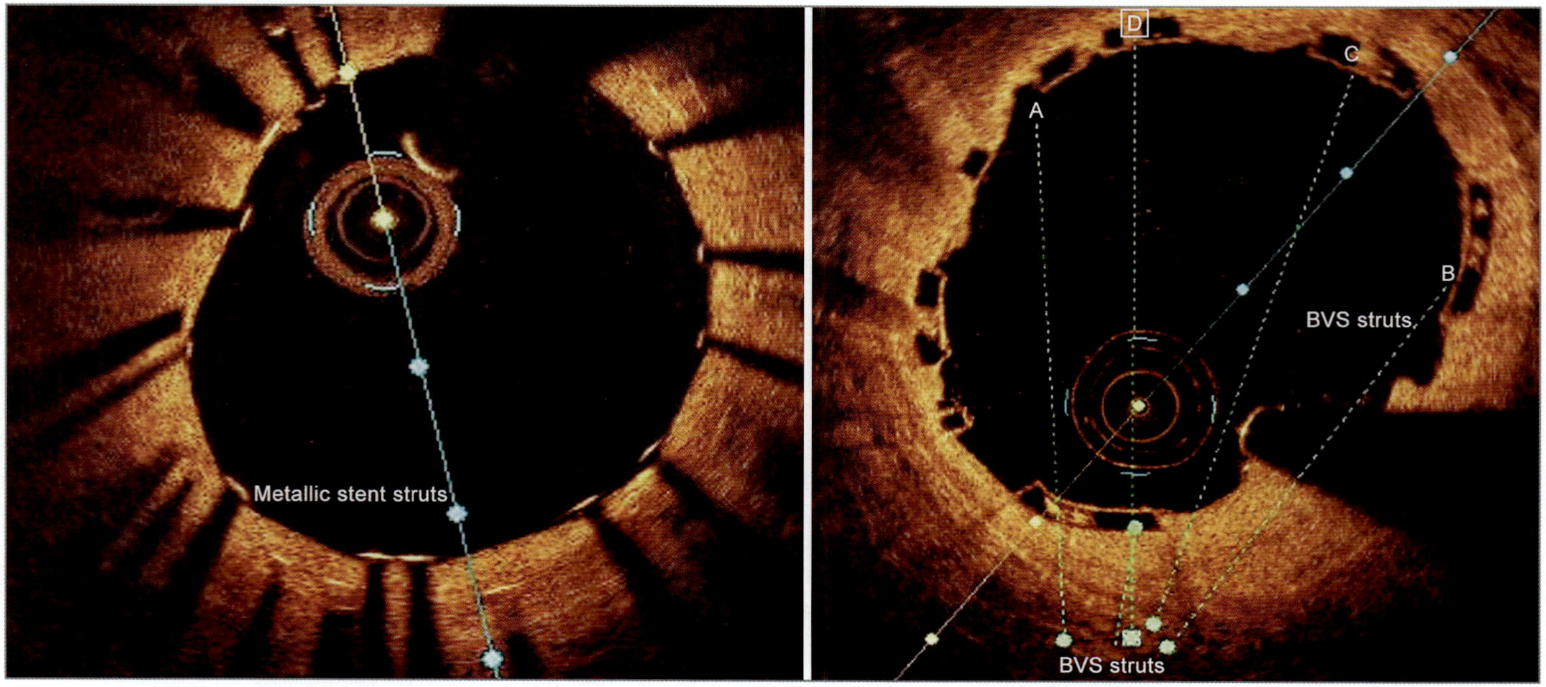

Fig. 6: Metallic and biodegradable vascular scaffold (BVS) stent struts.

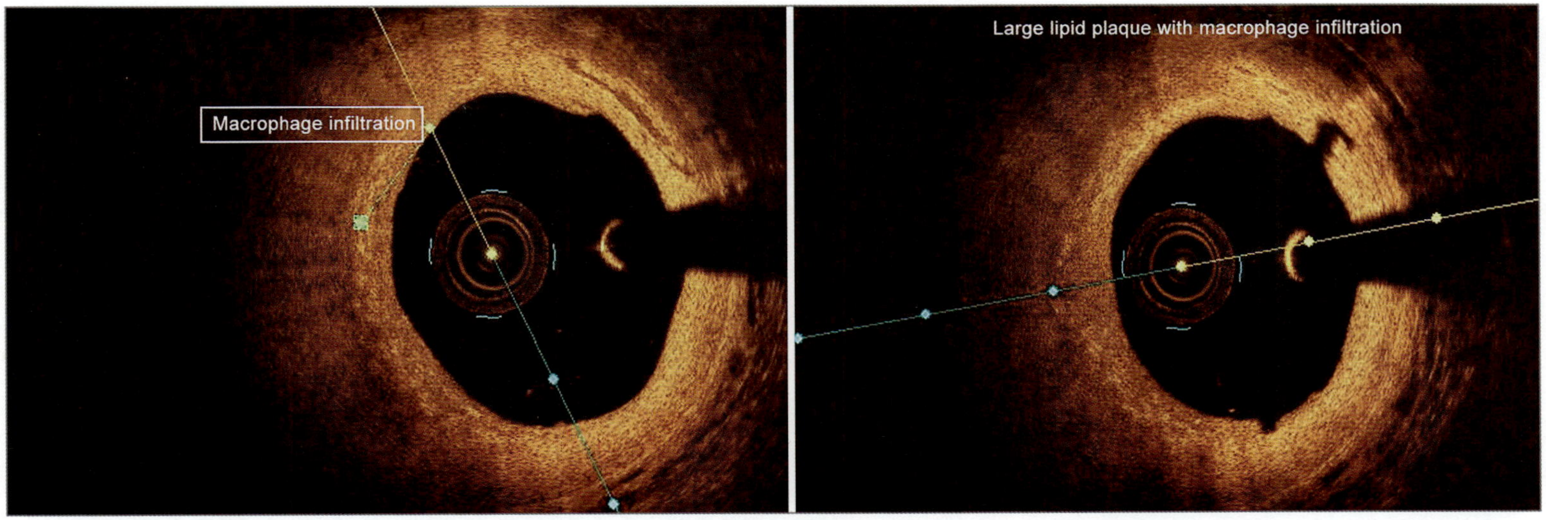

Fig. 7: Macrophages.

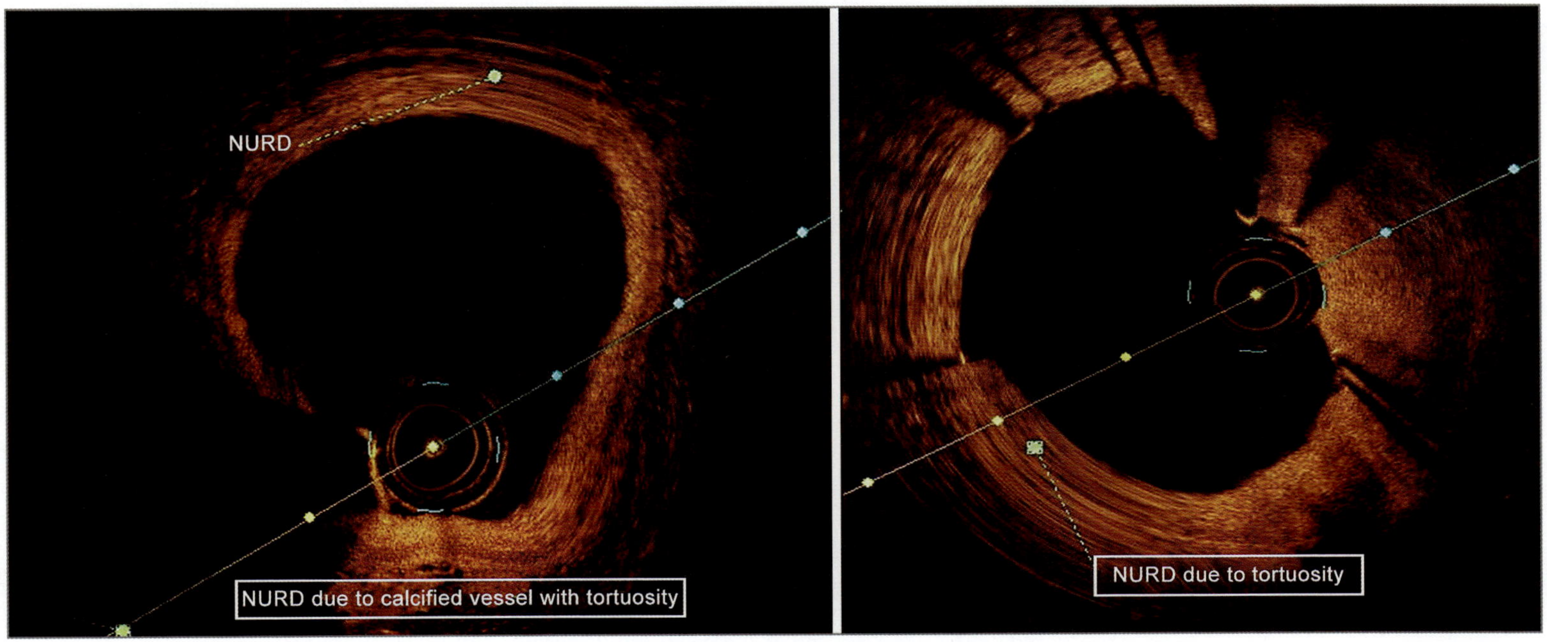

Fig. 8: Nonuniform rotational deformity (NURD).

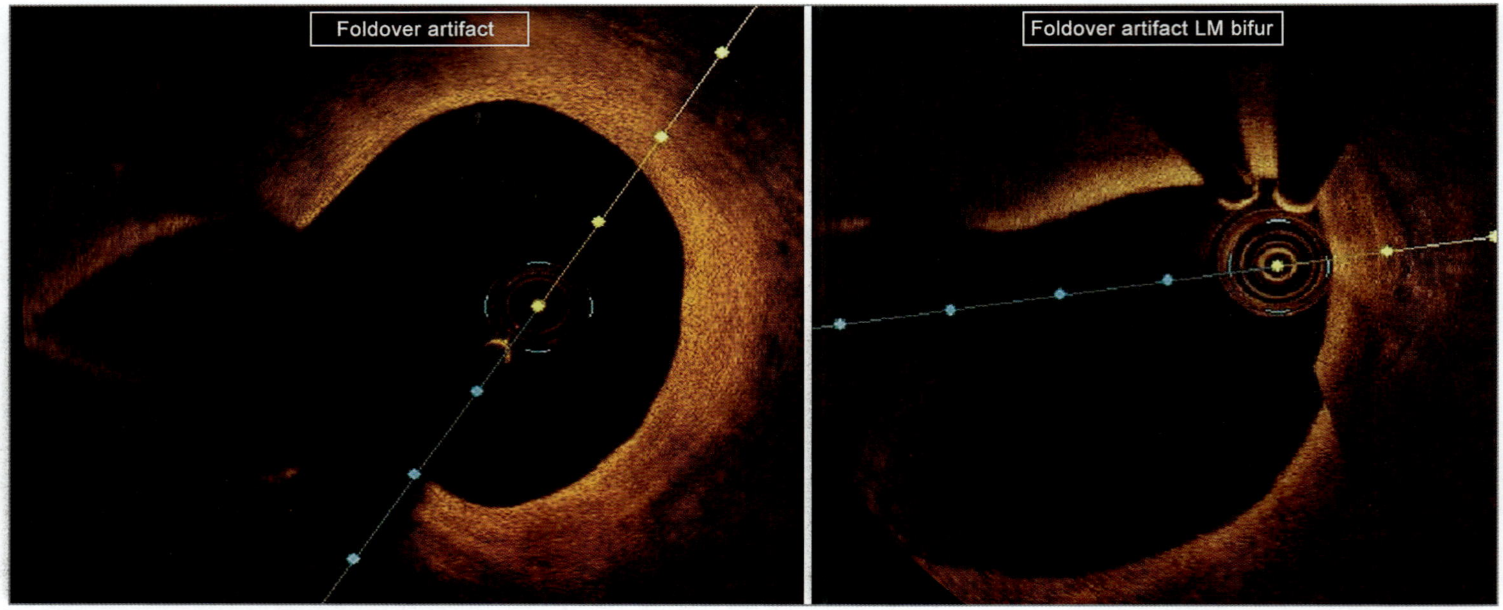

Fig. 9: Foldover artifact.

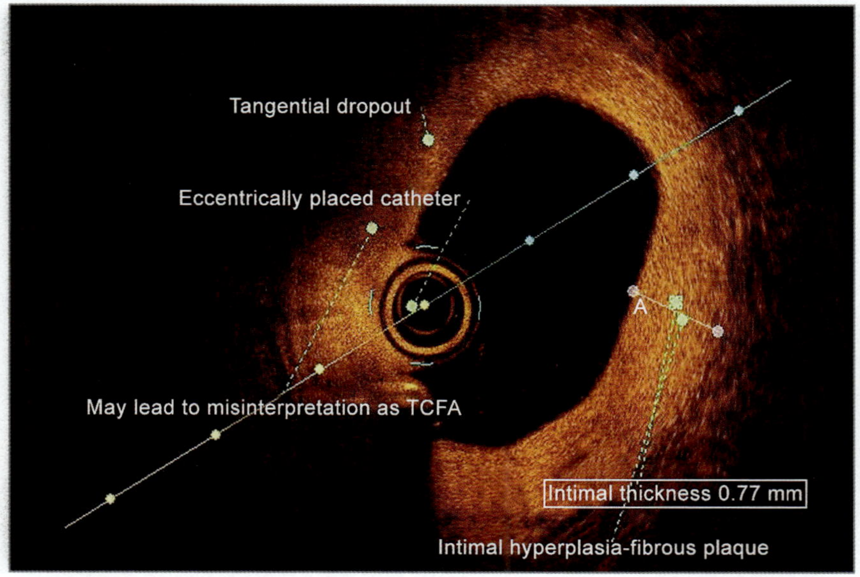

Fig. 10: Tangential light dropout. (TCFA: thin-capped fibroatheroma)

MOTION ARTIFACTS—SEW-UP OR SEAM ARTIFACT

Motion artifacts are seen as discontinuity in luminal surface as a result of artery motion that occurs during the time between the first and last A line of a cross-sectional image. Rapid artery or imaging wire movement leading to misalignment of the luminal border produces this artifact **(Fig. 11)**.[6]

OBLIQUITY/ECCENTRICITY

When the imaging catheter is centered and parallel to a cylindrical vessel, the luminal wall in OCT images will appear circular; however, when the catheter is oblique to the vessel axis, which places it closer to the artery wall in some longitudinal positions and further in others, a circular vessel will appear elliptical. This makes the measurements inaccurate **(Fig. 12)**.[4]

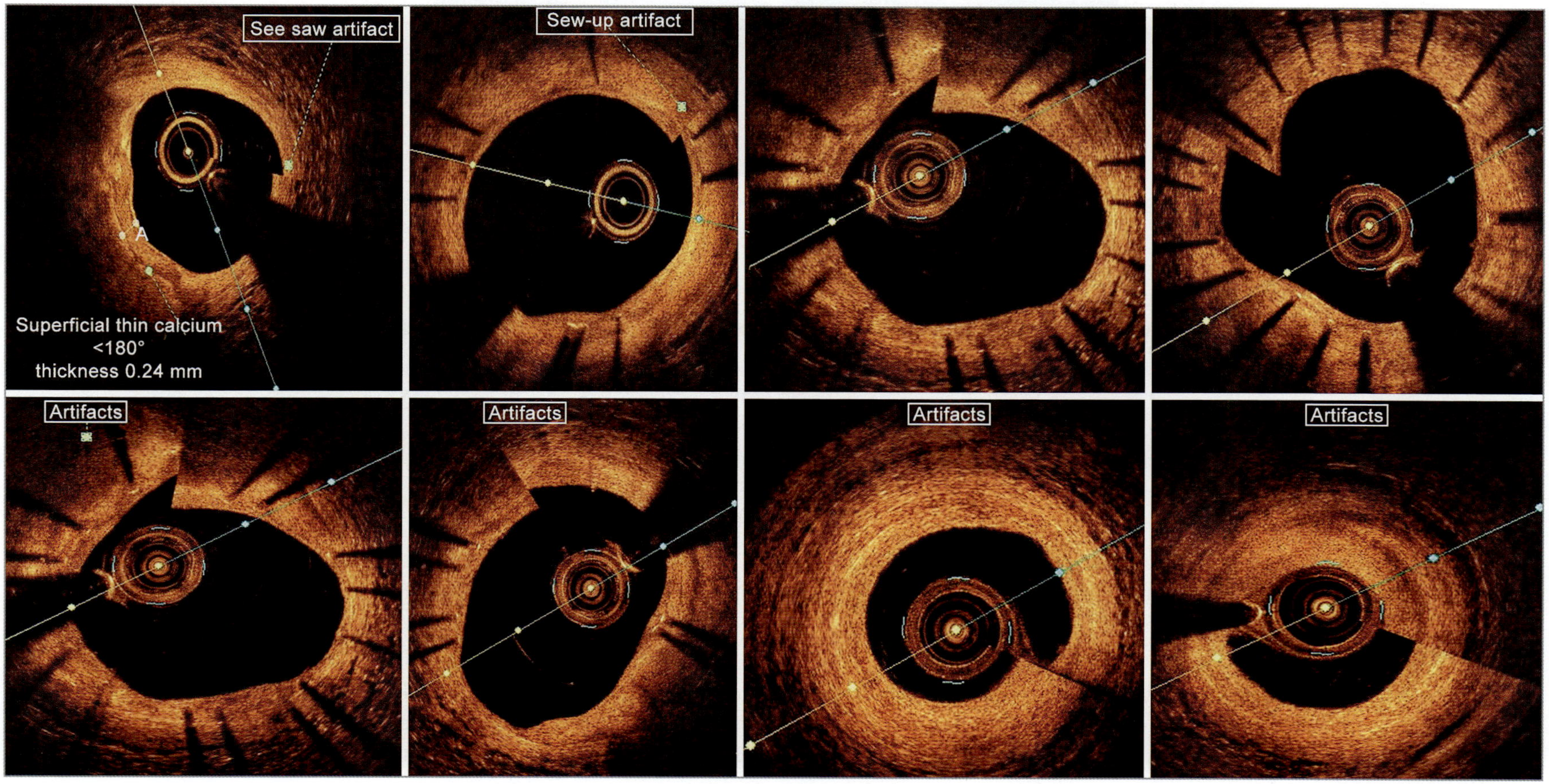

Fig. 11: Sew-up or seam artifacts.

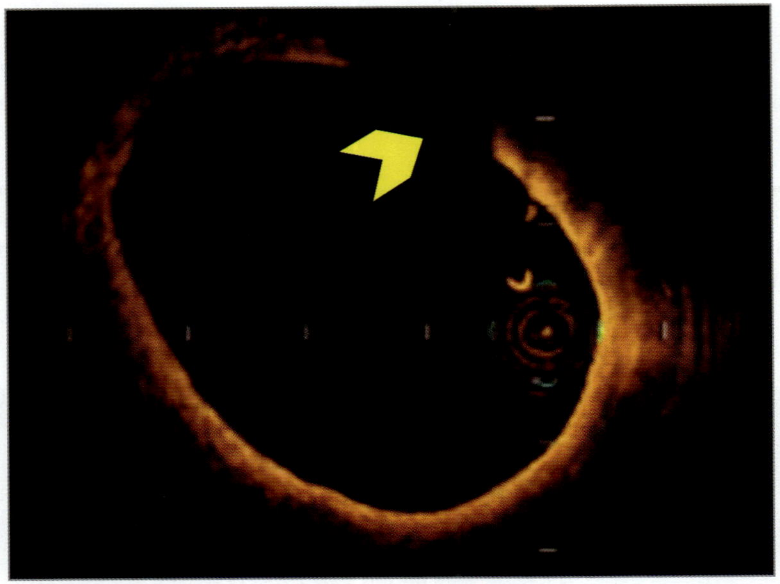

Fig. 12: Obliquity artifact, yellow arrowhead indicates shadowing artifact from guidewire.

CARROUSEL PHENOMENON

Artifact caused by eccentricity of the guidewire; **Figure 13** shows the elongation of the struts caused by the loss of resolution, illustrating the so-called carrousel phenomenon.

MERRY-GO-ROUND ARTIFACT

Merry-go-round artifact occurs when the small bright line segments that represent a stent strut appear elongated in the lateral direction **(Fig. 14)**.[4]

BLOOMING

Blooming is the increase in strut reflection thickness in the axial direction of OCT images, causing the small, bright line segment that represents the leading edge of a stent strut to appear thicker than normal, making it difficult to locate the true leading edge of the strut **(Fig. 15)**.[4]

SATURATION ARTIFACT

When a high reflector is encountered by OCT light, it may be backscattered at too high an intensity to be accurately detected by the detector.

Radial extent of the bright line can extend beyond the strongly backscattering object deep into the arterial wall. Stent struts, the guide wire, microcalcifications, and cholesterol crystals may produce these artifacts **(Fig. 16)**.[5] Saturation artifact due to air bubbles in the OCT catheter due to in proper flashing of OCT catheter.

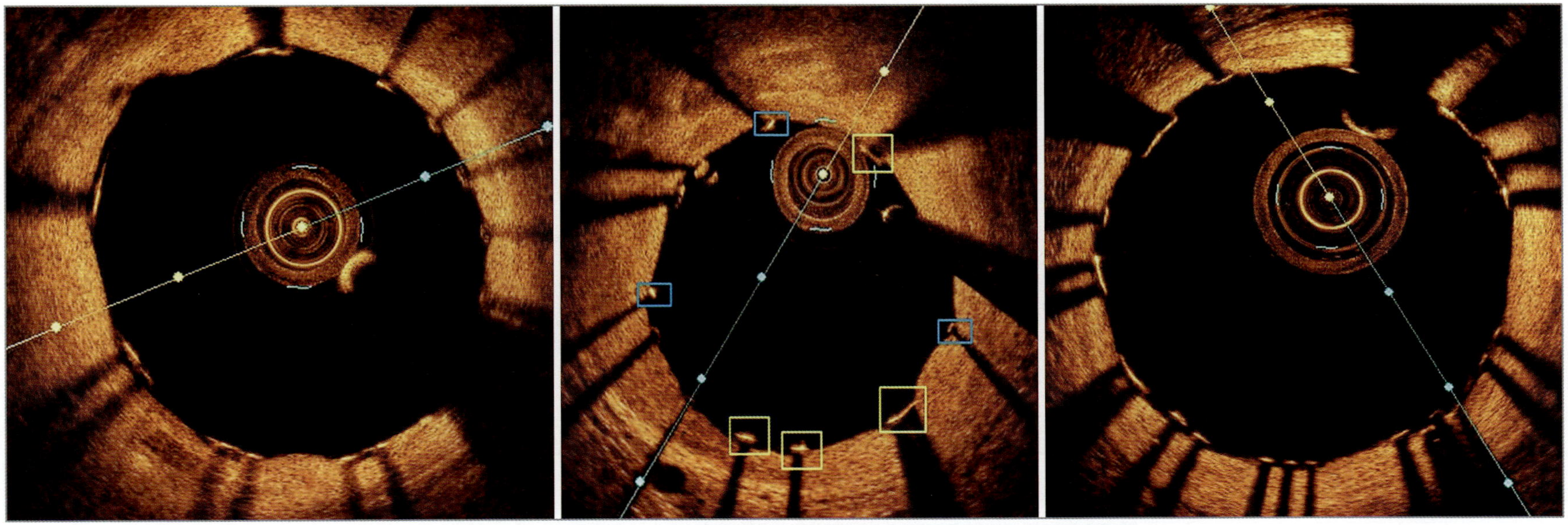

Fig. 13: Carrousel phenomenon.

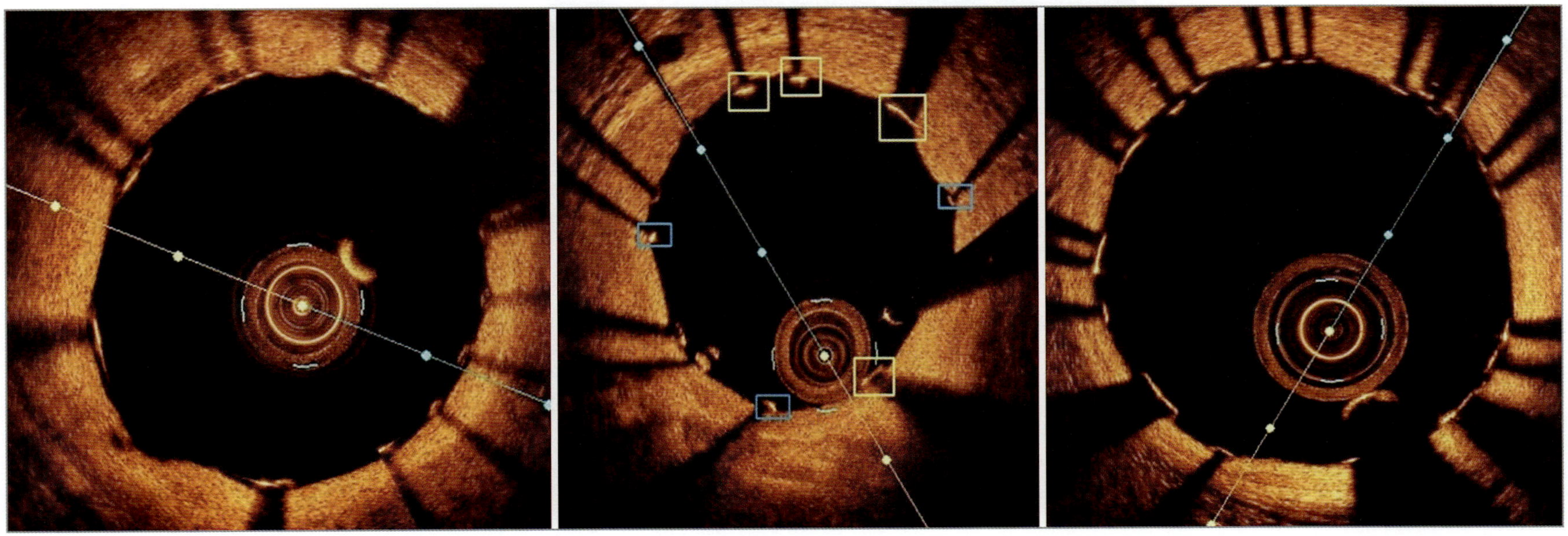

Fig. 14: Merry-go-round artifact.

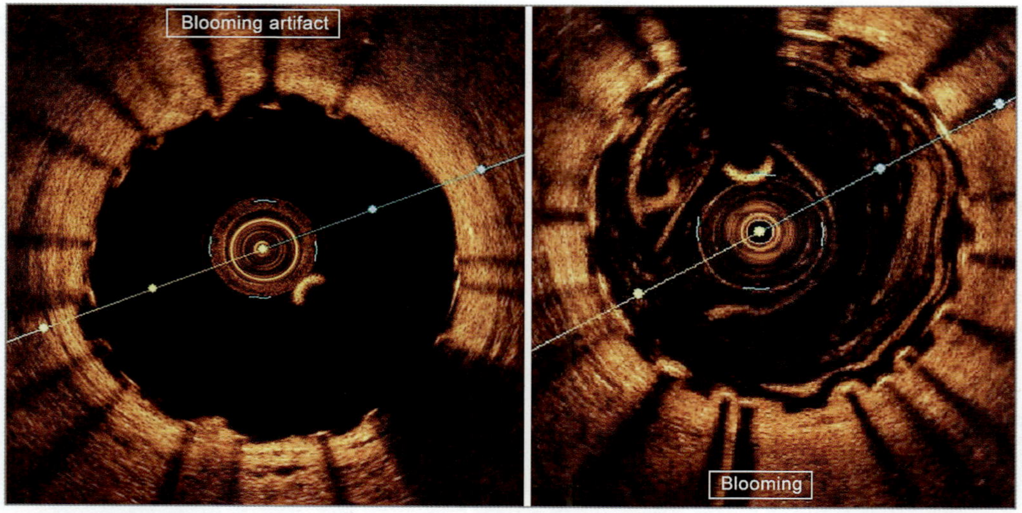

Fig. 15: Blooming.

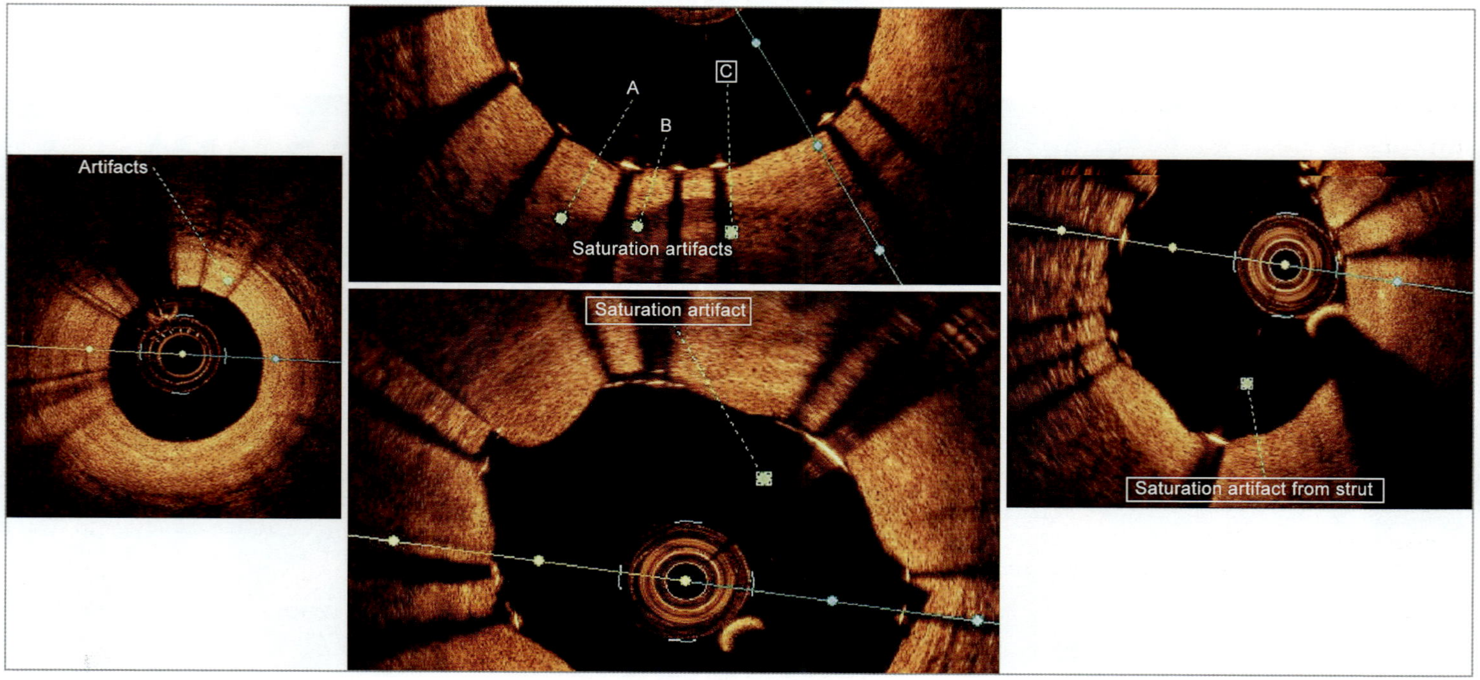

Fig. 16: Saturation artifact.

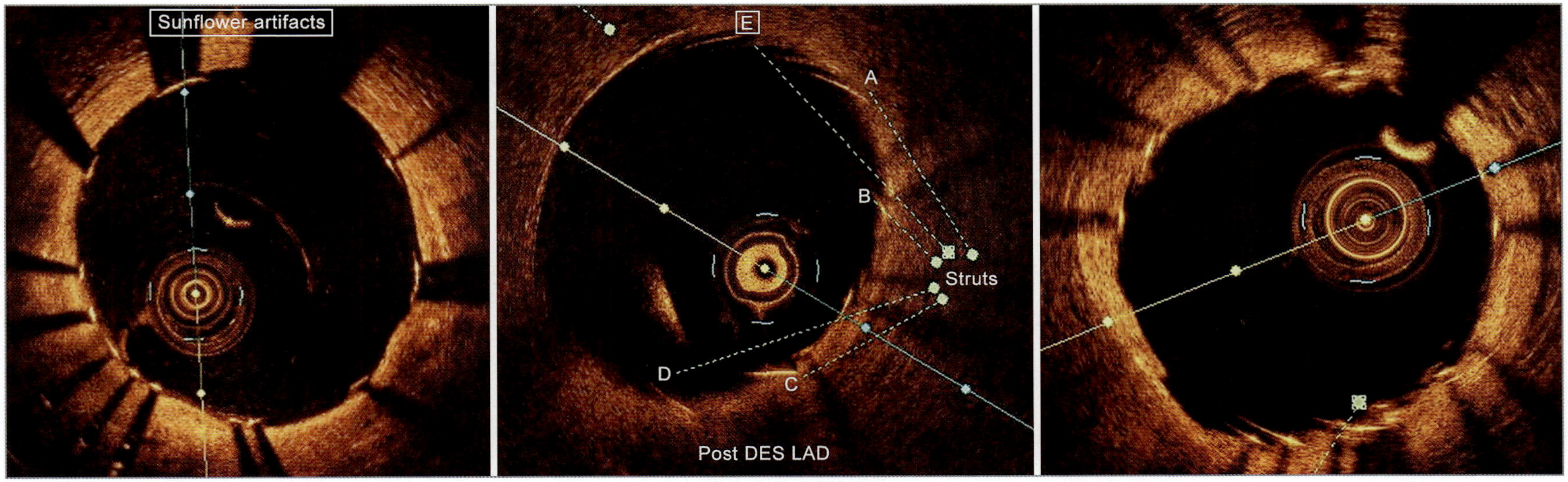

Fig. 17: Sunflower artifact.

SUNFLOWER ARTIFACT

When the OCT catheter is located in an eccentric position in the presence of metallic stent struts, the sunflower artifact can occur. Sunflower artifact occurs when stent struts appear to bend towards the OCT catheter as sunflowers grow toward the sun **(Fig. 17)**.[4]

REFERENCES

1. Herrero-Garibi J, Cruz-González I, Parejo-Díaz P, Jang IK. Optical coherence tomography: its value in intravascular diagnosis today. Revista Española de Cardiología. 2010;63(8):951-62.
2. Niida T, Murai T, Lee T, Kanaji Y, Matsuda J, Usui E, et al. Guidewire shadow artifacts in optical coherence tomography. Minerva cardioangiologica. 2017;65(2):126-33.
3. Mancuso JJ, Halaney DL, Elahi S, Ho D, Wang T, Ouyang Y, et al. Intravascular optical coherence tomography light scattering artifacts: merry-go-rounding, blooming, and ghost struts. J Biomed Opt. 2014;19(12):126017.
4. Phipps JE, Hoyt T, Halaney DL, Mancuso JJ, Milner TE, Feldman MD. Intravascular OCT Imaging Artifacts. In: Jang IK (Ed). Cardiovascular OCT Imaging. Switzerland: Springer, Cham; 2015.
5. Radiology Key. Intravascular OCT Imaging Artifacts. Available from https://radiologykey.com/intravascular-oct-imaging-artifacts/ [Last accessed February, 2024].
6. Subban V, Raffel OC, Vasu N, Victor SM, Sankardas MA. Intravascular ultrasound and optical coherence tomography for the assessment of coronary artery disease and percutaneous coronary intervention optimization: Specific lesion subsets. Indian Heart J Interv. 2018;1(2):95.

CHAPTER 28

Review of Current Update on Clinical Trials of Intravascular Imaging

Yasutsugu Shiono, Takashi Akasaka

INTRODUCTION

Coronary angiography has served as a standard imaging modality in order to visualize coronary anatomy and guide percutaneous coronary interventions (PCI) for decades. However, it has inherent limitations as a lumenogram that it can only depict vessel lumen geometry but provide little information about coronary artery walls and then it does not allow to assess vessel dimensions, plaque characteristics, and results after stent implantation in detail.

Intracoronary imaging such as intravascular ultrasound (IVUS) or optical coherence tomography (OCT) has been used to complement these shortcomings of the angiography. Intravascular imaging has been proven to be useful in variety of clinical settings such as vulnerable plaque, bifurcation, calcified lesions, poststent assessments, and so on as discussed elsewhere in this textbook.

The latest guidelines recommend IVUS as Class IIa for the severity assessment and treatment optimization in unprotected left main (LM) lesions and both IVUS and OCT for the detection of stent-related mechanical problems in a stent restenosis and for stent optimization.[1] For the stent optimization in particular, OCT has been upgraded from IIb in the previous version of guidelines to IIa in the current version, which shows that the indication of intravascular imaging is expanding.[2] Needless to say, these recommendations are based on an enormous number of previous clinical studies, but the recommendations do not cover all situations where intravascular imaging are being used in clinical practices.

To narrow this gap between the clinical practice and the guidelines recommendation, several studies are underway. In this chapter, we will introduce and summarize some of the ongoing pivotal clinical trials relevant to intravascular imaging.

IMAGING-GUIDED VERSUS ANGIOGRAPHY-GUIDED PERCUTANEOUS CORONARY INTERVENTION

Intracoronary imaging-guided PCI has proven to be superior to angiography-guided PCI mostly in IVUS studies. IVUS randomized controlled trials (RCTs) showed significant reduction in major adverse cardiac events (MACE) by IVUS-guided PCI than angiography-guided PCI, which was driven mainly by a reduction of repeat revascularization for stent restenosis.[3,4] Meta-analysis of IVUS studies[5-7] also showed a reduction of cardiovascular mortality and stent thrombosis as well as repeat revascularization.

With regard to OCT-guided PCI, the ILUMIEN III and OPINION trial showed the noninferiority of OCT-guided PCI to IVUS-guided PCI in terms of acute procedural results and midterm clinical outcomes.[8,9] Given these noninferiority studies of OCT-guided versus IVUS-guided PCI, we might be able to presume that OCT-guided PCI would be superior to angio-guided PCI. However, there has been no RCT comparing OCT-guided versus angiography-guided PCI, so some RCTs are underway.

ILUMIEN IV: OPTIMAL PCI (NCT03507777)

The Optical Coherence Tomography (OCT) Guided Coronary Stent Implantation Compared to Angiography: a Multicenter Randomized TriaL in PCI (ILUMIEN IV: OPTIMAL PCI) is a prospective, multicenter, single-blind, randomized study to compare OCT-guided coronary stent implantation versus angiography-guided coronary stent implantation.[10] The objective of this study is to show the superiority of OCT-guided PCI as compared with angiography-guided PCI in terms of post-PCI lumen dimensions and clinical cardiovascular outcomes. Post-PCI minimum stent area (MSA) and target vessel failure (TVF) defined as cardiac death, target vessel myocardial infarction (MI), or ischemia-driven target vessel revascularization (TVR) at a minimum of 1 year and up to 2 years are going to be assessed as the primary endpoints. A total of 3,656 subjects with high-risk clinical characteristics and angiographic lesions are expected to be enrolled from 125 global sites in North America (US and Canada), Europe, Middle East, and Asia–Pacific.

OCTOBER (NCT03171311)

The European Trial on Optical Coherence Tomography Optimized Bifurcation Event Reduction (The OCTOBER Trial) is an investigator initiated and investigator sponsored, randomized, controlled, prospective, multicenter, superiority trial comparing OCT-guided versus angio-guided revascularization in patients requiring complex bifurcation stent implantation.[11] This study is designed to show the superiority of OCT-guided PCI as compared with angiography-guided PCI in terms of 2-year clinical outcome in patients who have bifurcation stenting. Major adverse cardiovascular events (MACE) that consist of cardiac death, target lesion MI, and ischemic-driven target lesion revascularization (TLR) at 24 months are going to be assessed as primary endpoints. A total of 1,200 patients who require bifurcation stenting are going to be enrolled from the European centers.

COCOA (NCT03176810/UMIN000026021)

The Comparison between Optimal Coherence tomography guidance and Angiography Guidance in percutaneous coronary intervention (COCOA) study is a multicenter, prospective, randomized, controlled, open-label, parallel group study.[12] The purpose of this study is to demonstrate the superiority of OCT-guided PCI compared with angiography-guided PCI in terms of MSA immediately after stent implantation. The patient enrollment has been finished and 550 patients who had de novo coronary lesions were enrolled in Japan. Primary endpoint is MSA measured by OCT immediately after index PCI.

RENOVATE-COMPLEX-PCI (NCT03381872)

Intravascular Imaging versus Angiography-Guided Percutaneous Coronary Intervention for Complex Coronary Artery Disease (RENOVATE) study is a multicenter, prospective, randomized, controlled, open-label, parallel group study.[13] This study aims to compare clinical outcomes between intravascular imaging-guided versus angiography-guided PCI in complex lesions. A total of 1,620 subjects with complex coronary artery disease such as a true bifurcation lesion, chronic total occlusion (CTO), unprotected LM disease, lesions requiring long or multiple stenting, multi-vessel PCI, in-stent restenosis, and severely calcified lesions are enrolled in Korea. Unique feature of this study is that choice of intravascular imaging modalities by means of IVUS or OCT in the imaging-guided PCI arm is left to the operator's discretion to maximize the advantage of intravascular imaging according to the types of complex lesions. The TVF which consists of cardiac death and target vessel MI and TVR at 1-year after PCI is going to be assessed as the primary endpoint.

POTENTIAL VALUE OF VULNERABLE PLAQUE DETECTION AND INTERVENTIONAL PLAQUE PASSIVATION

One of the strengths of intravascular imaging is the detection of vulnerable plaques which potentially lead to coronary artery thrombosis and cause cardiovascular events including acute coronary syndrome (ACS) or sudden cardiac death. It has been shown that vulnerable plaques detected by intravascular imaging is associated with cardiovascular events. For example, the PROSPECT study showed features such as a minimum lumen area (MLA)

≤4 mm^2, a plaque burden ≥70%, and thin-cap fibroatheroma (TCFA) were predictors of subsequent MACE and the more of these features patients have, the more likely they have MACE, and those with all of the three high-risk features have 11 times risk of MACE compared with those without them.[14] At the same time, the positive predictive value (PPV) of these three high-risk features is as low as about 18.2% within a 3.4-year follow-up. Several studies using IVUS, near-infrared spectroscopy (NIRS)–IVUS, and OCT have demonstrated similar results that intravascular imaging-detected vulnerable plaque is associated with higher rate of cardiovascular events, but their PPV is low (17–23%) despite its high negative predictive value (NPV) (93–98%).[15-17]

Some studies are underway to test the potential value of vulnerable plaque detection by intravascular imaging and further the value of interventional passivation of vulnerable plaque to prevent future coronary events.

COMBINE OCT-FFR (NCT02989740)

The Combined Optical Coherence Tomography Morphologic and Fractional Flow Reserve Hemodynamic Assessment of Non-Culprit Lesions to Better Predict Adverse Event Outcomes in Diabetes Mellitus Patients COMBINE (OCT-FFR) Prospective Register (COMBINE OCT-FFR) is a prospective natural history registry.[18] The purpose of this study is to investigate the natural evolution of patients with at least one intermediate angiographic but nonhemodynamic significant stenotic lesion, in two subgroups of patients, with TCFA versus no TCFA as detected by OCT and to compare these two groups of patients with each other as well as with patients with fractional flow reserve (FFR)-positive and PCI-treated intermediate lesions on MACE. A total of 550 patients are expected to be enrolled. The primary endpoint is the per-patient incidence of the target lesion-related composite MACE defined as cardiac death, MI, clinically driven TLR, or hospitalization due to unstable or progressive angina at 18 months.

PROSPECT II and PROSPECT ABSORB (NCT02171065)

This study consists of two components: A Multicenter Prospective Natural History Study Using Multimodality Imaging in Patients With Acute Coronary Syndromes—PROSPECT II (Natural History Study) and Combined With a Randomized, Controlled, Intervention Study—PROSPECT ABSORB (randomized trial).[19] Firstly, PROSPECT II is a prospective observational study using multimodality imaging to examine the natural history of patients with unstable atherosclerotic coronary artery disease with the specific goal to establish the utility of IVUS and NIRS to identify plaques prone to future rupture and clinical events. Secondly, the randomized PROSPECT ABSORB is a randomized, open label, prospective, parallel study to examine whether treatment of vulnerable plaques with the ABSORB bioresorbable vascular scaffold (BVS) plus guideline-directed medical therapy (GDMT) safely increase the minimal lumen diameter (MLD) at 25 months compared with GDMT alone.

A total of 902 ACS (ST-elevation MI or non-ST-elevation MI) patients who required PCI have been enrolled. The primary endpoint is patient level nonculprit lesion-related nonculprit MACE through 2 years.

PREVENT (NCT02316886)

The Preventive Coronary Intervention on Stenosis with Functionally Insignificant Stenosis with Vulnerable Plaque Characteristics (PREVENT) is a parallel, open-label, randomized study to determine whether preventive coronary intervention on functionally insignificant coronary stenosis with vulnerable plaque characteristics plus optimal medical therapy reduces the incidence of cardiovascular events compared with optimal medical therapy alone.[20] Patients who have at least a coronary stenosis with >50% diameter stenosis with functionally nonsignificant FFR (>0.80) and meeting two of the following vulnerable features: MLA <4 mm^2, plaque burden >70%, lipid-rich plaque on NIRS defined as max lipid-core burden index $(\text{LCBI})_{4\text{mm}}$ >315, TCFA defined by OCT or virtual histology (VH)-IVUS are going to be enrolled and randomized. A total of 1,600 participants are expected to be enrolled. TVF at 2 years defined as a composite of cardiac death, target vessel-related MI, ischemia-driven TVR, or unplanned hospitalization for angina are assessed as the primary endpoint.

BIFURCATION LESIONS

Coronary bifurcations are frequently encountered in daily practice that account for 15–20% of all PCIs and are still one of the most challenging lesions in interventional cardiology in terms of early procedural success as well as long-term outcomes. Despite careful assessment by multiple projections, angiography can only provide limited information in bifurcation lesions. Bifurcation lesions are thought to be one of the lesions that interventional cardiologists benefit most from intravascular imaging that can provide crucial information in planning and optimizing stent treatments.

Many IVUS studies have reported its usefulness in bifurcation lesions, mainly in LM bifurcation and a consensus statement has been published in IVUS.[21] There is no such consensus document dedicated to OCT use in bifurcation. But OCT has nearly 10 times the spatial resolution of IVUS and its excellent image quality enables the construction of vivid three-dimensional (3D) images of coronary arteries and implanted stents. This excellent piece of intracoronary OCT engineering is expected to provide clinical benefits through planning to optimizing stages of stent implantation. One prospective registry of 3D-OCT in bifurcation lesions is going on.

Japanese 3D-OCT Bifurcation Registry (UMIN000026759)

The Japanese prospective observational study of 3D-OCT guided bifurcation PCI (Japanese 3D-OCT Bifurcation Registry) is a prospective multicenter observational study which is aimed to assess the link between initial results of 3D-OCT-guided bifurcation PCI and subsequent clinical outcomes and to investigate the clinical benefit of 3D-OCT-guided PCI in bifurcation lesions.[22] This study is going to enroll 600 patients who have de novo bifurcation lesions and require bifurcation stentings. Primary endpoint is going to be assessed by the incidence of side branch restenosis within 1 year after the initial PCIs among those who had optimal side branch dilatation, suboptimal side branch dilatation, and no side branch dilatation.

SEVERELY CALCIFIED LESIONS

Severely calcified coronary artery disease is another challenging lesion and is often encountered in patients who undergo PCI. Calcified plaques are often underappreciated by angiography alone, but their accurate assessments are crucial for planning the treatment strategy in PCI. Intracoronary imaging helps to detect, localize, and quantify coronary calcification, and thus can provide indispensable information for PCI. In particular, OCT has advantages over IVUS because OCT can penetrate calcium to a certain depth, measure its thickness, and then assess calcified plaques more quantitatively than IVUS.

In many cases with heavily calcified lesions, debulking or lesion modification are performed by means of cutting balloons, rotational or orbital atherectomy, laser therapy, and lithotripsy. These treatments are effective in calcified lesions, but their risks of procedure-related complications are not negligible. Intravascular imaging can be used to enable safe and effective deliveries of these treatments and also assess their results immediately after the procedures. So intravascular imaging has the potential to improve the outcome of PCIs in severely calcified lesions.

ECLIPSE (NCT03108456)

The Evaluation of Treatment Strategies for Severe CaLcIfic Coronary Arteries: Orbital Atherectomy vs. Conventional Angioplasty Technique Prior to Implantation of Drug-Eluting StEnts (ECLIPSE) trial is a prospective, multicenter, open-label, parallel assignment, randomized trial which aims at evaluating orbital atherectomy compared to conventional balloon angioplasty technique for the treatment of severely calcified lesions prior to implantation of drug-eluting stents (DES).[23] A total of 2,000 patients are expected to be enrolled. MSA measured by OCT at the end of the index procedure is going to be assessed as a primary endpoint and also TVF at 1 year defined as a composite of cardiac death, target vessel-related MI, or ischemia-driven TVR at 1 year after PCI are to be assessed.

DISRUPT CAD III (NCT03595176)

Prospective, Multicenter, Single-Arm, Global IDE Study of the Shockwave Coronary Intravascular Lithotripsy (IVL) System With the Shockwave C2 Coronary IVL Catheter in Calcified Coronary Arteries (DISRUPT CAD III) is a prospective, multicenter, single-arm, global investigational device exemption (IDE) study to evaluate the safety and effectiveness of the shockwave medical coronary intravascular lithotripsy (IVL) system in de novo, calcified, stenotic coronary arteries prior to stenting.[24] A total of 392 patients with severely calcified de novo lesions are to be enrolled. A 30-day MACE defined as a composite of cardiac death, MI, and TVR and number of patients who had a successful index procedure and without inhospital MACE are to be assessed.

CONCLUSION

Several studies are underway in many situations where intravascular imaging will provide benefits for coronary artery disease patients and interventional cardiologists who treat them as aforementioned and summarized in **Table 1**. When the results of these trials come out and prove the benefits as expected, the future versions of guidelines will be revised more in favor of the imaging-guided PCI, change our practice, and eventually lead to improvement of patients outcome.

TABLE 1: Ongoing studies in intravascular imaging.

Study	*Estimated number*	*Population*	*Design*	*Primary endpoint*
OCT-guided versus angiography-guided PCI				
ILUMIEN IV[10]	3,656	Patients with high-risk clinical and angiographic characteristics	RCT	Post-PCI MSA and TVF at 1 year and up to 2 years
OCTOBER[11]	1,200	Patients requiring complex bifurcation stenting	RCT	MACE at 24 months
COCOA[12]	550	Patients with de novo coronary lesions	RCT	MSA by OCT after index PCI
RENOVATE COMPLEX PCI[13]	1,620	Patients with complex coronary artery disease	RCT	TVF at 1 year
Vulnerable plaque detection and plaque sealing				
COMBINE OCT-FFR[18]	550	Patients with angiographic intermediate but nonhemodynamically significant lesions	Prospective observational study	Target lesion-related composite MACE at 18 months
PROSPECT II[19]	902	Patients with STEMI or NSTEMI	Prospective observational study	Patient level nonculprit lesion-related nonculprit MACE through 2 years
PROSPECT ABSORB[19]	902	Patients with STEMI or NSTEMI	RCT	Patient level nonculprit lesion-related nonculprit MACE through 2 years
PREVENT[20]	1,600	Patients who have coronary stenosis with >50% DS with nonsignificant FFR and vulnerable features	RCT	TVF at 2 years

Contd...

Contd...

Study	Estimated number	Population	Design	Primary endpoint
Bifurcation				
Japanese 3D-OCT Bifurcation Registry[22]	600	Patients who have de novo bifurcation lesions and require bifurcation stentings	Prospective observational study	The incidence of side branch restenosis within 1 year
Severely calcified lesions				
ECLIPSE[23]	2,000	Patients with severely calcified lesions	RCT	MSA by OCT at the end of the index procedure and TVF at 1 year
DISRUPT CAD III[24]	392	Patients with severely calcified de novo lesions	RCT	A 30-day MACE and number of patients who had a successful index procedure and without inhospital MACE

(DS: diameter stenosis; FFR: fractional flow reserve; MACE: major adverse cardiovascular event; MSA: minimal stent area; NSTEMI: non-ST-elevation myocardial infarction; OCT: optical coherence tomography; PCI: percutaneous coronary intervention; RCT: randomized controlled trial; STEMI: ST-elevation myocardial infarction; TVF: target vessel failure)

REFERENCES

1. Neumann FJ, Sousa-Uva M, Ahlsson A, Alfonso F, Banning AP, Benedetto U, et al. 2018 ESC/EACTS Guidelines on myocardial revascularization. Eur Heart J. 2019;40:87-165.
2. Windecker S, Kolh P, Alfonso F, Collet JP, Cremer J, Falk V, et al. Authors/Task Force members. 2014 ESC/EACTS Guidelines on myocardial revascularization: The Task Force on Myocardial Revascularization of the European Society of Cardiology (ESC) and the European Association for Cardio-Thoracic Surgery (EACTS) Developed with the special contribution of the European Association of Percutaneous Cardiovascular Interventions (EAPCI). Eur Heart J. 2014;35:2541-619.
3. Hong S-J, Kim B-K, Shin D-H, Nam CM, Kim JS, Ko YG, et al. Effect of intravascular ultrasound-guided vs angiography-guided everolimus-eluting stent implantation: the IVUS-XPL Randomized Clinical Trial. JAMA. 2015;314:2155-63.
4. Kim B-K, Shin D-H, Hong M-K, Park HS, Rha SW, Mintz GS, et al. Clinical impact of intravascular ultrasound-guided chronic total occlusion intervention with zotarolimus-eluting versus biolimus-eluting stent implantation: randomized study. Circ Cardiovasc Interv. 2015;8:e002592.
5. Elgendy IY, Mahmoud AN, Elgendy AY, Bavry AA. Outcomes with intravascular ultrasound-guided stent implantation: a meta-analysis of randomized trials in the era of drug-eluting stents. Circ Cardiovasc Interv. 2016;9:e003700.
6. Shin D-H, Hong S-J, Mintz GS, Kim JS, Kim BK, Ko YG, et al. Effects of intravascular ultrasound-guided versus angiography-guided new-generation drug-eluting stent implantation: meta-analysis with individual patient-level data from 2,345 Randomized Patients. JACC Cardiovasc Interv. 2016;9:2232-9.
7. Bavishi C, Sardar P, Chatterjee S, Khan AR, Shah A, Ather S, et al. Intravascular ultrasound-guided vs angiography-guided drug-eluting stent implantation in complex coronary lesions: meta-analysis of randomized trials. Am Heart J. 2017;185:26-34.
8. Ali ZA, Maehara A, Généreux P, Shlofmitz RA, Fabbiocchi F, Nazif TM, et al. Optical coherence tomography compared with intravascular ultrasound and with angiography to guide coronary stent implantation (ILUMIEN III: OPTIMIZE PCI): a randomised controlled trial. Lancet. 2016;388:2618-28.
9. Kubo T, Shinke T, Okamura T, Hibi K, Nakazawa G, Morino Y, et al. Optical frequency domain imaging vs. intravascular ultrasound in percutaneous coronary intervention (OPINION trial): one-year angiographic and clinical results. Eur Heart J. 2017;38:3139-47.
10. ClinicalTrials.gov. (2023). ILUMIEN IV: OPTIMAL PCI. Available from https://clinicaltrials.gov/ct2/show/NCT03507777 [Last accessed February, 2024].
11. ClinicalTrials.gov. (2023). The OCTOBER Trial - European Trial on Optical Coherence Tomography Optimized Bifurcation Event Reduction (OCTOBER) (OCTOBER). Available from https://clinicaltrials.gov/ct2/show/NCT03171311 [Last accessed February, 2024].

12. Kubo T, Shinke T, Okamura T, Hibi K, Nakazawa G, Morino Y, et al. Comparison between Optical Coherence tomography guidance and Angiography guidance in percutaneous coronary intervention (COCOA): study protocol for a randomized controlled trial. J Cardiol. 2018;72(2):170-5.
13. ClinicalTrials.gov. (2023). Intravascular Imaging- Versus Angiography-Guided Percutaneous Coronary Intervention For Complex Coronary Artery Disease (RENOVATE). Available from https://clinicaltrials.gov/ct2/show/NCT03381872 [Last accessed February, 2024].
14. Stone GW, Maehara A, Lansky AJ, de Bruyne B, Cristea E, Mintz GS, et al. A prospective natural-history study of coronary atherosclerosis. N Engl J Med. 2011;364:226-35.
15. Cheng JM, Garcia-Garcia HM, de Boer SP, Kardys I, Heo JH, Akkerhuis KM, et al. In vivo detection of high-risk coronary plaques by radiofrequency intravascular ultrasound and cardiovascular outcome: results of the ATHEROREMO-IVUS study. Eur Heart J. 2014;35:639-47.
16. Oemrawsingh RM, Cheng JM, Garcia-Garcia HM, van Geuns RJ, de Boer SP, Simsek C, et al. Near-infrared spectroscopy predicts cardiovascular outcome in patients with coronary artery disease. J Am Coll Cardiol. 2014;64:2510-8.
17. Waksman R. (2018). Assessment of coronary near-infrared spectroscopy imaging to detect vulnerable plaques and vulnerable patients. The Lipid-Rich Plaque Study. Available from https://www.tctmd.com/slide/lrp-assessment-coronary-near-infrared-spectroscopy-imaging-detect-vulnerable-plaques-and-vulnerable-patients [Last accessed February, 2024].
18. ClinicalTrials.gov. (2021). Optical Coherence Tomography Morphologic and Fractional Flow Reserve Assessment in Diabetes Mellitus Patients (COMBINE). Available from https://clinicaltrials.gov/ct2/show/NCT02989740 [Last accessed February, 2024].
19. ClinicalTrials.gov. (2021). PROSPECT II & PROSPECT ABSORB - an Integrated Natural History Study and Randomized Trial. (P2). Available from https://clinicaltrials.gov/ct2/show/NCT02171065 [Last accessed February, 2024].
20. ClinicalTrials.gov. (2023). Preventive PCI or Medical Therapy Alone for Vulnerable Atherosclerotic Coronary Plaque (PREVENT). Available from https://clinicaltrials.gov/ct2/show/NCT02316886 [Last accessed February, 2024].
21. Mintz GS, Lefèvre T, Lassen JF, Testa L, Pan M, Singh J, et al. Intravascular ultrasound in the evaluation and treatment of left main coronary artery disease: a consensus statement from the European Bifurcation Club. EuroIntervention. 2018;14:e467-74.
22. UMIN-CTR Clinical Trial. (2021). Japanese prospective observational study of 3D-OCT guided bifurcation PCI. Available from https://upload.umin.ac.jp/cgi-open-bin/ctr_e/ctr_view.cgi?recptno=R000030721 [Last accessed February, 2024].
23. ClinicalTrials.gov. (2023). Evaluation of Treatment Strategies for Severe CaLcIfic Coronary Arteries: Orbital Atherectomy vs. Conventional Angioplasty Technique Prior to Implantation of Drug-Eluting StEnts: The ECLIPSE Trial (ECLIPSE). Available from https://clinicaltrials.gov/ct2/show/NCT03108456 [Last accessed February, 2024].
24. ClinicalTrials.gov. (2023). Disrupt CAD III With the Shockwave Coronary IVL System. Available from https://clinicaltrials.gov/ct2/show/NCT03595176 [Last accessed February, 2024].

Optical Coherence Tomography New Algorithm

CHAPTER 29

INTRODUCTION

New Algorithm of OCT is a simple way but effective way of optimization of DES implantation by acquiring at least two runs of OCT imaging. Each optical coherence tomography (OCT) run serves a separate purpose. The pre-PCI (percutaneous coronary intervention) run helps determine the PCI strategy, and the post-PCI run allows for optimization of the stent as needed **(Fig. 1)**.

PRE-PCI OCT—STRATEGIZE (MLD) (FIG. 2A)

Morphology (Fig. 2B)

The morphology of the normal coronary artery and the plaque characterization has been discussed earlier in the Chapter 1. This new algorithm helps a beginner to interpret in a simple way. According to this classification, pre-OCT run and assessment has to do plaque modification of the vessel before stenting. The morphology of a coronary artery includes lipid plaque, fibrotic plaque, and calcium (mild, moderate, and severe) or sometimes any of the combination to decide direct stenting or plaque modification with complaint or noncompliant (NC) balloons (regular NC/OPN NC), atherectomy (rotational/orbital) or intravascular lithotripsy (IVL) followed by stenting.

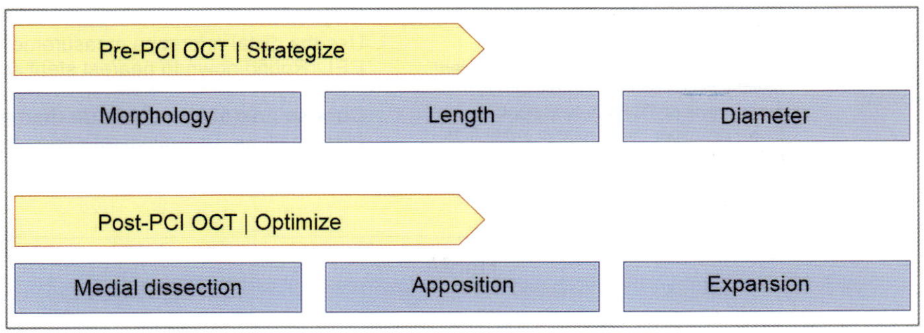

Fig. 1: Modern OCT-guided PCI workflow. (OCT: optical coherence tomography; PCI: percutaneous coronary intervention)

Length (Figs. 2C and D)

Selecting the landing zones—visually scan for largest luminal area, place landing zones in healthy tissue [i.e., external elastic lamina (EEL) visualization]. In the absence of EEL to represent healthy tissue find the largest lumen to avoid areas of thin-cap fibroatheroma (TCFA) or lipid pools so as to not land your stent edge in these high-risk areas.

Diameter (Figs. 2E and F)

To measure vessel diameter, take EEL measurements at each reference (lumen if EEL not visible). To choose stent diameter, use the distal reference measurement to select stent diameter.

External elastic lamina—Round down to nearest stent size; lumen—round up. To choose postdilation balloon diameter, for distal balloon, use distal reference measurement and for proximal balloon use proximal reference measurement.

EEL measurements:

- Average two perpendicular EEL measurements.
- Round down to the next quarter size, unless already at a stent size.

Lumen measurements:

- Use automatic measurements at distal reference.
- Round up to the next quarter size, even if already at a stent size.

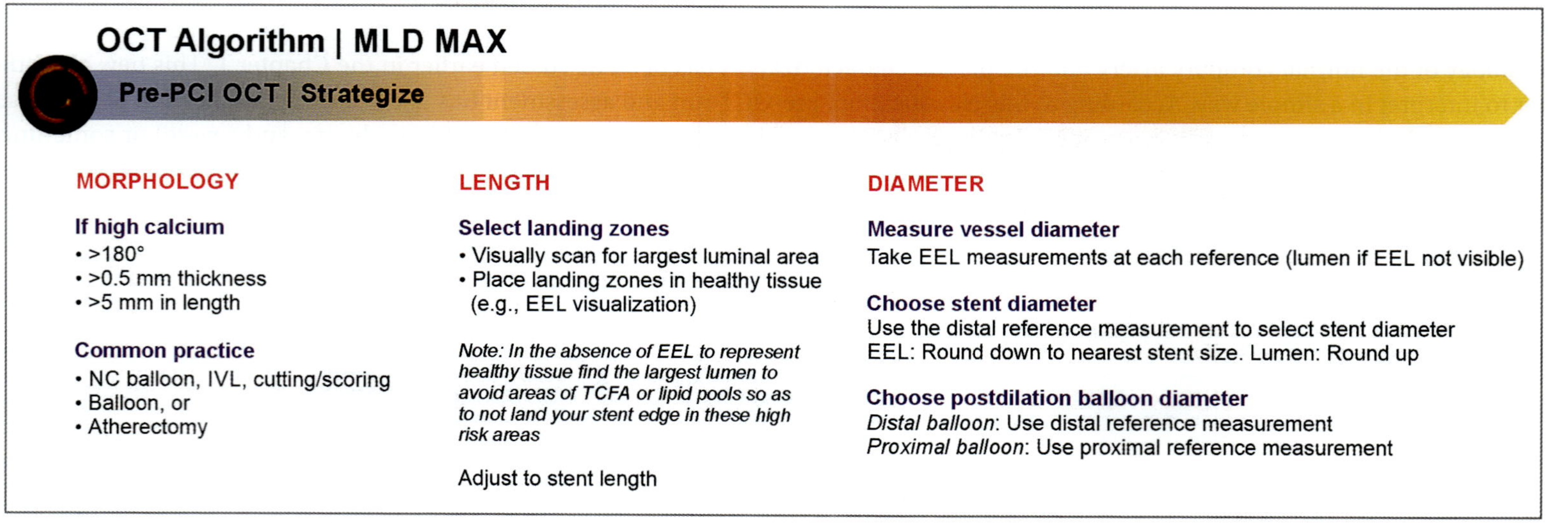

Fig. 2A

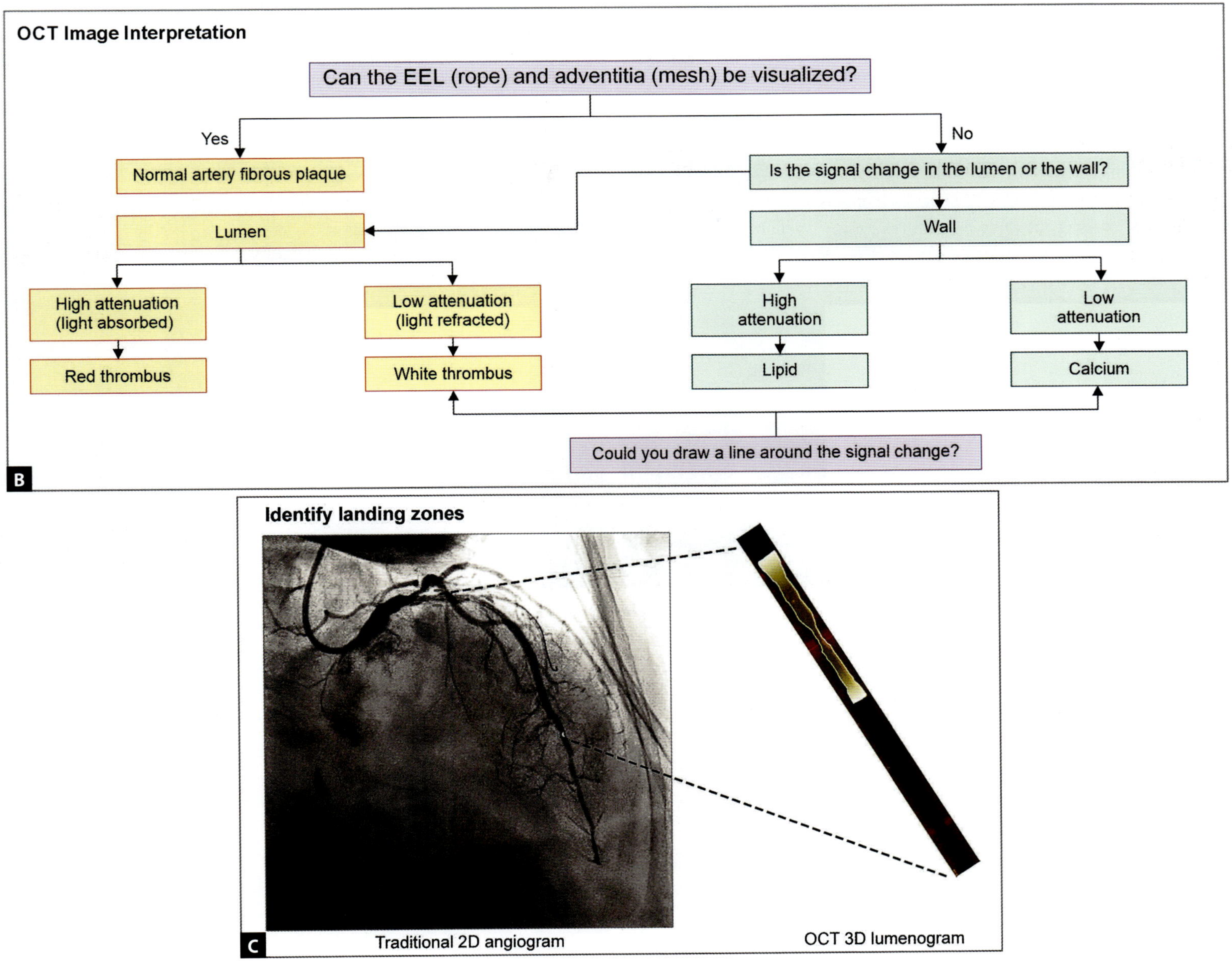
OCT Image Interpretation
Can the EEL (rope) and adventitia (mesh) be visualized?
Yes
No
Normal artery fibrous plaque
Is the signal change in the lumen or the wall?
Lumen
Wall
High attenuation (light absorbed)
Low attenuation (light refracted)
High attenuation
Low attenuation
Red thrombus
White thrombus
Lipid
Calcium
Could you draw a line around the signal change?
B
Identify landing zones
Traditional 2D angiogram
OCT 3D lumenogram
C

Figs. 2B and C

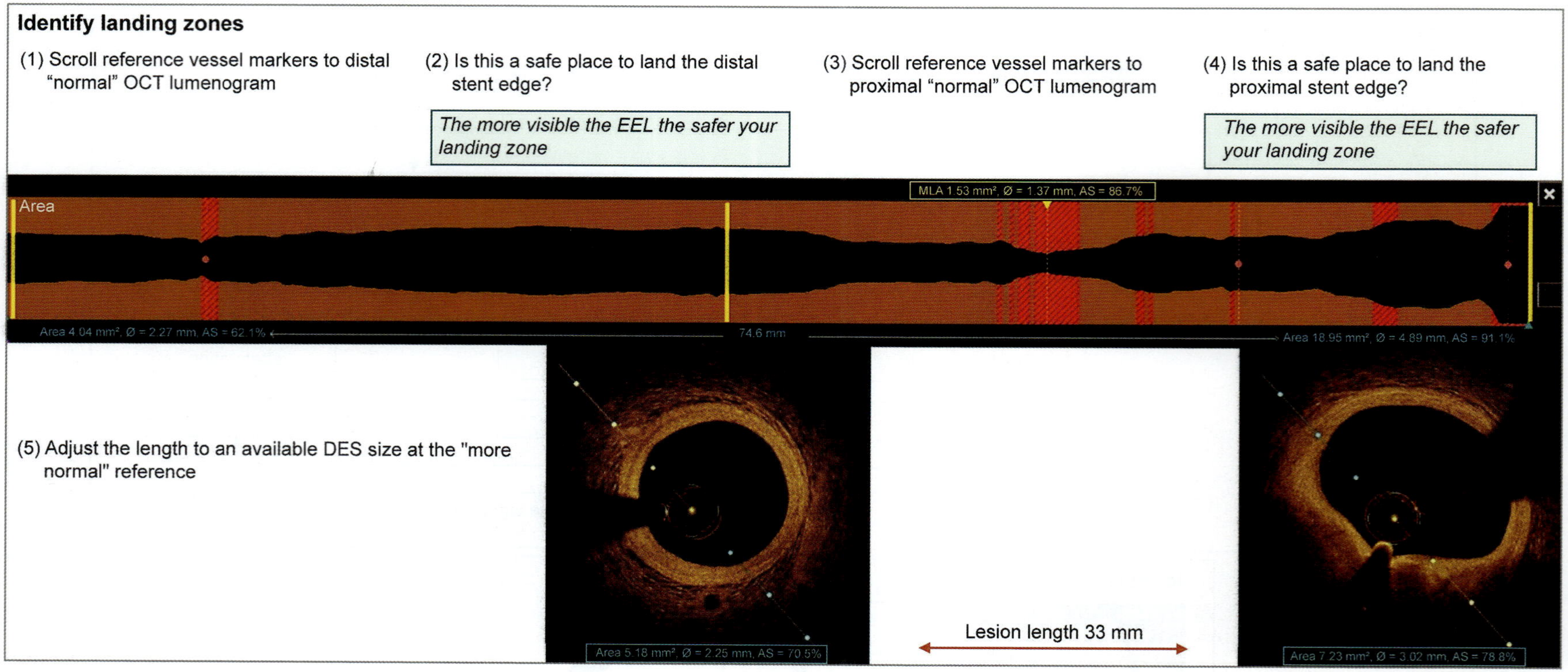
Identify landing zones
(1) Scroll reference vessel markers to distal "normal" OCT lumenogram
(2) Is this a safe place to land the distal stent edge?
The more visible the EEL the safer your landing zone
(3) Scroll reference vessel markers to proximal "normal" OCT lumenogram
(4) Is this a safe place to land the proximal stent edge?
The more visible the EEL the safer your landing zone
MLA 1.53 mm², Ø = 1.37 mm, AS = 86.7%
Area
Area 4.04 mm², Ø = 2.27 mm, AS = 62.1%
74.6 mm
Area 18.95 mm², Ø = 4.89 mm, AS = 91.1%
(5) Adjust the length to an available DES size at the "more normal" reference
Area 5.18 mm², Ø = 2.25 mm, AS = 70.5%
Lesion length 33 mm
Area 7.23 mm², Ø = 3.02 mm, AS = 78.8%

Fig. 2D

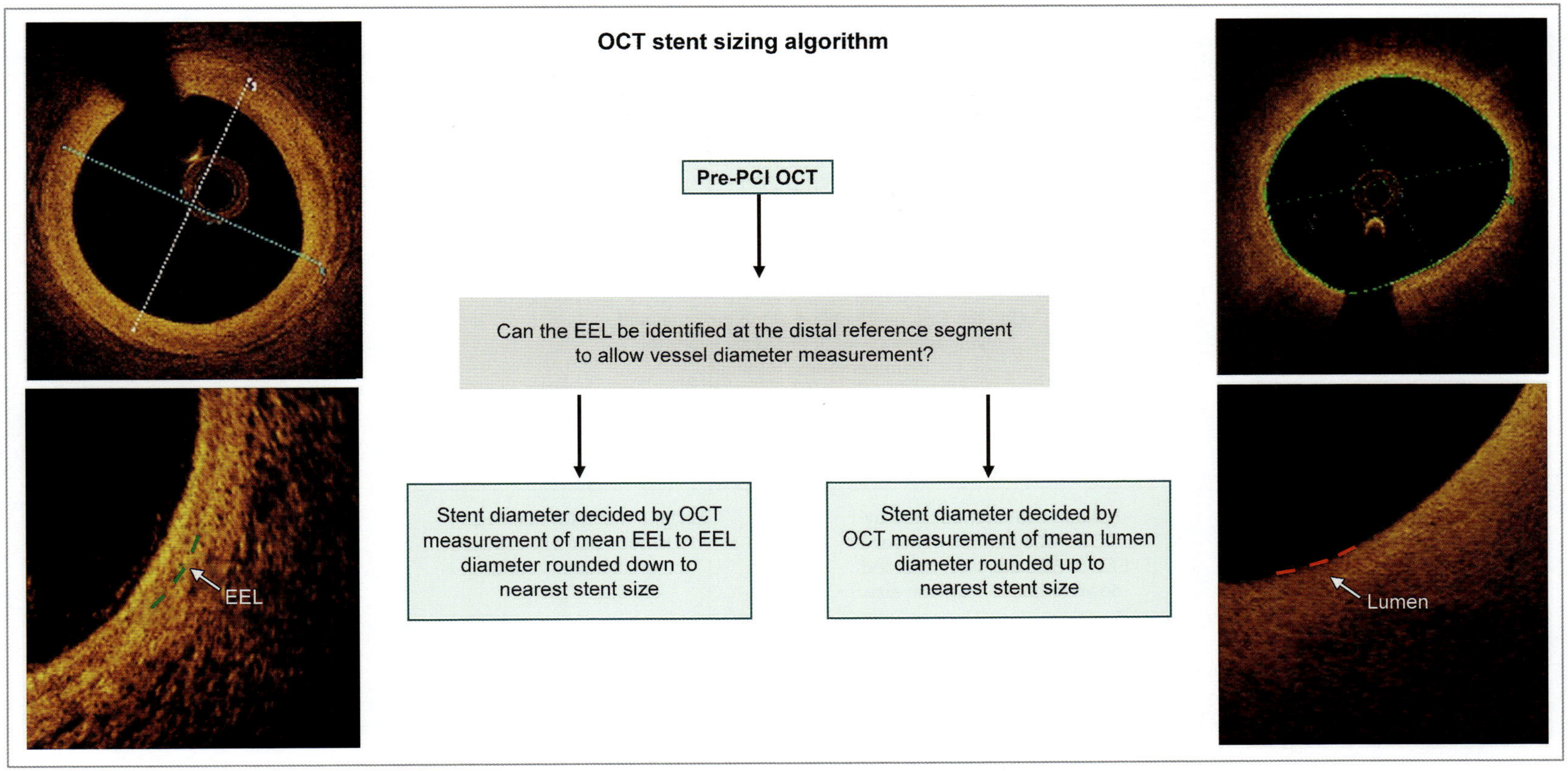
OCT stent sizing algorithm
Pre-PCI OCT
Can the EEL be identified at the distal reference segment to allow vessel diameter measurement?
Stent diameter decided by OCT measurement of mean EEL to EEL diameter rounded down to nearest stent size
Stent diameter decided by OCT measurement of mean lumen diameter rounded up to nearest stent size
EEL
Lumen

Fig. 2E

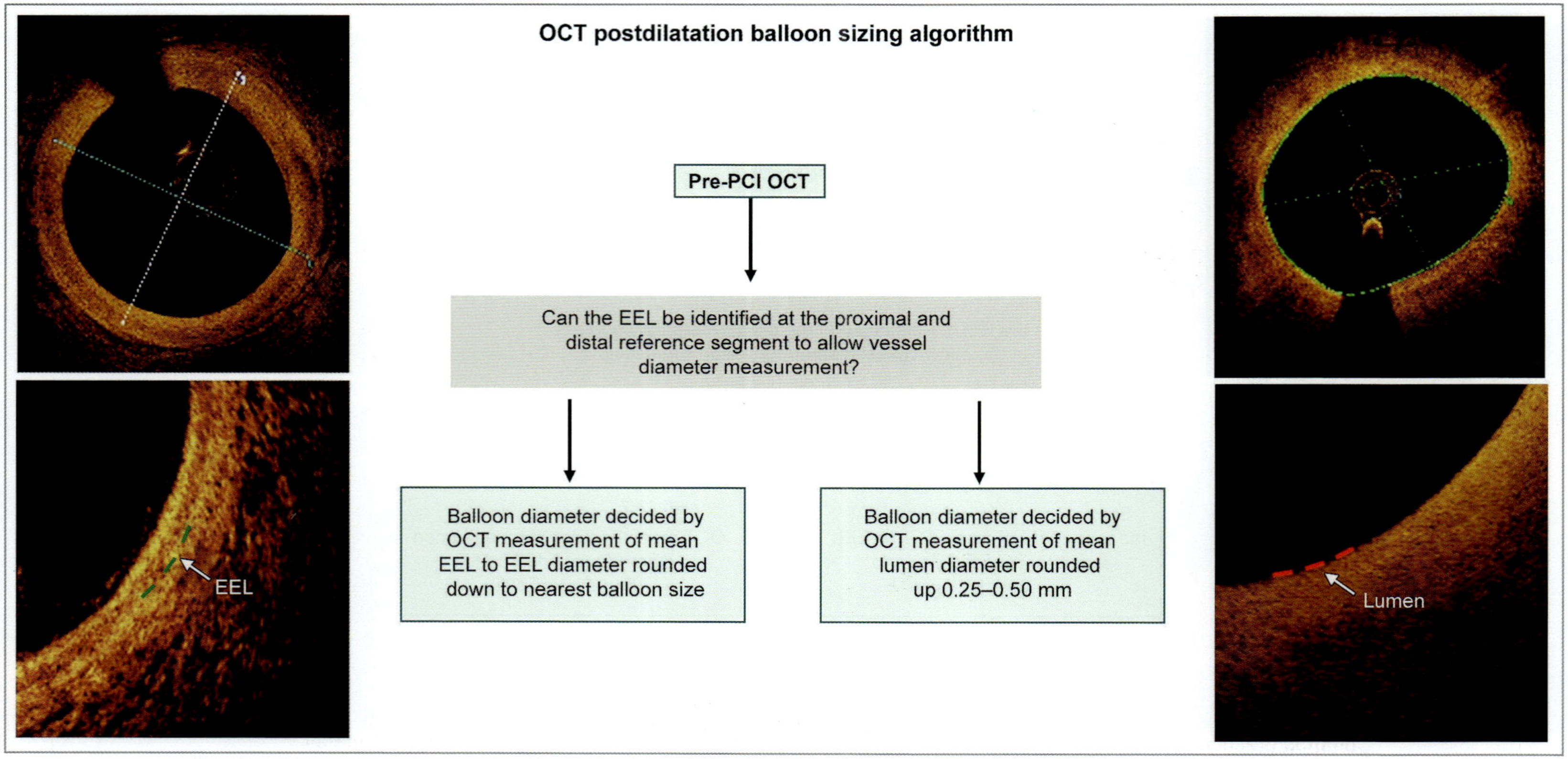

Fig. 2F

Figs. 2A to F: (A) New optical coherence tomography (OCT) algorithm pre-PCI (percutaneous coronary intervention) OCT strategize; (B) Plaque morphology; (C and D) Identifying landing zones; (E) Stent sizing algorithm; (F) Dilatation balloon sizing algorithm. (DES: drug-eluting stents; EEL: external elastic lamina; IVL: intravascular lithotripsy)

POST-PCI OCT—OPTIMIZE (MAX) (FIG. 3A)

Medial Dissection (Fig. 3B)

If dissection penetrates medial layer and is >1 quadrant arc that to be corrected by placing additional stent [particularly in left main (LM) or ostial left anterior descending (LAD)/left circumflex (LCX) or distal dissections].

Apposition (Fig. 3C)

If the gross malapposition is ≥0.3 mm from wall and longer than 3 mm, it should be corrected by dilating with semicompliant balloon at low pressure.

eXpansion (Fig. 3D)

More than or equal to 80% expansion of the stent is acceptable and ≥90% expansion is optimal with reference to proximal and distal diameters. If not achieved, postdilate with NC balloon.

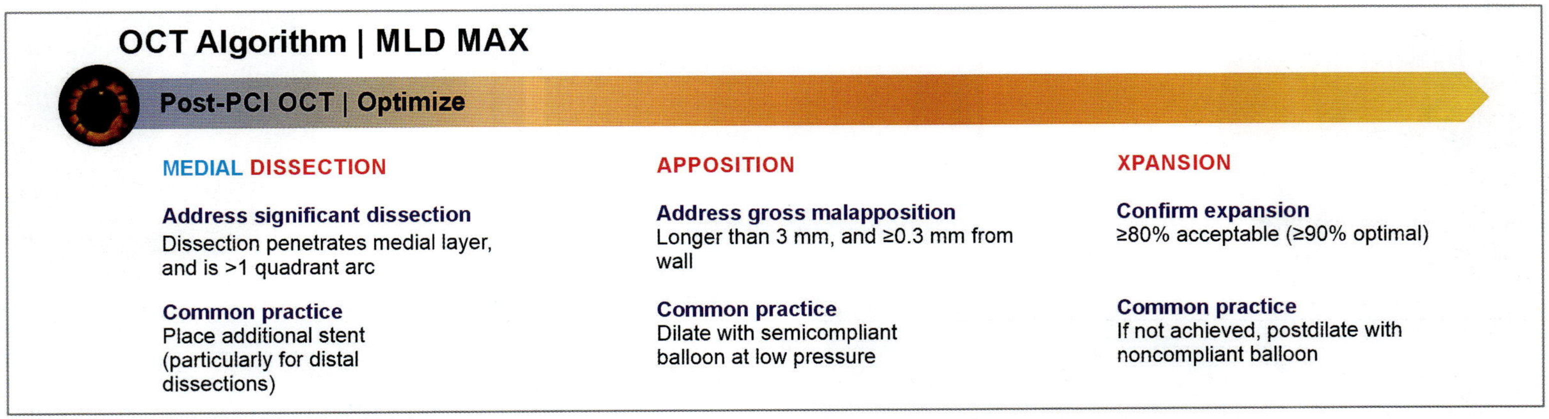

Fig. 3A

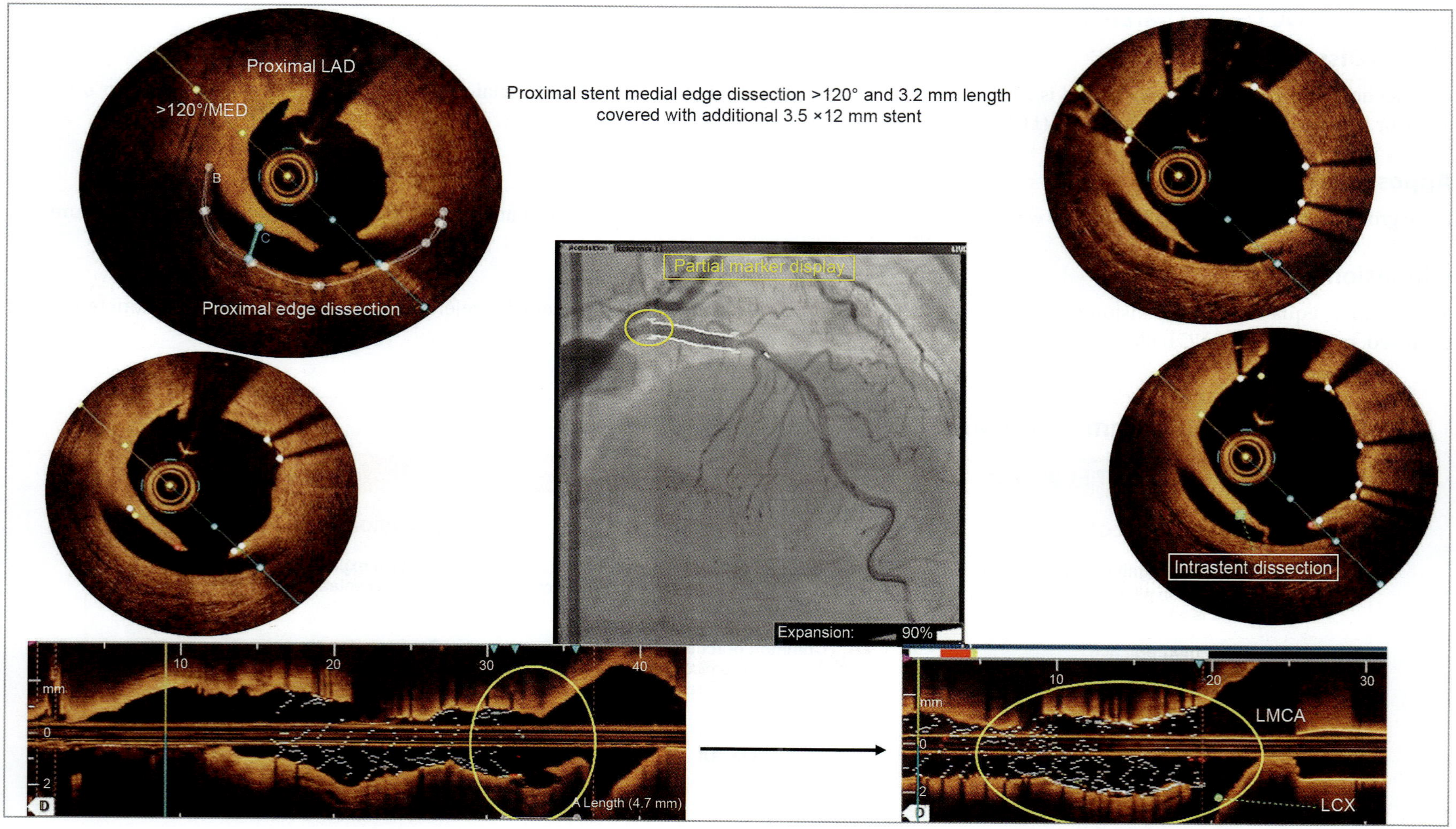
Proximal LAD
>120°/MED
B
C
Proximal edge dissection
Proximal stent medial edge dissection >120° and 3.2 mm length covered with additional 3.5 ×12 mm stent
Partial marker display
Expansion: 90%
Intrastent dissection
10
20
30
40
mm
0
2
Length (4.7 mm)
D
10
20
30
mm
0
2
LMCA
LCX
D

Fig. 3B

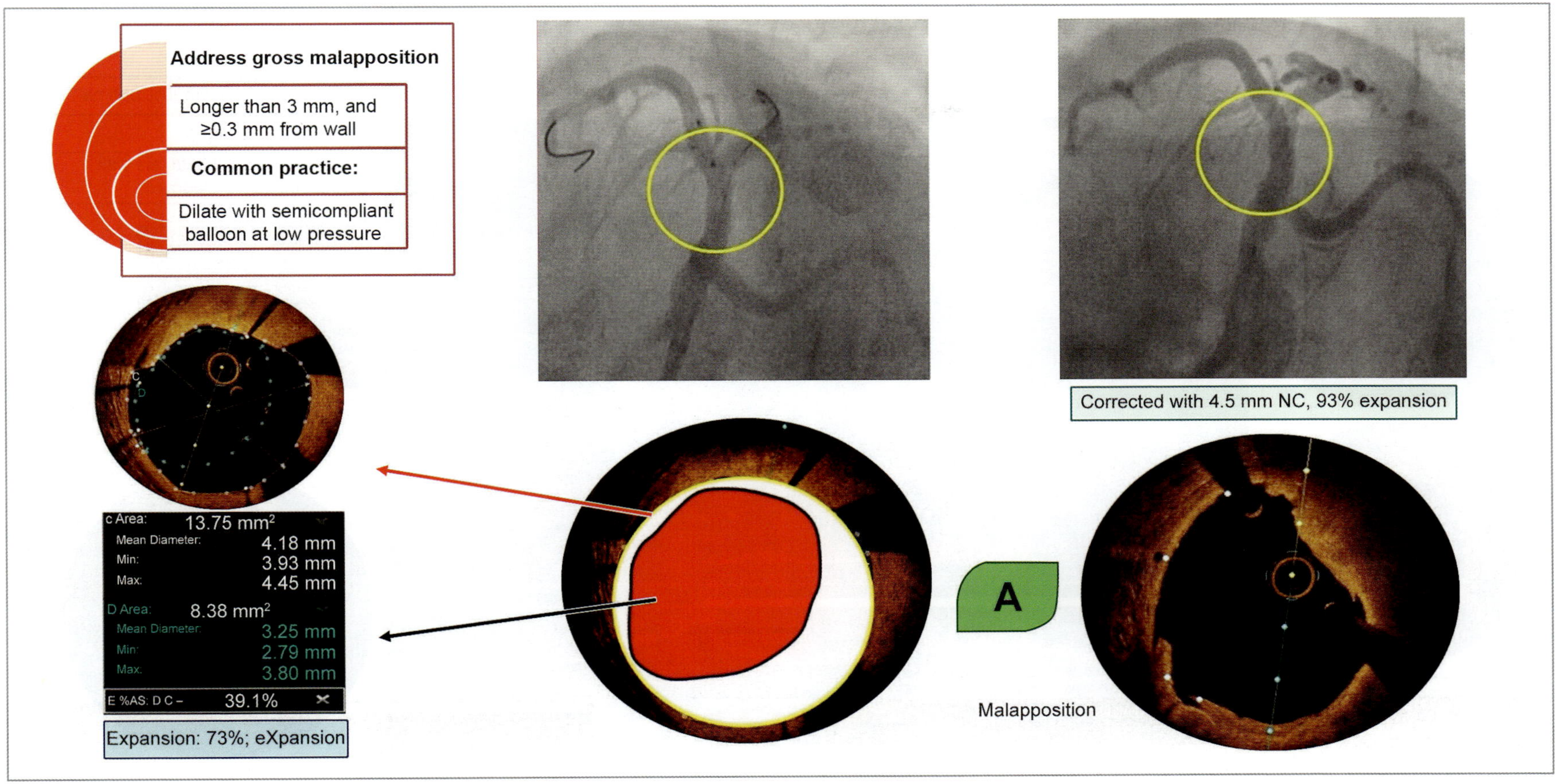

Address gross malapposition
Longer than 3 mm, and ≥0.3 mm from wall
Common practice:
Dilate with semicompliant balloon at low pressure
Corrected with 4.5 mm NC, 93% expansion
c Area: 13.75 mm²
Mean Diameter: 4.18 mm
Min: 3.93 mm
Max: 4.45 mm
D Area: 8.38 mm²
Mean Diameter: 3.25 mm
Min: 2.79 mm
Max: 3.80 mm
E %AS: D C – 39.1%
Expansion: 73%; eXpansion
A
Malapposition

Fig. 3C

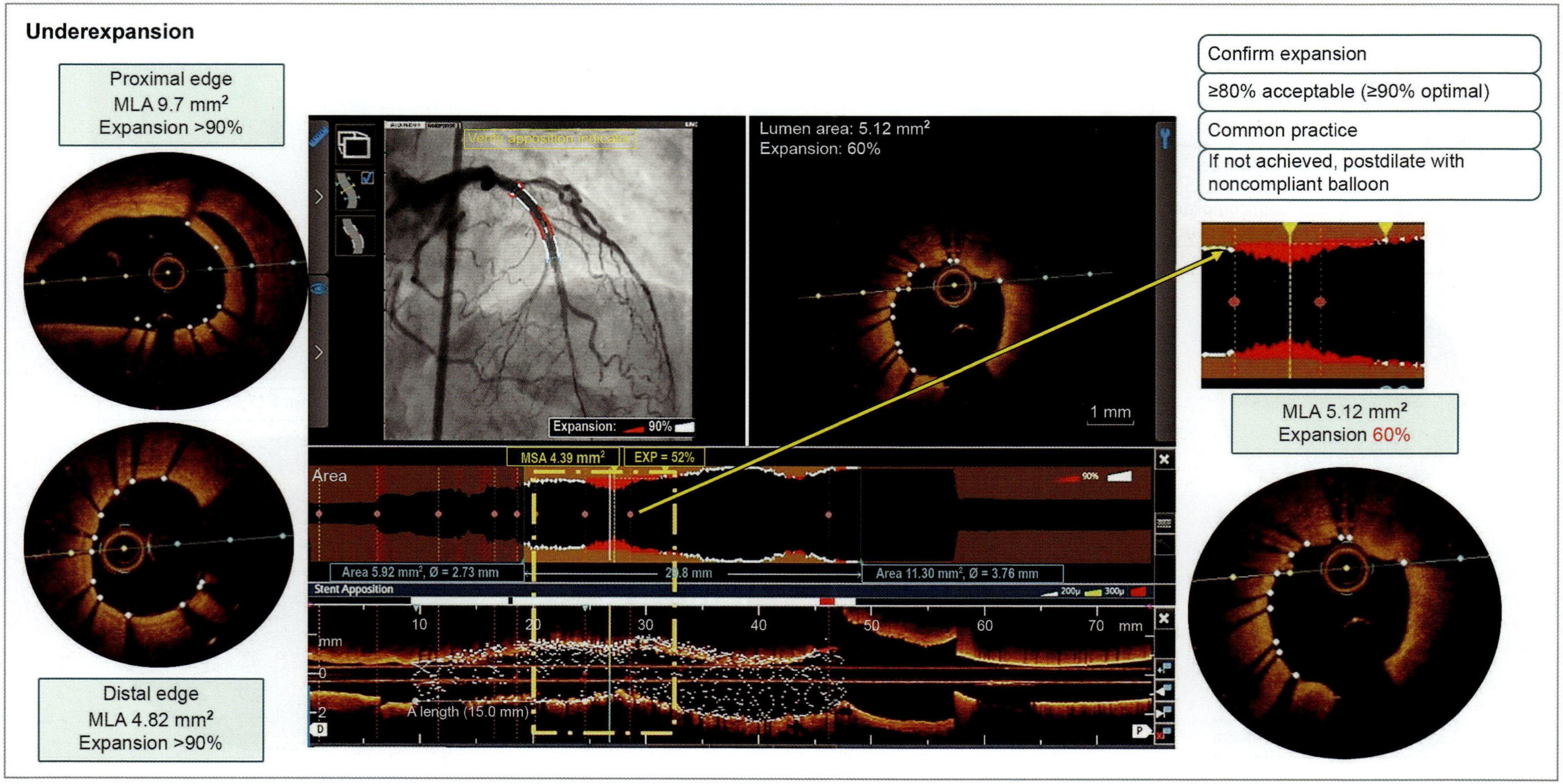

Fig. 3D

Figs. 3A to D: New optical coherence tomography (OCT) algorithm post-PCI (percutaneous coronary intervention) OCT optimize. (LAD: left anterior descending; LCX: left circumflex; LMCA: left main coronary artery; MLA: minimal lumen area; NC: noncompliant)

CASE 1

OCT + IVUS (intravascular ultrasound)-guided bifurcation stenting of LM–LAD, LAD and D1.

CLINICAL HISTORY

A 54-year-old presented with acute coronary syndrome (ACS)—evolved inferior STEMI (ST segment elevation myocardial infarction) [window period (WP) >24 h] **(Fig. 4A)**, coronary angiogram (CAG)—left main coronary artery (LMCA) + double-vessel disease (DVD), 2D ECHO showed hypokinesia of inferior wall, mild left ventricular (LV) dysfunction, ejection fraction (EF)—46%, on investigation (O/I): hemoglobin (Hb)—10. g/dL, random blood sugar (RBS)—128 mg/dL, serum creatinine—0.63 mg/dL, estimated glomerular filtration rate (eGFR)—112 mL/min. CAG—LAD/D1 bifurcation lesion, right coronary artery (RCA) distal critical lesion **(Figs. 4B to D)**.

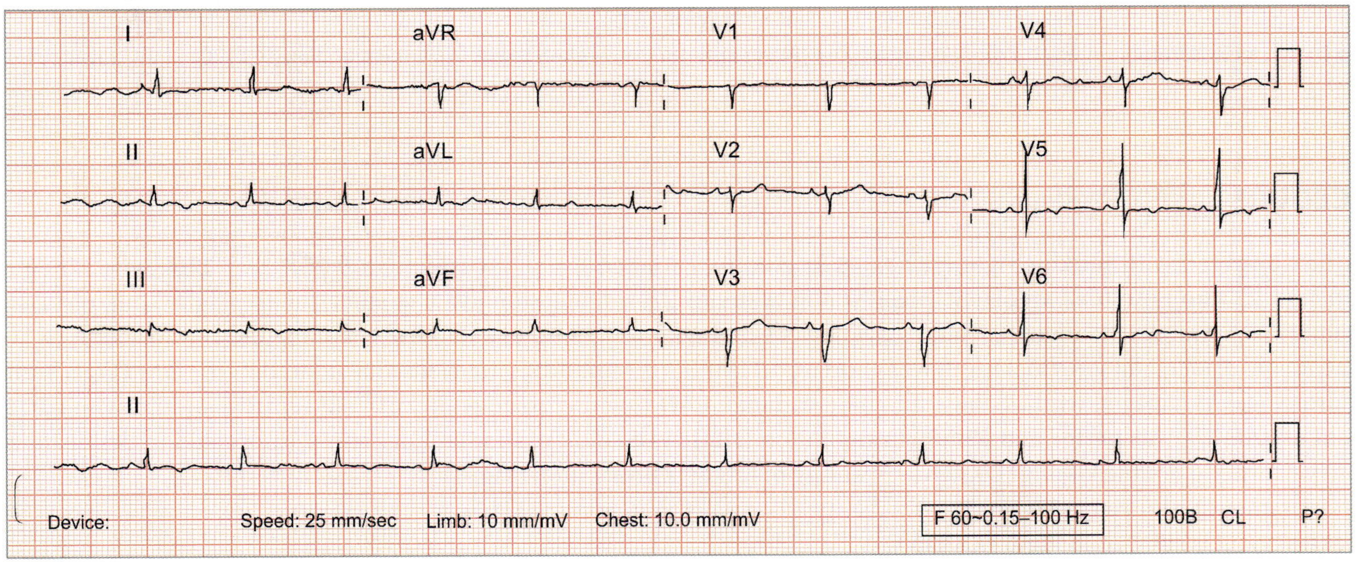

Fig. 4A

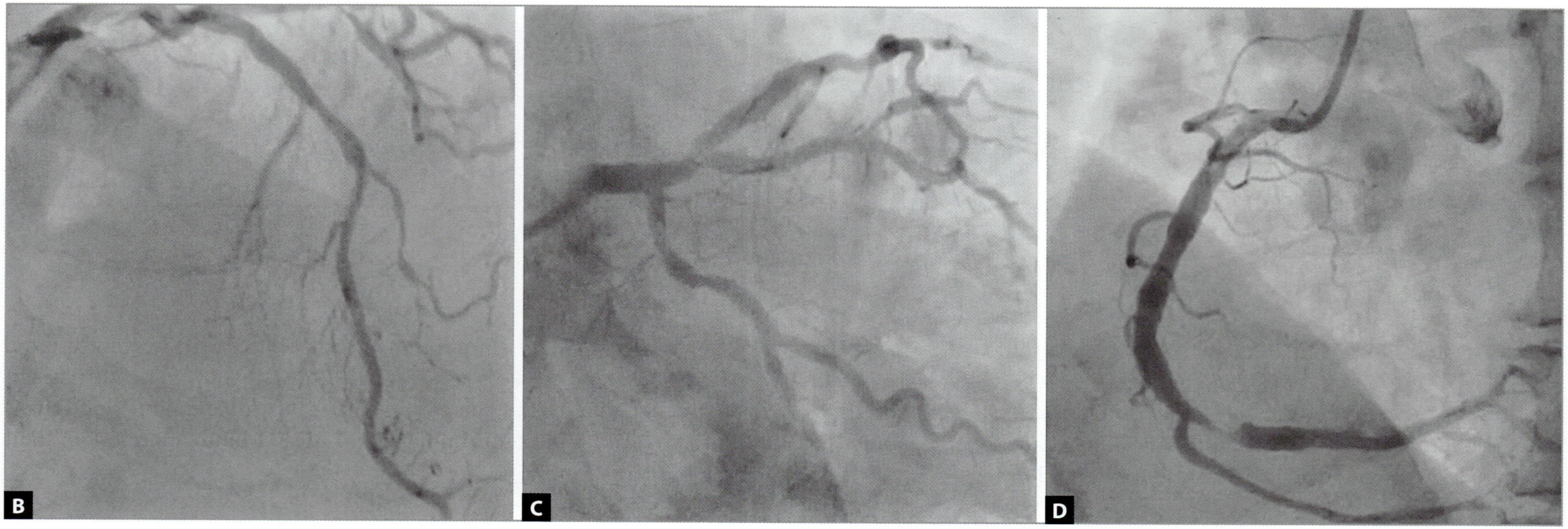

Figs. 4B to D

Figs. 4A to D: (A) Electrocardiogram (ECG), coronary angiogram (B) left anterior descending (LAD); (C) Left circumflex (LCX); (D) Right coronary artery (RCA).

PROCEDURE

Right coronary artery engaged with Judkins right (JR) 3.5–6 Fr guiding catheter, lesion crossed with 0.014″ Sion blue wire. Then distal RCA direct stenting done with 4.5 × 22 mm Resolute Onyx stent, postdistal RCA stenting residual lesion distal to stent due to plaque shift, distal stenting done with 3.5 × 22 mm Resolute Onyx and check angio revealed slow flow treated with intracoronary (IC) Inj. Nikoran, and nitroglycerin (NTG), postdilatation done with 5.0 × 12 mm NC Apollo balloon, final result was good with TIMI III (thrombolysis in myocardial infarction III) flow **(Figs. 5A to E)**.

Left coronary artery (LCA) engaged with XB 3.5–7 Fr guide catheter, LAD lesion crossed with 0.014″ BMW wire and D1 with 0.014″ Sion blue wire. Pre-PCI assessment of LAD-D1 was performed with high-definition (HD)-IVUS and OCT for comparison purpose and to delineate features of plaque morphology before performing double kissing (DK) crush stenting of LAD-D1 bifurcation **(Fig. 6)**.

Prestent IVUS assessment is showed in **Figure 7**.

Prestent OCT assessment is showed in **Figures 8A to C**.

Mid-LAD and D1 predilated with 3.5 × 10 mm angio-sculpt balloon. Postangio-sculpt OCT of LAD-LM is shown in **Figure 9**.

D1 side branch (SB) stenting done with 3.5 × 15 mm Resolute Onyx and Crushing stent with 4.0 × 12 mm NC Apollo balloon in LAD, D1 struts opened after crossing SB with 1.5 × 10 mm Tazuna. First kissing balloon dilatation with 4.0 × 12 mm NC Apollo balloon in LAD and 3.5 × 15 mm in D1 **(Figs. 10A to D)**.

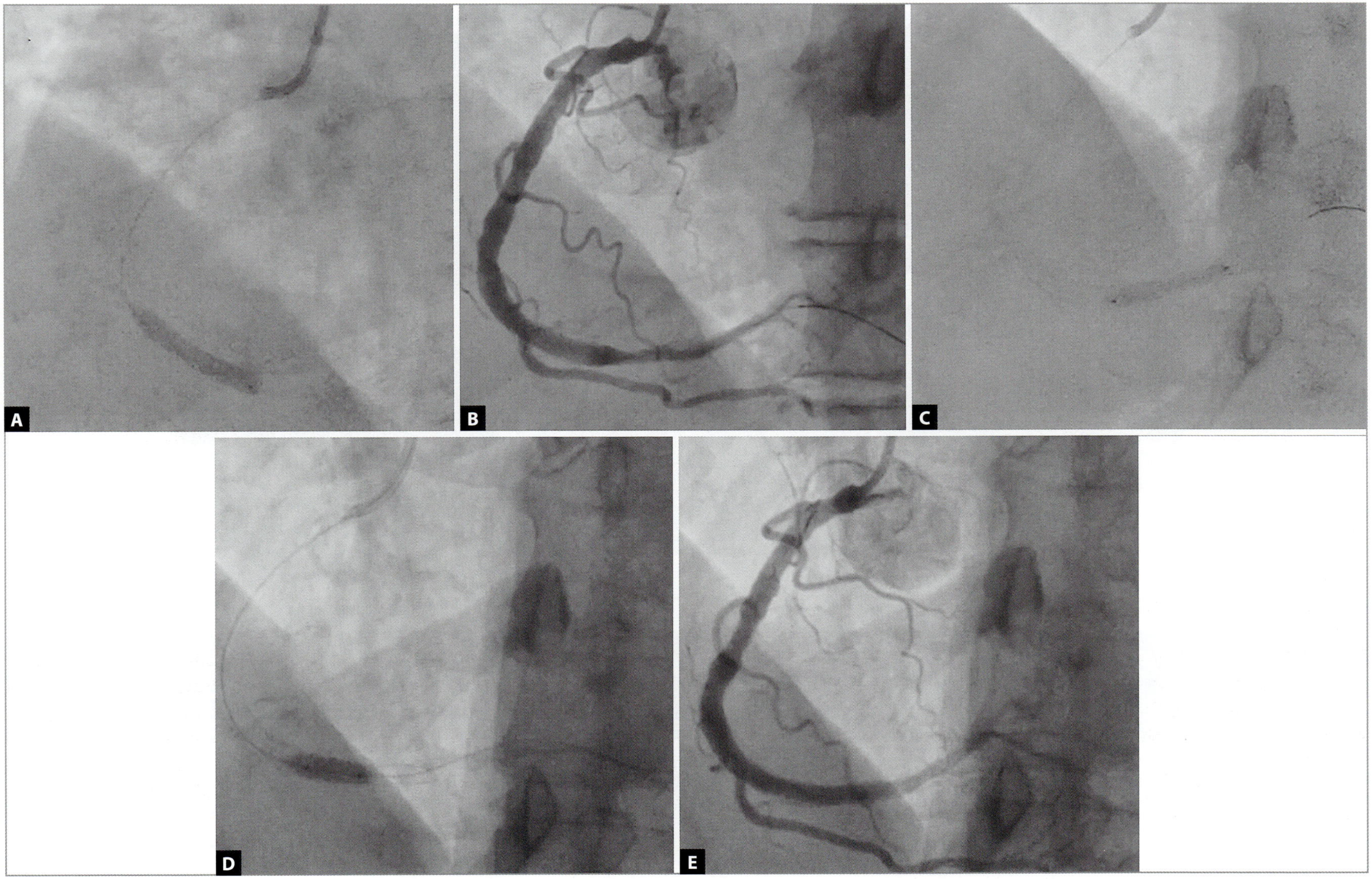

Figs. 5A to E: Coronary angioplasty of right coronary artery (RCA) vessel.

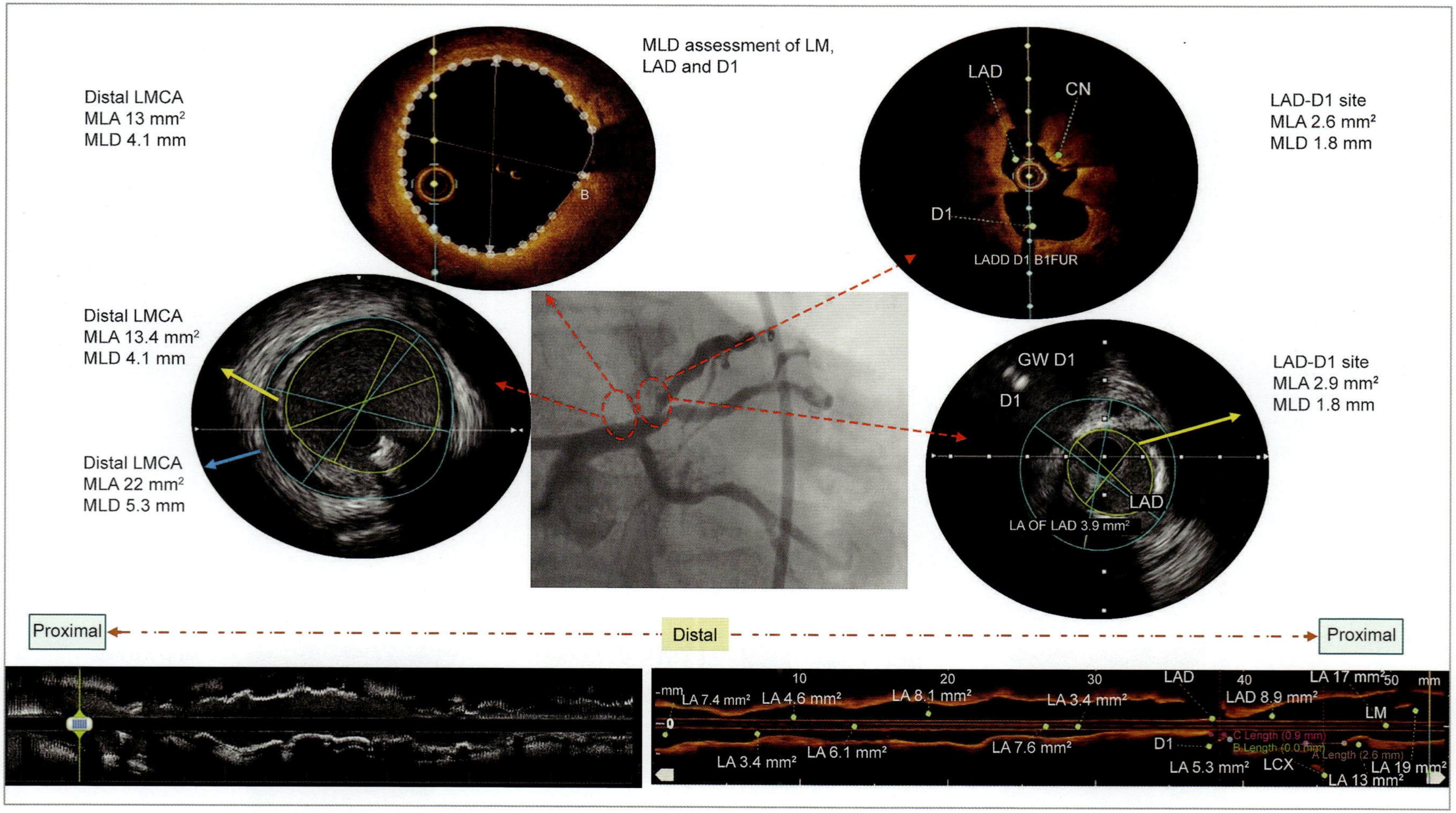

Fig. 6: Prestent IVUS and OCT assessment of LM and LAD-D1 bifurcation zones. (IVUS: intravascular ultrasound; LAD: left anterior descending; LMCA: left main coronary artery; OCT: optical coherence tomography; MED: medial edge dissection; MLA: minimal lumen area; MLD: minimal lumen diameter)

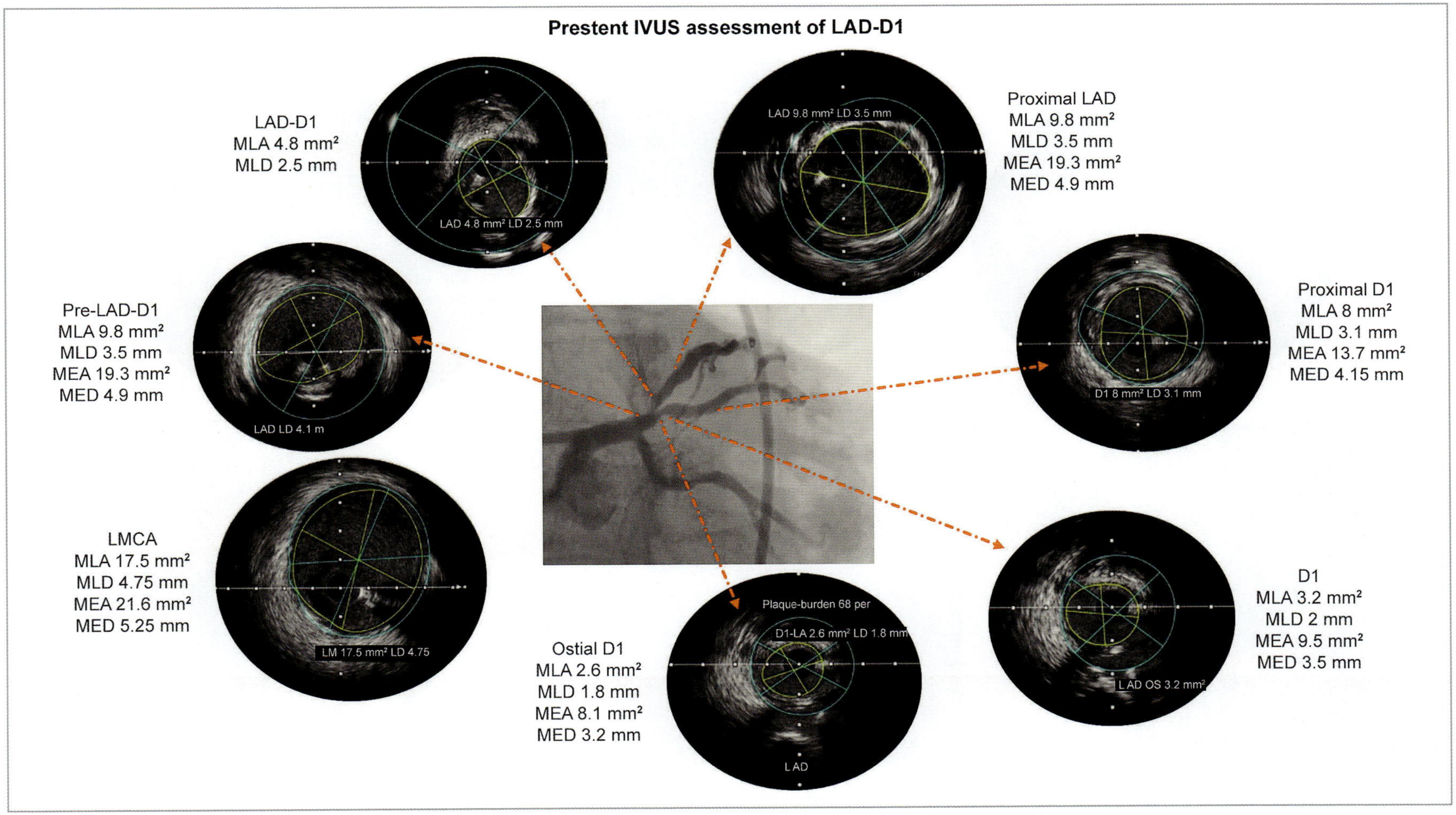

Fig. 7: Prestent IVUS assessment of LAD-D1 bifurcation. (IVUS: intravascular ultrasound; LAD: left anterior descending; MEA: mean external elastic area; MED: medial edge dissection; MLA: minimal lumen area; MLD: minimal lumen diameter)

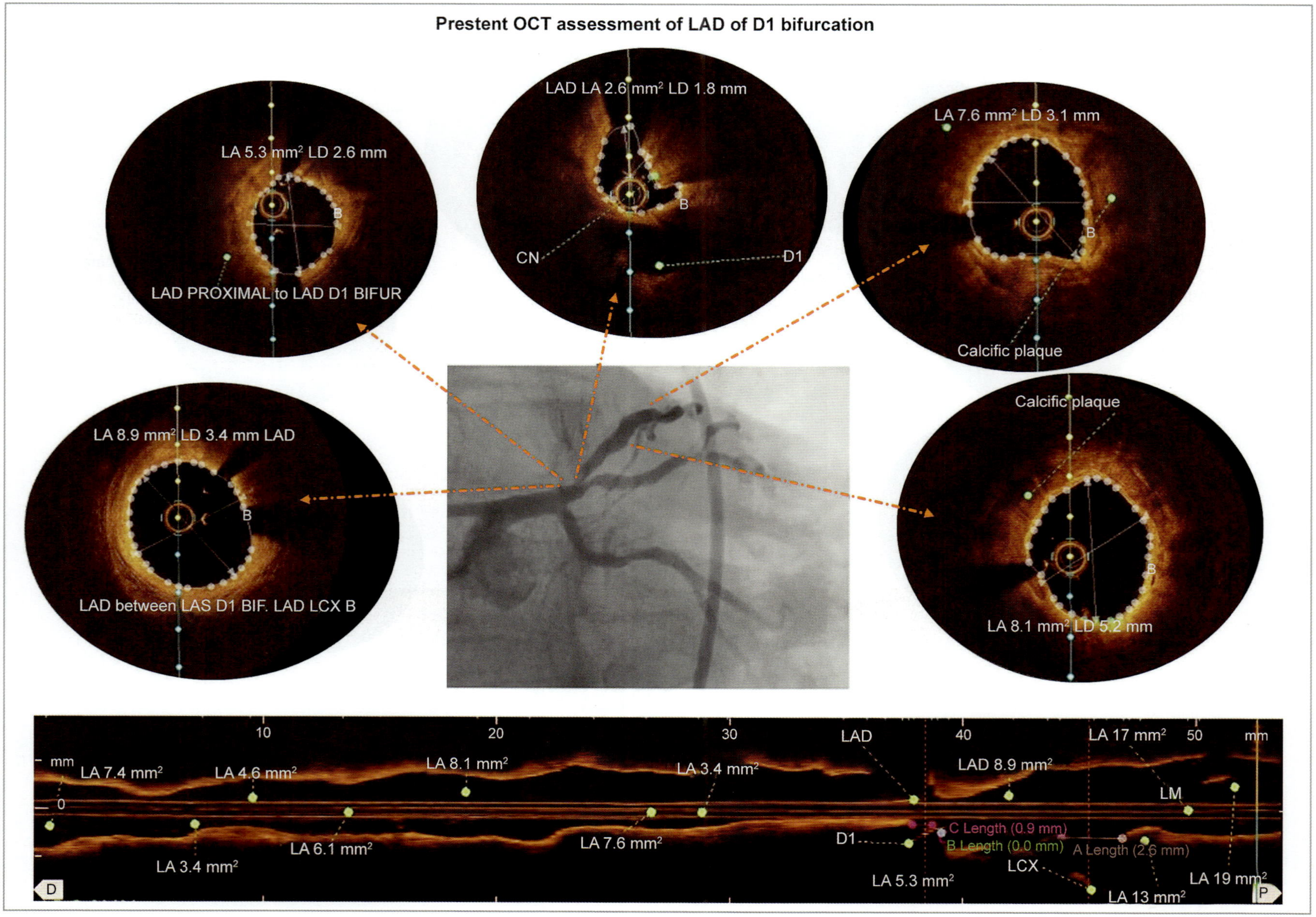

Prestent OCT assessment of LAD of D1 bifurcation
LA 5.3 mm² LD 2.6 mm
LAD PROXIMAL to LAD D1 BIFUR
LAD LA 2.6 mm² LD 1.8 mm
CN
D1
LA 7.6 mm² LD 3.1 mm
Calcific plaque
LA 8.9 mm² LD 3.4 mm LAD
LAD between LAS D1 BIF. LAD LCX B
Calcific plaque
LA 8.1 mm² LD 5.2 mm
mm
LA 7.4 mm²
LA 4.6 mm²
LA 8.1 mm²
LA 3.4 mm²
LAD
LAD 8.9 mm²
LA 17 mm²
LM
LA 3.4 mm²
LA 6.1 mm²
LA 7.6 mm²
D1
C Length (0.9 mm)
B Length (0.0 mm)
A Length (2.6 mm)
LCX
LA 5.3 mm²
LA 13 mm²
LA 19 mm²
D
P

Fig. 8A

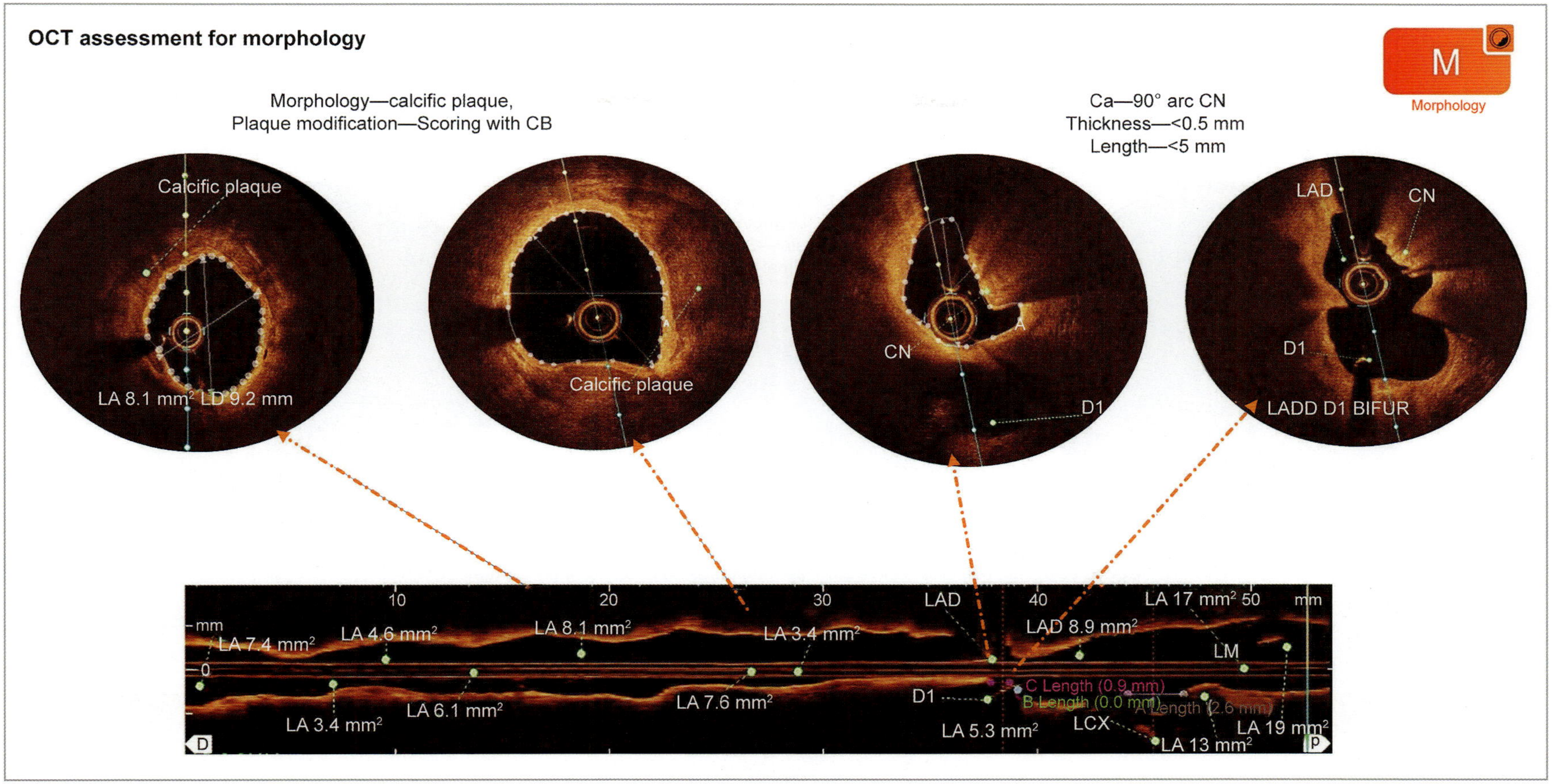
OCT assessment for morphology
M
Morphology
Morphology—calcific plaque,
Plaque modification—Scoring with CB
Ca—90° arc CN
Thickness—<0.5 mm
Length—<5 mm
Calcific plaque
LA 8.1 mm² LD 9.2 mm
Calcific plaque
CN
D1
LAD
CN
D1
LADD D1 BIFUR
10
20
30
40
50
mm
LAD
mm
0
LA 7.4 mm²
LA 4.6 mm²
LA 8.1 mm²
LA 3.4 mm²
LAD 8.9 mm²
LA 17 mm²
LM
LA 3.4 mm²
LA 6.1 mm²
LA 7.6 mm²
D1
C Length (0.9 mm)
B Length (0.0 mm)
A Length (2.6 mm)
LA 5.3 mm²
LCX
LA 13 mm²
LA 19 mm²
D
P

Fig. 8B

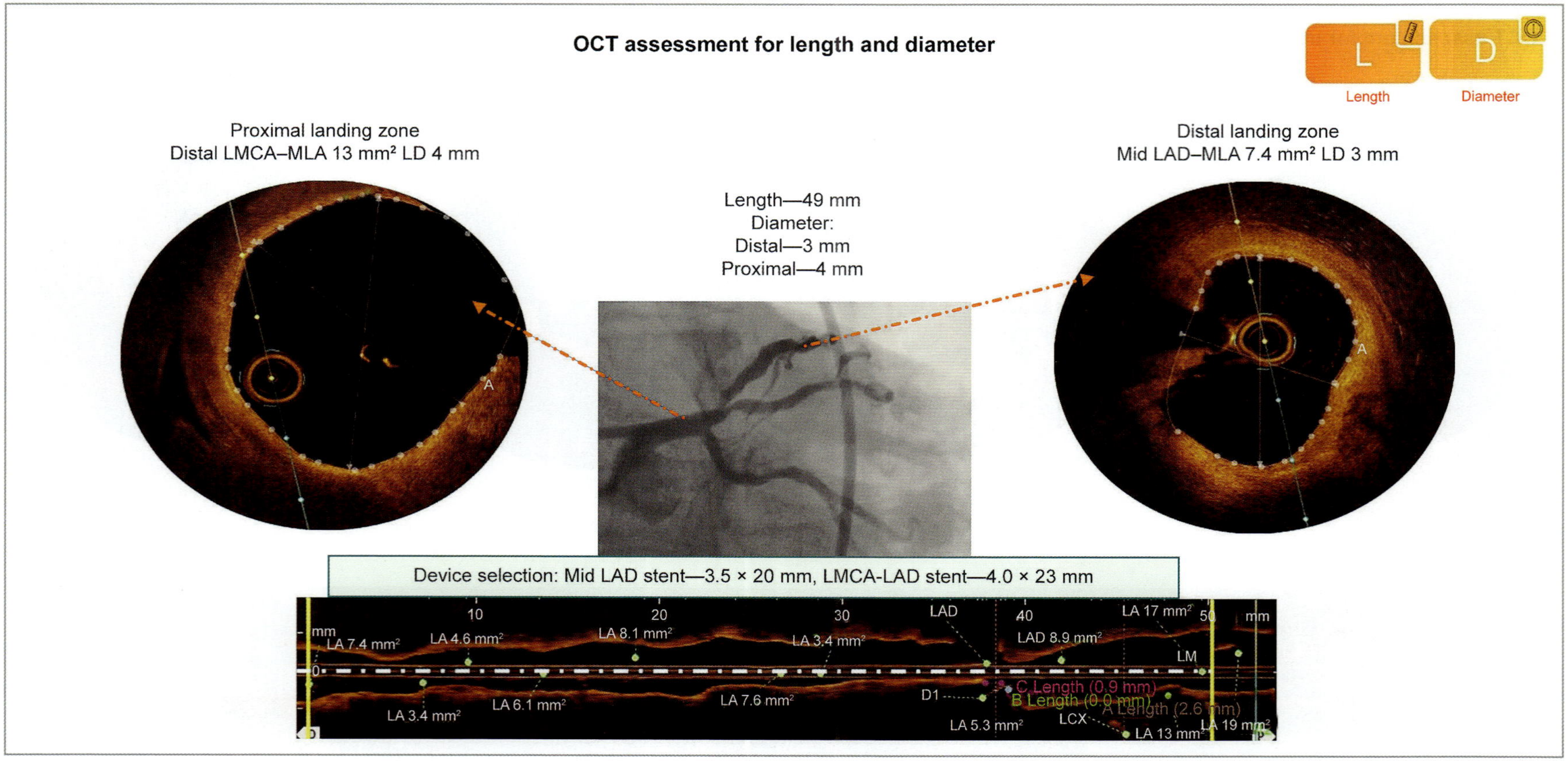

Fig. 8C

Figs. 8A to C: (A) MLD assessment of LAD-D1 bifurcation; (B) Plaque morphology; (C) Device selection (length and diameter). (CB: cutting balloon; LA: lumen area; LD: lumen diameter; LAD: left anterior descending; LCX: left circumflex; LMCA: left main coronary artery MLA: minimal lumen artery)

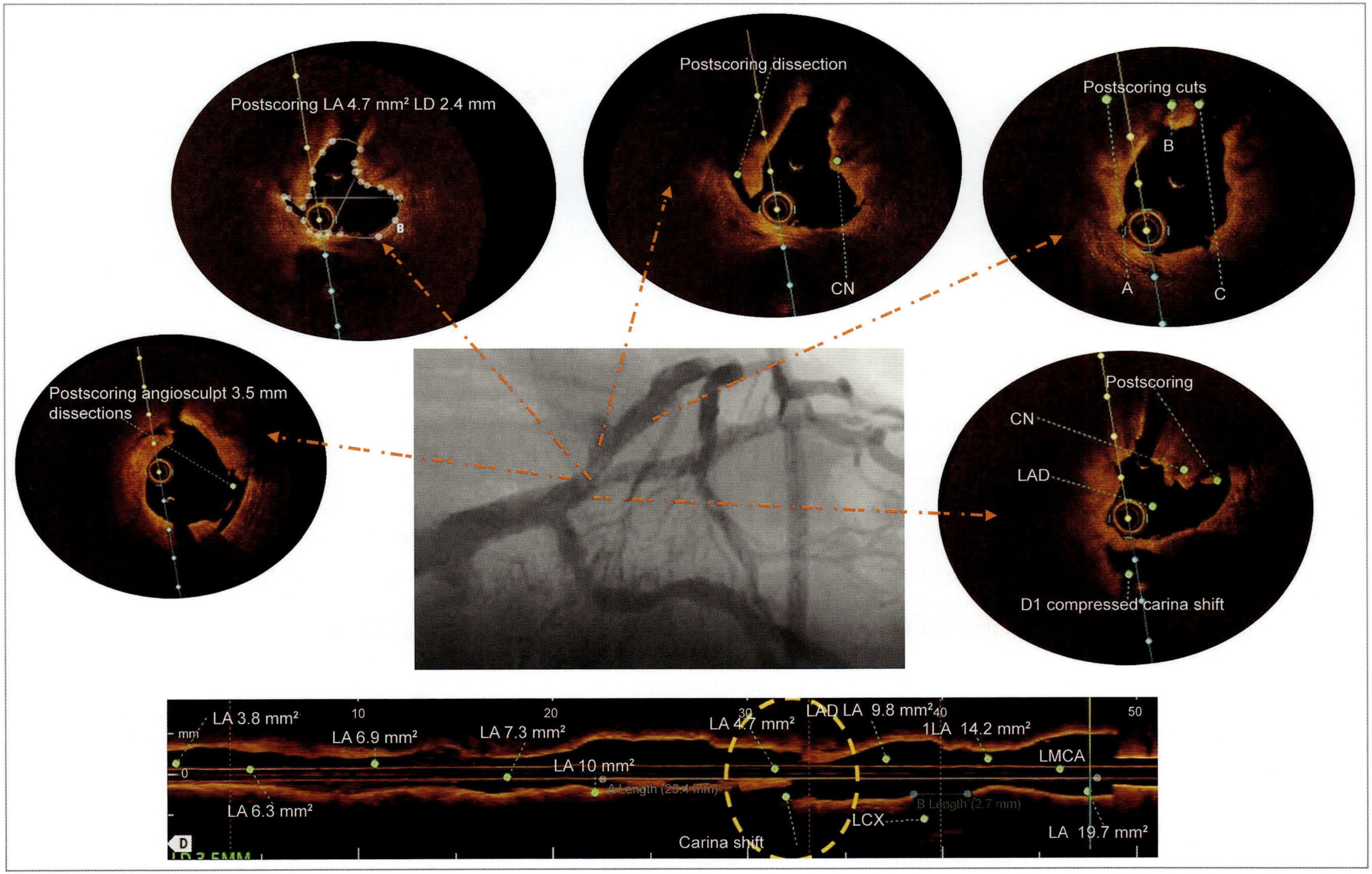

Fig. 9: Postscoring optical coherence tomography (OCT) assessment—Evidence of fractures suggestive of adequate modification.

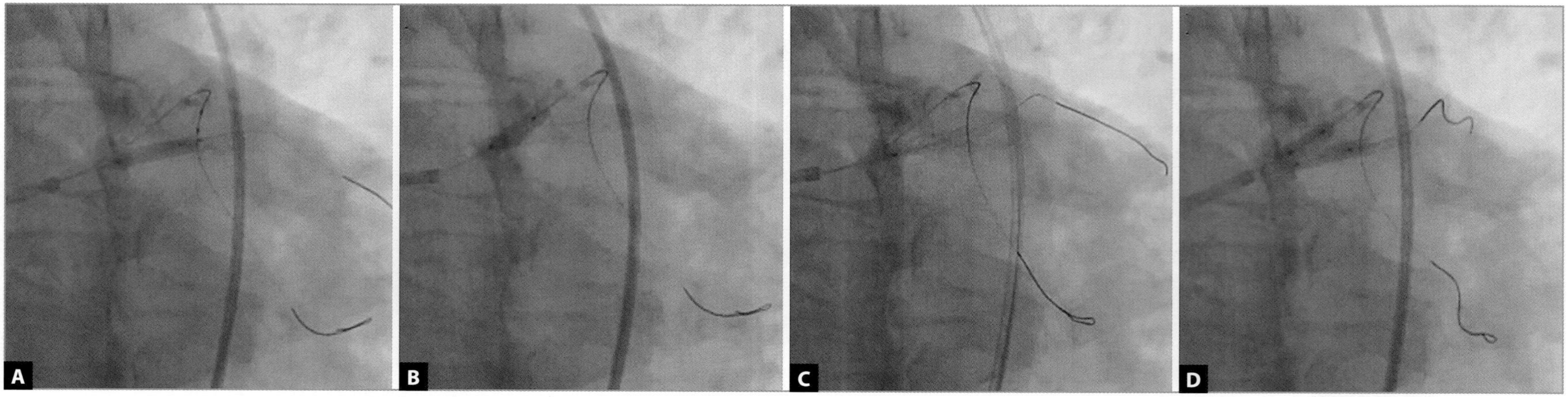

Figs. 10A to D: Side branch stenting, postdilatation, struts opening and first kissing balloon dilatation.

Post-D1 stent and post-FKB (final kissing balloon) OCT for crush evaluation ***(Fig. 11):*** Mid LAD stenting done with 3.5 × 30 mm Resolute Onyx, LMCA–LAD stenting done with 4.0 × 23 mm Xience Xpedition. Proximal optimization technique (POT) to LMCA with 4.5 × 0.8 mm NC Apollo balloon; later D1 wire recrossed through stent struts, opened with 2.0 × 10 mm Tazuna and postdilatation of LAD stent was done. Second kissing done with 4.0 × 10 mm NC Apollo balloon and 3.5 × 12 mm in D1, RePOT of LMCA with 4.5 × 0.8 mm NC Apollo, pinching of D1 Branch, opening with 1.5 × 10 mm, third kissing with 4.0 × 10 mm NC Apollo and 3.5 × 12 mm in D1. Final result was good with TIMI III flow **(Figs. 12A to F)**.

Poststent HD-IVUS and OCT showed well-expanded and apposed stent struts with no medial edge dissections ***(Figs. 13A to C):*** Optical coherence tomography images compared to IVUS images delineates luminal borders more accurately, specially in situations with critically narrowed lesions. OCT clearly demonstrated calcium nodule at the LAD-D1 bifurcation site with exact luminal dimensions and borders compared to vague borders of HD-IVUS, though images of HD-IVUS resolution is far better compared to regular IVUS images. HD-IVUS due to its high-resolution image can show calcium thickness, length, and arc more clearly and postplaque modification fractures of calcium. Delineation of adventitial border for measuring diameter of the vessel is more accurate with HD-IVUS compared to OCT due to its poor resolution of adventitia in the presence of large lipid pool and severe deep calcium. OCT can identify TCFA, plaque rupture (PR), plaque erosion (PE), recanalized thrombus, differentiating red thrombus from white thrombus and spontaneous coronary artery dissection (SCAD) more clearly compared to IVUS.

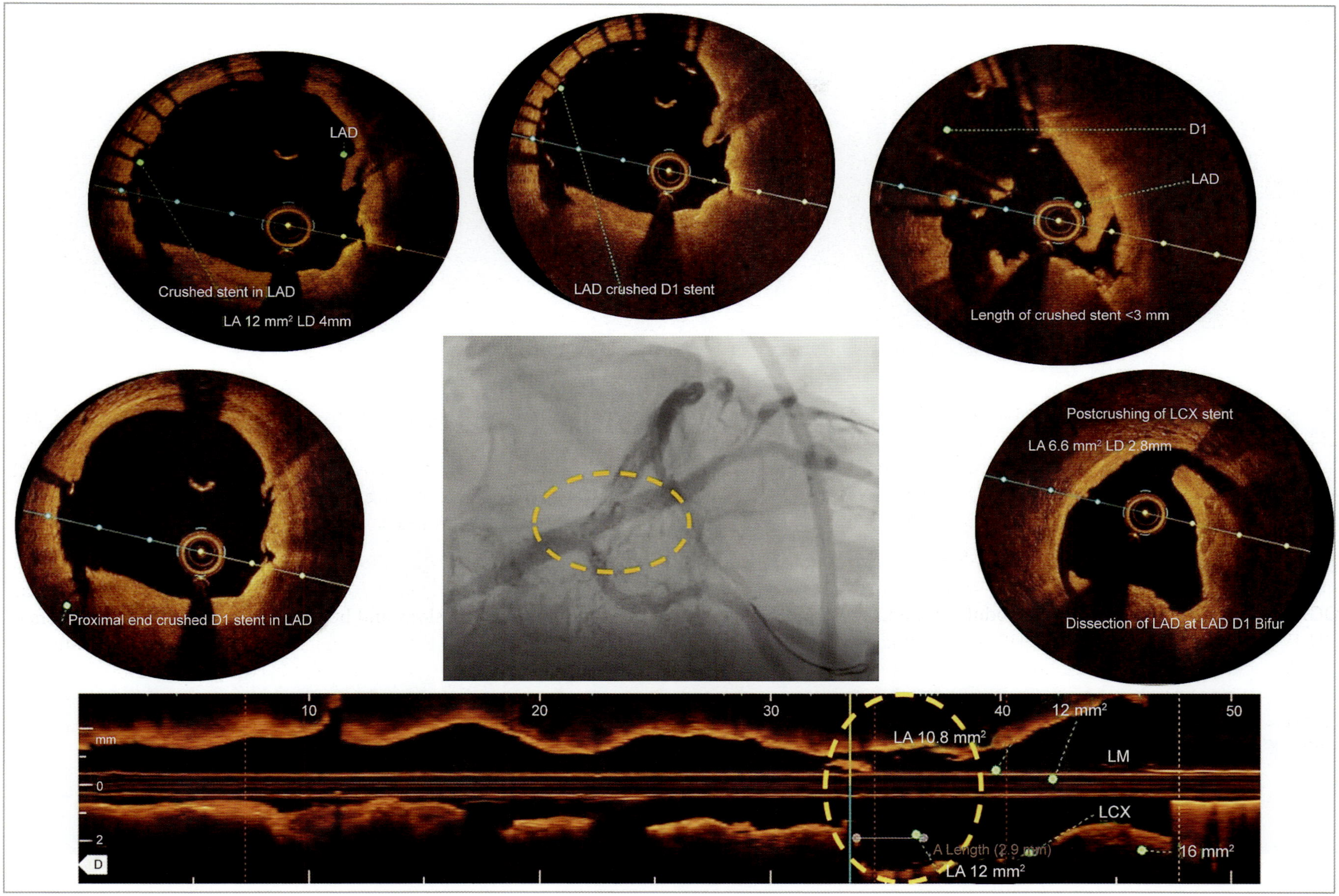

Fig. 11: Adequately crushed of proximal portion D1 stent in the LAD.

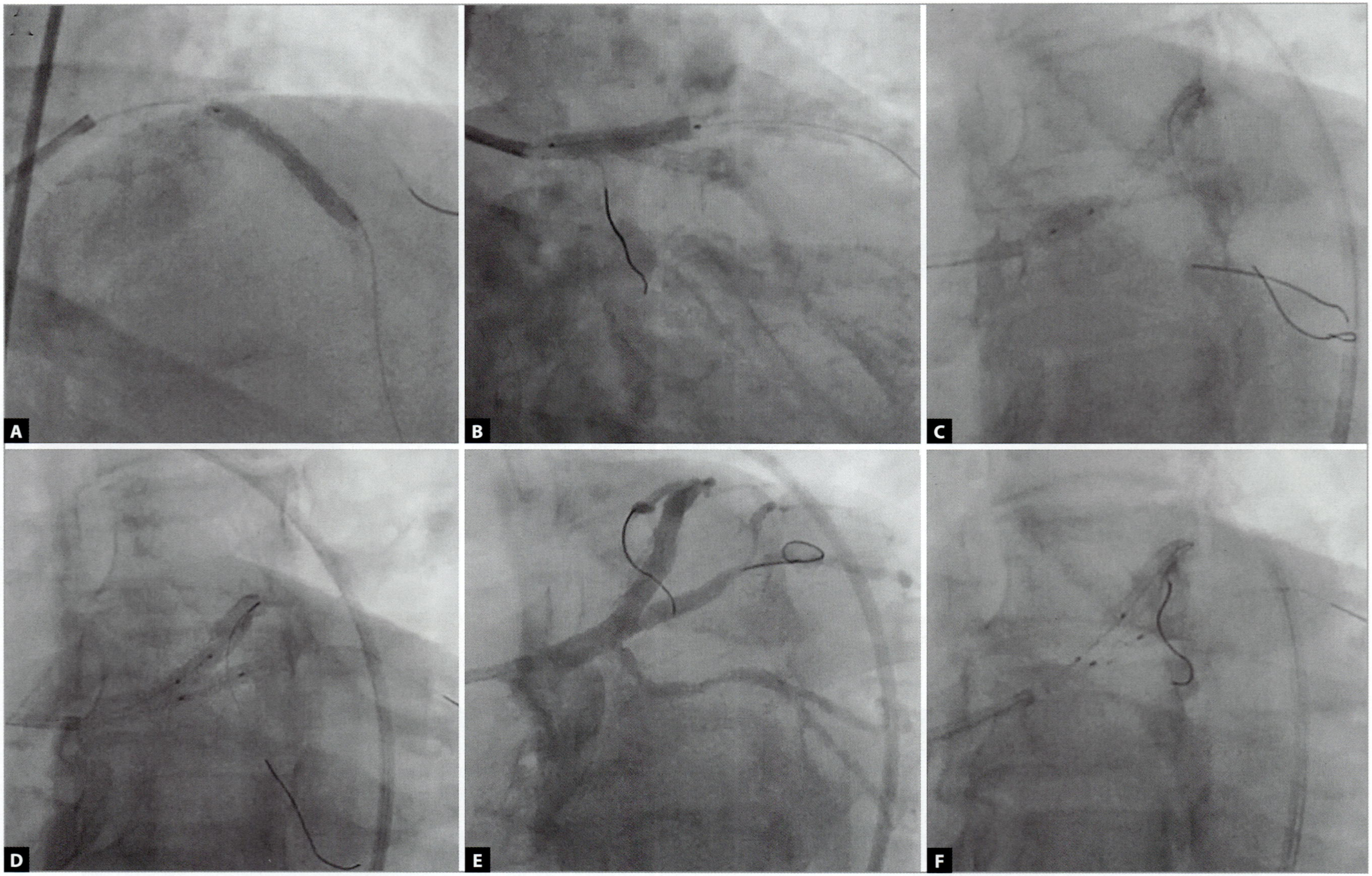

Figs. 12A to F: Main branch stenting, postdilatation, side branch crossing, and final kissing balloon dilatation.

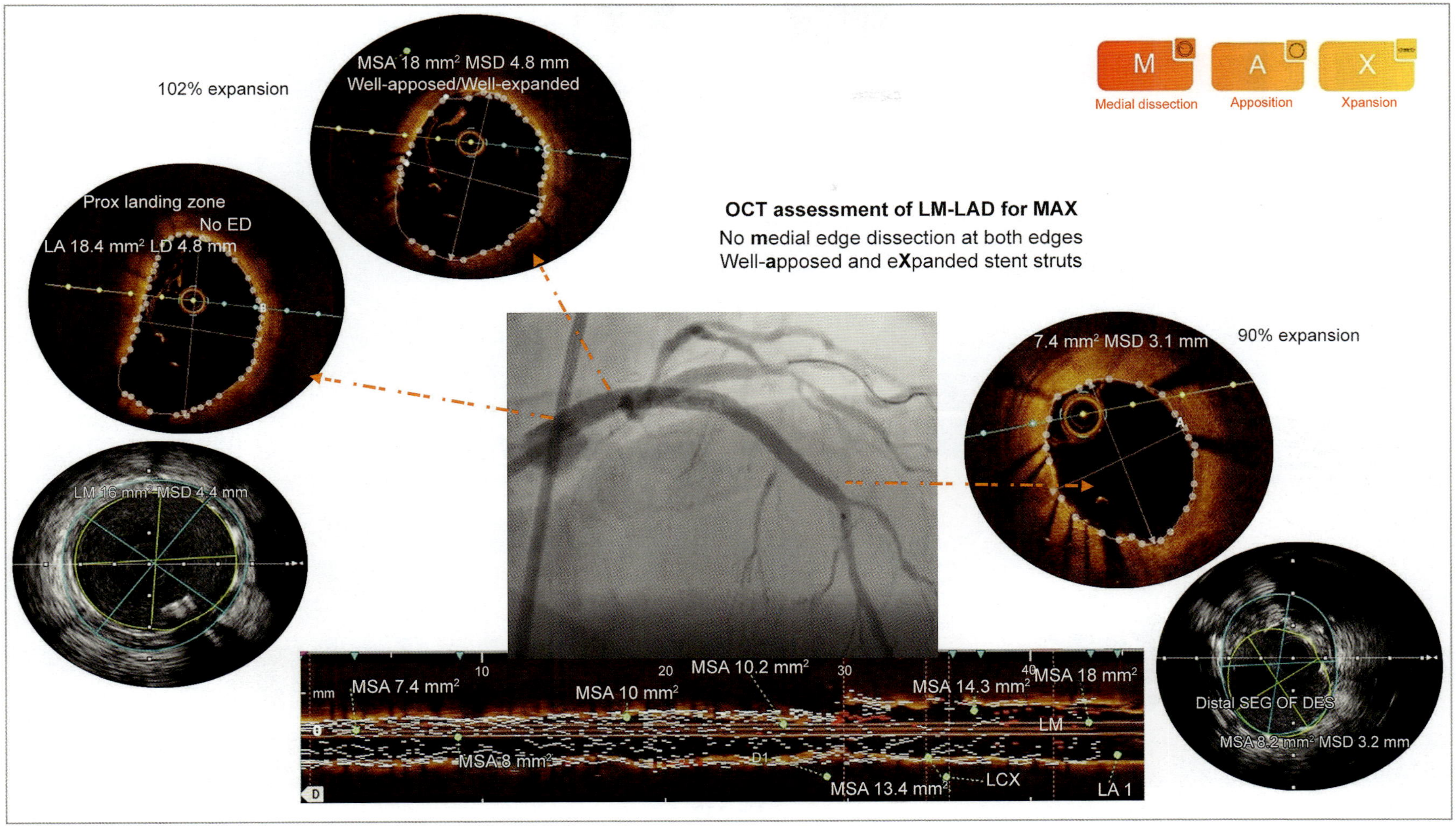
Medial dissection
Apposition
Xpansion
MSA 18 mm² MSD 4.8 mm
Well-apposed/Well-expanded
102% expansion
Prox landing zone
No ED
LA 18.4 mm² LD 4.8 mm
LM 16 mm² MSD 4.4 mm
OCT assessment of LM-LAD for MAX
No medial edge dissection at both edges
Well-apposed and eXpanded stent struts
7.4 mm² MSD 3.1 mm
90% expansion
Distal SEG OF DES
MSA 8.2 mm² MSD 3.2 mm
MSA 7.4 mm²
MSA 10 mm²
MSA 10.2 mm²
MSA 14.3 mm²
MSA 18 mm²
MSA 8 mm²
MSA 13.4 mm²
LM
LCX
LA 1
D1

Fig. 13A

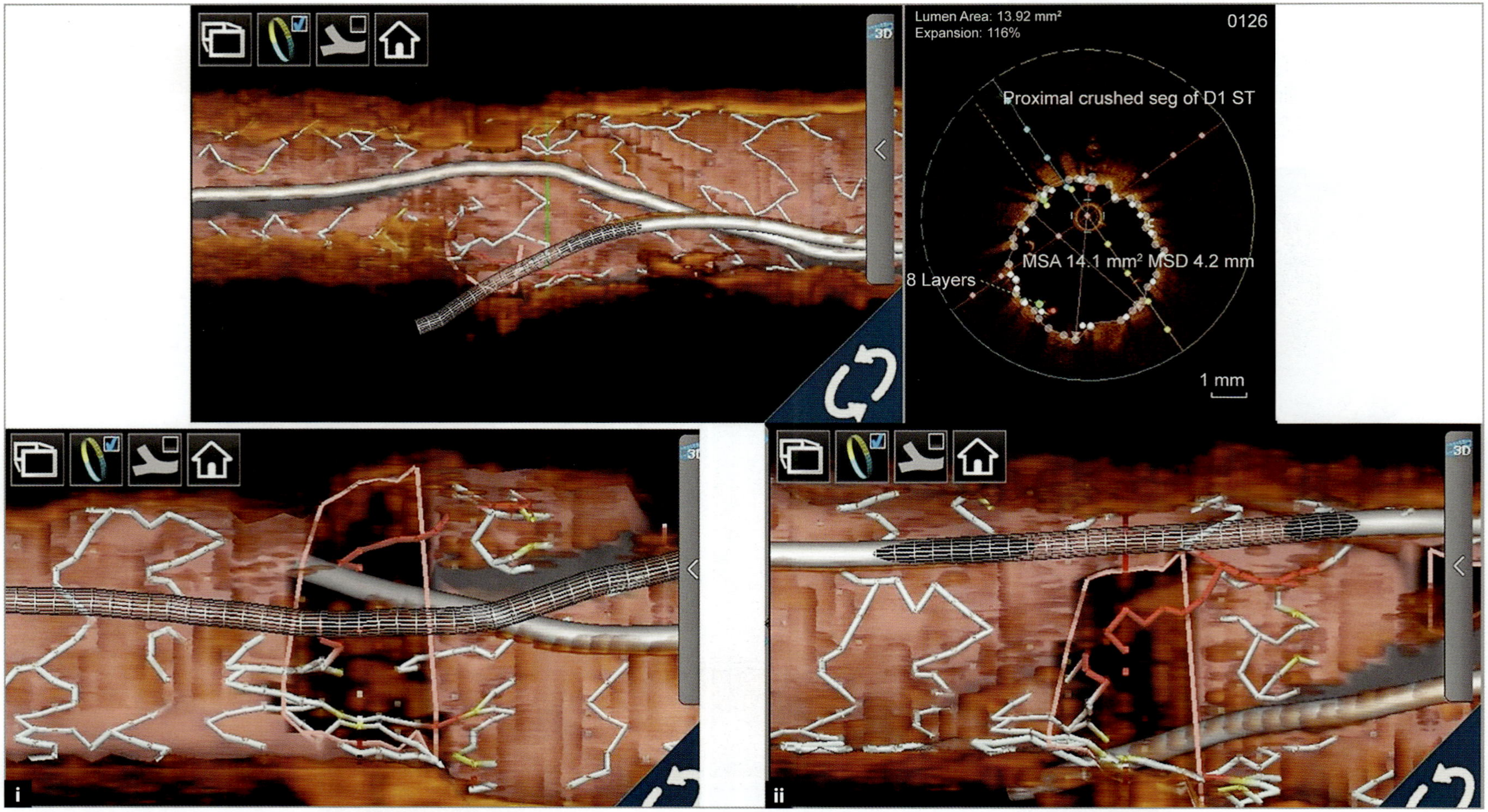
Lumen Area: 13.92 mm²
Expansion: 116%
0126
Proximal crushed seg of D1 ST
MSA 14.1 mm² MSD 4.2 mm
8 Layers
1 mm
i
ii

Fig. 13B

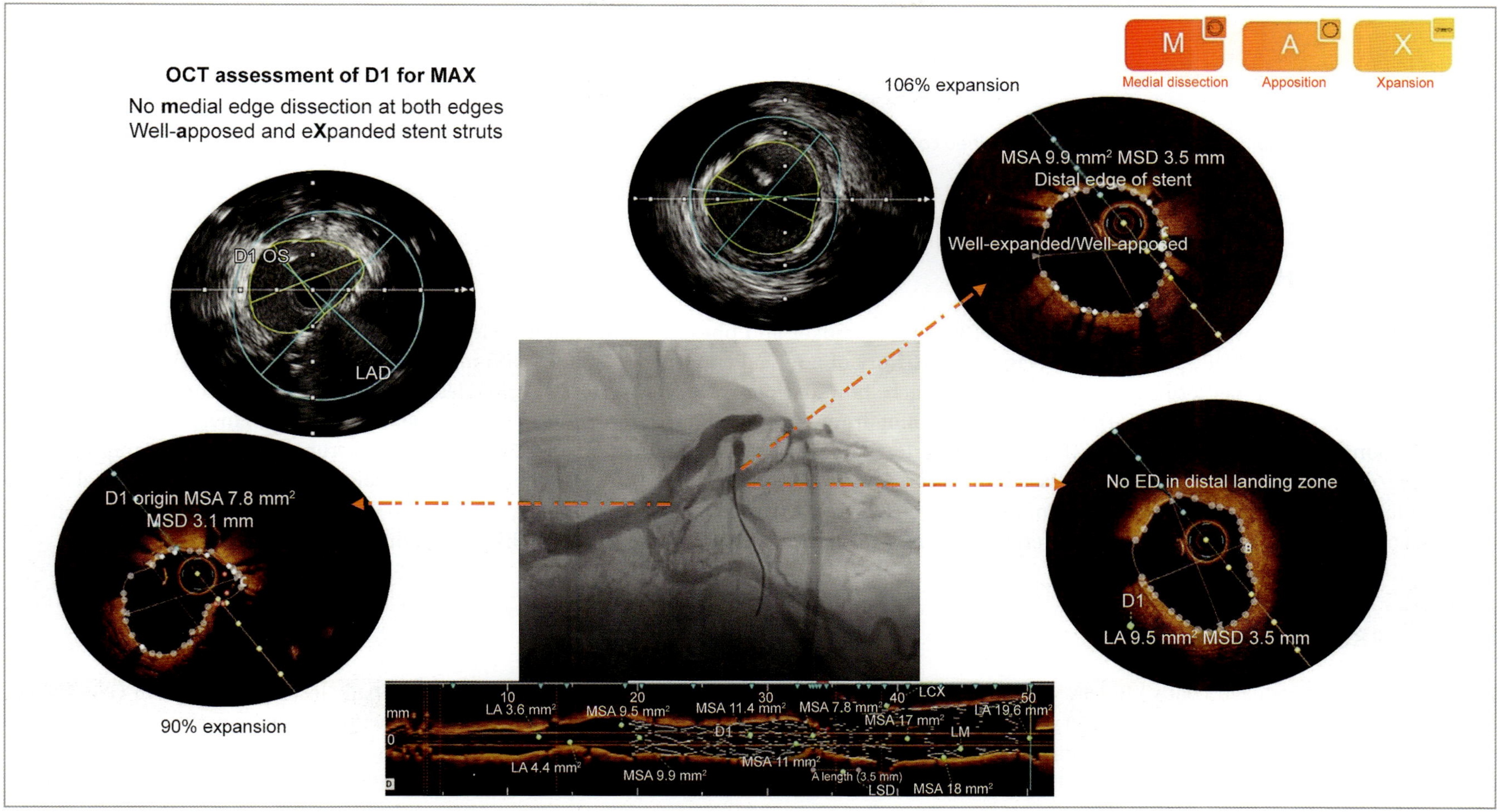

Fig. 13C

Figs. 13A to C: Poststent (A) MAX assessment with IVUS and OCT; (B) OCT assessment of SB ostium (i) GW crossing distal strut, (ii) GW crossing through proximal strut; (C) Side branch IVUS and OCT assessment. (IVUS: intravascular ultrasound; LA: lumen area; LCX: left circumflex; LM: left main; MSA: minimal stent area; OCT: optical coherence tomography)

CASE 2

OPN NC for plaque modification of PCI of severely calcified coronaries.

CLINICAL HISTORY

A 76-year-old male, known diabetic, hypertensive (30 years), smoker and obese with obstructive sleep apnea (OSA), presented with effort angina and shortness of breath (SOB) since 15 days **(Fig. 14A)**. History of nonhealing ulcer on left foot with mild cellulitis, and past history of angiographic evaluation in 2015 in another tertiary care hospital (AH) which showed triple-vessel disease (TVD)—mild lesion of LAD, borderline long segment of LCX, mid RCA chronic total occlusion (CTO) with retrograde filling from left system for which medical management was advised. Investigations: 2D Echo showed regional wall motion abnormality (RWMA) in RCA territory with mild LV dysfunction, EF—50%, Hb 13.4 g , serum creatinine 1.21 mg/dL, blood urea 29 mg/dL, eGFR 94, RBS 365 mg/dL, present admission CAG-TVD, long segment proximal to mid LAD 70% calcified lesion, LCX—proximal diffuse severe calcific lesion with mid total occlusion, mid RCA-CTO **(Figs. 14B to D)**, peripheral angiogram (PAG)—severe disease of tibioperoneal trunk, long total occlusion and severely calcified posterior tibial artery, and severe diffuse long segment of distal anterior tibial artery **(Fig. 14E)**.

PROCEDURE

Left coronary artery engaged with XB 3.5-7 Fr guiding catheter, initially tried with Sion blue, and Fielder XT, finally lesion crossed with Gaia I using Corsair support and predilated with 1.5 × 10 mm and 2 × 10 mm Tazuna balloons **(Fig. 15)**. Gaia I was exchanged with BMW wire multiple predilatations with 2.5 × 10 mm NC, lesion was not yielding with 2.5 × 15 mm NC **(Fig. 15)**. Initial plan was to do rotablation for plaque modification which was differed due to crossing of the lesion with 1.5 and 2.5 mm Tazuna balloons. Calcified lesion was unyielding with 2.5 mm NC balloon and there was difficulty in repositioning same NC balloon due to loss of profile. Hence, OPN NC 2.5 × 10 mm was opted for plaque modification using Guidezilla and entire disease segment of LCX (proximal-distal) was dilated up to 40 atm—due to difficulty in placing Guidezilla prior to placing OPN NC balloon and before acquiring OCT image Inchworm technique was used, for placing OPN NC and OCT catheter. Plan was to use ROTA, if there is no adequate plaque modification despite using OPN NC balloon which was to be confirmed with OCT imaging **(Fig. 15)**.

Postplaque modification with OPN NC OCT assessment of LCX of severely calcified LCX using Guidezilla support to place OCT catheter after deeply intubating Guidezilla up to mid LCX. Subsequently OCT run showed severe calcific plaque with expansion index (CVI score) of 4—thickness >0.5 mm, arc >180° and length >5 mm with multiple OPN-induced multiple fractures of calcium and dissection of plaque **(Fig. 16)**. Evidence of calcium fracture on OCT image indicates adequately modified calcium plaque and predicts better expansion of the stent with low target lesion revascularization (TLR) rate.

2.5 × 38 mm Xience Xpedition stent placed in distal LCX and 2.5 × 38 mm Xience Xpedition stent deployed in distal LCX, proximal LCX stenting done with 3.0 × 23 mm Xience Xpediton Stent using Guidezilla support, and postdilatation with 3.0 × 12 mm NC Trek **(Fig. 17)**. With inching technique

Guidezilla placed in distal LCX and OCT catheter was placed in distal LCX through Guidezilla to acquire poststent OCT run **(Fig. 18)**, as there is residual underexpansion. Further postdilatations were carried out with 3.0 × 10 mm OPN NC balloon up to 40–45 atm for adequate expansion—bigger the better. Final angio view showed well-implanted without any residual stenosis, and TIMI III flow **(Fig. 17)**.

PCI of LAD was done 2 days later to avoid contrast-induced nephropathy (CIN) after adequate hydration. LCA engaged with XB 3.5–6 Fr guiding catheter, LAD lesion was crossed with 0.014″ BMW wire. Predilatation done with 2.5 × 15 mm NC.

Prestent OCT analysis showed morphology—long segment fibrocalcific lesion with mild calcific plaque with arc 90°, thickness >0.5 mm, and length <5 mm, hence plaque modification using ROTA differed. Lesion length was 55 mm with healthy landing zones **(Fig. 19)**. After adequate predilatations with high-pressure NC balloon inflations, 2.75 × 48 mm Xience Xpedition stent deployed in mid LAD, ostioproximal LAD stenting done with 3.0 × 15 mm Xience Xpedition stent using Guidezilla support. Postdilatation done with 3.0 × 15 mm NC Trek. Final result good with TIMI III flow **(Fig. 20)**.

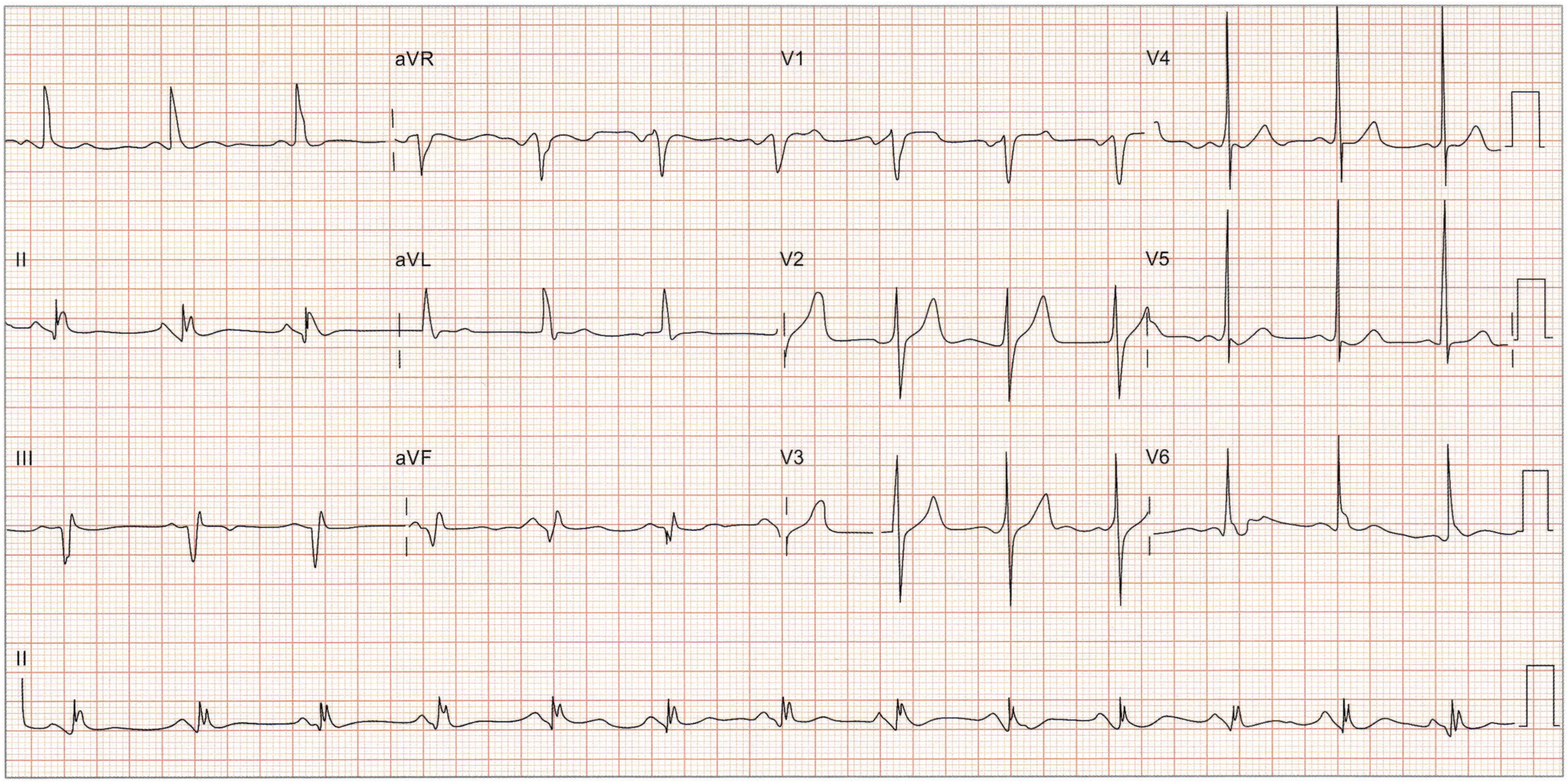

Fig. 14A

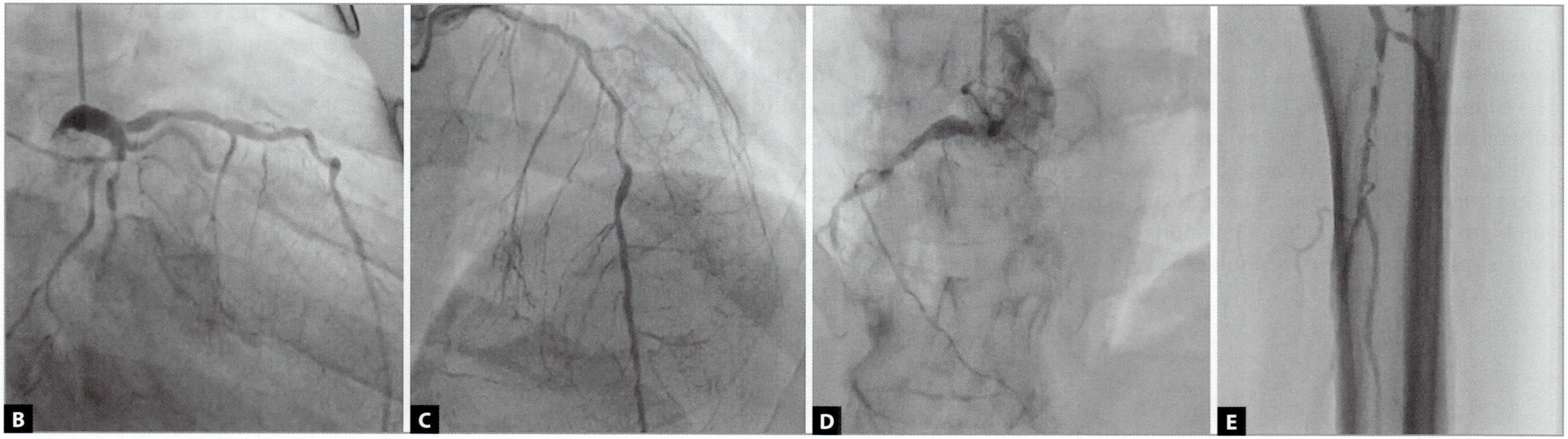

Figs. 14B to E

Figs. 14A to E: (A) ECG, coronary angiogram; (B) LCX; (C) LAD; (D) RCA; (E) Peripheral angiogram of left leg. (ECG: electrocardiogram; LAD: left anterior descending; LCX: left circumflex; RCA: right coronary artery)

Post-OCT assessment of LAD showed no medial edge dissection with well-apposed and eXpanded stent struts **(Fig. 21)**.

On fifth day, below knee angioplasty was performed through antegrade technique from left femoral artery approach using 7 Fr long sheath. Tibioperioneal trunk and posterior tibial artery was crossed with straight tip Terumo and Approach CTO wire using CXI microcatheter support, after placing wire predilated with 2.5 × 150 mm Hemoteg AG Ranger. Subsequently, drug-eluting balloon (DEB) of tibioperoneal trunk and posterior tibial artery was performed up to the level of ankle using 3.5 × 80 mm Lutonix balloon proximally and 2.5 × 150 mm Hemoteg AG Ranger distally. Distal anterior tibial artery angioplasty was done with 2.5 × 210 mm ev3 NanoCross Elite drug eluting balloon. Postballoon angioplasty angio view showed good antegrade flow of tibioperoneal trunk, posterior and anterior tibial artery **(Fig. 22)**.

It would be very difficult to place an OCT catheter in a tortuous calcified coronary artery for acquiring images. Many times forceful manipulations of OCT catheter may lead to kinking of the shaft, damage of light source resulting in failure of acquiring images. Guideliner/Guidezilla-assisted placement of OCT catheter will be very useful to cross tortuous bends and to place the catheter distal to the lesion to be examined. Severely calcified lesions are associated with artifacts of OCT imaging due to calcium-limiting rotation of OCT catheter and improper clearance of blood due to undilated critical lesions limiting contrast flow during injections. This case demonstrates usefulness of Guidezilla for acquiring OCT images in severely calcified coronary arteries.

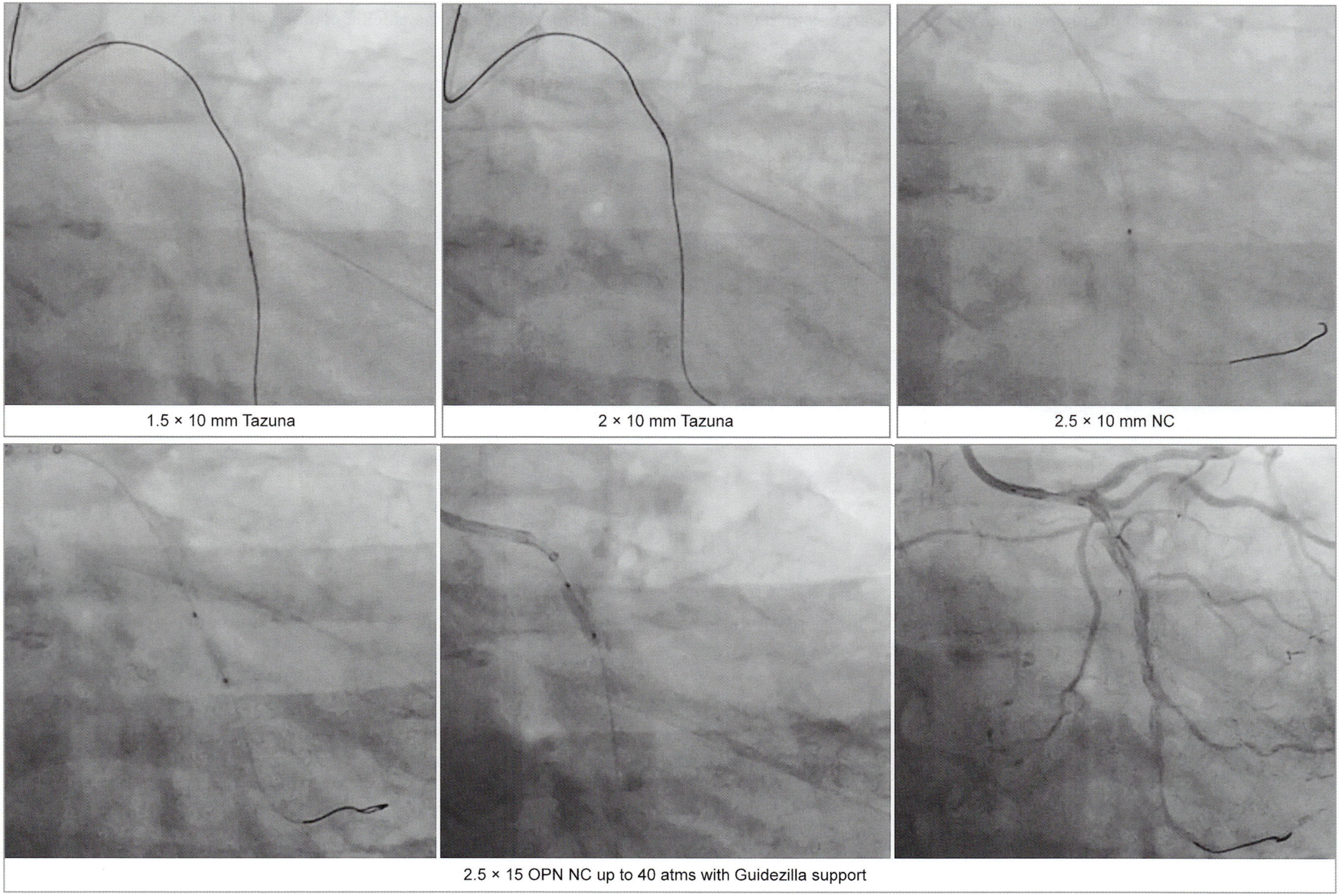

Fig. 15: Sequential predilations of left circumflex (LCX) vessel. (NC: noncompliant)

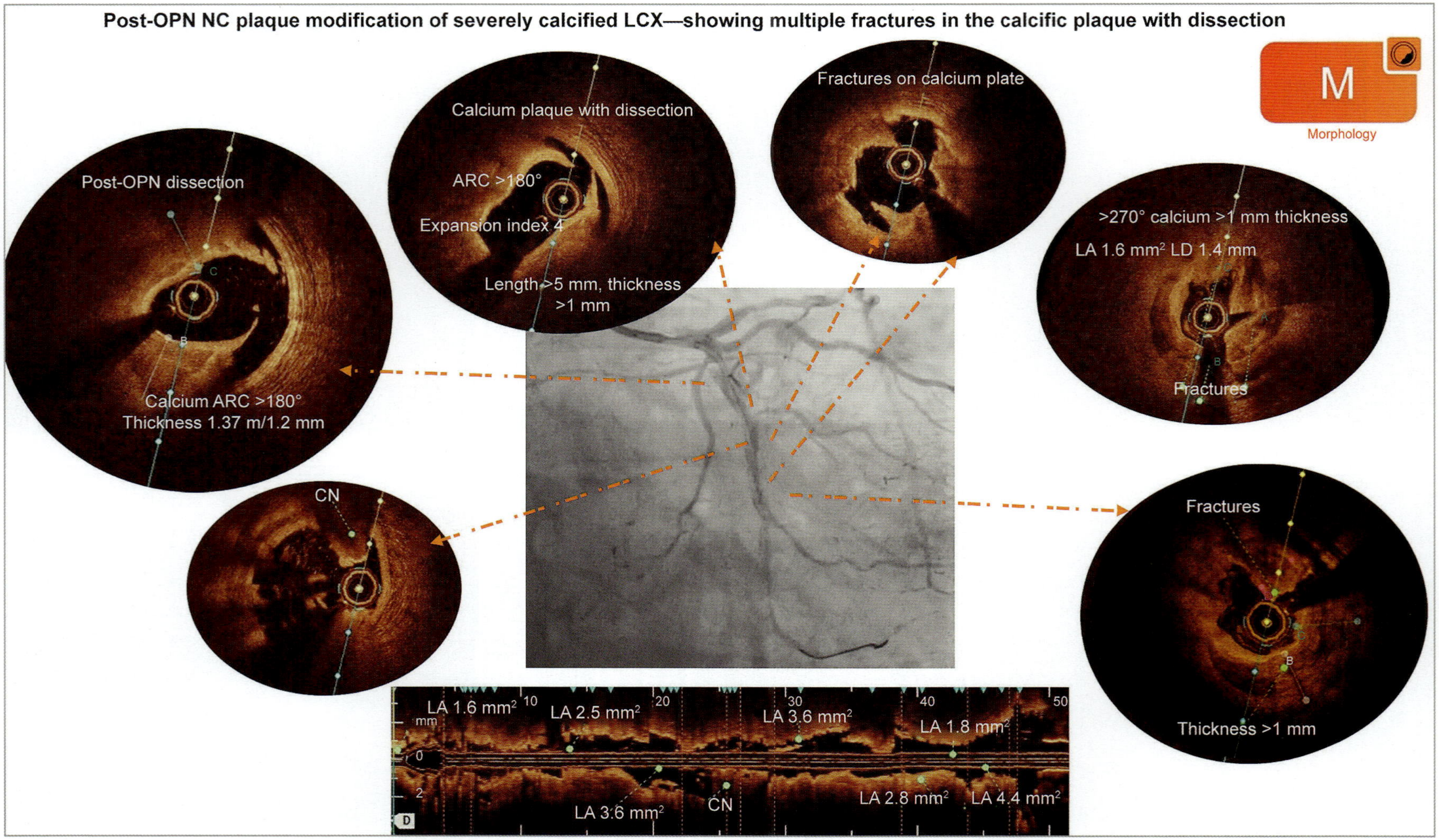

Fig. 16: Pre-PCI OCT assessment showed calcium fractures in entire LCX diseased segment. (LCX: left circumflex; OCT: optical coherence tomography; PCI: percutaneous coronary intervention)

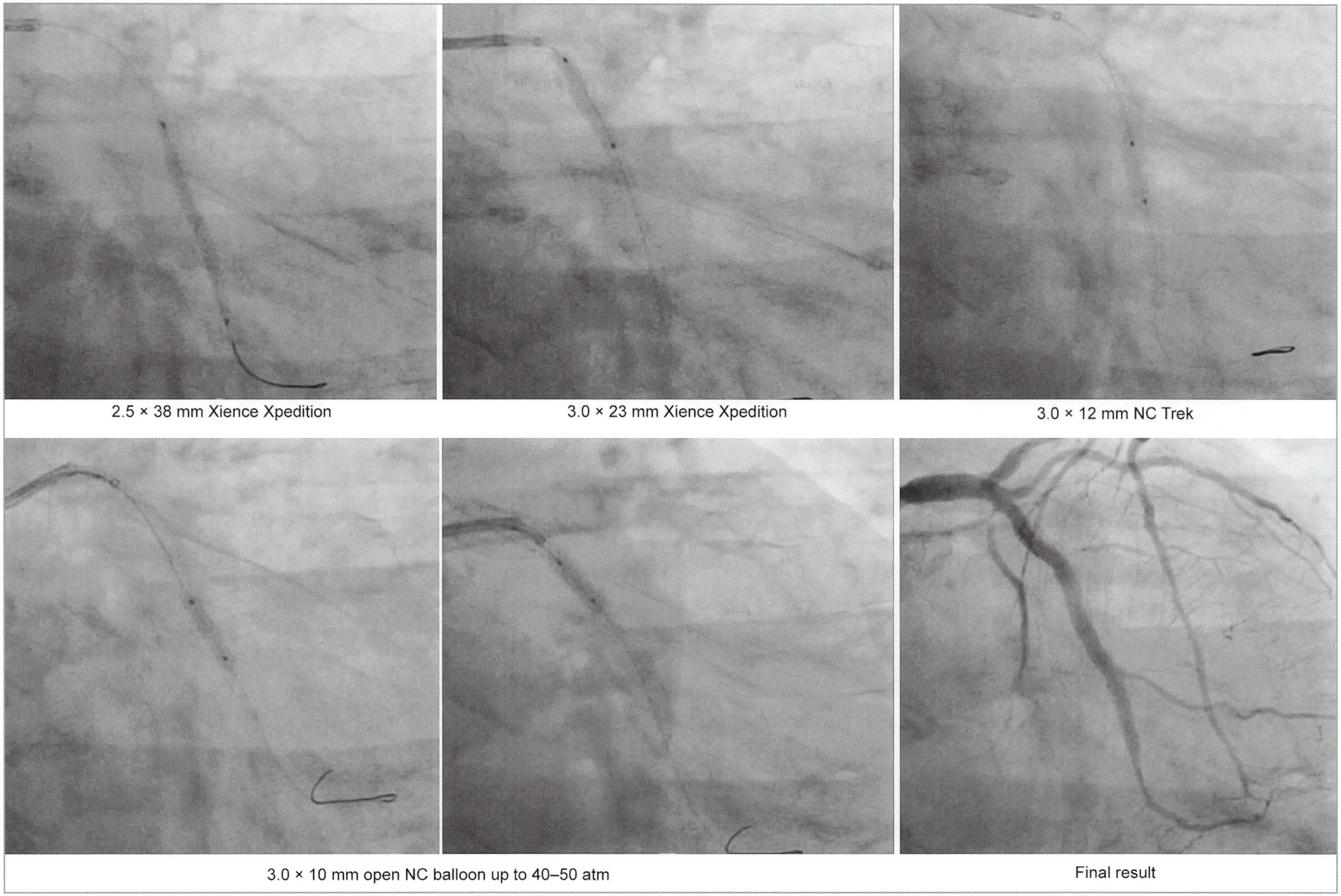

Fig. 17: Stenting, postdilatations with high pressure balloon in left circumflex (LCX) segment.

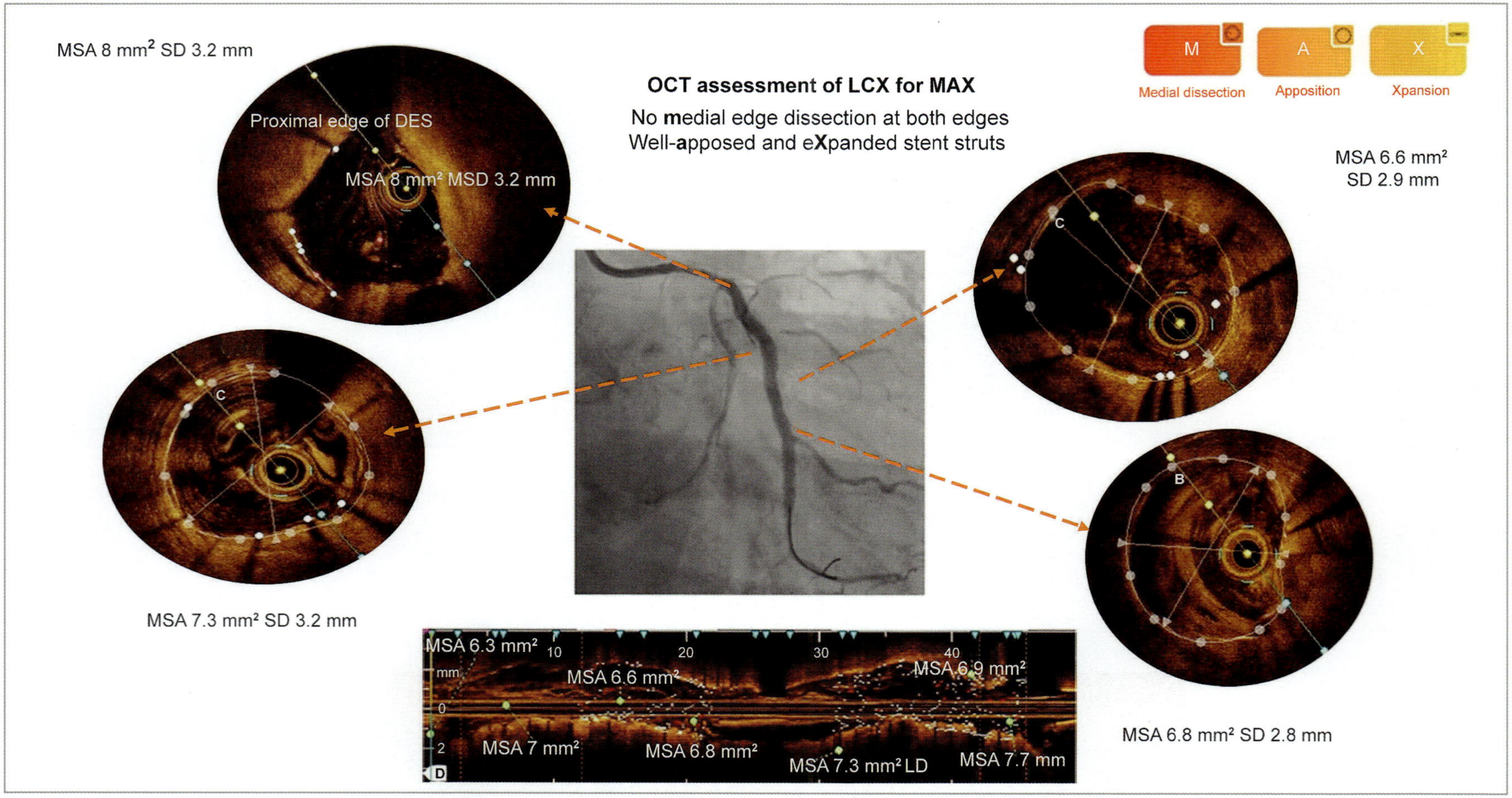

Fig. 18: Post-PCI OCT assessment of LCX showed well-expanded and apposed stent struts with no medial dissections. (LCX: left circumflex; MSA: minimal stent area; OCT: optical coherence tomography; PCI: percutaneous coronary intervention; SD: stent diameter)

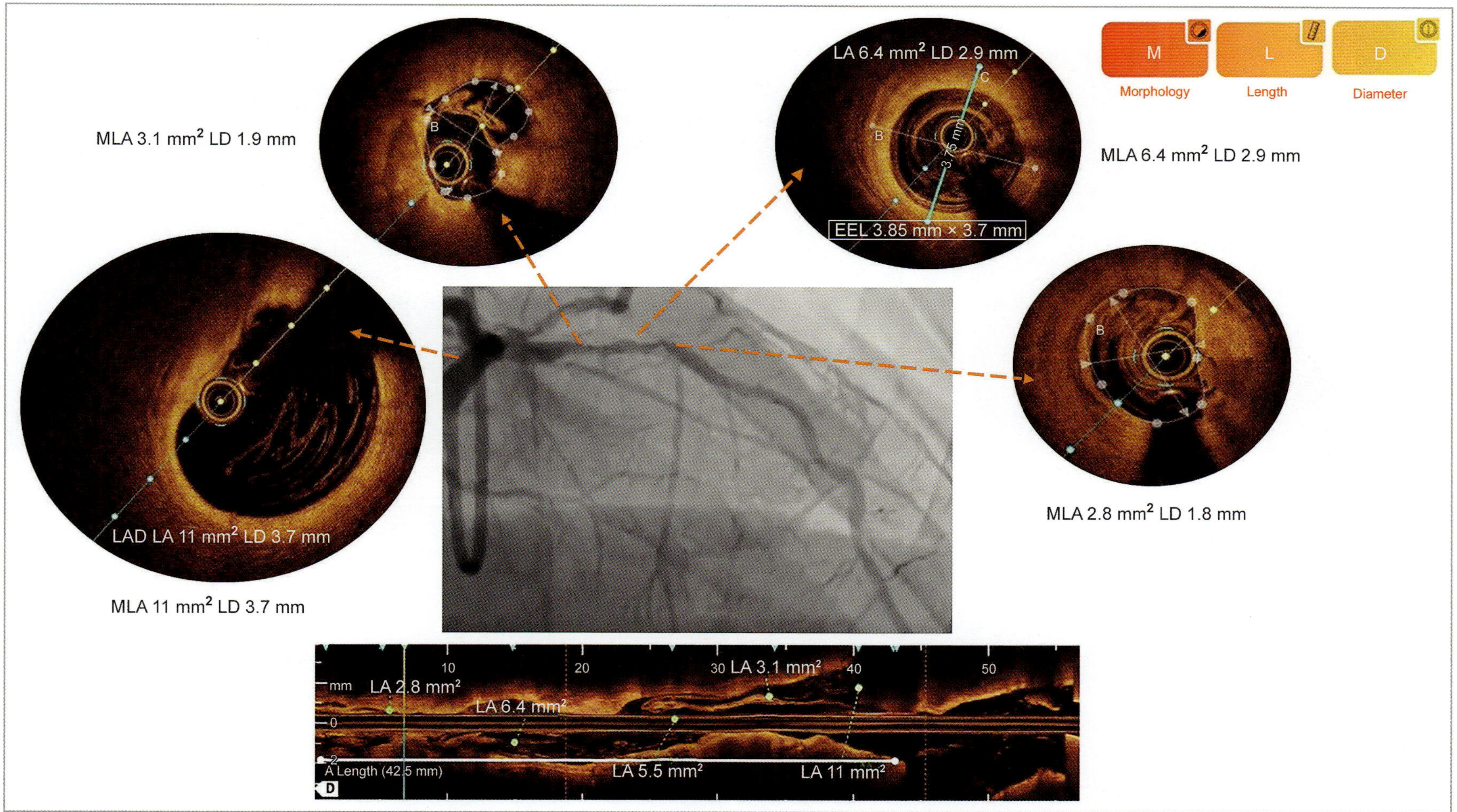

Fig. 19: Pre-PCI OCT assessment of LAD segment for plaque morphology and device selection. (LAD: left anterior descending; OCT: optical coherence tomography; PCI: percutaneous coronary intervention)

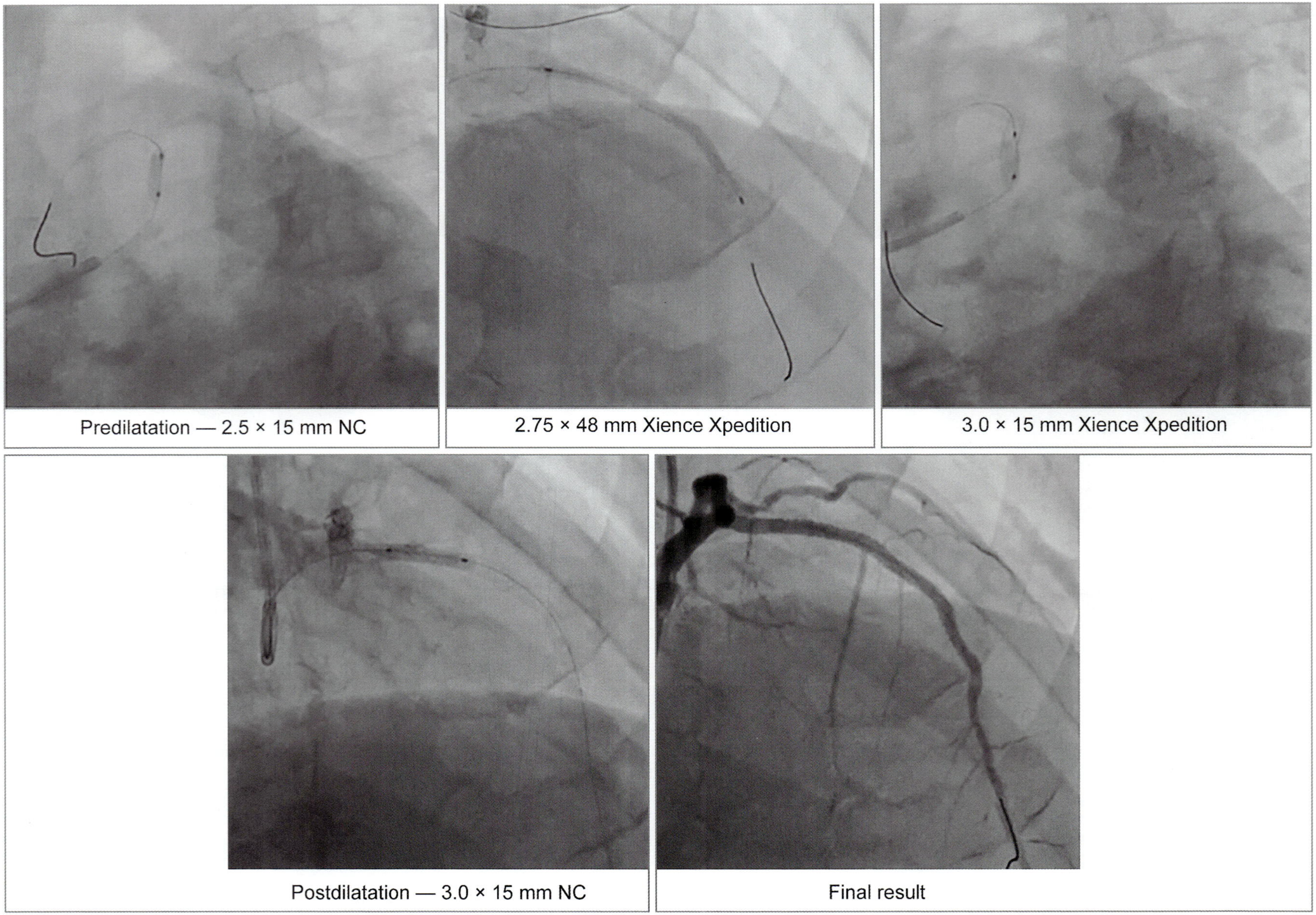

Fig. 20: Coronary angioplasty of left anterior descending (LAD) vessel. (NC: noncompliant)

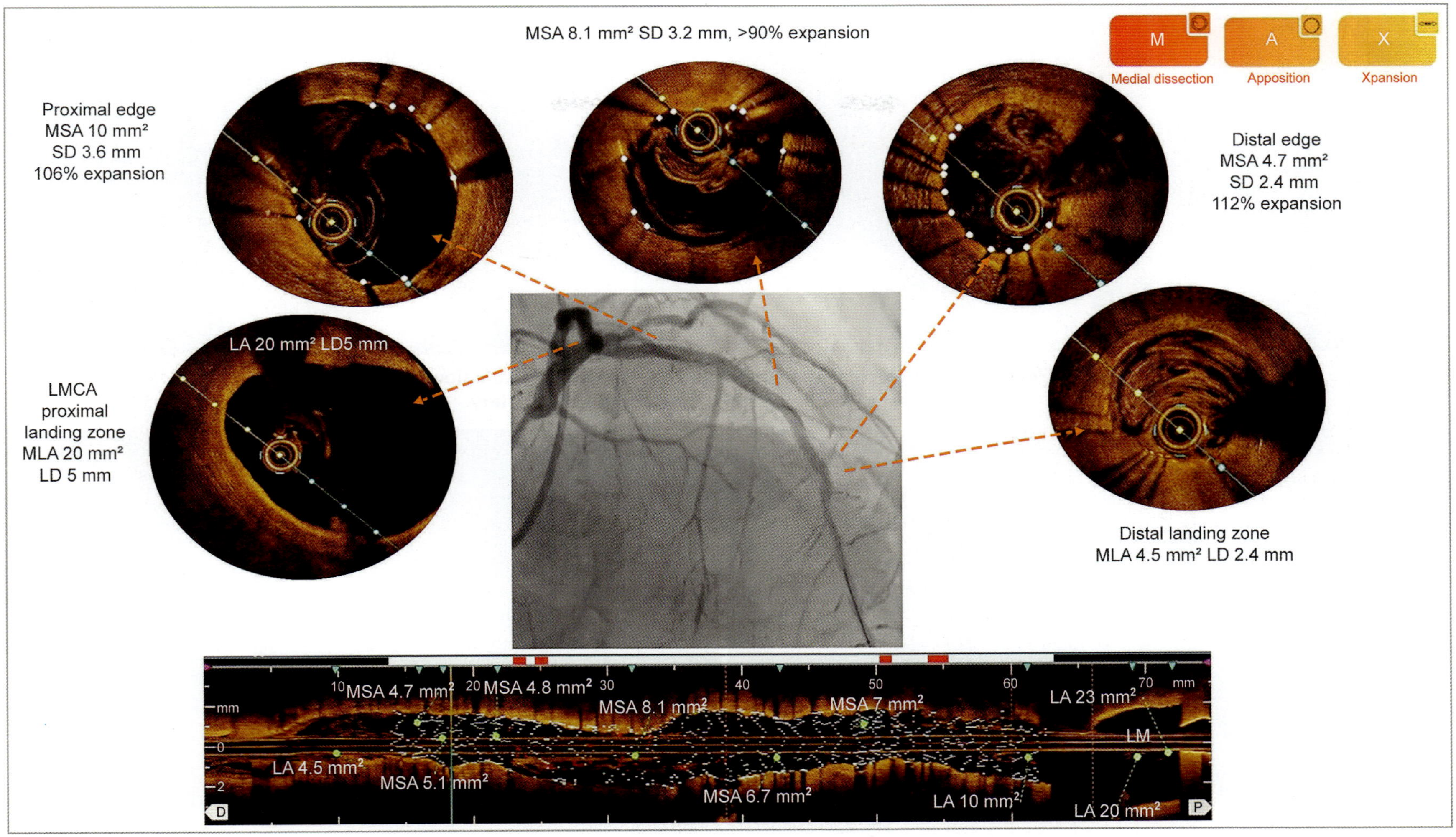

Fig. 21: Post-PCI OCT assessment showed well-expanded and apposed stent struts with no medial edge dissections. (LA: lumen area; LD: lumen diameter; MLA: minimal lumen area; MSA: minimal stent area; OCT: optical coherence tomography; PCI: percutaneous coronary intervention; SD: stent diameter)

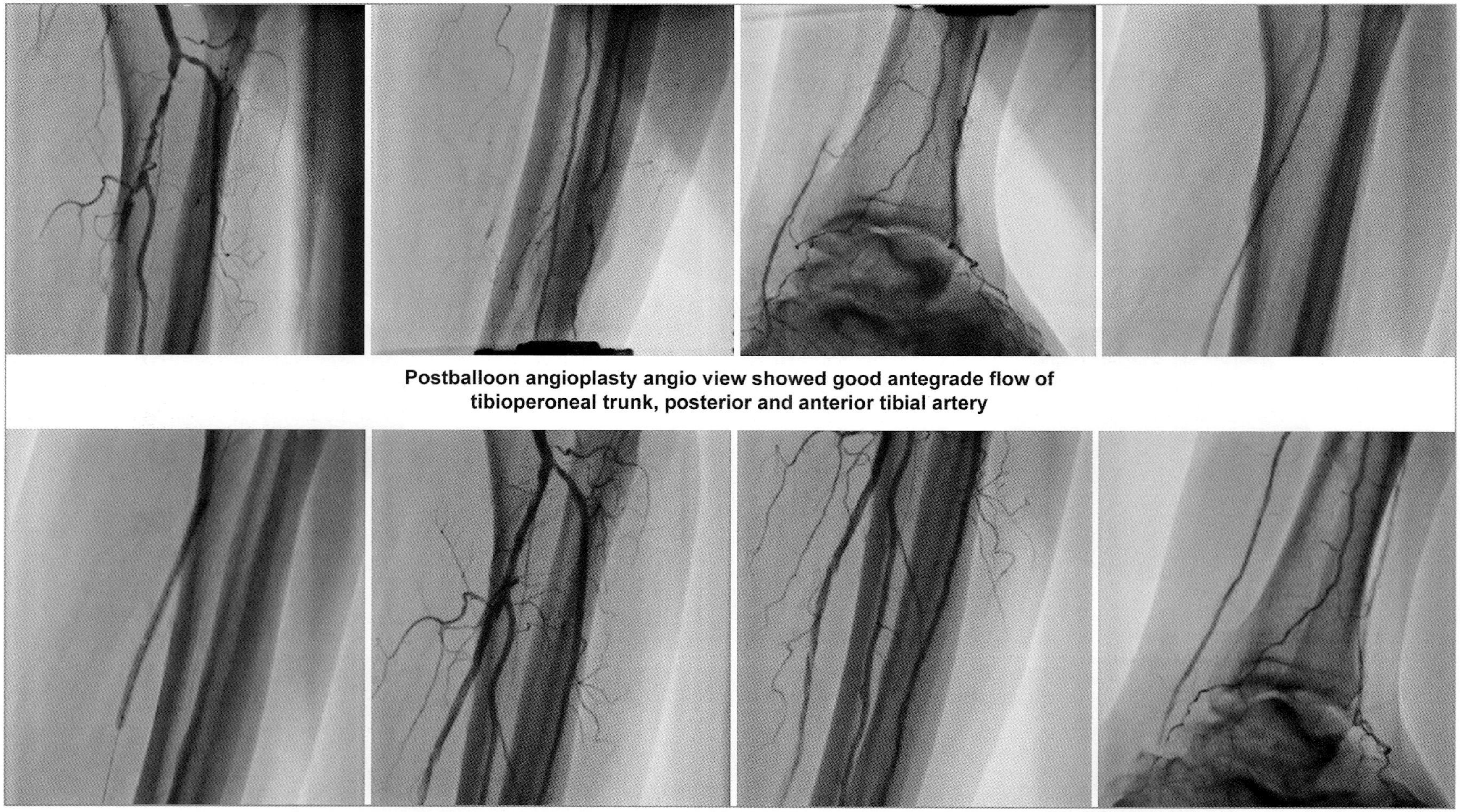

Fig. 22: Peripheral balloon angioplasty.

CASE 3

OCT for making complex situation simpler.

CLINICAL HISTORY

A 45-year-old female known diabetic, with acute kidney injury (AKI), presented with CAD-ACS—evolved anterior wall myocardial infarction (AWMI), electrocardiogram (ECG)—ST elevation and T inversion in V1-V4 leads, 2D ECHO—bilateral (B/L) pleural effusion, RWMA in LAD territory, mild LV dysfunction, EF—45%. Investigations: Hb—10.2 g/dL, TROP I -0.14 ng/mL, RBS—124 mg/dL, serum creatinine—1.15 mg/dL, eGFR—58 mL/min. CAG-LMCA—normal, LAD—proximal mild lesion with significant lesion of mid LAD, LCX—60%-70% ostioproximal lesion, RCA—mid to distal mild narrowing **(Fig. 23)**.

PROCEDURE

Left coronary artery engaged with EBU 3.5-6 Fr guiding catheter, fractional flow reserve (FFR) study of LCX was done to decide significance of LCX lesion which was negative, hence LCX stenting was avoided **(Fig. 23)**. LAD lesion crossed with 0.014″ Runthrough and D1 crossed with 0.014″ BMW.

Prestent OCT showed ***(Fig. 24A to C):***

Morphology: Lipid-rich plaque with macrophages and micro calcification in proximal LAD

Length: Lesion length is 27 mm

Diameter: Distal-LD—1.7 mm, external elastic lamina diameter (EELD)—2.4 × 2.3 mm, proximal—EELD—4 × 3.7 mm

Proximal to Mid LAD stenting done with 2.5 × 38 mm Xience Xpedition, postdilatation done with 2.75 × 12 mm NC Trek **(Fig. 25)**. Poststent OCT showed no medial dissection well-apposed and eXpanded stent struts **(Fig. 26)**.

Right coronary artery engaged with JR 3.5-6 Fr guiding catheter, lesion crossed with 0.014″ Runthrough wire, RCA—stenting done with 2.5 × 28 mm Xience Xpedition, and postdilatation done with 3.0 × 12 mm NC Trek. Final result was good with TIMI III flow **(Fig. 25)**.

Optical coherence tomography makes complex situations simpler by assessing severity of SB lesion, lesion length and any need for plaque modification. This patient has ostioproximal LCX lesion, and proximal LAD lesion without any significant involvement of LMCA on angiographic study. OCT run showed significant plaque burden of LMCA with luminal area of 6.9 mm^2, LCX ostial luminal area was good without any significant narrowing, no spiky carina, SB, and CT angles are >80° which indicate less chances of SB closure prior to provisional stenting (PS). LCX lesion was interrogated with FFR which indicated functionally insignificant lesion. In view of LMCA area is 6.9 mm^2, LM stenting was differed and LAD stenting was opted extending from ostium of LAD to cover entire disease segment of proximal to mid LAD. OCT guided us in avoiding LM, and SB stenting, thereby reducing the number and unnecessary additional stents.

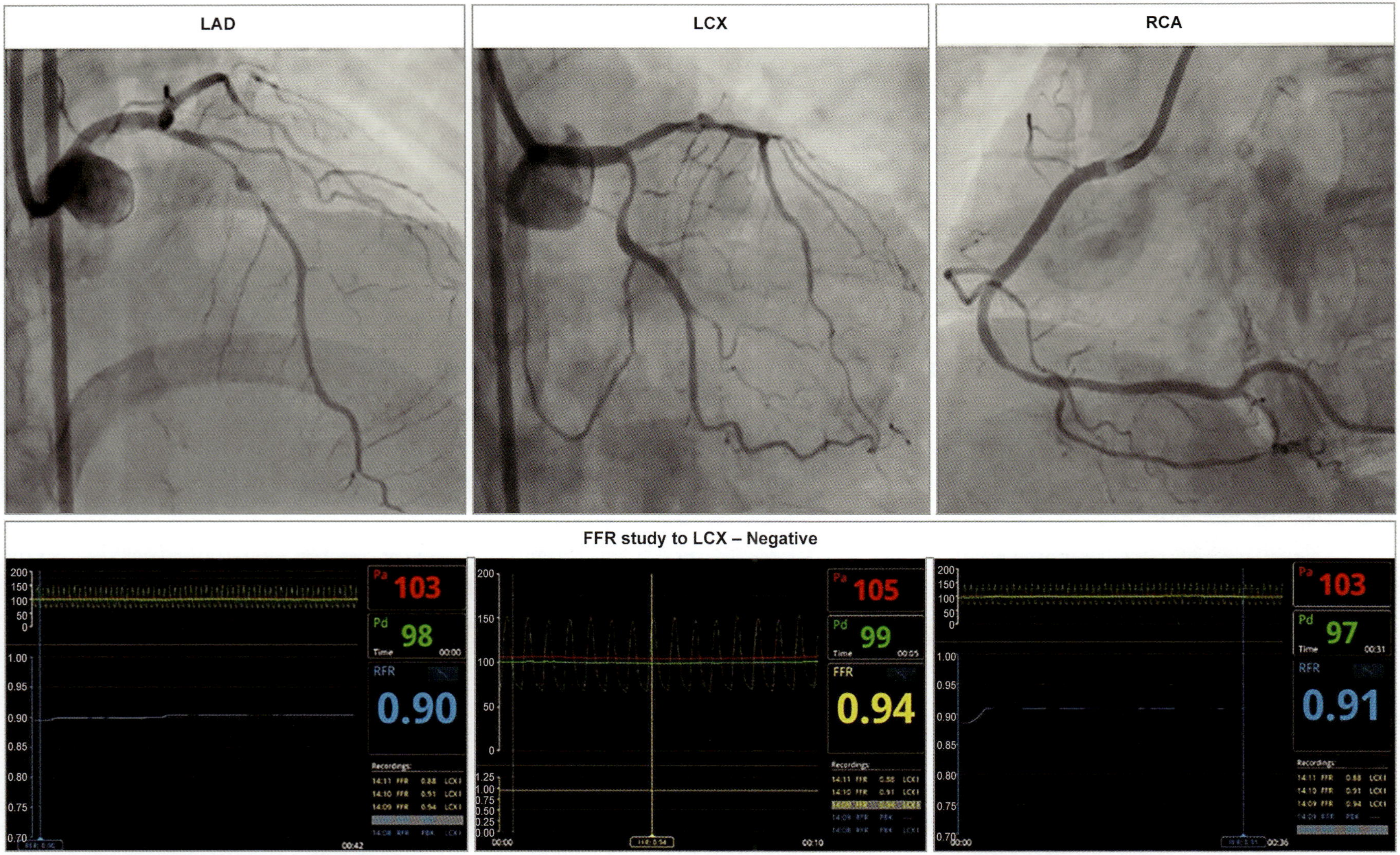

Fig. 23: Coronary angiogram and fractional flow reserve (FFR) study to left circumflex (LCX) vessel. (LAD: left anterior descending; RCA: right coronary artery)

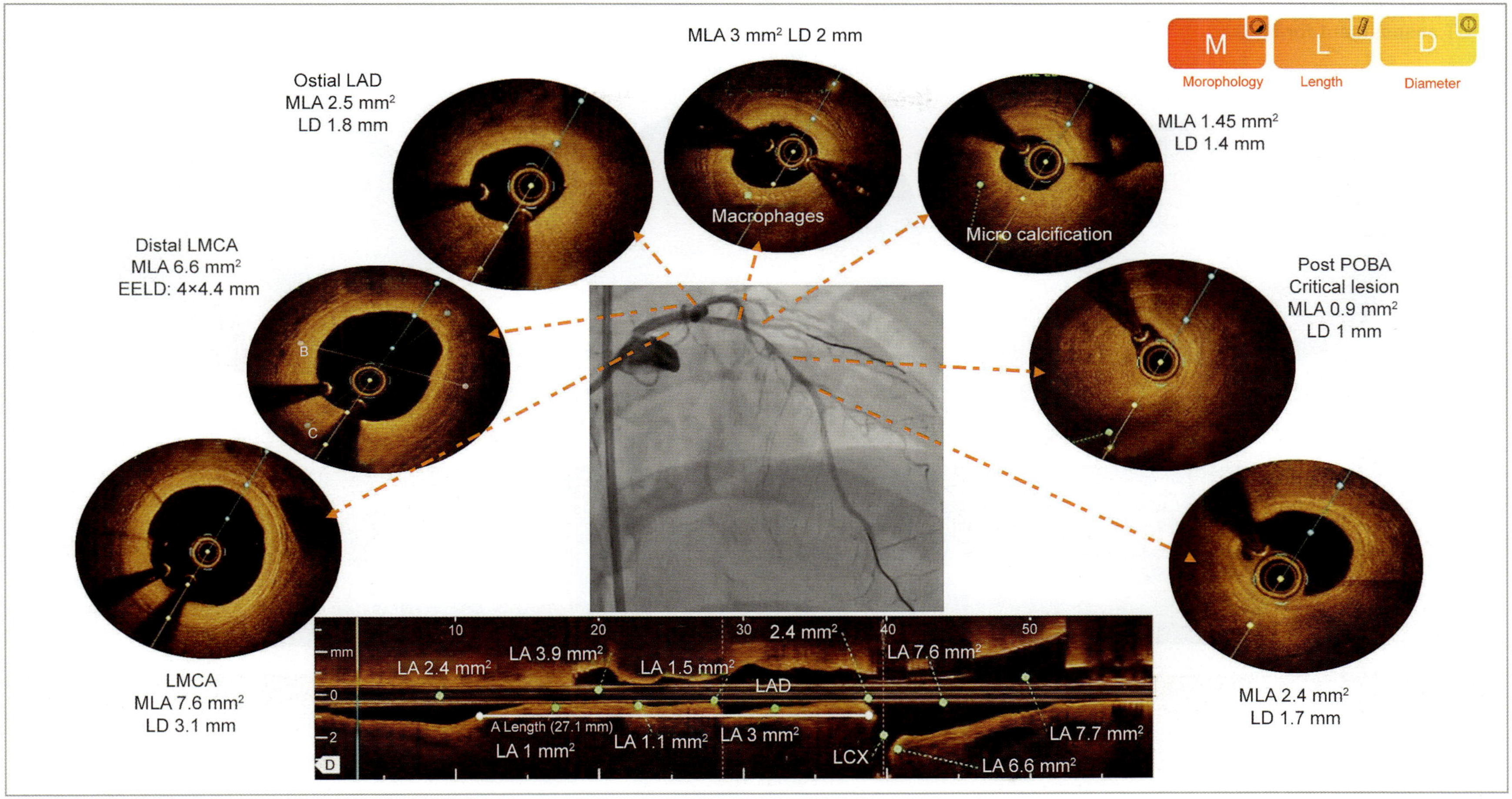
MLA 3 mm² LD 2 mm
M Morophology
L Length
D Diameter
Ostial LAD
MLA 2.5 mm²
LD 1.8 mm
MLA 1.45 mm²
LD 1.4 mm
Macrophages
Micro calcification
Distal LMCA
MLA 6.6 mm²
EELD: 4×4.4 mm
Post POBA
Critical lesion
MLA 0.9 mm²
LD 1 mm
LMCA
MLA 7.6 mm²
LD 3.1 mm
MLA 2.4 mm²
LD 1.7 mm
LA 2.4 mm²
LA 3.9 mm²
LA 1.5 mm²
2.4 mm²
LA 7.6 mm²
LAD
A Length (27.1 mm)
LA 1 mm²
LA 1.1 mm²
LA 3 mm²
LCX
LA 7.7 mm²
LA 6.6 mm²

Fig. 24A

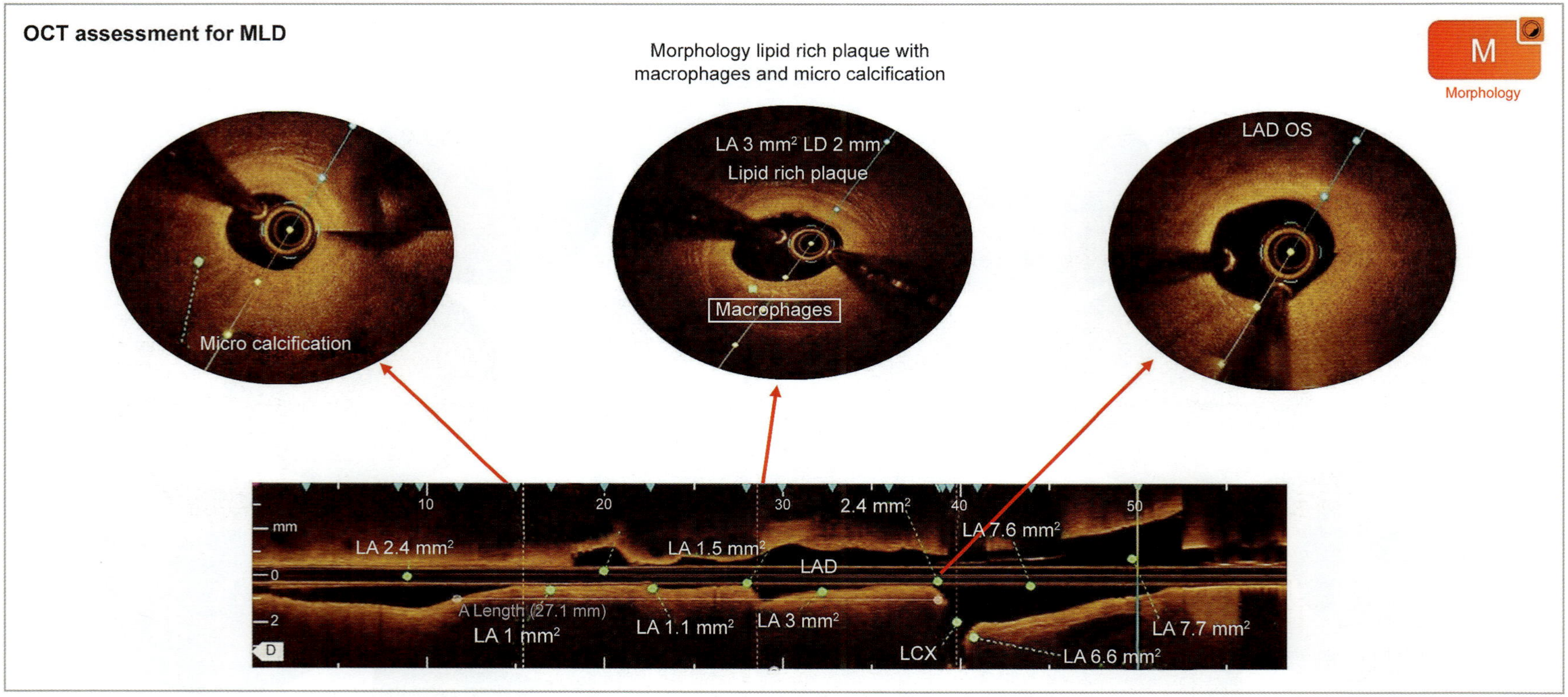

OCT assessment for MLD
Morphology lipid rich plaque with macrophages and micro calcification
M
Morphology
Micro calcification
LA 3 mm² LD 2 mm
Lipid rich plaque
Macrophages
LAD OS
mm
LA 2.4 mm²
LA 1.5 mm²
2.4 mm²
LA 7.6 mm²
LAD
A Length (27.1 mm)
LA 1 mm²
LA 1.1 mm²
LA 3 mm²
LCX
LA 7.7 mm²
LA 6.6 mm²
D

Fig. 24B

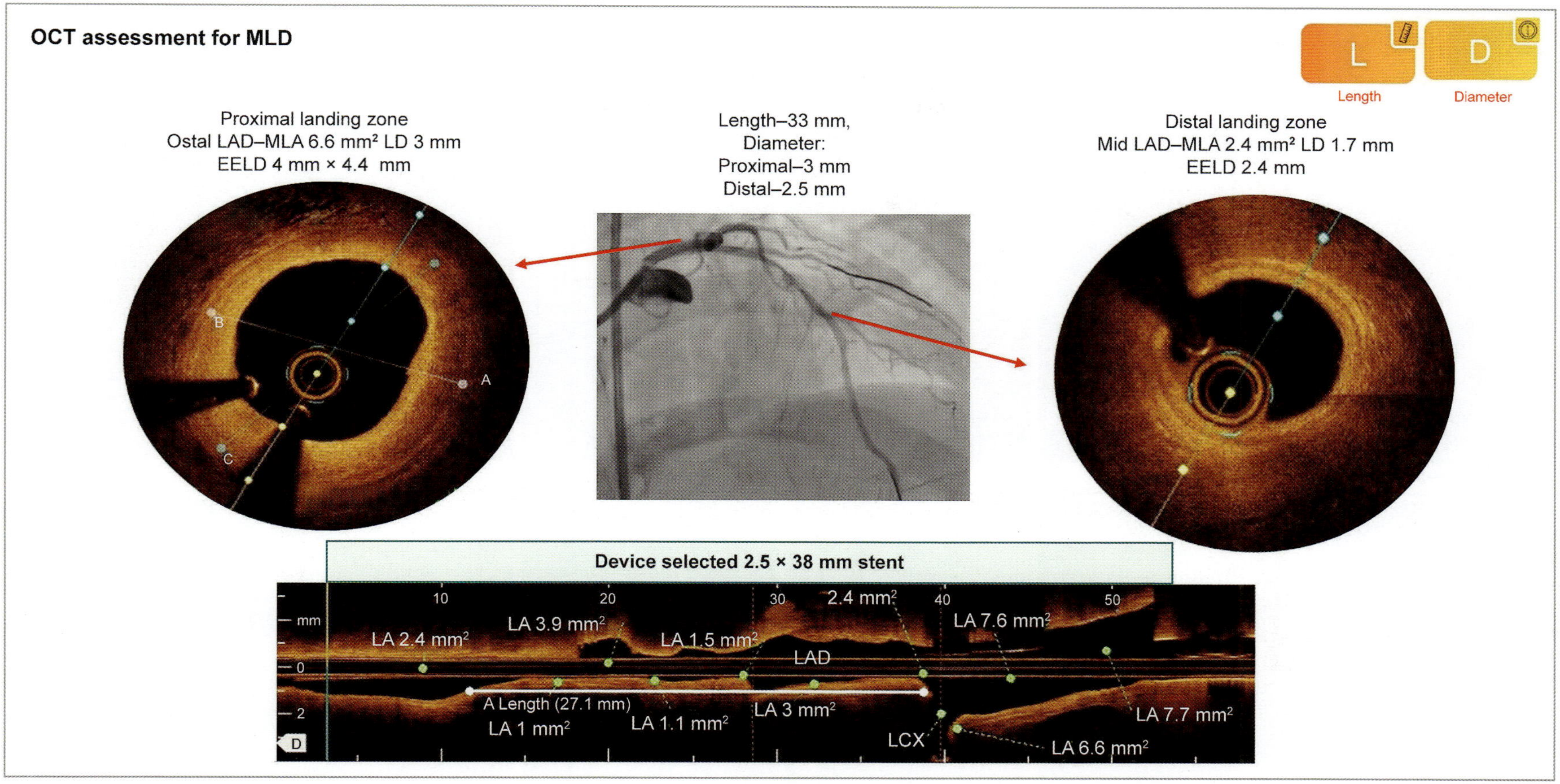

Fig. 24C

Figs. 24A to C: Pre-PCI OCT assessment. (A) MLD assessment of LM and LAD-Fibro-lipid plaque; (B) morphological assessment; (C) OCT assessment for device selection. (EELD: external elastic lamina diameter; LA: lumen area; LAD: left anterior descending; LCX: left circumflex; LD: lumen diameter; LMCA: left main coronary artery; MLA: minimal lumen area)

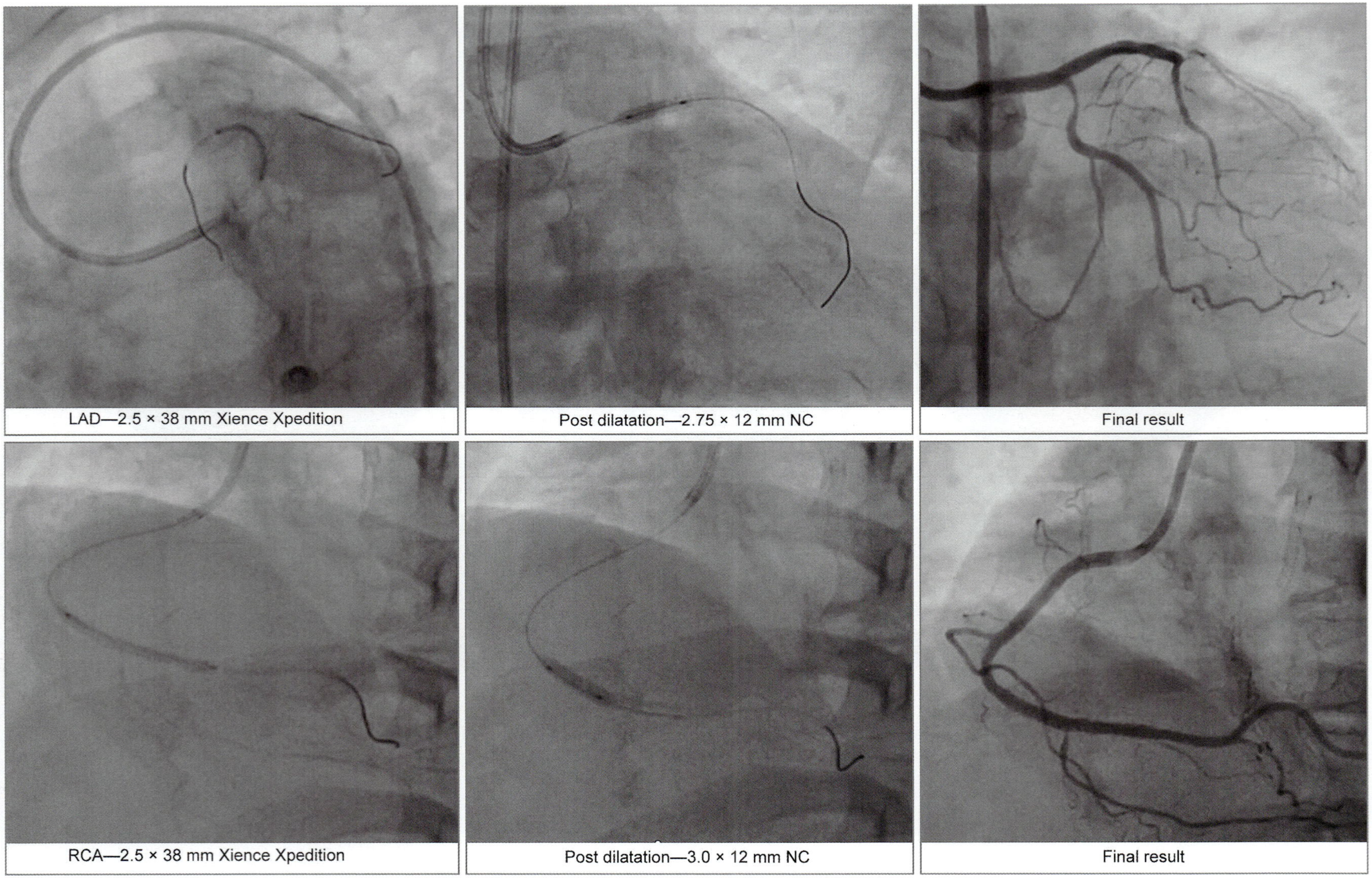

Fig. 25: Coronary angioplasty of left anterior descending (LAD) and right coronary artery (RCA) vessels. (NC: noncompliant)

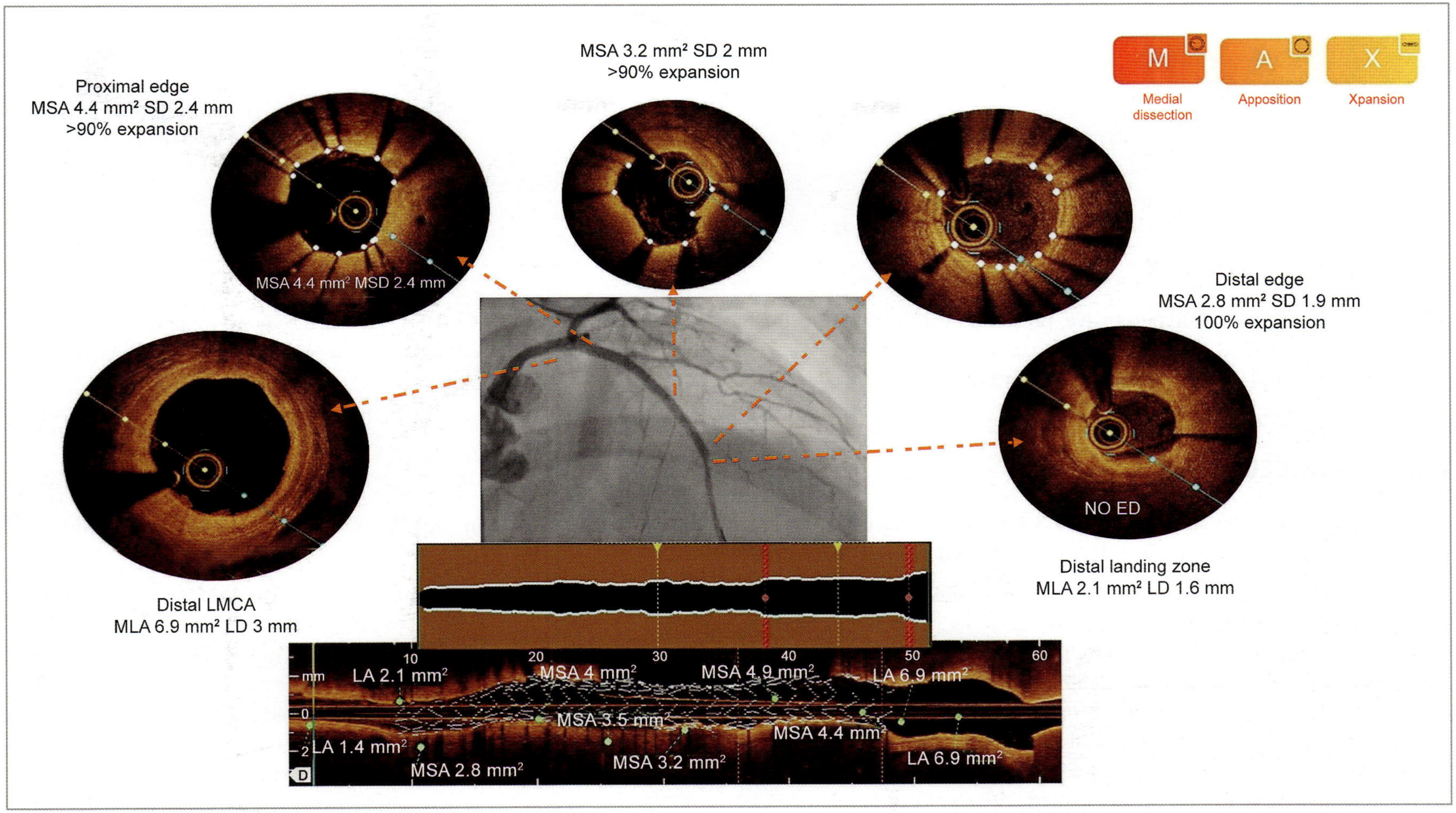

Fig. 26: Post-PCI OCT assessment of LAD showed well-expanded and apposed stent struts with no medial edge dissections. (LA: lumen area; LAD: left anterior descending; LD: lumen diameter; LMCA: left main coronary artery; MLA: minimal lumen area; MSA: minimal stent area; OCT: optical coherence tomography; PCI: percutaneous coronary intervention; SD: stent diameter)

CASE 4

Thick fibrotic plaque—unyielding to regular NC balloons.

CLINICAL HISTORY

A 70-year-old male known hypertensive, presented with complaints of chest pain for 5 days, CAD -ACS-USA, 2D ECHO—good LV function, EF—60%. Investigations: Hb—13.4 g/dL, RBS—92 mg/dL, serum creatinine—0.97 mg/dL, eGFR—79 mL/min. CAG-LAD—mid 95% tight lesion, RCA—proximal 70%–80% lesion. mid (CTO), filling retrogradely from left system **(Fig. 27)**.

PROCEDURE

Left coronary artery engaged with EBU 3.5–7 Fr guiding catheter, lesion crossed with 0.014″ Sion blue, D2 crossed with 0.014″ BMW, multiple predilatations were done to LAD and D2 at origin with 2.0 × 10 mm Tazuna **(Fig. 27)**.

Post-plain old balloon angioplasty (POBA) OCT showed: Morphology—fibrocalcific plaque, lesion length—34 mm, distal EELD—2.4 mm, proximal EELD—4.2 × 4.5 mm **(Fig. 28A)**.

Further dilated with 2.5 × 10 mm Tazuna, prestent OCT showed fibrocalcific plaque required OPN NC, minimal lumen area (MLA) 3.5 mm^2 **(Fig. 28B)**. Regular balloons were unable to open the lesion hence 2.5 × 10 mm OPN NC balloon dilated up to high pressure (40–45 atm). LAD—stenting done with 2.75 × 38 mm Resolute Onyx and postdilated done with 3.0 × 12 mm NC Apollo **(Fig. 29)**. Poststent OCT showed no medial edge dissection well-apposed and eXpanded stent. Final result was good with TIMI III flow **(Fig. 30)**.

Sometimes thick fibrotic lesions without significant calcium are associated with difficult to cross and expand with high inflation pressures of NC balloons. These lesions are associated with significant underexpansion with increased in-stent restenosis (ISR), stent thrombosis (ST), and major adverse cardiac events (MACE) rate during acute and long-term follow-up. Adequate predilatation high-pressure inflations at 40–45 atm with 1:1 size OPN NC balloons will result in adequate expansion improving acute and long-term outcomes.

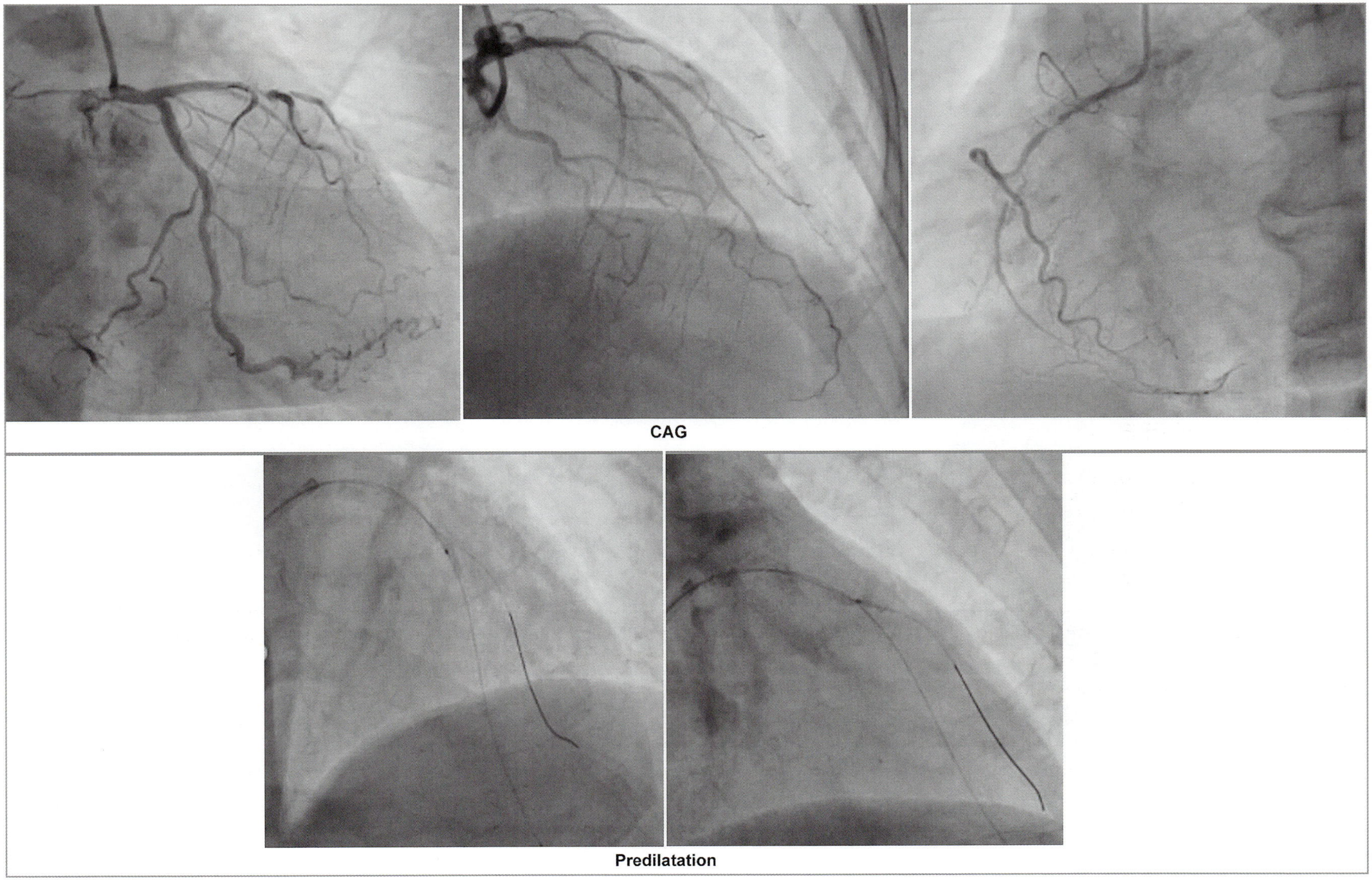

Fig. 27: Coronary angiogram (CAG) and predilatation of left anterior descending (LAD) lesion.

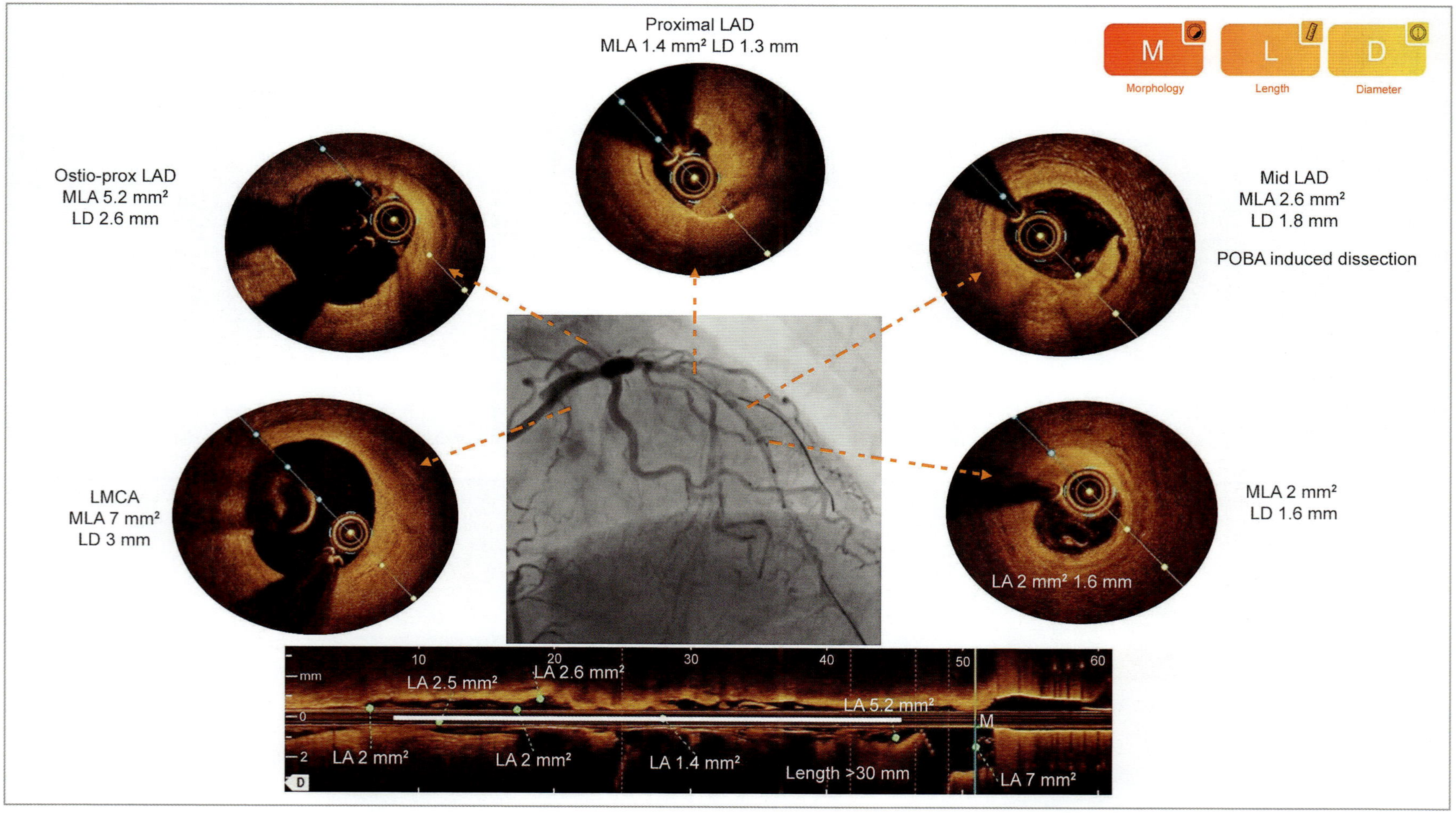
Proximal LAD
MLA 1.4 mm² LD 1.3 mm
M
Morphology
L
Length
D
Diameter
Ostio-prox LAD
MLA 5.2 mm²
LD 2.6 mm
Mid LAD
MLA 2.6 mm²
LD 1.8 mm
POBA induced dissection
LMCA
MLA 7 mm²
LD 3 mm
MLA 2 mm²
LD 1.6 mm
LA 2 mm² 1.6 mm
LA 2.5 mm²
LA 2.6 mm²
LA 5.2 mm²
LA 2 mm²
LA 2 mm²
LA 1.4 mm²
Length >30 mm
LA 7 mm²

Fig. 28A

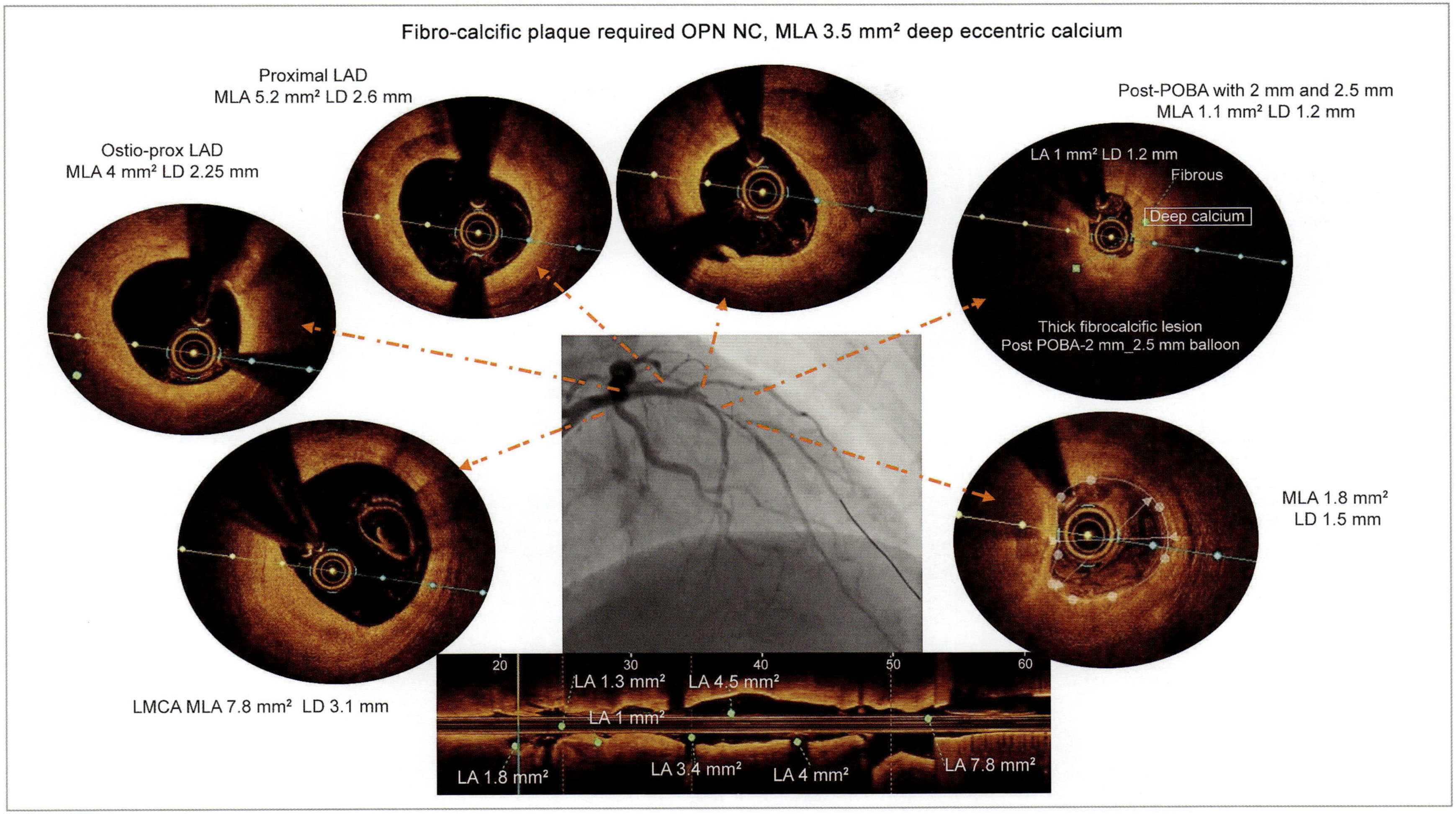

Fig. 28B

Figs. 28A and B: Pre-PCI OCT assessment. (A) MLD assessment of LAD-fibrotic plaque and (B) for plaque morphology. (LA: lumen area; LD: lumen diameter; LMCA: left main coronary artery; MLA: minimal lumen area; NC: noncompliant; OCT: optical coherence tomography; POBA: plain old balloon angioplasty; PCI: percutaneous coronary intervention)

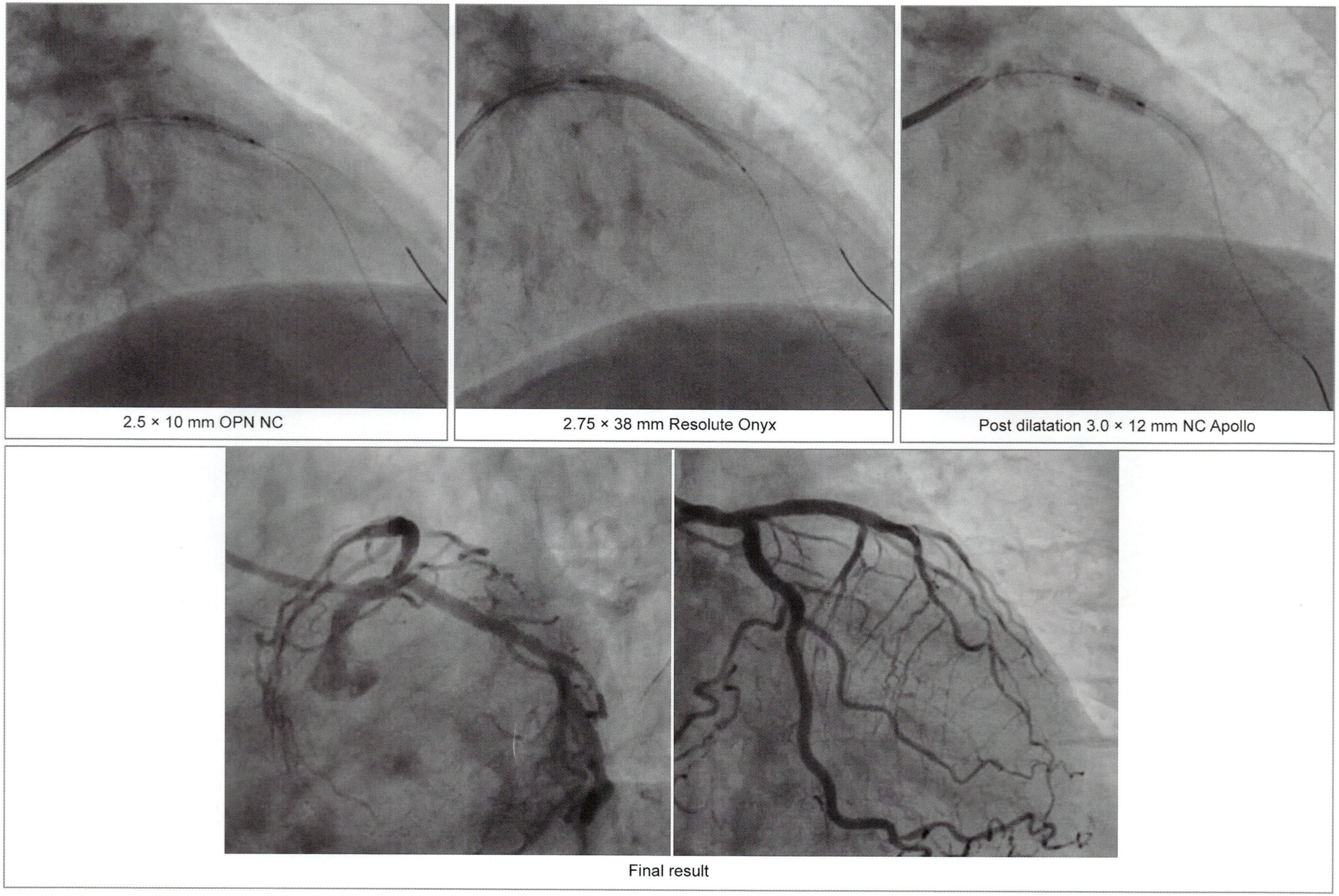

Fig. 29: Coronary angioplasty of diseased segment. (NC: noncompliant)

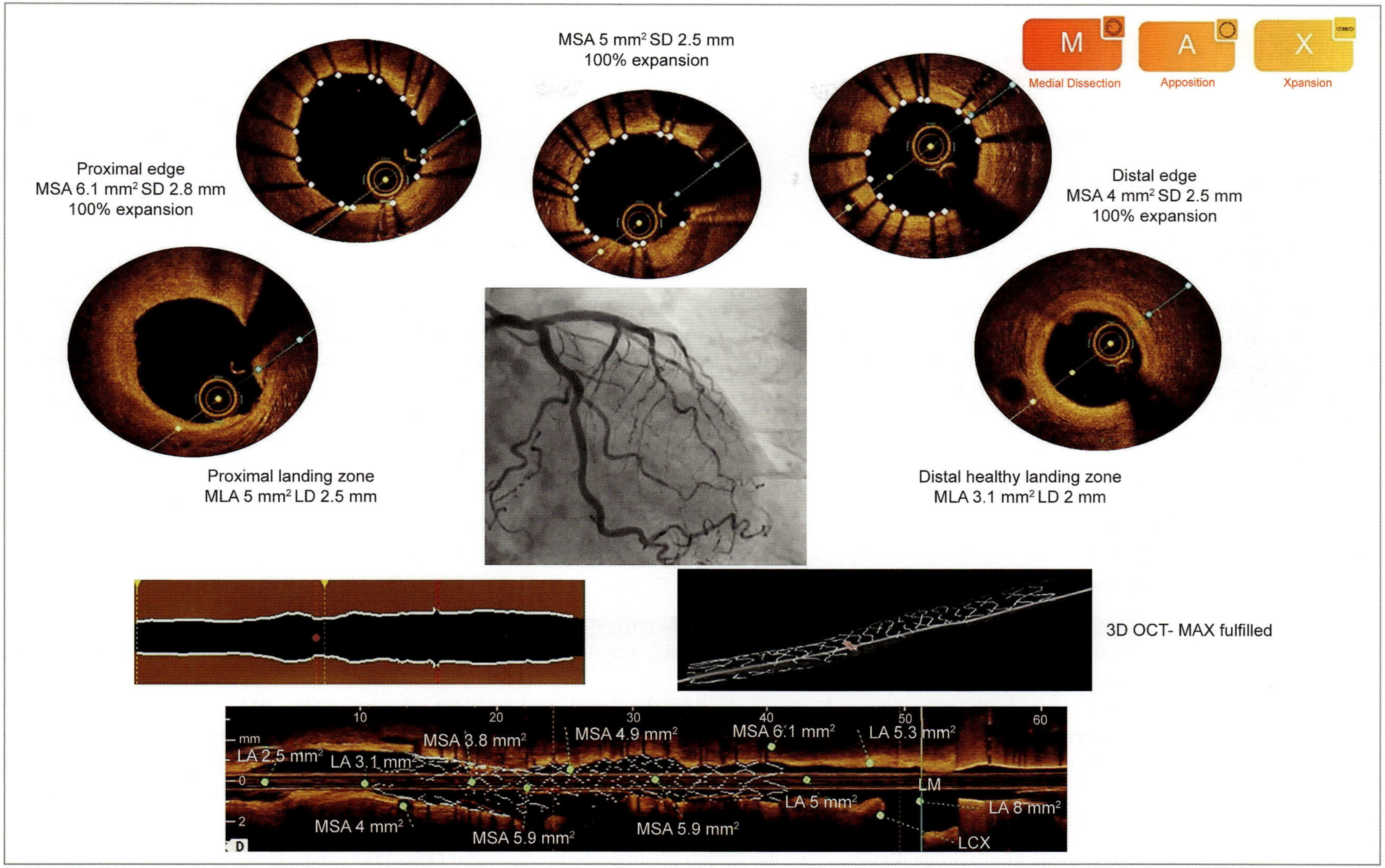

Fig. 30: Post-PCI OCT assessment showed well-expanded and apposed stent struts with no medial edge dissections. (OCT: optical coherence tomography; LA: lumen area; LD: lumen diameter; LCX: left circumflex; LM: left main; MLA: minimal lumen area; MSA: minimal stent area; PCI: percutaneous coronary intervention)

CASE 5

OCT-guided PCI of LM-LAD in acute AWMI.

CLINICAL HISTORY

A 50-year-old female known case of diabetic and hypertension, presented with typical angina for 2 days, ACS—evolved AWMI **(Fig. 31)**, CAG-LMCA + DVD, 2D ECHO—RWMA in LAD territory, moderate LV dysfunction, mild mitral regurgitation (MR), EF—38%. Investigations: Hb—12.6 g/dL, RBS—200 mg/dL, serum creatinine—1.22 mg/dL, eGFR—52 ml/min. CAG—LMCA distal 20%-30%, LAD—proximal total occlusion, major obtuse marginal (OM)—proximal 50% lesion **(Fig. 31)**.

PROCEDURE

Left main coronary artery engaged with EBU 3.5-7 Fr guiding catheter, LAD lesion crossed with 0.014″ BMW wire with microcatheter support. LCX crossed with 0.014″ Sion blue wire; check angio after predilatation of LAD ostium with 2.0 × 10 mm Tazuna—diffusely diseased LAD (proximal, mid, and distal segments) and diffusely diseased D2 **(Fig. 31)**.

Prestent OCT assessment: Morphology—long segment fibrolipid plaque with plaque rupture **(Fig. 32A)**.

Lesion length—48 mm, diameter: proximal—MLD: 2.8 mm, EELD—4.1 × 4.2 mm, Distal—MLD: 2.2 mm, EELD—3 × 2.9 mm. Device selected distal with stent 2.75 × 38 mm and proximal with 3.5 × 23 mm **(Fig. 32B)**.

Proximal to mid LAD stenting done with 2.75 × 28 mm Xience Xpedition—landing before LAD-D2 bifurcation **(Fig. 31)**, jailed balloon technique was used by jailing of 2 mm Tazuna balloon into the LCX with PS of LM-LAD for maintaining SB patency. LMCA to LAD stenting done with 3.5 × 23 mm Xience Xpedition, subsequently jailed balloon was removed from LCX, distal optimization technique (DOT) of LAD was done with 3.0 × 12 mm NC Trek balloon, jailed wire removed, POT of LMCA was done with 4.0 × 12 mm NC Trek balloon, check angio showed distal LAD and diagonal are small caliber, diffusely diseased vessels. RePOT done with 4.0 × 12 mm NC Trek **(Fig. 33)**.

Poststent OCT assessment: without any medial edge dissection, well-eXpanded and well-apposed stent **(Fig. 34A)**. Distal landing zone showed lipid rich plaque with more plaque burden **(Fig. 34B)**. Hence, treated with DEB instead of DES in view of small caliber vessel.

D2 and distal LAD dilated with 1.5 × 15 mm Tazuna, distal LAD dilated with DEB 2.25 × 25 mm MagicTouch balloon twice for 1 minute each, postdilatation of LAD stent was further optimized with 3.0 × 12 mm NC Trek postdilatation. Final result was good with TIMI III flow **(Fig. 35)**.

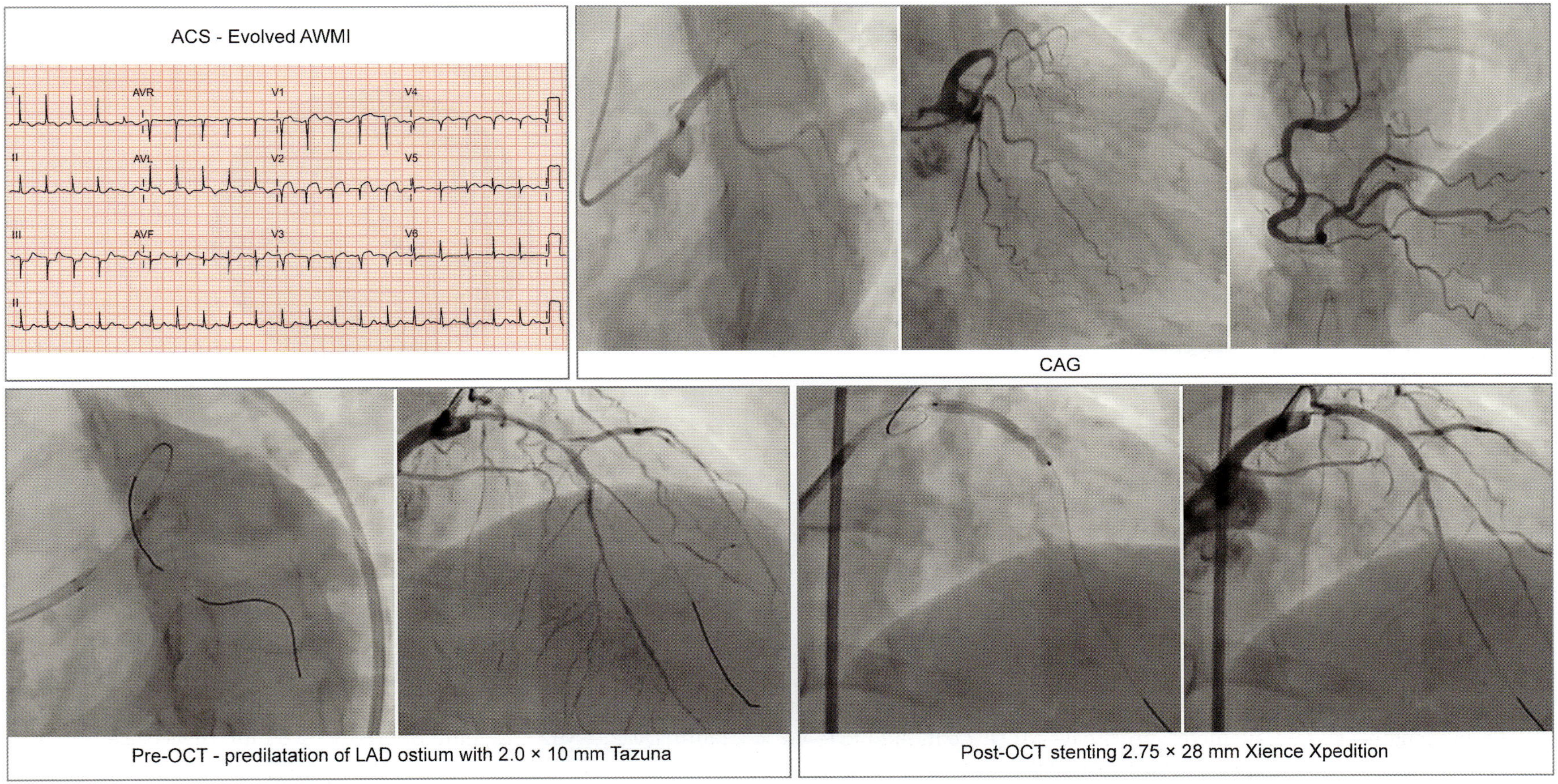

Fig. 31: PCI with Stenting of LAD for Anterior STEMI. Electrocardiogram (ECG), coronary angiogram (CAG), predilatation, and angioplasty. (ACS: acute coronary syndrome; AWMI: anterior wall myocardial infarction; OCT: optical coherence tomography)

Optical coherence tomography is very useful in assessing lesion length and severity in patients with diffusely diseased vessels. This case illustrates how OCT helped in choosing correct size of devise, and landing zones. OCT LM bifurcation view showed distal LM bifurcation angle 90° without any spiky carina suggestive of low chance SB closure after stenting. Provisional stenting (PS) of LM to LAD was opted because of its better long-term results of single stent over two-stent technique. Distal landing zone of LAD showed large lipid-rich plaque burden with small caliber vessel which was managed with DEB.

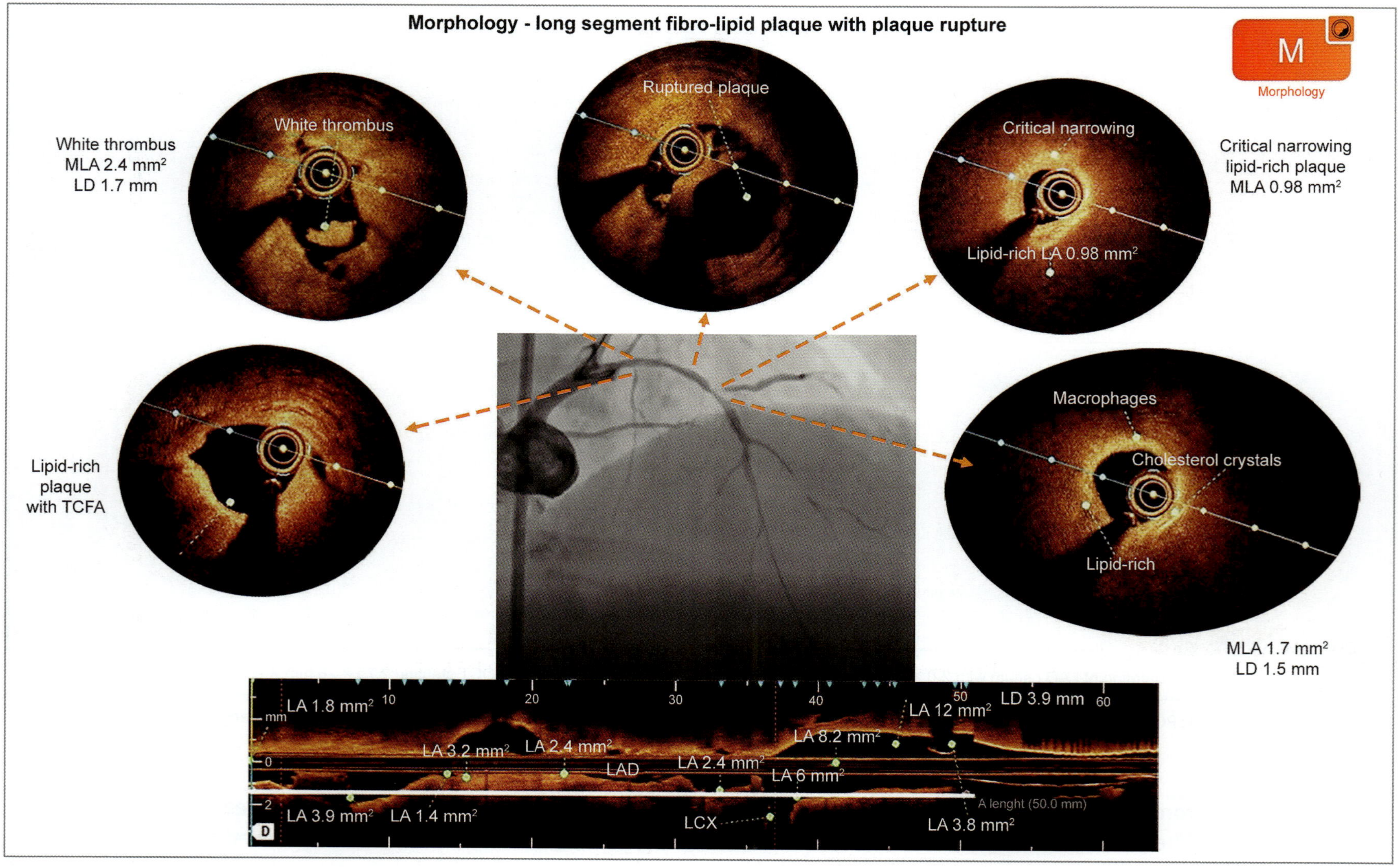

Morphology - long segment fibro-lipid plaque with plaque rupture
M
Morphology
White thrombus
MLA 2.4 mm²
LD 1.7 mm
White thrombus
Ruptured plaque
Critical narrowing
Lipid-rich LA 0.98 mm²
Critical narrowing
lipid-rich plaque
MLA 0.98 mm²
Lipid-rich
plaque
with TCFA
Macrophages
Cholesterol crystals
Lipid-rich
MLA 1.7 mm²
LD 1.5 mm
LA 1.8 mm²
LA 3.2 mm²
LA 2.4 mm²
LAD
LA 2.4 mm²
LA 8.2 mm²
LA 6 mm²
LA 12 mm²
LD 3.9 mm
LA 3.9 mm²
LA 1.4 mm²
LCX
A lenght (50.0 mm)
LA 3.8 mm²

Fig. 32A

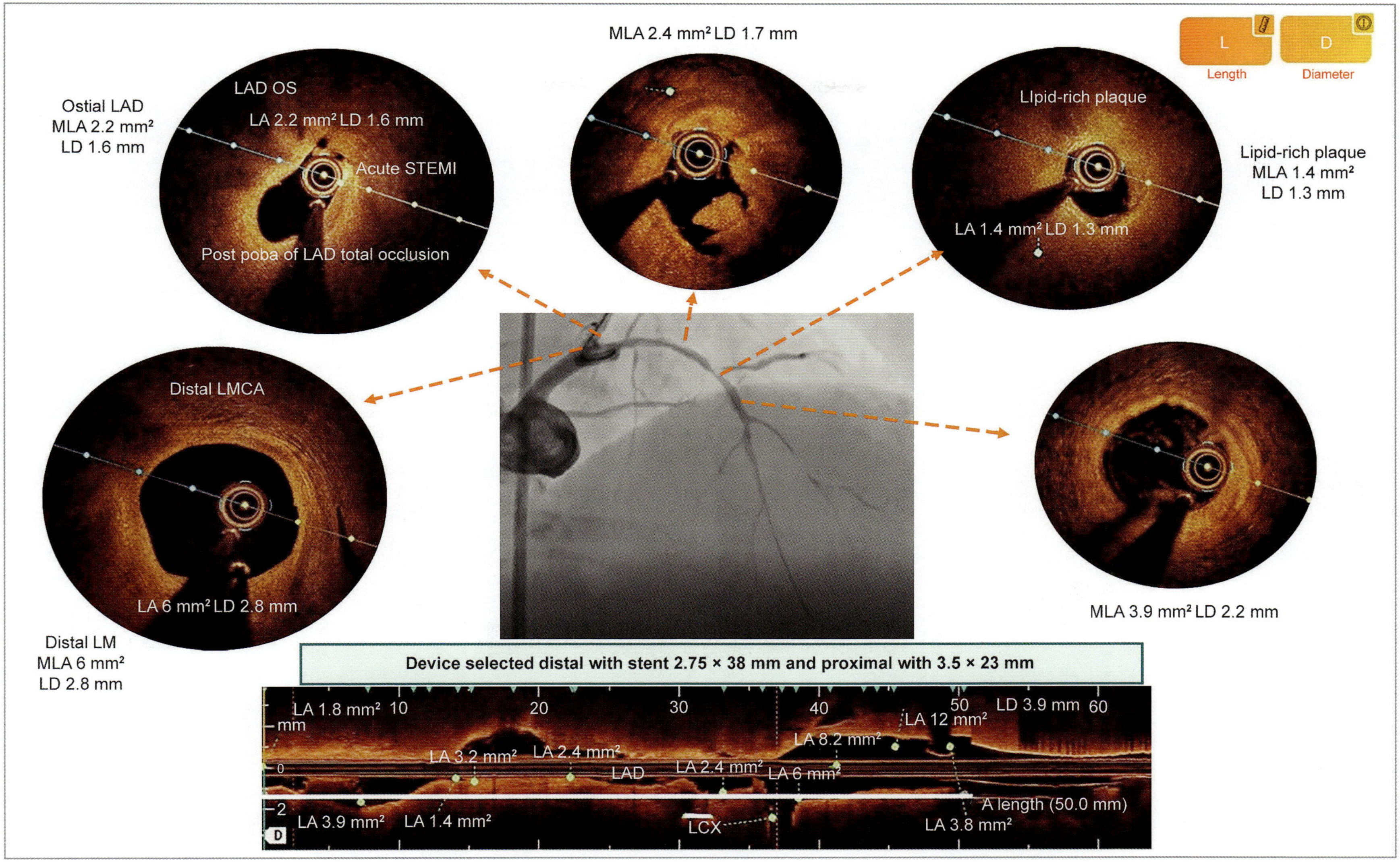

Fig. 32B

Figs. 32A and B: Pre-PCI OCT assessment. (A) for device selection; (B) for plaque morphology. (LAD: left anterior descending; LD: lumen area; LM: left main; MLA: minimal lumen area; OCT: optical coherence tomography; PCI: percutaneous coronary intervention)

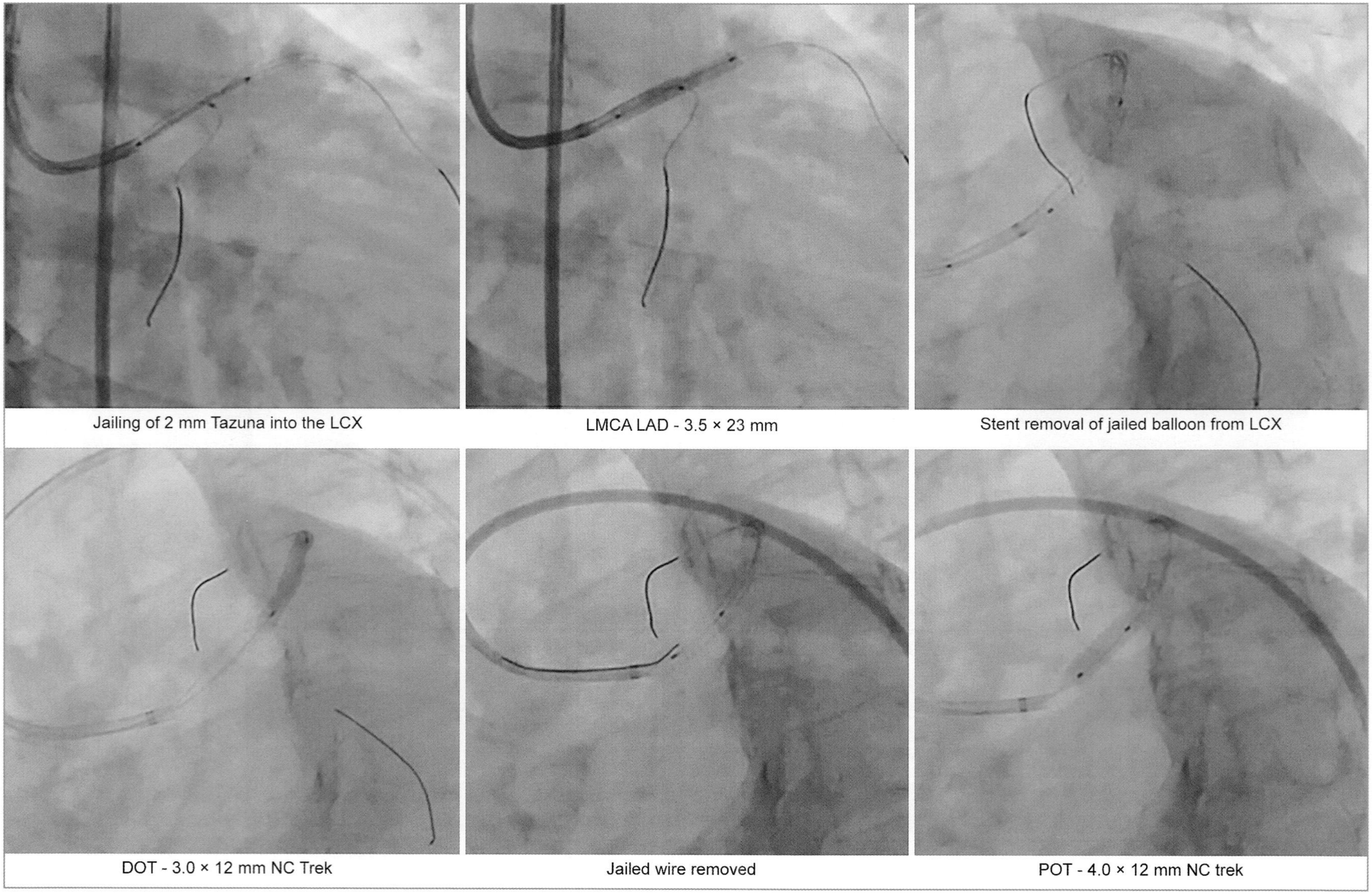

Fig. 33: Jailed balloon technique. (DOT: distal optimization technique; LAD: left anterior descending; LCX: left circumflex; LMCA: left main coronary artery; NC: noncompliant; POT: proximal optimization technique)

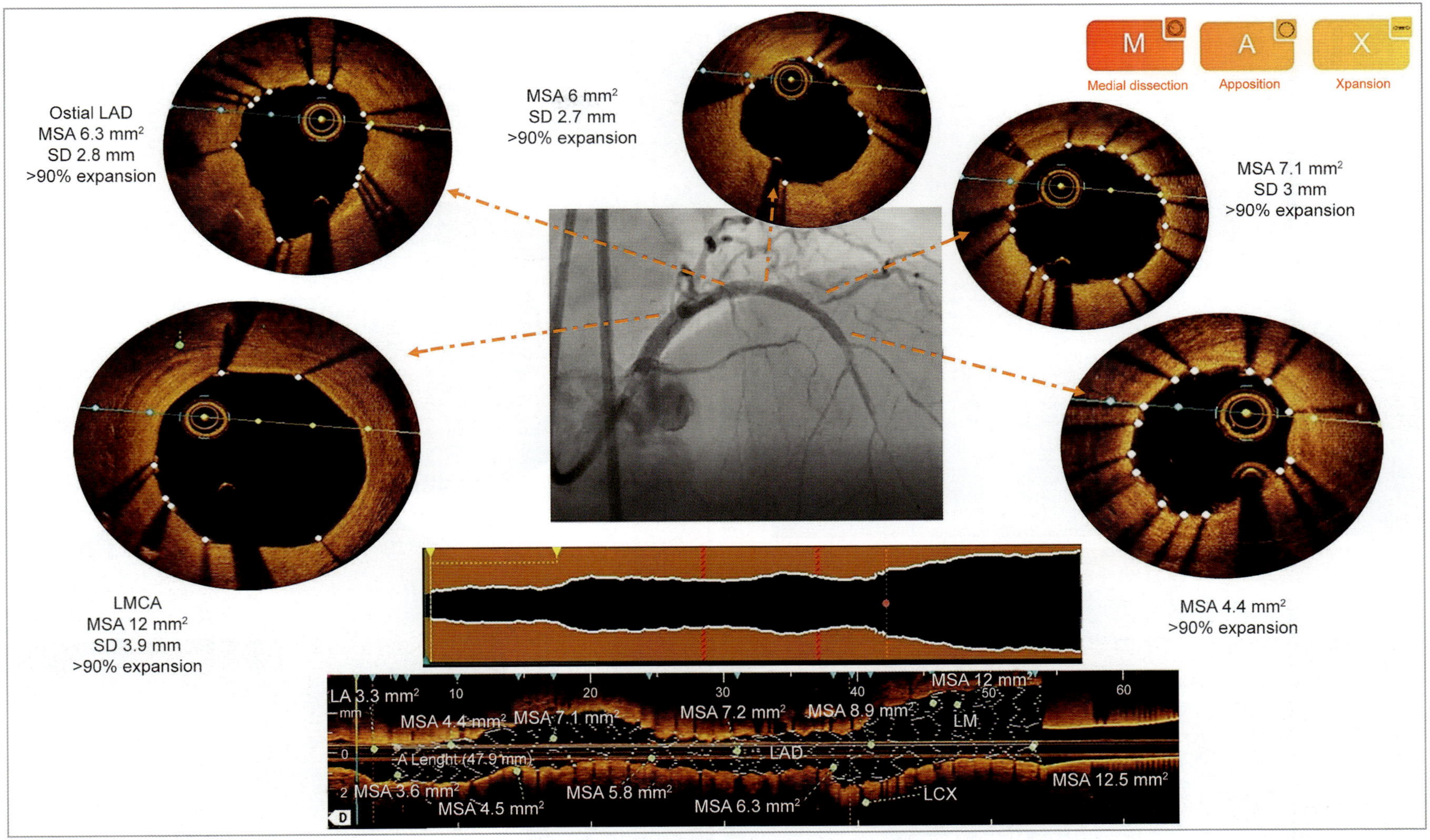
M
Medial dissection
A
Apposition
X
Xpansion
Ostial LAD
MSA 6.3 mm²
SD 2.8 mm
>90% expansion
MSA 6 mm²
SD 2.7 mm
>90% expansion
MSA 7.1 mm²
SD 3 mm
>90% expansion
LMCA
MSA 12 mm²
SD 3.9 mm
>90% expansion
MSA 4.4 mm²
>90% expansion
LA 3.3 mm²
MSA 4.4 mm²
MSA 7.1 mm²
MSA 7.2 mm²
MSA 8.9 mm²
MSA 12 mm²
LM
LAD
A Lenght (47.9 mm)
MSA 3.6 mm²
MSA 4.5 mm²
MSA 5.8 mm²
MSA 6.3 mm²
LCX
MSA 12.5 mm²

Fig. 34A

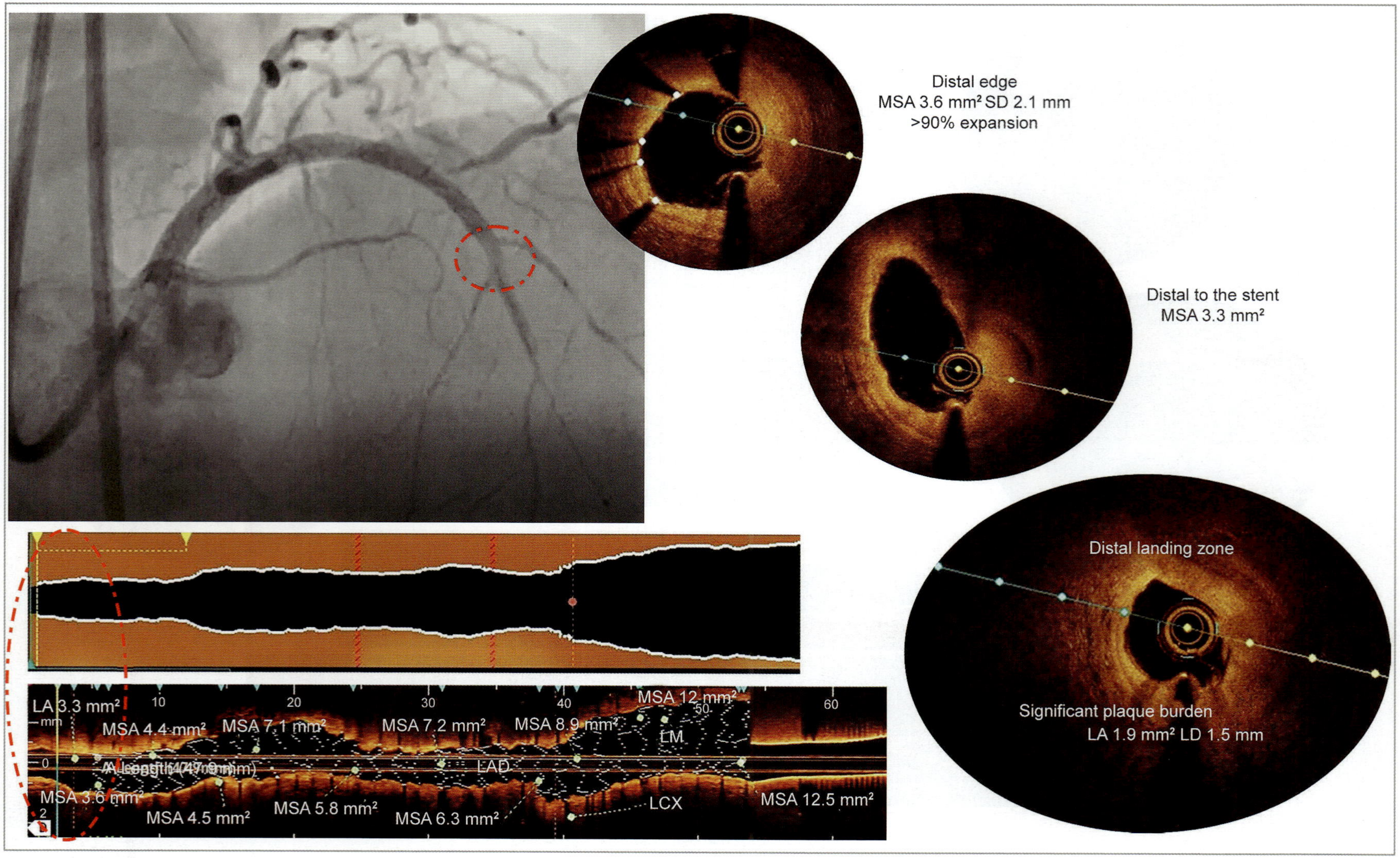

Fig. 34B

Figs. 34A and B: Poststent optical coherence tomography (OCT) assessment. (A) MAX assessment of LM and LAD; (B) distal to the distal stent edge showed significant plaque burden. (LA: lumen area; LCX: left circumflex; LD: lumen diameter; LM: left main; MSA: minimal stent area; SD: stent diameter)

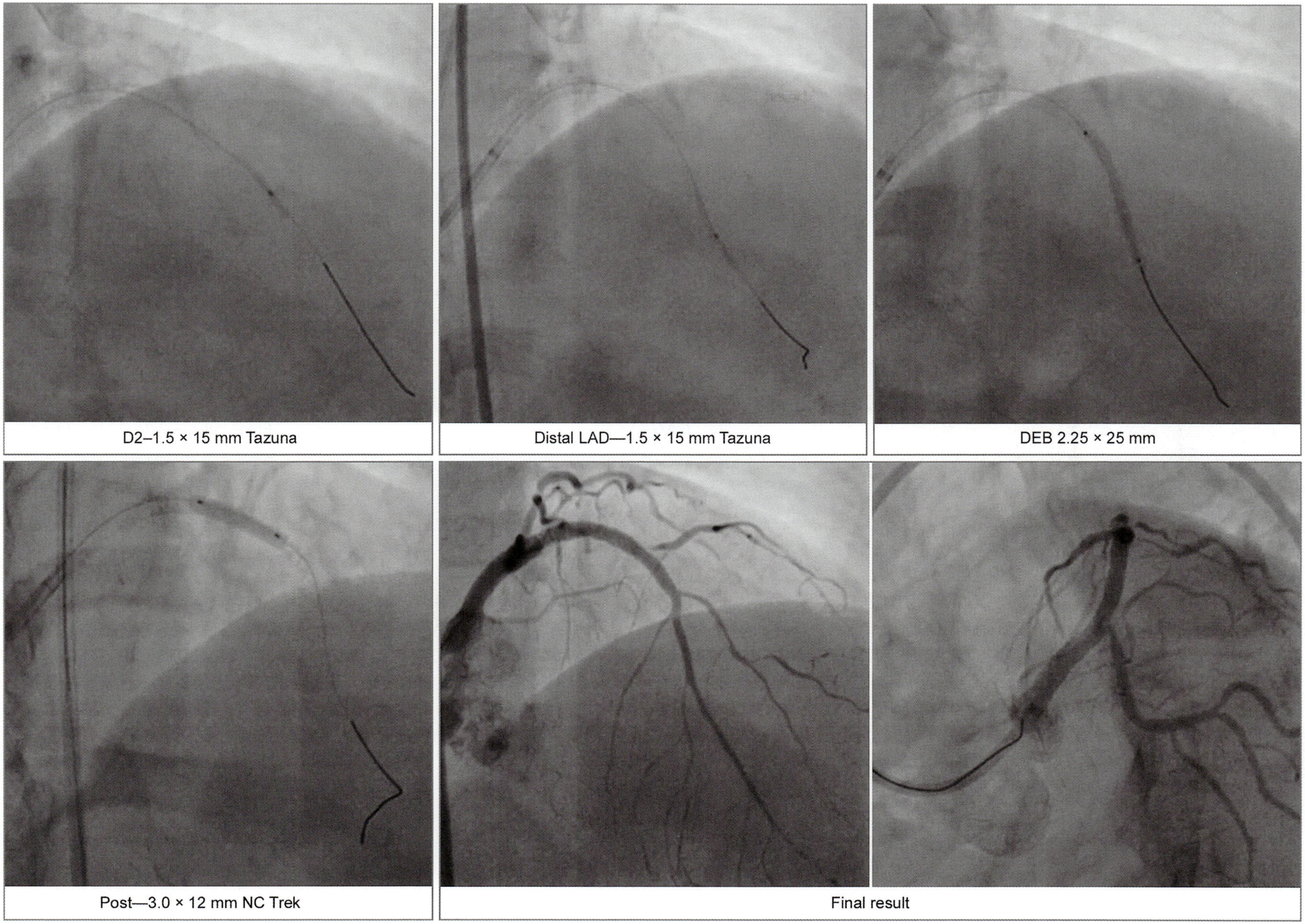

Fig. 35: Balloon angioplasty of the distal left anterior descending (LAD) lesion with drug-eluting balloon (DEB). (NC: noncompliant)

CASE 6

Underexpansion of the ostial LM stent.

CLINICAL HISTORY

A 65-year-old male known diabetic presented with ACS—evolved AWMI, S/P percutaneous transluminal coronary angioplasty (PTCA) (2009), 2D ECHO—mild LV dysfunction, EF—45%, CAG—borderline LMCA lesion, LAD: ostioproximal 90% lesion, mid 80% ISR, LCX, and RCA—normal **(Fig. 36)**; investigations: Hb—13.8 g/dL, RBS—205 mg/dL, serum creatinine—0.80 mg/dL, eGFR—94 mL/min.

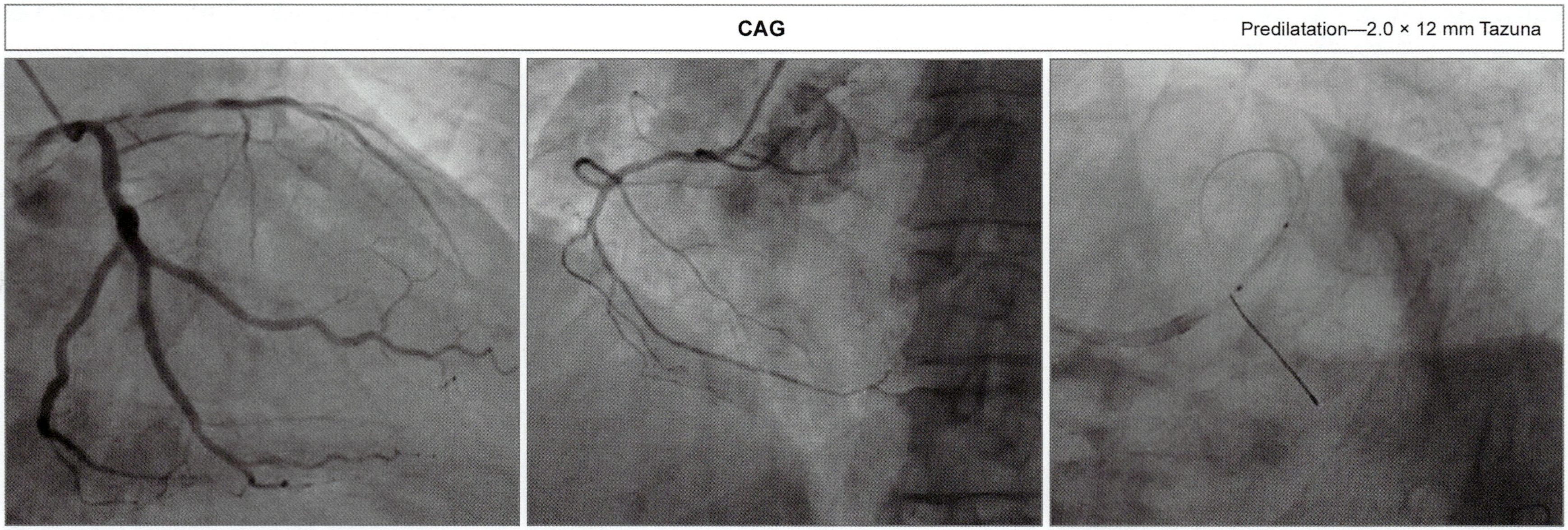

Fig. 36: Coronary angiogram (CAG) and predilatation.

PROCEDURE

Left coronary artery engaged with JL 3.5–7 Fr guiding catheter, LAD lesion crossed with 0.014 Runthrough wire, LCX crossed with 0.014" BMW wire, LAD was predilated with 2.0 × 12 mm Tazuna **(Fig. 36)**.

Post-POBA OCT assessment: MLD **(Fig. 37A)**
Morphology: Proximal edge ISR due to atherosclerosis—lipid-rich plaque, significant lipid-rich plaque lesion distal to the previously implanted stent with significant luminal narrowing
Lesion length and diameter: 60 mm long lesion, distal landing zone LA—2.6 mm^2 EELD—2.6 × 2.9 mm, proximal landing zone: lumen area (LA) 7.8 mm^2, lumen diameter (LD) 3 mm. Device selected: 66 mm, proximal stent 3 × 33 mm and distal 2.75 × 33 mm.

Scoring was opted for ISR lesion of LAD with 2.5 × 15 mm angio-sculpt, postscoring OCT assessment showed well-scored proximal LAD and ISR lesion **(Fig. 37B)**.

Mid-LAD stenting done with 2.75 × 33 mm Xience Xpedition and 3.0 × 33 mm Xience Xpedition stent deployed in LM—proximal LAD. POT of LMCA was done with 4.5 × 12 mm NC Trek and postdilatation of LAD was done with 3.0 × 15 mm NC Trek **(Fig. 38)**.

Poststenting OCT assessment well-expanded and apposed stent struts without any medial edge dissection of the LAD and LM stents **(Fig. 39A)** except ostioproximal portion of LM stent, which showed significant malapposition and underexpansion **(Fig. 39B)**. Hence, re-POT of ostioproximal LMCA was done with 4.5 × 12 mm NC Trek to rectifying malapposed and underexpanded proximal edge of LM stent **(Fig. 38)**.

Intravascular ultrasound of LM ostium was performed which showed well-expanded and apposed proximal portion of LM stent covering ostium of LMCA without any edge dissection **(Fig. 39C)**. Postdilatation of LAD was done for further optimization with 3.5 × 12 mm NC Trek. Final result was good with TIMI III flow.

In-stent restenosis lesion is due to progression of atherosclerotic plaque at the proximal and distal edges of stents leading to edge restenosis which requires PCI with DES implantation to cover entire diseased segment to avoid the future increased restenosis rate. ISR of stent is usually associated with thick fibrotic lesions which require adequate scoring with cutting balloon prior to restenting. Sometimes it would be very difficult to assess LM ostium with OCT due to many artifacts as a result of improper clearance of blood from LM ostium. This case illustrated malapposition, and underexpansion of ostial segment of LM stent which was rectified flaring of LM ostial stent with additional POT. Post-POT IVUS was performed because of its better delineation and visualization of LM ostium compared to OCT which confirmed well-expanded and apposed LM ostial stent.

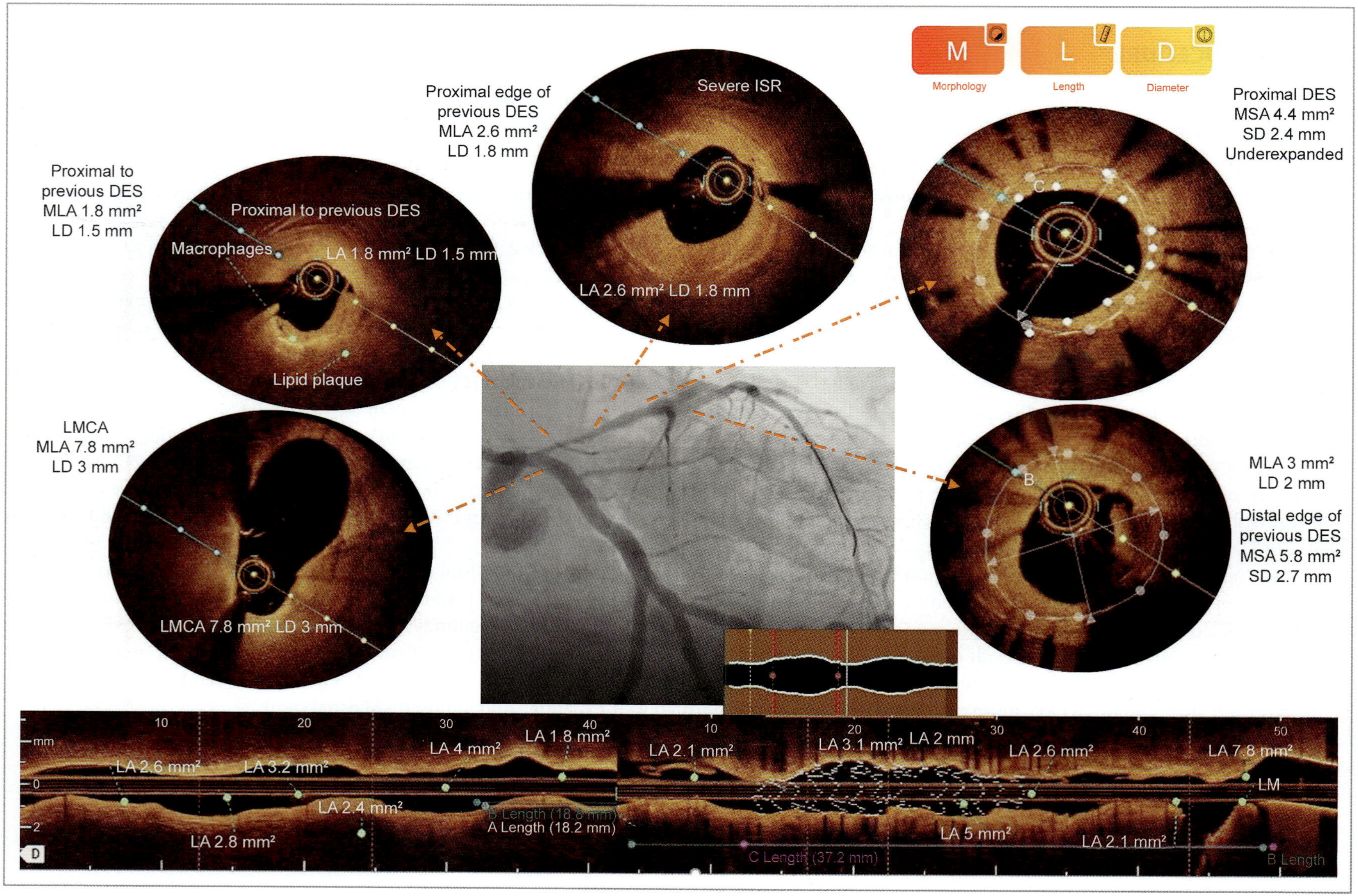
M
Morphology
L
Length
D
Diameter
Proximal to previous DES MLA 1.8 mm² LD 1.5 mm
Proximal to previous DES
Macrophages
LA 1.8 mm² LD 1.5 mm
Lipid plaque
Proximal edge of previous DES MLA 2.6 mm² LD 1.8 mm
Severe ISR
LA 2.6 mm² LD 1.8 mm
Proximal DES MSA 4.4 mm² SD 2.4 mm Underexpanded
LMCA MLA 7.8 mm² LD 3 mm
LMCA 7.8 mm² LD 3 mm
MLA 3 mm² LD 2 mm
Distal edge of previous DES MSA 5.8 mm² SD 2.7 mm
LA 2.6 mm²
LA 3.2 mm²
LA 4 mm²
LA 1.8 mm²
LA 2.4 mm²
LA 2.8 mm²
A Length (18.2 mm)
LA 2.1 mm²
LA 3.1 mm²
LA 2 mm
LA 2.6 mm²
LA 7.8 mm²
LM
LA 5 mm²
LA 2.1 mm²
C Length (37.2 mm)
B Length

Fig. 37A

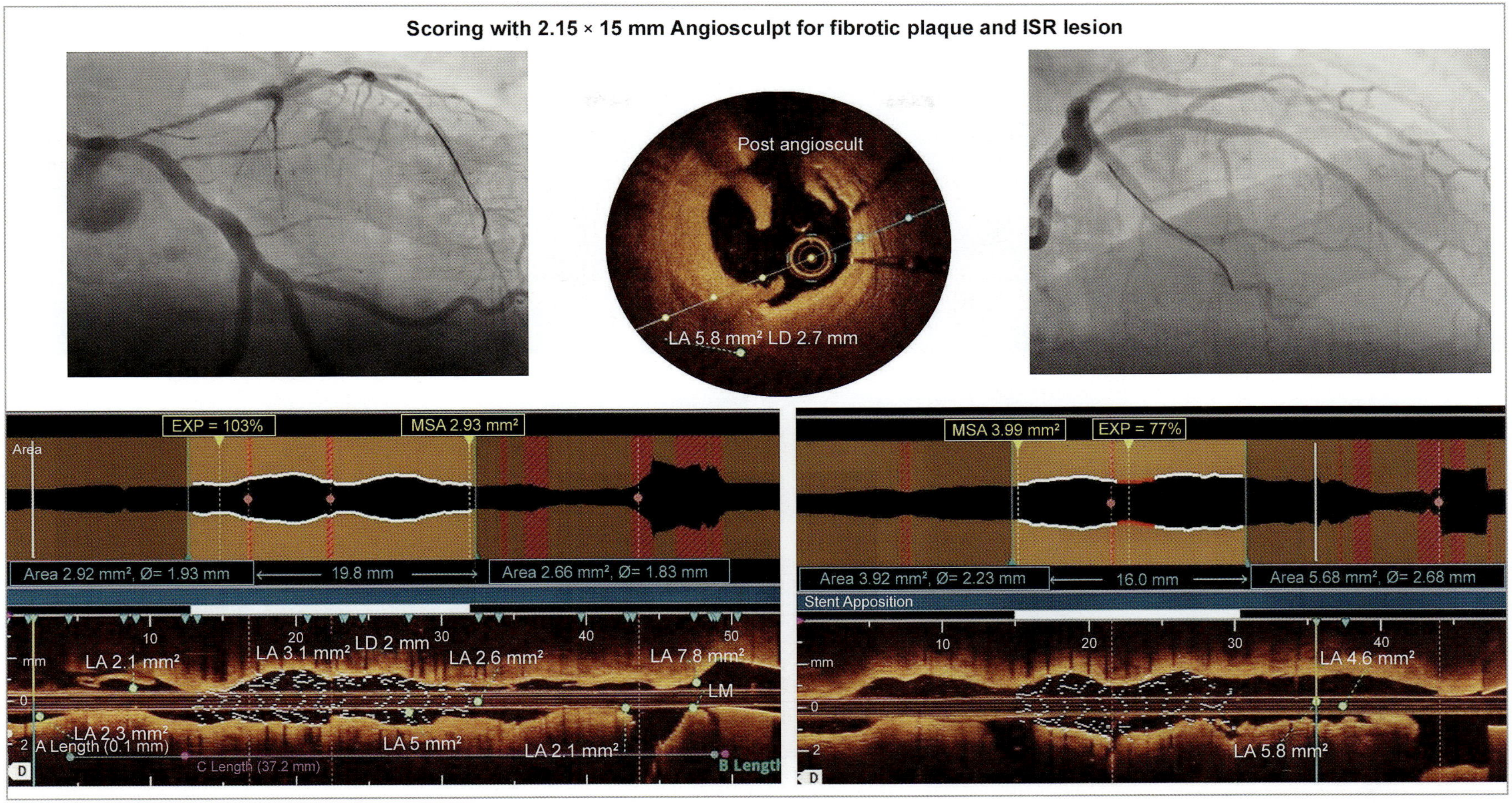

Fig. 37B

Figs. 37A and B: A Pre-PCI OT assessment for plaque morphology and plaque modification. (A) MLD assessment of LM and LAD-severe ISR and proximal edge restenosis; (B) postscoring OCT assessment. (LA: lumen area; LD: lumen diameter; OCT: optical coherence tomography; MLA: minimal luminal diameter; MSA: minimal stent area; PCI: percutaneous coronary intervention)

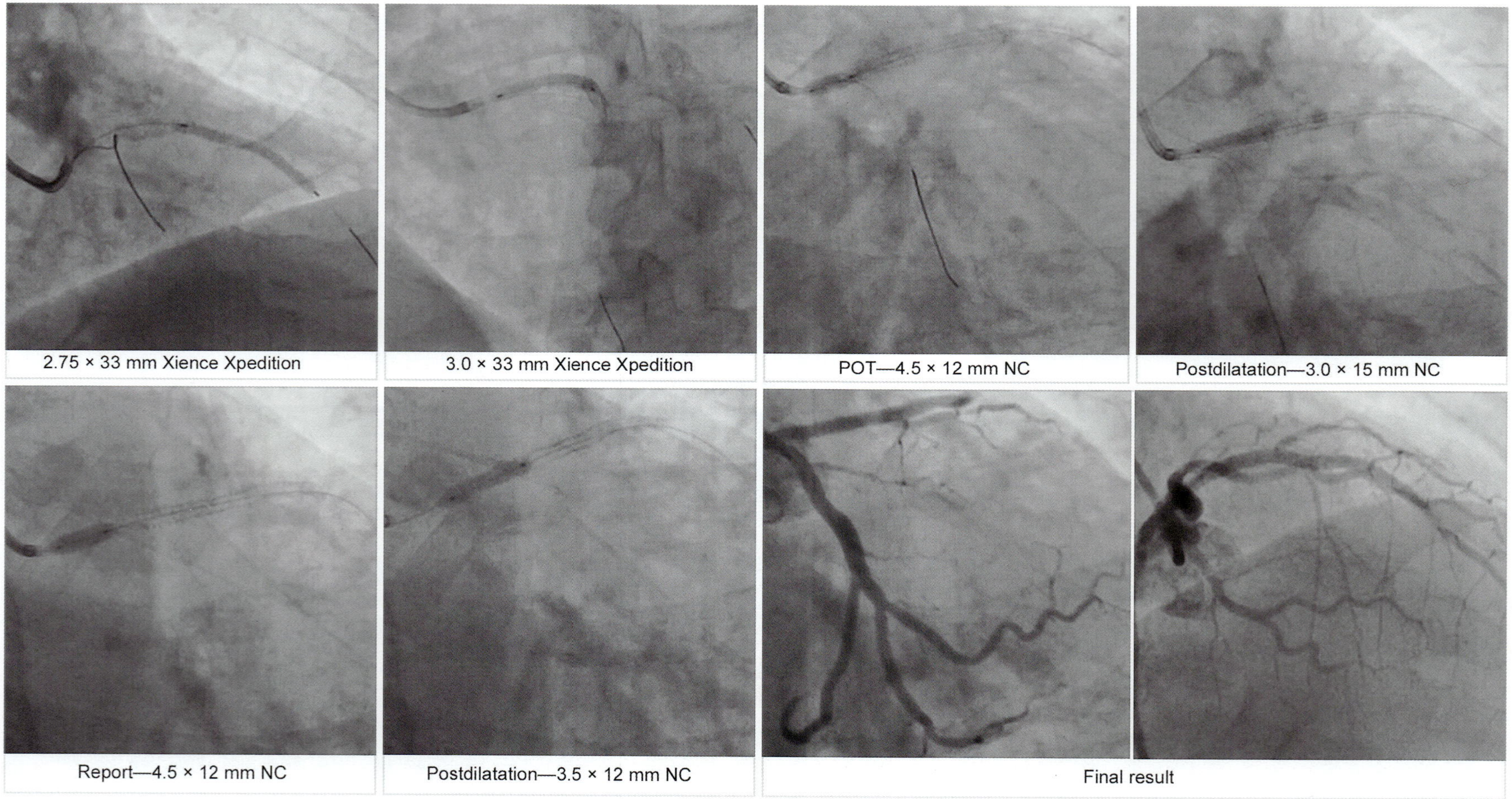

Fig. 38: PCI of LAD. Coronary angioplasty of the diseased vessel. (NC: noncompliant)

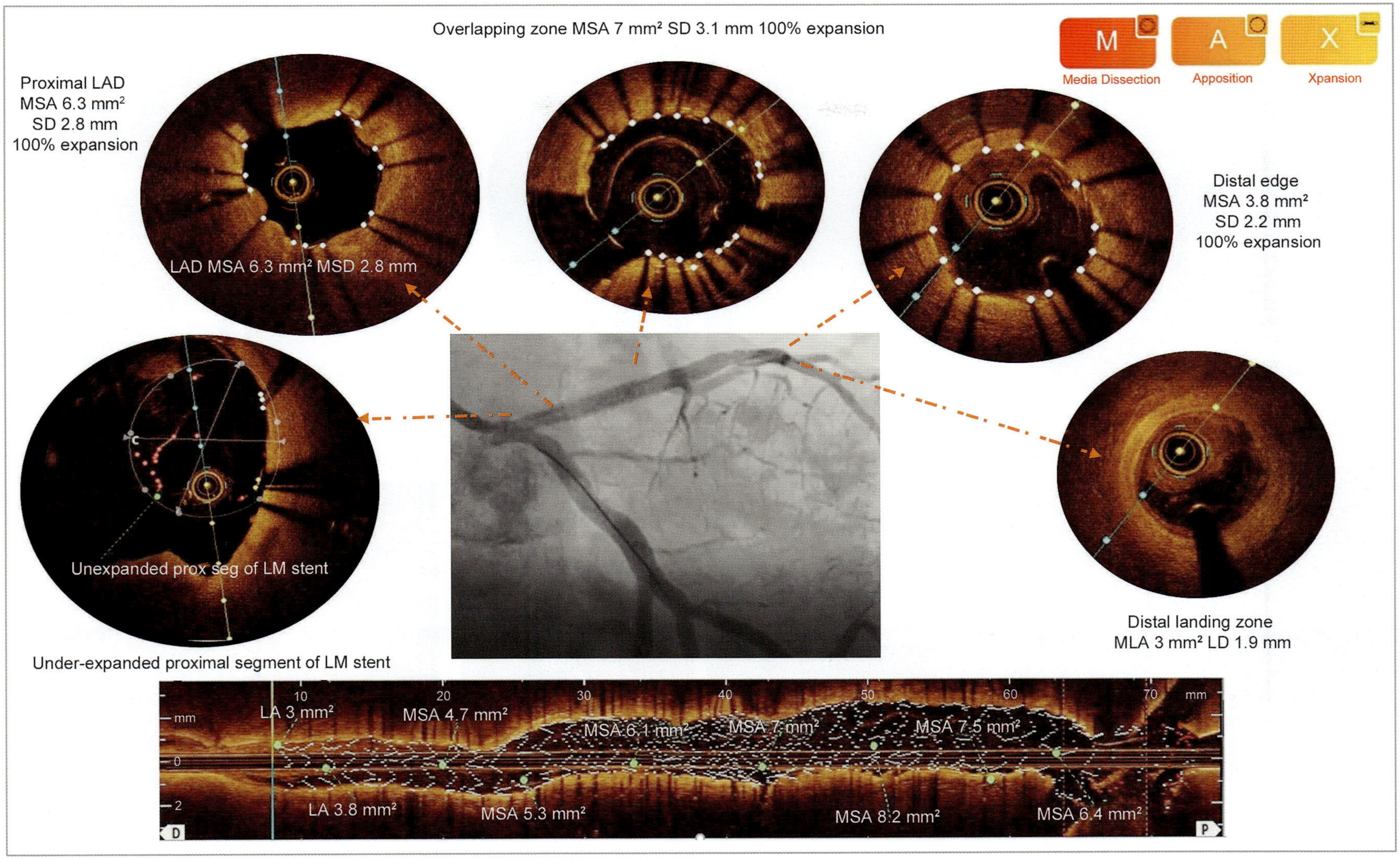
Overlapping zone MSA 7 mm² SD 3.1 mm 100% expansion
M
Media Dissection
A
Apposition
X
Xpansion
Proximal LAD
MSA 6.3 mm²
SD 2.8 mm
100% expansion
LAD MSA 6.3 mm² MSD 2.8 mm
Distal edge
MSA 3.8 mm²
SD 2.2 mm
100% expansion
Unexpanded prox seg of LM stent
Under-expanded proximal segment of LM stent
Distal landing zone
MLA 3 mm² LD 1.9 mm
LA 3 mm²
MSA 4.7 mm²
MSA 6.1 mm²
MSA 7 mm²
MSA 7.5 mm²
LA 3.8 mm²
MSA 5.3 mm²
MSA 8.2 mm²
MSA 6.4 mm²
mm
D
P

Fig. 39A

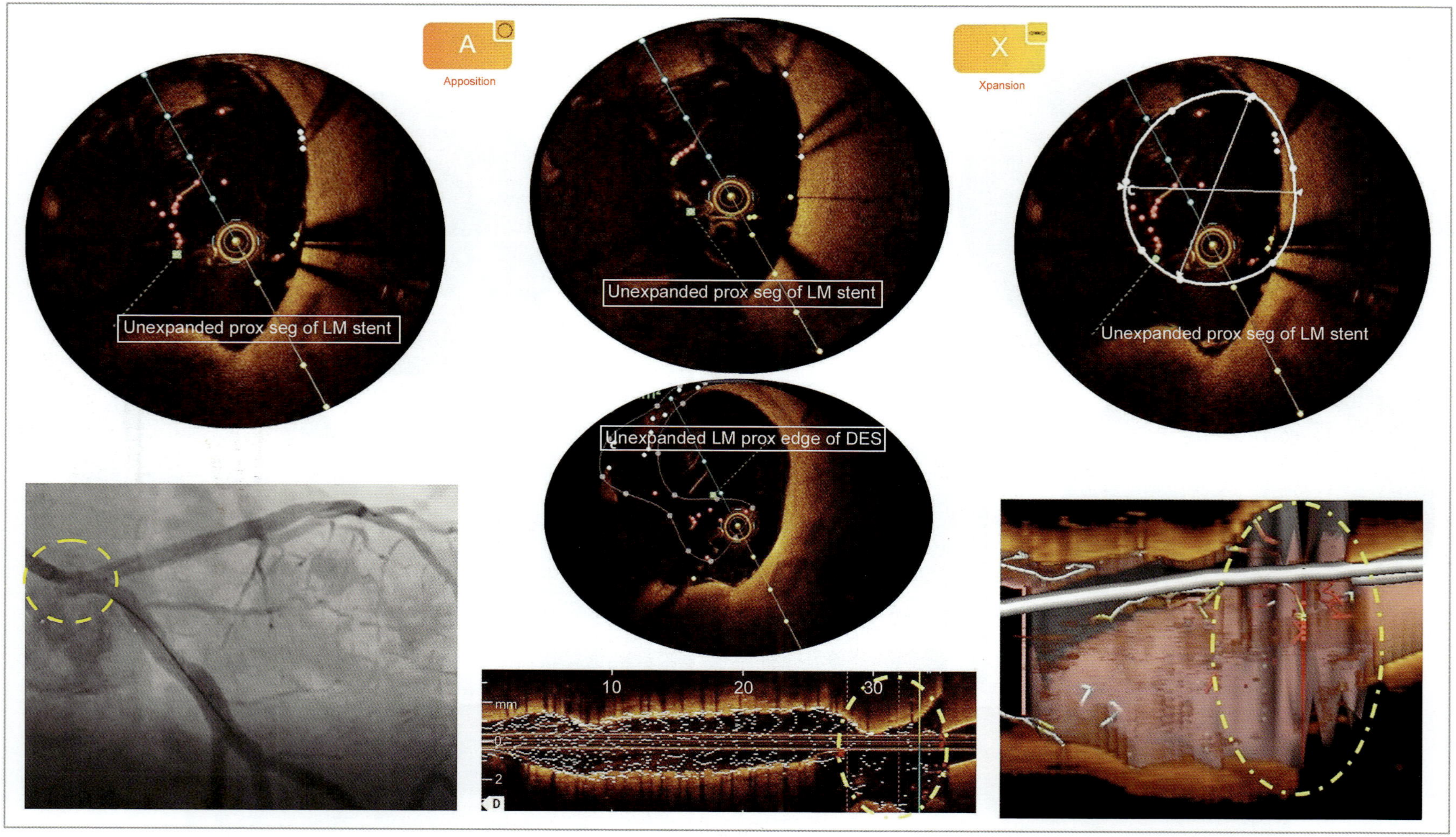
A
Apposition
X
Xpansion
Unexpanded prox seg of LM stent
Unexpanded prox seg of LM stent
Unexpanded prox seg of LM stent
Unexpanded LM prox edge of DES
10
20
30
mm
0
2
D

Fig. 39B

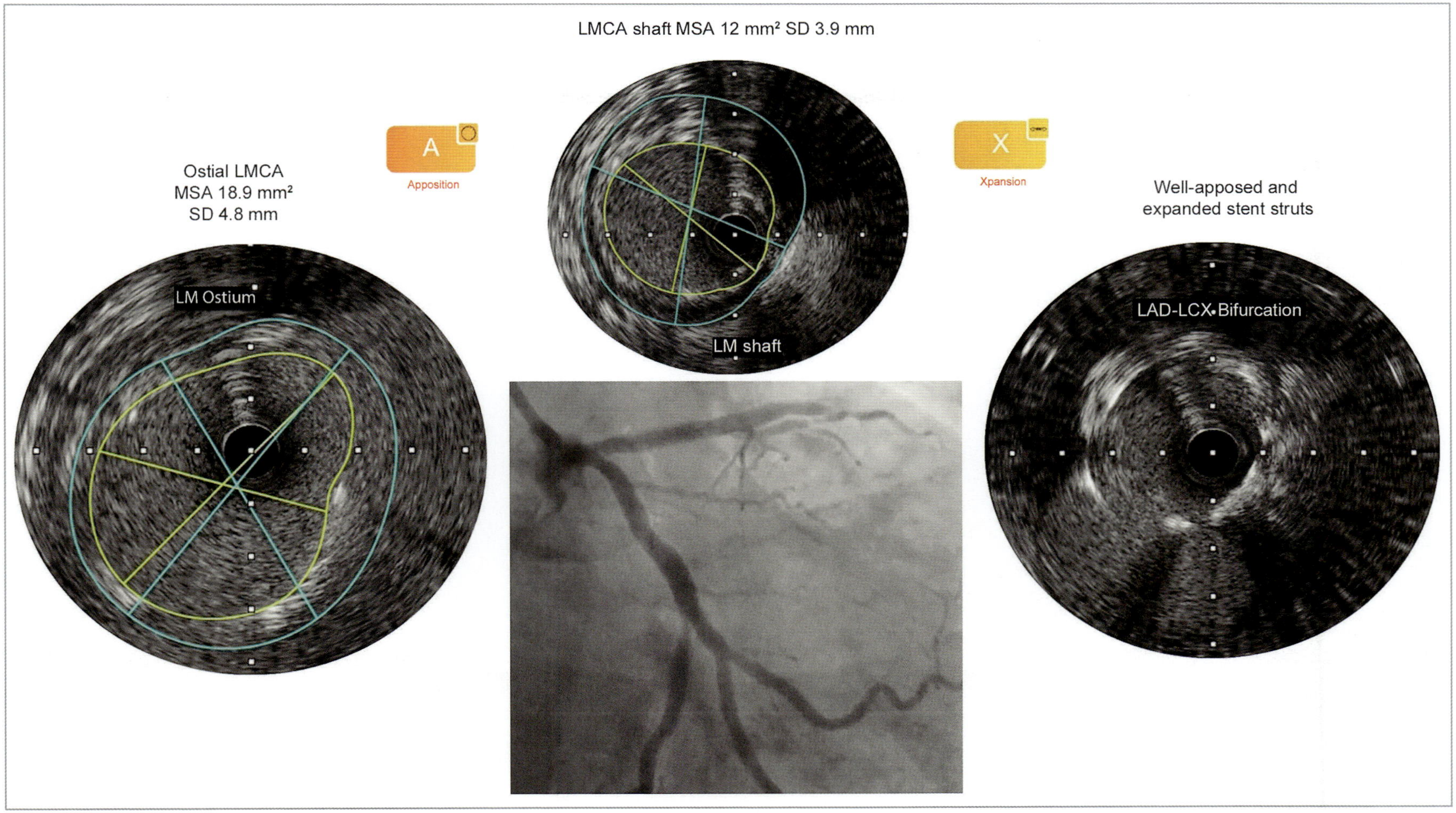

Fig. 39C

Figs. 39A to C: (A) MAX assessment of LAD-underexpanded and mal apposition of the proximal edge of LM stent; (B) Artifacts of OCT at the ostium of LM leading to improper assessment; (C) Post-POT IVUS showed well-expanded and apposed stent struts with no medial edge dissection at proximal portion. (IVUS: intravascular ultrasound; LMCA: left main coronary artery; MSA: minimal stent area; PCI: percutaneous coronary intervention; POT: proximal optimization technique; SD: stent diameter)

Index

Page numbers followed by *b* refer to box, *f* refer to figure, *fc* refer to flowchart, and *t* refer to table.

A

B

C

D

E

Q

R

S